Cardiovascular Interventions in Clinical Practice

Cardiovascular Interventions in Clinical Practice

EDITED BY

Jürgen Haase MD, PhD, FESC, FACC
Professor of Medicine, Consultant Cardiologist
Kardiocentrum Frankfurt
Klinik Rotes Kreuz
Frankfurt/Main, Germany

Hans-Joachim Schäfers MD, PhD
Professor of Surgery
Chair, Department of Thoracic and Cardiovascular Surgery
University Hospital Saarland
Homburg/Saar, Germany

Horst Sievert MD, FESC, FACC
Professor of Medicine
Head, Department of Cardiology
CardioVascular Center Frankfurt
Frankfurt, Germany

Ron Waksman MD, FACC
Professor of Medicine
Associate Director, Division of Cardiology
Director, Experimental Cardiology
Washington Hospital Center
Washington, DC, USA

WILEY-BLACKWELL
A John Wiley & Sons, Ltd., Publication

This edition first published 2010 © by Blackwell Publishing Ltd

Blackwell Publishing was acquired by John Wiley & Sons in February 2007. Blackwell's publishing program has been merged with Wiley's global Scientific, Technical and Medical business to form Wiley-Blackwell.

Registered office: John Wiley & Sons Ltd, The Atrium, Southern Gate, Chichester, West Sussex, PO19 8SQ, UK

Editorial offices: 9600 Garsington Road, Oxford, OX4 2DQ, UK

The Atrium, Southern Gate, Chichester, West Sussex, PO19 8SQ, UK

111 River Street, Hoboken, NJ 07030-5774, USA

For details of our global editorial offices, for customer services and for information about how to apply for permission to reuse the copyright material in this book please see our website at www.wiley.com/wiley-blackwell

Wiley also publishes its books in a variety of electronic formats. Some content that appears in print may not be available in electronic books.

Designations used by companies to distinguish their products are often claimed as trademarks. All brand names and product names used in this book are trade names, service marks, trademarks or registered trademarks of their respective owners. The publisher is not associated with any product or vendor mentioned in this book. This publication is designed to provide accurate and authoritative information in regard to the subject matter covered. It is sold on the understanding that the publisher is not engaged in rendering professional services. If professional advice or other expert assistance is required, the services of a competent professional should be sought.

The contents of this work are intended to further general scientific research, understanding, and discussion only and are not intended and should not be relied upon as recommending or promoting a specific method, diagnosis, or treatment by physicians for any particular patient. The publisher and the author make no representations or warranties with respect to the accuracy or completeness of the contents of this work and specifically disclaim all warranties, including without limitation any implied warranties of fitness for a particular purpose. In view of ongoing research, equipment modifications, changes in governmental regulations, and the constant flow of information relating to the use of medicines, equipment, and devices, the reader is urged to review and evaluate the information provided in the package insert or instructions for each medicine, equipment, or device for, among other things, any changes in the instructions or indication of usage and for added warnings and precautions. Readers should consult with a specialist where appropriate. The fact that an organization or Website is referred to in this work as a citation and/or a potential source of further information does not mean that the author or the publisher endorses the information the organization or Website may provide or recommendations it may make. Further, readers should be aware that Internet Websites listed in this work may have changed or disappeared between when this work was written and when it is read. No warranty may be created or extended by any promotional statements for this work. Neither the publisher nor the author shall be liable for any damages arising herefrom.

Library of Congress Cataloging-in-Publication Data
Cardiovascular interventions in clinical practice / edited by Jürgen Haase. — 1st ed.
     p. ; cm.
   Includes bibliographical references and index.
   ISBN 978-1-4051-8277-5 (hardcover : alk. paper)
   1. Cardiovascular system—Diseases—Treatment. 2. Heart—Surgery. I. Haase, Jürgen, Prof. Dr.
   [DNLM: 1. Cardiovascular Diseases—therapy. 2. Cardiac Surgical Procedures. 3. Cardiovascular Diseases—diagnosis. 4. Cardiovascular Diseases—pathology. WG 166 C2663 2009]
   RC669.C2863 2009
   616.1′06—dc22

                                                                              2009032166

ISBN: 9781405182775

A catalogue record for this book is available from the British Library.
Set in 9/12pt Meridien by Graphicraft Limited, Hong Kong
Printed and bound in Singapore by Fabulous Printers Pte Ltd

1   2010

Contents

Contents

List of Contributors

Suhny Abbara MD
Assistant Professor, Harvard Medical School
Director of Cardiovascular Imaging Section,
    Massachusetts General Hospital
Director of Education, Cardiac MR/PET/CT
    Program
Boston, MA, USA

Pierfrancesco Agostoni MD
Department of Cardiology
University Medical Center Utrecht
Utrecht, The Netherlands

Diana Aicher MD
Department of Thoracic and Cardiovascular
    Surgery
University Hospital of Saarland
Homburg/Saar, Germany

Ibrahim Akin MD
Department of Medicine
Division of Cardiology at the University Hospital
    Rostock
Rostock School of Medicine
Rostock, Germany

Seth Assar MD
St. Luke's Medical Center
Phoenix, AZ
University of Arizona
Tucson, AZ, USA

Birgit Assmus MD
Division of Cardiology
University Hospital Frankfurt/Main
Frankfurt/Main, Germany

Anirban Banerjee MD
Center for Cardiovascular Imaging
Tufts University Medical Center
Boston, MA, USA

Peter Barlis MD
Department of Cardiology
Royal Brompton Hospital
London, UK

Thomas Bartel MD
Cardiology Division
Department of Internal Medicine III
Medical University of Innsbruck
Innsbruck
Austria

Philipp Beerbaum MD
Senior Clinical Lecturer
King's College London
Consultant Paediatric Cardiologist
The Evelina Children's Hospital
London, UK

Robert H. Boone MD
Interventional Cardiology
St. Paul's Hospital
University of British Columbia
Vancouver, Canada

Marc Bosiers MD
Department of Vascular Surgery
AZ St-Blasius
Dendermonde, Belgium

Jagdish Butany MD
McLaughlin Centre for Molecular Medicine
University of Toronto
Department of Pathology
University Health Network
Toronto, Ontario, Canada

Sara D. Collins MD
Washington Hospital Center
Division of Cardiology
Washington, DC, USA

Stefano De Castro MD
Center for Cardiovascular Imaging
Tufts University Medical Center
Boston, MA, USA

Koen Deloose MD
Department of Vascular Surgery
AZ St-Blasius
Dendermonde, Belgium

Carlo Di Mario MD, PhD
Professor of Medicine
Consultant Cardiologist
Royal Brompton Hospital
London, UK

Mirko Doss MD
J.W. Goethe University
Frankfurt/Main, Germany

Maria Drakopoulou MD
Department of Cardiology
Hippokration Hospital
Athens Medical School
Athens, Greece

Savio D'Souza MD
Department of Cardiology
Royal Brompton Hospital
London, UK

Anthony L. Estrera MD
Department of Cardiothoracic and Vascular
    Surgery
University of Texas at Houston Medical
    School
Memorial Hermann Heart and Vascular
    Institute
Houston, TX, USA

Antonietta Evangelista MD
Center for Cardiovascular Imaging
Tufts University Medical Center
Boston, MA, USA

Francesco F. Faletra MD
Center for Cardiovascular Imaging
Tufts University Medical Center
Boston, MA, USA

Paul Fefer MD
The Schulich Heart Programme
Sunnybrook Research Institute
Sunnybrook Health Sciences Centre
Toronto, Ontario, Canada

Wolfgang Fehske MD
Associate Professor of Medicine
Head, Department of Cardiology
St. Vinzenz-Hospital
Cologne, Germany

Ted Feldman MD, FACC, FSCAI
Professor of Medicine
Chair, Interventional Cardiology
Evanston Northwestern Health Care
Cardiovascular Institute
Mt View, CA, USA

Giuseppe Ferrante MD
Department of Cardiology
Royal Brompton Hospital
London, UK

Michael C. Fishbein MD
Piansky Professor of Pathology and
    Medicine
Department of Pathology and Laboratory
    Medicine
David Geffen School of Medicine at UCLA
Los Angeles, CA, USA

Jennifer Franke MD
CardioVascular Center Frankfurt
Frankfurt, Germany

Hector M. Garcia-Garcia MD, MSc
Thoraxcenter
Erasmus Medical Center
Rotterdam, The Netherlands

Nikolaus Gassler MD, MA
Professor of Pathology
Institute of Pathology
RWTH Aachen University
Aachen, Germany

Anne L. Gaster MD, PhD
Thoraxcenter
Erasmus Medical Center
Rotterdam, The Netherlands

Ramil Goel MD
Banner Good Samaritan Medical Center
Phoenix, AZ, USA

Nieves Gonzalo MD
Thoraxcenter
Erasmus Medical Center
Rotterdam, The Netherlands

Kevin L. Greason MD
Department of Cardiovascular Surgery
Mayo Clinic
Rochester, MN, USA

Matthias Gutberlet MD, PhD
Professor of Radiology
Director of the Department of Diagnostic and
    Interventional Radiology
University Leipzig/Leipzig Heart Center
Leipzig, Germany

Juan Luis Gutiérrez-Chico MD,
PhD, FESC
Interventional Cardiology Unit
Vigo University Hospital
Vigo, Spain

Jürgen Haase MD, PhD, FESC, FACC
Professor of Medicine, Consultant Cardiologist
Kardiocentrum Frankfurt
Klinik Rotes Kreuz
Frankfurt/Main, Germany

Markus K. Heinemann MD, PhD
Professor of Pediatric Cardiac Surgery
University Hospital
Johannes Gutenberg University Mainz
Mainz, Germany

Esther Herpel MD
Institute of Pathology
University Clinics Heidelberg
Germany

Richard R. Heuser MD, FACC, FACP,
FESC, FASCI
Director of Cardiology St. Luke's Hospital and
    Medical Center
Clinical Professor of Medicine, University of
    Arizona College of Medicine
Phoenix, AZ, USA

Siew Yen Ho PHD, FRCPath, FESC
Professor and Head of Cardiac Morphology Unit
Royal Brompton Hospital and Imperial College
    London
London, UK

L. Nelson Hopkins MD
Professor and Chairman of Neurosurgery and
    Professor of Radiology
Department of Neurosurgery and Radiology and
    Toshiba Stroke Research Center
School of Medicine and Biomedical Sciences
University of Buffalo, State University of New York
Department of Neurosurgery, Millard Fillmore
    Gales Hospital, Kaleida Health
Buffalo, NY, USA

Christian Ihling MD
Professor of Medicine
Gemeinschaftspraxis für Pathologie
Frankfurt/Main
Germany

Hüseyin Ince MD
Department of Medicine
Division of Cardiology at the University Hospital
    Rostock
Rostock School of Medicine
Rostock, Germany

Ignacio Inglessis MD
Adult Congenital Heart Disease Program
Department of Cardiology
Massachusetts General Hospital
Boston, MA, USA

Pascal Jabbour MD
Department of Neurosurgery
Thomas Jefferson University Hospital
Jefferson Hospital for Neuroscience
Philadelphia, PA, USA

Saibal Kar MD, FACC, FSCAI
Evanston Northwestern Health Care
Cardiovascular Institute
Mt View, CA, USA

Osamu Katoh MD
Director of Research Center
Toyohashi Heart Center
Toyohashi, Aichi, Japan

Martin G. Keane MD
Cardiovascular Division
Department of Medicine
University of Pennsylvania School of Medicine
Philadelphia, PA, USA

Prafulla G. Kerkar MD
Professor and Head
Department of Cardiology
Seth GS Medical College and KEM Hospital
Mumbai, India

Kourosh Keyhani MD
Department of Cardiothoracic and Vascular
    Surgery
The University of Texas at Houston Medical
    School
Memorial Hermann Heart and Vascular Institute
Houston, TX, USA

Carey Kimmelstiel MD
Center for Cardiovascular Imaging
Tufts University Medical Center
Boston, MA, USA

Stephan Kische MD
Department of Medicine
Division of Cardiology at the University Hospital
    Rostock
Rostock School of Medicine
Rostock, Germany

List of Contributors

Michael J. Kostal MD
Cardiovascular Division
Department of Medicine
University of Pennsylvania School of Medicine
PA, USA

Neville Kukreja MA, MRCP
Thoraxcenter
Erasmus Medical Center
Rotterdam, The Netherlands

Takashi Kunihara MD, PhD
Department of Thoracic and Cardiovascular
    Surgery
University Hospital of Saarland
Homburg, Germany

Chi K. Lai MD, FRCPC
Assistant Professor of Pathology
Department of Pathology and Laboratory
    Medicine
David Geffen School of Medicine at UCLA
Los Angeles, CA, USA

Katharina Lehn
Cardiovascular Center Frankfurt
Frankfurt, Germany

Elad I. Levy MD
Associate Professor of Neurosurgery and
    Radiology
Departments of Neurosurgery and Radiology and
    Toshiba Stroke Research Center
University at Buffalo, State University of New York
Department of Neurosurgery
Millard Fillmore Gates Hospital, Kaleida Health
Buffalo, NY, USA

Faqian Li MD, PhD
Assistant Professor
Department of Pathology and Laboratory
    Medicine
University of Rochester Medical Center,
    Rochester, NY, USA

Artur Lichtenberg MD, PhD
Clinic for Cardiovascular Surgery
University of Düsseldorf
Düsseldorf, Germany

Christos Lioupis MD
Department of Vascular Surgery
AZ St-Blasius
Dendermonde, Belgium

Joachim Lotz MD
Institute of Radiology
Hannover Medical School
Hannover, Germany

Suntharo Ly MD
St. Luke's Medical Center
Phoenix, AZ
University of Arizona
Tucson, AZ, USA

Shawn McMahon PA, MPH
Center for Vascular Care
Washington Hospital Center
Washington, DC, USA

Pedro Marcos-Alberca MD, PhD
Cardiovascular Imaging Unit
Hospital Clinico San Carlos
Madrid, Spain

Charles C. Miller III PhD
Department of Cardiothoracic and Vascular
    Surgery
The University of Texas Medical School at
    Houston
Memorial Hermann Heart and Vascular Institute
Houston, TX, USA

Michael de Moor MBBCh, FACC,
FSCAI
Pediatric Cardiology Division
Floating Hospital for Children
Tufts University Medical Center
Boston, MA, USA

Anton Moritz MD, PhD
J.W. Goethe University
Frankfurt/Main, Germany

Sabareesh K. Natarajan MD, MS
Endovascular Research Fellow and Voluntary
    Assistant Professor, Health Sciences
Department of Neurosurgery and Toshiba Stroke
    Research Center
University at Buffalo
State University of New York
Buffalo, NY, USA

Christoph A. Nienaber MD, PhD
Professor of Medicine Chair, Division of
    Cardiology
University Hospital Rostock
Rostock, Germany

Uwe Nixdorff MD, FESC
Professor of Medicine
European Prevention Center
Duisburg, Germany

Sean O'Donnell MD, FACS
Director of Vascular and Endovascular Surgery
Center for Vascular Care
Washington Hospital Center
Washington, DC, USA

Yoshinobu Onuma MD
Thoraxcenter
Erasmus Medical Center
Rotterdam, The Netherlands

Adytia Pandey MD
Assistant Professor, Neurosurgery
University of Michigan
Michigan, USA

Natesa G. Pandian MD
Professor of Medicine
Center for Cardiovascular Imaging
Tufts University Medical Center
Boston, MA, USA

Patrick Peeters MD
Department of Cardiovascular and Thoracic Surgery
Imelda Hospital
Bonheiden, Belgium

Milind S. Phadke MD
Senior Registrar, Department of Cardiology
Seth GS Medical College and KEM Hospital
Mumbai, India

Tina L. Pinto Slottow MD
Division of Cardiology
Washington Hospital Center
Washington, DC, USA

Shakeel A. Qureshi MD
Department of Congenital Heart Disease
Evelina Children's Hospital
London, UK

Jörg Radermacher MD
Professor of Medicine
Head, Department of Nephrology
Johannes Wesling Klinikum Minden
Minden, Germany

Steve Ramcharitar BM BCh
DPhil MRCP
Thoraxcenter
Erasmus Medical Center
Rotterdam, The Netherlands

Tim C. Rehders MD
Department of Medicine
Division of Cardiology at the University Hospital
    Rostock
Rostock School of Medicine
Rostock, Germany

Wolfgang Roggendorf MD
Professor of Medicine
Department of Neuropathology
Institute of Pathology
University of Würzburg
Würzburg, Germany

Dieter S. Ropers MD, FESC, FACC
Assistant Professor of Medicine
Department of Cardiology
University of Erlangen
Erlangen, Germany

Hazim J. Safi MD
Department of Cardiothoracic and Vascular
    Surgery
The University of Texas at Houston Medical
    School
Memorial Hermann Heart and Vascular
    Institute
Houston, TX, USA

Frederick St. Goar MD, FACC, FSCAI
Evanston Northwestern Health Care
Cardiovascular Institute
Mt View, CA, USA

Volker Schächinger MD
Professor of Medicine
Head, Department of Cardiology
Klinikum Fulda
Fulda, Germany

Hans-Joachim Schäfers MD, PhD
Professor of Surgery
Chair, Department of Thoracic and Cardiovascular
    Surgery
University Hospital of Saarland
Homburg/Saar, Germany

Hartzell V. Schaff MD
Professor of Surgery
Chair, Department of Cardiovascular Surgery
Mayo Clinic
Rochester, MN, USA

Dierk Scheinert MD
Professor of Medicine
Clinical Director of the Parkhospital Liepzig
Medical Clinic I, Angiology, Cardiology and Heart
    Center Leipzig, Department for Angiology
Leipzig, Germany

Andrej Schmidt MD
Parkhospital Leipzig
Medical Clinic I, Angiology, Cardiology and Heart
    Centre Leipzig, Department for Angiology
Leipzig, Germany

Philipp A. Schnabel MD
Professor of Medicine
Institute of Pathology
University Clinics Heidelberg
Heidelberg, Germany

Juerg Schwitter MD, FESC
Director, Cardiac MR Center of the University
    Hospital Lausanne—CHUV
Associate Professor, Cardiology Section
Lausanne, Switzerland

Patrick W. Serruys MD, PhD,
FESC, FACC
Professor of Medicine
Head, Department of Interventional
    Cardiology
Thoraxcenter
Erasmus Medical Center
Rotterdam, The Netherlands

Leon D. Shturman MD
Cardiac MR/PET/CT Program
Massachusetts General Hospital
MA, USA

Adnan H. Siddiqui MD PhD
Assistant Professor of Neurosurgery and
    Radiology
Departments of Neurosurgery and Radiology and
    Toshiba Stroke Research Center
University at Buffalo, State University of
    New York
Department of Neurosurgery
Millard Fillmore Gates Hospital, Kaleida Health
Buffalo, NY, USA

Horst Sievert MD, FESC, FACC
Professor of Medicine
Head, Department of Cardiology
Cardiovascular Center Frankfurt
Frankfurt, Germany

Kenneth V. Snyder MD, PhD
Department of Neurosurgery and Toshiba Stroke
    Research Center
University at Buffalo, State University of
    New York
Buffalo, NY, USA

Torsten Sommer MD
Professor of Medicine
Head, Department of Radiology
DRK Krankenhaus Neuwied
Neuwied, Germany

Christodoulos Stefanadis MD
Professor of Cardiology
Chair, Department of Cardiology
Hippokration Hospital
Athens Medical School
Athens, Greece

Bradley H. Strauss MD, PhD, FACC
Professor of Cardiology
The Schulich Heart Programme
Sunnybrook Research Institute
Sunnybrook Health Sciences Centre
McLaughlin Centre for Molecular Medicine,
    University of Toronto
Toronto, Ontario, Canada

Asmir I. Syed MD
Professor of Medicine
Associate Director, Division of Cardiology
Director, Experimental Cardiology
Washington Hospital Center
Washington, DC, USA

Rabih G. Tawk MD
Endovascular Neurosurgery Fellow
Department of Neurosurgery and Toshiba Stroke
    Research Center
School of Medicine and Biomedical Sciences
University at Buffalo, State University of New York
Department of Neurosurgery
Millard Fillmore Gates Hospital, Kaleida Health
Buffalo, NY, USA

Daniel Thomas MD
Department of Radiology
University Hospital Bonn
Bonn, Germany

John D.R. Thomson MD
Department of Congenital Heart Disease
Leeds General Infirmary
Leeds, UK

Konstantinos Toutouzas MD
Department of Cardiology
Hippokration Hospital
Athens Medical School
Athens, Greece

Jurgen Verbist MD
Department of Cardiovascular and Thoracic
    Surgery
Imelda Hospital
Bonheiden, Belgium

Frank E.G. Vermassen MD, PhD
Professor of Medicine
Department of Vascular Surgery
Ghent University Hospital
Ghent, Belgium

Paul Vermeersch MD
Antwerp Cardiovascular Institute Middelheim
Ziekenhuis Netwerk Antwerpen
Antwerp, Belgium

List of Contributors

Erol Veznedaroglu MD
Director, Stroke and Cerebrovascular Center of
    New Jersey
Chief Cerebrovascular and Endovascular
    Neurosurgery
Trenton, NJ, USA

Ron Waksman MD, FACC
Professor of Medicine
Associate Director, Division of Cardiology
Director, Experimental Cardiology
Washington Hospital Center
Washington, DC, USA

Arne Warth MD
Institute of Pathology
University Clinics Heidelberg
Germany

John G. Webb MD
Director, Cardiac Catheterization Laboratory
St. Paul's Hospital
McLeod Professor of Heart Valve Intervention
University of British Columbia
Canada

Susan E. Wiegers MD
Cardiovascular Division
Department of Medicine
University of Pennsylvania School of Medicine
Philadelphia, PA, USA

Neil Wilson MB BS DCH FRCP FRCP(CH)
Consultant Paediatric Cardiologist
Director, Paediatric Cardiac Catheter Laboratory
Department of Paediatrics
John Radcliffe Hospital
University of Oxford
Oxford, UK

Nina Wunderlich MD
Department of Cardiology
Cardiovascular Center Frankfurt
Frankfurt, Germany

José Luis Zamorano MD, PhD, FESC
Professor of Medicine
Chair, Cardiovascular Institute
Hospital Clinico San Carlos
Madrid, Spain

Thomas Zeller MD
Professor of Medicine
Head, Department of Angiology
Heart Centre Bad Krozingen
University of Freiburg
Krozingen, Germany

Preface

Since the introduction of percutaneous transluminal coronary angioplasty by Andreas Grüntzig in 1977, interventional cardiology has offered a variety of less invasive approaches for the treatment of cardiovascular disease compared with surgery with less morbidity, but more competitive regarding long-term clinical outcome.

Modalities like percutaneous coronary interventions, percutaneous closure techniques for the treatment of atrial septal defects, and peripheral vascular interventions are widely used as alternatives to the respective surgical procedures. More recently, percutaneous techniques for aortic valve replacement and mitral valve reconstruction have been introduced. By this expansion of indications for catheter-based interventions a traditional domain of cardiovascular surgery is touched.

In the face of the enthusiasm for less invasive treatment modalities by the interventionalists and the skepticism of many surgeons, we believe that interventional and surgical procedures do represent complementary rather than competitive approaches and that the currently available armamentarium has the potential to offer well-tailored management options for the individual patient.

The idea of this textbook is to discuss the potential clinical benefit of interventional versus surgical modalities for adult patients with cardiovascular disease requiring either an interventional or a surgical procedure and in particular for those patients who might be candidates for both strategies. This discussion is based on the detailed description of the individual pathology, pathophysiology, imaging, and clinical outcome which may be required or helpful when comparing the various treatment options.

Thus, *Cardiovascular Interventions in Clinical Practice* represents a new comprehensive concept designed to aid students, residents, general practitioners, cardiologists, neurologists, and surgeons in understanding the potential clinical benefit of both interventional and surgical management on the grounds of the individual pathology and prognosis.

Jürgen Haase
Hans-Joachim Schäfers
Horst Sievert
Ron Waksman

November 2009

1 Septal Defects and Valvular Heart Disease

1 Pathology of Atrial and Ventricular Septal Defects

Siew Yen Ho

Royal Brompton Hospital and Imperial College London, London, UK

Introduction

Congenital deficiencies of the atrial and ventricular septa are among the most common of congenital cardiac lesions. Ventricular septal defects occur in 24–35% while atrial septal defects occur in 4–11% of liveborn babies with congenital heart disease [1]. These defects can occur in isolation, in combination, or in association with many other defects. A ventricular septal defect is an integral part of tetralogy of Fallot, double-outlet ventricles, and common arterial trunk. It is also frequently encountered in association with complete and congenitally corrected transposition, pulmonary atresia, univentricular atrioventricular connections and coarctation, or interruption, of the aortic arch. When occurring in isolation, diagnosis may be delayed, sometimes well into adult life or later decades. In this chapter, we focus on these septal defects occurring as isolated lesions and discuss some of the complicating anomalies. For a better understanding of the anatomy of atrial and ventricular septal defects, it is pertinent to begin with a review of the normal cardiac septum.

Normal septal structures

Atrial septum

A cursory look from the right atrium gives the impression of an extensive septal structure. In particular, anterosuperior to the oval fossa, the seemingly vast expanse of "atrial septum" is the right atrial wall overlying the aortic root (Fig. 1.1a). Sectional cuts demonstrate the septum limited to the floor of the foramen ovale and the muscular rim immediately around it (Fig. 1.1b). The peripheral structures are the infolded right atrial wall anterosuperiorly, superiorly, posteriorly, and inferiorly, and the fibrofatty sandwich of the atrial and ventricular musculature anteroinferiorly [2]. The superior and posterior parts of the rim, often called the "septum

Cardiovascular Interventions in Clinical Practice. Edited by Jürgen Haase, Hans-Joachim Schäfers, Horst Sievert and Ron Waksman. © 2010 Blackwell Publishing.

secundum," are mainly the infolded right atrial wall between the base of the superior caval vein and the insertion of the right pulmonary veins to the left atrium. This infolding from the epicardial aspect is known to surgeons as "Waterston's groove," through which the left atrium can be accessed without entering the right atrium. Posteroinferiorly, the rim is continuous with the wall of the inferior caval vein. The true septal component is formed by the floor of the foramen ovale ("septum primum"), which functions like a flap valve by closing against the muscular rim in postnatal life when pressure in the left atrium exceeds that in the right atrium (Fig. 1.1c). In the normal heart, the valve is adequate to overlap the muscular rim so that there is no potential for interatrial shunts. The valve is completely adherent to the rim but there is an adhesion gap, or probe patency, in approximately one-fourth of the population, and this provides the potential for right-to-left shunting through the foramen ovale [3–5]. The rim is an infolding of the muscular wall of the right atrium, and the flap valve is a thin sheet of fibromuscular tissue that is usually 0.5–1.5 mm thick. Fatty tissues of the interatrial groove fill the epicardial side of the fold of the muscular rim. The extent of fatty tissue varies, and when it appears excessive in the normal heart it can give the erroneous impression of lipomatous septal hypertrophy. In young adults, the upper limit of normal fat deposit is defined as 1.5 cm in the transverse dimension on echocardiography [6].

Ventricular septum

In the majority of hearts, the right ventricle is in its anticipated location relative to the left ventricle. When the heart is seen from the front, there is considerable overlapping of the ventricular chambers. The anteriorly situated right ventricle curves over the left ventricle such that the right ventricular outflow tract passes cephalad and a little leftward, crossing over the rightward-directed left ventricular outflow tract (Fig. 1.2a and b). The ventricular septum looks very different when viewed from the right and left ventricular aspects. Significantly, the inlet part on the right side is covered over by the septal leaflet of the tricuspid valve, whereas the corresponding part on the left side borders the aortic outflow tract and is devoid of septal attachments to the

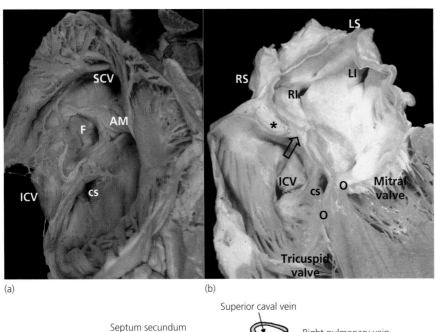

(a)   (b)

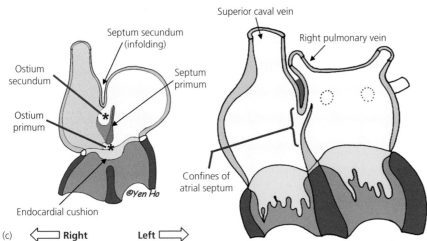

(c) ⟵ **Right**   **Left** ⟹

Figure 1.1 (a) The right atrium opened and displayed in right anterior oblique orientation to show the septal aspect *en face*. The oval fossa (F) is surrounded by a muscular rim. The anterior component of the rim extends to the anterior wall lying just behind the aorta (aortic mound; AM). In this heart, the eustachian valve guarding the entrance of the inferior caval vein (ICV) is like a fishnet (Chiari network). (b) A four-chamber cut of a heart shows the atrial septum in profile. The flap valve (open arrow) is thin. The infolding of the right atrial wall enclosing epicardial fat (asterisk) is well seen in this section. The circles mark the offset attachments of the mitral and tricuspid valves. (c) These diagrams represent the change from embryonic to definitive pattern at the atrial septum. The infolded septum secundum with epicardial fat (blue shape) is shown on the right-hand panel. cs, Coronary sinus; LI, LS, RI, and RS, orifices of the pulmonary veins (left inferior, left superior, right inferior, right superior); SCV, superior caval vein.

mitral valve (Fig. 1.2c and d). This is because the acute angulation between inflow and outflow tracts in the left ventricle places the outflow tract between the septum and the "anterior" leaflet of the mitral valve. The septal attachment of the mitral valve is confined to the hinge line (also known as the annulus) of its leaflets, and this is seen only in the posteroinferior parts of the left ventricle close to the cardiac crux. The simulated echocardiographic four-chamber section displays the difference in levels of attachments of the hinge lines of the mitral and tricuspid valves at the septum (Fig. 1.1b). This offset arrangement between the two valves results in a part of the muscular ventricular septum being situated between the right atrium and the left ventricle. Although previously termed the muscular atrioventricular septum, its composition is a sandwich of right atrial wall on one side, crest of the muscular ventricular septum on the other, with intervening fibrofatty tissue from the inferior atrioventricular groove,

which ingresses from the epicardium at the crux of the heart. Adjoining the "sandwich" anterosuperiorly is the central fibrous body together with the membranous component of the cardiac septum. The central fibrous body contains the penetrating bundle of His. Its continuation, the atrioventricular conduction bundle, is sandwiched between the crest of the muscular septum and the membranous septum (Fig. 1.3a). This feature is particularly relevant when considering holes in the vicinity of the membranous septum (Fig. 1.3b). The hinge line of the tricuspid valve crosses the membranous septum, effectively dividing it into atrioventricular and interventricular components (Fig. 1.3a). Viewed from the left ventricular aspect, the membranous septum is adjacent to the aortic valve. It adjoins the interleaflet fibrous triangle that lies in between the right and the noncoronary leaflets. Thus, the landmark for the course of the atrioventricular conduction bundle is the septal area between the

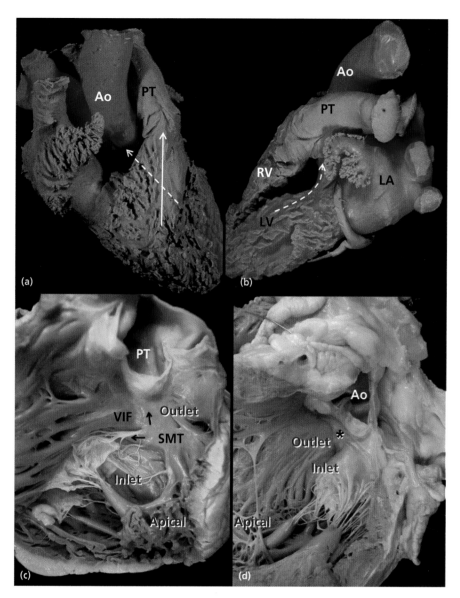

Figure 1.2 (a) This endocast of a normal heart viewed from the front shows the right ventricular outflow tract (solid arrow) crossing over the left ventricular outflow tract (broken arrow). (Note that the pulmonary valve is at a higher level than the aortic valve.) (b) The endocast viewed from the left side shows the relationship of the left ventricular outflow tract (broken arrow) to that of the right. The right ventricle is opened to show the septum and the three portions of the ventricle. (c) The limbs (arrows) of the septomarginal trabeculation (SMT) cradle the ventriculoinfundibular fold (VIF). (d) Dissection into the left ventricular outflow tract shows the proximity of the inlet and outlet portions. The asterisk marks the membranous septum. Ao, aorta; LA, left atrium; LV, left ventricle; PT, pulmonary trunk; RV, right ventricle.

right and noncoronary aortic sinuses. From there, the atrioventricular bundle branches into the right and left bundle branches (Fig. 1.3a). The cord-like right bundle branch passes through the muscular part of the septum to emerge subendocardially close to the insertion of the medial papillary muscle of the tricuspid valve. On the left side of the septum, the left bundle branch descends in the subendocardium to branch into three main radiating and interconnecting fascicles. The branching bundle and the proximal portion of the left bundle branch are, therefore, closely related to the septal aspect of the outflow tract immediately beneath the aortic valve (Fig. 1.3b).

Anterosuperior to the membranous septum is the pulmonary outflow tract exiting from the right ventricle. The musculature anterior to the membranous septum is the supraventricular crest, comprising the ventriculoinfundibular fold and its insertion into the septomarginal trabeculation at the septum (Fig. 1.2c). The septomarginal trabeculation is a characteristic muscle band looking like a tree trunk flattened against the ventricular septum in the right ventricle. It branches into two limbs that cradle the ventriculoinfundibular fold. One limb points anterosuperiorly to blend into the musculature of the subpulmonary infundibulum. The other limb points posteroinferiorly, and it is from this limb that the medial papillary muscle (also known as the conal muscle or muscle of Lancisi) arises to support the anteroseptal commissure of the tricuspid valve. The distal part of the septomarginal trabeculation extends into the moderator band that crosses the right ventricular cavity. The apical portion of the right ventricle bears coarse trabeculations that can obscure the presence of muscular septal defects.

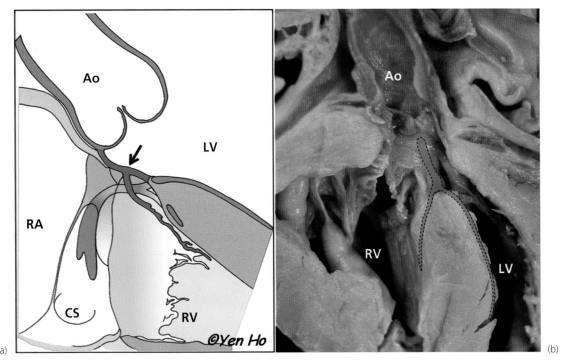

Figure 1.3 (a) Location of the atrioventricular conduction system (orange) in a normal heart. The atrioventricular conduction bundle penetrates through the central fibrous body to pass between the membranous septum and the crest of the ventricular septum, and continues as the branching bundle. The membranous septum (arrow) is crossed by the hinge line of the tricuspid valve. (b) Longitudinal cut through a heart with a perimembranous ventricular septal defect has the atrioventricular conduction bundle (orange shape) superimposed to show the bundle emerging from the area of tricuspid–aortic–mitral valvar fibrous continuity and the close relationship between the bundle and the margin of the septal defect. Ao, aorta; cs, coronary sinus; LV, left ventricle; RA, right atrium; RV, right ventricle.

In the outflow portion of the right ventricle, the conical sleeve of subpulmonary infundibulum is continuous with the ventriculoinfundibular fold. The infundibulum elevates the pulmonary valve away from the septum. Thus, in the normal heart, it is not possible to define a discrete muscular structure equivalent to an outlet septum separating aortic and pulmonary outflow tracts. The outlet septum is expressed in malformations of the outflow tract such as in hearts with Fallot's tetralogy, in which it is an exclusively right ventricular structure.

For convenience in describing the location of holes in the ventricular septum, the right ventricle can be considered as having three portions, although there are no anatomic lines that would allow division of the muscular septum into three parts (Fig. 1.2c). Thus, the inlet portion of the right ventricle is taken to be the portion receiving the tricuspid valve while the outlet portion is the part leading to the semilunar valves, and is mainly musculature proximal to the subpulmonary infundibulum. The remaining portion, the trabecular portion, is the most extensive. Owing to the configuration of the left ventricular inflow and outflow tracts, with the aortic outlet wedged between the septum and the mitral valve, much of the inlet portion of the right ventricle overlaps the outlet portion of the left ventricle (Fig. 1.2d).

Atrial septal defects

Although generally categorized as atrial septal defects (ASDs), some of the defects commonly referred to as ASDs are interatrial communications rather than deficiencies of the atrial septum. This is because the extent of the atrial septum is rather limited when a *septum* is defined as a partition that separates two adjacent chambers, and passage through the septum will not exit the heart (see Atrial septum). Strictly speaking, the septum that separates the two atrial chambers is the valve that is circumscribed by the muscular rim of the foramen ovale (Fig. 1.1a). Defects within this area, usually termed "secundum defects," are true atrial septal defects (Fig. 1.4a). By contrast, sinus venosus defects, coronary sinus defects, and "ostium primum" defects are outside the confines of the true atrial septum although, unequivocally, they permit interatrial shunting (Fig. 1.4a) [3].

Patent foramen ovale

As discussed above, the patent foramen ovale (PFO) is very common. It exists because of an incomplete circumferential adhesion of the *septum primum* (the flap valve of the foramen) to the *septum secundum* (the rim of the fossa). The gap, the last

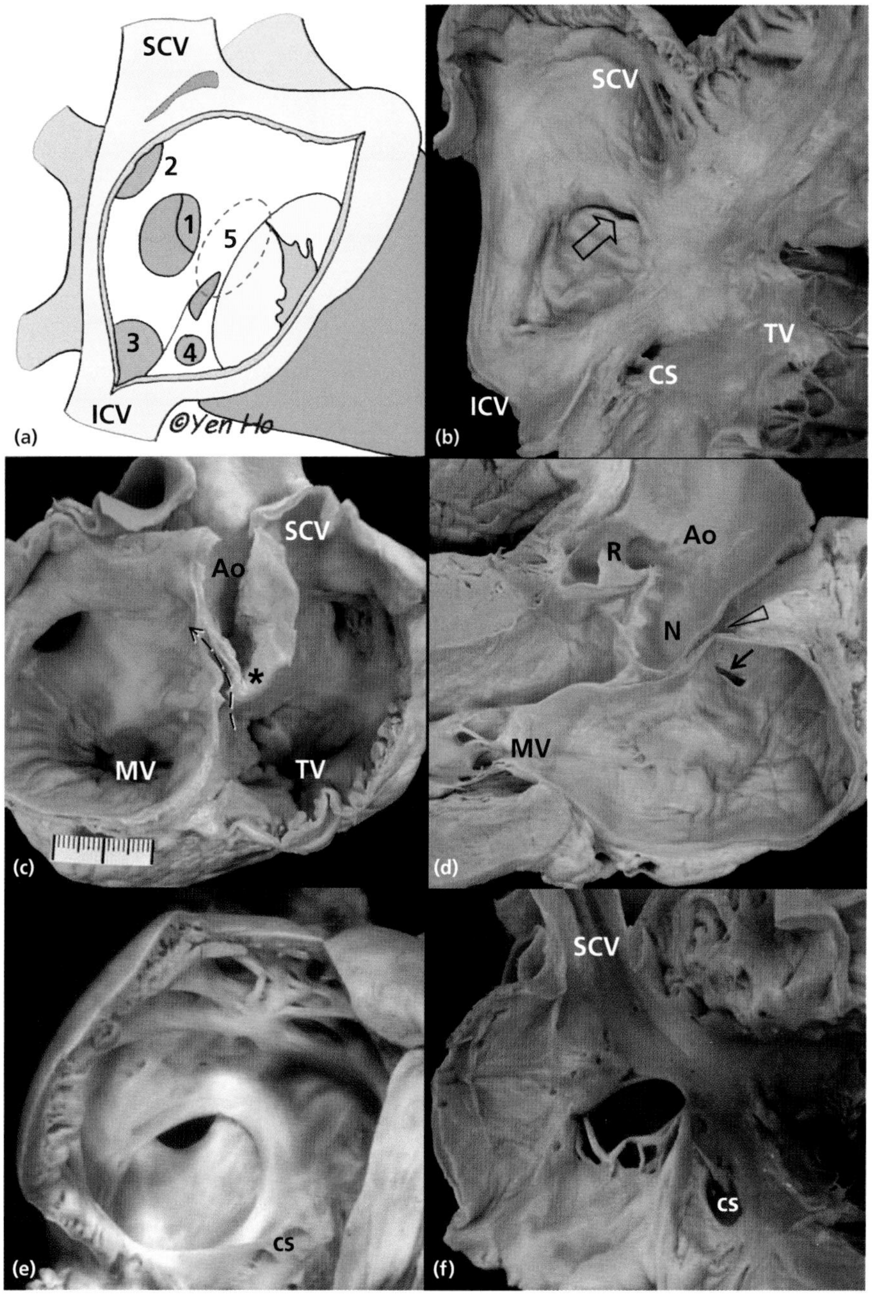

Figure 1.4 Locations of various interatrial communications in the right atrium. (a) The oval fossa defect (1) is the true atrial septal defect. The superior (2) and inferior (3) sinus venosus defects are related to the entrances of the corresponding caval veins. The coronary sinus defect (4) is at the site of the coronary sinus orifice. The atrial component of the atrioventricular septal defect (broken line) is indicated by the number 5. The orange shapes represent the sinus and atrioventricular nodes. (b) The patent foramen ovale (arrow) lies at the anterocephalad margin of the oval fossa. (c) Cut through the atria viewed from behind shows the infolded right atrial wall (asterisk) forming the right margin of the tunnel-like patent foramen ovale (arrow). (Note the aortic root emerging immediately anteriorly.) (d) Long-axis cut through the left heart shows the proximity of the exit (arrow) of the patent foramen ovale to the anterior wall of the left atrium. This part of the atrial wall can be exceedingly thin and it borders the transverse pericardial sinus (triangle) and the noncoronary aortic sinus (N). (e) Right atrial view shows an oval-shaped defect in the atrial septum owing to deficiency of the flap valve. (f) The valve of the oval fossa is lacking and only a few strands remain in the fossa. Ao, aorta; cs, coronary sinus; ICV, inferior caval vein; LV, left ventricle; MV, mitral valve; PT, pulmonary trunk; R, right coronary aortic sinus; SCV, superior caval vein; TV, tricuspid valve.

part of the valve to become adherent, is located at the antero-cephalad margin of the rim (if viewing the right atrium in a simulated right anterior oblique projection; Fig. 1.4b). The adhesion gap leaves a slit-like tunnel that allows a probe to be passed obliquely from the right atrium into the left atrium in approximately 25% of cadaver hearts. The length of the tunnel depends on the extent of overlap between the flap valve and the rim [7,8]. In the left atrium the exit site of the probe is at the crescentic margin of the flap valve, and this is closely related to the anterior wall of the left atrium

(Fig. 1.4c). This part of the wall can be exceedingly thin, and perforations can lead to the transverse pericardial sinus and the aortic root (Fig. 1.4c and d).

Morphologically, there are two forms of PFO [7]. The first is the valve-competent form in which, under normal circumstances, the valve is large enough to overlap the muscular rim, much like a door closing against a door frame. Although forming a perfect seal, some of these valves are aneurysmal in appearance and bow into the right and left atrial chambers with the respiratory phases. The second form is the valve-incompetent form, which probably results from stretching of the muscular rim in atrial dilation and/or retraction of the aneurysmal valve, allowing the flap valve to herniate markedly leftward or rightward, reducing the extent of overlap. It is arguable whether this form is due to deficiency of valvar tissues and is a true defect of the oval fossa ("secundum defect").

Defects within the oval fossa

Usually these so-called "secundum" defects are located at the site of the embryonic "ostium secundum" rather than a deficiency of the "septum secundum" since the septum secundum is largely the infolded right atrial wall. Deficiencies, perforations, or complete absence of the valve guarding the foramen ovale (the embryonic "septum primum") are the most common types of interatrial communications with a spectrum of sizes. The simplest form is one resulting from the valve being too small to overlap the muscular rim and so leaving an oval-shaped aperture between the rim and the edge of the valve (Fig. 1.4e). This form is most amenable to transcatheter repair providing there are adequate muscular borders without impinging upon the orifices of the pulmonary veins, the atrioventricular valves, the caval veins, or the coronary sinus [9–11]. Even so, the location of the valve is variable [9]. In some cases, it may be more anteriorly situated or more posteriorly situated. The valve itself may be perforated with single or multiple fenestrations. Sometimes, it appears like a net or is represented by a filigreed remnant (Fig. 1.4f).

When the valve is completely absent, or nearly completely absent, the defect is the hole surrounded by the muscular rim of the fossa. If the anterior rim is deficient, it is worth bearing in mind the proximity of the anterior margin to the transverse sinus and the aortic root. The right coronary and noncoronary aortic sinuses are in the immediate neighborhood. A deficient posterior rim reduces the distance to the orifices of the right pulmonary veins and also increases the proximity to the epicardium due to effacement of the infolding. Occasionally, the defect may extend toward the inferior caval vein or toward the atrioventricular junction. In the case of the latter situation, the distance of the defect from the annular attachment of the mitral valve may become reduced, increasing the risk of damaging the mitral valve during device closure. Although defects in the oval fossa do not alter the basic disposition of the sinus and atrioventricular nodes of the conduction system, these very large defects will reduce the distances between the margin of the defects and the atrioventricular node or the orifice of the coronary sinus.

In cases associated with persistent left superior caval vein draining into the coronary sinus, the coronary sinus is usually enlarged. In these cases, the muscular margin between the coronary sinus orifice and the defect needs to be evaluated carefully. Cases of successful device closure without obstructing coronary venous return have been reported [11].

Sinus venosus defects

These defects are usually located in the mouth of the superior caval vein and described as superior sinus venosus defects. The inferior sinus venosus defects are related to the inferior caval vein and are far less common. The key feature of sinus venosus defects is that they exist outside the confines of the true atrial septum (see Atrial septum). This is not to say that they cannot become confluent, or coexist, with deficiency of the oval fossa.

In the case of a superior sinus venosus defect, the mouth of the superior caval vein typically overrides the atrial septum above the superior rim of the oval fossa (Fig. 1.4a) [12]. Anomalous insertion of the right pulmonary veins into the wall of the superior caval vein is usual in this situation. The defect, therefore, has a well-defined inferior border, the superior rim of the oval fossa, which encloses epicardial fat. Roofing the defect is the overriding caval vein. Owing to the lack of a superior rim for anchorage, currently available devices for closing atrial septal defects are unsuitable. Surgical repair of this defect should take account of potential obstruction to the superior caval pathway following restoration of pulmonary venous return to the left atrium. Also at risk is the sinus node and its arterial supply should there be the need to widen the cavoatrial junction [13].

Sinus venosus defects related to the mouth of the inferior caval vein have similar features to those of superior sinus venosus defects. In the inferior position, the defect's roof is delineated by the posteroinferior rim of the oval fossa and the orifice of the inferior caval vein opens to both left and right atria (Fig. 1.4a). The lower right pulmonary vein can attach anomalously to the wall of the inferior caval vein. This type of defect is remote from the anticipated locations of the sinus and atrioventricular nodes but it lacks an inferior rim for device anchorage.

Coronary sinus defects

Defects termed "coronary sinus defects" cover a spectrum ranging from a hole at the site of the orifice of the coronary sinus and absence of the coronary sinus itself, to a single or multiple fenestrations along the course of the coronary sinus, allowing it to communicate directly with the left atrium. Absence of the wall of the coronary sinus together with the adjoining portion of the left atrial wall results in the deficiency described as unroofing of the coronary sinus [14]. The defect usually leaves the persistent left superior caval vein connecting directly to the left atrium. When existing as a hole at the orifice of the coronary sinus, it may be amenable to device closure [15]. However, closing a large defect at the site of the orifice of the coronary sinus may jeopardize the atrioventricular node because the triangle of Koch becomes foreshortened.

"Ostium primum" defects

This type of defect, although producing an interatrial shunt, is not a true atrial septal defect (Fig. 1.4a). Hearts with

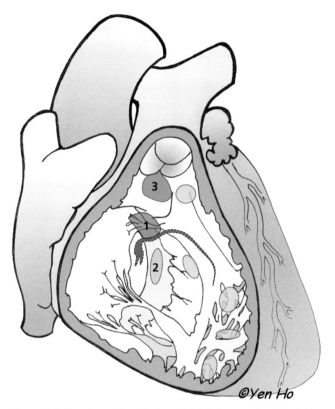

Figure 1.5 Three types of ventricular septal defect as seen from the right ventricle. The atrioventricular conduction bundle (red line) is shown skirting close to the posteroinferior margin of the perimembranous defect (1). By contrast, the bundle is related to the superior margin of a muscular inlet defect (2). Muscular defects can be located anywhere in the muscular septum and are represented by the yellow ovals. The doubly committed and juxtaarterial defect (3) are intimately related to the arterial valves.

this type of defect belong to the spectrum of hearts with atrioventricular septal defect since they have the same characteristic anatomic feature of a common atrioventricular junction [16]. In many cases, the oval fossa is intact and the so-called atrial septal defect exists between the free margin of the atrial septum and the atrial aspect of the conjoined leaflets of the atrioventricular valves. The septal component of the left and right atrioventricular junctions are at the same level (lack of offset between the atrioventricular valves). Owing to the valvar leaflets forming a significant part of the margin of the defect and the displaced atrioventricular node and atrioventricular conduction bundle being in the immediate vicinity, it will be exceedingly difficult to close this type of defect using current transcatheter devices without incurring complications.

Ventricular septal defects

This is one of the most common congenital heart malformations. The incidence is much higher when the defect exists

in isolation as most require little if any attention. A major determinant of outcome is the size of the defect. The majority become proportionally smaller with time. Spontaneous closure of the defect occurs in up to half of cases recognized in childhood [17,18], and it has been suggested may also occur in adult life. Generally, those who are asymptomatic are likely to have small defects.

This review of the morphology is restricted to isolated ventricular septal defects. For reasons already discussed, the ventricular component of atrioventricular septal defects will not be included. Also excluded are septal defects following myocardial infarction.

Description of ventricular septal defects

Over the decades, there have been many classifications of ventricular septal defects. In more recent decades, however, three main categories of ventricular septal defects are recognized: *perimembranous* (or membranous/infracristal), *muscular* (or trabecular), and *doubly committed and juxtaarterial* (or infundibular/supracristal/subpulmonary) (Fig. 1.5). These descriptions are applicable to defects existing in isolation as well as in association with other malformations. The distinction between perimembranous and muscular septal defects highlights the relationship of the defect's margins to the atrioventricular conduction system [19].

The location of any hole in the septum between ventricles can be described relative to the three portions of the normal right ventricle, i.e., inlet, apical trabecular, and outlet, with the approach by the surgeon usually from the right side of the heart. Furthermore, the size of the defect and any associated misalignment of septal structures need to be considered in any treatment strategy.

Muscular defects

The muscular defect is characterized by having completely muscular borders. Reportedly, it accounts for 5% of all ventricular septal defects, but its true incidence may be considerably higher as small muscular defects tend to close spontaneously. They can be described as being located in the inlet, outlet, or apical trabecular portions of the right ventricle. Muscular defects, especially those in the apical portion, may be multiple, giving the septum a Swiss cheese appearance, but these are rare. The thick right ventricular trabeculations overlying the septum may make it difficult to visualize or approach these defects from the right side. Some defects appear very small on the right ventricular side but actually form a large confluent defect when examined from the left side (Fig. 1.6a and b).

Muscular defects located in the inlet portion may be partially hidden by the septal leaflet of the tricuspid valve. A rim of muscle separates the border of the defect from the hinge of the tricuspid valve, distinguishing it from a perimembranous defect located in the inlet portion (Fig. 1.5). By virtue of its location, the atrioventricular conduction bundle is related to

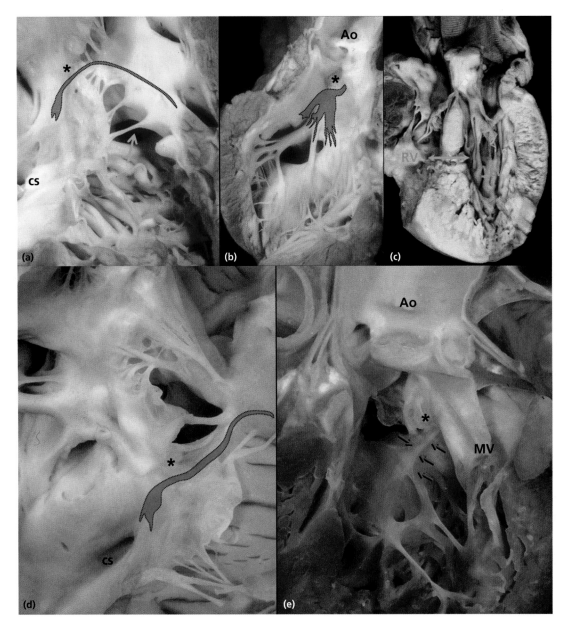

Figure 1.6 (a) Right and (b) left ventricular views of the same heart. The locations of the atrioventricular conduction bundles are superimposed (red) and the membranous septum is marked by an asterisk. The defect (arrow) is small on the right ventricular side but considerably larger on the left side where it is crossed by several muscle bundles. (c) Long-axis cut profiles a muscular defect (arrow) and shows its muscular borders suitable for device closure. (d) Right and (e) left views of the same heart with a perimembranous ventricular septal defect. The defect excavates toward the inlet portion of the right ventricle and is partially covered by the septal leaflet of the tricuspid valve. A remnant of the membranous septum (asterisk) is seen at the posteroinferior border. The atrioventricular node and bundle (red line) pass in this margin. The bundle emerges on the left side and is seen as a white streak (arrows).

the superior margin of the muscular defect. This is in distinct contrast to perimembranous defects (see below). When a muscular inlet defect co-exists with a perimembranous defect, the atrioventricular conduction bundle runs in the muscle bar separating the two defects (Fig. 1.5).

Muscular defects high in the outlet portion are very rare. Seemingly safe from the pulmonary valve, they may be sited close to the aortic valve on the left ventricular side. When the muscular rim in the superior border is narrow, such defects may be difficult to distinguish from doubly committed and juxtaarterial defects (see below).

The majority of muscular defects are not round [20]. They range from being slit-like to the more usual oval shape or D shape (Fig. 1.6a–c). Furthermore, the defects tend to "burrow" through the septum such that their opening on the right side of the septum is offset from that on the left side. In some cases the opening on one side is larger than on the other side and in others the hole is crossed by muscle bars on one side (Fig. 1.6a and b).

Perimembranous defects

This is the most common type of ventricular septal defect. Being in the environs of the membranous septum, it is related to several important structures. As these defects usually involve a more extensive area than that occupied by the normal membranous septum, they are best described as perimembranous. The key feature of perimembranous defects in all hearts with concordant atrioventricular connections is either a remnant of the membranous septum or fibrous continuity between the atrioventricular valves at the posteroinferior border (Fig. 1.6d and e). It is at this part of the border that the atrioventricular conduction bundle emerges from the central fibrous body to become subendocardial and, in most cases, the branching portion of the bundle appears on the left side of the septal crest.

Perimembranous defects vary in shapes and sizes and can extend toward the inlet, outlet, or apical trabecular portions. Large defects have been described as confluent. In our pathological series [20], the majority of perimembranous defects were oval or round in shape when the septum was viewed *en face* from the right side. When located in the inlet, they are partially, or even entirely, covered over by the septal leaflet of the tricuspid valve (Fig. 1.6d and e). Cords tethering the leaflet usually cross the defect on the right ventricular aspect but in some cases are inserted to the septal crest or to the left side of the septum. In this location, the defect tends to be oval shaped with its long axis parallel to the valvar hinge line. The tricuspid and mitral valves lose their "offset" relationships and their hinge lines form the "roof" of the defect in long-axis echocardiographic sections. Owing to there being a defect, the atrioventricular conduction bundle is displaced more posteroinferiorly than normal, but it is still related to the area of fibrous valvar continuity in the posteroinferior margin of the defect. The medial papillary muscle is located in its anterosuperior border. Perimembranous inlet defects have been described as *atrioventricular canal type* defects [21] but differ in not having the hallmark of a common atrioventricular junction that characterizes atrioventricular septal defects [16].

Perimembranous defects that excavate toward the outlet portion are close to the semilunar valves. Although variable in shape, they tend to be more circular than the other forms of perimembranous defects. In hearts with normal arterial relationships, the aortic valve minimally overrides the septal crest. Aortic, mitral, and tricuspid valvar continuity forms the fibrous posteroinferior border (Fig. 1.3b). Again, it is this fibrous border that harbors the atrioventricular conduction bundle. The medial papillary muscle supporting the tricuspid valve is close to this quadrant of the hole. The distance of the rim of the defect from the conduction bundle depends on the size of the remnant of the membranous septum.

Some perimembranous defects excavate toward the trabecular portion. These tend to be oval or triangular with their long axis directed toward the cardiac apex. In these, the medial papillary muscle is located at the apical quadrant of the defect. Again, the atrioventricular conduction bundle runs in the posteroinferior border. On the left ventricular side of the septum there may be a rim of muscle between the defect and the aortic valve.

Tissue tags adjacent to perimembranous defects can be accessory tissues from the tricuspid valve or the membranous septum. Also described as ventricular septal aneurysms, these are involved in spontaneous closure or diminution in size of the defects [22]. True membranous septal defects are very rare and they are small. Even rarer are defects (described as Gerbode defects) that arise owing to the absence of the atrioventricular component of the membranous septum, resulting in shunting from the left ventricle to the right atrium. Shunts at this level are more often a result of perimembranous defects that are associated with a deficiency in the septal leaflet of the tricuspid valve.

Doubly committed and juxtaarterial defects

These defects account for 5–10% of ventricular septal defects and are more commonly found in the Orient and in Latin America. The feature that characterizes doubly committed and juxtaarterial defects is the lack of muscular separation between the arterial valves in the superior borders. These defects are *roofed* by the pulmonary and aortic valves. Only a fibrous raphe runs between the adjoining valvar leaflets. In some cases, the right coronary leaflet of the aortic valve prolapses into the defect. In many, the posteroinferior margin of doubly committed and juxtaarterial defects is muscular, owing to the fusion between the inferior limb of the septomarginal trabeculation and the ventriculoinfundibular fold. In others, the posteroinferior margin extends to the remnant of the membranous septum and becomes perimembranous. By the nature of their immediate proximity to the semilunar valves, these types of defects are unsuitable for closure using currently available devices. There is hardly any superior margin for safe anchorage without interfering with mobility of the semilunar valves or creating outflow obstruction.

Atrioventricular septal defect

As discussed above, the so-called primum ASD form is unlikely to be suitable for device closure. The form with a common valvar orifice (so-called complete form or atrioventricular canal defect) with both atrial and ventricular defects is also unsuitable. The bridging leaflets of the atrioventricular valve can be compromised. The rarest form that has only a ventricular component of the defect, when carefully selected, may be amenable to device closure. A 4-year-old patient underwent successful implantation of a device with good outcome (Dr. Michael Rigby, personal communication, 2007).

In this child, there was accessory valvar tissue at the margin of the defect.

Malalignment of septal structures

Descriptions of ventricular septal defects are not complete without considering whether the septal components are aligned. Malalignment between atrial and ventricular septa or between components of the muscular ventricular septum have important consequences on the structures in the vicinity of the septal defect. Perhaps the best-known situation of septal malalignment is anterocephalad deviation of the outlet septum in hearts with Fallot's tetralogy. In Fallot, the outlet septum is entirely in the right ventricle and its malalignment produces overriding of the aortic valve as well as subpulmonary stenosis. In contrast, malalignment of the outlet septum into the left ventricular outflow is associated with obstructive lesions of the aortic arch.

Malalignment between atrial and ventricular septa is exemplified by cases with straddling and overriding of the tricuspid valve. Whether existing with isolated ventricular septal defects or with other intracardiac defects, the cardinal feature is that the muscular septum does not extend to the crux of the heart but inserts to the right of the crux. The malalignment results in an abnormally located atrioventricular conduction axis with the atrioventricular node situated in the posterolateral margin of the tricuspid orifice and the bundle penetrating at the point at which the ventricular septum meets the right atrioventricular junction.

Conclusions

A good understanding of the morphological substrates and variations of atrial and ventricular septal defects is particularly relevant in the era of interventional cardiology [10]. An appreciation of the limited extent of the atrial septum helps in distinguishing true atrial septal defects from all other forms of interatrial communications, and also in identifying the ideal site for trans-septal puncture. Interatrial communications that are suitable for transcatheter device closure must be sufficiently remote from the atrioventricular valves, coronary sinus, pulmonary and caval veins, and the aortic root. To minimize the risk of complications, some of these defects, either because of their very large size, or because of their close relationship to these vital structures, require very careful evaluation before considering transcatheter device closure.

Description of ventricular septal defects need not rely on developmental concepts. The categorization described above draws attention to the location of the defect and the proximity of the defect margins to crucial cardiac structures. When considering transcatheter device closure of perimembranous ventricular septal defects, the size of the defect relative to the heart size is important on account of the locations of the aortic valve and the atrioventricular conduction bundle in

the immediate vicinity. Ventricular septal defects roofed by the arterial valves and those associated with malalignment of the septal components are unlikely to be suitable for percutaneous device closure without risking damage to adjacent valvar structures.

Acknowledgments

The Cardiac Morphology unit headed by Professor Ho receives funding from the Royal Brompton and Harefield Hospital Charitable Fund.

References

1. Hoffman J.I. (1990) Congenital heart disease: incidence and inheritance. *Pediatr Clin North Am* **37**:25–43.
2. Ho S.Y., Sanchez-Quintana D., Cabrera J.A., *et al.* (1999) Anatomy of the left atrium: implications for radiofrequency ablation of atrial fibrillation. *J Cardiovasc Electrophysiol* **10**:1525–1533.
3. Patten B.M. (1931) The closure of the foramen ovale. *Am J Anat* **48**:19–44.
4. Schroeckenstein R.F., Wasenda G.J., & Edwards J.E. (1972) Valvular competent patent foramen ovale in adults. *Minn Med* **55**:11–13.
5. Hagen P.T., Scholz D.G., & Edwards W.D. (1984) Incidence and size of patent foramen ovale during the first 10 decades of life: an autopsy study of 965 normal hearts. *Mayo Clin Proc* **59**:17–20.
6. Pochis W.T., Saeian K., & Sagar K.B. (1992) Usefulness of transesophageal echocardiography in diagnosing lipomatous hypertrophy of the atrial septum with comparison to transthoracic echocardiography. *Am J Cardiol* **70**:396–398.
7. Ho S.Y., McCarthy K.P., & Rigby M.L. (2003) Morphological features pertinent to interventional closure of patent ovale foramen. *J Interven Cardiol* **16**:1–6.
8. Marshall A.C. & Lock J.E. (2000) Structural and compliant anatomy of the patent foramen ovale in patients undergoing transcatheter closure. *Am Heart J* **140**:303–307.
9. Ferreira S.M.A.G., Ho S.Y., & Anderson R.H. (1992) Morphologic study of defects of the atrial septum within the oval fossa: implications for transcatheter closure of left-to-right shunt. *Br Heart J* **67**:316–320.
10. Rigby M.L. (1999) The era of transcatheter closure of atrial septal defects. *Heart* **81**:227–228.
11. Carlson K.M., Johnston T.A., Jones T.K., & Grifka R.G. (2004) Amplatzer™ septal occluder closure of secundum atrial septal defects in the presence of persistent left superior vena cava to coronary sinus. *Pediatr Cardiol* **25**:686–689.
12. Oliver J.M., Gallego P., Gonzalez A., Dominguez F.J., Aroca A., & Mesa J.M. (2002) Sinus venosus syndrome: atrial septal defect or anomalous venous connection? A multiplane transesophageal approach. *Heart* **88**: 634–638.
13. Busquet J., Fontan F., Anderson R.H., Ho S.Y., & Davies M.J. (1984) The surgical significance of the atrial branches of the coronary arteries. *Int J Cardiol* **6**:223–234.

14. Raghib G., Ruttenberg H.D., Anderson R.C., *et al.* (1965) Termination of left superior vena cava in left atrium, atrial septal defect, and absence of coronary sinus; a developmental complex. *Circulation* **31**:906–918.

15. Di Bernado S., Fasnacht M., & Berger F. (2003) Transcatheter closure of a coronary sinus defect with an Amplatzer septal occluder. *Catheter Cardiovasc Interv* **60**:287–290.

16. Becker A.E. & Anderson R.H. (1982) Atrioventricular septal defects. What's in a name. *J Thorac Cardiovasc Surg* **83**:461–469.

17. Alpert B.S., Mellitis E.D., & Rowe R.D. (1973) Spontaneous closure of small ventricular septal defects; probability rates in the first five years of life. *Am J Dis Child* **125**:194–196.

18. Corone P., Doyen F., Gaudeau S., *et al.* (1997) Natural history of ventricular septal defect. A study involving 790 cases. *Circulation* **55**:908–915.

19. Milo S., Ho S.Y., Wilkinson J.L., & Anderson R.H. (1980) The original anatomy and atrioventricular tissues of hearts with isolated ventricular septal defects. *J Thorac Cardiovasc Surg* **79**:244–255.

20. McCarthy K.P., Leung P.K.C., & Ho S.Y. (2005) Perimembranous and muscular ventricular septal defects—morphology revisited in the era of device closure. *J Interven Cardiol* **18**:507–513.

21. Neufeld H.N., Titus J.L., DuShane J.W., *et al.* (1961) Isolated ventricular septal defect of the persistent common atrioventricular canal type. *Circulation* **23**:685–696.

22. Ramaciotti C., Keren A., & Silverman N.H. (1986) Importance of (perimembranous) ventricular septal aneurysms in the natural history of isolated perimembranous ventricular septal defect. *Am J Cardiol* **57**:268–272.

2 Echocardiography of Atrial and Ventricular Septal Defects

Natesa G. Pandian[1], Antonietta Evangelista[1], Francesco F. Faletra[2], Stefano De Castro[1], Siew Yen Ho[1], Anirban Banerjee[1] & Carey Kimmelstiel[1]

[1]Center for Cardiovascular Imaging, Tufts University Medical Center, Boston, MA, USA
[2]Cardiocentro, Lugano, Switzerland

Introduction

Atrial septal defects (ASDs) and ventricular septal defects (VSDs) represent 10% and 25–40%, respectively, of all congenital heart diseases diagnosed at birth. ASDs, in particular, constitute around 30% of the congenital heart defects diagnosed in adults [1]. Although the primary method of therapy for closure of the ASD and VSD has been surgical repair for many decades, approaches that employ catheter-based devices have emerged as the method of choice for many lesions in recent decades [2]. The development and spread of those new interventional techniques have generated the need for appropriate selection of patients for this therapeutic approach [3]. The purposes of the diagnostic examination in patients with these lesions include detection and delineation of the site, size, and geometry of the defect, recognition of the spatial relationship of the lesion to adjacent structures, assessment of the hemodynamic impact of the lesion, and unmasking of associated lesions. This chapter will review the anatomy, pathophysiology, echocardiographic diagnosis, and treatment of atrial and ventricular septal defects, with emphasis on features that have a bearing on percutaneous interventions for both disorders.

Atrial septal defects

Embryology and anatomy of the atrial septum

At the fourth and fifth weeks of gestation, the division of the atria begins with the formation of the septum primum, creating a temporary communication between the two atria—the ostium primum. Before complete closure of the ostium primum, numerous perforations appear in the superior part of the septum primum. The coalescence of these perforations results in the formation of the ostium secundum. At this point of embryologic development, the superior rim of the atrial septum evolves, formed by extensive infolding of the atrial wall between the venous component of the right atrium and the right pulmonary veins. This, called the septum secundum, overlaps the ostium primum, creating the foramen ovale.

The atrial septum from the right atrial septal surface is formed by the fossa ovalis and its surrounding rim. The rim often appears as thicker or raised muscle that surrounds an oval-shaped depression (the fossa) that is covered over by a thin valve that lies on the left atrial aspect. The fossa ovalis is completely overlapped by its valve, a flap of tissue that is continuous with the left atrial wall. During fetal life, the valve opens leftward, allowing blood to flow from the right atrium into the left atrium through its aperture (foramen ovale). After birth, higher pressure in the left atrium pushes the valve rightward onto its rim, closing the foramen ovale. The fossa ovalis is anatomically closed in about two-thirds of adults as a result of complete adhesion of the valve to its rim. In the remaining one-third it remains patent at the site of the previous foramen ovale. A patent foramen ovale remains a potential source for right-to-left shunt. A redundant valve tissue may form an aneurysm of the fossa ovalis. It is the valve of the fossa ovalis that is the target for trans-septal crossing when interventions are performed. Although the right aspect of the septum is often characterized by the crater-like structure of the fossa ovalis, the atrial septum is relatively featureless when viewed from the left atrium [4].

Pathophysiology and management

Clinical effects of isolated ASDs are usually related to left-to-right shunting. The magnitude of the shunt is related to the size of the defect and to the relative compliance of the left- and right-sided cardiac chambers, and indirectly related to the resistance of the pulmonary and systemic circulation [5]. Approximately 15% of ostium secundum ASDs spontaneously close by 4 years of age. If left untreated, patients with hemodynamically significant ASDs will develop symptoms of right-sided heart failure secondary to pulmonary hypertension (due to the pulmonary vascular obstructive disease caused by increased right-sided flow). Certain types of ASDs (sinus venosus and

Cardiovascular Interventions in Clinical Practice. Edited by Jürgen Haase, Hans-Joachim Schäfers, Horst Sievert and Ron Waksman. © 2010 Blackwell Publishing.

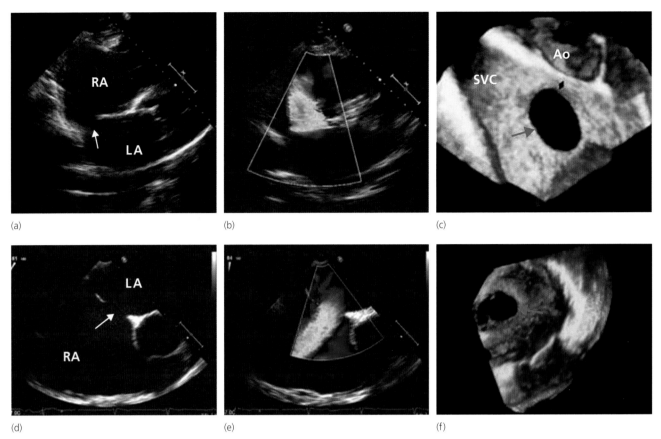

Figure 2.1 2-D and 3-D echocardiographic images of secundum ASDs. (a) A subcostal 2-D echocardiographic image displaying a large ASD. (b) The shunt flow through the defect. (d, e) The defect and shunt flow in TEE recordings. (c, f) 3-D echocardiographic *en face* images of ASDs: (c) the right atrium; (f) the left atrium. The *en face* images are useful in measuring the size of the defect and that of the surrounding rims. RA, right atrium; LA, left atrium; SVC, superior vena cava; Ao, Aorta.

primum varieties) do not close spontaneously. Their location and the presence of concomitant lesions preclude transcatheter closure. Surgery is recommended for patients with these types of ASDs [6]. In patients with patent foramen ovale (PFO) after a cryptogenic stroke, closure of the interatrial communication with surgery or a catheter-delivered device should be considered if the cerebral events are prolonged or recurrent, or if they are followed by residual neurologic deficit [7].

As a general rule, adults with a significant ASD with evidence of right heart dilation should be offered elective closure soon after the diagnosis is established, irrespective of age, whereas in children, device closure is often performed at 5 years of age. Current indications for ASD closure are [8] right atrial and right ventricular dilation, ASD minimum diameter >10 mm, and/or pulmonary to systemic flow ratio (Q_p/Q_s) of >1.5:1.0. Transcatheter device closure of secundum atrial septal defects now represents the standard of care for this abnormality. Indications for catheter closure are the same as for surgical closure, but patient selection criteria are more narrowly defined [9]. Patients in whom the stretched secundum ASD is >36 mm, the atrial septal rims are inadequate (<4–5 mm) to permit stable device deployment, the defect is in close proximity to

the atrioventricular valves, the coronary sinus, or the venae cavae, or in whom other cardiac conditions requiring surgical repair are present are usually referred for surgical repair [10].

Echocardiographic anatomy and diagnosis of atrial septal defects

There are four major types of ASDs: ostium secundum, ostium primum, sinus venosus and coronary sinus septal defect (Figs. 2.1 and 2.2). Two- and three-dimensional echocardiography (2-DE and 3-DE) provide direct noninvasive visualization of all types of ASD (Fig. 2.3). Doppler techniques aid in the detection and quantitation of the shunt flow (Fig. 2.3). Although the lesions are identified as interruptions in the linear image of the atrial septum on a 2-D echocardiographic image, 3-DE can display the hole in the septum in *en face* views and allow for the measurement of the geometry of the defect and its rim. The presence of an ASD is generally suspected by indirect echocardiographic findings: enlargement of the right ventricle, septal flattening, and paradoxical motion of the interventricular septum (Fig. 2.3). These findings suggest right ventricular volume overload and represent grounds for suspicion of a defect.

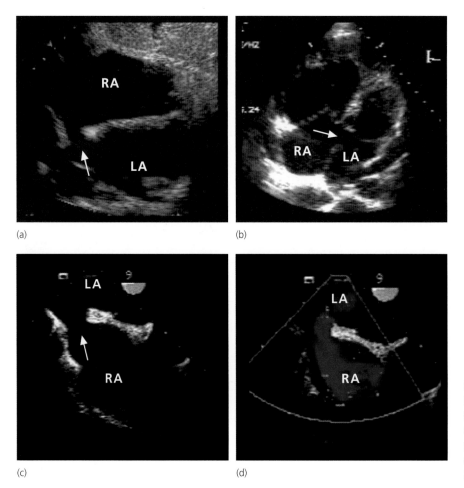

Figure 2.2 Various types of ASDs are shown in these 2-D echocardiographic images. (a) A subcostal transthoracic view showing a sinus venosus type ASD (arrow). (b) An ostium primum defect. (c, d) TEE images of a sinus venosus defect. RA, right atrium; LA, left atrium.

The *ostium secundum* defect, located in the area of the fossa ovalis, is the most common type of ASD, accounting for about 75% of all cases. The shape of the defect varies from circular to oval. Less often, strands of tissue cross the defect, creating a fenestrated appearance that suggests multiple defects. Rarely, a defect can extend posteriorly and inferiorly, approaching the site of inferior vena cava entry into the right atrium. Transthoracic 2-DE views in the parasternal short axis, as well as apical and subcostal four-chamber views, allow for the detection of ASDs. Ostium secundum ASD is visualized in the middle portion of the septum in the fossa ovalis area (Fig. 2.1). Modified views that place the interatrial septum as perpendicular to the imaging plane as possible are often needed to delineate the defect and measure the dimensions. When transthoracic examination is suboptimal, transesophageal echocardiography (TEE) provides crisp definition of the lesion (Fig. 2.1). The ostium secundum defect lies centrally and the sinus venosus more superiorly, with the mouth of the superior vena cava overriding its superior margin. It is important to interrogate the entire atrial septum to ensure that small defects at the margins of the septum are not missed [11].

Color Doppler displays the presence and direction of the shunt flow across the ASD. From transthoracic 2-DE and 3-DE images, the following measurements can be made: dimensions, area and circumference, and the extent of the rim surrounding the defect. 3-DE, particularly by TEE approach, provides excellent images of all four rims of the atrial septum surrounding the ASD. The tissue surrounding the defect is measured as follows: the superior–anterior rim is the distance from the anterior border of the defect to the outer aortic wall closest to the defect; the inferior–anterior rim is from the inferior border of the defect to the tricuspid valve annulus; the superior–posterior rim is between the superior border of the defect to the midpoint of the inlet orifice diameter of the superior vena cava; and the inferior–posterior rim is from the inferior border of the defect to the midpoint of the inlet orifice diameter of the inferior vena cava [12]. These measurements greatly aid in the selection of patients for transcatheter device closure.

Ostium primum defect

The *ostium primum* defect accounts for about 15% of ASDs, and is located in the lower part (or septum primum) of the interatrial septum (Fig. 2.2). This ASD presumably results from failure of the endocardial cushion to close the ostium primum. This is sometimes termed a partial atrioventricular septal defect. Ostium primum defects involve the common

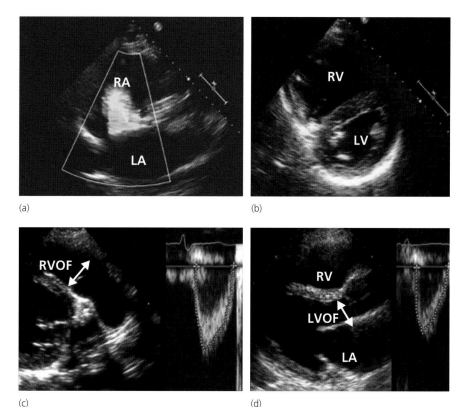

(a)

(b)

(c)

(d)

Figure 2.3 (a) A large ASD. (b) A short-axis recording that shows an enlarged right ventricle and flattening of the interventricular septum secondary to volume overload. (c) This image depicts the method of right ventricular outflow dimension measurement and pulsed Doppler recording of flow in that region necessary for quantitation of pulmonary blood flow. (d) Left ventricular outflow tract measurement and flow recording, necessary for quantitation of systemic blood flow. RA, right atrium; LA, left atrium; RV, right ventricle; LV, left ventricle; RVOF, right ventricular outflow tract; LVOF, left ventricular outflow tract.

atrioventricular septum, and are associated with deformity of the alignment of the atrioventricular valves and often with defects of the adjacent interventricular septum. One diagnostic hallmark of the disorder is the absence of the inferior part of the atrial septum (septum primum), which is adjacent to the atrioventricular valves. In contrast to secundum defects, primum defects are more easily visualized from the apical as well as the subcostal approach, with atrioventricular valve tissue forming their lower margin, and the secundum septum forming their upper margin. Ostium primum defects most commonly coexist with a cleft in the anterior leaflet of the mitral valve. Parasternal short-axis 2-D imaging displays a cleft as a gap in the anterior leaflet. The whole span of the cleft is better seen on a 3-D image. Color Doppler often shows a mitral regurgitation jet in various views.

Sinus venosus defect

The *sinus venosus* defect, which accounts for 10% of ASDs, usually involves the superior interatrial septum near the superior vena cava (SVC), and is almost always accompanied by partial anomalous pulmonary venous connection of the right upper pulmonary vein. Less commonly, the defect may occur at the junction of the right atrium and inferior vena cava (IVC) and be associated with an anomalous connection of the right lower pulmonary vein to the IVC. Sinus venosus defects may be difficult to detect by transthoracic 2-DE as they are located superiorly in the interatrial septum near its junction with the superior vena cava. Often nonconventional views should be attempted to image the superior portion of the septum (Fig. 2.2). With TEE, sinus venosus defects,

as well as the anomalous pulmonary vein(s), are easily identified. From the upper esophageal window when rotating the imaging plane to about 90°, the distal SVC and the superior atrial septum are visible in their long axis. In the sinus venosus ASD, the SVC often overrides the atrial septum, best seen in the biatrial view.

Coronary sinus defect

Coronary sinus defects are exceedingly rare, difficult to detect with certainty, and are associated with anomalous insertion of a left-sided superior vena cava into the coronary sinus. Modified four-chamber views are necessary to see the coronary sinus and the adjoining atrial septum. In the coronary sinus defect, injection of saline contrast in the left arm reveals transient entry of contrast bubbles into the left atrium, followed by rapid filling of the left ventricle.

All the Doppler modalities form an integral part of the echocardiographic examination of ASDs. Color Doppler displays the shunt flow and direction. From pulsed Doppler recordings of pulmonary and aortic valve flow recordings and 2-D echocardiographic measurement of right ventricle and left ventricle outflow dimensions, the pulmonary (Q_p)–systemic blood flow (Q_s) ratio can be measured by multiplying the cross-sectional area derived from the diameter by the time velocity integral of the flow in the outflow tract (Fig. 2.3). Continuous-wave Doppler provides recordings of tricuspid regurgitation jet velocity from which right ventricle to right atrium systolic pressure gradient is derived. This gradient, added to the estimated right atrium pressure, yields a measurement of right ventricle systolic pressure, and from this posterior–anterior

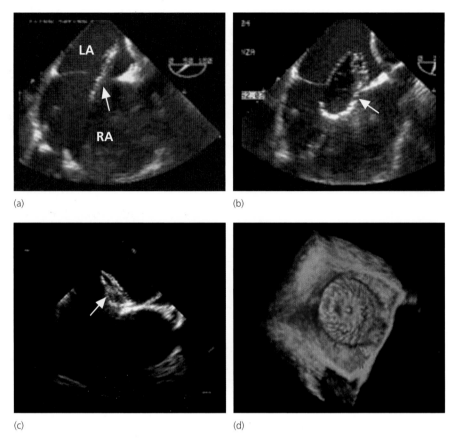

(a)

(b)

(c)

(d)

Figure 2.4 Transesophageal echocardiographic images during percutaneous closure of an ASD with an Amplatzer device. (a) A catheter is seen crossing the atrial septum through the ASD. (b) Balloon inflation (arrow) to measure the stretched diameter of the defect. (c) Image after both discs have been deployed (arrow). (d) 3-D echocardiographic image (*en face* view from the left atrium) showing a deployed device. RA, right atrium; LA, left atrium.

systolic pressure. From recordings of pulmonary regurgitation jet, pulmonary artery diastolic pressure can be estimated as well. Although color Doppler images easily reveal the shunt flow of an ASD, contrast echocardiography using agitated saline is helpful in patients with technically suboptimal acoustic windows to unmask a shunt. In the setting of a shunt, microbubbles are seen in the left atrium with systemic venous injection. However, the same finding may be seen in patients with pulmonary arteriovenous fistulae. In the latter, the bubbles arrive in the left atrium after a few heart beats, rather than appearing almost simultaneously in the right and left atria, as is noted in the former condition. An echocardiographic examination is also used to confirm the presence or absence of coexisting disorders, such as mitral valve prolapse, cleft mitral valve, anomalous pulmonary venous drainage, shunt lesions such as a VSD and patent ductus arteriosus (PDA), and stenotic and regurgitant valve lesions.

Patent foramen ovale

The possible role of a PFO in cryptogenic strokes has been well documented [13]. PFO differs from ostium secundum in its tunnel-like morphology. Contrast echocardiography is particularly useful in recognizing PFO, which is too small to be directly seen by conventional transthoracic imaging. Saline contrast examination by TEE coupled with the Valsalva maneuver is a sensitive method to confirm or exclude a PFO.

Guidance during percutaneous closure of atrial septal and patent foramen ovale defects

While transthoracic imaging may provide sufficient guidance during percutaneous closure of ASDs in children, TEE is often needed during such a procedure in adults (Fig. 2.4). Before closure, TEE is used to determine the size of the defect and to measure the ASD rim, as outlined earlier. For closure of ostium secundum ASDs, a 4- to 5-mm rim between the defect and the atrioventricular valves, the superior and inferior caval veins, and the entry of the pulmonary veins into the left atrium [14] is considered to be necessary for the use of closure devices. Additional information is provided about the stretched dimension of the ASD during balloon sizing, the position of the sheath and occluder during and after deployment, the outcome of the procedure after release, the presence of residual shunting, obstruction to systemic or pulmonary venous pathways, and interference with atrioventricular valve function. Under TEE guidance, the left atrial portion of the device is released, and drawn tight. After ensuring that the left atrium side device is well placed and not prolapsing through the defect, the right atrium portion of the device is released. With the closure device in an optimal position, pulling and pushing on the delivery wire or catheter then confirms that the device is secure. After deployment of the device and before disengaging, color Doppler and saline contrast injection are used to interrogate the atrial septum for residual shunt or other secondary defects. 3-DE

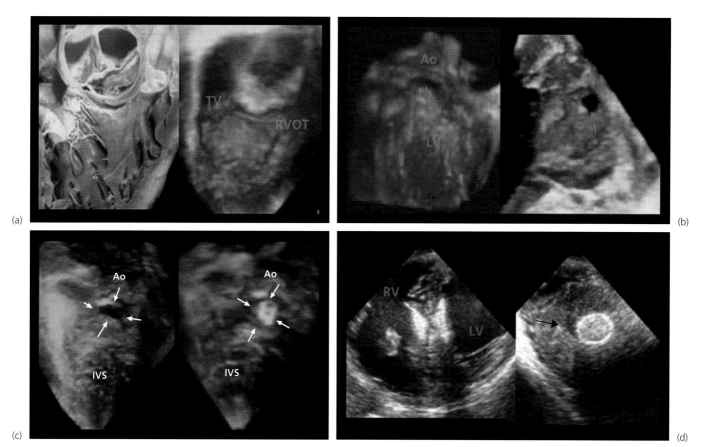

Figure 2.5 (a) Anatomic and 3-D echocardiographic images of a normal interventricular septum seen in an *en face* view from the right ventricle. (b) 3-D echocardiographic images of a membranous VSD (left) and muscular VSD (right). (c) 3-D echocardiographic image of a large VSD before and after closure. (d) An occluder device is seen deployed in a patient with post-infarct VSD; the occluder and a residual defect (arrow) are seen. AO, aortic valve; IVS, interventricular septum; LV, left ventricle; RV, right ventricle; RVOT, right ventricular outflow tract; TV, tricuspid valve.

can also provide valuable information on the mechanism of any residual shunt after device deployment [12,15]. When multiple openings are present, 2-D TEE may fail to detect the exact number of smaller (<2 mm) openings in 25% of cases, but these can be successfully detected by 3-DE. 3-D TEE plays a vital role in preselection of patients with multiple defects for double device closure [16]. Intracardiac echocardiography, imaging with a catheter-based transducer, is another modality helpful in guiding interventions. The advantage of this technique is that the interventionist can perform the procedure whereas TEE requires another operator to introduce and manipulate the TEE probe. However, the imaging plans provided by intracardiac imaging are limited compared with TEE.

Ventricular septal defects

Embryology and anatomy of ventricular septum
The interventricular septum is a highly complex, 3-D structure formed from a number of morphologically distinct subunits. The ventricular septum is formed by contributions from the primitive ventricle and bulbus, the endocardial cushions, and the conal cushions (part of the tissue that develops into the pulmonary artery and aorta). Although the ventricular septum is being formed, the position of the ventricles and the atrioventricular canal region shifts to align each atria and its valve over the correct ventricle. The left ventricle emerges from the primitive left ventricle, and the right ventricle from the bulbus cordis. The major division of the ventricles occurs as a ridge of muscular tissue that folds up into the ventricle and the two sides of the ridge fuse into the muscular or trabecular septum [17]. The remaining part of the ventricular septum is formed by contributions from the endocardial and conal cushion tissue.

The ventricular septum can be divided into two morphological components, the membranous septum and the muscular septum (Fig. 2.5). The membranous septum is small and is located at the base of the heart between the inlet and outlet components of the muscular septum and below the right and noncoronary cusps of the aortic valve. The muscular septum is a nonplanar structure that can be divided into inlet, trabecular, and infundibular components. The inlet portion is inferior–posterior to the membranous septum. It begins at the level of the atrioventricular valves and ends at their chordal attachments apically. The outlet or infundibular septum separates the right and left ventricular outflow tracts. It is called an "outlet" because it forms the outflow part of the right ventricle, or "infundibular" because it forms the area below the pulmonary artery. Defects occur anywhere along the ventricular septum, and their size and location determine the different types of VSD. When viewed from the right ventricular aspect, VSDs can be described as located at the membranous, inlet, muscular, or outlet portions of the septum. A subarterial (supracristal) VSD is a unique type of VSD in the superior margin of the outlet septum.

Another type of VSD is the acquired VSD, such as post-traumatic ventricular septal rupture or postinfarction VSD (PIVSD) (Fig. 2.5). Despite a reduction in the frequency of PIVSD with the regular use of thrombolysis, the incidence remains as high as 0.2% [18]. Two types of PIVSD exist: simple and complex [19]. Simple ruptures are direct through-and-through defects. Complex ruptures are associated with serpiginous dissection tracts remote from the primary site of tear of the ventricular septum. Complex ruptures occur mostly in the inferior acute myocardial infarction and less in the anterior infarction. Ruptures that involve the inferior–basal portion of the septum are much more likely to be complex than ruptures in all other locations. Septal rupture defects can be either very large or multiple, with the possibility of expanding in size over time. Ventricular septal rupture usually occurs within 1 week after the initial myocardial infarction, but can be a catastrophic complication even within the first 24 h [20].

Pathophysiology and management

The functional disturbance caused by a VSD depends on the magnitude of the shunt. A small VSD with high resistance to flow permits only a small left-to-right shunt, whereas large interventricular communication allows a large left-to-right shunt, if there is no pulmonic stenosis. Quantifying the shunt by the ratio of pulmonary–systemic circulation (Q_p/Q_s) is useful. The severity of pulmonary vascular disease correlates with the size of the shunt. In time, as pulmonary vascular resistance increases, irreversible histologic changes may occur within the pulmonary vascular bed. Untreated, a reversal of the flow occurs, leading to a right-to-left shunt with the development of cyanosis (Eisenmenger complex). The natural history of VSDs encompasses a wide spectrum, ranging from spontaneous closure to congestive cardiac failure and death in early infancy. Muscular VSDs can undergo spontaneous closure as a result of muscular occlusion. Perimembranous defects can close by formation of accessory tissue from the tricuspid valve. Subarterial (supracristal) defects can close by prolapse of the right aortic cusp, sometimes with deleterious effects on the aortic valve. A reduction in the size of the defect by any of these mechanisms results in changes in the hemodynamic significance of the defect. Other defects, such as malalignment

ventricular septal defects and the atriovenous canal type or inlet ventricular septal defect, are unlikely to close spontaneously.

Patients with VSD with evidence of significant left ventricular volume overload or progressive aortic valve disease require closure of the defect [21]. Endocarditis is a lifelong risk in unoperated patients and those with residual defects [22]. Proper prophylaxis and periodic follow-up are indicated. Patients with PIVSD are generally in an unstable clinical position, with acute hemodynamic changes that are poorly tolerated because of a reduction in ventricular function. The optimal treatment strategy is still under discussion [23]. Percutaneous closure during the acute phase after the infarction is a high-risk procedure with a high likelihood of failure, as is also the case with surgical repair [24]. Another additional risk involves the theoretical formation of a systemic or pulmonary embolism of fragile parts of necrotic tissue.

Location has been used as an indication for surgical closure regardless of the need for medical management in the case of infundibular defects [25]. Chamber enlargement is another measure of the degree of shunting and may indicate the need for closure. Generally, a change in Q_p/Q_s from 1.5:1.0 to 2:1 [26] or evidence of increased pulmonary arteriolar resistance is an indication for closure. A pulmonary–systemic vascular resistance ratio greater than 0.9:1.0 or pulmonary arteriolar resistance greater than 12 Wood units is regarded as a contraindication to surgery. Multiple "Swiss cheese" defects refractory to medical management may require a palliative pulmonary artery banding procedure.

At the present time, suitable candidates for percutaneous closure are those with a muscular VSD or a residual defect at the patch margins following cardiac surgery, and those who have suffered a myocardial infarction [27] (Fig. 2.5). Because of their close proximity to the aortic and tricuspid valves, perimembranous VSDs are generally considered unsuitable for transcatheter device closure unless there is a contraindication to open heart surgery. Even then, only perimembranous defects opening to the inlet of the right ventricle may be suitable [28]. Other defects unsuitable for device closure include those that are doubly committed and those associated with aortic valve prolapse, a straddling atrioventricular valve, or a distance of less than 4 mm between the border and semilunar or atrioventricular valve [29].

Echocardiographic anatomy and diagnosis of ventricular septal defects

Two- and three-dimensional echocardiographic imaging provides direct noninvasive visualization of all types of ventricular septal defect. Long- and short-axis views and modified apical views can display these defects on 2-DE (Fig. 2.6). A survey of the whole septum from base to apex in various views is necessary to detect and delineate the location, size, and shape of the defects. 3-DE can portray the defect in *en face* projections [30] (Fig. 2.5). Color Doppler imaging aids in the detection by displaying the shunt flow. Continuous-wave Doppler

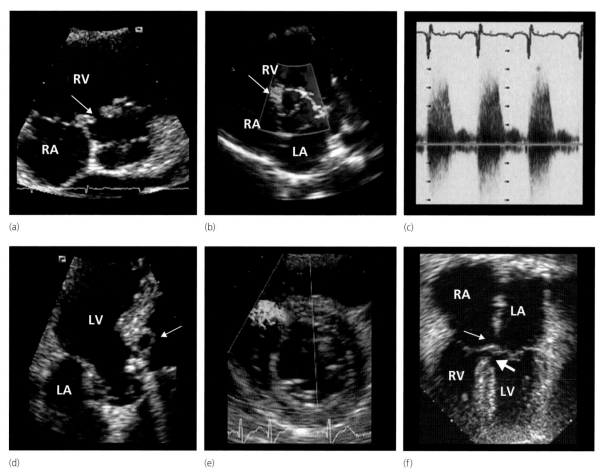

(a)　　　　　　　　　(b)　　　　　　　　　(c)

(d)　　　　　　　　　(e)　　　　　　　　　(f)

Figure 2.6 Various types of ventricular septal defects are depicted in these 2-D echocardiographic images. (a) A perimembranous VSD in the parasternal short-axis view. (b) Color Doppler displaying a left-to-right shunt through the VSD. (c) Pulsed Doppler recording of the shunt velocity. (d) A VSD and aneurysm of the membranous septum. (e) A muscular type of VSD with shunt flow. (f) Both a VSD (thick arrow) and an ASD (thin arrow) are seen in this patient with the atrioventricular septal defect. RA, right atrium; LA, left atrium; RV, right ventricle; LV, left ventricle.

allows for determination of the gradient between the ventricles (Fig. 2.6).

True defects of the membranous septum are surrounded by fibrous tissue without extension into adjacent muscular septum (Fig. 2.6). Such defects are rare. Defects that involve the membranous septum and extend into one of the three muscular components are called perimembranous VSDs, and are more common. These defects can be associated with the formation of pseudoaneurysm tissue along the right ventricular side of the septum, which can be seen in 2-D and 3-D echocardiographic images. A perimembranous inlet VSD has no muscular rim between the defect and the atrioventricular valve annulus. Defects in the inlet septum can include abnormalities of the tricuspid and mitral valves. Sometimes called common atrioventricular canal defect, they should not be mistaken for the VSD component in hearts with an atrioventricular septal defect. The latter entity has the distinctive morphologic feature of a common atrioventricular junction, which is not seen in hearts with perimembranous inlet VSD. A defect in the trabecular septum is called a muscular VSD if

the defect is completely rimmed by muscle (Fig. 2.6). Such defects may be singular and small, and the incidence of spontaneous closure tends to be high; alternatively, they can be multiple with significant hemodynamic effects. In the most severe manifestation, the septum displays a "Swiss cheese" appearance. Color Doppler imaging displays the shunt flow when the septum is scanned in various projections.

Defects in the infundibular septum are called infundibular, outlet, supracristal, conal, conoventricular, subpulmonary, or doubly committed subarterial defects. A deficient infundibular septum may be present with corresponding degrees of misalignment of the infundibular septum and the remainder of the ventricular septum. Although this defect may exist in isolation, it is most frequently associated with other defects such as tetralogy of Fallot.

Three-dimensional echocardiography presents an accurate view of the anatomy of the VSD (Fig. 2.5). Planes that show the VSD from its right aspect reproduce the surgical viewpoint of a right ventriculotomy (right ventricle *en face* view). From these images it is possible to define the morphologic nature of the margins of the defect, its shape, and the direction in which the defect extends into the ventricular septum. Other anatomic structures such as the tricuspid valve leaflet, the right ventricular outflow tract, and the aortic valve can be displayed in their realistic spatial distribution [31]. Similar to a surgeon's perspective, direct 3-D echocardiographic visualization of certain membranous and muscular VSDs from the right ventricle *en face* view can be obscured by overlying tissue or cardiac structures. In particular, perimembranous VSDs, on the right ventricle side, may be obscured by either tricuspid valve tissue or remnants of the membranous septum; they are best seen from a three-chamber view, which includes the left atrium, left ventricle, and aorta. The perimembranous VSDs are either circular or oval and can consistently be seen immediately below the aortic valve. However, in about 15% of patients, a small, thin rim of tissue, 2 mm in length, is interposed between the aortic valve and superior rim of the defect. From the left ventricle cut plane, certain large perimembranous defects can be seen extending posteriorly to the atrioventricular septum or inferiorly to the muscular septum [30].

The outlet defects are best visualized on parasternal long-axis and short-axis views. In the parasternal short-axis view, they can be differentiated into supracristalis and infracristalis, based on their position above or below the crista supraventricularis. The 3-D echocardiographic *en face* projection from the left side shows doubly committed VSDs to be directly sub-aortic, albeit slightly more anterior than the typical perimembranous defect. The right ventricle *en face* projection portrays the defects directly subpulmonic, away from the membranous septum and adjacent tricuspid valve. After the diagnosis of an outlet VSD, it is important to thoroughly evaluate these patients for any evidence of aortic valve prolapse (specifically of the right coronary cusp) and for aortic regurgitation. 3-DE not only allows accurate assessment of the VSD size and degree of valve prolapse but also provides enhanced spatial appreciation of the commitment of the defect to both great arteries.

Muscular VSDs can be more difficult to visualize by 3-DE. Like the perimembranous VSDs, the cut plane should be initially oriented parallel to the left ventricle septal surface. However, the cut plane should be then rotated in various directions to better visualize the muscular defects, dependent on their location within the ventricular septum. For example, the cut plane should be rotated to include the aorta to best visualize high muscular defects. A two-chamber view, including only the left atrium and left ventricle, is best used to depict more posterior and/or inferior defects. The 3-D echocardiographic left ventricle *en face* projections provide unobstructed evaluation of the defects, their borders, surrounding structures, and their complex shapes [30]. Defects of the posterior inlet septum are usually best seen from the apical four-chamber and the subcostal view, both of which image the posterior cardiac structures. The septal leaflet of the tricuspid valve may partially obscure these defects, making them appear smaller than they actually are.

Small ventricular septal defects could be difficult to be visualized by 2-D or 3-D imaging alone; color Doppler demonstration of flow through the ventricular septum into the right ventricle aids in the detection of such defects. Doppler estimation of the pressure gradient between the two ventricles is best achieved with the Doppler interrogation beam parallel to the flow from the left to right ventricle. The spectral Doppler signal shows a rapid early systolic rise to a midsystolic peak and rapid late systolic fall; its shape is rather similar to that of atrioventricular valve regurgitation. The maximum velocity of flow through the defect provides a relatively accurate measurement of the pressure difference between the ventricles. The smaller the VSD, the higher is the flow velocity across the defect. The right ventricular pressure can theoretically be estimated by subtracting the interventricular pressure gradient from systolic aortic blood pressure, which is used as a surrogate for left ventricular pressure. A high velocity indicates low right ventricular and pulmonary artery pressure (small VSDs), whereas a low velocity indicates a high right ventricle pressure (usually in the presence of large VSDs). If the jet velocity progressively increases it means that the VSD is likely to close. In patients with Eisenmenger's syndrome, the signal is of low velocity and shows bidirectional flow.

When limitations in image quality prevent evaluation of these aspects of the VSDs by transthoracic echocardiography, transesophageal 2-D and 3-D examinations are useful. From the mid-esophageal window (0°), flexion displays the left ventricular outflow tract and the thin membranous part of the septum. Advancing the probe reveals the muscular/trabecular part of the septum (see muscular VSD), but it may be impossible to fully interrogate the apex in this view. Having performed the 2-D echo sweep, this is repeated using color flow mapping. Although it may be difficult to align the Doppler beam parallel to VSD flow, it is important to look out for turbulence within the right ventricle cavity and a flow convergence zone within the left ventricle cavity. In sub-arterial (supracristal) VSD and in rarer perimembranous VSDs, TEE is valuable in identifying the prolapse of the right aortic cusp into the defect resulting in aortic regurgitation. Such prolapse may potentially cause permanent damage to the aortic valve leaflets.

Guidance during percutaneous closure of ventricular septal defects

Size and the position and relationship with contiguous cardiac structures are crucial parameters that need to be accurately evaluated for the preoperative description of VSD for planning and performing percutaneous device closure or surgical closure of VSD. Although 2-DE is helpful in the detection of VSD lesions, 3-DE offers a better description of the geometry of VSDs and thus is useful in the selection of patients for surgery or device closure. Because the *en face* projection allows delineation of the shape and of the entire diameters and area, running the images frame by frame enables the dynamic change of the defect to be observed, and allows the maximum anterior–posterior and superior–inferior diameters and the largest and smallest areas of defect to be measured. This advantage of 3-D imaging is even more apparent when measurements of crescentric and triangular muscular defects are required, and in the case of any VSD with an asymmetric shape. One can also accurately define the location of the VSD in the septum, its relationship with other anatomic structures such as the tricuspid valve, the attachment of the tricuspid valve chordae to the right ventricular wall, the right ventricular outflow tract, and the aortic valve, and the margins of the VSD [32] (Fig. 2.5). Knowledge of the precise relationship to other anatomic landmarks helps avoid complications from device closure such as damage to the aortic or tricuspid valves. The presence of a 2 mm or more rim of tissue between the perimembranous defect and the aortic valve is generally required for device closure of perimembranous VSDs [33], or a distance of more than 4 mm between the border and semilunar or atrioventricular valve for device closure of muscular VSDs [34].

Precise delineation of the size, shape, and position of the VSD helps in appropriate preselection of patients and in planning optimal percutaneous or surgical approaches for defect repair. Criteria for the transcatheter closure of the ventricular septal defects are thought to be single muscular ventricular septal defect (maximal diameter <12 mm and distance >5 mm from the margins of the defect to the mitral valve, aortic valve, and apex) [29]. Balloon sizing of the defect is useful, but the type of closure device selected will depend on many factors, including the preference and experience of the operator, the thickness of the ventricular septum, and the exact morphology of the defect. The preference in the case of solitary defects is to use one of the various Amplatzer occluders (Amplatzer, Plymouth, MN, USA).

The *en face* 3-D echocardiographic view of ventricular septum is particularly useful in patients with PIVSD in deciding whether to use a surgical or percutaneous approach. The location of the PIVSD and the size of the margins of the VSD from the apex or semilunar or atrioventricular valves need to be considered when assessing the apppropriateness of a surgical patch or device closure. In some selected cases, the use of contrast echocardiography can be useful in the detection of PIVSD, in particular for smaller septum rupture or PIVSD with serpiginous aspect. The irregular edges of the PIVSD can be the cause of any residual shunt. The most commonly used device for PIVSD closure is the Amplatzer septal occluder [24] (Fig. 2.5).

VSD closure cannot be performed safely without the use of TEE. This mode of imaging is essential to provide information about the position of the wire, sheath, and occluder during and after deployment, particularly any interference with atrioventricular or semilunar valve function before release. There is a significant risk of a periprocedural hemopericardium which can be recognized immediately. The procedure is technically much more difficult than closure of an ASD. After

VSD device closure, the 3-D views can illustrate the geometric profile (flat or mushrooms profile due to oversizing) of the device from both the left and right sidse and can determine if it protrudes in the left or right ventricular outflow tract. Color Doppler imaging is useful to estimate the presence of any residual shunt. Real-time 3-D TEE may reduce radiation exposure from fluoroscopic guidance and also potentially shorten the procedure time for interventions [35].

Conclusion

Various modalities of echocardiography are necessary to recognize atrial and ventricular septal defects, to delineate precisely the size and geometry of the defects as well as the size of their rims, to estimate the shunt flow and pulmonary artery pressures, and to assess the hemodynamic effects on the cardiac chambers. 3-D echocardiography is particularly useful in the selection of patients for surgery and the use of closure devices. 2-D and 3-D TEE have become valuable tools both in the operating room and in the interventional laboratory to guide the corrective procedure, assess the efficacy of closure, and facilitate the immediate detection of complications.

References

1. Dave KS, Pakrashi BC, Woolder GH, *et al.* (1973) Atrial septal defect in adults: clinical and hemodynamic results of surgery. *Am J Cardiol* **31**:7–14.
2. Connelly MS, Webb GD, Sommerville J, *et al.* (1988) Canadian consensus conference on adult congenital heart defects. *Can J Cardiol* **14**:395–452.
3. Konstantinides S, Geibel A, Olschewski M, *et al.* (1995) A comparison of surgical and medical therapy for atrial septal defect in adults. *N Engl J Med* **333**:469–473.
4. Faletra F, Pandian NG, & Ho SY. (2008) The cardiac septum. In: Faletra F, Pandian NG, Ho SY (eds). *Anatomy of the Heart by Multislice Computed Tomography*. Oxford, UK: Wiley-Blackwell, pp. 81–87.
5. Mas MS & Bricker JT. (1990) Clinical physiology of left-to-right shunts. In: Garson A Jr., Bricker JT, McNamara DG (eds). *The Science and Practice of Pediatric Cardiology*. Pennsylvania: Lea & Febiger, pp. 999–1001.
6. Murphy GJ, Gersh BJ, McGoon MD, *et al.* (1990) Long-term outcome after surgical repair of isolated atrial septal defect: follow-up at 27–32 years. *N Engl J Med* **323**:1644–1650.
7. Meissner I, Khandheria BK, Heit JA, *et al.* (2006) Patent foramen ovale: innocent or guilty? Evidence from a prospective population-based study. *J Am Coll Cardiol* **47**:440–445.
8. Webb G & Gatzoulis MA. (2006) Atrial septal defects in the adult: recent progress and overview. *Circulation* **114**:1645–1653.
9. Carminati M, Hausdorf G, Tynan M, *et al.* (1997) Initial clinical experience of transcatheter closure of secundum atrial septal defect with a septal occlusion device. *Eur Heart J* **19**(Suppl.):136.

10. Vida VL, Barnoya J, O'Connell M, *et al.* (2006) Surgical versus percutaneous occlusion of ostium secundum atrial septal defects: results and cost-effective considerations in a low-income country. *J Am Coll Cardiol* **47**:326–331.

11. Masani ND. (2001) Transoesophageal echocardiography in adult congenital heart disease. *Heart* **86**(Suppl. 2):II30–II40.

12. Magni G, Hijazi Z, Pandian NG, *et al.* (1997) Two- and three-dimensional transesophageal echocardiography in patient selection and assessment of atrial septal defect closure by the new DAS-Angel wings device: initial clinical experience. *Circulation* **96**:1722–1728.

13. De Castro S, Cartoni D, Fiorelli M, *et al.* (2000) Morphological and functional characteristics of patent foramen ovale and their embolic implications. *Stroke* **31**:2407–2413.

14. Acar P, Saliba Z, Bonhoeffer P, *et al.* (2001) Assessment of the geometric profile of the Amplatzer and Cardioseal septal occluders by three dimensional echocardiography. *Heart* **85**(4):451–453.

15. Marx GR, Fulton DR, Pandian NG, *et al.* (1995) Delineation of site, relative size and dynamic geometry of atrial septal defect by real-time three-dimensional echocardiography. *J Am Coll Cardiol* **25**:482–490.

16. Cao Q, Radtke W, Berger F, *et al.* (2000) Transcatheter closure of multiple atrial septal defects. Initial results and value of two- and three-dimensional transoesophageal echocardiography. *Eur Heart J* **21**:941–947.

17. Van Mierop LH & Kutsche LM. (1985) Development of the ventricular septum of the heart. *Heart Vessels* **1**:114–119.

18. Crenshaw BS, Granger CB, Birnbaum Y, *et al.* (2000) Risk factors, angiographic patterns, and outcomes in patients with ventricular septal defect complicating acute myocardial infarction: GUSTO-I trial investigators. *Circulation* **101**:27–32.

19. Edwards BS, Edwards WD, & Edwards JE. (1984) Ventricular septal rupture complicating acute myocardial infarction: identification of simple and complex types in 53 autopsied hearts. *Am J Cardiol* **54**:1201–1205.

20. Menon V, Webb JG, Hillis LD, *et al.* (2000) Outcome and profile of ventricular septal rupture with cardiogenic shock after myocardial infarction: a report from the SHOCK trial registry. *J Am Coll Cardiol* **36**:1110–1116.

21. Minette MS & Sahn DJ. (2006) Ventricular septal defects. *Circulation* **114**:2190–2197.

22. Gersony WM, Hayes CJ, Driscoll DJ, *et al.* (1993) Bacterial endocarditis in patients with aortic stenosis, pulmonary stenosis, or ventricular septal defect. *Circulation* **87**(Suppl. I):I121–I126.

23. Topaz O. (2003) The enigma of optimal treatment for acute ventricular septal rupture. *Am J Cardiol* **92**:419–420.

24. Bialkowski J, Szkutnik M, Kusa J, *et al.* (2007) Transcatheter closure of postinfarction ventricular septal defects using Amplatzer devices. *Rev Esp Cardiol* **60**:548–551.

25. Lun K, Li H, Leung MP, *et al.* (2001) Analysis of indications for surgical closure of subarterial ventricular septal defect without associated aortic cusp prolapse and aortic regurgitation. *Am J Cardiol* **87**:1266–1270.

26. Backer CL, Winters RC, Zales VR, *et al.* (1993) Restrictive ventricular septal defect: how small is too small to close? *Ann Thorac Surg* **56**:1014–1018.

27. Pesonen E, Thilen U, Sandstrom S, *et al.* (2000) Transcatheter closure of post-infarction ventricular septal defect with the Amplatzer septal occluder device. *J Scand Cardiovasc* **34**:446–448.

28. Rigby M & Redington A. (1995) Primary transcatheter umbrella closure of perimembranous ventricular defect. *Br Heart J* **73**:368–371.

29. Acar P, Abdel-Massih T, Douste-Blazy MY, *et al.* (2002) Assessment of muscular ventricular septal defect closure by transcatheter or surgical approach: a three-dimensional echocardiographic study. *Eur J Echocardiogr* **3**:185–191.

30. Kardon RE, Cao QL, Masani N, *et al.* (1998) New insights and observations in three-dimensional echocardiographic visualization of ventricular septal defects. *Circulation* **98**:1307–1314.

31. Chen FL, Hsiung MC, Nanda N, *et al.* (2006) Real time three-dimensional echocardiography in assessing ventricular septal defects: an echocardiographic-surgical correlative study. *Echocardiography* **23**:562–568.

32. De Castro S, Caselli S, Papetti F, *et al.* (2006) Feasibility and clinical impact of live three-dimensional echocardiography in the management of congenital heart disease. *Echocardiography* **23**:553–561.

33. Acar P, Abadir S, & Aggoun Y. (2007) Transcatheter closure of perimembranous ventricular septal defects with Amplatzer occluder assessed by real-time three-dimensional echocardiography. *Eur J Echocardiogr* **8**:110–115.

34. Thanopoulos BD & Rigby ML. (2005) Outcome of transcatheter closure of muscular ventricular septal defects with the Amplatzer ventricular septal defect occluder. *Heart* **91**:513–516.

35. Balzer J, Kühl H, Rassaf T, *et al.* (2008) Real-time transesophageal three-dimensional echocardiography for guidance of percutaneous cardiac interventions: first experience. *Clin Res Cardiol* **97**:565–574.

3 MRI of Atrial and Ventricular Septal Defects

Philipp Beerbaum

Evelina Children's Hospital, and King's College, London, UK

Introduction

The intention of this chapter is to review current applications of cardiac MRI in the evaluation of septal defects, which represent the most common form of congenital heart disease if bicuspid aortic valve is excluded [1]. Cardiac septal defects include atrial and ventricular septal defects, endocardial cushion defects (partial/complete atrioventricular septal defects), and residual defects (also including intraatrial baffle leaks in more complex congenital heart defects such as atrial-switch in transposition of the great arteries).

This chapter will not address ventricular septal rupture after myocardial infarction as MRI has no practical role in the management of these acutely ill patients, which rather is based on echocardiography [2]. Moreover, the role of cardiac MRI in the diagnosis of patent foramen ovale (PFO) will not be discussed because it is not used in clinical management, although it is possible to use dynamic first-pass contrast agent signal–time studies to demonstrate rapid recirculation and PFO shunting [3].

The specific *anatomical features* of any given septal defect may be identified readily using cardiac MRI methods [4]. Both dark-blood spin-echo MRI and bright-blood gradient-echo two-dimensional (2-D) MRI are helpful to identify anatomy, i.e., to delineate the specific septal defect morphology and location in relation to relevant adjacent structures [5]. Flow-sensitive phase-contrast cine sequences are particularly useful to image shunts across septal defects [6–8]. More recently, 2-D steady-state free precession (2-D SSFP) cine MRI has become the "work horse" imaging technique for many cardiac MRI applications, such as quantitative ventricular volumetrics and valve imaging, as it combines excellent blood–myocardium contrast and rapid scanning [9]. Contrast-enhanced 3-D MR angiography and 3-D bright-blood SSFP "whole-heart" volume imaging are especially useful when septal defects are combined with associated lesions in more complex congenital heart disease [10,11].

Cardiovascular Interventions in Clinical Practice. Edited by Jürgen Haase, Hans-Joachim Schäfers, Horst Sievert and Ron Waksman. © 2010 Blackwell Publishing.

In routine clinical practice, the *hemodynamic effect* of a given septal defect may be easily quantified using volumetric techniques assessing ventricular output [12]. Thus, end-diastolic and end-systolic ventricular volumes are usually assessed using 2-D SSFP cine imaging, and stroke volume and ejection fraction are calculated, with inter- and intraobserver quality being satisfactory for both the right and the left ventricle [13,14]. Hence, cardiac MRI is now regarded as the gold standard method to obtain quantitative ventricular volumes [9]. Moreover, blood flow in the great vessels may be quantified using phase-contrast cine MRI. The "MR flow" technique allows both volume flow rates to be obtained and peak velocities to be estimated to quantify valvular gradients and valvular regurgitation. Pulmonary–systemic blood flow ratios (Q_p/Q_s) may be calculated noninvasively by comparing the pulmonary artery flow with the aortic flow measurement [15]. Moreover, pulmonary vascular resistance may be quantified precisely by combining MR phase-contrast flow with pressure measurements obtained by MR-guided cardiac catheterization [16,17].

Atrial septal defects

Classification and pathophysiology

The various atrial septal defects (ASDs) represent a relatively frequent lesion (accounting for 6–10% of all congenital heart disease [18]) and may be classified according to their location, relative to the fossa ovalis, and their embryology. *Secundum ASD* is the most frequent type of ASD (~80% of all ASDs). It represents a substantial defect in the fossa ovalis as opposed to a persistent foramen ovale (PFO), which is a communication between the atria resulting from the nonfusion of the primum and secundum part of the atrial septum.

Sinus venosus ASD represent approximately 5–10% of all ASDs. The septal defect is usually posterosuperior to the fossa ovalis and is associated with anomalous pulmonary drainage to the right atrium or to the superior vena cava close to its entrance into the right atrium [19]. The left-sided pulmonary veins usually join the left atrium normally. Rarely, the defect is located posteroinferiorly such that the inferior vena cava may join both atria, resulting in some cyanosis [18].

The amount and direction of shunting across any large enough atrial septal defect depends on the difference between the compliances of the right ventricle, supporting the low-resistance pulmonary vascular system, and the left ventricle, supporting the high-resistance systemic vascular bed. In isolated ASDs there is usually *left-to-right (L/R) shunting* from the left atrium to the right atrium, imposing an increased volume load for the right-sided cardiovascular structures and resulting in their dilation. Smaller defects have a high rate of spontaneous closure during the first 4 years of life [20]. In growing children two-thirds of secundum ASDs may enlarge with time, and there is the potential for secundum ASDs to outgrow transcatheter closure with specific devices [21]. This is an important observation guiding the timing of transcatheter ASD closure as some devices are not applicable beyond a certain defect size. Defects anteroinferior to the fossa are termed as "primum ASDs" (~5–10% of all ASDs) and belong to the group of endocardial cushion defects [22] as discussed below (see under Atrioventricular septal defects).

Although very rare, an ASD may allow for atrial-level right-to-left shunting, resulting in cyanosis:

• secundum ASD or PFO associated with complex congenital heart disease such as with obstruction of the right-sided cardiovascular structures or with total anomalous pulmonary venous return (in which the systemic perfusion depends completely on the atrial septal communication);

• ASD associated with idiopathic or secondary severe pulmonary hypertension (Eisenmenger's syndrome) [23];

• An "unroofed coronary sinus" is a rare cardiac anomaly in which communication occurs between the coronary sinus and the left atrium as a result of the partial or complete absence of the roof of the coronary sinus. It is associated with a persisting left superior vena cava being connected to the left atrial roof. This lesion causes left-to-right shunting owing to the septal defect but also moderate right-to-left shunt resulting from the anomalous left persisting vena cava connection to the left atrium roof [24,25];

• Cor triatriatum dextrum, caused by remnants of the right sinus venosus valve in which there has been failure in the regression of the cranial part of the valve, leads to membranes attached to the crista terminalis. Thus, an obstruction in right atrium is present that may eventually cause atrial level right-to-left shunting, and so causing cyanosis in the presence of an ASD [26]; and

• Very rarely, a large defect in the inferior–posterior part of the atrial septum may be associated with partial drainage of blood from the inferior vena cava to the left atrium, resulting in cyanosis [27]. Similar hemodynamics may occasionally result from ASD repair when inappropriate positioning of the patch directs inferior vena cava blood to the left atrium.

Treatment

Although most patients with isolated secundum ASD are nowadays successfully managed using transcatheter techniques, all other forms of ASD usually require surgical patch closure [28,29]. For the high sinus venous defects associated with partial anomalous pulmonary venous connection to the superior vena cava, surgical repair consists of the construction of a tunnel using an autologous pericardial patch to redirect the right upper lobe pulmonary venous blood across the former sinus venosus septal defect and toward the left atrium [18]. The overall risk of mortality and morbidity from transcatheter and surgical treatment is extremely low in experienced centers [30]. The management usually occurs in the pediatric age group, although the diagnosis may occasionally only be made in adulthood as clinical symptoms may be only subtle. The rationale for transcatheter or surgical defect closure following diagnosis, regardless of the patient's age, is based on evidence that the defect is associated with a long-term risk of atrial fibrillation and heart failure, an increased risk of stroke in patients treated at an older age, and a reduction in life expectancy of nontreated patients [31–33]; in addition, there is evidence that even older patients benefit clinically from defect closure [29].

The role of cardiac magnetic resonance imaging before and after atrial septal defect treatment

The diagnosis of an ASD is most frequently made by transthoracic echocardiography (TTE) in childhood. In *secundum ASD* the most usual approach is TTE in the outpatient setting, followed in many patients by transesophageal echocardiography (TEE) in the catheterization laboratory if it is deemed suitable for transcatheter closure based on the TTE findings of right ventricle dilation and anatomical defect characteristics [34]. The goal is to correctly assess the defect's size, shape, and spatial relations to adjacent structures, such as the aortic root, the atrioventricular valves, the caval veins, and the atrial roof/free wall. Also important information to obtain is the presence or absence of multiple septal fenestrations, floppy or aneurysmal septal tissue, and/or oversized eustachian valve or Chiari's network tissue, which may possibly interfere with devices during interventional treatment [35]. Moreover, detection of associated anomalies, such as partial pulmonary venous anomalies, is necessary [36,37]. All such information is vital in deciding whether or not a particular patient should proceed to transcatheter device closure or whether he or she should undergo surgical closure. In younger children, echocardiography is the leading imaging modality, and there is little need for cardiovascular MRI in the management of secundum ASD patients.

However, a number of survey studies on clinical ASD management have revealed that in older children or adults, and when the defect is large, many centers do in fact use cardiac MRI to fully characterize an ASD prior to closure [28,29]. Table 3.1 summarizes the *goals* and suggested *scan protocols* when investigating an ASD both prior to and after repair of the defect by cardiovascular MRI. MRI has been shown to facilitate determination of the defect size and shape using

Table 3.1 Atrial septal defects.

Goals of the MRI examination	Suggested MRI protocol
Morphology	Localizer and 2-D cine SSFP in four-chamber view
Detect native or residual ASD and evaluate size, shape, and distance to adjacent structures	Multislice 2-D cine SSFP stack in short axis covering the ventricles to quantitatively evaluate right and left ventricular volumes and mass
Determine pulmonary and systemic venous connections	Gadolinium-enhanced 3-D MR angiography to detect pulmonary/ systemic venous anomalies and exclude vascular anomalies;
Exclude associated cardiovascular defects and valvular disease	alternatively axial multislice 2-D inflow MR angiography, or 3-D SSFP
Determine hemodynamic relevance (Q_p/Q_s)	volume scan covering the mediastinum
	Flow velocity-encoded cine MRI to assess defect size, shape, and
Function	distance to adjacent structures
Assess quantitative ventricular function	Through-plane flow velocity-encoded cine MRI for left-to-right shunt
Exclude evidence for pulmonary hypertension, such as right ventricular hypertrophy	quantitation (pulmonary arteries, ascending aorta)

phase-contrast MRI [6–8], enable assessment of ventricular volumes and mass [38] as well as pulmonary and systemic venous connections [39], and enable quantitation of the magnitude of left-to-right shunting [15]. Cardiac MRI is also very helpful in the differential diagnosis of a dilated right ventricle in older children with poor acoustic windows in whom an atypical pretricuspid left-to-right shunt lesion is suspected [38].

In *sinus venosus ASD,* the size, location, and shape of the defect can be assessed by phase-contrast MRI slices across the defect, or by using an *en face* 2-D phase-contrast slice obtained in the atrial septal plane. The through-plane flow encoding value may be set to a low value, such as 50–70 cm/s, in which case there will be aliasing, demonstrating nicely the position and shape of the superior septal defect; additional slices may be planned if they are deemed necessary (Fig. 3.1) [7,40]. Alternatively, a stack of axial 2-D steady-state free precession (2-D SSFP) cine slices from across the defect (obtained in a series of breath-holds) may be used, and these will show both defect size and topographical anatomy of pulmonary venous connections [41]. The course of the pulmonary and systemic veins may also be determined easily using 2-D inflow MR angiography (Fig. 3.2) or contrast-enhanced 3-D MR angiography [10,39]. Novel 3-D SSFP volume-scanning techniques gated to the diastole are less useful for ASD evaluation because the delineation of very thin and potentially mobile septal tissue may not be possible, and the dynamic information is not available using this approach although, on the other hand, associated pulmonary or systemic anomalous connections are nicely depicted [11].

As with secundum ASD evaluation using MRI, quantitative through-plane phase-contrast flow measurement in the great arteries will demonstrate the increased stroke volume in the main pulmonary artery (MPA) compared with the stroke volume measured in the ascending aorta (AAO). Thus, the MPA/AAO blood flow ratio represents the Q_p/Q_s ratio (Fig. 3.3), which is a well-known quantitative expression of

cardiac shunting, traditionally obtained by invasive cardiac catheterization using oximetry [42]. Cardiac MRI, however, has been demonstrated to be superior to oximetry in quantifying cardiac shunting in infants and children [15].

In the occasional patient with suspected pulmonary hypertension, MR-guided cardiac catheterization has been shown to enable precise determination of pulmonary vascular resistance, thereby successfully guiding a decision of whether or not closure is warranted [16]. This is discussed in more detail below (see section on late-presentation cardiac septal defect at risk for obstructive pulmonary vascular disease).

Cardiac MRI is less important after defect closure except in patients after atrial baffle procedures, such as atrial switch in transposition of the great arteries or higher sinus venosus ASD. MRI can nicely demonstrate any local residual septal defect (e.g., baffle leak) and quantify the resulting residual shunt. Moreover, MRI can detect any possible stenosis of the baffle resulting in pulmonary venous congestion, or stenosis of the superior vena cava, when the patch tunnel may produce a narrowing of its entrance into the right atrium. In the rare patient with cyanosis after ASD repair, MRI can detect intracardiac right-to-left shunting such as resulting from inadequate connections between systemic veins and the left atrium, or provide evidence for pulmonary hypertension associated with residual atrial-level shunting.

Atrioventricular septal defects

Classification and pathophysiology

In this group of so-called "endocardial cushion" defects, there is great variability in the morphology of atrial and ventricular septal defects, as well as of the atrioventricular valves, and a detailed discussion is beyond the scope of this chapter. In all forms of atrioventricular septal defects (AVSDs), however, the atrioventricular valves have the same septal insertion level, in contrast to the leaflet arrangements in the normal

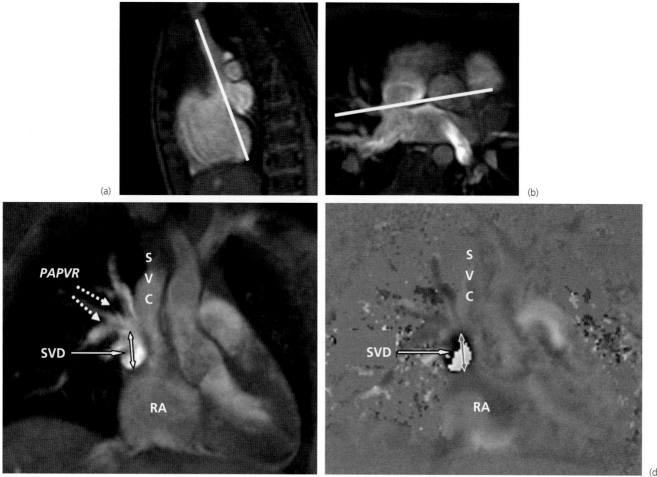

(a)

(b)

(c)

(d)

Figure 3.1 *En face* projection of superior sinus venosus atrial septal defect (SVD). *En face* phase-contrast MR imaging section prescribed in the plane of the atrial septum, as planned from a sagittal survey scan (a) and a transverse inflow MRA slice at the level of the defect (b). Phase-contrast MR images of an SVD in the coronal plane: defect size (double-headed arrows (c) and (d)) and shape can be estimated on the coronal phase image (d), which displays maximum flow, whereas anatomic information (e.g., adjacent structures) can be gleaned from the corresponding magnitude image (c). Note: the partial anomalous pulmonary venous return (PAPVR; dotted arrows) from the right upper lobe and middle lobe to the superior vena cava (SVC) (c). RA, right atrium.

heart, in which the septal tricuspid leaflet is positioned more toward the apex than the mitral valve. Hence, the distance from the cardiac crux to the left ventricular apex is foreshortened, and the distance from the apex to the aortic valve is increased. This results in anterior displacement of the left ventricular outflow tract (LVOT, goose-neck deformity). After surgical repair, progressive LVOT obstruction may occur. It is not uncommon that further cardiovascular defects are associated with partial and complete AVSD, as summarized in Table 3.2, and this is relevant to the use of cardiac MRI as an

Table 3.2 Atrioventricular septal defects (AVSDs): associated defects.

Partial AVSD	Complete AVSD
Prone to:	Prone to:
Left ventricular hypoplasia	Tetralogy of Fallot
Atrioventricular valve abnormalities: parachute valve, double-orifice valve, left atrioventricular valve	Double-outlet right ventricle (DORV)
	Complex atrial isomerism defects
Progressive left-ventricular outflow tract obstructions	Coarctation of the aorta
Coarctation of the aorta	

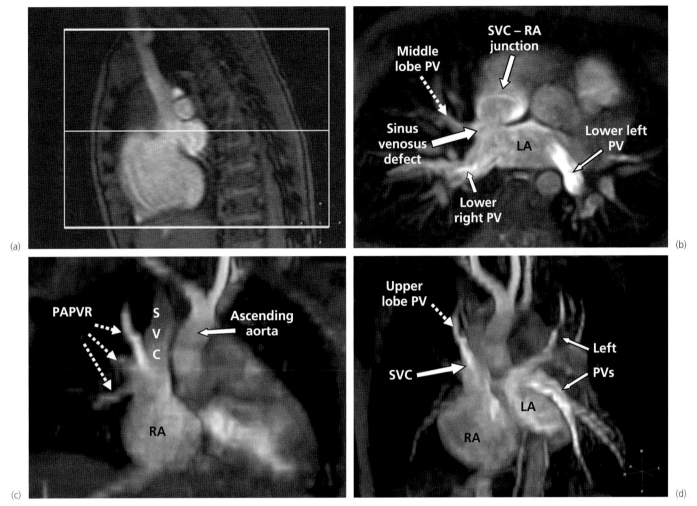

Figure 3.2 Sinus venosus ASD and partial anomalous pulmonary venous return. Inflow MR angiography (MRA) displaying a partial anomalous pulmonary venous return to the superior vena cava in sinus venosus atrial septal defect. (a) Lateral plan scan with borders of the multislice inflow MRA stack. (b) Transverse thin-slab maximal intensity projection of the inflow MR angiography, displaying a large sinus venous ASD at the level of the superior vena cava as well as pulmonary venous connections. (c) Angulated (RAO) coronal thin-slab maximal intensity projection of the inflow MRA displaying anomalous right pulmonary venous connections to the superior vena cava. (d) Angulated (LAO) coronal thin-slab maximal intensity projection of the inflow MR angiography displaying normal left pulmonary venous connections to the left atrium. LA, left atrium; PAPVR, partial anomalous pulmonary venous return [dotted arrows in (c)]; PV, pulmonary vein; RA, right atrium; SVC, superior vena cava.

imaging tool for the evaluation of AVSD prior to treatment and also after repair.

Partial AVSD includes a primum ASD, resulting in a purely atrial-level left-to-right shunt (as discussed above), and a transitional AVSD, in which a primum ASD is combined with a small and restrictive defect component of the ventricular inlet septum (Fig. 3.4), with ventricular-level left-to-right shunting that is of usually little hemodynamic significance. Both subtypes have *two separate* atrioventricular valves inserting at the *same level*, as opposed to the complete AVSD, in which there is always a common atrioventricular valve annulus. In partial AVSD, the anterior left atrioventricular valve leaflet invariably displays a cleft, which is most easily demonstrated in diastole by short-axis echocardiography, but may also be demonstrated by MRI.

In this subgroup, the predominant hemodynamic feature is atrial-level left-to-right shunting, with volume load and consequently dilation of the right heart and the pulmonary vessels.

Complete AVSD is characterized by the presence of only *one common atrioventricular valve annulus* and a *large primum ASD* continuous with a *large inlet VSD*. About 40–45% of children with Down syndrome have congenital heart disease, and, of these, approximately 40% have an AVSD (usually the complete form) [22]. The classical complete AVSD has only one atrioventricular valve orifice, whereas a subtype named "intermediate AVSD" is characterized by two separate atrioventricular valve orifices within one common atrioventricular valve annulus. Hence, in complete AVSD there is combined atrial and ventricular left-to-right shunting with both right

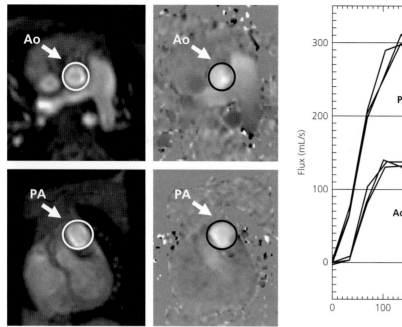
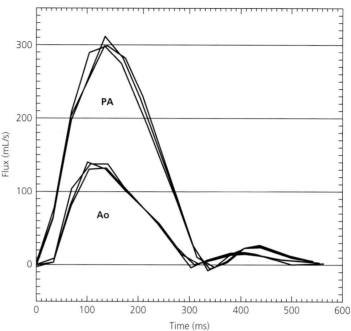

Figure 3.3 Left-to-right shunt quantification by phase-contrast cine MRI. Phase-contrast MR imaging section prescribed perpendicular to the ascending aorta (Ao) and main pulmonary artery (PA). Left: magnitude images; Right: phase images with velocity encoding. From the phase images the velocity is measured in each pixel within the region of interest (vessel lumen, circles). The mean velocity (cm/s) in the marked area (cm^2) yields the instantaneous flow volume (cm^3/s). As this is done over multiple time points over a reconstructed cardiac cycle in cine phase-contrast MRI this yields stroke volumes per reconstructed heart beat in both the PA and aorta, as displayed on the right panel. The difference represents the absolute left-to-right shunt per heart beat. Multiplication of each stroke volume with the heart rate results in the respective cardiac output, the ratio of which derives the Q_p/Q_s ratio as a traditional parameter of shunt magnitude. Q_s, systemic cardiac output; Q_p, pulmonary cardiac output.

heart and left heart dilation; there is also free pressure transmission across the large VSD, and this results in exposure of the pulmonary vasculature to both high pressure and high blood flow. These patients are at high risk of developing pulmonary obstructive vascular disease, resulting in Eisenmenger's syndrome should surgical treatment be delayed much beyond the first year of life without palliative pulmonary arterial banding [43].

Treatment

In all forms of AVSD the treatment is surgical. Anticongestive medication is often needed before the procedure. *Partial AVSD* repair consists of primum ASD closure, using autologous pericardial patch tissue, and atrioventricular valve reconstruction, involving cleft suture of the anterior leaflet of the left atrioventricular valve. The operation is usually delayed into the second or third year of life if no pulmonary hypertension is suspected [22,29]. For patients with *complete AVSD*, primary corrective surgery usually involves single-patch closure of the atrioventricular septal defect and atrioventricular valve separation/reconstruction of the common atrioventricular valve. The operation is usually undertaken in infancy to prevent the development of obstructive pulmonary vascular disease [22,44]. Alternatively, in more complex cases, or those with associated comorbidity that precludes early repair,

intermediate protection of the pulmonary vascular bed in infancy may be achieved by placement of a pulmonary band, with elective repair performed later in childhood under improved conditions [22]. However, a small subset of patients will present at an advanced age, or may have other respiratory comorbidities, such as lung disease of prematurity, which predisposes them to pulmonary hypertension [43]. This can be associated with increased perioperative mortality from elevated pulmonary vascular resistance, and when there is severe obstructive PVD surgical repair of the defect may even be contraindicated [45,46].

The role of cardiac magnetic resonance imaging pre- and post repair of atrioventricular septal disease

Although TTE and TEE are more commonly used in children with partial and complete AVSD *prior to repair*, cardiac MRI can nicely demonstrate all important diagnostic features, such as defect size and extension (Fig. 3.4), ventricular dilation and involvement of any atrioventricular valve pathology, and can quantitatively assess left-to-right shunt using phase-contrast MR flow. Table 3.3 summarizes the *goals* and suggested *scan protocols* when investigating AVSD both before and after repair by cardiovascular MRI. Cine 2-D SSFP MRI allows volumetric assessment in combination with phase-contrast MR flow,

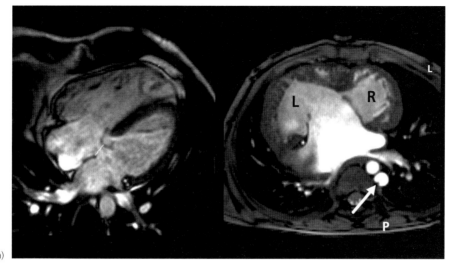

(a)   (b)

Figure 3.4 Partial and complete atrioventricular septal defect. (a) A four-chamber view using 2-D cine MRI in a 4-year-old girl with a *"transitional" atrioventricular septal defect* (AVSD; see text for further details on definitions). In this patient, the AVSD is mainly composed of a large primum atrial septal defect which causes relevant atrial-level left-to-right shunting. As a result, the right ventricle is exposed to increased volume load and hence is enlarged, as apparent on this image. In addition, there is a small ventricular septal defect (VSD) component of the AVSD located in the inlet portion of the ventricular septum. As this communication is restrictive, there is only little ventricular-level left-to-right shunting and hence—in the presence of a competent left atrioventricular valve—the left ventricle is of normal size. The restrictive nature of the ventricular AVSD component also explains why there is no right ventricular hypertrophy. (b) A four-chamber view using 2-D cine MRI (SSFP) in an infant with *complete AVSD,* which is in this particular case part of a very complex cardiac defect, including ambiguous cardiac situs (left atrial isomerism) with dextrocardia, pulmonary stenosis, and interruption of the intrahepatic portion of the inferior vena cava with vena azygos continuation (white arrow) to a left superior vena cava. Note: unlike in the previous example there is no atrial septum left and also a huge ventricular component of the AVSD. This results in biventricular enlargement and right ventricular hypertrophy. L, morphological left ventricle, R, morphological right ventricle.

which can precisely quantify any atrioventricular valve regurgitation and left ventricle–left atrium dilation. In those patients with initial palliative procedure is placement of a pulmonary artery band, cardiac MRI can demonstrate the band position and any obstruction of the branch pulmonary

arteries [47] that may necessitate patching during the definitive repair of the AVSD.

Cardiac MRI is particularly useful in the evaluation of residual problems *after* surgical repair, and is often used for this purpose in older children and young adults, in whom

Table 3.3 Atrioventricular septal defects.

Goals of the MRI examination	Suggested MRI protocol
Morphology Detect native or residual primum ASD and evaluate size and position Detect native or residual Inlet VSD component and evaluate size and position Assess atrioventricular valve morphology (including papillary muscles) Assess left ventricular outflow tract and aortic valve Determine pulmonary and systemic venous connections Exclude associated defects, such as tetralogy of Fallot, double-outlet right ventricle (DORV), aortic coarctation, or situs anomalies (e.g., left or right atrial isomerism)	Localizer and 2-D cine SSFP in four-chamber view Multislice 2-D cine SSFP stack in short axis covering the ventricles to quantitatively evaluate right and left ventricular volumes and mass Gadolinium-enhanced 3-D MR angiography to detect pulmonary/systemic venous anomalies and exclude vascular anomalies 3-D SSFP volume scan covering the mediastinum Through-plane flow velocity-encoded cine MRI for left-to-right shunt quantitation (pulmonary arteries, ascending aorta)
Function Determine left-to-right shunt (Q_p/Q_s) Assess quantitative ventricular function and quantify regurgitation volumes of atrioventricular valves Exclude evidence for pulmonary hypertension, such as right ventricular hypertrophy	Targeted single 2-D cine SSFP slices to delineate the native or residual septal defect; alternatively in-plane flow velocity-encoded cine MRI to assess defect size, shape, and distance to adjacent structures Targeted single 2-D cine SSFP slices for left and right ventricular outflow tracts and valvular anatomy and aortic arch Targeted single 2-D black-blood slices in case of associated defects

there may be suboptimal acoustic windows. Although surgical repair yields excellent long-term results in terms of mortality, as many as 20–25% of all AVSD patients experience reoperation at some point during their lifetime, with progressive left atrioventricular valve regurgitation being the predominant lesion. Its quantitation by cardiac MRI provides important information that is highly valuable for guiding conservative treatment (e.g., angiotensin-converting enzyme [ACE] inhibitors) and for the timing of surgical left atrioventricular valve reconstruction or replacement. The regurgitation is quantified by a combination of volumetry and quantitative flow: the left ventricular stroke volume is measured from a stack of 2-D cine SSFP slices covering both of the ventricles in the short axis. The effective aortic stroke volume (or pulmonary stroke volume in case of aortic valve incompetence) is assessed by MR flow. The difference constitutes the absolute amount of left atrioventricular regurgitant volume, which is commonly expressed as a fraction of the total left ventricular stroke volume (the regurgitant fraction). Alternatively, regurgitation is the difference in volumetric left and right ventricular stroke volume if the tricuspid and pulmonary valves are competent. Any residual septal defects may also be readily displayed and analyzed in terms of their significance by cardiac MRI. Importantly, progressive obstruction of the left ventricular outflow tract may occur. In this constellation, TEE is the leading imaging modality but cardiac MRI may be particularly helpful by providing quantitative data on left ventricular volumetric function and mass and by precisely delineating the exact morphology of the outflow obstruction.

Ventricular septal defects

Classification and pathophysiology

Defects of the interventricular septum are the most common congenital heart defect, accounting for 15–20% of all congenital heart disease excluding ventricular septal defects (VSD) occurring as part of a more complex condition. All parts of the ventricular septum may be involved. The septum may be divided into a small membranous portion and a large muscular portion; the latter has an inlet, a trabecular component, and an outlet component. The trabecular muscular part may be further subdivided into a central, marginal, and apical portion. VSDs are named and classified anatomically according to the site of their appearance. In ~70% of cases, the VSD occurs in the perimembranous region immediately below the aortic valve (Fig. 3.5a). Larger perimembranous VSDs may extend into the inlet septum, trabecular septum, or outlet septum. Inlet VSDs occur in the same portion of the septum that is affected in complete AVSD (see above). Very often, a VSD is part of a more complex cardiac defect, such as tetralogy of Fallot (Fig. 3.5d) or double-outlet right ventricle (Fig. 3.5c).

In patients with an isolated VSD, the clinical manifestation will be determined by the magnitude of the left-to-right shunt. In small defects with flow restriction, the shunt is negligible and hence the patient is asymptomatic. However, in larger defects, the clinical scenario is determined not only by the defect size, but by the degree of pulmonary artery restriction and pulmonary vascular resistance. In patients with pulmonary artery restriction, such as pulmonary valve stenosis, flow obstruction may be sufficient to protect the pulmonary vascular bed and hence the patient will be asymptomatic. In those with no flow restriction, the shunt will be modulated by the pulmonary vascular resistance. In the case of low resistance, shunt magnitude is high and heart failure will eventually develop. As the resistance increases (in response to high pulmonary pressure and flow), the pulmonary flow decreases and symptoms of heart failure may resolve. In the extreme situation, called Eisenmenger's syndrome, the pulmonary resistance exceeds the systemic resistance such that the shunt is reversed, resulting in cyanosis.

Treatment

Treatment is usually surgical and most commonly involves patch closure. However, more recently, new transcatheter techniques have been developed for the closure of selected defects in the catheterization laboratory [2,48,49]. This has been demonstrated to be a particularly useful alternative to surgery in single midmuscular VSD (Fig. 3.5a) [48] but also in smaller perimembranous VSD, provided there is a sufficient rim of tissue present below the aortic valve [49,50]. Some patients with multiple VSDs or an eccentrically located muscular VSD may benefit from hybrid closure techniques, combining avoidance of cardiopulmonary bypass with good accessibility in the operating room. Also, for a number of postsurgical residual defects, transcatheter closure may be a useful alternative to a reoperation [51].

The role of cardiac magnetic resonance imaging before and after treatment of ventricular septal disease

Prior to repair, TTE and TEE are the leading imaging modalities. However, particularly when there are difficulties in delineating associated cardiovascular lesions, there may be a role for cardiac MRI prior to an intervention or operation. Table 3.4 summarizes *diagnostic goals* and suggested *protocols* when performing cardiac MRI in patients with VSDs. In the case of multiple VSDs, 3-D cardiac MRI may be helpful preoperatively to determine the precise anatomy. Moreover, in patients with doubly committed subarterial VSD, problems such as asymmetry of the aortic root, partial valve prolapse, and associated aortic regurgitation can be easily assessed. Occasionally, after defect closure any residual shunting needs to be quantified precisely, and in this case MR phase-contrast flow studies are useful. Moreover, any persisting volume load may be determined by quantifying the ventricular volumes and mass and any associated postoperative problem, such as obstruction

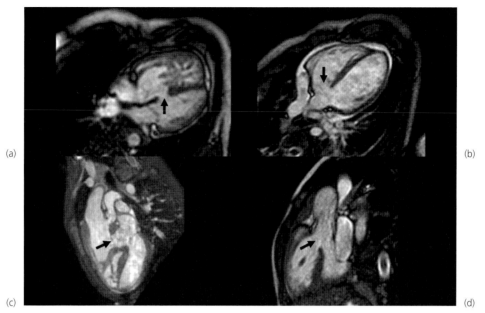

Figure 3.5 Different types of ventricular septal defects (VSDs). This composite figure demonstrates VSDs from four different patients to provide a selection of examples of possible anatomical locations of a VSD in an individual patient. Understanding of the size and anatomical position is of paramount importance when choosing the appropriate treatment modality. (a) A large *midmuscular VSD* in a 5-month-old infant, imaged with 2-D cine SSFP (steady-state free precession) in a four-chamber projection. Of note is the hypertrophied and enlarged right ventricle, suggesting free transmission of the systemic pressure through the defect. This defect is a possible candidate for closure by a muscular VSD occluder, deployed either percutaneously using a transcatheter approach or during a hybrid procedure in theatre. (b) A *perimembranous VSD* of moderate size, which sits below the aortic valve annulus, with no muscular tissue between the crest of the VSD and the aortic valve. In contrast to (a) there is no hypertrophy of the right ventricle, suggesting the restrictive nature of the defect with normal right ventricular and pulmonary pressures. The left ventricle is enlarged as a result of relevant left-to-right shunting in this 5-year-old boy. MRI was performed using an angulated 2-D cine SSFP slice to display the defect. (c) An example of a constellation, in which the *VSD is part of a more complex congenital cardiovascular defect*. There is malposition of the aorta, such that both great arteries arise from the right ventricle (double-outlet right ventricle [DORV]), with the aorta positioned anteriorly and to the right of the pulmonary artery. The VSD is the only outlet for the left ventricle, which appears hypoplastic, with overriding of the mitral valve inlet over the large VSD. There is a marked muscular subpulmonary obstruction in this patient, and hence the main pulmonary artery is hypoplastic. The MRI was performed using a 3-D single-phase SSFP volume scan with off-line reformatting during image post-processing, which is particularly useful in such complicated lesions. (d) An example of overriding of the aortic root over a large *outlet VSD* in a 15-month-old boy with Tetralogy of Fallot. This type of VSD is characteristic for tetralogy of Fallot and is called "misalignment VSD" as there is anterior and rightward deviation of the outlet part of the ventricular septum. MRI was performed using an angulated 2-D cine SSFP slice to display the defect.

of the left ventricular outflow tract or acquired aortic valve incompetence, can be evaluated in great detail.

Late-presentation cardiac septal defect at risk for obstructive pulmonary vascular disease

In the small but important subgroup of patients who present late with a large VSD or complete AVSD [43], there will be a need to assess the level of pulmonary vascular resistance in more detail than is possible by estimating the systolic right ventricular pressure using Doppler echocardiography. This is necessary to exclude patients in whom surgical repair is contraindicated owing to progression of obstructive pulmonary vascular disease, eventually resulting in Eisenmenger's syndrome. In clinical practice, the presence and severity of obstructive pulmonary vascular disease are usually assessed by measuring the pulmonary vascular resistance (PVR) in the cardiac catheterization laboratory. Traditionally, invasive pressures and oximetry for flow quantitation are performed at baseline and with the administration of pulmonary vasodilators to lower the PVR to assess the reactivity of the pulmonary arteriolar system [1]. This approach, however, is limited by the well-known weaknesses of the oximetric method of flow quantitation at high pulmonary flow conditions [52,53].

X-ray and MRI cardiac catheter in the assessment of obstructive pulmonary vascular disease

The advent of noninvasive *in vivo* measurement of pulmonary blood flow by phase-contrast magnetic resonance imaging (PC-MRI) [54] has enabled highly precise quantitation of pulmonary and systemic blood flows and, thus, the measurement of

Table 3.4 Ventricular septal defects.

Goals of the MRI examination	Suggested MRI protocol
Morphology	Localizer and 2-D cine SSFP in four-chamber view
Detect native or residual VSD and evaluate size and position	Multislice 2-D cine SSFP stack in short axis covering the ventricles to quantitatively evaluate right and left ventricular volumes and mass
Assess left ventricular outflow tract and aortic valve geometry and function	Gadolinium-enhanced 3-D MR angiography to detect pulmonary/systemic venous anomalies and exclude vascular anomalies
Determine pulmonary and systemic venous connections	3-D SSFP volume scan covering the mediastinum
Exclude associated defects	Through-plane flow velocity-encoded cine MRI for left-to-right shunt quantitation (pulmonary arteries, ascending aorta)
	Targeted single 2-D cine SSFP slices to delineate the native or residual VSD alternatively in-plane flow velocity-encoded cine MRI to assess defect size, shape and distance to adjacent structures
Function	
Determine quantitative left-to-right shunt (Q_p/Q_s)	*Consider additional scans*
Assess quantitative ventricular and valvular function	Targeted single 2-D cine SSFP slices for left and right ventricular outflow tracts and valvular anatomy and aortic arch
Exclude evidence of pulmonary hypertension, such as right ventricular hypertrophy	Targeted single 2-D black-blood slices in instances of associated defects
	Flow velocity-encoded cine MRI to assess defect size and distance to adjacent structures

Table 3.5 Late-presentation septal defects.

XMR cardiac catheter procedure
General anesthetics to ensure optimal steady-state conditions and minimal motion artifacts using breath-hold scans
Outside the scanner: Insert appropriate femoral venous and atrial sheaths, heparinize, and place MRI-compatible Swan–Ganz catheters to obtain transpulmonary mean pressure gradients as well as trans-systemic mean pressure gradients
Inside the scanner: Determine baseline morphology and function, as summarized in Tables 3.3 and 3.4 for AVSD and VSD MRI evaluation
Hemodynamic cardiac MRI investigation (MR-compatible catheters in position):
Determine **baseline left-to-right shunt (Q_p/Q_s)** by quantitative MR flow in the pulmonary artery and ascending aorta
Determine **total pulmonary vascular resistance level (R_p)** by quantitative MRI flow in the pulmonary artery, *plus* simultaneous mean pressures in the main pulmonary artery and left atrium (or pulmonary wedge):
at rest
under pulmonary vasodilators such as nitric oxide, 100% oxygen, or prostacyclin
Determine **differential pulmonary vascular resistance levels (R_{RPA}/R_{LPA})** by measuring the quantitative MR flow *plus* simultaneous mean pressures separately in each branch pulmonary artery when there are multiple *different sources of pulmonary blood supply*
Determine **systemic vascular resistance (R_s)** by measuring MRI quantitative flow in the ascending aorta and the mean aortic systemic venous (right atrial) pressure to express the R_p/R_s **ratio** as a clinically well-known parameter of pulmonary vascular resistance

LPA, left pulmonary artery; RPA, right pulmonary artery.

shunts in infants and children with congenital heart disease [15]. Using this unique MRI advantage over conventional flow quantitation techniques, it was recently demonstrated that flow quantitation by phase-contrast MRI can be performed alongside with invasive pressure measurements in the setting of a combined X-ray and MRI (XMR) cardiac catheterization laboratory [16] to more accurately quantify the PVR [17]. Table 3.5 summarizes diagnostic *goals* and suggested *protocols* when performing "XMR" cardiac catheterization in patients at risk of obstructive pulmonary vascular disease. This technique overcomes the inherent problems associated with measure-ment of left-to-right shunt and PVR by oximetry and the Fick method, allowing accurate determination of PVR even in the presence of high pulmonary artery flow rates and oxygen saturations [17]. Additionally, with XMR there is much less exposure to ionizing radiation [16]. In Fig. 3.6 the increasing discrepancy is displayed when adding pulmonary vasodilators during PVR assessment in a left-to-right shunt cardiac septal defect. This approach is clinically feasible, as recently demon-strated for assessment of pulmonary vascular disease [40]. Moreover, XMR cardiac catheterization has been shown to allow the determination of differential pulmonary vascular

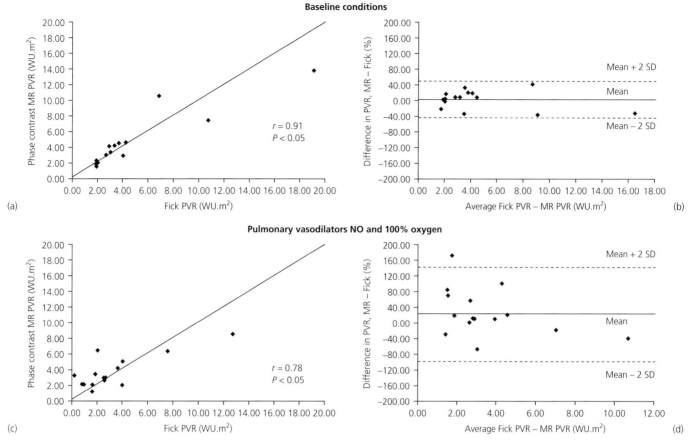

Figure 3.6 Determination of pulmonary vascular resistance (PVR) by use of MRI flow quantification versus oximetric shunt estimation using the Fick method. This graph displays a comparison of MR flow-based PVR versus Fick flow-based PVR [17]. (b) and (d) show the correlation and (a) and (c) show the agreement between both methods to obtain PVR. In (a) and (b) PVR was assessed at baseline, whereas in (c) and (d) PVR was measured during pulmonary vasodilation using 100% oxygen and nitric oxide in ventilated patients with late-presentation cardiac septal defects. Of note is the fair agreement at baseline as opposed to the considerable disagreement between measurements taken during pulmonary vasodilation, which is thought to be a result of bias of the oximetry method in the presence of high pulmonary flow and high pulmonary oxygen concentration [17].

resistance (in each lung separately) in the setting of both cardiac septal defects and in single-ventricle physiology [55].

Summary and perspective

In the management of patients with cardiac septal defects, cardiac MRI is increasingly recognized as a versatile and useful clinical tool. The ability to morphologically display associated lesions and to quantify hemodynamic severity renders the method an attractive tool even when good characterization of intracardiac anatomy is available from echocardiography. The noninvasiveness of the technique and fact that radiation exposure is not required make the technique particularly invaluable in children and young adults.

The unique method of flow quantitation has been successfully combined with invasive pressure recordings to yield accurate assessment of PVR in patients with late-presentation cardiac septal defect at risk for obstructive pulmonary vascular disease. Novel techniques of 3-D imaging [17] are being developed and it is foreseeable that 3-D time-resolved imaging of structure and flow will help to make cardiac MRI operator independent and improve time efficiency. Image fusion techniques may allow for regular use of overprojected 3-D MRI pictures to assist with interventions for VSD closure in the cardiac catheterization laboratory.

References

1. McDaniel NL & Gutgesell HP. (2008) Ventricular septal defects. In: Allen HD, Driscoll DJ, Shaddy RE, Feltes TF (eds). *Moss and Adams' Heart Disease in Infants, Children, and Adolescents*, Vol. 1, 7th edn. Philadelphia: Lippincott Williams & Wilkins, pp. 667–681.

2. Holzer R, Balzer D, Amin Z, *et al.* (2004) Transcatheter closure of postinfarction ventricular septal defects using the new Amplatzer muscular VSD occluder: results of a U.S. Registry. *Catheter Cardiovasc Interv* **61**:196–201.

3. Mohrs OK, Petersen SE, Erkapic D, *et al.* (2007) Dynamic contrast-enhanced MRI before and after transcatheter occlusion of patent foramen ovale. *AJR Am J Roentgenol* **188**:844–849.

4. Colletti PM. (2005) Evaluation of intracardiac shunts with cardiac magnetic resonance. *Curr Cardiol Rep* **7**:52–58.

5. Wang ZJ, Reddy GP, Gotway MB, Yeh BM, & Higgins CB. (2003) Cardiovascular shunts: MR imaging evaluation. *Radiographics* **23**(Spec No.):S181–194.

6. Holmvang G, Palacios IF, Vlahakes GJ, *et al.* (1995) Imaging and sizing of atrial septal defects by magnetic resonance. *Circulation* **92**:3473–3480.

7. Beerbaum P, Korperich H, Esdorn H, *et al.* (2003) Atrial septal defects in pediatric patients: noninvasive sizing with cardiovascular MR imaging. *Radiology* **228**:361–369.

8. Thomson LE, Crowley AL, Heitner JF, *et al.* (2008) Direct en face imaging of secundum atrial septal defects by velocity-encoded cardiovascular magnetic resonance in patients evaluated for possible transcatheter closure. *Circ Cardiovasc Imaging* **1**:31–40.

9. Keenan NG & Pennell DJ. (2007) CMR of ventricular function. *Echocardiography* **24**:185–193.

10. Greil GF, Powell AJ, Gildein HP, & Geva T. (2002) Gadolinium-enhanced three-dimensional magnetic resonance angiography of pulmonary and systemic venous anomalies. *J Am Coll Cardiol* **39**:335–341.

11. Sorensen TS, Korperich H, Greil GF, *et al.* (2004) Operator-independent isotropic three-dimensional magnetic resonance imaging for morphology in congenital heart disease: a validation study. *Circulation* **110**:163–169.

12. Pennell DJ. (2002) Ventricular volume and mass by CMR. *J Cardiovasc Magn Reson* **4**:507–513.

13. Karamitsos TD, Hudsmith LE, Selvanayagam JB, Neubauer S, & Francis JM. (2007) Operator induced variability in left ventricular measurements with cardiovascular magnetic resonance is improved after training. *J Cardiovasc Magn Reson* **9**:777–783.

14. Mooij CF, de Wit CJ, Graham DA, Powell AJ, & Geva T. (2008) Reproducibility of MRI measurements of right ventricular size and function in patients with normal and dilated ventricles. *J Magn Reson Imaging* **28**:67–73.

15. Beerbaum P, Korperich H, Barth P, Esdorn H, Gieseke J, & Meyer H. (2001) Noninvasive quantification of left-to-right shunt in pediatric patients: phase-contrast cine magnetic resonance imaging compared with invasive oximetry. *Circulation* **103**:2476–2482.

16. Razavi R, Muthurangu V, & Baker E. (2003) Cardiac catheterisation guided by MRI in children and adults with congenital heart disease. *Lancet* **362**(9399):1877–1882.

17. Muthurangu V, Taylor A, Andriantsimiavona R, *et al.* (2004) Novel method of quantifying pulmonary vascular resistance by use of simultaneous invasive pressure monitoring and phase-contrast magnetic resonance flow. *Circulation* **110**:826–834.

18. Porter CJ & Edwards WD. (2008) Atrial septal defects. In: Allen HD, Driscoll DJ, Shaddy RE, & Feltes TF (eds). *Moss and Adams' Heart Disease in Infants, Children, and Adolescents.* Vol. 1, 7th edn. Philadelphia: Lippincott Williams & Wilkins, pp. 632–645.

19. Van Praagh S, Carrera ME, Sanders SP, Mayer JE, & Van Praagh R. (1994) Sinus venosus defects: unroofing of the right pulmonary veins—anatomic and echocardiographic findings and surgical treatment [see comments]. *Am Heart J* **128**:365–379.

20. Cockerham JT, Martin TC, Gutierrez FR, Hartmann AF, Goldring D, & Strauss AW. (1983) Spontaneous closure of secundum atrial septal defect in infants and young children. *Am J Cardiol* **52**:1267–1271.

21. McMahon CJ, Feltes TF, Fraley JK, *et al.* (2002) Natural history of growth of secundum atrial septal defects and implications for transcatheter closure. *Heart* **87**:256–259.

22. Cetta F, Minich LL, Edwards WD, Dearani JA, & Puga FJ. (2008) Atrioventricular septal defects. In: Allen HD, Driscoll DJ, Shaddy RE, & Feltes TF (eds). *Moss and Adams' Heart Disease in Infants, Children, and Adolescents.* Vol. 1, 7th edn. Philadelphia: Lippincott Williams & Wilkins, pp. 646–667.

23. Engelfriet PM, Duffels MG, Moller T, *et al.* (2007) Pulmonary arterial hypertension in adults born with a heart septal defect: the Euro Heart Survey on adult congenital heart disease. *Heart* **93**:682–687.

24. Hahm JK, Park YW, Lee JK, *et al.* (2000) Magnetic resonance imaging of unroofed coronary sinus: three cases. *Pediatr Cardiol* **21**:382–387.

25. Kong PK & Ahmad F. (2007) Unroofed coronary sinus and persistent left superior vena cava. *Eur J Echocardiogr* **8**:398–401.

26. Sarikouch S, Blanz U, Sandica E, & Beerbaum P. (2006) Adult congenital heart disease: cor triatriatum dextrum. *J Thorac Cardiovasc Surg* **132**:164–165.

27. Burri H, Vuille C, Sierra J, Didier D, Lerch R, & Kalangos A. (2003) Drainage of the inferior vena cava to the left atrium. *Echocardiography* **20**:185–189.

28. Rigatelli G, Cardaioli P, & Hijazi ZM. (2007) Contemporary clinical management of atrial septal defects in the adult. *Expert Rev Cardiovasc Ther* **5**:1135–1146.

29. Kharouf R, Luxenberg DM, Khalid O, & Abdulla R. (2008) Atrial septal defect: spectrum of care. *Pediatr Cardiol* **29**:271–280.

30. Du ZD, Hijazi ZM, Kleinman CS, Silverman NH, & Larntz K. (2002) Comparison between transcatheter and surgical closure of secundum atrial septal defect in children and adults: results of a multicenter nonrandomized trial. *J Am Coll Cardiol* **39**:1836–1844.

31. Campbell M. (1970) Natural history of atrial septal defect. *Br Heart J* **32**:820–826.

32. Murphy JG, Gersh BJ, McGoon MD, *et al.* (1990) Long-term outcome after surgical repair of isolated atrial septal defect. Follow-up at 27 to 32 years. *N Engl J Med* **323**:1645–1650.

33. Engelfriet P, Meijboom F, Boersma E, Tijssen J, & Mulder B. (2008) Repaired and open atrial septal defects type II in adulthood: an epidemiological study of a large European cohort. *Int J Cardiol* **126**:379–385.

34. Magni G, Hijazi ZM, Pandian NG, *et al.* (1997) Two- and three-dimensional transesophageal echocardiography in patient selection and assessment of atrial septal defect closure by the new DAS-Angel Wings device: initial clinical experience. *Circulation* **96**:1722–1728.

35. Cooke JC, Gelman JS, & Harper RW. (1999) Chiari network entanglement and herniation into the left atrium by an atrial septal defect occluder device. *J Am Soc Echocardiogr* **12**:601–603.

36. Stumper O, Vargas-Barron J, Rijlaarsdam M, *et al.* (1991) Assessment of anomalous systemic and pulmonary venous connections by transoesophageal echocardiography in infants and children. *Br Heart J* **66**:411–418.

37. Pascoe RD, Oh JK, Warnes CA, Danielson GK, Tajik AJ, & Seward JB. (1996) Diagnosis of sinus venosus atrial septal defect with transesophageal echocardiography. *Circulation* **94**:1049–1055.

38. Greil GF, Beerbaum P, Razavi R, & Miller O. (2008) Imaging the right ventricle: non-invasive imaging. *Heart* **94**:803–808.

39. Grosse-Wortmann L, Al-Otay A, Goo HW, *et al.* (2007) Anatomical and functional evaluation of pulmonary veins in children by magnetic resonance imaging. *J Am Coll Cardiol* **49**:993–1002.

40. Beerbaum P, Parish V, Bell A, Gieseke J, Koerperich H, & Sarikouch S. (2008) Atypical atrial septal defects in pediatric patients: non-invasive evaluation by cardiovascular magnetic resonance. *Pediatr Radiol* **38**: 1188–1194.

41. Valente AM, Sena L, Powell AJ, Del Nido PJ, & Geva T. (2007) Cardiac magnetic resonance imaging of sinus venosus defects. *Pediatr Cardiol* **28**:51–56.

42. Hillis LD, Winniford MD, Jackson JA, & Firth BG. (1985) Measurements of left-to-right intracardiac shunting in adults: oximetric versus indicator dilution techniques. *Cathet Cardiovasc Diagn* **11**:467–472.

43. Massin MM & Dessy H. (2006) Delayed recognition of congenital heart disease. *Postgrad Med J* **82**:468–470.

44. Yamaki S, Yasui H, Kado H, *et al.* (1993) Pulmonary vascular disease and operative indications in complete atrioventricular canal defect in early infancy. *J Thorac Cardiovasc Surg* **106**:398–405.

45. Friedli B, Langford K, Mustard W, & Keith J. (1974) Ventricular septal defect with increased pulmonary vascular resistance: late results of surgical closure. *Am J Cardiol* **33**:403–409.

46. Neutze JM, Ishikawa T, Clarkson PM, Calder AL, Barratt-Boyes BG, & Kerr AR. (1989) Assessment and follow-up of patients with ventricular septal defect and elevated pulmonary vascular resistance. *Am J Cardiol* **63**:327–331.

47. Geva T, Greil GF, Marshall AC, Landzberg M, & Powell AJ. (2002) Gadolinium-enhanced 3-dimensional magnetic resonance angiography of pulmonary blood supply in patients with complex pulmonary stenosis or atresia: comparison with x-ray angiography. *Circulation* **106**:473–478.

48. Arora R, Trehan V, Thakur AK, Mehta V, Sengupta PP, & Nigam M. (2004) Transcatheter closure of congenital muscular ventricular septal defect. *J Interv Cardiol* **17**:109–115.

49. Holzer R, de Giovanni J, Walsh KP, *et al.* (2006) Transcatheter closure of perimembranous ventricular septal defects using the amplatzer membranous VSD occluder: immediate and midterm results of an international registry. *Catheter Cardiovasc Interv* **68**:620–628.

50. Arora R, Trehan V, Kumar A, Kalra GS, & Nigam M. (2003) Transcatheter closure of congenital ventricular septal defects: experience with various devices. *J Interv Cardiol* **16**:83–91.

51. Holzer RJ, Chisolm J, Hill SL, & Cheatham JP. (2006) Transcatheter devices used in the management of patients with congenital heart disease. *Expert Rev Med Devices* **3**:603–615.

52. Cigarroa RG, Lange RA, & Hillis LD. (1989) Oximetric quantitation of intracardiac left-to-right shunting: limitations of the Qp/Qs ratio. *Am J Cardiol* **64**:246–247.

53. Hillis LD, Firth BG, & Winniford MD. (1985) Analysis of factors affecting the variability of Fick versus indicator dilution measurements of cardiac output. *Am J Cardiol* **56**:764–768.

54. Firmin DN, Nayler GL, Klipstein RH, Underwood SR, Rees RS, & Longmore DB. (1987) In vivo validation of MR velocity imaging. *J Comput Assist Tomogr* **11**:751–756.

55. Bell A, Tangcharoen T, Hegde S, *et al.* (2008) *MRI Cardiac Catheter Assessment of Total and Differential Pulmonary Vascular Resistance in the Context of Single Ventricle Physiology*. Paper presented at the 11th Annual Scientific Sessions. Society for Cardiovascular Magnetic Resonance (SCMR); Rome, Italy.

4 Catheter Closure of Atrial and Ventricular Septal Defects

Ignacio Inglessis[1], Neil Wilson[2] & Michael de Moor[3]

[1]Massachusetts General Hospital, Boston, MA, USA
[2]John Radcliffe Hospital, University of Oxford, Oxford, UK
[3]Floating Hospital for Children, Tufts University Medical Center, Boston, MA, USA

Atrial septal defect closure

Historical background

King and Mills [1] reported the first successful transcatheter closure of atrial septal defects (ASDs) in 1974. However, the devices utilized were rigid and required a very large introducer, limiting their widespread use. Lock *et al.* [2] modified the Rashkind patent ductus arteriosus (PDA) occluder into a double-hinged device, the Clamshell Septal Occluder™ (C.R. Bard Inc., Billerica, MA, USA), and successfully closed small to moderate-sized ASDs in animal models.

Following these early encouraging results, the Clamshell device was extensively tested in humans, proving to be a safe and effective alternative to surgical ASD closure [3,4]. Nevertheless, the risk for device embolization, high incidence of arm fracture, and the >50% incidence of residual shunt observed with the use of the Clamshell at late follow-up promoted its subsequent redesigning and improvement. The next generation of devices, the CardioSEAL and its self-centered modification, the STARFlex Septal Occluders™ (NMT, Boston, MA, USA), proved to be more resistant to metal fatigue and less susceptible to fractures and embolization.

Further variations of the concept of one or two umbrellas with attached polyurethane or Dacron fabric produced the ASDOS™ (Sulzer-Osypka, Rheinfelden, Germany), AngelWing™ (Microvena Corporation, White Bear Lake, MN, USA), and Sideris Buttoned™ (Custom Medical Devices, Athens, Greece) devices in the 1990s. These devices were tested in clinical trials, but resulted in a higher than acceptable implantation failure and rate of residual shunt [5–7]. The ePTFE-covered Helex™ (W.L. Gore™ & Associates, Flagstaff, AZ, USA) device has gained popularity as a biocompatible, retrievable, and low-profile device.

The Amplatzer Septal Occluder™ (AGA Medical Corporation, Plymouth, MN, USA) device was introduced in the late 1990s. With its basic design of a double disk with a connecting waist made of nitinol, the Amplatzer Septal Occluder became the first fully retrievable and self-centered device, gaining acceptance for transcatheter closure of small to large ASDs in the pediatric and adult population and is currently the most widely used device worldwide.

Morphology and pathophysiology

Atrial septal defects are relatively frequent, with an estimated incidence of 941 per million births [8]. ASDs may be single or multiple, and they can be located anywhere in the septum. Depending on their location in the septum, ASDs have been traditionally categorized as ostium primum, ostium secundum, sinus venosus, and coronary sinus defects. We will focus on ostium secundum defects in this chapter, as they are the only ASDs amenable to transcatheter closure.

Ostium secundum ASDs are located in the fossa ovalis, although they frequently extend beyond its limits, and they usually result from deficient development of the septum primum or, less frequently, the septum secundum. ASDs are frequently associated with other cardiac malformations. Worth considering is the incidence of myxomatous degeneration of the mitral valve, with varied degrees of insufficiency [9], and the anomalous pulmonary venous return to the right side of the heart, as both of these abnormalities might preclude transcatheter ASD closure, if significant.

The size of the left-to-right shunt, and its consequent hemodynamic burden on the heart and lungs, depends partly on the size of the defect, but also on the relative right and left ventricular compliance and the ratio of pulmonary to systemic vascular resistance [10–12]. Early in life, right ventricular compliance and pulmonary vascular resistance (PVR) are higher than the corresponding left ventricular compliance and systemic vascular resistance (SVR). Consequently, the size of the left-to-right shunt and hemodynamic burden is minimal, and, not infrequently, large ASDs can be missed in infancy and early childhood. With aging, the expected increase in SVR associated with hypertension and decrease in left ventricular compliance secondary to left ventricular diastolic dysfunction

Cardiovascular Interventions in Clinical Practice. Edited by Jürgen Haase, Hans-Joachim Schäfers, Horst Sievert and Ron Waksman. © 2010 Blackwell Publishing.

leads to a further increase in left-to-right shunting. Right ventricular dilation/failure, pulmonary hypertension and increased PVR, tricuspid and/or pulmonary valve insufficiency, and supraventricular arrhythmias are the late consequences of unrepaired ASDs with large left-to-right shunts.

If the PVR exceeds the SVR, then, eventually, a right-to-left shunt develops, cyanosis ensues, and the diagnosis of Eisenmenger's syndrome is established, typically in early adulthood.

Indications for transcatheter arterial septal defect closure

Treatment for an ASD is normally instituted if imaging reveals the presence of right ventricular volume overload. This is usually associated with a pulmonary–systemic flow ratio (Q_p/Q_s) >1.5, the threshold associated with the potential for right ventricular dysfunction, progressive pulmonary vascular disease, and arrhythmias, even in asymptomatic patients.

Caution should be exercised in patients with severe pulmonary hypertension, especially those with right-to-left shunt and cyanosis, as this may exacerbate right ventricular failure or even result in death by eliminating the "pop-off" valve for the right ventricle once the ASD is closed. Nevertheless, closure should still be considered an option for such patients if the net Q_p/Q_s is >1.5, which typically is associated with a PVR of less than 8–10 Wood units and a PVR/SVR of less than 0.2–0.4, even though the pulmonary pressures and resistance may remain elevated post closure. Transient ASD balloon occlusion at the time of catheterization may aid in the assessment of the acute hemodynamic response to device closure, although the long-term predictive value of such maneuvers remains unclear. Complex strategies aiming to identify appropriate candidates for closure based on the predictive value of the pulmonary vasodilatory reserve, as determined by the response to pulmonary vasodilators, such as inhaled nitric oxide [13], or the use of customized fenestrated closure devices have been reported to be of value in patients with bidirectional shunt, severe pulmonary hypertension, and/or right ventricular failure [14]. Paradoxical embolism is an indication for closure, even in patients with nonhemodynamically significant ASDs.

Transcatheter closure is possible for ASDs with a maximum stretched diameter of 40 mm using the Amplatzer closure device. Ideally, rims greater than 5 mm are required for placement of ASD closure devices (see below).

Technical aspects of transcatheter atrial septal defect closure

General anesthesia is mandatory for pediatric patients and, in general, for adults in whom transesophageal echocardiography (TEE) guidance is contemplated. However, intracardiac echocardiography (ICE), which is increasingly common, allows many procedures to be performed under conscious sedation.

Accurate evaluation of several morphologic features of the interatrial septum is important in determining the feasibility and safety of transcatheter closure, including the dimensions, shape, and number of defects, size of the surrounding rims, and proximity to adjacent structures, i.e., right-sided pulmonary veins, venae cavae, atrioventricular valves, prominent eustachian valves or Chiari network, and the coronary sinus. Although single-plane or biplanar fluoroscopic and angiographic guidance alone is possible, most operators favor echocardiography guidance, as it offers a more complete and accurate evaluation of the interatrial septum and surrounding structures. Both TEE and ICE have proven to be useful and effective in guiding procedures [15,16]. Three-dimensional echocardiography (Fig. 4.1) is emerging as a very useful tool for the accurate evaluation of the anatomy and geometry of ASDs and their relationship to surrounding structures [17,18]. Irrespective of the technique, echocardiographic evaluation should be performed before catheter crossing of the ASD to avoid catheter-induced distortions.

All intravenous lines should be filtered to avoid air embolization. Femoral venous access is the preferred route for all of the currently available ASD closure devices; however, device delivery is also possible via the internal jugular or hepatic veins (transhepatic access) in cases of femoral/inferior vena cava obstruction, albeit this technique is more technically challenging [19,20]. The left femoral vein is the preferred route for advancing the ICE probe into the heart using a 30-cm-long sheath, leaving the right femoral vein for delivery of the closure device. Arterial access is required only for those patients in need of left-sided catheterization. Once all access is obtained, the patient receives a full dose of intravenous heparin (100 U/kg) with an activated clotting time (ACT) goal of approximately 250 for the duration of the procedure. Intravenous antibiotics, usually a first-generation cephalosporin or vancomcyin, are prescribed at the time of implant and for the next 24 h. Complete hemodynamic evaluation is mandatory before attempting transcatheter closure, with careful assessment of pulmonary pressure and intracardiac shunt, and pulmonary vascular resistance (PVR) calculation. Routine right pulmonary vein angiography in the left anterior oblique (LAO) cranial projection is advocated by some operators to further evaluate the septal anatomy, rule out anomalous venous return, and help determine the best fluoroscopic angulation for device deployment.

Atrial septal defects are usually easily crossed via the femoral vein/inferior vena caval approach with the use of 45° angled catheters, such as the MP-2 or Goodale–Lubin. Catheters with tighter angulations, such as the AL-1 or JL4, are frequently required for the internal jugular vein/superior vena cava approach. The catheter is best positioned in the left upper pulmonary vein and exchanged for a heavy 0.035-inch wire such as the Amplatzer super stiff™, which allows for stable delivery of a sizing balloon. Although balloon sizing to obtain the stretched maximum diameter of centrally located small ASDs (<10 mm) is not always required, it is mandatory for

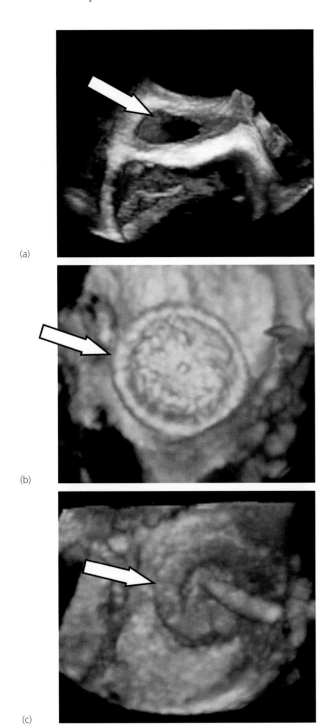

(a)

(b)

(c)

Figure 4.1 Three-dimensional TEE images of an ostium secundum ASD revealing (a) adequate surrounding rims (white arrow). The (b) left (white arrow) and (c) right retention disks of an Amplatzer ASD closure device are visualized while deployed (white arrow).

34 mm diameters, while the NuMED balloon is available in diameters between 20 and 40 mm, in 5 mm increments. The balloon is inflated across the ASD with diluted contrast under fluoroscopic (usually in the LAO cranial projection) and echocardiographic guidance. Although initially it was proposed to inflate the balloon until a noticeable waist was evident, this technique frequently resulted in defect oversizing by overstretching a thin and pliable septum. Consequently, the current recommendation is to inflate the balloon until disappearance of shunt around the balloon is observed by color Doppler ("stop-flow technique"), ideally assessed in two orthogonal echocardiographic views, i.e., bicaval and short-axis views. The maximum obtained diameter is used to select the device.

The currently available ASD closure devices in the USA include the Amplatzer, CardioSEAL (and its STARFlex modification), and Helex devices (Fig. 4.2). The Amplatzer closure device is the most widely used device and is constructed by a continuous weave of nitinol, forming a self-expanding double-disk device joined by a connecting waist, with polyester fabric sewed to each individual component. The Amplatzer device is available is sizes from 4 to 40 mm (38 mm in the USA), as determined by the diameter of the connecting waist, with 1 mm increments up to 20 mm and 2 mm increments between 20 and 40 mm. The left atrial disks are 12–16 mm larger in diameter than the connecting waist (depending on device size), providing a circumferential device rim around the defect to increase stability. For ASDs with sufficient rims, a device 2 mm larger than the obtained maximum balloon diameter is selected. For ASDs with a deficient anterior (aortic) rim, it had been proposed to choose a device 4 mm greater than the maximum diameter, with portions of the retaining disks "hugging" the aortic wall and effectively eliminating the shunt. However, recent reports of device erosions in patients (Fig. 4.3) with such deficient anterior rims raised concerns in the interventional community [21]. Consequently, it is now recommended that a smaller device is chosen, at the expense of an increased risk for residual shunts. It is recommended that the device should not be greater than 50% of the ASD diameter before balloon sizing and only 2 mm greater than the diameter of the ASD by balloon sizing measured by the "stop-flow technique". The size of the Amplatzer delivery sheath ranges from 6F for devices <10 mm to 14F for the 40-mm device, all with a 45° angled tip. Alternatively, the Hausdorf-Lock™ (Cook Inc, Bloomington, IN, USA) curved sheath allows for a more parallel alignment of the closure device to the septum and is particularly useful in patients with large defects and deficient anterior rims.

Once the delivery sheath is advanced to the right pulmonary vein, particular attention should be paid to avoid air embolization as the dilator is retrieved. The right atrial disk is screwed to the delivery cable and introduced to a loading sheath, which eventually is screwed to the end of the Amplatzer delivery sheath or pushed through the bleeding valve of the Hausdorf-Lock sheath.

larger and elliptically shaped defects, facilitating precise device selection. The most frequently used balloons are the Amplatzer™ (AGA Medical Corporation, Plymouth, MN, USA) and the NuMED (NuMED Inc., Hopkinton, NY, USA) sizing balloons. The Amplatzer sizing balloon is available in 24 and

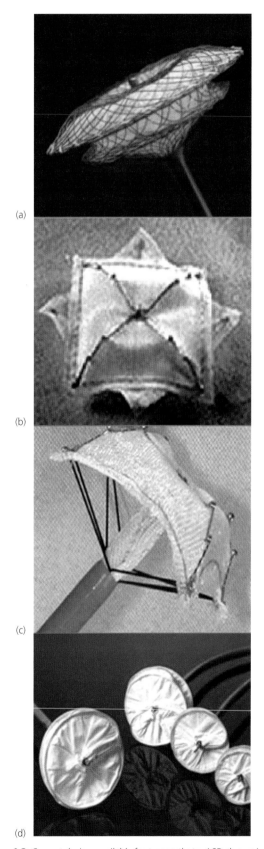

(a)

(b)

(c)

(d)

Figure 4.2 Current devices available for transcatheter ASD closure in the USA. (a) Amplatzer, (b) CardioSEAL, (c) STARFlex, (d) Helex.

The standard technique for delivery of the Amplatzer closure device calls for sheath withdrawal to the middle of the left atrium, followed by deployment of the left atrial disk by simultaneous pushing of the delivery cable and further withdrawing of the delivery sheath, carefully avoiding puncture of the left atrium wall. Special attention needs to be paid to the ACT and prevention of any development of thrombus at the end of the sheath. Further withdrawal of the sheath exposes the midconnecting waist, which allows for self-centering, once the device makes contact with the interatrial septum. Following careful echocardiographic evaluation to ensure absence of left atrial disk prolapse into the right atrium, the delivery sheath is further withdrawn, while simultaneously gently pulling the delivery cable, and the right atrial disk is deployed. Once more, careful echocardiographic evaluation is required at this point to assure proper device deployment and avoid compromise of surrounding structures, such as the right-sided pulmonary veins, venae cavae, atrioventricular valves, and coronary sinus.

The great advantage of the Amplatzer closure device is its complete retrievability while still attached to the delivery cable by virtue of the "metal memory" properties of nitinol. In cases of unsatisfactory deployment, device retrieval is easily accomplished by pulling on the delivery cable, while the device reintroduces itself into the delivery sheath. If proper deployment is confirmed on echocardiography, then device release is accomplished by counterclockwise rotation of the delivery cable.

More recently, the Amplatzer Multifenestrated Septal Occluder™ (AGA Medical Corporation, Golden Valley, MN, USA) became available for the closure of multifenestrated (cribriform) ASDs. The device is available in 18, 25 and 35 mm diameters, with both retention disks having the same size.

Device embolization is rare and usually occurs during the first 24 h post deployment. It is usually well tolerated, unless the device aligns in parallel with the plane of any heart valve. Percutaneous retrieval is usually successful by using a sheath that is at least 2 French larger than the one used for device delivery, in conjunction with a 10-mm Microvena snare catheter system. Nevertheless, surgical removal is still required in many cases.

The same basic technical principles described for the percutaneous deployment of the Amplatzer™ closure device apply to the CardioSEAL, STARFlex and Helex devices. However, important differences are pertinent.

The CardioSEAL device consists of two joined square-shaped umbrellas, manufactured from a cobalt alloy wire skeleton, to which a knitted Dacron fabric is attached. The wire skeleton of each umbrella consists of four wires with three separate articulations, each responsible for the device flexibility and radial strength. The addition of a unique self-centered mechanism via a microcoil spring yielded the next-generation device, the STARFlex. Both umbrellas are the same size in both devices, with the CardioSEAL available in 17, 23, 28, and 33 mm and the STARFlex in 23, 28, and 33 mm (38 mm

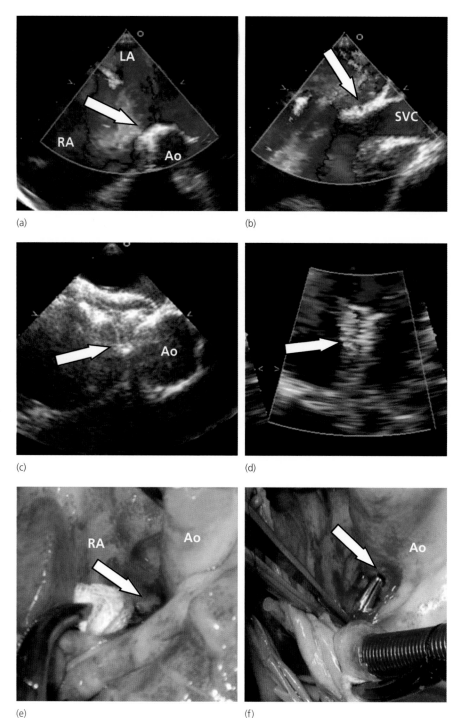

Figure 4.3 A 28-year-old pregnant woman underwent transcatheter ASD closure for severe right-sided heart failure. (a) TEE revealed a deficient anterior rim (white arrow) but (b) an adequate superior rim (white arrow). (c) An oversized Amplatzer ASD occluder was deployed, overlapping the anterior surface of the aorta (white arrow). (d) TTE the next day revealed no pericardial effusion; however, a new left-to-right shunt through the device was detected by color Doppler (white arrow). The patient developed pericardial tamponade 48 h after the procedure and was taken urgently to the operating room, where (e) the right atrial disk of the Amplatzer device was seen protruding through the roof of the right atrium (white arrow) and (f) eroding the anterior surface of the aorta (white arrow). Ao, aorta; LA, left atrium; RA, right atrium; SVC, superior vena cava.

available in Europe only). The self-centering mechanism makes the STARFlex a more suitable device than the CardioSEAL for transcatheter ASD closure; however, it has yet to be approved in the USA for such use.

Balloon sizing of the ASD is also mandatory when using the CardioSEAL and STARFlex devices, and a device/maximum balloon size ratio of 2:1 is recommended for device selection. The recommended sheath size is 11F and 10F for CardioSEAL and STARFlex devices, respectively. Although the left sided disk is easily retrievable by pulling back the device into the delivery sheath, complete device retrieval requires the use of a snare system and a larger sheath once the right disk is deployed. Therefore, the 10 or 11Fr delivery sheath should be advanced inside a short 14Fr sheath (which could be left outside the body) before being introduced into the body, in case device retrieval is required.

The Helex closure device is a nonself-centered double disk device manufactured from a continuous nitinol wire to which a hydrophilic ePTFE (Gore-Tex™, W.L. Gore™ & Associates, Flagstaff, AZ, USA) is attached. The Helex device achieves a low profile once deployed, with the added advantage of the long proven biocompatibility of Gore-Tex™ in the cardiovascular system. The Helex ™ device is available in 15, 20, 25, 30, and 35 mm, with a device/maximum balloon size ratio of 2:1 recommended for device selection. The Helex device is supplied with its own delivery sheath and it is introduced only via a short 10 or 12F venous sheath. It has a unique deployment mechanism, with a "push, pinch, and pull" sequence required under fluoroscopic and echocardiographic guidance. Of note, Gore-Tex™ is more echogenic than Dacron and polyester and, therefore, echoscatter on the early Helex™ devices hindered visualisation.

Irrespective of the device used, ASA therapy (81–325 mg/day) and prophylaxis against subacute bacterial endocarditis is prescribed for 6 months post closure. Routine transthoracic echocardiography should be performed at 24 h, 6–8 weeks, 6 months, and yearly for at least 5 years post closure.

Results

Most centers favor percutaneous closure, if the anatomy is suitable, as transcatheter closure has been reported to be associated with fewer complications than surgery [22,23]. The phase II trial of the Amplatzer ASOD™ found that transcatheter closure was associated with fewer complications than surgery [22].

Percutaneous closure of ASD has been shown to improve right ventricular dilation and function, as well as exercise capacity measured by cardiopulmonary exercise testing in nonrandomized uncontrolled studies [24,25].

The largest reported series of transcatheter ASD closure in children and adults is from the worldwide Amplatzer registry [26]. Immediate success, defined as complete closure or trivial/small residual shunt, was reported in 97% of cases, with 100% meeting the same criteria at 3 years. Although there were no procedural deaths, complications such as device embolization, cardiac arrhythmias, and thrombus formation occurred in a small number of patients. As mentioned above, late device erosion occurring as late as 3 years post closure has been recently reported in patients with deficient anterior and/or superior rims [21]. Therefore, patients with such anatomy who undergo transcatheter ASD closure with the Amplatzer device should be followed closely.

Although earlier nonrandomized studies reported greater safety and efficacy with the use of the Amplatzer device compared with the Clamshell and CardioSEAL devices for transcatheter closure of ASDs [27,28], success with the self-adjusting STARFlex modification is reported to be equal to that achieved with the Amplatzer septal occluder [29,30]. Late device arm fractures without clinical consequences have been reported in a small proportion of patients, particularly with the use of large CardioSEAL devices. Similar success rates of more than 95% have been reported with the Helex device, with device embolization or wire fracture also occurring in only a small proportion of cases [23,31].

Device thrombosis rates in patients undergoing transcatheter closure of ASD or patent foramen ovale with the CardioSEAL, STARFlex, Helex, and Amplatzer devices have been reported to be 7.1%, 5.7%, 0.8%, and 0%, respectively, when TEE was performed between 4 weeks and 6 months post closure [32]. Most cases resolved with anticoagulation; however, surgical removal was required in a small number of patients.

Summary

Transcatheter closure is a time-tested, safe, and effective alternative to surgery for the treatment of children and adults with ASD in experienced hands. Although randomized controlled studies comparing transcatheter versus surgical closure of ASDs may never be completed, there is growing consensus in the medical community that transcatheter closure is preferred, if the anatomy is suitable. Several devices are available, all with their own pros and cons, and training is required in their particular deployment technique. As with any new technique applied in medicine, long-term follow-up of patients undergoing transcatheter closure is mandatory in order to better understand and prevent potential complications, in particular the risk for late erosion.

Ventricular septal defect closure

Historical background

The first transcatheter closures of small congenital muscular ventricular septal defects (VSDs) were reported in 1988 by James Lock *et al.* [33] using Rashkind™ (C.R. Bard Inc., Billerica, MA, USA) patent ductus arteriosus occluding devices [33]. In 1991, the results of larger muscular VSD transcatheter closure using the Clamshell™ ASD device was reported in the *New England Journal of Medicine* from Children's Hospital Boston [34]. The development of transcatheter VSD closure was originally and historically hampered by large delivery sheaths, high rate of residual shunt, and inability to recapture and reposition the device, because the original devices such as the Clamshell, Sideris Button Device™, and even coils, were not intended for VSD closure.

The complexity and often high risk associated with the surgical closure of muscular VSD stimulated progress in transcatheter VSD occlusion. The evolution of the Clamshell device to the CardioSEAL, and its FDA approval under high-risk protocol for closure of muscular VSDs, meant that several centers have persisted with transcatheter VSD closure using this device [35]. Other PDA devices, ASD devices, coils, and the StarFLEX device have been used by various investigators in Europe [36]. The new technology of the Amplatzer device came to be tested and reported in 1999 [37]. The Amplatzer

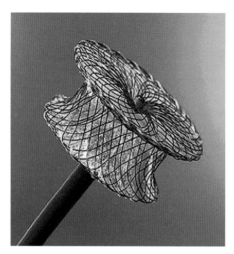

Figure 4.4 Amplatzer muscular VSD occluder.

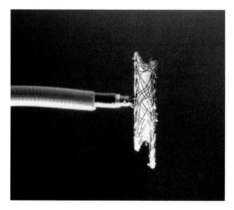

Figure 4.5 Amplatzer membranous VSD occluder.

device can often be deployed through a smaller sheath. Its retrievability allows it to be repositioned or redeployed if the initial appearance is unsatisfactory; thus, residual shunting may be less of a problem. Further design changes meant the Amplatzer Muscular device (Fig. 4.4) could also be used for postmyocardial infarction VSD closure. Alterations in the rims and waist thickness, and in the delivery cable, lead to the further evolution of the Amplatzer device for closure of perimembranous VSDs (Fig. 4.5) [38].

Morphology and pathophysiology

Ventricular septal defects are not uncommon, and in fact account for approximately 24–35% of all congenital heart disease [39]. Acquired VSD is uncommon and may be secondary to a myocardial infarction with ischemic rupture of a focal part of the ventricular septum, or to sharp trauma such as a stab wound.

Symptoms depend on the degree of left-to-right shunt and pulmonary hypertension (PHT), which depends on the size of the defect. A large nonrestrictive VSD will cause a large left-to-right shunt with flow-related PHT. If left unoperated,

the excessive pulmonary blood flow will lead to injury of the pulmonary vascular bed and pulmonary vascular occlusive disease (PVOD), elevated pulmonary vascular resistance (PVR), and eventually Eisenmenger's syndrome. A moderate-sized VSD may be associated with a large left-to-right shunt with less pulmonary hypertension, but with symptoms of pulmonary overcirculation and left ventricular overload. A patient with a small VSD may be asymptomatic but develop complications of infective endocarditis or aortic insufficiency if the VSD lies beneath the aortic valve and an aortic cusp is unsupported.

Neonates and infants with large left-to-right shunt, pulmonary overcirculation, and low pulmonary vascular resistance present with failure to thrive, poor feeding, diaphoresis, tachypnea, increased work of breathing, and recurrent pulmonary infections. On examination there is tachypnea, intercostal and subcostal retractions, tachycardia, hepatomegaly, and clinical cardiomegaly. The constellation of symptoms and signs of pulmonary overcirculation is somewhat erroneously referred to as "heart failure" in neonates and infants. The intensity of the heart murmur depends on the size of the defect, the degree of left-to-right shunt, PHT, and PVOD [39].

Left unoperated, as the PVR increases and the left-to-right shunt decreases, the symptoms and signs of "heart failure" resolve. Resolution of symptoms may also occur if the VSD diminishes in size or closes spontaneously. Spontaneous closure occurs more frequently in small to moderate-sized apical or midseptal congenital muscular VSDs than in perimembranous VSDs.

Postmyocardial infarct VSD is less common than congenital defects, and it usually occurs in the midapical region of the muscular ventricular septum as a result of rupture of necrotic septal myocardial tissue. Affected patients are usually hemodynamically unstable, presenting with a new murmur and hypotension after myocardial infarct. Whether treated surgically or by transcatheter device, the prognosis is frequently poor. The new infarct evolves with increasing necrosis around the edges of the VSD, so that either a surgical patch or a transcatheter device is unstable, developing residual shunting or even late embolization of the device [40].

Sharp trauma resulting in a VSD may present with symptoms of pulmonary overcirculation, such as dyspnea or diminished exercise capacity. A new murmur and heart failure may be appreciated either as a result of these symptoms or coincidentally.

Ventricular septal defects can be classified [41] according to the morphology of their borders, as viewed from the right ventricle. Viewed from the right ventricle, the interventricular septum can be divided into three areas: the inlet, the trabeculum or body, and the outlet. The septum is divided into a small membranous region below the atrioventricular valves and a muscular region that becomes thicker toward the apex of the heart.

Perimembranous VSDs have fibrous continuity between the atrioventricular valves. The atrioventricular conduction tissue traverses the posteroinferior margin. A membranous flap representing the remnant of the membranous septum may be seen. Perimembranous defects in the outlet portion of the right ventricle are related to the aortic valve in the left ventricular outlet. Perimembranous defects may extend toward the outlet portion, toward the apical portion, or toward the inlet portion. Large confluent perimembranous VSDs extend to all three ventricular portions.

Muscular defects have completely muscular borders when viewed from the right ventricular aspect. The proximity of muscular defects to the tricuspid valve and atrioventricular conduction bundles depends on the location of the defect in the septum. Muscular VSDs occur in the inlet, apical, midseptal, anterior, or outlet septum. Multiple muscular VSDs sometimes create a "Swiss Cheese" interventricular septum.

Doubly committed and juxtaarterial defects (also known as supracristal defects) are defined as VSD in which arterial valves form the roof and there is lack of muscular separation between the aortic and pulmonary valves. These defects are more prevalent in Asians. With doubly committed subarterial VSD, device closure risks damaging the aortic and pulmonary valves.

Many VSDs are oval or irregular in shape, rather than circular. Some are triangular, quadrangular, teardrop shaped or slit like. Muscular VSDs tend to burrow through the septum or be divided by small muscle bars on one side [9].

The distance of the defect from the anticipated site of the atrioventricular conduction bundle is variable and is usually greater with muscular VSDs [41]. The distance from the rim of the VSD to the atrioventricular valve and ventriculoarterial valves is usually well appreciated on echocardiography.

Postmyocardial infarction VSDs are most commonly located in the midapical region of the ventricular septum [42].

Indications for transcatheter ventricular septal defect closure

Several patients with muscular VSD deemed suitable for surgical closure can be considered for transcatheter closure. Access to muscular VSDs is frequently difficult for the surgeon because of the trabeculation of the right ventricle. A large muscular VSD in infancy causes pulmonary overcirculation, tachypnea, and failure to thrive. The initial palliative operation while the child is very small may be insertion of a pulmonary artery band to limit pulmonary blood flow and prevent pulmonary hypertension. For corrective surgery of the VSD, left or right ventriculotomy is often necessary, but is associated with subsequent hemodynamic instability, morbidity, and mortality. Transcatheter devices are most suitable when the VSD is in the midseptal, apical, or anterior muscular interventricular septum. Devices may also be placed at the time of open heart surgery or by perventricular technique so that cardiopulmonary bypass is not necessary. Smaller muscular VSDs commonly close spontaneously. A persistent muscular VSD causing a significant left-to-right shunt (symptoms, or

left atrial and left ventricular dilation by echo) should be carefully evaluated and considered for transcatheter VSD closure, even if there is no pulmonary hypertension.

Residual VSD at the patch margins following open heart surgery or an intentional fenestration left in a patch (for example for staged repair of tetralogy of Fallot in patients with diminutive pulmonary arteries) may be amenable to device closure [43,44].

Large perimembranous VSDs in neonates or infants are generally surgically corrected with relatively low mortality even when associated with other anomalies such as transposition of the great arteries or aortic arch abnormalities. Transcatheter VSD closure is considered more feasible in patients over 8 kg with restrictive, moderate-sized perimembranous VSD, with at least a 2-mm rim between the VSD margin and the aortic valve. Indications for VSD closure in these older patients would be any evidence of pulmonary hypertension, symptoms or asymptomatic signs on echo of left atrial and left ventricular dilation, and volume overload. The FDA has not approved any device for closure of perimembranous VSD and there remains concern regarding development of late heart block after transcatheter device closure of perimembranous VSD [45].

Doubly committed VSD is not suitable for transcatheter closure because of the proximity of the aortic and pulmonary valves.

Postmyocardial infarction VSD almost always causes hemodynamic instability, usually severe; thus intervention is usually indicated, although the risks are high.

Technical aspects of transcatheter ventricular septal defect closure

In the USA, only the Amplatzer muscular VSD device and the CardioSEAL are approved for transcatheter closure of muscular VSDs. A full echocardiogram is required to evaluate the exact size, position, and number of VSDs and to determine the relationship of the VSD to the valves and whether or not the valves are normal. The procedure is usually done under general anesthesia and using transesophageal echocardiography (TEE) in a catheterization laboratory, preferably with biplane fluoroscopy. The femoral vein and femoral artery are accessed and a full hemodynamic study is done. Access through the right internal jugular vein (RIJV) is the best approach for muscular VSDs in the midmuscular, posterior muscular, or apical muscular septum [42]. The patient is heparinized to keep the ACT over 200, and intravenous antibiotics are given. The systemic and pulmonary blood flows are calculated, pulmonary artery pressure measured, and pulmonary vascular resistance assessed. Associated defects and VSD(s) size and location and relationship to the valves are assessed on TEE and angiography. The size of the VSD can be measured either by TEE and angiography [42] or by balloon sizing [40], enabling the correct device size to be chosen. Access to the muscular VSD can either be from the femoral or internal jugular vein directly from the right ventricle (when the muscular VSD is large), or perventricular through a median sternotomy [46].

Most commonly, access to the muscular VSD can be achieved retrogradely by advancing a Judkins right coronary catheter or Cobra catheter from the left ventricle across the VSD to the right ventricle. A soft-tipped wire is advanced through the catheter to the right ventricle up to the pulmonary arteries. The catheter is advanced over the wire and the existing guide wire replaced with either an Amplatzer "Noodle" wire or a 0.035-inch regular exchange length wire. From the pulmonary artery, this wire is snared using a Gooseneck snare (ev3, Plymouth, MN, USA) and pulled back to the femoral vein or RIJV. This creates an arteriovenous through-and-through loop over which a large sheath from the femoral vein can be positioned in the left ventricle.

Alternatively, a venovenous through-and-through loop from the femoral vein may be created through the atrial septum via a long trans-septal sheath. Accessing the VSD via the left atrium and left ventricle, the VSD is then crossed with a Swan–Ganz™ balloon catheter [40], which is directed up to the pulmonary artery, where an exchange length wire through the Swan–Ganz™ catheter is snared and brought out to the femoral vein or RIJV. This step should be performed with caution in order to prevent the catheter floating from the right ventricle to the right atrium and snaring in the right atrium, which may occur if the catheter passes through the chordae of the tricuspid valve, causing rupture of the chordae and severe tricuspid insufficiency [40]. A large Mullins-type sheath can then be passed over the wire from the vein to the right atrium, right ventricle and through the VSD to the left ventricle.

Kinks may develop in the large sheath with any method described above. This can be circumvented with a 0.018-inch glide wire left inside the sheath as the device is advanced. The small wire is removed once the device reaches the end of the sheath in the left ventricle [42].

If an Amplatzer muscular VSD device is used, then a device 1–2 mm greater than the VSD size is chosen (there are eight different sizes, between 4 and 18 mm in 2-mm increments, which are delivered through a 6F to 9F sheath). The waist of the device measures 7 mm in length and the diameter of the disks is usually 8 mm greater (i.e., 4-mm rims) than the waist, except in the case of the smallest 4-mm device, the rims of which are 2.5 mm greater than the waist. A CardioSEAL device should be 2–2.5 times the size of the VSD. The CardioSEAL is made of two disks connected by a central post and comes in five different sizes (17, 23, 28, 33, and 40 mm) The CardioSEAL is not a self-centering device and is deployed through a larger sheath (10F and 11F). The smaller sheath of the Amplatzer device is a significant advantage in small children. The Amplatzer device is also more easily retrievable should the need arise for it to be repositioned or redeployed. With the end of the sheath in the mid-left ventricle (but away from the left ventricular free wall) the dilator and wire are slowly removed. Great attention to detail is required to ensure that no clots or air

develop in the sheath. The device is passed through the sheath and then the left ventricular disk gently pushed past the end of the sheath into the left ventricular cavity. With the left ventricular disk free in the left ventricular cavity, the sheath, delivery cable, and device are pulled back gently so that the left ventricular disk is now in apposition with the left ventricular aspect of the septum. The waist of the device and the right ventricular disk are now exposed by retracting the sheath back over the cable. The position of the device is now evaluated by angiography and TEE. If the position or device does not appear to be satisfactory, then the device can be retracted back into the sheath and repositioned or replaced by a different size or type of device. If the device appears satisfactory on TEE and angiography, then it can be deployed by releasing it from the delivery cable. Repeat evaluation by TEE and left ventricular angiography is done again with the device deployed.

Perventricular muscular VSD closure is done in small or hemodynamically unstable patients or where vascular access is a problem. The procedure is either done in the operating room with TEE guidance or in a "hybrid room." Through a median sternotomy a purse-string suture is placed by the surgeon on the right ventricular wall opposite the VSD. The exact details of this procedure are beyond the scope of this text; the reader is referred to a more detailed description of the technique [14]. Suffice it to say the device is deployed in a similar manner across the VSD using a short sheath advanced from the right ventricular free wall.

Postmyocardial infarction VSD transcatheter closure maybe attempted in a similar manner as for congenital muscular VSDs. The VSD is accessed from the left ventricle with a Judkins right coronary catheter (or similar), and the through-and-through wire brought out via the right internal jugular vein. Affected patients are usually critically ill, in cardiogenic shock, and receiving ventilatory, inotropic, and balloon pump support. The VSD with its necrotic edges may become larger with balloon sizing or pull-through of the device. A large (40 mm) CardioSEAL or STARFlex (NMT, Boston, MA, USA) device may be deployed via a large (12F) sheath. Dr. Kurt Amplatz and AGA (Plymouth, MN, USA) have developed a specific postinfarction Amplatzer muscular VSD occluder (PIMVSD) in sizes from 16 to 24 mm in diameter (again available in 2-mm increments) of the waist and 5-mm rims on the right ventricular and left ventricular side. The waist is 10 mm long. The device can be deployed through an Amplatzer TorquVue™ sheath size 9F or 10F. Closure of larger postmyocardial VSDs can be attempted using large Amplatzer atrial septal occluders [47].

Restrictive perimembranous VSDs have been reported to be closed by transcatheter Sideris, Rashkind, and even coil devices. More recently, the Amplatzer membranous VSD occluder (AGA Medical Corp., Plymouth, MN, USA) has been used in some large centers with acceptable results, provided there is at least a 2-mm rim of tissue between the aortic valve

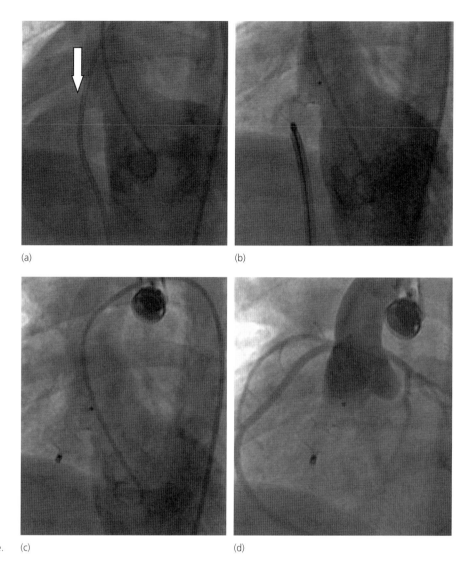

Figure 4.6 (a) Left ventricular angiogram showing perimembranous VSD (arrowed). (b) Amplatzer device still attached to cable, positioned in VSD. (c) Amplatzer device deployed in VSD. (d) Aortogram showing relationship of Amplatzer device to aortic valve.

(a)

(b)

(c)

(d)

and the VSD. The device has a waist which is 1.5 mm in length (compared with 7 mm for the Amplatzer muscular VSD device) and ranges from 4 to 18 mm in diameter. The left ventricular disk is eccentric with only 0.5 mm at the cephalad margin of the device but a 5-mm rim around the rest of the waist. There is a platinum radiopaque marker at the inferior end of the device to direct the position of the device. The right ventricular disk has a symmetrical 2-mm rim. The VSD is crossed with a Judkins right coronary catheter and a through-and-through wire from right femoral artery to the right femoral vein is created in a similar way as for an anterior muscular VSD. The Amplatzer membranous VSD occluder is delivered through a specific Amplatzer TorquVue™ delivery system (AGA, Plymouth, MN, USA), which has a special delivery pusher catheter with a metal ring fixed at its tip. The pin vice on the right ventricular disk has a flattened part, which coincides with a flat part inside the metal ring, so that the occluder is deployed in the correct orientation (Fig. 4.6).

The deployment procedure is complex and the reader is referred to more detailed and specific text [40,48] for more specific procedural details.

Results

The largest reported series of congenital VSD transcatheter closure in 430 patients (until July 2005) is from the European Registry [49]. There were 119 muscular and 250 perimembranous VSD transcatheter closures reported from 23 centers. A 95% success rate was reported. There was one death. Aortic insufficiency occurred in 14 patients, device embolization in five cases, and complete heart block following perimembranous VSD closure occurred in 5% (6.7% heart block for residual VSD postsurgery device occlusion). Young age and low weight were significant risk factors.

A CardioSEAL VSD registry from 18 centers for high-risk muscular VSD device closure in 55 patients reported no deaths but an 8% event rate, 4% embolization rate, and 6%

explant rate. Ninety-two percent of intended VSD device implants were judged to be successful [50].

Postinfarction VSD using the Amplatzer device has been reported as procedurally successful in 16 out of 18 patients, but the 30-day mortality rate was 28% [51].

Other complications and problems that can occur from ventricular device closure include hemolysis, residual shunt, hemodynamic instability, and arrhythmias during the procedure caused by large sheaths in the heart and across valves, bleeding requiring blood transfusion, device entanglement in the mitral or tricuspid valves and chordae, pericardial tamponade, kinking of the sheath, and air embolism or thromboembolism causing neurological deficit.

Summary

Only a small proportion of individuals with a VSD are candidates for device closure. Transcatheter closure of VSD is a technically difficult procedure: an experienced team of cardiologists, anesthesiologists, catheter laboratory staff and surgeons needs to be available to ensure that device closure can be performed with adequate safety. The possibility of severe complications is very real. Even so, current results are good, especially for muscular VSD, and support increasing use of this technique in appropriate patients. Early and late complete heart block after transcatheter perimembranous VSD closure remains a major concern.

References

1. King TD & Mills NL. (1974) Nonoperative closure of atrial septal defects. *Surgery* **75**:383–388.
2. Lock JE, Rome JJ, Davis R, *et al.* (1989) Transcatheter closure of atrial septal defects. Experimental studies. *Circulation* **79**:1091–1099.
3. Boutin C, Mesewe NN, Smallhorn JF, *et al.* (1993) Echocardiographic follow up of atrial septal defects after catheter closure by double umbrella device. *Circulation* **88**:621–627.
4. Prieto LR, Foreman CK, Cheatham JP, & Latson LA. (1995) Intermediate-term outcome of transcatheter secundum atrial septal defect closure using the Bard Clamshell Septal Umbrella. *Am J Cardiol* **76**:695–698.
5. Babic UU, Grujicic S, Popovic Z, *et al.* (1991) Double-umbrella device for transvenous closure of patent ductus arteriosus and atrial septal defect: first experience. *J Interv Cardiol* **4**:283–296.
6. Rao PS & Sideris EG. (2001) Centering-on demand buttoned device: its role in transcatheter occlusion of atrial septal defects. *J Interv Cardiol* **14**:81–89.
7. Rickers C, Hamm C, Stern H, *et al.* (1998) Percutaneous closure of secundum atrial septal defect with a new self centering device ("angel wings"). *Heart* **80**:517–521.
8. Hoffman JE & Kaplan S. (2002) The incidence of congenital heart disease. *J Am Coll Cardiol* **39**:1890.
9. Joy J, Kartha CC, & Balakrishnan KG. (1993) Structural basis for mitral valve dysfunction associated with ostium secundum atrial septal defects. *Cardiology* **82**:409–414.
10. Fuse S, Tomita H, Hatakeyama K, *et al.* (2001) Effects of size of an atrial septal defect on shunt volume. *Am J Cardiol* **88**:1447–1450.
11. Craig RJ & Selzer A. (1968) Natural history and prognosis of atrial septal defect. *Circulation* **37**:805–815.
12. Dalen JE, Haynes FW, & Dexter L. (1967) Life expectancy with atrial septal defect. Influence of complicating pulmonary vascular disease. *JAMA* **200**:442–446.
13. Balzer D, Kort H, Day R, *et al.* (2002) Inhaled Nitric Oxide as Preoperative Test (INOP test I): the INOP Test Study Group. *Circulation* **106**:I76–81.
14. Bruch L, Winkelmann A, Sonntag S, *et al.* (2007) Fenestrated occluders for treatment of ASD in elderly patients with pulmonary hypertension and/or right heart failure. *J Interv Cardiol* **21**:44–49.
15. Boccalandro F, Baptista E, Muench A, *et al.* (2004) Comparison of intracardiac echocardiography versus transesophageal guidance for percutaneous transcatheter closure of atrial septal defect. *Am J Cardiol* **93**:437–440.
16. Rigateli G, Cardaioli P, Braggion G, *et al.* (2007) Transesophageal echocardiography and intracardiac echocardiography differently predict technical challenges or failures of interatrial shunts catheter based closure. *J Interv Cardiol* **20**:77–81.
17. Passeri J, Inglessis I, Palacios I, & Picard M. (2007) Initial experience with real time three-dimensional transesophageal echocardiography in patients undergoing transcatheter atrial septal defect closure. *Circulation* **116**:II_401 (abs.).
18. Balzer J, Kuhl H, Rassaf T, *et al.* (2008) Real-time transesophageal three-dimensional echocardiography for guidance of atrial septal defect closures. *Eur Heart J* **97**:565–574.
19. Sader M, De Moor M, Pomenrantsev E, & Palacios I. (2003) Percutaneous transcatheter patent foramen closure using the right internal jugular venous approach. *Catheter Cardiovasc Interv* **60**:536–539.
20. Shim D, Lloyd T, & Beekman R III. (1999) Transhepatic therapeutic cardiac catheterization: a new option for the pediatric interventionalist. *Catheter Cardiovasc Interv* **4**:41–45.
21. Divekar A, Gaamangwe T, Shaikh N, *et al.* (2005) Cardiac perforations after device closure of atrial septal defects with the Amplatzer septal occluder. *J Am Coll Cardiol* **45**:1213–1218.
22. Du ZD, Hijazi ZM, Kleinman CS, *et al.* (2002) Amplatzer investigators. Comparison between transcatheter and surgical closure of secundum atrial septal defect in children and adults: results of a multicenter non randomized trial. *J Am Coll Cardiol* **39**:1836–1844.
23. Jones T, Latson L, Zahn E, *et al.* (2007) Results of the US Multicenter Pivotal Study of the Helex septal occluded for percutaneous closure of secundum atrial septal defects. *J Am Coll Cardiol* **49**:2215–2221.
24. Veldtman GR, Razack V, Siu S, *et al.* (2001) Right ventricular form and function after percutaneous atrial septal defect closure. *J Am Coll Cardiol* **37**:2108–2113.
25. Brochi MC, Baril JF, Dore A, *et al.* (2002) Improvement in exercise capacity in asymptomatic and mildly symptomatic adults after atrial septal defect percutaneous closure. *Circulation* **106**:1821–1826.
26. Omeish A & Hijazi ZM. (2001) Transcatheter closure of atrial septal defects in children and adults using the Amplatzer Septal Occluder. *J Interv Cardiol* **14**:37–44.
27. Butera G, Caminati M, Chessa M, *et al.* (2004) CardioSEAL/STARFlex versus Amplatzer devices for percutaneous closure of

small to moderate (up to 18 mm) atrial septa defects. *Am Heart J* **148**:507–510.

28. Post M, Suttorp M, Jaarsma W, & Plokker T. (2006) Comparison of outcome and complications using different types of devices for percutaneous closure of a secundum atrial septal defect in adults: a single center experience. *Catheter Cardiovasc Interv* **67**:438–443.

29. Carminati M, Chessa M, Buter G, *et al.* (2001) Transcatheter closure of atrial septal defects with the STARFlex device: early results and follow up. *J Interv Cardiol* **14**:319–324.

30. Nugent AW, Britt A, Gauvreau K, *et al.* (2006) Device closure rates of simple atrial septal defects optimized by the STARFlex device. *J Am Coll Cardiol* **48**:538–544.

31. Zahn E, Wilson N, Cutright W, & Latson L. (2001) Development and testing of the Helex septal occluder, a new expanded polytetrafluoroethylene atrial septal defect occlusion system. *Circulation* **104**:711–716.

32. Krumsdorf U, Ostermayer S, Billinger K, *et al.* (2004) Incidence and clinical course of thrombus formation on atrial septal defect and patent foramen ovale closure devices in 1,000 consecutive patients. *J Am Coll Cardiol* **21**:302–309.

33. Lock JE, Block PC, McKay RG, Bain DS, & Keane JF. (1988) Transcatheter closure of ventricular septal defects. *Circulation* **82**:1681–1685.

34. Bridges N, Perry S, Keane J, *et al.* (1991) Preoperative transcatheter closure of congenital muscular ventricular septal defects. *N Engl J Med* **324**:1312–1317.

35. Lims DS, Forbes TJ, Rothman A, Lock JE, & Landzburg MJ. (2007) Transcatheter closure of high risk muscular ventricular septal defects with the CardioSEAL occluder: initial report from the CardioSEAL VSD registry. *Catheter Cardiovasc Interv* **70**:740–744.

36. Carminati M, Butera G, Chessa M, for the Investigators of the European VSD Registry (2007) Transcatheter closure of congenital ventricular septal defects: results of the European Registry. *Eur Heart J* **28**:2361–2368.

37. Amin Z, Gu X, Berry JM, *et al.* (1999) New device for closure of muscular ventricular septal defects in a canine model. *Circulation* **100**:320–328.

38. Hijazi ZM, Hakim F, Haweleh AA, *et al.* (2002) Catheter closure of perimembranous ventricular septal defects using the new Amplatzer membranous VSD occluder. *Catheter Cardiovasc Interv* **56**:508–515.

39. Hoffman JIE. (1987) Incidence, mortality and natural history. In Anderson RH, Macartney FJ, Shinebourne EA, & Tynan M (eds). *Pediatric Cardiology*. Edinburgh: Churchill Livingstone, pp. 3–13.

40. Mullins CE. (2006) Ventricular septal defect occlusions. In: Mullins CE (ed). *Cardiac Catheterization in Congenital Heart Disease*. Oxford: Blackwell Publishing, pp. 803–841.

41. McCartthy KP, Leung PKC, & Ho SY. (2005) Perimembranous and muscular ventricular septal defects—morphology revisited in the era of device closure. *J Interv Cardiol* **18**:507–513.

42. Hijazi ZM. (2003) Device closure of ventricular septal defects. *Catheter Cardiovasc Interv* **60**:107–114.

43. Knauth A, Lock JE, Perry SB, *et al.* (2004) Transcatheter device closure of congenital and postoperative residual ventricular septal defects. *Circulation* **110**:501–507.

44. Marshall AC, Love BA, Lang P, *et al.* (2003) Staged repair of Tetralogy of Fallot and diminutive pulmonary arteries using a fenestrated ventricular septal defect patch. *J Thorac Cardiovasc Surg* **126**:1427–1433.

45. Sullivan I. (2007) Transcatheter closure of perimembranous ventricular septal defect: is the risk of heart block too high? *Heart* **93**:284–286.

46. Bacha EA, Galantowicz ME, Cheatham JP, *et al.* (2005) Multicenter experience with perventricular device closure of muscular ventricular septal defects. *Pediatr Cardiol* **26**:169–175.

47. Lowe HC, Jang IK, Yoerger DM, MacGillivray TE, de Moor M, & Palacios IF. (2003) Compassionate use of the Amplatzer ASD closure device for residual postinfarction ventricular septal rupture following surgical repair. *Catheter Cardiovasc Interv* **59**:230–233.

48. Hijazi ZM, Hakim F, Haweleh AA, *et al.* (2002) Catheter closure of perimembranous ventricular septal defects using the new Amplatzer membranous VSD occluder. *Catheter Cardiovasc Interv* **56**:508–515.

49. Carminati M, Butera G, Chessa M, *et al.* Investigators of the European VSD Registry. (2007) Transcatheter closure of congenital ventricular septal defects: Results of the European Registry. *Eur Heart J* **28**:2361–2368.

50. Lim DS, Forbes TJ, Rothman A, Lock JE, & Landzburg MJ. (2007) Transcatheter closure of high risk muscular ventricular septal defects with the CardioSEAL occluder: initial report from the CardioSEAL VSD Registry. *Catheter Cardiovasc Interv* **70**:740–744.

51. Holzer R, Balzer D, Amin Z, *et al.* (2004) Transcatheter closure of postinfarction ventricular septal defects using the new Amplatzer muscular VSD occluder: Results of a U.S. Registry. *Catheter Cardiovasc Interv* **61**:196–201.

5   Catheter Closure of Patent Foramen Ovale

Nina Wunderlich[1], Katharina Lehn[1], Neil Wilson[2] & Horst Sievert[1]

[1]Cardiovascular Center Frankfurt, Frankfurt, Germany
[2]John Radcliffe Hospital, Oxford, UK

Historical background

The patent foramen ovale (PFO) (Fig. 5.1), with its potential pathologic importance as an intracardiac right-to-left shunt, has gained attention over the last two decades as a culprit implicated in embolic stroke and migraine. Interventional closure of the PFO with catheter-delivered devices is an innovative and expanding field of interventional cardiology. Percutaneous PFO closure was first performed by Bridges *et al.* in 1992 [1], who used a double-umbrella clamshell device (Bard, USCI, Billerica, MA, USA) in 36 patients after presumed paradoxical embolism.

Transcatheter closure of interatrial septal defects is now a routine procedure that can be performed using different devices and is associated with low rates of complications and recurrence. Many of the devices used were adapted from devices designed to close atrial septal defects (ASDs). The right and left anchor arms are rigidly connected to each other at a fixed distance. Unlike an ASD, which is a hole in the interatrial septum, a PFO has a tunnel of variable length that can vary from 0 to 20 mm. Thus, the current devices, in which the distance between the right and left disks is rigid and fixed, may distort the septal anatomy and, in rare instances, may even cause the PFO to remain open. Despite continuing progress in occluder design, materials, and implantation technique, most of the devices used today are still based on the two-disk principle.

Despite the limitations, transcatheter closure of PFO with devices is a very safe and effective technique associated with high closure rates. It has repeatedly been shown to reduce the risk of recurrent stroke significantly, from as high as 56% before closure to about 4% after closure [2–4], although the results from randomized trials are still pending. As mentioned above, in many centers worldwide transcatheter closure of PFOs with devices has become a standard of care for patients suffering from cryptogenic stroke.

Cardiovascular Interventions in Clinical Practice. Edited by Jürgen Haase, Hans-Joachim Schäfers, Horst Sievert and Ron Waksman. © 2010 Blackwell Publishing.

Morphology and pathophysiology of patent foramen ovale

The foramen ovale plays a vital role in embryonic development; it allows oxygenated blood from the inferior vena cava to bypass the fluid-filled lungs and to pass directly to the systemic circulation via the left ventricle.

Post partum, left atrial pressure exceeds right atrial pressure, pushing the overlapping parts of septum primum and secundum together, thus causing functional closure of the foramen ovale. However, in up to 35% of the general population, this is not followed by anatomical closure, leaving a potential pathway for venous thrombi to enter systemic circulation [5]. Others suspect that the PFO itself promotes clot formation or instigates paroxysmal atrial fibrillation, hence increasing the risk of cardioembolic events [6,7].

Although the actual mechanism seems difficult to demonstrate, the incidence of PFO among patients with cryptogenic stroke varies between 45% and 54%, compared with only 9–27% of control groups or 23% of those who have experienced a stroke with a determinant cause [8–10]. In young patients the PFO is particularly suspected to play a major role in stroke genesis, as concomitant diseases such as arrhythmia or atherosclerosis are less frequent [8,9,11]. More recently, it was proven that there is also an association between the presence of a PFO and cryptogenic stroke in elderly patients [12].

The prevalence of a PFO decreases with increasing age, from 34% in patients aged 30–35 to 20% in patients over 80 years. This may imply that the defect closes over time, but it may also be that the younger patients with PFO die earlier [5]. Interestingly, the size of the PFO increases with age from 3.4 mm in patients aged 10 years to 5.8 mm in patients over the age of 90 years. The annual recurrence rate of cerebral ischemic events ranges from 2.3% to 14.4%, despite blood-thinning therapy [13–18], and the annual recurrence for stroke and death is 1.2–7.2% [13,14,18].

The risk of another embolic event increases further with a larger PFO size and when the PFO is associated with an atrial septal aneurysm (ASA) [12,14,19–21]. Mas *et al.* [20] found that the risk of a transient ischemic attack (TIA) or stroke was

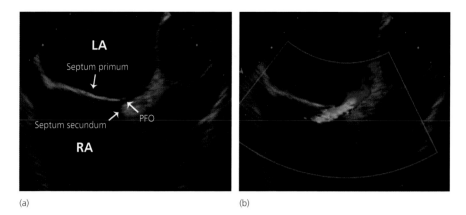

Figure 5.1 Typical PFO in transesophageal echocardiography (long-axis view, 109°) with a relatively short tunnel. (a) PFO in two-dimensional echocardiography. (b) PFO with color Doppler.

(a)

(b)

significantly higher (19.2% higher at 4 years) in patients with a PFO in combination with an atrial septal aneurysm than in patients with a PFO only. Atrial septal aneurysm alone, however, is not a risk factor for stroke. It is also important to remember that, in the general population, a PFO by itself does not appear to be a risk factor for cerebrovascular events [22,23]. Only the combination of a PFO with a thrombogenic disorder is potentially hazardous.

Interatrial communications are also suspected to play an important role in the pathogenesis of migraine, especially migraine with aura [20,24]. The pathological mechanism is suspected to be similar to that in stroke patients. Instead of venous thrombi entering the systemic circulation, vasoactive substances such as serotonin cross the PFO without being metabolized in the lungs [25].

Indications for patent foramen ovale closure

Transcatheter closure is usually considered for an otherwise unexplained embolic stroke, a transient neurological event (e.g., TIA), or a peripheral embolism [14,26]. Because of the high incidence of a PFO in healthy subjects, all other potential sources for the embolic event, such as atrial fibrillation or carotid stenosis, need to be excluded. Other indications are decompression sickness in divers [27] and platypnea–orthodeoxia [28]. To date, there are no controlled randomized trials that prove this approach is better than medical therapy. On the other hand, there are no randomized trials showing that medical therapy, which is frequently considered as standard of care and recommended according to most guidelines [29,30], is effective in preventing recurrent events. Some studies are under way to determine whether there is an indication for PFO closure in patients with migraine headaches with aura [31,32].

Technical aspects

A number of occlusion devices have been developed over the years. All ASD occlusion systems are also suitable for PFO closure.

Only the Amplatzer Septal Occluder (AGA Medial, Golden Valley, MN, USA) comes in two versions: an ASD and a PFO device.

The most commonly implanted interatrial septal closure devices today are the Amplatzer® Septal Occluder, the Amplatzer® PFO Occluder (AGA Medical Corp., Golden Valley, MN, USA), the CardioSEAL®/STARFlex® (NMT Medical, Boston, MA, USA), and the Helex Septal Occluder (W.L. Gore & Associates, Flagstaff, AZ, USA). For these frequently used devices, implantation techniques and management of peri-interventional complications will be presented.

For all PFO closure procedures we recommend transesophageal echocardiography (TEE) to confirm the diagnosis, exclude thrombi, and assess anatomic characteristics, such as the exact location of the PFO, tunnel length, thickness and morphology of the atrial septum, additional defects, and presence of an ASA, which can play an important role for device selection. A high-quality transesophageal echocardiogram helps to avoid most of the potential pitfalls and complications. Conscious sedation may be helpful when the TEE probe is not well tolerated. Alternatively, intracardiac echocardiography (ICE) may be used. Before intervention, intravenous antibiotic is administered. Institutional use varies on this point; some centers repeat this intravenous administration some hours later. Vascular access is gained through the right or left femoral vein. After sheath placement 10 000 units of unfractured heparin is given.

We perform balloon sizing of all defects because the size of the PFO is unpredictable by TEE. The defect size may vary between 1 and 26.3 mm. The PFO is crossed with a multipurpose catheter, which is advanced in the left upper pulmonary vein. A stiff guidewire is introduced and the catheter is exchanged for a sizing balloon [NuMED, Inc., Hopkinton, NY, USA or AGA Medical Corp., Golden Valley, MN, USA). It is inflated with dilute contrast medium. The pressure in the balloon should be monitored during inflation and should not exceed 0.05 atmospheres to avoid overstretching of the PFO. The sizing balloon is then withdrawn into the PFO and the stretched diameter is measured by calibrated biplane fluoroscopy or by TEE/ICE. The same guidewire is used to advance the specific introducer sheaths to facilitate device delivery.

After sheath removal manual pressure is maintained on the femoral vein and a compression bandage is applied for 12 h. After implantation, aspirin (100 mg/day) is prescribed for 6 months and clopidogrel (75 mg/day) for 3 months. Prophylaxis against endocarditis is recommended for 6 months.

We perform TEE at 1 and 6 months after the implantation to exclude complications and to confirm complete closure.

Current devices and results

CardioSEAL®, STARFlex®, and BioSTAR®

The CardioSEAL septal occluder (Fig. 5.2a) is a modified version of the original clamshell device. It is the current US version. Two square Dacron patches are straightened by four wire spring arms composed of a cobalt-based alloy. The device is available in sizes from 17 mm to 40 mm. The current version, the CardioSEAL STARFlex septal occluder, represents a further revision of the CardioSEAL occluder. It has small micro-

springs attached at the end of each opposing arm of the left and right atrial disk. These interconnecting springs are designed to facilitate centering of the device and to provide closer adaption to the septum, thereby decreasing the device profile. For larger ASDs, there is a version with six arms with a device diameter of 38 mm.

Patients with paradoxical embolism and PFO ($n = 272$) were involved in the prospective FORECAST (The Foramen Occlusion for Paradoxical Embolism Using the Cardioseal and Starflex Occluders Registry) and underwent closure with the CardioSEAL or STARFlex devices. There was a successful device implantation in 99.3% of the patients and an intra-procedural complication rate of 6.6% (such as stroke or TIA in 1.8%, and device embolization in 0.7%). A trace of residual shunt was observed in 95.2%, and complete closure of the PFO in 72.2% of the patients [33].

Kiblawi *et al.* [34] reported on 456 patients with cryptogenic stroke or TIA and PFO who underwent closure with the

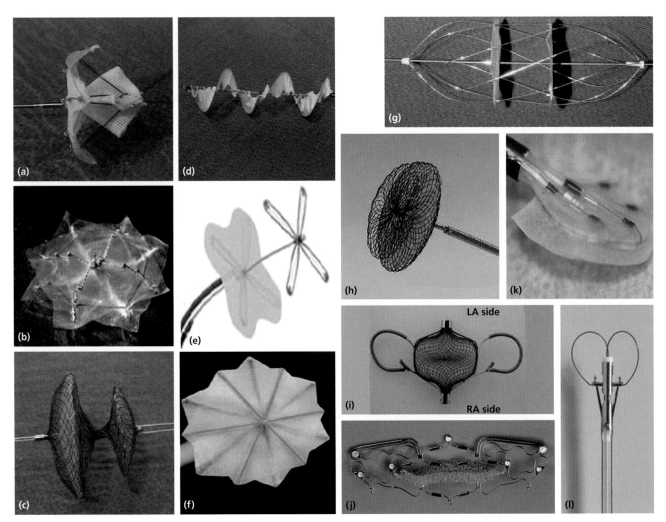

Figure 5.2 Occluders: (a) STARFlex, (b) BioSTAR, (c) Amplatzer, (d) Helex, (e) Premere, (f) Cardia, (g) Solysafe, (h) OccluTech, (i) SeptRX, (j) Coherex, (k) PFx, and (l) Heart Stitch.

CardioSEAL device. Implantation was successful in all patients and none experienced a recurrent embolic event during the procedure or during their hospital stay. There were 32 acute procedural complications (7.1%), device retrieval complications in eight patients, arrhythmia in seven patients, and hematoma in six patients. At a mean follow-up of 17.8 ± 11.1 months, seven patients experienced a recurrent embolic event, with five of these events occurring within 6 weeks of the procedure. Interestingly, six of these patients had a complete closure and no thrombus formation at the time of follow-up, using TEE. The most common complications on follow-up were atrial arrhythmia in 19%, which resolved spontaneously or after treatment in all patients, and headache or migraine in 1.5%, which resolved in most patients within 6 months. Echocardiography 6 months post procedure was adequate for analysis in a total of 276 patients. Of these, six patients had residual shunting (2.2%) and only one patient had more than mild shunting [34].

A multicenter, randomized, controlled trial (CLOSURE-1) investigating the STAR-Flex device compared with best medical therapy (aspirin, warfarin, or both) in 800 patients with stroke or TIA due to presumed paradoxical embolism stopped enrolling in late 2008. Data are not yet published.

Regarding migraine headaches, The Migraine Intervention with STARFlex (MIST) Trial was a multicenter, prospective, randomized trial evaluating the STARFlex device in 147 patients with a history of migraine with aura and a PFO with a moderate to large right-to-left shunt. Patients underwent either implantation of a STARFlex device or sham procedure, in an attempt to minimize placebo effect in the control group. Patients were followed for 6 months with a primary end point of cure of migraine. The study failed to demonstrate a difference in the primary end point, but patients in the closure group reached the secondary end point with a 50% reduction in headache days (42% closure vs. 23% sham; $P = 0.038$) [35].

The BioSTAR® septal occluder (Fig. 5.2b) (NMT Medical, Inc., Boston, MA, USA) is an advanced version of the CardioSEAL–STARFlex devices. It has a bioabsorbable fabric mounted on the STARFlex double-umbrella system. The device consists of a heparin-coated, acellular tissue-engineered collagen matrix derived from the submucosal layer of the porcine small intestine (Organogenesis Inc., Canton, MA, USA). The matrix allows absorption and replacement of the membranes with native human tissue of up to 95%, leaving almost only the metal spring arms behind, which are eventually endothelialized [36,37].

The BioSTAR® Evaluating Study (BEST) evaluated 58 patients with a history of cryptogenic stroke, decompression sickness, or platypnea–orthodeoxia who had a clinically significant ASD or PFO. Fifty-three of these patients had a PFO. Device implantation was successful in all patients who had a PFO. Device retrieval was necessary in one patient because intra-procedural TEE revealed that the device position was in-

appropriate. A larger device was placed successfully during the same procedure. Complications were limited to atrial arrhythmias in five patients. There was a complete closure rate of more than 96% and there were no device-related adverse events [38].

Implantation technique

Patent foramen ovale closure with a CardioSEAL/StarFLEX and the BioSTAR device is a straightforward, simple, and safe procedure in the context of appropriate training and proctoring.

The 10F trans-septal delivery sheath used for the placement of the device is advanced over the same wire used for balloon sizing after the balloon is withdrawn. Once the tip of the sheath's dilator is placed across the defect, the sheath alone is advanced into the left atrium while holding the dilator and wire in place. The dilator and wire are then withdrawn from the sheath.

It is advisable to have the 10F sheath introduced through a short 11F sheath. This stays outside the patient and is introduced into the vein only in the case of device retrieval being required.

It is essential to remove air that might have entered the sheath during removal of the dilator and wire.

Normally, a CardioSEAL device size and a STARFlex device size, which are, respectively, about 2 times and 1.6–2 times the measured stretched PFO diameter, are selected.

The occluder is prepared by immersing it in a bowl of heparinized saline. The delivery catheter is prepared by loosening the Tuohy–Borst adapter and the locking nut at the back end and advancing the inner catheter 4–5 cm beyond the end of the outer catheter. The following steps of preparing the occluder for implantation differ slightly between CardioSEAL and StarFLEX devices.

For the securement of CardioSEAL, the pin lock is released and the locking pin is advanced 2–3 mm out of the locking pod. The Tuohy–Borst adapter is tightened after flushing the catheter with heparinized saline. The locking nut remains loose, permitting the inner catheter to move toward the outer sheath. The locking pins of the device and the catheter are then brought into contact by crossing them. The occluder is then reoriented so that the device's locking pin aligns it as near parallel as possible to the pin on the catheter. Once the device pin is slid into the locking pod, the catheter locking pin is withdrawn into the pod, securing the device to the catheter. To confirm securement, the locking tab on the end of the inner catheter is engaged, and a gentle tug on the occluder is performed.

The securement mechanism for the STARFlex occluder does not consist of overlapping ball-tipped pins within the locking pod; rather it has forceps that grasp the ball-tipped pin on the device and retract it within the pod. This allows greater freedom of movement and less distortion of the device before release.

Once the occluder is connected to the delivery catheter, the umbrellas are collapsed by pulling the sutures away from the catheter as it enters the funnel. Continued pulling on the suture retracts the device into the end of the loading tube and once the device in position one suture is cut and removed from the occluder. The protective housing around the loading tube is then removed and diskarded. The flushing Tuohy–Borst adapter is then connected to the loader. A heparinized saline flush evacuates air from the introducer sheath. Finally, the tip of the delivery catheter is advanced toward the occluder by withdrawing the inner catheter through the locking nut. The tip of the outer catheter should be advanced 3–4 mm from the tip of the right umbrella within the introducer tube, secured by tightening the locking nut.

During continuous flushing with heparinized saline, the introducer tube is inserted through the hemostatic valve of the delivery sheath, having the locking tab engaged and the locking nut tightened. The delivery catheter is then advanced 20–30 cm while the delivery sheath is held in place, advancing the occluder out of the introducer tube and into the sheath. The introducer assembly is withdrawn from the sheath and positioned at the rear of the delivery catheter, which is then advanced to bring the collapsed occluder to the high inferior vena cava or low right atrium. The locking nut is loosened and the inner catheter is advanced from the outer catheter to position the distal ends of the occluder at the tip of the delivery sheath. The locking nut is then retightened. At this time, the sheath should be rotated clockwise under TEE or ICE control to bring it into a more perpendicular position in relation to the interatrial septum. After confirming that the delivery sheath is still positioned in the left atrium, the device is deployed under fluoroscopy and transesophageal control.

The deployment is made by slowly withdrawing the sheath until passing the central hub marker and making sure the occluder does not move relatively to landmarks. Sheath withdrawal is performed until the tip of the sheath just passes the central hub marker on fluoroscopy. The left atrial umbrella should then be unsheathed and fully opened. The delivery sheath and the delivery catheter can be slowly withdrawn together, bringing the left atrial disk close to the septum. Withdrawal is continued until slight left atrial umbrella eversion is seen. Then only the sheath is withdrawn, being careful to maintain tension and eversion on the left atrial umbrella. When the tip of the sheath is withdrawn beyond the tips of the right atrial umbrella, this umbrella opens.

The occluder position is confirmed by TEE and fluoroscopy before release. The delivery catheter is retracted, ensuring that full release and disengagement from the occluder are achieved.

The delivery catheter is completely withdrawn from the sheath followed by withdrawal of the sheath, which stays in the inferior vena cava. After a final assessment of the occluder position the delivery sheath is removed.

Amplatzer® patent foramen ovale and atrial septal defect occluder

The Amplatzer family of devices (Fig. 5.2c) (AGA Medical, Golden Valley, MN, USA), including the Amplatzer PFO occluder and the Amplatzer septal occluder, are the most commonly implanted devices for interatrial septal defects worldwide. The Amplatzer PFO occluder is similar to the Amplatzer ASD occluder. The devices are both composed of a self-expanding nitinol (nickel–titanium alloy) wire frame mesh, forming two disks that are covered by Dacron patches that facilitate device endothelialization. The ASD and PFO occluder are very similar, except for two important differences between them: first, the left atrial disk of the ASD occluder is larger than the PFO occluder and the right atrial disk of the PFO occluder is larger than the ASD occluder (an exception to this is the 18-mm device in which both disks are the same size); second, there are differences in the diameter of the waist connecting the two disks. With the ASD occluder, the connecting waist varies in diameter depending on the size of the occluder (up to 40 mm). In contrast, the PFO occluder is designed with a 3-mm connecting waist for every currently available size (18, 25, and 35 mm).

Masura et al. [39] introduced the Amplatzer ASD occluder in 1997 as a new device for ASD closure. In 1999, Berger et al. [40] used this device for PFO closure and reported their experiences in 68 patients. Complete closure was achieved in all enrolled patients without any adverse events. In the same year, Han et al. [41] introduced the PFO version of the Amplatzer device, and in 2000 Waight et al. [42] reported the first clinical experiences in two PFO patients.

A number of trials have reported great procedural success (93–100%) and a low incidence of periprocedural complications [43–48].

In 2006, Thanopoulus et al. [49] reported a small, non-randomized, prospective series of 92 patients with a history of cryptogenic stroke or TIA and PFO. Forty-eight of the patients underwent PFO closure with a PFO device, whereas 44 patients declined the intervention and were treated with aspirin and clopidogrel. In the device group, all patients underwent successful implantation, with periprocedural complications reported in six patients. Five patients had atrial arrhythmia and one patient had a hemopericardium. A 100% closure rate was confirmed by transthoracic contrast echocardiography within 6 months. A 2-year clinical follow-up revealed no recurrent ischemic events in the device group compared with 30% in the medically treated group ($P < 0.001$) [49]. The excellent mid- and long-term outcomes in the described series are encouraging but require confirmation in large, randomized, prospective, multicenter trials. Currently ongoing trials which will evaluate the efficacy and safety of the Amplatzer PFO device compared with medical therapy for the treatment of migraine headaches include the PC-Trial (currently enrolling in Europe and Canada); the Randomized Evaluation of Recurrent Stroke comparing PFO Closure to

Established Current Standard of Care Treatment (RESPECT) for patients with cryptogenic stroke or TIA; and the Prospective, Randomized Investigation to Evaluate Incidence of Headache Reduction in Subjects with Migraine and PFO Using the Amplatzer PFO Occluder to Medical Management (PREMIUM).

Implantation technique

The guidewire is positioned preferably in a left pulmonary vein, which facilitates support of the sizing balloon catheter and advancement of the deployment sheath into the left atrium.

An 8F or 9F Amplatzer introducer set is used (9F for a 35-mm PFO or a larger ASD occluder). A 35-mm PFO occluder may become necessary, if a selected 25-mm occluder is pulled through the PFO with normal traction force during an attempt to place it at the septum. A larger device may also be desirable in the context of a large atrial septum aneurysm when embolization is feared or in the presence of an extremely long tunnel for fear of running out of material on the right disk. A very thick septum secundum or a large aortic root protruding close to the fossa ovalis may also be better treated with a large diameter device.

Some centers do not perform balloon sizing routinely when using Amplatzer devices; this practice carries the risk of pull-through of the 25-mm occluder. The pusher cable is screwed into the thread of the right atrial disk. The screw is not completely tightened to ensure proper unscrewing at the time of release. With the device and loader submersed in saline solution, the device is pulled backwards into the short loader sheath. To get rid of air bubbles, the device is pushed out and retracted once or twice and the system flushed thoroughly. Once the delivery sheath has reached the inferior vena cava according to the instructions for use, the dilator is removed to allow back-bleeding to purge all air from the system. Alternatively, the sheath and dilator are introduced into the pulmonary vein and the dilator removed, slowly encouraging bleed back through the sheath.

After connecting the hemostasis valve and flushing with a syringe, the left atrium is entered. The sheath is advanced over the guidewire through the PFO and into the left atrium. Correct position of the delivery sheath is verified by a test injection of contrast medium. Once in a satisfactory position, the guidewire should be removed and the sheath flushed with saline. The loader is then introduced to the delivery sheath and the device is advanced into the sheath by pushing (not rotating) the delivery cable. Under fluoroscopy and echocardiographic guidance (a left oblique cranial projection and a 30–50° angle on TEE is normally ideal for device positioning), the left atrial disk is deployed by pulling firmly against the atrial septum, which can be felt and observed via echocardiography. The sheath and pusher cable are then pulled back together under fluoroscopic control. When the left disk reaches the PFO, it will pull the valve closed and

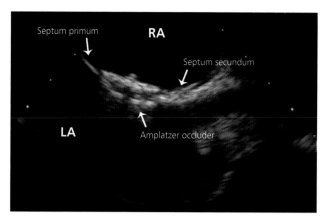

Figure 5.3 Accurate position of an 18-mm Amplatzer PFO occluder in transesophageal echocardiography (113°). The two disks embrace the septum secundum properly.

change its position to one parallel to the interatrial septum. Maintaining tension on the pusher cable, the sheath is then further withdrawn until the right-sided disk is open. Fluoroscopy and TEE controls in several views are needed to prove that the septum secundum is embraced by the two disks of the occluder (Fig. 5.3) and to ascertain a correct and secure device position. When the position is satisfactory, the device can be released. The plastic vice is attached to the delivery cable, the screw is tightened and the device can be unscrewed from the cable by turning the cable counterclockwise (Fig. 5.3; indicated by an arrow on the vice). In the unlikely event that this should not be possible, the sheath can be advanced against the right atrial disk to fix the device, which facilitates detachment.

Helex® septal occluder

The Helex Septal Occluder (Fig. 5.2d) (W.L. Gore & Associates, Flagstaff, AZ, USA) is composed of a superelastic, spiral-shaped single-strand nitinol wire covered with a biocompatible membrane composed of expanded polytetrafluoroethylene (ePTFE). After release from the sheath, the wire assumes a spiral shape. It consists of two circular equal-sized disks, fixed by an integral locking system passing through the center of the device from left to right. This locking system connects the atrial disks at their centers and stabilizes the occluder in the defect. A radiopaque eyelet mechanism ensures good visibility and therefore easy positioning by fluoroscopy guidance. Device diameter ranges from 15 to 35 mm.

Billinger *et al.* [50] reported multicenter experience in 128 patients with previous paradoxical embolism undergoing PFO closure with the Helex device. Device implantation was successful in all but one patient. Two patients experienced device embolization (in one patient 24 h after the procedure), and in 32 patients the initial device required removal during the procedure and replacement by a new one. There were no device-related, major adverse events acutely or in the follow-up period, and the two embolized occluders were successfully retrieved without further complications. Complete closure was achieved in 90% of patients at a mean follow-up of 21 ± 11 months with no recurrent embolic events and no device-related thrombus formation [50].

Implantation technique

When choosing the appropriate device size, the occluder-to-defect diameter ratio must be at least 1.6:1.0. After unpacking the Helex system, the occluder is withdrawn into the integral green delivery catheter. This should be performed with the occluder and the distal portion of the delivery catheter submerged in heparinized saline solution. A 20-ml syringe containing heparinized saline is connected to the red retrieval cord cap. After tightening of the mandrel luer and loosening of the control catheter luer, the control catheter can be flushed. When this is completed, the gray control catheter with the attached syringe is withdrawn until only 3 cm of the device is outside the delivery catheter. Doing so will cause the mandrel to bend slightly. Now the mandrel luer is loosened and the occluder is completely withdrawn into the delivery catheter by pulling the gray control catheter. The mandrel will exit the side port of the y-hub and protrude by a few centimeters. To avoid air embolism, it is important to keep the syringe with heparinized saline attached to the red retrieval cord cap at all times.

After loading the delivery catheter into the 10F introducer sheath, the syringe is removed from the retrieval cord cap. It is important to ensure that this cap is securely attached to the control catheter as it secures the retrieval cord. The distal tip of the delivery catheter has a radiopaque marker. Under fluoroscopy and TEE control, it is advanced into the left atrium. This may be facilitated by using a monorail technique. The integral Helex delivery catheter has a monorail port close to the distal tip, which can be used to run the system over the previously placed wire in the pulmonary vein. In this case the access sheath at the groin should be 12F. The monorail wire is obviously removed once the system is in the left atrium.

Device deployment is easier when the delivery catheter is more perpendicular to the septum. Thus, the delivery catheter usually has to be rotated clockwise.

The left atrial disk is deployed by repeating the following steps. Fixing the delivery catheter, the gray control catheter is advanced in the left atrium until the tan mandrel luer engages the side port of the y-hub. However, the tip of the control catheter should not touch the atrial wall. If space in the left atrium is inadequate, the control catheter should be advanced in smaller steps. Fixing the delivery and the control catheter, the mandrel is pulled back approximately 2 cm so the left atrial disk is gradually configured. These steps are repeated until the central eyelet of the occluder exits the delivery catheter, indicating that the left atrial disk is completely deployed. The tan mandrel may be slightly withdrawn to ensure that it is apposed closely to the atrial septum.

To allow the right atrial disk deployment, the gray control catheter is fixed while the delivery catheter is pulled back until the mandrel luer touches the side port of the y-hub. The mandrel luer is then tightened. The right atrial disk is configured by fixing the delivery catheter and advancing the control catheter until it stops at the y-arm hub, where the control catheter luer is then tightened.

The position and configuration of the disks should be controlled by TEE and fluoroscopy. If the device is well positioned, the red retrieval cord cap is removed and the mandrel luer is loosened. The locking mechanism is activated by sharply pulling the mandrel, while keeping the delivery catheter in place. If the device position is satisfactory, the whole delivery system is removed from the patient. The retrieval cord will move through the right atrial eyelet of the occluder, thereby releasing it completely.

Repositioning of the device is an option when the position is suboptimal. This is possible only before engaging the locking mechanism. If the occluder is already locked but is judged to be in an unsatisfactory position, it may be recaptured (see below). For repositioning, the red retrieval cord cap and the mandrel luer need to be tightened first. Gently pulling back the gray control catheter, the device is completely withdrawn into the delivery catheter as it was during the initial loading procedure. The delivery catheter is then repositioned within the left atrium and the device is redeployed following the steps mentioned above. If increased force is necessary during repositioning, the Helex system may be damaged or kinked. In that case, we recommend removing the whole system and replacing it with a new one.

Recapture of the occluder may be necessary in the case of an unacceptable occluder position after lock release or if repositioning cannot be easily performed. The mandrel luer needs to be open. With the red retrieval cord cap removed, the retrieval cord is gently withdrawn until the control catheter meets the right atrial eyelet of the device. The retrieval cord cap is firmly attached and the control catheter is withdrawn, causing the device to return into the delivery catheter in its linear form. Interference of the device eyelet with the tip of the delivery sheath may lead to frame fracture of the occluder or snapping of the retrieval cord so careful manipulation in the latter stages of recapture is required to avoid this complication.

Premere™ occluder

The Premere™ occluder (Fig. 5.2e) (St Jude Medical, Inc., St. Paul, MN, USA) is exclusively designed for PFO closure. Two cross-shaped nitinol anchors are positioned between two layers of knitted polyester and linked by a flexible polyester braided tether. The variable tether length allows adjustment according to the thickness of the interatrial septum and tunnel length. This device is suitable for long tunnel-type PFOs.

Another important feature of this device is the reduction of foreign material and the decrease of the device profile owing to the fact that only the right atrial anchor is covered with the knitted polyester membrane. The anchors are retrievable and can be repositioned until the tether is cut. The Premere occluder is available in diameters of 20 and 25 mm. A 30-mm device is currently under evaluation.

The Premere occluder was evaluated in the CLOSEUP (PFO Closure Using Premere) trial in 73 patients with a history of TIA or cryptogenic stroke and a PFO. The device (15 mm and 20 mm) was successfully implanted in 67 patients (92%), but anatomic considerations precluded successful deployment in six patients. Complete closure on contrast echocardiography was noted in 86% of the patients at 6 months. There was no evidence of device-related thrombi. One patient experienced transient atrial fibrillation (resolved at 3-month follow-up); no other events have been reported [51].

In the currently enrolling multicenter, prospective, randomized ESCAPE (Effect of Septal Closure of Atrial PFO on Events of Migraine with the Premere™ migraine trial) migraine trial, the effect of septal closure of atrial PFO on events of migraine refractory to medical treatment is evaluated with the Premere occluder. The phase II trial is currently enrolling with a primary efficacy endpoint of a reduction in headache frequency and primary safety endpoint of the rate of major complications.

Cardia patent foramen ovale occluder

The Cardia PFO occluder family (Fig. 5.2f) (Cardia, Burnsville, MN, USA) consists of four device generations built of two Ivalon disks mounted on nitinol arms. The first two device generations have tetragonal disks on four nitinol arms. The third- and fourth-generation devices comprise hexagonal disks on six nitinol arms. Unique to the current version (Intrasept) is a dual articulating sail at the center, which enables the device to align with the individual septum configuration and concurrently reduces tissue distortion. This occluder system is available in 20, 25, 30, and 35 mm diameters. It can be delivered through 9–11F sheath and is fully retrievable throughout the procedure.

Spies *et al.* [52] reported on 403 patients with presumed paradoxical embolism and PFO who underwent closure with the first three generations of this device. Successful implantation was performed in all patients. A 2% periprocedural complication rate included transient ST-segment elevation, pericardial effusion and device embolization. A residual shunting at 6 months' follow-up was detected in 39 out of 361 patients (10.8%) by TEE. Thrombus formation was detected on 10 devices with no associated adverse events on Coumadin (warfarin) treatment. The annual risk for recurrent stroke was 0.8% and for recurrent TIA 1.2% after 645 patient-years of follow-up. Encouraging results have been reported from using the Intrasept device [53].

Newer devices and approaches

Solysafe® septal occluder

The Solysafe® Septal Occluder (Fig. 5.2g) (Swissimplant AG, Solothurn, Switzerland) can be used for ASD and for PFO closure. A major advantage of this new self-centering device is that it is delivered over a guidewire, superseding a long transseptal sheath. The device consists of two centering foldable polyester patches that are attached to eight phynox wires. Phynox is a cobalt–chromium–nickel alloy. The material is similar to nitinol with properties of elasticity and memory retention. Each end of the device has a wire holder, which is attached to the eight wires. The wire holders can be moved toward each other to position the device. By moving the wire holders toward each other, the eight wires snap into a second stable position. The patches that are attached to the wires are stretched out and cover the defect. By a clicking system, the wire holders are kept together and the device is held in position. Until the guidewire is removed the device can be readjusted.

Ewert *et al.* evaluated the Solysafe occluder in 29 patients. Twenty-five of these patients received a 15-mm device and two patients each received 20- and 25-mm devices. The only peri-interventional complication was the occurrence of atrial fibrillation in one patient, which was successfully treated medically. At discharge, closure was complete, or only trivial residual shunt remained, in 97% patients; at 6 months' follow-up complete closure was noted in all patients [54].

Occlutech®

The Occlutech® device (Fig. 5.2h) (Occlutech, Jena, Germany) is technically very similar to the Amplatzer Septal occluder. Unlike the Amplatzer devices, there is no hub on the left atrial side. The device comes in two different sizes (25-mm right atrial disk/23-mm left atrial disk and 30-mm right atrial disk/27-mm left atrial disk). At this time the first in-human trials have been concluded with encouraging results [55].

SeptRX™ occluder

The SeptRX device (Fig. 5.2i) (Cordis Cooperation, Miami, FL, USA) is based on a unique concept: it targets only the PFO tunnel as opposed to the right and left atrial surfaces. The small device is implanted directly into the flap of the PFO and is stabilized by two left atrial anchors that adjust to the tunnel length without significantly changing the configuration of the septum primum. By implanting the device in the tunnel, the defect is stretched out in the anterior–posterior direction, causing an approximation of septum primum and secundum. Minimizing foreign material in the atria reduces the risk of thrombus formation on the device, and the fact that it does not significantly change the configuration of septum primum may be a potential advantage of this approach.

We recently completed the first human trial involving 13 patients (with successful device implantation achieved in 11); there were no procedural complications. Preliminary results at 6 months' follow-up are encouraging, with a closure rate of 100% as determined by transcranial Doppler and TEE (W. Zimmerman, unpublished data).

Coherex flat stent

The first human implantation of the Coherex FlatStent™ PFO occluder (Fig. 5.2j) (Coherex Medical, Inc., Salt Lake City, UT, USA) was performed on 2 October 2007. The occluder consists of a superelastic nitinol lattice containing polyurethane foam in the intratunnel cells of the device. The foam stimulates tissue growth inside the tunnel. This innovative device leaves only a minimal surface exposed in the atria.

The device body expands within the PFO tunnel, drawing the septum primum and the septum secundum into contact without a significant change in the structure of the septum primum. Proximal anchors open into the right atrium, and strategically placed microtines are designed to ensure that the device does not migrate or embolize. The device can be resheathed and repositioned as necessary until it is detached.

At present, one size of the FlatStent is available within clinical trials for stretched diameters of 4–10 mm. A larger device is under development. Preclinical trials in animals have been successfully completed, and a clinical trial for CE Marking is under way in Europe with excellent results to date [56].

Cierra PFx™ closure system

The PFx closure system (Fig. 5.2k) (Cierra, Inc., Rodwood City, CA, USA) was the first percutaneous PFO closing system which did not employ an implantable device.

After entering the right atrium with the PFx catheter, which is introduced over a guidewire through a 16F sheath, the tip of the system is advanced to the overlapping part of septum primum and septum secundum. Correct positioning of the closure system is ensured by fluoroscopy and TEE. A vacuum is applied through the catheter shaft to keep the two components of the septum in position. Monopolar radiofrequency energy is applied over an electrode on the overlapping part of the septa. This process fuses the tissue of septum primum and septum secundum by denaturation of proteins with heat. PFO closure is achieved by inflammation and subsequent fibrosis.

After the process the whole system is removed from the right atrium and no foreign material is left in the heart. The results of the Paradigm I study, published in 2007, demonstrated the feasibility of closing PFO without implantation [57].

Although closure rates with the PFx System were lower than with implantable occluders, with a primary closing rate <80%, the study showed potential success of closing PFO without device-related complications, such as atrial fibrillation, thrombus formation, TIA, or device fracture.

Despite these promising results, Cierra recently had to shut down its business for financial reasons.

Heart Stitch™

Heart Stitch™ (Fig. 5.2l) (Sutura Inc., Fountain Valley, CA, USA) is a transcatheter polyprophylene suture system for closing PFOs that is based on the SuperStitch technology (utilized as a closure technique for femoral vessels). The device consists of individually deployable needles, and its sutures pose no risk of erosion or embolization. The procedure is relatively simple: the HeartStitch system is introduced and deployed into the left atrium. Sequentially, the septum primum and secundum are then sutured and the HeartStitch system is withdrawn. Early investigation is under way.

Complications owing to patent foramen ovale closure with devices

In principle, most complications are best managed by prevention rather than treatment after the complication has occurred. Complications resulting from vessel injury can be avoided by using a careful and judicious technique of wire insertion under fluoroscopy. If access to the left atrium cannot be gained via the PFO, trans-septal puncture using standard techniques can be performed.

In the case of embolization or malposition, the device can be removed usually by snaring and retrieval using a loop snare. A long, large-caliber sheath (up to 16F) should be positioned close to the device to allow complete retraction. Amplatzer devices should be snared at the screw. If parts of the device remain outside the long sheath, then the occluder, snare, and sheath should be removed together. Alternatives would be to use a Dotter basket or forceps.

Frame fractures are rare and usually do not require treatment as they do not affect the function of the device. Atrial thrombi after transcatheter PFO closure are also a rare complication. Krumsdorf *et al.* [58] reported on the incidence of thrombus formation on nine different devices in 1000 consecutive patients. Thrombus formation was more common on older devices (ASDOS [Osypka, BmbH, Grenzach-Wyhlen, Germany], Buttoned device [Custom Medical Devices, Athens]), but newer devices also demonstrated the potential to develop thrombus formation after 4 weeks. The document incidence of thrombus formation was 7.1% for the CardioSEAL occluder, 5.7% for the StarFLEX, 6.6% for the PFO-Star (first and second generation), 0.8% for the Helex occluder, and 0% for the Amplatzer device. This is a significant advantage, especially for the Amplatzer and Helex devices. Newer devices tend to minimize the material in the atria and are therefore less thrombogenic. Thrombus formation on these devices is expected to be extremely rare. If thrombi are identified, medical treatment (most commonly, anticoagulation is used, but also clopidogrel and aspirin, or low-molecular-weight heparin) solves the problem in most cases. It is recommended that control TEE is performed monthly until the thrombus has resolved. Very few patients require surgery to remove the thrombotic clots and the device.

Erosion of the superior atrial wall into the pericardium or into the aorta has been described with some devices [59,60]. This may be a result of the size of the device. On the other hand, small devices may be associated with a higher incidence of incomplete closure.

In patients with a very long PFO tunnel we recommend using a Premere occluder as the first choice because this occluder allows adjustment according to the tunnel length. An alternative would be to implant an intratunnel device (Coherex or SeptRX).

Septal aneurysms do not influence the choice of the device very much, because it is not intended to straighten or to cover the aneurysm. Therefore, every occluder can be used for PFO closure in patients with septal aneurysms.

Summary

The association of cryptogenic stroke with PFO is well established. There is also an association between migraine headache and PFO. However, a PFO should be considered more of a contributing factor to migraine rather than a cause. The treatment of patients with cryptogenic stroke and PFO is still controversial. Possible treatments are blood-thinning therapy (antiplatelet or anticoagulation), surgery, or transcatheter closure of the defect. Numerous devices, both currently available and in development, have demonstrated that PFO closure can be performed safely and effectively and that the rates of complication and recurrence of embolic events are low. We also have to consider that most patients prefer to have their PFO closed by catheter techniques than to have lifelong anticoagulation treatment or undergo surgery.

Data from randomized, controlled studies comparing PFO closure with conventional therapy are still pending. The conduction and completion of appropriately designed, randomized, controlled trials may enable us to establish the precise population who are at greatest risk and who would benefit the most from PFO closure.

The major limitation of all ongoing randomized trials is a very short follow-up of 2–5 years; they run the risk of remaining underpowered if enrolment is terminated too early or the follow-up interval is not adequate. The purpose of this very safe but nevertheless invasive procedure is to prevent stroke in the long term.

However, the trend of interventional treatment of intracardiac shunts is leading toward defect-specific systems and new devices minimizing the amount of foreign material left in the atria. These device refinements will undoubtedly improve the safety and efficacy of PFO closure in the future.

References

1. Bridges ND, Hellenbrand W, Latson L, Filiano J, Newburger JW, & Lock JE (1992) Transcatheter closure of patent foramen ovale after presumed paradoxical embolism. *Circulation* **86**:1902–1908.
2. Sievert H, Trepels T, Zadan E, *et al.* (2001) Catheter closure of PFO for prevention of recurrent embolic stroke and TIA: acute results and follow-up in 400 patients. *Am J Cardiol* **88**(Suppl. 1): 118–120.
3. Sievert H, Ostermayer S, Billinger K, *et al.* (2002) Transcatheter closure of PFO for prevention of paradoxical embolism and recurrent embolic stroke with the CardioSeal STARFlex occluder. *Am J Cardiol* **90**(Suppl. 1):H37–H39.
4. Sommer RJ, Kramer PH, Sorensen SG, *et al.* (2002) Closure of PFO with CardioSeal Septal Occluder: highly effective intervention. *Am J Cardiol* **90**(Suppl. 1):H37.
5. Hagen PT, Scholz DG, & Edwards WD (1984) Incidence and size of patent foramen ovale during the first 10 decades of life: An autopsy study of 967 normal hearts. *Mayo Clin Proc* **59**:17–20.
6. Mas JL (1994) Patent foramen ovale, atrial septal aneurysm and ischemic stroke in young adults. *Eur Heart J* **15**:446–449.
7. Berthet K, Lavergne T, Cohen A, *et al.* (2000) Significant association of the atrial vulnerability with atrial septal abnormalities in young patients with ischemic stroke of unknown cause. *Stroke* **31**:398–403.
8. Lechat P, Mas J, & Laseault G (1988) Prevalence of patent foramen ovale in patients with stroke. *N Engl J Med* **318**:1148–1152.
9. Webster M, Chancellor A, & Smith H (1988) Patent foramen ovale in young stroke patients. *Lancet* **2**:11–12.
10. Steiner M, Di Tuillio MR, Rundek T, *et al.* (1998) Patent foramen ovale size and embolic brain imaging findings among patients with ischemic stroke. *Stroke* **29**:944–948.
11. Harvey JR, Teague SM, Anderson JL, Voyles WF, & Thadani U (1986) Clinically silent atrial septal defects with evidence of cerebral embolizaton. *Ann Intern Med* **105**:695–697.
12. Handke M, Harloff A, Olschewski M, *et al.* (2007) Patent foramen ovale and cryptogenic stroke in older patients. *N Engl J Med* **357**:2262–2268.
13. Bogousslavsky J, Garazi S, Jeanrenaud X, Aebischer N, & Van Melle G (1996) Stroke recurrence in patients with patent foramen ovale. The Lausanne study. Lausanne stroke with paradoxical embolism study group. *Neurology* **46**:1301–1305.
14. Mas JL & Zuber M (1995) Recurrent cerebrovascular events in patients with patent foramen ovale, atrial septal aneurysm, or both and cryptogenic stroke or transient ischemic attack. French study group on patent foramen ovale and atrial septal aneurysm. *Am Heart J* **130**:1083–1088.
15. De Castro S, Cartoni D, Fiorelli M, *et al.* (2000) Morphological and functional characteristics of patent foramen ovale and their embolic implications. *Stroke* **31**:2407–2413.
16. Nedeltchev K, Arnold M, Wahl A, *et al.* (2002) Outcome of patients with cryptogenic stroke and patent foramen ovale. *J Neurol Neurosurg Psychiatry* **72**:347–350.
17. Homma S, Sacco RL, Di Tullio MR, Sciacca RR, & Mohr J; PFO in Cryptogenic Stroke Study (PICSS) Investigators. (2002) Effect of medical treatment in stroke patients with patent foramen ovale in Cryptogenic Stroke Study. *Circulation* **5**:2625–2631.

18. Stone DA, Godard J, Coretti MC, *et al.* (1996) Patent foramen ovale: association between the degree of shunt by contrast transesophageal echocardiography and the risk of future ischemic neurological events. *Am Heart J* **131**:158–161.

19. Overell JR, Bone I, & Lees KR (2000) Interatrial septal abnormalities and stroke: a meta-analysis of case–control studies. *Neurology* **55**:1172–1179.

20. Mas JL, Arquizan C, Lamy C, *et al.*; for the patent foramen ovale and atrial septal aneurysm study group. (2001) Recurrent cerebrovascular events associated with patent foramen ovale, atrial septal aneurysm, or both. *N Engl J Med* **345**:1740–1746.

21. Schuchlenz HW, Weihs W, Horner S, & Quehenberger F (2000) The association between the diameter of a patent foramen ovale and the risk of embolic cerebrovascular events. *Am J Med* **109**: 456–462.

22. Meissner I, Khandheria BK, Heit JA, *et al.* (2006) Patent foramen ovale: innocent or guilty? Evidence from a prospective population-based study. *J Am Coll Cardiol* **47**:440–445.

23. Di Tullio MR, Sacco RL, Sciacca RR, Jin Z, & Homma S (2007) Patent foramen ovale and the risk of ischemic stroke in a multiethnic population. *J Am Coll Cardiol* **49**:797–802.

24. Anzola GP, Magoni M, Guindani M, Rozzini L, & Dalla Volta G (1999) Potential source of cerebral embolism in migraine with aura: a transcranial Doppler study. *Neurology* **52**:1622–1625.

25. Pitt BR, Hammond GL, & Gillis CN (1982) Comparison of pulmonary and extrapulmonary extraction of biogenic amines. *J Appl Physiol* **52**:1330–1332.

26. Kerut EK, Norfleet WT, Plotnick GD, & Giles TD (2001) Patent foramen ovale: a review of associated conditions and the impact of physiological size. *J Am Coll Cardiol* **38**:613–623.

27. Germonpre P, Hashi F, Dendale P, *et al.* (2005) Evidence for increasing patency of the foramen ovale in divers. *Am J Cardiol* **95**:912–915.

28. Chen GP, Goldberg SL, & Gill EA Jr. (2005) Patent foramen ovale and platypnea-orthodeoxia syndrome. *Cardiol Clin* **23**:85–89.

29. Sacco RL, Adams R, Albers G, *et al.* (2006) Guidelines for prevention of stroke in patients with ischemic stroke or transient ischemic attack: a statement for healthcare professionals from the American Heat Association/American Stroke Association Council on Stroke: co-sponsored by the Council on Cardiovascular Radiology and Intervention: The American Academy of Neurology affirms the value of this guideline. *Circulation* **113**:409–449.

30. Messe SR, Siverman IE, Kizer JR, *et al.* (2004) Practice parameter: recurrent stroke with patent foramen ovale and atrial aneurysm: report of the Quality Standards Subcommittee of the American Academy of Neurology. *Neurology* **62**:1042–1050.

31. Schwerzmann M, Nedeltcher K, Lagger F, *et al.* (2005) Prevalence and size of directly detected patent foramen ovale in migraine with aura. *Neurology* **65**:1415–1418.

32. Reisman M, Christofferson RD, Jesurum J, *et al.* (2005) Migraine headache relief after transcatheter closure of patent foramen ovale. *J Am Coll Cardiol* **45**:493–495.

33. Alameddine F & Block PC (2004) Transcatheter patent foramen ovale closure for secondary prevention of paradoxical embolic events: acute results from the FORECAST registry. *Catheter Cardiovasc Interv* **62**:512–516.

34. Kiblawi FM, Sommer RJ, & Levchuck SG (2006) Transcatheter closure of patent foramen ovale in older adults. *Catheter Cardiovasc Interv* **68**:136–143.

35. Dowson A, Wilmshurst P, Muir KW, Mullen M, & Nightingale S (2006) A prospective, multicenter, randomized, double blind, placebo-controlled trial to evaluate the efficacy of patent foramen ovale closure with the STARFlex septal repair implant to prevent refractory migraine headaches: the MIST Trial. *Neurology* **67**:185.

36. Jux C, Bertram H, Wohlsein P, Bruegmann M, & Paul T (2006) Interventional atrial septal defect closure using a totally bioresorbable occluder matrix: development and preclinical evaluation of the BioSTAR device. *J Am Coll Cardiol* **48**:161–169.

37. Jux C, Wohlsein P, Bruegmann M, Zutz M, Franzbach B, & Bertram H (2003) A new biological matrix for septal occlusion. *J Interv Cardiol* **16**:149–152.

38. Mullen MJ, Hildick-Smith D, De Giovanni JV, *et al.* (2006) BioSTAR Evaluation Study (BEST): a prospective, multicenter, phase I clinical trial to evaluate the feasibility, efficacy, and safety of the BioSTAR bioabsorbable septal repair implant for the closure of atrial-level shunts. *Circulation* **114**:1962–1967.

39. Masura J, Gavora P, Formanek A, & Hijazi ZM (1997) Transcatheter closure of secundum atrial defects using the new self-centering Amplatzer septal occluder: initial human experiences. *Catheter Cardiovasc Diagn* **42**:388–393.

40. Berger F, Ewert P, Bjornstad PG, *et al.* (1999) Transcatheter closure as standard treatment for most interatrial defects: experience in 200 patients treated with the Amplatzer septal occluder. *Cardiol Young* **9**:468–473.

41. Han YM, Gu X, Titus JL, *et al.* (1999) New self-expanding patent foramen ovale occluder device. *Catheter Cardiovasc Interv* **47**:370–376.

42. Waight DJ, Cao QL, & Hijazi ZM (2000) Closure of patent foramen ovale in patients with orthodeoxia-platypnea using the amplatzer devices. *Catheter Cardiovasc Interv* **50**:195–198.

43. Wahl A, Meier B, Haxel B, *et al.* (2001) Prognosis after percutaneous closure of patent foramen ovale for paradoxical embolism. *Neurology* **57**:1330–1332.

44. Sievert H, Horvath K, Zadan E, *et al.* (2001) Patent foramen ovale closure in patients with transient ischemic attack/stroke. *J Interv Cardiol* **14**:261–266.

45. Braun M, Gliech V, Boscheri A, *et al.* (2004) Transcatheter closure of patent foramen ovale (PFO) in patients with paradoxical embolism. Periprocedural safety and mid-term follow-up results of three different device occluder systems. *Eur Heart J* **25**:424–430.

46. Hong TE, Thaler D, Brorson J, Heitschmidt M, & Hijazi ZM; Amplatzer PFO Investigators. (2000) Transcatheter closure of patent foramen ovale associated with paradoxical embolism using the Amplatzer PFO occluder: initial and intermediate-term results of the U.S. multicenter clinical trial. *Catheter Cardiovasc Interv* **60**:524–528.

47. Khositseth A, Cabalka AK, Sweeney JP, *et al.* (2004) Transcatheter Amplatzer device closure of atrial septal defects and patent foramen ovale in patients with presumed paradoxical embolism. *Mayo Clin Proc* **79**:35–41.

48. Chatterjee T, Petzsch M, Ince H, *et al.* (2005) Interventional closure with Amplatzer PFO occluder of patent foramen ovale in patients with paradoxical cerebral embolism. *J Interv Cardiol* **18**:173–179.

49. Thanopoulos BV, Dardas PD, Karanasios E, & Mezilis N (2006) Transcatheter closure versus medical therapy of patent foramen ovale and cryptogenic stroke. *Catheter Cardiovasc Interv* **86**:741–746.

50. Billinger K, Ostermeyer S, Carminati M, *et al.* (2006) HELEX Septal Occluder for transcatheter closure of patent foramen ovale: multicenter experience. *Euro Interv* **1**:465–471.

51. Buschek F, Sievert H, Kleber F, *et al.* (2006) Patent foramen ovale closure using the Premere device: the results of the CLOSEUP trial. *J Interv Cardiol* **19**:328–333.

52. Spies C, Doshi R, Timmermanns I, & Schrader E (2006) Closure of patent foramen ovale in patients with cryptogenic thromboembolic events using the Cardia PFO occluder. *Eur Heart J* **37**:365–371.

53. Spies C, Timmermanns I, Reissmann U, van Essen J, & Schräder R (2008) Patent foramen ovale closure with the Intrasept occluder: Complete 6–56 months follow-up of 247 patients after presumed paradoxical embolism. *Catheter Cardiovasc Interv* **71**:390–395.

54. Ewert P, Söderberg B, Dähnert I, *et al.* (2008) ASD and PFO closure with the Solysafe septal occluder—results of a prospective multicenter pilot study. *Catheter Cardiovasc Interv* **71**:398–402.

55. Krizanic F, Sievert H, Pfeiffer D, *et al.* (2008) Clinical evaluation of a novel occluder device (Occlutech) for percutaneous transcatheter closure of patent foramen ovale (PFO). *Clin Res Cardiol* **97**:872–877.

56. Reiffenstein I, Majunke N, Wunderlich N, *et al.* (2008) Percutaneous closure of patent foramen ovale with a novel FlatStent. *Expert Rev Med Devices* **5**:419–425.

57. Sievert H, Fischer E, Heinisch C, Majunke N, Roemer A, & Wunderlich N (2007) Transcatheter closure of patent foramen ovale without an implant: initial clinical experience. *Circulation* **116**:1701–1706.

58. Krumsdorf U, Ostermayer S, Billinger K, *et al.* (2004) Incidence and clinical course of thrombus formation on atrial septal defect and patent foramen ovale closure devices in 1000 consecutive patients. *J Am Col Cardiol* **43**:302–309.

59. Trepels T, Zeplin H, Sievert H, *et al.* (2003) Cardiac perforation following transcatheter PFO closure. *Catheter Interven* **58**:111–113.

60. Palma G, Rosapepe F, Vicchio M, Russolillo V, Cioffi S, & Vosa C (2007) Late perforation of right atrium and aortic root after percutaneous closure of patent foramen ovale. *J Thorac Cardiovasc Surg* **134**:1054–1055.

6 Surgical Closure of Atrial and Ventricular Septal Defects

Markus K. Heinemann

University Hospital, Johannes Gutenberg University, Mainz, Germany

Introduction

This chapter deals with the surgical closure of isolated atrial or ventricular septal defects. In contrast to corresponding chapters on interventional techniques, atrioventricular septal defects (also known as atrioventricular canal defects) affecting both levels of the cardiac partition to various extents and for which interventional treatment options do not exist are excluded.

Atrial septal defects

Historical background

The apparent relative ease of surgical access made atrial septal defects the primary target of surgeons considering operations on the heart. After several ingenious attempts to gain entry into the right atrium by means of hypothermia and inflow occlusion or through the so-called "atrial well" by Gross *et al.* [1], it was Gibbon [2] who performed surgical closure of an atrial septal defect under extracorporeal circulation using a "pump oxygenator" in 1953. This procedure can be considered the first ever successful open heart operation, setting the foundation for the development of cardiac surgery as we know it today. Fifty-five years on, this specialty has undergone enormous transformations, both in techniques as well as in the spectrum of diseases treated. It should, however, always be remembered that the first and foremost motivation to operate upon the heart was the treatment of congenital heart disease, starting off with closure of an atrial septal defect.

Morphology and pathophysiology

An atrial septal defect (ASD) is defined as a communication of variable size between the left and the right atrium, commonly caused by arrested development of a part of the interatrial

Cardiovascular Interventions in Clinical Practice. Edited by Jürgen Haase, Hans-Joachim Schäfers, Horst Sievert and Ron Waksman. © 2010 Blackwell Publishing.

septal structures. Simplifying cardiogenesis very briefly, the septum primum is of thin connective tissue origin and arises from the area of the inferior vena cava of the primitive, undivided heart, growing toward the roof of the then common atrium. On its way, it overlaps the free, crescent-shaped edge of the more muscular septum secundum coming from above. This overlap occurs on the left atrial side, thereby facilitating fetal blood flow from the right atrium across the "foramen ovale" into the left atrium, providing relatively highly oxygenated blood from the umbilical cord to the left ventricle and ascending aorta. This communication closes after birth with the rise of left atrial pressure and increased pulmonary blood flow. If it can still be probed postnatally it is considered a patent foramen ovale (PFO).

Underdevelopment of the septum primum results in a hole within the fossa ovalis. This is the most common atrial septal defect, called "secundum type" (ASD II) because of the persistence of the ostium secundum, the chronologically second atrial communication during embryologic development.

Persistence of the first interatrial communication on the atrioventricular level of the primitive heart is often and somewhat confusingly called a "primum type ASD (ASD I)." This is not merely an atrial communication but represents a particular form of atrioventricular septal defect, unfailingly involving one or both of the atrioventricular valves. It should better be considered a "partial atrioventricular septal defect." For this reason it shall not be dealt with in this chapter.

A sinus venosus defect is caused by incomplete fusion of a part of the right horn of the sinus venosus with the atrial wall between what is to become the superior and inferior vena cava. Most common is the superior type close to the upper cavoatrial junction. This being a defect of the wall of the primitive common venous system, it is >90% associated with partial anomalous pulmonary venous connection (PAPVC) of the right (upper) pulmonary veins into the superior vena cava or right atrium. Inferior sinus venosus defects involve the inferior vena cava and sometimes the right lower pulmonary veins. They are extremely rare.

A coronary sinus septal defect represents deficiencies in the wall of the left horn of the sinus venosus which is to become the (affected) coronary sinus. Persistence of a left

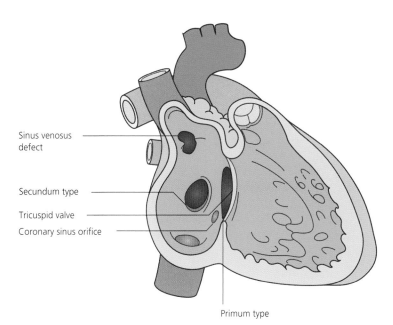

Sinus venosus
defect

Secundum type

Tricuspid valve

Coronary sinus orifice

Primum type

Figure 6.1 Anatomic classification of ASDs. Anatomy of the right atrium; sinus venosus and secundum type defects are shown. A coronary sinus defect is in the area of the coronary sinus orifice involving it (normal orifice shown). A "primum" type defect is shown in a different hue because it should be regarded as an atrioventricular septal defect.

superior vena cava is commonly associated. Again, these defects are rare.

Interatrial communications (Fig. 6.1) result in blood flow from the left to the right atrium, a left-to-right shunt, causing an increased volume load of the right ventricle. The amount of shunting is determined by the right ventricular compliance in diastole. As this is normally quite high, if somewhat unpredictable over time, isolated atrial septal defects usually remain asymptomatic for a number of years or even decades. Symptoms of heart failure can occur when the ratio of pulmonary/systemic blood flow (Q_p/Q_s) is larger than 1.5:1.0. A decrease in right or left ventricular compliance, acquired mitral valve lesions, or systemic hypertension may lead to an increase in left-to-right shunting, even late in life.

The development of pulmonary hypertensive disease in an isolated, untreated ASD is very uncommon. It may occasionally occur after decades but its natural course and morphology are clearly different from the disease encountered in ventricular or atrioventricular septal defects much earlier in life (see below) [3]. Spontaneous closure of atrial septal defects is rare because they represent structural deficiencies in thin cardiac walls not undergoing major postnatal changes. Chronic distension of the atrial chambers may lead to the development of atrial fibrillation over time. Because of the interatrial communication there is the risk of paradoxical embolization of a small venous thrombus across the hole into the systemic circulation. This is also true for hemodynamically insignificant small PFOs.

Indications

An undisputed indication for closure of an atrial septal defect is the presence of symptoms. The debate remains when to close asymptomatic ASDs. A Q_p/Q_s ratio of more than 1.5 and/or signs of right ventricular volume overload are universally agreed upon.

If surgery is the method of choice in an asymptomatic child, the timing of the operation can usually be delayed until the age of 4 or 5 years, rendering it technically easy and completely safe. The insult of extracorporeal circulation is better tolerated at this age, and the transfusion of blood products should be avoidable. Psychologically, it makes sense to "cure" the heart defect before the child enters school.

Although the closure of an ASD used to be a very common operation for decades, the development of safe interventional devices has reduced the indication for the surgical approach dramatically. In the most common form, ASD II, surgery is to be preferred if the boundaries of the defect are close to important neighboring structures, such as the mitral, tricuspid, or aortic valve, the coronary sinus orifice, or the venae cavae. The size of the patient must also be taken into account. In the rare case of a symptomatic infant with a large ASD II, surgery may be preferable because of limited vascular access. Moreover, a rim of tissue is required to anchor the interventional devices used; thus, a mismatch may result between the amount of foreign material to be implanted and a small heart with a lot of growth potential.

For sinus venosus defects and coronary sinus defects, with their very special anatomic particularities and frequently associated venous malformations, surgery remains the method of choice.

An ASD I, as explained above, represents an atrioventricular lesion involving the atrioventricular valves. Its treatment is always surgical but shall not be discussed further.

Technical aspects

For the surgical closure of an ASD, access to the heart can be gained in two ways. A median sternotomy with cannulation of the ascending aorta and both venae cavae is the conventional method. Because the tissue of children is elastic and

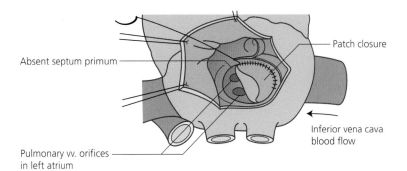

Patch closure

Absent septum primum

Inferior vena cava
blood flow

Pulmonary vv. orifices
in left atrium

Figure 6.2 ASD II patch closure. Surgeon's view of the opened right atrium. Patch closure is begun from near the orifice of the inferior vena cava (right-hand corner).

the right atrium and aorta are readily accessible, the skin incision can usually be kept very limited, starting below the sternomanubrial junction and ending above the xyphoid. If a midline approach is to be avoided, this is usually done for cosmetic reasons. A right anterior thoracotomy with a sub-mammary skin incision is a commonly used alternative, especially in girls from puberty onwards, in whom the breast buds are already discernible. Other approaches have also been used [4–6]. Lateral incisions require the division of intercostal muscle, spreading of the rib cage, and the opening of the right pleural space to reach the right lateral aspect of the pericardium. Although both venae cavae can be cannulated comparatively easily, the aorta may pose a challenge. If it is not safely reachable, one has to revert to femoral arterial cannulation, with all of its potential disadvantages, especially when performed on children. If the aorta can be cannulated but not clamped, the repair can be done during a period of ventricular fibrillation. Great care must then be taken to minimize the risk of air embolism in an otherwise safe procedure. Totally robotic approaches remain highly controversial and shall not be discussed here.

Irrespective of the mode of thoracotomy, the closure of the defect itself is a straightforward procedure [7,8]. The right atrium is incised obliquely, starting from the base of its appendage and continuing toward the inferior vena cava. The septal situs is inspected and the relevant anatomic structures, as well as the defect, are identified.

In a very large ASD II, resulting from agenesis of the septum primum, the lower rim of the defect will merge with the posterior wall of the inferior vena cava. Size and shape of the defect determine the mode of closure. A direct closure with a running, nonabsorbable monofilament suture can be chosen if the defect is of moderate size and slit-like configuration. Tension on this suture must be avoided by all means because it will eventually result in its dehiscence, rendering the operation void.

Surgical closure of most secundum-type defects requires a patch of appropriate size and shape. In the low-pressure system of the atria, foreign material should be avoided. Autologous pericardium is the material of choice for most groups, because it is easily accessible, free of charge, pliable, and robust enough. Better handling properties can be achieved by pretreating it after harvesting with 0.6% glutaraldehyde solution over a period of 10 min, followed by consecutive rinsing. The patch is tailored according to the borders of the defect and sutured into place with a nonabsorbable monofilament suture. The suture line starts at the lowest point toward the inferior cava and is led upward, first posteriorly and then anteriorly along the rim of the defect (Fig. 6.2). Before tying the knot, ventilation of the lungs will help to de-air the left atrium. In friable tissue, anchoring stitches can be added. The right atriotomy is closed with a monofilament suture (absorbable in children, nonabsorbable in adults), the heart is de-aired through the cardioplegia incision, and coronary circulation is then re-established by taking off the cross-clamp. Weaning from cardiopulmonary bypass should be uneventful and the formerly volume-overloaded right atrium will already have returned to normal dimensions by the end of the procedure.

In the case of sinus venosus defects, care must be taken to insert the upper venous cannula high into the superior vena cava at its junction with the innominate vein. This guarantees enough space for the concomitant repair of a partial anomalous pulmonary venous connection. Because these aberrant veins can be overlooked preoperatively, it is the duty of the surgeon to inspect the upper caval axis thoroughly. The azygos vein must be identified because it marks the highest level at which a connection of an anomalous right pulmonary vein can be expected. This technical requirement may render lateral access techniques inappropriate.

The incision on the right atrium is led from the base of the atrial appendage upward and, in the case of anomalous venous connections, into the posterolateral aspect of the superior vena cava beyond the level of the highest anomalous vein. At the cavoatrial junction, care must be taken not to injure the sinus node, which can usually be identified on the anteromedial aspect. In children, its blood supply is also clearly visible; this is of particular importance in the horseshoe type of sinus node, which tends to lie more at the posterior aspect of the vena cava and may receive small branches of the right coronary artery, both from the medial and from the lateral side. Atrial anatomy is then identified. The actual sinus venosus defect may be surprisingly small and is to be found high in the dorsal interatrial wall. It may be accompanied by an additional ASD II

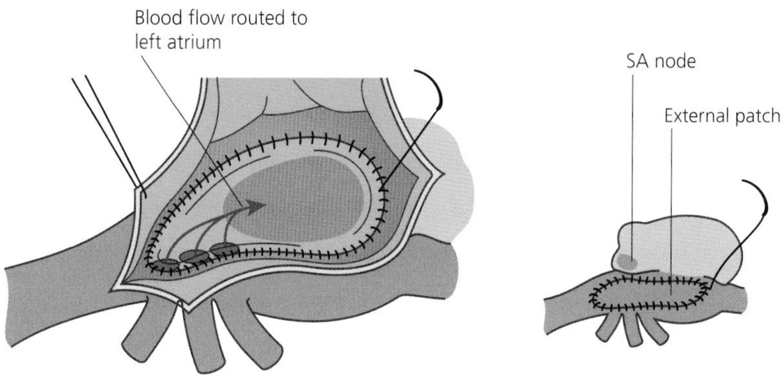

Figure 6.3 Repair of sinus venosus defect with PAPVC (partial anomalous pulmonary venous connection). The teardrop-shaped patch is already implanted, tunneling the blood from the (three) anomalously connecting pulmonary veins through the (enlarged) defect into the left atrium (arrow). Inset: the cavoatrial incision is shown being closed with an additional patch.

or PFO. A significant left-to-right shunt is often caused by the anomalous venous drainage rather than the atrial communication. All the aberrant veins are then identified, and a complete assessment of the venous drainage of the right lung must be performed. The concept of the preferred technique for correction is to lead the pulmonary venous blood behind a baffle through the septal defect into the left atrium [7]. If the ASD is smaller than the combined diameter of the anomalous veins, it must be enlarged into the fossa ovalis so that it is not restrictive. An additional ASD can be incorporated to accomplish this. A tear-shaped baffle is then tailored, ideally from autologous pericardium. It is sutured into the posterior wall of the superior vena cava with a fine (6.0 or 7.0) nonabsorbable monofilament suture beginning at the highest point. The aim is to guide unobstructed blood flow along the backside of the baffle. The patch is then led around the inferior rim of the ASD (Fig. 6.3). Upon closing the incision in the vena cava, it must be judged if a direct closure will not lead to a relative stenosis obstructing systemic venous return from the upper half of the body. In case of doubt, an additional patch is used to close this incision.

Coronary sinus defects are approached in a similar way as for an ASD II. Usually the defects are circular in shape and pericardial patch closure is required. Care must be taken not to obstruct the orifice of the coronary sinus. The atrioventricular node lies hidden, close to the anterior aspect of the defect. Accordingly, shallow suture bites in this area must be taken. A left persistent superior vena cava can be cannulated additionally, drained with an intraluminal vent catheter, or clamped intermittently. In the common absence or hypoplasia of an interconnecting vein, ligation is inappropriate.

The complex but rare entity of unroofed coronary sinus, which can also be encountered with coronary sinus defects, shall not be discussed here.

Results

Closure of an ASD is a safe procedure with mortality approaching zero [9]. Cross-clamping times are short and ventricular function is usually very good, with the immediate effect of the volume load being taken off the right ventricle. Significant morbidity may result from transient supraventricular tachycardias. In adults presenting with atrial flutter, this can persist postoperatively depending on its duration and severity [10], calling for additional ablation maneuvers.

When performing the operation under ventricular fibrillation without application of an aortic cross-clamp, as is often done through a lateral approach, the main danger is that of air embolism. Extreme care must be taken to avoid this deleterious complication. Vigorous de-airing must be performed and intrapericardial insufflation of carbon dioxide can be considered to replace the room air with a totally soluble gas. Careful blood gas management by the pump technician is required, because an increase of P_{CO_2}, resulting from absorption via the pump suction devices may lead to hyperperfusion of the brain.

Caval stenosis is a dreaded complication after repair of sinus venosus defects, but is usually a result of inappropriate technique being used [11]. Particularly in such a seemingly simple operation, the responsibility of the surgeon is immense because he or she has to provide the assumed security for the patient, which is taken for granted. Operations on children should therefore be performed only in specialized centers. Nevertheless, attention to detail is just as important in the adult. A thorough knowledge of the intricacies of congenital heart defects is required.

Summary

Atrial septal defects cause a left-to-right shunt on the atrial level with consequent volume loading of the right ventricle. Before planning closure either interventionally or surgically, the correct anatomic variant must be identified. Special forms of the secundum-type defect (ASD II) and all cases of sinus venosus, as well as coronary sinus defects, remain indications for surgical treatment. Patch closure can be performed extremely safely. It is, however, fraught with technical detail, as is common for congenital heart defects.

Ventricular septal defects

Historical background

Soon after successful closure of atrial septal defects, surgeons embarked on the task to reach the innermost part of the

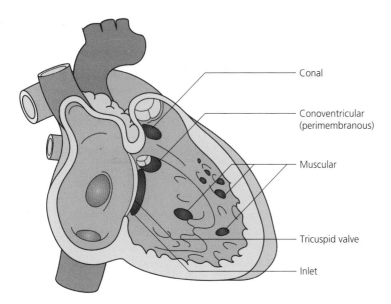

Conal

Conoventricular
(perimembranous)

Muscular

Tricuspid valve

Inlet

Figure 6.4 Anatomic classification of VSDs. Right ventricular anatomy: inlet, muscular, conoventricular, and conal defect sites are shown.

heart, the ventricular chambers. On 26 March 1954, Lillehei *et al.* [12] were the first to close a ventricular septal defect (VSD), utilizing a parent as circulatory support for the operated child by means of what was called "cross-circulation." Within 2 years, a total of 27 patients had been treated this way, 19 of whom survived [12]. At the same time, Kirklin *et al.* [14], in 1955, closed the first VSD with the help of extracorporeal circulation, which had been further refined at the Mayo Clinic [13,14]. Even the elegant transatrial approach, the routine method used to repair most defects today, was described as early as 1957 by Stirling, again of Lillehei's group [15].

In fact, the vigorous parallel development of techniques to cure congenital heart disease, at the University of Minnesota in Minneapolis and at Rochester's Mayo Clinic (two institutions only 70 miles apart in the same state), quickly established cardiac surgery as a medical field of its own. The historic reports still make fascinating reading today, especially when one realizes that those pioneers already raised scientific questions to which we have yet to provide the answers.

Even before the advent of open-heart surgery the deleterious natural history of untreated ventricular septal defects had inspired the surgical community to think of palliative measures. In 1952, Muller and Dammann [16] described the method of pulmonary artery banding to protect the pulmonary vascular bed from pressure overload and to postpone the onset of pulmonary vascular obstructive disease. Although this operation has almost completely lost its place in the treatment of VSD, it still remains a surgical tool for the therapy of certain forms of complex univentricular heart disease with unrestricted pulmonary blood flow.

Morphology and pathophysiology

By analogy with ASDs, a VSD is defined as a communication of variable size between the left and the right ventricle, commonly caused by arrested development of a part of the interventricular septal structures. Simplifying cardiogenesis, again very briefly, the ventricular partition is formed by a large muscular part, originally perforated by numerous fenestrations, and a small membranous section consisting of fibrous tissue. The membranous section is situated cephalad in the heart in the outflow part of the ventricles, and is connected to the septum of the former truncus arteriosus communis, which is to separate into the aorta and the pulmonary trunk. This uppermost part is called the conal or conotruncal septum.

The most common site of VSDs is the zone in which muscular and membranous parts merge. Failure of fusion results in a hole, called a perimembranous or conoventricular defect. Unfortunately, different nomenclatures are used for the classification of VSDs [14,17,18]. If one is to divide the right ventricle into an inlet, a trabecular, and an outlet part, VSDs can be encountered in each section, called inlet (atrioventricular canal type) VSD (6%), muscular VSD (10%), conoventricular (perimembranous) VSD (80%), and conal VSD (4%) accordingly (Fig. 6.4). With the location determining surgical technique, this is the classification chosen for use in this chapter. Anatomic descriptions are given together with the surgical technique.

The natural history of a VSD is dependent on its size and anatomy. Depending on the extent of left-to-right shunt and the resulting pulmonary blood flow, a defect is classified as restrictive or nonrestrictive. In the latter, right ventricular systolic pressure equals that of the left ventricle. The correcting variable determining pulmonary blood flow is the pulmonary vascular resistance (R_p), which is physiologically increased postnatally. The true hemodynamic significance of a VSD may therefore become apparent only after several weeks of life, with the R_p decreasing along with lung differentiation. A restrictive VSD has a Q_p/Q_s flow ratio of less than 1.5:1.0. Nonrestrictive defects commonly have a diameter at least that of the aortic valve, with Q_p/Q_s ratios reaching 3:1 and more. Large shunt volumes cause the rapid development of congestive heart failure in the infant, provoking symptoms such as dys-/tachypnea, sweating, feeding problems, and failure to thrive. The onset of symptoms determines the time of surgery, although it must be emphasized that elective closure before manifestation of cardiac failure is the goal, independent of age or weight. Thus, most hemodynamically significant VSDs are to be closed within the first months of life.

Untreated VSDs with pulmonary arterial hypertension will lead to remodeling of the pulmonary arterial walls [19–21]. This will eventually become irreversible and cause a massive increase in its R_p. When the ratio of pulmonary to systemic resistance, R_p/R_s, exceeds 1:1, reversal of shunt flow into a right-to-left direction and diminished pulmonary perfusion will occur, with the patients becoming cyanotic. This is known as the Eisenmenger reaction [22].

Small, apical muscular VSDs, on the other hand, show a tendency for spontaneous closure at the time of postnatal differentiation of the ventricular myocardium. In the membranous part of the septum, defects can be partially or even totally pseudo-occluded by a prolapse of accessory connective tissue in conjunction with the neighboring tricuspid valve. The misleading term "aneurysm VSD" is often used.

The direct relationship with the aortic valve in conoventricular VSDs may lead to aortic insufficiency. The noncoronary leaflet of the valve prolapses into the defect and becomes deformed over time, complicating repair if the operation has been postponed [23,24].

Even very small VSDs without any hemodynamic significance but with turbulences irritating the endocardial surface may trigger endocarditis, necessitating prophylactic regimens in the untreated lesion. This is an argument in favor of closing a small VSD [25].

Indications

As has been outlined above, a large VSD ($Q_p/Q_s > 1.5:1$) should be closed before the onset of symptoms of congestive heart failure. This is usually the case within the first months of life. In smaller, restrictive defects, repair may be postponed until later in life. VSDs affecting the aortic valve should be operated upon before the valve tissue undergoes structural changes. Close observation is warranted. Other collateral damage to be observed along with untreated VSDs is the development of subaortic stenosis or of right ventricular hypertrophy in the shape of a "double-chambered right ventricle" [26]. The matter of threatening endocarditis has been discussed. All these secondary effects further complicate simple VSD closure and can be avoided by a timely operation.

Technical aspects

The standard access to the heart for closure of a VSD is via a median sternotomy with cannulation of the distal ascending aorta and both venae cavae. Reports of so-called minimally invasive techniques have been published. These techniques do compromise exposure of the defect. Furthermore, an appropriate closure of a VSD requires much more time and technical expertise than that of an ASD, for which the limitations have been discussed above. Therefore, those approaches should be discussed critically and must be restricted to surgeons with great experience and to elder patients [27,28]. After aortic cross-clamping and induction of cardioplegic arrest, the VSD is exposed via a cardiac incision according to its localization.

The closure techniques described in the following paragraphs unequivocally involve the utilization of patch material. For this, Dacron is strongly recommended because of its handling and physical properties with PTFE as an alternative. Autologous pericardium is used by a few groups but bears the disadvantage of relative friability. The suture techniques mentioned are explicitly advocated for a safe closure. Individual experience may diverge from this, as is so often the case with surgical techniques. However, direct closure, even of a seemingly small defect, is definitely advised against; the enormous tension on such sutures caused by the contracting myocardium places them at an unacceptably high risk of dehiscence.

Conoventricular ventricular septal defects

The most common form of VSD, also known as perimembranous, is generally reached via a transatrial approach. The right atrium is incised longitudinally, and the tricuspid valve leaflets are retracted into the atrium with a blunt retractor or stay sutures. This exposes the right ventricular aspect of the interventricular septum with a conoventricular defect usually visible in the cephalad corner of the tricuspid valve ring. If visualization of the upper rim of the VSD is compromised, partial detachment of the anterosuperior leaflet of the tricuspid valve can become necessary.

With the circumference of the defect exposed and completely visualized, sutures are placed around it. Double armed, non-absorbable, braided sutures buttressed with small felt pieces are recommended. The first suture is placed in the anteroinferior aspect of the muscular septum. Continuing in a clockwise direction, and taking care not to compromise any chordae of the tricuspid valve, the inferoposterior area is reached in which the conduction system lies hidden within the septum. Here, sutures must be placed more superficially on the right ventricular surface, somewhat apart from the rim of the defect (Fig. 6.5). When approaching the tricuspid valve ring, the sutures can be placed from the right atrial side with the pledgets positioned in the atrium. At this point, traction is employed on the sutures in a caudad direction, thereby exposing the upper rim of the VSD. The next sutures are applied anteriorly and counterclockwise, again in the muscular septum. Upon reaching the aortic valve, which must be clearly visualized in order not to injure it, the border of tissue in which to anchor the sutures may become extremely limited. Longitudinal stitches,

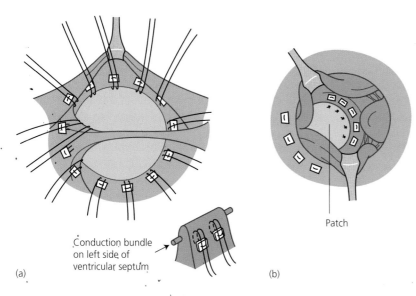

Patch

Figure 6.5 Transatrial/transtricuspid closure of conoventricular VSD. (a) Interrupted, buttressed sutures are placed around the rim of the VSD with four of the pledgets situated within the right atrium. Inset: The course of the conduction bundle toward the left-sided surface of the ventricular septum is shown. (b) The patch is anchored into place, again with four pledgets situated within the right atrium.

optionally monofilament and not buttressed, may help to overcome this delicate zone along the undersurface of the valve. The sutures are then completed posteriorly, mostly from the right atrium again. The patch, preferably of woven Dacron fabric, is tailored according to the size and shape of the VSD. The sutures are then passed through the patch, which, upon completion, is lowered onto the right ventricular aspect of the septum. Only then all are sutures tied. Tricuspid valve function is tested by instillation of fluid into the right ventricle. Rarely, reconstructive measures are necessary. The right atrium is closed with an absorbable running suture and the operation is concluded in the usual fashion as described for ASD closure above.

Inlet ventricular septal defects

Inlet VSDs can be reached very effectively via the transatrial approach because they are in continuation with the tricuspid valve ring. For this reason, they are also called atrioventricular canal-type VSDs. There is no tissue between the rim of the defect and the valve annulus. All posterior sutures must therefore be placed from within the right atrium. A maze of atypical chordae may obscure the lower rim. A continuous monofilament suture can be passed more easily around these obstacles in a mattress fashion. The conduction system is usually relatively superficial inferoposteriorly. In this zone, carefully placed interrupted sutures are recommended. Thus, a combination of suture techniques is often helpful.

Conal ventricular septal defects

These defects high up in the outflow region are very close to the pulmonary valve. They are often associated with more complex forms of congenital heart disease of the conotruncal region such as truncus arteriosus communis. Isolated conal VSDs can be reached through a limited infundibulotomy of the right ventricle or, more elegantly, through the pulmonary valve.

The risk of injuring the conduction system is low, because it is far away from the borders of these defects. A transvalvular approach may offer only limited exposure if the VSD is not of the usual shallow crescent shape but extends deep into the muscular septum. A longitudinal incision in the anterior wall of the outflow tract facilitates safe repair.

Muscular ventricular septal defects

Isolated, midmuscular, inferior, or posterior defects can usually be closed through the tricuspid valve. The further they are located in the trabecularized part of the right ventricle toward the apex, the more difficult exposure can become. Muscle bundles may even create the impression of multiple defects. Their partial transection will improve visualization. By definition, the complete circumference of a muscular VSD is formed by myocardium. Interrupted, buttressed sutures are therefore recommended throughout. The surgeon has to bear in mind that the muscular part of the interventricular septum plays an important role in cardiac contraction, applying a great deal of tension on sutures anchored within it.

Anterior or apical defects can be exposed only through a ventriculotomy. Although an apical left ventriculotomy provides excellent exposure because of the lack of trabeculations, its long-term sequelae are dreaded [29]. The development of appropriate interventional closure techniques has rendered this approach almost obsolete [30]. When catheter techniques are still not an option, a right ventriculotomy can be done relatively safely [31]. Hybrid solutions with catheter devices delivered through cardiac incisions also seem to offer promising alternatives [32,33].

Swiss-cheese ventricular septal defects

This somewhat casually named entity describes a profound lack of differentiation of the muscular interventricular septum in its trabecularized part. Multiple muscular defects result. When these defects are small and localized in the more apical region, spontaneous closure may occur. Extension of larger defects into the mid-muscular septum will lead to early hemodynamic relevance. As surgical access is limited and traumatic, interventional methods offer a reasonable alternative [34,35]. Under certain circumstances, preliminary pulmonary artery banding via sternotomy early in life can be a sensible strategy for this formidable disease.

Results

Primary closure of an isolated VSD has yielded excellent results in centers specializing in surgery of congenital heart disease. Mortality, as in ASD, approaches zero, and significant morbidity also should be almost nonexistent [7,8]. It remains arguable if this standard, which must be offered to every patient, can be achieved in units with low-volume surgery. Rigid quality control is essential.

Observed morbidity is closely related to the type of defect. In conoventricular VSDs the proximity of the aortic valve endangers its integrity. Perfect visualization without compromise is the best protection. Complete atrioventricular block caused by damage to the conduction system is observed in up to 3% of patients [36]. Mostly it is a transient phenomenon aided by tissue swelling and passes within a couple of days. Within the first 2 postoperative weeks, the indication for permanent pacemaker placement must be judged guardedly. Tricuspid valve insufficiency provoked by exposing measures should be detected and dealt with intraoperatively. Residual VSD can still be an issue in the closure of (multiple) muscular defects. Here, interventional methods have come to help. Routine intraoperative transesophageal echocardiography is a valuable tool to diagnose any kind of residual pathology in the operating room with the option to deal with it instantaneously.

The excellent standard of quality achieved by "conventional" surgery is the bar against which new developments must be measured. This is true both for alternative surgical techniques as well as for interventional devices. Recent models, such as the "Amplatzer membranous septal occluder," are designed with the surgeon's experience in mind, showing modifications of the superior rim to avoid aortic valve damage. The necessity for sufficient tissue in which to anchor the device has led to irritation of the conduction system followed by complete atrioventricular block and transvenous pacing over several weeks. All this must be taken into account when considering associated morbidity. Currently, closure of a VSD remains a surgical domain, with the use of interventional devices to be limited to strongly controlled study protocols [37–40].

Summary

A ventricular septal defect causes a left-to-right shunt on the ventricular level with consequent pressure load on the pulmonary vascular bed. Its natural history is determined by its size and location and is much more malignant than that of an ASD. If left untreated for too long, irreversible remodeling of the pulmonary vasculature or damage of related cardiac structures will ensue. Closure of a hemodynamically significant defect commonly becomes necessary within the first months of life. It is performed surgically with the aid of a fabric patch and meticulous suture techniques, depending on the anatomy. Results are excellent and remain the standard against which alternatives are to be measured.

References

1. Gross RE, Pomerantz AA, Watkins E Jr, *et al.* (1952) Surgical closure of defects of the interauricular septum by use of an atrial well. *N Engl J Med* **247**:455–460.

2. Gibbon JH (1954) Application of a mechanical heart and lung apparatus to cardiac surgery. *Minn Med* **37**:171–185.

3. Haworth SG (1983) Pulmonary vascular disease in secundum atrial septal defect in childhood. *Am J Cardiol* **51**:265–272.

4. Bichell DP, Geva T, Bacha EA, *et al.* (2000) Minimal access approach for the repair of atrial septal defect: the initial 135 patients. *Ann Thorac Surg* **70**:115–118.

5. Doll N, Walther T, Falk V, *et al.* (2003) Secundum ASD closure using a right lateral minithoracotomy: five-year experience in 122 patients. *Ann Thorac Surg* **75**:1527–31.

6. Tiete AAAR, Sachweh JS, Kozlik-Feldmann R, *et al.* (2002) Minimally invasive surgery for congenital heart defects in paediatric patients. *Thorac Cardiovasc Surg* **50**:271–275.

7. Castaneda AR, Jonas RA, Mayer JE, & Hanley FL (1994) *Cardiac surgery of the neonate and infant,* 1st edn. Philadelphia: WB Saunders.

8. Kirklin JW & Barratt-Boyes BG (1993) *Cardiac Surgery,* 2nd edn. New York: Churchill Livingstone.

9. Murphy JG, Gersh BJ, McGoon MD, *et al.* (1990) Long-term outcome after surgical repair of isolated atrial septal defect. Follow-up at 27 to 32 years. *N Engl J Med* **323**:1645–1650.

10. Brandenburg RO Jr, Holmes DR Jr, Brandenburg RO, *et al.* (1983) Clinical follow-up study of paroxysmal supraventricular tachyarrhythmias after operative repair of secundum type atrial septal defect in adults. *Am J Cardiol* **51**:273–276.

11. Stewart S, Alexon C, & Manning J (1986) Early and late results of repair of anomalous pulmonary venous connection to the superior vena cava with a pericardial baffle. *Ann Thorac Surg* **41**:498–501.

12. Lillehei CW, Cohen M, Warden HE, *et al.* (1955) The results of direct vision closure of ventricular septal defects in eight patients by means of controlled cross circulation. *Surg Gynecol Obstet* **101**:446–466.

13. DuShane JW, Kirklin JW, Patrick RT, *et al.* (1956) Ventricular septal defects with pulmonary hypertension: surgical treatment by means of a mechanical pump-oxygenator. *JAMA* **160**:950–953.

14. Kirklin JW, Harshbarger HG, Donald DE, & Edwards JE (1957) Surgical correction of ventricular septal defect: anatomic and technical considerations. *J Thorac Cardiovasc Surg* **33**:45–59.

15. Stirling GR, Stanley PH, & Lillehei CW (1957) Effect of cardiac bypass and ventriculotomy on right ventricular function; with report of successful closure of ventricular septal defect by use of atriotomy. *Surg Forum* **8**:433–438.

16. Muller WH Jr & Dammann JF Jr (1952) The treatment of certain congenital malformations of the heart by creation of pulmonic stenosis to reduce pulmonary hypertension and excessive

pulmonary blood flow: a preliminary report. *Surg Gynecol Obstet* **95**:213–219.

17. van Praagh R, Geva T, & Kreutzer J (1989) Ventricular septal defects: how shall we describe, name and classify them? *J Am Coll Cardiol* **14**:1298–1299.

18. Becker AE & Anderson RH (1982) *Cardiac pathology*. Edinburgh: Churchill Livingstone.

19. Heath D & Edwards JE (1958) The pathology of hypertensive pulmonary vascular disease: a description of six grades of structural changes in the pulmonary arteries with special reference to congenital cardiac septal defects. *Circulation* **18**:533–547.

20. Hislop A, Haworth SG, Shinebourne EA, *et al.* (1975) Quantitative structural analysis of pulmonary vessels in isolated ventricular septal defects in infancy. *Br Heart J* **37**:1014–1021.

21. Rabinovitch M, Keane JF, Norwood WI, *et al.* (1984) Vascular structure in lung tissue obtained at biopsy correlated with pulmonary hemodynamic findings after repair of congenital heart defects. *Circulation* **69**:655–667.

22. Eisenmenger V (1897) Die angeborenen Defekte der Kammerscheidewand des Herzens. *Z Klin Med Suppl.* **32**:1–28.

23. Tatsuno K, Konno S, Ando M, *et al.* (1973) Pathogenetic mechanisms of prolapsing aortic valve and aortic regurgitation associated with ventricular septal defect. *Circulation* **48**:1028–1037.

24. Trusler GA, Moes CAF, & Kidd BSL (1973) Repair of ventricular septal defect with aortic insufficiency. *J Thorac Cardiovasc Surg* **66**:394–403.

25. Backer CL, Winters RC, Zales VR, *et al.* (1993) Restrictive ventricular septal defect: how small is too small to close? *Ann Thorac Surg* **56**:1014–1019.

26. Eroglu AG, Oztunc F, Saltik L, *et al.* (2003) Evolution of ventricular septal defect with special reference to spontaneous closure rate, subaortic ridge and aortic valve prolapse. *Pediatr Cardiol* **24**:31–35.

27. Kadner A, Dodge-Khatami A, Dave H, *et al.* (2006) Closure of restrictive ventricular septal defects through a right axillary thoracotomy. *Heart Surg Forum* **9**:E836–839.

28. Mavroudis C, Backer CL, Stewart RD, *et al.* (2005) The case against minimally invasive cardiac surgery. *Semin Thorac Cardiovasc Surg Pediatr Card Surg Annu* 193–197.

29. Hanna B, Colan SD, Bridges ND, *et al.* (1991) Clinical and myocardial status after left ventriculotomy for ventricular septal defect closure. *J Am Coll Cardiol* **17**(Suppl.):110A.

30. Lock JE, Block PC, McKay RG, *et al.* (1988) Transcatheter closure of ventricular septal defects. *Circulation* **78**:361–368.

31. Myhre U, Duncan BW, Mee RB, *et al.* (2004) Apical right ventriculotomy for closure of apical ventricular septal defects. *Ann Thorac Surg* **78**:204–208.

32. Bacha EA, Cao QL, Galantowicz ME, *et al.* (2005) Multicenter experience with periventricular device closure of muscular ventricular septal defects. *Pediatr Cardiol* **26**:169–175.

33. Okubo M, Benson LN, Nykanen D, *et al.* (2001) Outcomes of intraoperative device closure of muscular ventricular septal defects. *Ann Thorac Surg* **72**:416–423.

34. Seddio F, Reddy VM, McElhinney DB, *et al.* (1999) Multiple ventricular septal defects: how and when should they be repaired? *J Thorac Cardiovasc Surg* **117**:134–140.

35. Waight DJ, Bacha EA, Kahana M, *et al.* (2002) Catheter therapy of Swiss cheese ventricular septal defects using the Amplatzer muscular VSD occluder. *Cathet Cardiovasc Intervent* **55**:355–361.

36. Andersen HO, deLeval MR, Tsang VT, *et al.* (2006) Is complete heart block after surgical closure of ventricular septal defects still an issue? *Ann Thorac Surg* **82**:948–956.

37. Butera G, Chessa M, & Carminati M (2007) Percutaneous closure of ventricular septal defects. State of the art. *J Cardiovasc Med* **8**:39–45.

38. Hirsch R, Lorber A, Shapira Y, *et al.* (2007) Initial experience with the Amplatzer membranous septal occluder in adults. *Acute Card Care* **9**:54–59.

39. Michel-Behnke I, Le TP, Waldecker B, *et al.* (2005) Percutaneous closure of congenital and acquired ventricular septal defects—considerations on selection of the occlusion rate. *J Interv Cardiol* **18**:89–99.

40. Xunmin C, Shisen J, Jianbin G, *et al.* (2007) Comparison of results and complications of surgical and Amplatzer device closure of perimembranous ventricular septal defects. *Int J Cardiol* **120**:28–31.

7   Pathology of Aortic Stenosis

Nikolaus Gassler[1] & Philipp A. Schnabel[2]

[1]Institute of Pathology, RWTH Aachen University, Aachen, Germany
[2]Institute of Pathology, University Clinics Heidelberg, Heidelberg, Germany

Types of aortic stenosis

The term aortic stenosis includes three different forms of left ventricular outflow obstruction; true stenosis of the aortic valvular orifice must be distinguished from subvalvular and supravalvular aortic stenosis. Supravalvular aortic stenosis is very rare and is frequently found in patients with Williams–Beuren syndrome. The stenosis is morphologically characterized by focal hypoplasia of the ascending aorta. A supravalvular diaphragm with a central orifice is a rare variant.

Subvalvular aortic stenosis is characterized by obstruction of the left ventricular outflow tract below the aortic valve. In many cases, a fibromuscular diaphragm develops, narrowing the outflow tract between the septum and the anteroseptal leaflet of the mitral valve. Fusion of the diaphragm and leaflet has been observed. This variant of subvalvular aortic stenosis differs from the muscular conus stenosis proposed by Schmincke, which is also known as the muscular variant of the disease. The muscular variant is probably due to focal cardiomuscular hypertrophy. Combination of different types of aortic stenosis has been recorded [1].

True aortic valve stenosis (AVS) is found at a higher frequency than either of the other types. In AVS three major diagnostic considerations have to be made: degenerative, congenital bi- or monocuspid, and postinflammatory (postrheumatic) valve disease.

Pathologic evaluation of the aortic valve

Gross anatomy of the aortic valve

The aortic valve is normally composed of three semilunar cusps which are fixed to the annulus fibrosus of the aorta. The aortic cusps are called valvulae semilunaris posterior, dextra, or sinistra. In the center of the free margin of each semilunar cusp lies a fibrocartilaginous nodule, the nodulus Arantius.

Fibrous thickened strands originating from the annulus fibrosus cross the fundus of the semilunar cusps and finally reach the noduli Arantii. The free margins of the cusps at both sides of the noduli Arantii are very thin and form semilunar tracts, lunulae. Above each aortic cusp lies a bulge of the aortic root called the aortic sinus or sinus of Valsalva.

Microscopic anatomy of the aortic valve

Histologically, aortic valve cusps comprise a well-defined layered structure with fibrosa, spongiosa, and ventricularis. The major structural component is the collagen-dense fibrosa, which extends to the free cusp edge and which is found in contact with the surface-lining endothelium. Densely packed collagen bundles of the fibrosa layer interact with the valvular ring in the region of the commissures. The collagen bundles are intermingled with some fibroblasts and very fine elastic fibers. The central position in the valve cusps is occupied by the spongiosa, which is best developed in the basal third. It does not extend to the free edge where fibrosa and ventricularis are exclusively found. The spongiosa is composed of large amounts of proteoglycans in association to loosely arranged collagen fibrils and some fibroblasts. Adjacent to the spongiosa layer, the ventricularis is found in direct contact with the surface endothelium. This layer is characterized by its richness in elastic fibers, which are larger and more numerous than in the fibrosa. The arrangement of fiber bundles varies with the state of stress. In the stressed state bundles are wavy and the inflow surface is smoother than in the relaxed state. Aortic valve cusps become thicker, more opaque, and less pliable with age due to an increase in the collagen content.

Clinical data

Clinicians have to keep in mind that interpretation of morphologic findings is improved by providing relevant clinical data. The questionnaire must include data for probe identification and a correct and well-defined description of resected materials. The emphasis placed on clinical data differs between clinicians and clinical pathologists. From the morphologic point of view, important anamnestic data include the time course of asymptomatic and symptomatic aortic valve disease, diagnosis of infectious/non-infectious acute or chronic valve endocarditis,

Cardiovascular Interventions in Clinical Practice. Edited by Jürgen Haase, Hans-Joachim Schäfers, Horst Sievert and Ron Waksman. © 2010 Blackwell Publishing.

or establishment of any systemic disease. Further interest is given to application of cardiotoxic therapeutics, such as doxorubicin, daunorubicin, chloroquine, or anthracycline. In such cases, special fixation of small myocardial probes from septal myomectomy and ultrastructural examination is recommended. However, septal myomectomy is performed for hemodynamically significant hypertrophy of the ventricular septum in fewer than 10% of AVS patients.

Owing to heavy valve calcification, valve cusps may be removed in numerous small pieces, which can impair pathologic (gross) examination. In such cases, clinicians should provide additional statements concerning commissural fusion, location of bulky nodules, occurrence of a median raphe, the number of valve cusps, and aortic valve mobility.

Gross pathology of the aortic valve

Important macromorphologic criteria are the number of valve cusps, the topography of calcified nodules, the structure of commissures, and the establishment of raphes. The term raphe is used to describe the conjoint or so-called fused area of two injured or underdeveloped cusps, turning into a malformed commissure. These raphes can be established partially or totally. In contrast to raphes, commissure of the aortic valve describes the space between two lateral and parallel attachments of adjacent valve cusps to the aortic wall, normally not adhering to each other. Commissures are different from the appositional zone between free edges of adjacent cusps.

Unicuspid aortic valve stenosis results in a "teardrop-shaped" valve, usually with two raphes and only one commissure. Bicuspid aortic stenosis is characterized by two leaflets, nodular calcification at the aortic surface, and a median raphe. However, bicuspid aortic valve includes different morphologic phenotypes presenting with different hemodynamic conditions [2]. AVS with calcified nodules on the aortic surface of structured valve cusps is indicative of senile calcific aortic stenosis. It is suggested that the presence of heavily calcified valves, probably removed in numerous small pieces, favors the diagnosis of degenerative aortic stenosis. Often there is a combined aortic stenosis and insufficiency (see Chapter 12).

Evaluation of commissures is of great importance because fusion of one, two, or all three commissures is the most important diagnostic feature in aortic valves removed for postinflammatory stenosis. In such cases, the calcifying process begins at the commissures and extends on to the cuspal surface. Bulky nodules at the base of valve cusps are found less often in postinflammatory AVS than in degenerative aortic valve disease. In postrheumatic AVS, mitral valve changes are frequently found because the susceptibility of mitral leaflets to rheumatic disease is higher (see Chapters 16 and 21). It has been suggested that the weight of operatively excised stenotic aortic valves is a relevant parameter in valve stenosis [3].

Valvular vegetations indicative of infectious valve endocarditis may be present anywhere on the valve surface, but are often attached to the line of closure. Their appearance varies from soft reddish to ginger to brownish. In chronic or smoldering valve endocarditis, fibrotic valve thickening, calcification, and/or transvalvular perforation may be found.

Histopathology of the aortic valve

Brownish, ginger, or erythroid-colored valve tissues deserve closer attention for the diagnosis or exclusion of valve endocarditis, especially of the chronic or smoldering type. Histomorphologic investigation includes description of the valve cusps basic structure (intact vs. fibrosis vs. necrosis), distribution of calcified particles, occurrence and morphology of blood vessels (neovascularization), quality and quantity of inflammatory cellular infiltrates, and establishment of fibrin aggregates at the valve cusps surface. However, acute fibrin platelet thrombi may be found on the valve cusps surface secondary to the operative procedure and not indicative for mural thrombi or valve endocarditis. The histologic feature of a raphe is a ridge with abundant elastic fibers [4].

Etiology and pathogenesis of aortic valve stenosis

Two major groups of AVS can be defined, congenital and acquired. These groups comprise further entities and special pathophysiologic mechanisms, as detailed below.

It is suggested that the prevalence of AVS in the Western world has risen in recent years because of a growing elderly population and improved diagnostic procedures [5]. Morphologic features of AVS such as calcification and stiffening of the valve cusps can be found in about 50% of people aged 75–80 years and in up to 75% of those over 85 years old [6]. Patients with clinically significant AVS constitute approximately 2% of unselected individuals over 65 years or 5.5% of those over 85 years [6–8]. There is consent that in the last decades there has been a remarkable shift in the primary cause of AVS in the elderly from rheumatic heart disease to degenerative calcification of tricuspid aortic valve [9]. However, there is a discrepancy in the frequency of degenerative calcification of tricuspid and congenital uni- or bicuspid aortic valves. Some studies in Western populations have found the leading cause of AVS to be degenerative calcification of tricuspid aortic valves, followed by calcification of bicuspid valves [10,11]. However, in another study comprising 465 patients, bicuspid calcified aortic valves (63.7%) were the predominant cause of isolated AVS, followed by tricuspid calcified AVS (26.9%) [12]. This latter point of view is further underlined by a US multicenter study comprising 1849 patients and reviewing four decades (1960–2005) [13]. In this study, congenitally malformed aortic valves were found to be more common than tricuspid aortic valves. A more detailed US study including 932 patients (mean age 70 years) provides further support that an underlying congenitally malformed valve (either uni- or bicuspid) is more common than a tricuspid aortic valve, at least in men [14]. A study by Stephan and co-workers [15] included 115 patients suffering from AVS (mean age 70 years), of whom half had congenitally malformed valves and half had tricuspid aortic valves. Collins and co-workers [16] suggested that a tricuspid, bicuspid, and unicuspid aortic valve may represent a phenotypic continuum of a similar disease process.

It has been suggested by several observers that the frequency of different mechanisms in AVS etiology is influenced by geographic and demographic/sociologic factors. This point of view is supported by the observation that the common causes of AVS in Asia are postinflammatory disease (56%) and degenerative calcification with coincidence of hypertension, dyslipoproteinemia, and/or diabetes mellitus, but not congenitally malformed aortic valve cusps [17].

The timing of interventional treatment or surgical replacement of AVS depends on the underlying disease [14]. There are three treatment options for AVS: balloon dilatation in noncalcified congenital AVS (normally carried out in childhood), surgical replacement, and interventional replacement, which is a new treatment option for patients with "end-stage" AVS and/or severe comorbidities. Unicuspid aortic valve replacement is frequently performed in the fourth and fifth decades of life. Replacement of sclerotic bicuspid valve is typically indicated in the seventh decade. Women who undergo surgical excision of stenotic aortic malformed valves are about one decade older than men. Numerous surgical aortic valve replacements due to degenerative calcification of tricuspid valves are performed in both sexes in about the eighth decade. Timing of aortic valve replacement is predominantly dependent on the functional severity, which is mainly determined by aortic valve area; an aortic valve area of $<0.75\,cm^2$ in adults normally results in symptoms, and necessitates valve replacement to prevent the development of left ventricular failure.

Congenital aortic valve disease

The bicuspid aortic valve is the most common congenital aortic valve abnormality, occurring in 0.9–2% of the population, and frequently results in AVS [4,18]. This malformation may be found in about 49% of patients with AVS [14]. Unicuspid aortic valve is the next most important congenital cause of AVS. Quadricuspid aortic valves are very rare and are typically associated with the development of aortic regurgitation, not AVS [19]. In addition, congenital pentacuspid aortic valve without stenosis or regurgitation has been reported [20].

In a genome-wide scan, linkage of bicuspid aortic valve and/or associated cardiovascular abnormalities to chromosomes 18q, 5q, and 13q was found, indicating the inheritance of malformed aortic valve cusps [21]. True valve abnormalities must be distinguished from pseudo-bicuspid or pseudo-unicuspid aortic valves resulting from inflammatory cusps damage in infectious valve endocarditis or rheumatic fever.

It has to be stressed that congenital bicuspid aortic valve disease is made up of a spectrum of different morphologic phenotypes presenting with different hemodynamic conditions. Malformation of a commissure and the adjacent parts of the two corresponding valve cusps forming a raphe are central to the description and classification of congenital bicuspid aortic valve [22]. Thus, the morphologic variants include a spectrum from completely missing commissures leading to two valve cusps, sinuses, and commissures, to a greater or lesser malformation of one or two commissural structures and the adjacent valve cusps. The most frequent variants consist of three developmental cusp and commissure formations and are different from the true bicuspid aortic valve composed of two cusps. Following the morphologic criteria mentioned above, the proposed classification system consists of three characteristics, with the number of raphes (types 0–2) as the major characteristic and two supplementary characteristics (spatial position of valve cusps or raphes and functional valve status) [23].

It is thought that mechanical stress, the phenomenon of "wear and tear", plays a greater role in AVS resulting from malformed aortic valves than from tricuspid valves. This point of view is supported by the observation that bicuspid aortic valve predisposes to earlier manifestation of AVS (Fig. 7.1). The view that AVS due to malformed aortic valves is a passive, age-related degenerative disease simply caused by imbalance of tissue resistance and mechanical load is obsolete. Several recent studies have shown that AVS pathogenesis is an active process, resembling in some essentials atherosclerosis (see below); however, the basal pathogenetic mechanisms appear to be similar in both bicuspid and tricuspid aortic valves [24].

Acquired aortic valve disease

Inadequate mechanical stress was previously assumed to be the most important and basic functional aspect in development of AVS. It is now recognized, however, that the etiology and pathogenesis of AVS involve an active inflammatory, atherosclerotic process similar to that in (coronary) artery disease, and some risk factors for calcific AVS are identical to those of atherosclerosis, including hypertension, smoking, increased age, male gender, diabetes mellitus, and disturbances in high- and low-density lipoprotein levels [7,25]. However, the association of AVS calcification with dyslipidemia or diabetes mellitus is not always proven [26]. Despite the similarities between AVS and atherosclerosis, there are some important differences in their etiology and pathogenesis. For example, fibrocalcific thickening and calcification are more extensive in AVS than atherosclerosis, and are the main causes of the clinical manifestations of valve dysfunction in the former (Fig. 7.2). Severe atherosclerosis and AVS do not always coincide, and the role of medical therapy, which is helpful in atherosclerosis, is not established in AVS. Furthermore, the prevalence of coexisting AVS and coronary artery disease is discrepant: half of patients with AVS have significant coronary artery disease, but most patients with coronary artery disease do not have AVS [27]. The low concordance appears to be the result of other genetic or metabolic factors more specific for

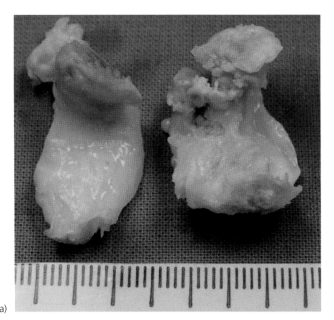

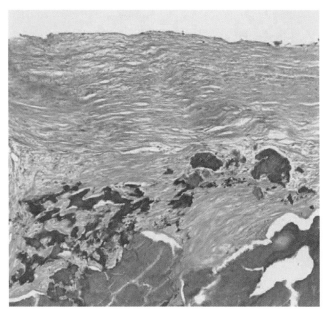

Figure 7.1 Congenital bicuspid aortic valve of a 38-year-old woman. (a) Severe calcification and increased thickness of valve tissues is visible. (b) Histologic section of the calcified aortic valve cusp (left). Note the fine fragmented deposits in the calcification front (Alcian/periodic acid Schiff [PAS] staining).

calcification processes. In this scenario, AVS should not be considered a simple degenerative disease [28].

Different mechanisms probably involved in AVS development are discussed elsewhere [29,30]. The sequence of interacting pathophysiologic events includes endothelial injury, accumulation and deposition of lipids/lipoproteins, complement system activation, generation of advanced glycation end products, influx and activation of inflammatory cells associated with extracellular matrix remodeling, and neovascularization, which intensifies the inflammatory cellular influx and calcification (Fig. 7.2). Current understanding of AVS pathogenesis is discussed further below, specifically the newly identified molecular pathways that could be of interest for medical approaches. There is some evidence that AVS represents a systemic inflammatory condition involving elevated serum levels of molecules such as C-reactive protein and soluble E-selectin [31].

Endothelial damage

The initiating event in AVS pathogenesis is considered to be endothelial damage. This endothelial injury occurs more often on the aortic side of the valve cusps, especially in valve commissures, and is probably due to an increased mechanical or complex shear stress across the valve surface endothelium [32–34]. Asymmetric endothelial lesions indicate that systemic pressure and abnormal blood rheology predispose to AVS [35]. *In vitro* experiments show that endothelial cells are sensitive to flow direction and align perpendicular or parallel to flow direction [36]. However, additional mechanisms are assumed to promote endothelial damage, including external risk factors. Establishment of endothelial damage and first tissue remodeling are probably coordinated by infiltration of different types of inflammatory cells, especially macrophages and T cells, and accumulation of lipoproteins. This pathologic sequence of early aortic valve injury appears similar to initial changes in atherosclerotic lesions. An association of AVS with systemic endothelial dysfunction has been suggested [37,38].

Recently, the role of complement activation as an important mechanism in exacerbation of early valve damage to AVS has been described [39]. Importantly, in this study, upregulation of C3aR in valve tissues was found to be caused by external risk factors also, such as cigarette smoke. In addition, receptors for the anaphylatoxins C3a and C5a are expressed in coronary artery atherosclerotic plaques in humans, providing further evidence of similarities in the pathogenesis of AVS and arteriosclerosis [40]. In addition, decreased availability of nitric oxide and prostacyclin in AVS endothelial cells favors the view that a link between endothelial damage and inflammation exists [41].

Expression of adhesion molecules by endothelial cells is found in AVS but not in normal aortic valve cusps [42]. The phenomenon is suggested to be a molecular mechanism for recruitment of inflammatory cells. In patients with AVS, increased expression of E-selectin has been found in surface lining endothelium of damaged valve cusps and in serum. Soluble E-selectin serum levels depend on the presence of AVS and decrease after AVS replacement. Endothelial damage is additionally found in established AVS and frequently associated with calcification (Fig. 7.3).

Inflammation

The observation that normal aortic valve tissues are almost devoid of inflammatory cells, whereas AVS tissues are

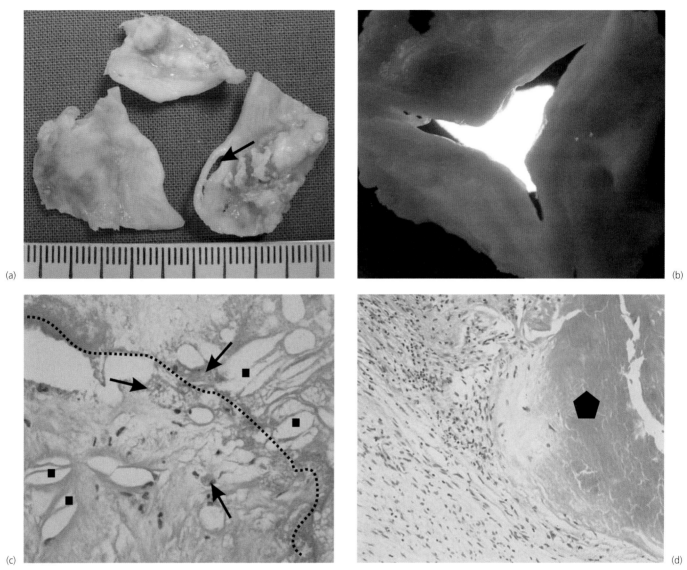

Figure 7.2 Degenerative aortic valve stenosis. (a) Explanted aortic valve cusps with strong calcification and tissue rigidity in a 75-year-old man. The arrow indicates valve tissue perforation. (b) Transillumination of explanted aortic valve with lumen stenosis from strong calcification and partly fused commissures (69-year-old woman). Calcified lesions predominantly expanded into the aortic side of the valve. (c) Histomorphologic features of aortic valve calcification. Lymphocytes and lipid-loaded macrophages (arrows) are found adjacent to extracellular lipids and cholesterol clefts (black squares). The dotted line denotes fine granular tissue calcifications. (d) An increased number of lymphocytes and strong tissue calcification (black pentagon) are shown. Between the components, extracellular lipids and macrophages are visible.

infiltrated by macrophages and lymphocytes to various degrees, favors the hypothesis of chronic aortic valve damage as an active inflammatory process. Different types of inflammatory cells, including solitary T-cells, mast cells, macrophages, and foam cells, are regularly found in early AVS lesions [32,43,44]. The active role of such inflammatory cells in AVS pathogenesis is visible by expression of interleukin types, interleukin receptors, cytokines (e.g., transforming growth factor β1 [TGF-β1]), and other substances by the cells. T-cells in the vicinity of calcifications express interleukin 2 receptors, demonstrating their activated state [45]. An

important role for aortic valve interstitial cells is assumed from their expression of Toll-like receptors (TLR2 and TLR4). Stimulation of interstitial cells by receptor agonists such as peptidoglycan and lipopolysaccharide induces the expression of proinflammatory mediators as well as upregulation of osteogenesis-associated factors [46]. It has now been proven that *Chlamydophila pneumoniae* is not involved in AVS pathogenesis as a significant inflammation-associated pathogen [47].

Experimental evidence is accumulating that mast cells play an important role in AVS pathogenesis [48]. This view is

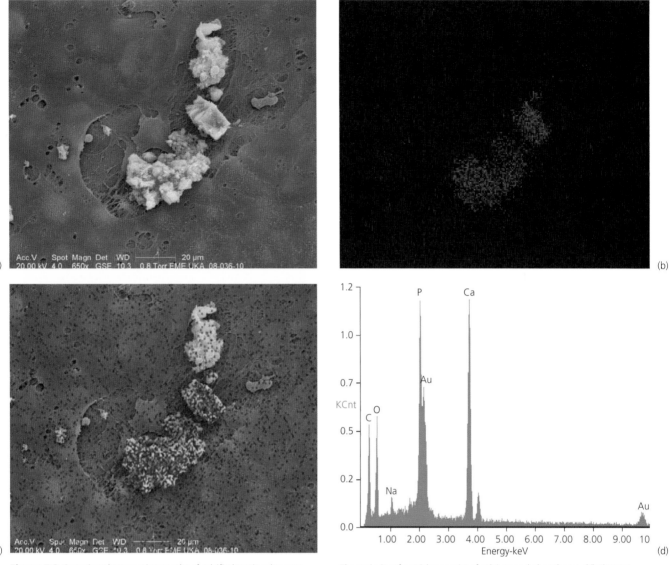

Figure 7.3 Scanning electron micrographs of calcified aortic valve cusp. (a) Endothelial denudation in association with crystalloid particles is found. Note the microvilli on the endothelial surface. (b) Subtraction technique for visualizing the prevalent elements, which are calcium and phosphorus. (c) Overlay from the particle surface (A) and element analysis results (B). The majority of particles consist of calcium and phosphorus. (d) Element analysis diagram of particles clearly demonstrates predominance of the two elements, calcium and phosphorus. Investigations and images courtesy of Dipl.-Ing. M. Bovi (Electron Microscopic Facility, RWTH Aachen University, Germany).

substantiated by the observation of a high number of degranulated CD117-expressing mast cells in fibrotic but not in normal aortic valve cusps. Since mast cell granules include several bioactive substances, such as histamine, proinflammatory cytokines, heparin, and proteases, mast cell activation is suggested as an important step in tissue remodeling and activation of other inflammatory cells. This issue is further elucidated by our improved knowledge of pathways associated with certain mast cell-derived products such as tumor necrosis factor α (TNFα) [49], vascular endothelial growth factor [50], and matrix metalloproteinases (MMPs) [51].

Lipid accumulation

An important role for lipids in AVS pathogenesis and atherosclerosis is widely accepted [29,52–55]. However, the molecular mechanisms and pathways associated with increased lipid deposition, different types of lipids, and secondary modification of lipids are only partly elucidated. The concept of "valvulometabolic risk" for AVS development and progression is an attempt to overcome this limitation by interactive studies in the field of lipid metabolism, molecular biology, and epidemiology. In this setting it has been shown that, in addition to local lipid accumulation in aortic valve tissues, visceral obesity, with its attendant metabolic complications, is a risk factor in the development and progression of AVS [52]. Technical procedures and equipment for lipid analysis have recently improved considerably. Important innovative analytical approaches are liquid chromatography and mass spectrometry, which is useful for analyzing the level of lipids and their interacting partners in multicellular structures [56].

Extracellular accumulations of plasma-derived apolipoproteins and "structural lipids" are present in aortic valve lesions [57]. The important role of apolipoproteins in AVS pathogenesis has been shown in several experiments [58]. In addition, different types of lipid modifications are reported to accelerate AVS pathology and tissue calcification (see below). Oxidized cholesterol and/or low-density lipoprotein (LDL) can be found abundantly in degenerated aortic valve cusps and sometimes in association with T-cell infiltrates, suggesting that such LDL particles promote local inflammation and tissue remodeling [59]. In addition to LDL, hypercholesterolemia is assumed to favor the development of AVS by causing thickening of valve cusps [60]. This phenomenon is probably due to a cholesterol-associated increase in interstitial valve cusp cells with deposition of extracellular matrix [29].

There is evidence for an interacting role of lipids as a stimulating component in vascular and valve tissue calcification [61,62].

Extracellular matrix remodeling and loss of flexibility

Tissue remodeling is assumed to be one important mechanism resulting in valve thickening and abnormal aortic valve function. In physiologic conditions, valve tissues, especially the extracellular matrix, are maintained by a strictly controlled balance between synthesis and degradation of its component proteins. There is evidence that in vascular and valve tissues a disequilibrium of this balance leads to pathologic remodeling and tissue valve cusp rigidity [63]. Interdependence of lipid metabolism and fibrocalcific remodeling of valve tissues plays an active pathologic role in this process [64]. Moreover, mechanical stress, bioactive substances, and inflammation have been shown to modify the composition of extracellular matrix by regulation of aortic valve interstitial cells [65]. It is suggested that an altered extracellular matrix architecture associated with compromised valve function accelerates valve cusp degeneration and calcification [66]. Remodeling of valve tissues is influenced by MMPs (e.g., MMP-1, MMP-2, MMP-3, and MMP-9), which are expressed by endothelial cells, smooth muscle cells, and macrophages. MMPs are endopeptidases with conserved functional domains, and their proteolytic action degrades extracellular matrix components in diverse tissue types, including vascular and valve tissues [67,68]. Levels expression of and enzymatic activities of different types of MMPs are increased in AVS tissues and AVS calcification compared with unaffected valves [69,70]. This disequilibrium is assumed to be an important factor in the development and progression of extracellular matrix remodeling [71]. Expression of MMPs is influenced by various contributors involved in AVS pathogenesis, including RANKL (receptor activator for nuclear factor κB ligand), tenascin-C, elastolytic cathepsins, TNFα, and receptor of advanced glycation end products [72]. MMP activity is further regulated by their tissue inhibitors (tissue inhibitors of metalloproteinase, TIMPs), which are also found in cardiac tissues [73]. It is assumed that an imbalance between MMPs and TIMP exists [51,74], which is further modified by reactive oxygen species, migration and activation of T-cells, tenascin C expression, expression of adhesion molecule 1, alkaline phosphatase activity, and cytokine activation [75].

There is experimental evidence that fibrosa layer interstitial cells play an important role in valve tissue remodeling [76]. Interstitial cells are able to differentiate into myofibroblasts expressing smooth muscle actin, vimentin, desmin, and HLA-DR. The switch of antigen expression is considered as a state of chronic activation, with production of collagen and interstitial substances leading to fibrosis and functional interference. An elevated collagen–elastin ratio, which further contributes to valve stiffening, has been proposed as an indicator of valve tissue remodeling [48,77]. Exaggeration of tissue injury results in ongoing valve cusp calcification, sometimes associated with bone formation, which further inhibits valve function by loss of flexibility. It is hypothesized that AVS pathology is promoted by so-called replicative senescence of valve tissue cells, demonstrated by decreased telomere length [78]. Recently, repression of Smad-mediated myofibroblast activation in aortic valve interstitial cells by fibroblast growth factor 2 was recorded [79]. The newly discovered pathway has been suggested as a promising tool in engineering effective AVS therapeutics.

Components of the renin–angiotensin system (RAS) have identified in aortic valve tissues, and their expression was found to parallel AVS development and lipid storage [80]. It is suggested that angiotensin-converting enzyme (ACE) is provided to the leaflets by circulating LDL–ACE mixed particles and a subset of macrophages. Colocalization of angiotensin II and profibrotic angiotensin II type 1 receptors (AT-R1) in diseased valve tissues has been reported [80]. The proinflammatory and profibrocalcific properties of angiotensin II are assumed to play an important role in AVS pathogenesis [81]. Inhibition of antifibrotic effector molecules, which is also found in stenotic aortic valve tissues, results in promotion of profibrotic RAS activity [82].

Calcification/ossification

Valve tissue calcification is a very common and prominent lesion and contributes substantially to leaflet rigidity and valve dysfunction (Fig. 7.3). There is a strong correlation between a high degree of calcification in a valve cusp and rapid disease progression and poor outcome [83]. Initiation of calcification occurs primarily on the aortic side of the valve cusps, where blood flow is more turbulent, indicating that shear stress and its interaction with surface-lining endothelial cells is important in AVS pathogenesis. Progression of AVS calcification is linked to metabolic bone disease, which is characterized by increased bone tissue remodeling such as occurs in Paget's disease, osteopathy associated with renal disease, and secondary hyperparathyroidism [84–86].

It is assumed that aortic valve myofibroblasts, which are responsive to nitric oxide, angiotensin II, and local hormones [87], play a central role in aortic valve tissue calcification by phenotypic transdifferentiation into osteoblast-like cells [88]. Synthesis of a calcific nidus by such transdifferentiated valvular interstitial cells is inducible by application of bioactive substances and depends on alkaline phosphatase activity [89]. The pro-osteogenic activity of transdifferentiated myofibroblasts is promoted by macrophages endowed with osteogenic activity [90]. Recently, different types of TGF-β and bone morphogenic proteins, as well as TNFα, Sox9, Runx2/Cbfa1, thymosin, insulin-like growth factor I, transcription factor Egr-1, and extracellular nucleotides, were identified as bioactive substances playing a role in valve tissue calcification [91–95]. The mechanisms and pathways of cellular transdifferentiation are very complex and, apparently, not a simply spontaneous phenomenon, as previously assumed. This became clear through experiments with interstitial cells isolated from nonstenotic aortic valves. After stimulation with osteogenic mediators, these interstitial cells underwent phenotypic transdifferentiation into osteoblast-like cells. In addition to transdifferentiation effects, TGF-β1, upregulated by serotonin, is able to induce the expression of alkaline phosphatase and MMP-9, both of which are associated with matrix calcification [96–98]. In cultured cells, TGF-β1 mediates the procalcification activity of aortic valve interstitial cells through mechanisms involving apoptosis [99]. At present, however, aortic valve tissue calcification is recognized as a complex process involving plenty of additive factors and mechanisms.

C-reactive protein is detectable in damaged aortic valve tissues and has been suggested as a mediator in calcification [100]. This hypothesis is further substantiated by experimental procedures using aortic wall equivalents. In this *in vitro* model, increasing levels of C-reactive protein levels promote aortic wall calcification [101]. Calcification and ossification of aortic valve tissues are modified by molecules primarily identified in developing bone, such as osteopontin, osteonectin, osteocalcin, osterix, and tenascin [102,103]. Osteoprotegerin and its ligand RANKL, which are antagonists in bone remodeling, are expressed in aortic valve tissues and involved in valve cusp calcification [104]. It has been shown that RANKL is able to stimulate aortic valve myofibroblasts to express osteoblast-associated genes, resulting in matrix calcification and calcific nodule formation.

The role of circulating proteins as systemic regulators of dystrophic calcification is well established. Concentrations of serum calcium and phosphorus within the normal range are almost high enough to result in spontaneous precipitation, and inhibitors of calcification are therefore of great importance. In a recent study, serum concentrations of fetuin-A, a liver-derived protein that forms a complex with calcium and phosphorus, increasing their solubility, were investigated [105]. Among patients with AVS, an inverse association between fetuin-A and aortic stenosis was observed.

Accumulation of lipids, including oxidized cholesterols such as 25-hydroxycholesterol, was demonstrated to facilitate the establishment of a nidus for local calcium deposits and ongoing calcification [106]. The calcification process is further accelerated by reactive oxygen species (particularly hydrogen peroxide) [107] and oxidized LDL, and is modified by sympathetic nervous system activity. The important role of lipid accumulation in early aortic valve lesions and lipid accumulation in the progress of AVS calcification is well established [57]. Delipidation of valve tissues by experimental treatment with ethanol has been shown to reduce AVS calcification in various animal species [108,109].

Macrophages, which are regularly found in vascular and valve lesions, are assumed to be an important cell type in early lipid accumulation. Membrane scavenger receptors were discovered as conserved components in their molecular lipid enrichment profile [110]. The receptors are capable of binding oxidized lipids. Lipids and their modifications initiate immunologic activities that are cellular based as well as determined by serologic components, promoting tissue calcification. In this scenario, osteoprotegerin was recently suggested as a molecular link for calcification in atherosclerosis [111].

Formation of metaplastic lamellar bone, sometimes including various types of hematopoietic cells in different stages of maturation, is estimated to occur in about 13% of severely calcified aortic valves in patients with AVS [112]. Intravalvular bone trabeculae morphologically show remodeling, microfractures, and healing where endochondral ossification may occur. Interactions between bone marrow-derived mesenchymal stem cells and aortic valve matrix or serum-derived components/cells are assumed to be of importance in metaplastic osteogenesis [113]. Following this hypothesis, mesenchymal stem cells provided by the bloodstream can migrate into injured valvular tissues and then participate in valve cusp remodeling. Recently, a central role of LDL receptor-related protein 5 (Lrp5) in the osteoblastic differentiation process, causing valve thickening and ossification, has been described [114]. Lrp5, osteocalcin, and other osteochondrogenic differentiation markers were increased in calcified aortic valves, whereas Sox9, Lrp5 receptor, and osteocalcin were increased in myxomatous mitral valves. The distribution pattern is hypothesized to be an endochondral bone differentiation process that results in deposition of cartilage in the mitral valve and bone in the aortic valve [114]. Experimental findings suggest that canonical Wnt signaling acts to maintain an undifferentiated, proliferating progenitor mesenchymal stem cell population, whereas noncanonical Wnts facilitate osteogenic differentiation. Consequently, loss-of-function and gain-of-function mutations of Lrp5 would perturb Wnt signaling and would, respectively, depress and promote osteogenesis by affecting migrating mesenchymal stem cells [115,116].

Inflammatory cells are found adjacent to metaplastic bone tissues that may facilitate tissue calcification by secretion of cytokines and proteases. As detailed above, the secretion products are involved in transdifferentiation of a subpopulation of interstitial cells into osteoblast-like cells.

There is some evidence that AVS development is related to genetic factors, such as receptors for serotonin or vitamin D as well as mutations in the *NOTCH1* gene [117]. *NOTCH1* encodes a transcriptional factor that is involved in osteogenic differentiation and valve development. Functional *NOTCH1* mutations may increase osteoblast formation and valve tissue calcification [117,118]. The relationship between apolipoprotein E alleles and development of AVS is unclear. Although the importance of the apolipoprotein E4 allele to AVS calcification has been demonstrated [119], another large trial found no association between apolipoprotein E alleles and AVS [120]. A significant association of the vitamin D receptor B allele with AVS has been described [121]. Lipodystrophies are a heterogeneous group of diseases characterized by abnormal fat distribution and mutations in the *LMNA* gene, which occasionally show association with AVS [122].

Neovascularization

Formation of vascular structures in aortic valve tissues is suggested to be an important step in AVS pathogenesis. Intravalvular vessels may facilitate the continuous entry of inflammatory cells and serum-derived components into leaflet tissues. Vessel formation depends on the presence of angiogenic factors and their inhibitors. Important molecules involved in this scenario are VEGF (vascular endothelial growth factor), SPARC (secreted protein acidic and rich in cysteine), and chondromodulin [50,123,124]. The degree of tissue vascularization in AVS varies and probably depends on the underlying disease. It is recognized that the number of vascular structures is higher in AVS due to infectious valve endocarditis or rheumatic valve disease than in so-called degenerative valve disease. The morphology of intravalvular vessels varies, but thin-walled vascular structures may be more frequently found after valve endocarditis.

Pharmacologic intervention

An increasing number of experimental and clinical studies show that AVS is an actively regulated disease in which retardation or prevention of disease progression could be achieved by medical therapeutics. This section reports some promising approaches mentioned. A summary of retrospective and recent studies of medical therapy in AVS prevention is given by Goldbarg *et al.* [125].

Serum levels of C-reactive protein, which is assumed to play a role in tissue calcification, can be influenced by statins [88]. Hypercholesterolemia is assumed to favor the development of AVS by causing thickening of valve cusps [60]. This phenomenon, associated with increased proliferation of valve cusp cells, can be diminished by the application of atorvastatin [126]. Atorvastatin treatment downregulates levels of TGF, bone morphogenic proteins, alkaline phosphatase, and osteocalcin, which are key molecules in tissue calcification, and interferes with the Lrp5 receptor pathway [127,128]. In general, statins (3-hydroxy-3-methylglutaryl-coenzyme A reductase inhibitors) lower lipid levels, possess pleiotropic mechanisms, and disrupt some inflammatory pathways [125].

Extracellular ATP and the P2Y receptor cascade have been identified as important regulators of bone remodeling, whereas its breakdown product, adenosine, is known to have anti-inflammatory properties. In contrast to adenosine, ATP is able to increase alkaline phosphatase activity by an atorvastatin-sensitive pathway [129]. Recently, β_2-adrenergic receptors in the sympathetic nervous system were identified as an innovative target for pharmacologic intervention in valve tissue calcification. Receptor inhibition with salmeterol is able to diminish alkaline phosphatase activity [130]. Tissue calcification and AVS pathogenesis can be decelerated by inhibition of neovascularization. Several substances are identified to interfere in this process, including statins and modified tetracyclines [123].

As outlined above, the RAS was recently identified as playing a role in AVS pathogenesis and myocardial tissue remodeling. Consequently, AT-R1 antagonists and ACE inhibitors are promising candidates in the medical therapy of AVS [131]. In parallel, pharmacologic intervention in the serotonin system could be a powerful tool to decelerate AVS pathogenesis.

Pathophysiology of aortic valve stenosis

Tissue remodeling with valve thickening and calcification of the cusps, which are found particularly on the aortic side of the valve, obstructs opening of the valve during systole and impedes postsystolic closing. Mechanical disturbances of aortic valve function result in hemodynamic perturbation and reactive change in the left ventricular myocardium and the aorta. The classic symptom triad of AVS, including angina pectoris, syncope, and heart failure, as well as bystander symptoms such as dyspnea, exertional hypotension, and atrial or ventricular tachyarrhythmia, are a consequence. Pathophysiologic mechanisms in AVS are detailed below.

Left ventricular hypertrophy

Valve thickening and calcification are hallmarks of AVS and are associated with a reduction in valve area and normal

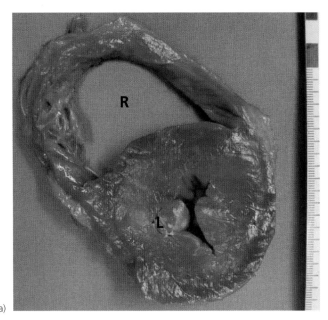

(a)

(b)

Figure 7.4 Left ventricular hypertrophy due to severe aortic valve stenosis in a 68-year-old man. (a) Strongly expanded left ventricular wall (L) with consecutive narrowing of the left ventricular cavity. Left myocardial tissues are differently colored, including some yellowish spots which indicate ischemic necrosis. Additionally, right ventricular enlargement (R) is seen as a consequence of long-standing compromised left ventricular function in severe aortic valve stenosis. (b) The schema illustrates discrepancy of the left (L) and right (R) ventricular cavity diameter (black areas). The gray area shows tangential parts of the right ventricular wall.

stroke volume. The relationship between left ventricular wall stress and ejection fraction is inverse. To maintain stroke volume and normalize left ventricular wall stress, the left ventricular myocardium shows concentric hypertrophy and increasing pump force. The ventricular myocardial hypertrophy is able to maintain normal wall stress despite the increased left ventricular pressure load. A compensated state is morphologically characterized by myocardial thickening without enlargement of the ventricular cavity (Fig. 7.4). In an ultrastructural view, replication of sarcomeres is the basis of myocardial hypertrophy.

In the compensatory state, the hypertrophied myocardium produces sufficiently high left ventricular pressures when contracting to force blood past the AVS. Consequently, a pressure gradient results between the left ventricle and the ascending aorta. Myocardial contractility is preserved until the late stages of AVS, when the obstruction becomes so severe that the pressure load overwhelms the myocardial ability to compensate. The increase in left ventricular wall thickness and development of symptoms, such as chest pain, shortness of breath, or syncope, are suggested to be critical determinants of ventricular performance in patients with AVS [132]. Significant hypertrophy of the ventricular septum can result in or aggravate hemodynamic perturbations in AVS.

Progress in myocardial hypertrophy takes many years as AVS obstruction becomes more severe. In congenital AVS, the increase in aortic valve obstruction occurs gradually because the valve orifice shows only little change as the child grows [133]. Impairment of left ventricular performance is due to inadequate development of myocardial hypertrophy, depression of myocardial contractility, or a combination of the two.

Aortic valve narrowing is associated with systolic and diastolic left ventricular dysfunction (afterload mismatch) because the left ventricle becomes less compliant [5]. It is assumed that diastolic dysfunction can occur earlier than systolic dysfunction and is a consequence of both impaired myocardial relaxation and decreased left ventricular compliance. Myocardial stiffness is partly a consequence of myocardial fibrosis, which develops with long-standing myocardial hypertrophy and remains even in the case of hypertrophy regression. Left ventricular filling is impaired due to poor diastolic relaxation and becomes increasingly reliant on left atrial function; elevated left ventricular end-diastolic pressures, left atrial enlargement, and pulmonary hypertension can result. As atrial contraction plays a particularly important role in filling of the left ventricle in AVS, development of atrial fibrillation is a catastrophe for the maintenance of normal forward stroke volume.

In AVS, left ventricular output often fails to rise adequately during cardiac exercise. This is a result of the diminishing ability to increase the stroke volume (elevated left ventricular mass-to-volume ratio) (Fig. 7.4). The additive mechanism, an increase in heart rate, is also limited. Acceleration in heart rate is physiologically characterized by a decreased systolic period, during which the stroke volume is maintained by an increase in the pressure gradient, the aortic valve flow rate, and a slight increase in the valve area [5]. This adaptive mechanism is more and more limited with AVS progression and results in terminal heart failure. Thus, progressive left ventricular ejection fraction reduction is suggested as a viable tool to identify a patient's risk of AVS and the best time for valve replacement surgery [134].

Hemodynamic perturbation

Severe AVS is associated with impairment of cardiac output and blood supply. These hemodynamic alterations affect blood flow across the ascending/thoracic aorta, the coronary arteries, and the mitral valve. In severe AVS, elevated left ventricular filling pressures may lead to secondary pulmonary artery hypertension.

Dilation of the thoracic aorta has been suggested as an important variable in AVS outcome, especially after aortic valve replacement [135] (compare with Chapter 12). Post-stenotic dilation is more severe in bicuspid AVS than in tricuspid valves, which may contribute to the increased frequency of aortic complications. Distances between aortic valve level and point of maximum ascending aorta diameter are significantly increased in bicuspid AVS compared with tricuspid AVS. Especially in bicuspid AVS, chronic hemodynamic perturbation can result in asymmetric dilation at the convexity of the vessel segment [136].

In AVS, coronary blood flow at rest is elevated in absolute terms but is normal when corrected for myocardial mass. Reduced coronary flow reserve may produce inadequate myocardial oxygenation in severe AVS, even in the absence of coronary artery disease. Increased left ventricular muscle mass, elevated intraventricular pressures, and the prolongation of left ventricular ejection contribute to an elevation of myocardial oxygen consumption. In turn, high intraventricular pressures, potentially exceeding coronary perfusion pressures, and the shortening of diastole impair coronary perfusion, leading to an imbalance between myocardial oxygen supply and demand. Myocardial perfusion is also diminished by the relative decline in myocardial capillary density in myocardial hypertrophy. In long-standing severe AVS, functional mitral regurgitation, as a consequence of left ventricular dilation, may further deteriorate the compromised hemodynamics (see Chapter 21). The prevention of hemodynamic perturbation in the presence of severe aortic stenosis can be achieved either by the conventional procedure of surgical valve replacement or, in the case of high operative risk, by transcatheter aortic valve implantation.

Acknowledgment

P. Akens is gratefully acknowledged for typing and proofreading the manuscript.

References

1. Patanè S, Marte F, & Di Bella G (2009) Asymptomatic double site of left ventricular outflow tract obstruction: subvalvular aortic stenosis associated with valvular aortic stenosis. *Int J Cardiol* **133**:e30–e32.
2. Fernandes SM, Sanders SP, Khairy P, *et al.* (2004) Morphology of bicuspid aortic valve in children and adolescents. *J Am Coll Cardiol* **44**:1648–1651.
3. Roberts WC & Ko JM (2003) Weights of operatively-excised stenotic unicuspid, bicuspid, and tricuspid aortic valves and their relation to age, sex, body mass index, and presence or absence of concomitant coronary artery bypass grafting. *Am J Cardiol* **92**:1057–1065.
4. Roberts WC (1970) The congenitally bicuspid aortic valve. A study of 85 autopsy cases. *Am J Cardiol* **26**:72–83.
5. Phillips D (2006) Aortic stenosis: a review. *AANA J* **74**:309–315.
6. Lindroos M, Kupari M, Heikkila J, *et al.* (1993) Prevalence of aortic valve abnormalities in the elderly: an echocardiographic study of a random population sample. *J Am Coll Cardiol* **21**:1220–1225.
7. Stewart BF, Siscovick D, Lind BK, *et al.* (1997) Clinical factors associated with calcific aortic valve disease. Cardiovascular Health Study. *J Am Coll Cardiol* **29**:630–634.
8. Chan KL (2003) Is aortic stenosis a preventable disease? *J Am Coll Cardiol* **42**:593–599.
9. Matsumura T, Ohtaki E, Misu K, *et al.* (2002) Etiology of aortic valve disease and recent changes in Japan: a study of 600 valve replacement cases. *Int J Cardiol* **86**:217–223.
10. Dare AJ, Veinot JP, Edwards WD, *et al.* (1993) New observations on the etiology of aortic valve disease: a surgical pathologic study of 236 cases from 1990. *Hum Pathol* **24**:1330–1338.
11. Butany J, Collins MJ, Demellawy DE, *et al.* (2005) Morphological and clinical findings in 247 surgically excised native aortic valves. *Can J Cardiol* **21**:747–755.
12. Davies MJ, Treasure T, & Parker DJ (1996) Demographic characteristics of patients undergoing aortic valve replacement for stenosis: relation to valve morphology. *Heart* **75**:174–178.
13. Roberts WC, Ko JM, & Hamilton C (2005) Comparison of valve structure, valve weight, and severity of the valve obstruction in 1849 patients having isolated aortic valve replacement for aortic valve stenosis (with or without associated aortic regurgitation) studied at 3 different medical centers in 2 different time periods. *Circulation* **112**:3919–3929.
14. Roberts WC & Ko JM (2005) Frequency by decades of unicuspid, bicuspid, and tricuspid aortic valves in adults having isolated aortic valve replacement for aortic stenosis, with or without associated aortic regurgitation. *Circulation* **111**:920–925.
15. Stephan PJ, Henry AC, Hebeler RF, *et al.* (1997) Comparison of age, gender, number of aortic valve cusps, concomitant coronary artery bypass grafting, and magnitude of left ventricular-systemic arterial peak systolic gradient in adults having aortic valve replacement for isolated aortic valve stenosis. *Am J Cardiol* **79**:166–172.
16. Collins MJ, Butany J, Borger MA, *et al.* (2008) Implications of a congenitally abnormal valve: a study of 1025 consecutively excised aortic valves. *J Clin Pathol* **61**:530–536.

17. Chuangsuwanich T, Warnnissorn M, Leksrisakul P, *et al.* (2004) Pathology and etiology of 110 consecutively removed aortic valves. *J Med Assoc Thai* **87**:921–934.

18. Ward C (2000) Clinical significance of the bicuspid aortic valve. *Heart* **83**:81–85.

19. Timperley J, Milner R, Marshall AJ, & Gilbert TJ (2002) Quadricuspid aortic valves. *Clin Cardiol* **25**:548–552.

20. Cemri M, Cengel A, & Timurkaynak T (2000) Pentacuspid aortic valve diagnosed by transoesophageal echocardiography. *Heart* **84**:E9.

21. Martin LJ, Ramachandran V, Cripe LH, *et al.* (2007) Evidence in favor of linkage to human chromosomal regions 18q, 5q and 13q for bicuspid aortic valve and associated cardiovascular malformations. *Hum Genet* **121**:275–284.

22. Osler W (1886) The bicuspid condition of the aortic valve. *Trans Assoc Am Physicians* **2**:185–192.

23. Sievers HH & Schmidtke C (2007) A classification system for the bicuspid aortic valve from 304 surgical specimens. *J Thorac Cardiovasc Surg* **133**:1226–1233.

24. Wallby L, Janerot-Sjöberg B, Steffensen T, *et al.* (2002) T lymphocyte infiltration in non-rheumatic aortic stenosis: a comparative descriptive study between tricuspid and bicuspid aortic valves. *Heart* **88**:348–351.

25. Mazzone A, Venneri L, & Berti S (2007) Aortic valve stenosis and coronary artery disease: pathophysiological and clinical links. *J Cardiovasc Med (Hagerstown)* **8**:983–989.

26. Agmon Y, Khandheria BK, Meissner I, *et al.* (2001) Aortic valve sclerosis and aortic atherosclerosis: different manifestations of the same disease? Insights from a population-based study. *J Am Coll Cardiol* **38**:827–834.

27. Otto CM & O'Brien KD (2001) Why is there discordance between calcific aortic stenosis and coronary artery disease? *Heart* **85**:601–602.

28. Hughes BR, Chahoud G, & Mehta JL (2005) Aortic stenosis; is it simply a degenerative process or an active atherosclerotic process? *Clin Cardiol* **28**:111–114.

29. Helske S, Kupari M, Lindstedt KA, *et al.* (2007) Aortic valve stenosis: an active atheroinflammatory process. *Curr Opin Lipidol* **18**:483–491.

30. Mazzone A, Epistolato MC, De Caterina R, *et al.* (2004) Neoangiogenesis, T-lymphocyte infiltration, and heat shock protein-60 are biological hallmarks of an immunomediated inflammatory process in end-stage calcified aortic valve stenosis. *J Am Coll Cardiol* **43**:1670–1676.

31. Sanchez PL, Santos JL, Kaski JC, *et al.* (2006) Relation of circulating C-reactive protein to progression of aortic valve stenosis. *Am J Cardiol* **97**:90–93.

32. Otto CM, Kuusisto J, Reichenbach DD, *et al.* (1994) Characterization of the early lesion of "degenerative" valvular aortic stenosis. Histological and immunohistochemical studies. *Circulation* **90**:844–853.

33. Aikawa E, Nahrendorf M, Sosnovik D, *et al.* (2007) Multimodality molecular imaging identifies proteolytic and osteogenic activities in early aortic valve disease. *Circulation* **23**:377–386.

34. Mirzaie M, Meyer T, Schwarz P, *et al.* (2002) Ultrastructural alterations in acquired aortic and mitral valve disease as revealed by scanning and transmission electron microscopical investigations. *Ann Thorac Cardiovasc Surg* **8**:24–30.

35. Thubrikar MJ, Aouad J, & Nolan SP (1986) Patterns of calcific deposits in operatively excised stenotic or purely regurgitant aortic valves and their relation to mechanical stress. *Am J Cardiol* **58**:304–308.

36. Butcher JT, Penrod AM, Garcia AJ, *et al.* (2004) Unique morphology and focal adhesion development of valvular endothelial cells in static und fluid flow environments. *Arterioscler Thromb Vasc Biol* **24**:1429–1434.

37. Poggianti E, Venneri L, Chubuchny V, *et al.* (2003) Aortic valve sclerosis is associated with systemic endothelial dysfunction. *J Am Coll Cardiol* **41**:136–141.

38. Goland S, Trento A, Czer LS, *et al.* (2008) Thoracic aortic arteriosclerosis in patients with degenerative aortic stenosis with and without coexisting coronary artery disease. *Ann Thorac Surg* **85**:113–119.

39. Helske S, Oksjoki R, Lindstedt KA, *et al.* (2008) Complement system is activated in stenotic aortic valves. *Atherosclerosis* **196**:190–200.

40. Oksjoki R, Laine P, Helske S, *et al.* (2007) Receptors for the anaphylatoxins C3a and C5a are expressed in human atherosclerotic coronary plaques. *Atherosclerosis* **195**:90–99.

41. Tedgui A & Mallat Z (2001) Anti-inflammatory mechanisms in the vascular wall. *Circ Res* **88**:877–887.

42. Ghaisas NK, Foley JB, O'Briain DS, *et al.* (2000) Adhesion molecules in nonrheumatic aortic valve disease: endothelial expression, serum levels and effects of valve replacement. *J Am Coll Cardiol* **36**:2257–2262.

43. Helske S, Lindstedt KA, Laine M, *et al.* (2004) Induction of local angiotensin II-producing systems in stenotic aortic valves. *J Am Coll Cardiol* **44**:1859–1866.

44. Wallby L, Steffensen T, & Broqvist M (2007) Role of inflammation in nonrheumatic, regurgitant heart valve disease. A comparative, descriptive study regarding apolipoproteins and inflammatory cells in nonrheumatic heart valve disease. *Cardiovasc Pathol* **16**:171–178.

45. Olsson M, Dalsgaard CJ, Haegerstrand A, *et al.* (1994) Accumulation of T lymphocytes and expression of interleukin-2 receptors in nonrheumatic stenotic aortic valves. *J Am Coll Cardiol* **23**:1162–1170.

46. Meng X, Ao L, Song Y, *et al.* (2008) Expression of functional Toll-like receptors 2 and 4 in human aortic valve interstitial cells: potential roles in aortic valve inflammation and stenosis. *Am J Physiol Cell Physiol* **294**:C29–C35.

47. Kaden JJ, Bickelhaupt S, Grobholz R, *et al.* (2003) Pathogenetic role of Chlamydia pneumoniae in calcific aortic stenosis: immunohistochemistry study and review of the literature. *J Heart Valve Dis* **12**:447–453.

48. Helske S, Syväranta S, Kupari M, *et al.* (2006) Possible role for mast cell-derived cathepsin G in the adverse remodelling of stenotic aortic valves. *Eur Heart J* **27**:1495–1504.

49. Kaden JJ, Kilic R, Sarikoc A, *et al.* (2005) Tumor necrosis factor alpha promotes an osteoblast-like phenotype in human aortic valve myofibroblasts: a potential regulatory mechanism of valvular calcification. *Int J Mol Med* **16**:869–872.

50. Soini Y, Salo T, & Satta J (2003) Angiogenesis is involved in the pathogenesis of nonrheumatic aortic valve stenosis. *Hum Pathol* **34**:756–763.

51. Fondard O, Detaint D, Iung B, *et al.* (2005) Extracellular matrix remodelling in human aortic valve disease: the role of matrix metalloproteinases and their tissue inhibitors. *Eur Heart J* **26**:1333–1341.

52. Mathieu P, Després JP, & Pibarot P (2007) The "valvulo-metabolic" risk in calcific aortic valve disease. *Can J Cardiol* **23** (Suppl. B): 32B–39B.

53. Yilmaz MB, Guray U, Guray Y, *et al.* (2004) Lipid profile of patients with aortic stenosis might be predictive of rate of progression. *Am Heart J* **147**:915–918.

54. Rossebo AB & Pedersen TR (2004) Hyperlipidaemia and aortic valve disease. *Curr Opinion Lipidol* **15**:447–451.

55. Otto CM (2004) Aortic stenosis and hyperlipidemia: establishing a cause-effect relationship. *Am Heart J* **147**:761–763.

56. Wenk MR (2005) The emerging field of lipidomics. *Nat Rev Drug Discov* **4**:594–610.

57. O'Brien KD, Reichenbach DD, Marcovina SM, *et al.* (1996) Apolipoproteins B, (a), and E accumulate in the morphologically early lesion of "degenerative" valvular aortic stenosis. *Arterioscler Thromb Vasc Biol* **16**:523–532.

58. Tanaka K, Sata M, Fukuda D, *et al.* (2005) Age-associated aortic stenosis in apolipoprotein E-deficient mice. *J Am Coll Cardiol* **46**:134–141.

59. Mohty D, Pibarot P, Després JP, *et al.* (2008) Association between plasma LDL particle size, valvular accumulation of oxidized LDL, and inflammation in patients with aortic stenosis. *Arterioscler Thromb Vasc Biol* **28**:187–193.

60. Drolet MC, Roussel E, Deshaies Y, *et al.* (2006) A high fat/high carbohydrate diet induces aortic valve disease in C57BL/6J mice. *J Am Coll Cardiol* **47**:850–855.

61. Demer LL (2001) Cholesterol in vascular and valvular calcification. *Circulation* **104**:1881–1883.

62. Abedin M, Lim J, Tang TB, *et al.* (2006) N-3 fatty acids inhibit vascular calcification via the p38-mitogen-activated protein kinase and peroxisome proliferator-activated receptor-gamma pathways. *Circ Res* **98**:727–729.

63. Jacob MP (2003) Extracellular matrix remodeling and matrix metalloproteinases in the vascular wall during aging and in pathological conditions. *Biomed Pharmacother* **57**:195–202.

64. Cote C, Pibarot P, Despres JP, *et al.* (2008) Association between circulating oxidised low-density lipoprotein and fibrocalcific remodelling of the aortic valve in aortic stenosis. *Heart* **94**:1175–1180.

65. Kaden JJ, Dempfle CE, Grobholz R, *et al.* (2005) Inflammatory regulation of extracellular matrix remodelling in calcific aortic valve stenosis. *Cardiovasc Pathol* **14**:80–87.

66. Merryman WD, Lukoff HD, Long RA, *et al.* (2007) Synergistic effects of cyclic tension and transforming growth factor-beta1 on the aortic valve myofibroblast. *Cardiovasc Pathol* **16**:268–276.

67. Galis ZS & Khatri JJ (2002) Matrix metalloproteinases in vascular remodeling and atherogenesis: the good, the bad, and the ugly. *Circ Res* **90**:251–262.

68. Wilton E, Bland M, Thompson M, *et al.* (2008) Matrix metalloproteinase expression in the ascending aorta and aortic valve. *Interact Cardiovasc Thorac Surg* **7**:37–40.

69. Satta J, Oiva J, Salo T, *et al.* (2003) Evidence for an altered balance between matrix metalloproteinase-9 and its inhibitors in calcific aortic stenosis. *Ann Thorac Surg* **76**:681–688.

70. Yeghiazaryan K, Skowasch D, Bauriedel G, *et al.* (2007) Could activated tissue remodeling be considered as early marker for progressive valve degeneration? Comparative analysis of checkpoint and ECM remodeling gene expression in native degenerating aortic valves and after bioprosthetic replacement. *Amino Acids* **32**:109–114.

71. Stephens EH & Grande-Allen KJ (2007) Age-related changes in collagen synthesis and turnover in porcine heart valves. *J Heart Valve Dis* **16**:672–682.

72. Basta G (2008) Receptor for advanced glycation endproducts and atherosclerosis: from basic mechanisms to clinical implications. *Atherosclerosis* **196**:9–21.

73. Ahmed SH, Clark LL, Pennington WR, *et al.* (2006) Matrix metalloproteinases/tissue inhibitors of metalloproteinases: relationship between changes in proteolytic determinants of matrix composition and structural, functional, and clinical manifestations of hypertensive heart disease. *Circulation* **113**:2089–2096.

74. Edep ME, Shirani J, Wolf P, *et al.* (2000) Matrix metalloproteinase expression in nonrheumatic aortic stenosis. *Cardiovasc Pathol* **9**:281–286.

75. Jian B, Jones PL, Li Q, *et al.* (2001) Matrix metalloproteinase-2 is associated with tenascin-C in calcific aortic stenosis. *Am J Pathol* **159**:321–327.

76. Olsson M, Rosenqvist M, & Nilsson J (1994) Expression of HLA-DR antigen and smooth muscle cell differentiation markers by valvular fibroblasts in degenerative aortic stenosis. *J Am Coll Cardiol* **24**:1664–1671.

77. Eriksen HA, Satta J, Risteli J, *et al.* (2006) Type I and type III collagen synthesis and composition in the valve matrix in aortic valve stenosis. *Atherosclerosis* **189**:91–98.

78. Kurz DJ, Kloeckener-Gruissem B, Akhmedov A, *et al.* (2006) Degenerative aortic valve stenosis, but not coronary disease, is associated with shorter telomere length in the elderly. *Arterioscler Thromb Vasc Biol* **26**:e114–117.

79. Cushing MC, Mariner PD, Liao JT, *et al.* (2008) Fibroblast growth factor represses Smad-mediated myofibroblast activation in aortic valvular interstitial cells. *FASEB J* **22**:1769–1777.

80. O'Brien KD, Shavelle DM, Caulfield MT, *et al.* (2002) Association of angiotensin-converting enzyme with low-density lipoprotein in aortic valvular lesions and in human plasma. *Circulation* **106**:2224–2230.

81. Mehta PK & Griendling KK (2007) Angiotensin II cell signaling: physiological and pathological effects in the cardiovascular system. *Am J Physiol Cell Physiol* **292**:C82–C97.

82. Helske S, Laine M, Kupari M, *et al.* (2007) Increased expression of profibrotic neutral endopeptidase and bradykinin type 1 receptors in stenotic aortic valves. *Eur Heart J* **28**:1894–1903.

83. Rosenhek R, Binder T, Porenta G, *et al.* (2000) Predictors of outcome in severe, asymptomatic aortic stenosis. *N Engl J Med* **343**:611–617.

84. Strickberger SA, Schulman SP, & Hutchins GM (1987) Association of Paget's disease of bone with calcific aortic valve disease. *Am J Med* **82**:953–956.

85. Palta S, Pai AM, Gill KS, *et al.* (2000) New insights into the progression of aortic stenosis: implications for secondary prevention. *Circulation* **101**:2497–2502.

86. Maher ER, Pazianas M, & Curtis JR (1987) Calcific aortic stenosis: a complication of chronic uraemia. *Nephron* **47**:119–122.

87. Rajamannan NM & Otto CM (2004) Targeted therapy to prevent progression of calcific aortic stenosis. *Circulation* **110**:1180–1182.

88. Skowasch D, Schrempf S, Preusse CJ, *et al.* (2006) Tissue resident C reactive protein in degenerative aortic valves: correlation

with serum C reactive protein concentrations and modification by statins. *Heart* **92**:495–498.

89. Mathieu P, Voisine P, Pépin A, *et al.* (2005) Calcification of human valve interstitial cells is dependent on alkaline phosphatase activity. *J Heart Valve Dis* **14**:353–357.

90. Aikawa E, Nahrendorf M, Fiqueiredo JL, *et al.* (2007) Osteogenesis associates with inflammation in early-stage atherosclerosis evaluated by molecular imaging *in vivo*. *Circulation* **116**:2841–2850.

91. Mohler ER (2004) Mechanisms of aortic valve calcification. *Am J Cardiol* **94**:1396–1402.

92. Radcliff K, Tang TB, Lim J, *et al.* (2005) Insulin-like growth factor-I regulates proliferation and osteoblastic differentiation of calcifying vascular cells via extracellular signal-regulated protein kinase and phosphatidylinositol 3-kinase pathways. *Circ Res* **96**:398–400.

93. Annes JP, Munger JS, & Rifkin DB (2003) Making sense of latent TGFbeta activation. *J Cell Sci* **116**:217–224.

94. Watson KE, Boström K, Ravindranath R, *et al.* (1994) TGF-beta1 and 25-hydroxycholesterol stimulate osteoblast-like vascular cells to calcify. *J Clin Invest* **93**:2106–2113.

95. Clark-Greuel JN, Connolly JM, Sorichillo E, *et al.* (2007) Transforming growth factor-beta1 mechanisms in aortic valve calcification: increased alkaline phosphatase and related events. *Ann Thorac Surg* **83**:946–953.

96. Jian B, Xu J, Connolly J, *et al.* (2002) Serotonin mechanisms in heart valve disease I: serotonin-induced up-regulation of transforming growth factor-beta1 via G-protein signal transduction in aortic valve interstitial cells. *Am J Pathol* **161**:2111–2121.

97. Xu J, Jian B, Chu R, *et al.* (2002) Serotonin mechanisms in heart valve disease II: the 5-HT2 receptor and its signaling pathway in aortic valve interstitial cells. *Am J Pathol* **161**:2209–2218.

98. Perco P, Wilflingseder J, Bernthaler A, *et al.* (2008) Biomarker candidates for cardiovascular disease and bone metabolism disorders in chronic kidney disease: a systems biology perspective. *J Cell Mol Med* **12**:1177–1187.

99. Jian B, Narula N, Li QY, *et al.* (2003) Progression of aortic valve stenosis: TGF-beta1 is present in calcified aortic valve cusps and promotes aortic valve interstitial cell calcification via apoptosis. *Ann Thorac Surg* **75**:457–465.

100. Guerraty M & Mohler ER (2007) Models of aortic valve calcification. *J Investig Med* **55**:278–283.

101. Warrier B, Mallipeddi R, Karla PK, *et al.* (2005) The functional role of C-reactive protein in aortic wall calcification. *Cardiology* **104**:57–64.

102. Satta J, Melkko J, Pöllänen R, *et al.* (2002) Progression of human aortic valve stenosis is associated with tenascin-C expression. *J Am Coll Cardiol* **39**:96–101.

103. Majumdar R, Miller DV, Ballman KV, *et al.* (2007) Elevated expressions of osteopontin and tenascin C in ascending aortic aneurysms are associated with trileaflet aortic valves as compared with bicuspid aortic valves. *Cardiovasc Pathol* **16**:144–150.

104. Kaden JJ, Bickelhaupt S, Grobholz R, *et al.* (2004) Receptor activator of nuclear factor kappaB ligand and osteoprotegerin regulate aortic valve calcification. *J Mol Cell Cardiol* **36**:57–66.

105. Ix JH, Chertow GM, Shlipak MG, *et al.* (2007) Association of fetuin-A with mitral annular calcification and aortic stenosis among persons with coronary heart disease: data from the heart and soul study. *Circulation* **115**:2533–2539.

106. Mohler ER, Chawla MK, Chang AW, *et al.* (1999) Identification and characterization of calcifying valve cells from human and canine aortic valves. *J Heart Valve Dis* **8**:254–260.

107. Liberman M, Bassi E, Martinatti MK, *et al.* (2008) Oxidant generation predominates around calcifying foci and enhances progression of aortic valve calcification. *Arterioscler Thromb Vasc Biol* **28**:463–470.

108. Shen M, Kara-Mostefa A, Chen L, *et al.* (2001) Effect of ethanol and ether in the prevention of calcification of bioprostheses. *Ann Thorac Surg* **71**:S413–S416.

109. Levy RJ (1997) Strategies to mitigate mineralization in the bioprosthetic or homograft cusp and aortic wall. *J Heart Valve Dis* **6**:7–8.

110. Li AC & Glass CK (2002) The macrophage foam cell as a target for therapeutic intervention. *Nat Med* **8**:1235–1242.

111. Morony S, Tintut Y, Zhang Z, *et al.* (2008) Osteoprotegerin inhibits vascular calcification without affecting atherosclerosis in ldlr(-/-) mice. *Circulation* **117**:411–420.

112. Mohler ER, Gannon F, Reynolds C, *et al.* (2001) Bone formation and inflammation in cardiac valves. *Circulation* **103**:1522–1528.

113. Leskelä HV, Satta J, Oiva J, *et al.* (2006) Calcification and cellularity in human aortic heart valve tissue determine the differentiation of bone-marrow-derived cells. *J Mol Cell Cardiol* **41**:642–649.

114. Caira FC, Stock SR, Gleason TG, *et al.* (2006) Human degenerative valve disease is associated with up-regulation of low-density lipoprotein receptor-related protein 5 receptor-mediated bone formation. *J Am Coll Cardiol* **47**:1707–1712.

115. Boland GM, Perkins G, Hall DJ, *et al.* (2004) Wnt 3a promotes proliferation and suppresses osteogenic differentiation of adult human mesenchymal stem cells. *J Cell Biochem* **93**:1210–1230.

116. Baksh D, Boland GM, & Tuan RS (2007) Cross-talk between Wnt signaling pathways in human mesenchymal stem cells leads to functional antagonism during osteogenic differentiation. *J Cell Biochem* **101**:1109–1124.

117. Garg V, Muth AN, Ransom JF, *et al.* (2005) Mutations in NOTCH1 cause aortic valve disease. *Nature* **437**:270–274.

118. O'Brien KD (2006) Pathogenesis of calcific aortic valve disease: a disease process comes of age (and a good deal more). *Arterioscler Thromb Vasc Biol* **26**:1721–1728.

119. Novaro GM, Sachar R, Pearce GL, *et al.* (2003) Association between apolipoprotein E alleles and calcific valvular heart disease. *Circulation* **108**:1804–1808.

120. Ortlepp JR, Pillich M, Mevissen V, *et al.* (2006) APOE alleles are not associated with calcific aortic stenosis. *Heart* **92**:1463–1466.

121. Ortlepp JR, Hoffmann R, Ohme F, *et al.* (2001) The vitamin D receptor genotype predisposes to the development of calcific aortic valve stenosis. *Heart* **85**:635–638.

122. Araújo-Vilar D, Lado-Abeal J, Palos-Paz F, *et al.* (2008) A novel phenotypic expression associated with a new mutation in LMNA gene, characterized by partial lipodystrophy, insulin resistance, aortic stenosis and hypertrophic cardiomyopathy. *Clin Endocrinol (Oxf.)* **69**:61–68.

123. Salo T, Soini Y, Oiva J, *et al.* (2006) Chemically modified tetracyclines (CMT-3 and CMT-8) enable control of the pathologic remodellation of human aortic valve stenosis via MMP-9 and VEGF inhibition. *Int J Cardiol* **111**:358–364.

124. Yoshioka M, Yuasa S, Matsumura K, *et al.* (2006) Chondromodulin-I maintains cardiac valvular function by preventing angiogenesis. *Nat Med* **12**:1151–1159.

125. Goldbarg SH, Elmariah S, Miller MA, *et al.* (2007) Insights into degenerative aortic valve disease. *J Am Coll Cardiol* **50**:1205–1213.

126. Rajamannan NM, Subramaniam M, Springett M, *et al.* (2002) Atorvastatin inhibits hypercholesterolemia-induced cellular proliferation and bone matrix production in the rabbit aortic valve. *Circulation* **105**:2660–2665.

127. Osman L, Yacoub MH, Latif N, *et al.* (2006) Role of human valve interstitial cells in valve calcification and their response to atorvastatin. *Circulation* **114**(1 Suppl.):I547–I552.

128. Rajamannan NM, Subramaniam M, Caira F, *et al.* (2005) Atorvastatin inhibits hypercholesterolemia-induced calcification in the aortic valves via the Lrp5 receptor pathway. *Circulation* **112**(9 Suppl.):I229–I234.

129. Osman L, Chester AH, Amrani M, *et al.* (2006) A novel role of extracellular nucleotides in valve calcification: a potential target for atorvastatin. *Circulation* **114**(1 Suppl.):I566–I572.

130. Osman L, Chester AH, Sarathchandra P, *et al.* (2007) A novel role of the sympatho-adrenergic system in regulating valve calcification. *Circulation* **116**(11 Suppl.):I282–I287.

131. Arishiro K, Hoshiga M, Negoro N, *et al.* (2007) Angiotensin receptor-1 blocker inhibits atherosclerotic changes and endothelial disruption of the aortic valve in hypercholesterolemic rabbits. *J Am Coll Cardiol* **49**:1482–1489.

132. Brown ML, Pellikka PA, Schaff HV, *et al.* (2008) The benefits of early valve replacement in asymptomatic patients with severe aortic stenosis. *J Thorac Cardiovasc Surg* **135**:308–315.

133. Han RK, Gurofsky RC, Lee KJ, *et al.* (2007) Outcome and growth potential of left heart structures after neonatal intervention for aortic valve stenosis. *J Am Coll Cardiol* **50**:2406–2414.

134. Avakian SD, Grinberg M, Ramires JA, *et al.* (2008) Outcome of adults with asymptomatic severe aortic stenosis. *Int J Cardiol* **123**:322–327.

135. Morgan-Hughes GJ, Roobottom CA, Owens PE, *et al.* (2004) Dilation of the aorta in pure, severe, bicuspid aortic valve stenosis. *Am Heart J* **147**:736–740.

136. Bauer M, Gliech V, Siniawski H, *et al.* (2006) Configuration of the ascending aorta in patients with bicuspid and tricuspid aortic valve disease undergoing aortic valve replacement with or without reduction aortoplasty. *J Heart Valve Dis* **15**:594–600.

8   Echocardiography of Aortic Stenosis

Michael J. Kostal & Susan E. Wiegers

University of Pennsylvania School of Medicine, Philadelphia, PA, USA

Anatomic evaluation of the aortic valve

Parasternal windows offer the clearest transthoracic echocardiographic assessment of the aortic valve. In the parasternal long-axis view, the aortic valve can be visualized anteriorly to the mitral valve. The right coronary cusp sits anteriorly, and the leaflet visualized posteriorly is typically the noncoronary cusp. These leaflets open in systole and approximate the walls of the aortic root, provided the stroke volume is normal (Fig. 8.1a). During diastole, the leaflets close, with the coaptation in the middle of the aortic root (Fig. 8.1b). The parasternal long axis usually affords the examiner the ability to visualize abnormalities of the valve leaflets such as calcification and thickening. This view also presents a good opportunity to see leaflet prolapse, vegetations, and aortic insufficiency with the assistance of color flow Doppler.

Rotation of the transducer by 90° shows an *en face* view of the valve in the parasternal short-axis view. The right coronary cusp is most anterior in this projection, with the left coronary cusp posterior and to the right and the noncoronary cusp to the left of the image, typically bisected by the interatrial septum (Fig. 8.2). The commissure between the left and right cusps lies adjacent to the pulmonic valve, and the commissure of the right and noncoronary cusps is found at the level of the tricuspid valve.

Apical five-chamber and long-axis views also show the aortic valve, but since the valve is in the far field in these views the anatomic information is often less robust. However, this view typically presents optimal alignment perpendicular to the valve and parallel to blood flow, which allows excellent Doppler ultrasound analysis of aortic stenosis and insufficiency.

Transesophageal echocardiography also plays an important role in assessment of the aortic valve. Midesophageal multiplanar imaging at an angle of roughly 130° creates a long-axis view of the valve (Fig. 8.3). This allows the best opportunity to make accurate measurements of the left ventricular outflow tract (LVOT), coronary sinuses, and the sinotubular junction. Placement of the probe in the midesophagus with an imaging angle of 35–50° reveals the short-axis view of the valve. As discussed later, this view often allows an opportunity to planimeter the area of the aortic valve opening. Transgastric placement of the probe reveals very little anatomic information about the valve but offers the best opportunity in a transesophageal study to perform Doppler interrogation of the aortic valve. Transesophageal echocardiography usually allows the crispest two-dimensional (2-D) imaging of the valve, whereas Doppler assessments are more reliable for transthoracic studies owing to the limitations of the esophagus that may prevent optimal alignment with the outflow jet [1].

Three-dimensional (3-D) echocardiography is a novel and exciting imaging modality that may enhance echocardiographic diagnosis of aortic stenosis. Both transthoracic and transesophageal imaging of the valve provide unique images that emphasize the nonplanar suspension of the commissures, despite the planar appearance of the valve on 2-D imaging. These modalities allow more detailed aortic planimetric assessments as well as volumetric assessments not currently available in traditional 2-D imaging [2–5].

Assessment of severity of aortic stenosis

Two-dimensional echocardiography

As aortic stenosis progresses, the valve leaflets become thickened and eventually exhibit decreased mobility. In patients with good acoustic windows, this can be appreciated in both the parasternal long- and short-axis views. By focusing on leaflet motion, left ventricular chamber dimensions, left ventricular wall thickness, and left ventricular function, one can gain a qualitative estimate of aortic stenosis severity [6]. In an attempt to provide more quantitative data, earlier studies measured maximal leaflet separation in the long axis as a percentage of the aortic root diameter and found a good correlation to aortic valve areas assessed by cardiac catheterization [7]. The excursion may be measured on M-mode or 2-D imaging. Other studies have suggested that an absolute leaflet excursion of less than 8 mm correlates with severe aortic stenosis [6,8].

Cardiovascular Interventions in Clinical Practice. Edited by Jürgen Haase, Hans-Joachim Schäfers, Horst Sievert and Ron Waksman. © 2010 Blackwell Publishing.

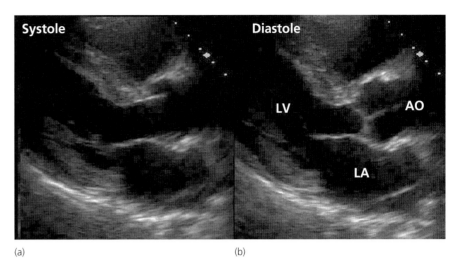

Figure 8.1 (a) Transthoracic parasternal long-axis view of the aortic root in systole. The aortic valve leaflets are opened and the ventricle has reached minimum size. The leaflets approximate the aortic root wall. The sinuses of Valsalva are evident. (b) Transthoracic parasternal long axis in diastole. The coaptation point of the valve lies in the middle of the aortic root. AO, ascending aorta; LA, left atrium; LV, left ventricle.

These methods have largely fallen to the wayside with the advent of more sophisticated Doppler-based measurements.

Planimetry

Imaging the aortic valve in short-axis views allows an examiner to attempt to planimeter maximal orifice in systole. Unfortunately, this can prove to be challenging as it requires good acoustic windows, ability to image in a plane exactly perpendicular to the valve, and the ability to select the correct level of imaging through the aortic valve (Fig. 8.2) [7,9–12]. However, some small studies have shown good correlation of transthoracic planimetry of aortic valve areas with catheter-derived aortic valve areas [11]. The improved imaging resolution of transesophageal echocardiography in concert with

the development of multiplane imaging represented a significant step forward in planimetric assessment of the aortic valve [13,14]. Multiple studies have demonstrated excellent correlation of transesophageal-based planimetry measurements with catheter-derived aortic valve areas, but not all studies have reached that conclusion [15–18].

The advent of 3-D echocardiography has advanced even further the echocardiographer's ability to obtain a precise planimetry measurement of the aortic valve area. The latest advance in 3-D echocardiography is the development of real-time image acquisition from both transthoracic and transesophageal approaches. This functionality particularly aids in definition of domed aortic valves and those with angulated orifices [2]. It also allows accurate planimetry of the aortic valve area in the presence of subvalvular or supravalvular lesions that may obfuscate traditional continuity equation calculations [2]. Real-time 3-D echocardiography enables

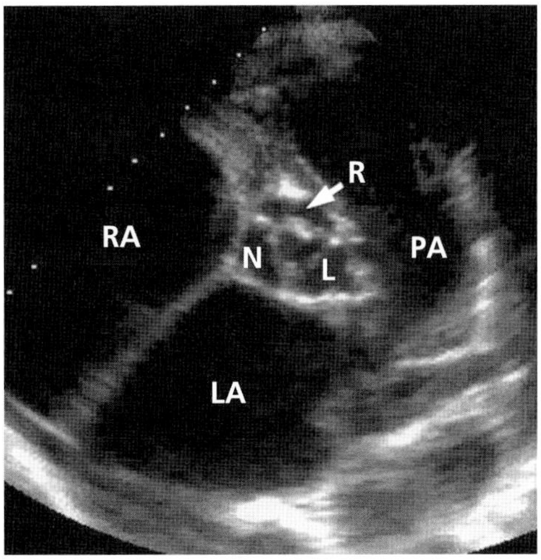

Figure 8.2 Transthoracic parasternal short axis in systole at the level of the aortic valve in a patient with rheumatic aortic stenosis. The commissures are fused and the orifice is visible in the center of the aortic root. The noncoronary cusp (N) is transected by the interatrial septum. The right coronary cusp (R) is the most anterior cusp. There is biatrial enlargement owing to severe mitral stenosis, which is not pictured here. LA, left atrium; PA, pulmonary artery; R, right coronary cusp; RA, right atrium.

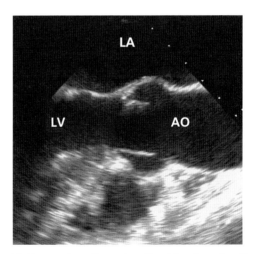

Figure 8.3 Transesophageal image from the midesophageal position: imaging angle 128°. The aorta (AO) is seen in the long axis view. In this case, the right coronary cusp is imaged at the bottom of the image. LA, left atrium; LV, left ventricle.

simultaneous visualization of parasternal long-axis and short-axis views, which in turn allows the examiner to select optimal positioning of imaging planes in which to perform planimetry [5,19]. Recent data suggest that this method of using 3-D echocardiography is feasible and accurate in assessment of aortic stenosis when compared with values derived by the continuity equation and transesophageal planimetry [19].

It is worth noting that planimetry, by definition, seeks to define a geometric assessment of aortic valve area in the setting of aortic stenosis. Doppler echocardiography and the continuity equation, discussed later in this chapter, measure an effective aortic valve area which represents the minimal cross-sectional area of the systolic jet downstream of the aortic valve [20]. Recent research has demonstrated *in vitro* that sequential increases in flow rates across simulated valves with fixed geometric orifice areas enable calculation of variable effective valve areas, as measured by the continuity equation [21]. Other authors have demonstrated significant differences between anatomic aortic valve area by planimetry and effective aortic orifice area in patients with bicuspid valves [22]. These discrepancies must be taken into consideration when assessing the severity of aortic stenosis, and they will be addressed further in subsequent sections of this chapter.

Doppler assessment of velocity and gradients

The advent of Doppler echocardiography allowed measurements of blood flow velocity and pressure gradients across the aortic valve. Blood traveling through the narrowed orifice of a stenotic aortic valve accelerates and becomes turbulent. Maximal aortic velocity is a reproducible measurement that is an excellent predictor of clinical outcome [23]. Velocities correlate with severity of aortic stenosis with the following parameters: mild 2.6–3 m/s, moderate 3–4 m/s, and severe >4 m/s [23].

The transvalvular pressure gradient is related to the transvalvular velocity by the modified Bernoulli equation:

$$\text{Pressure gradient} = 4(V_{AV}^2 - V_{LVOT}^2)$$

where V_{AV} is the velocity for the aortic valve.

The velocity in the LVOT (V_{LVOT}) is interrogated in the apical five-chamber view, with the sample volume on the ventricular side of the aortic valve (AV). The maximal gradient across the stenotic valve is recorded with continuous-wave Doppler from the apical five-chamber and apical long-axis views, as well as the second right intercostal space and the suprasternal notch. Use of a nonimaging probe with a small footprint probe (Pedhoff) in these positions usually provides the highest aortic valve velocity, but it is often the most technically demanding part of the study.

With velocities in the LVOT usually being <1 m/s, the V_{LVOT} term is typically negligible compared with the velocity jet across the obstruction. This permits further simplification of the Bernoulli equation to the following:

$$\text{Pressure gradient} = 4V_{AV}^2$$

Thus, for example, if the continuous-wave Doppler velocity across the aortic valve is 4 m/s, the calculated peak gradient across the aortic valve would be 64 mmHg. These Doppler-derived gradients usually correlate very well with catheter-derived gradients from invasive studies [24–27]. Other studies suggest that they reliably predict the risk of cardiac events over a 2-year period [28]. In general, mean gradients based on Doppler assessment can be used to stratify aortic stenosis as mild (<25 mmHg), moderate (25–40 mmHg), or severe (>40 mmHg) [29]. However, some practical and theoretical considerations must be taken into account when using this method.

Continuous-wave Doppler relies on the ultrasound beam remaining parallel to the direction of blood flow across the aortic valve. Measured velocity of the blood flow varies inversely with the cosine of the angle between the ultrasound beam and the direction of blood flow. Failure to align the ultrasound beam with the direction of blood flow will result in underestimation of the pressure gradient across the aortic valve. Older patients who present with aortic stenosis often have a more horizontal orientation of the aortic valve, rendering accurate measurements more difficult. The continuous-wave beam may also inadvertently cross other areas of high-velocity flow, such as mitral insufficiency or subclavian stenosis. This will "contaminate" the velocity recording and may lead to an overestimation of the peak and mean gradients across the aortic valve.

Aortic insufficiency imposes a volume load on the left ventricle that often results in higher flow velocities across the LVOT. This is a situation in which it may not be appropriate to discard the V_{LVOT} term, as doing so would lead to an overestimation of the aortic valve gradient. This can be remedied by including the proximal LVOT flow velocity in the Bernoulli relationship shown below:

$$P_1 - P_2 = 4(V_2^2 - V_1^2)$$

The peak gradient derived by Doppler echocardiography represents a peak instantaneous gradient, which is always higher than a catheter-derived peak–peak gradient. However, tracing the spectral envelope of the continuous-wave Doppler measurement generates a mean gradient that is similar to the mean gradient measured by invasive assessment. Recent *in vitro* research suggests that the catheter-based peak–peak gradients may be highly influenced by systemic arterial compliance, whereas peak instantaneous and mean gradients are not [30]. The catheters that cross the aortic valve in an invasive study may further obstruct a very small aortic valve orifice and artificially increase the transvalvular gradient; this does not occur in Doppler echocardiography [31].

The phenomenon of pressure recovery may explain cases in which Doppler gradients exceed invasive measurements.

The aortic stenosis ejection jet is moving fastest at the valve orifice, which is the site of greatest pressure change. The jet loses velocity as it enters the aortic root and kinetic energy is converted to potential energy. Because Doppler echocardiography measures maximal velocity across the valve and pressure catheters used in invasive studies are placed in the proximal aorta, the Doppler gradient tends to be higher. The catheter-based gradient is lower owing to pressure recovery that has occurred in the proximal aorta. The degree of pressure recovery may be significant [32–37]. An *in vitro* study that examined varying stenoses and varying amounts of jet eccentricity found that Doppler- and catheter-derived gradients correlated well with the combination of a small valve area and a large aorta [37]. However, Doppler measurements overestimated catheter-based gradients in the setting of less severe stenosis and a smaller aorta [37]. The authors assert that the magnitude of pressure recovery may be predicted and even corrected for [37]. Other researchers sought to validate a mathematical model that would predict where the aortic stenosis jet would reattach to the aortic wall, as this is the site of pressure recovery. The variables in the model included maximal jet velocity, aortic valve area, and aortic root area. The authors demonstrated that the location of pressure recovery could be accurately predicted by Doppler echocardiography *in vitro*, which could potentially allow for optimal placement of aortic pressure-sensing catheters in an invasive study [38]. Recent *in vivo* research sought to examine whether discrepancies between Doppler and catheter measurements of aortic valve gradients could be both predicted and corrected by the use of an energy loss coefficient equation, which takes into account the geometric diameter of the aorta [39,40]. When the gradients were used in the continuity equation to calculate the aortic valve area, corrected valve areas always correlated better with Gorlin-derived valve areas than with uncorrected Doppler-derived valve areas. This was particularly true at normal cardiac outputs, but correlations were slightly less robust at lower cardiac outputs [40]. Recent clinical studies have demonstrated that pressure recovery can be measured invasively and tends to be small in a majority of patients [41]. It is determined by the ratio of the aortic valve area to the ascending aorta cross-sectional area, with the combination of less severe aortic stenosis and a small aorta resulting in the greatest amount of pressure recovery, and consequently larger discrepancies between Doppler- and catheter-derived assessments of aortic stenosis severity [41].

Continuity equation

The continuity equation uses the principle of conservation of mass to calculate an aortic valve area based on Doppler echocardiography measurements [26,42–45]. The product of the velocity–time integral (VTI) at the LVOT and the cross-sectional area (CSA) of the LVOT represents the stroke volume. Conservation of mass mandates that the volume crossing the aortic valve must be the same, so the following equation can be derived:

$$CSA_{LVOT} \times VTI_{LVOT} = CSA_{AV} \times VTI_{AV}$$

The LVOT is assumed to be circular, and the area is obtained by measuring the diameter of the LVOT in the parasternal long-axis view in midsystole (Fig. 8.4a) [46]. The LVOT VTI is typically measured by pulse-wave Doppler in the apical five-chamber or long-axis view. The aortic valve VTI is obtained using continuous-wave Doppler in the same views (Fig. 8.4b). The final equation may be rearranged to solve for aortic valve area (AVA) as follows:

$$AVA = \pi (D/2)^2 \times VTI_{LVOT} / VTI_{AV}$$

where D is the diameter of the LVOT. Several studies have demonstrated excellent correlation between aortic valve areas calculated by the continuity equation and those derived by invasive studies using the Gorlin formula [16,43,44,47,48]. Previous research has established that aortic valve areas derived by the Gorlin equation are flow dependent, yielding high calculated valve areas at higher flow rates [49]. Initially, continuity-derived aortic valve areas were thought to be largely flow independent [50–52]. However, others have utilized exercise or pharmacologic methods to increase transvalvular flow and demonstrated that the aortic valve areas derived by the continuity equation are also flow dependent [53–55]. This will be particularly relevant in the discussion of low-gradient aortic stenosis to follow. Aortic valve areas are frequently classified as mild ($>1.5\,cm^2$), moderate (91.0–$1.5\,cm^2$), or severe ($<1.0\,cm^2$) aortic stenosis [29].

The continuity equation remains valid if maximal velocities in the LVOT and across the aortic valve are substituted for VTIs [23]. One may also use the velocities measured by Doppler echocardiography to generate the dimensionless index or velocity ratio, expressed as the following:

$$\text{Velocity ratio} = V_{LVOT} / V_{AS}$$

where V_{AS} is the velocity across the aortic valve, measured by continuous wave Doppler. This is particularly useful when imaging of the dimensions of the LVOT is suboptimal. A dimensionless index or velocity ratio of <0.25 suggests severe aortic stenosis [23].

The accurate measurement of the LVOT is crucial to obtaining accurate assessments of the aortic valve area via the continuity equation. The assumption that the LVOT is round and bisected by the parasternal long-axis view underpins the calculation of aortic valve area by the continuity equation. Accuracy of this measurement is particularly important as the value is squared in the continuity equation. An error in the measurement will propagate a substantial error [56,57]. Patients with normal aortic valves underwent examination by traditional transthoracic echocardiography (TEE) and 3-D echocardiography with planimetry of the LVOT. 3-D measurements allowed the authors to determine that approximately half of

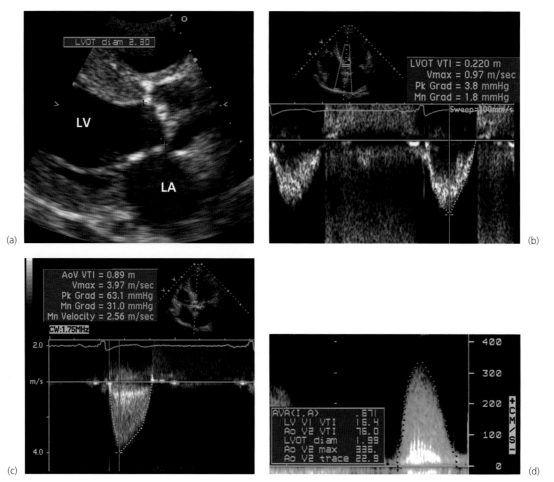

(a)

(b)

(c)

(d)

Figure 8.4 (a) Transthoracic parasternal long axis view in systole. The patient has severe calcific aortic stenosis and the leaflet motion is severely reduced. The LVOT diameter is properly measured immediately below the cusp insertions in this view. (b) Spectral display of pulse-wave Doppler at the level of the LVOT from the apical position. The modal velocity has been traced. The velocity–time integral (LVOT VTI) is 0.22 m. (c) Spectral display of continuous wave Doppler across the aortic valve from the apical position. The peak gradient is 63 mmHg and the mean gradient is 31 mmHg. The velocity time integral (AoV VTI) is 0.89 m. By the continuity equation (see text) this patient's aortic valve area is calculated as 1.0 cm². (d) From a different patient, spectral display of continuous-wave Doppler across the aortic valve from the suprasternal position is seen using a nonimaging (Pedhoff) catheter. LA, left atrium; LV, left ventricle.

the patients had elliptical LVOTs, in which major and minor diameters of the LVOT varied by 20% or greater in half of the patients. In the patients with elliptical LVOTs, the traditional 2-D calculations (πr^2) consistently underestimated LVOT area and aortic valve area compared with calculations based on 3-D planimetry of the elliptical LVOT [58]. Precise measurement of the LVOT is one area in which 3-D echocardiography may optimize noninvasive assessment.

There are other methods to circumvent the potential inaccuracies of measured LVOTs and VTIs. Recent clinical research investigated whether volumetric calculation of stroke volume by subtracting systolic volume from diastolic volume using Simpson's biplane rule could improve accuracy in assessing the aortic valve area [59–62]. They discovered that the volumetric approach correlated well with traditional continuity calculations but that it was slightly better correlated with Gorlin-based calculations, particularly in patients with

flow acceleration (velocity > 1.5 m/s) in the LVOT [63]. Other authors have focused on utilizing the ability of 3-D echocardiography to accurately assess left ventricular volume to establish a novel method of calculating aortic valve area that limits some of the potential inaccuracies of the continuity equation [64–66]. Instead of using the Doppler-derived stroke volumes described above, stroke volume was directly measured using real-time 3-D echo by subtracting end-systolic volume from end-diastolic volume. The value was then divided by the maximal aortic VTI to derive the aortic valve area. The authors then compared this value with those derived by the Gorlin equation, Hakki's formula, the Doppler continuity equation, and by deriving a stroke volume using Simpson's volumetric method. Although aortic valve areas derived by 3-D real-time echocardiography demonstrated the best linear correlation with Gorlin, they tended to consistently underestimate the aortic valve area by 0.084–0.193 cm² [57]. These volumetric-based calculations may be particularly useful in situations in which planimetry does not perform well, such as in patients with bicuspid aortic valves [22]. They are not applicable if there is significant mitral or aortic insufficiency.

Low-gradient aortic stenosis

Patients with aortic stenosis, decreased ejection fraction, and low transvalvular gradients present a unique challenge for clinicians. Its difficulty lies in determining if the patients' decreased ejection fraction is a result of inadequate left ventricular compensation (afterload mismatch) or of an independent cardiomyopathy. Surgery may be of some benefit for patients in the former group, but patients in the latter group may have a high operative risk with less expectation of improvement [67]. Dobutamine stress echocardiography plays a vital role in determining which patients have relative or "pseudo" stenosis, which have fixed aortic stenosis with left ventricular contractile reserve, and which have fixed aortic stenosis without contractile reserve [68,69]. Some authors have proposed that contractile reserve is manifested by an increase in peak velocity >0.6 m/s, an increase of >20% in stroke volume, and an increase of >10 mmHg in the mean transvalvular gradient [67].

In patients with low ejection fraction and relative or "pseudo" stenosis, a modest rise in transvalvular gradient and a more significant rise in calculated aortic valve area is to be expected [70]. Absolute increase in valve area is often >0.3 cm^2 with a final valve area >1 cm^2 [68,71,72]. In those with more severe or "fixed" stenosis and contractile reserve the rise in transvalvular gradient is more dramatic, with minimal change in aortic valve area [68,71–73]. Those with aortic stenosis and little contractile reserve often exhibit minimal change in mean pressure gradient or final aortic valve area [68,70–72,74]. Some authors recommend dobutamine stress echocardiography for any patient with aortic stenosis with a mean transvalvular gradient less than 30 mmHg [73].

It should be noted that clinical recommendations based on these findings remain difficult. Although most patients with relative or "pseudo" stenosis do not undergo surgery and do well, those in whom the valve area does not increase above 1.2 cm^2 and do not have an alternative diagnosis for left ventricular dysfunction may still benefit from surgery [70,73,75]. Patients with fixed aortic stenosis and evident contractile reserve are frequently referred for surgery; more than 75% of these patients show improvement in symptoms and left ventricular function [68,71,72]. The absence of left ventricular contractile reserve in the setting of fixed aortic stenosis predicts a poor prognosis whether surgical or medical therapy is pursued [68,71,72]. This group of patients has a higher operative mortality [71,74,76]. However, the presence or absence of contractile reserve may not reliably predict significant differences in postoperative symptoms, prognosis, and left ventricular function in those who survive surgery [67,71,77].

Variability of individual patient flow responses and the subsequent variability in transvalvular gradients and aortic valve areas may confound the attempt to delineate between relative or fixed aortic stenosis with dobutamine stress echocardiography [75,78,79]. Investigators in the TOPAS (True or Pseudo-Severe Aortic Stenosis) Study sought to establish a new parameter that could accommodate these variable responses to dobutamine stress echocardiography. They sought to derive the effective orifice area at a standardized flow rate of 250 mL/s, roughly the flow rate of patients with aortic stenosis and preserved left ventricular function. In the *in vitro* portion of the study, traditional continuity-derived effective orifice areas had good *sensitivity* for truly severe stenosis (95%) but suboptimal *specificity* (57%). The newly derived projected effective orifice area had sensitivity and specificity of 88% and 93%, respectively [75]. The parameter performed similarly well with *in vivo* studies, particularly when indexed to body surface area.

A body of literature suggests that dobutamine stress echocardiography is safe in assessing patients with low-gradient aortic stenosis [80–82]. However, it is worth noting that several studies have illuminated the increased risk of dangerous ventricular dysrhythmias with the use of dobutamine stress echocardiography in patients with aortic stenosis [80,81,83]. Furthermore, vasodilation resulting from dobutamine infusion may precipitate dangerous hypotension in patients with aortic stenosis because their stroke volume is relatively fixed, particularly in those without contractile reserve [83].

Dobutamine stress echocardiography remains the gold standard to diagnose aortic stenosis in patients with reduced ejection fraction. Recent work has sought to determine whether low-level exercise stress testing, frequently used to assess left ventricular reserve after ischemic insult, could satisfactorily answer the same question in patients with severe aortic stenosis (aortic valve area <0.75 cm^2), reduced ejection fraction (35%), and low transvalvular gradient [84,85]. Measuring the ejection fraction using Simpson's rule and the aortic valve area using the continuity equation, the authors determined that patients receiving dobutamine experienced a significant increase in ejection fraction (23%, $P < 0.001$), but patients who exercised experienced a significant decrease in ejection fraction. In contrast to the dobutamine group, those who undertook exercise could not demonstrate a significant increase in aortic valve area calculated by the continuity equation [84].

Exercise testing in asymptomatic aortic stenosis

Management of asymptomatic aortic stenosis has been a clinical conundrum for some time. The risks of operative morbidity and mortality must be weighed against the possibility of an adverse event without surgery; valve durability and the ability to sustain anticoagulation must also be considered [23]. Exercise testing has been advocated and evaluated in this setting and has demonstrated that reduced exercise tolerance, systolic blood pressure increase of <20 mmHg, and abnormal exertional symptoms favor referral for aortic valve replacement [23,86–88]. Recent investigation sought to determine whether the addition of Doppler echocardiography to exercise testing could add prognostic value to this patient population. The most robust predictors of an adverse cardiac event included an abnormal exercise test, increases in mean transvalvular gradient of ≥18 mmHg, and aortic valve area <0.75 cm^2 [89]. The study suggests that there is incremental prognostic information to be gained in adding Doppler echocardiography to exercise testing in asymptomatic patients with severe aortic stenosis.

Aortic valve resistance

Some authors have suggested that both noninvasive and invasive studies can utilize aortic valve resistance as a way to assess aortic stenosis severity in a fashion that may be less flow-dependent than methods described above [90–94]. Aortic valve resistance (R) is expressed by the following equation:

$$R = 1.333(4V_{AV}^2)/A_{LVOT} \times V_{LVOT}$$

where V_{AV} and V_{LVOT} are the velocities for the aortic valve and LVOT, respectively, and A_{LVOT} is the area of the LVOT. The conversion factor was 1.333 to dyne s/cm^{-5}. However, some studies suggested that aortic valve resistance added minimal additional information to echocardiographic assessments of the aortic valve, and that the measurement is also flow dependent [78,79,95–97].

Novel echocardiographic techniques

Severity index

Calcification of the aortic valve leaflets is readily assessed on TEE. Calcification of the valve predicts worse prognosis, and a score known as the severity index assesses and quantifies aortic leaflet calcification and mobility [98,99]. When calculated in patients undergoing invasive and echocardiographic assessment for aortic stenosis, the severity index was significantly different and increased with disease severity in patients determined to have aortic sclerosis, mild to moderate aortic stenosis, and severe aortic stenosis [100]. It also correlated well with the maximal aortic jet velocity [100]. This validation of the severity index suggests it may be a useful adjunctive tool in assessing aortic stenosis.

Contrast agents

A clinical scenario in which a patient with suboptimal transthoracic echocardiographic windows underwent cardiac catheterization but had an aortic valve that could not be crossed has been described [101]. Faced with evidence of potentially more severe aortic valve disease (heavy calcification and restricted leaflet movement) than suggested by the continuity equation, the authors administered intravenous contrast.

The enhanced Doppler measurements confirmed the clinical suspicion of severe aortic stenosis. Small studies of patients examined serially by TEE suggest that administration of intravenous contrast will improve interobserver variability for LVOT size and aortic valve area, and that it yields increased velocities at both prevalve and postvalve levels [102].

Biphasic Doppler patterns

Echocardiographic assessment of flow patterns in the aorta may also yield information regarding the severity of aortic stenosis. A series of 59 patients underwent standard TEE with measurement of Doppler flow in the descending thoracic aorta. Patients with left-sided valvular insufficiency, prosthetic aortic valves, hypertrophic cardiomyopathy, infra- or supra-aortic valvular lesions, and arrhythmia were excluded. The absence of a biphasic Doppler flow pattern in the descending aorta had a 96% negative predictive value for excluding severe stenosis in valve areas <1.5 cm^2 [103]. All patients with biphasic flow patterns and an S_1/S_2 ratio of <0.5 (where S_1 is peak velocity of the initial systolic profile and S_2 is the peak velocity of the secondary systolic profile) had severe aortic stenosis [103]. This method may assist in echocardiographic diagnosis of aortic stenosis when conventional methods are less feasible.

Peak to mean pressure decrease ratio

The observation that continuous-wave velocity envelopes are asymmetric in moderate aortic stenosis but more symmetric in severe aortic stenosis provided the stimulus for the creation of the peak to mean pressure decrease ratio [104]. The investigators demonstrated that the peak to mean pressure decrease ratio was 1.75 in mild, 1.66 in moderate, and 1.56 in severe aortic stenosis [73,104]. Researchers recently sought to validate these observations against Doppler continuity, Gorlin, and previously described echocardiography–cardiac magnetic resonance (CMR) hybrid approaches to calculating aortic valve area in small series patients who had undergone echocardiography, cardiac catheterization, and cardiac MRI [105,106]. Although ratios of <1.75 had good sensitivity (94%) and ratios <1.5 had good specificity (92%), the positive predictive value when compared with Gorlin ranged from 0.67 to 0.69, less than originally reported in previous studies [104,105]. The authors note that, although this ratio does not depend on accurate measurement of the LVOT, the ratio can vary significantly in a beat-to-beat fashion, even with well-defined Doppler envelopes [105].

Conclusion

Echocardiography provides an assessment of valvular morphology and hemodynamics that often obviates the need for invasive hemodynamic assessment. Of course, many of these patients are of an age to mandate coronary angiography before surgical valve replacement. TEE is essential for identifying the level of the obstruction, the severity of the obstruction, and associated cardiac pathology. TEE remains the mainstay of appropriate assessment of significant valve disease [107]. TEE and 3-D echocardiography are further advances in the noninvasive assessment of aortic stenosis.

References

1. Stoddard MF, Hammons RT, & Longaker RA (1996) Doppler transesophageal echocardiographic determination of aortic valve area in adults with aortic stenosis. *Am Heart J* **132**: 337–342.

2. Mallavarapu RK & Nanda NC (2007) Three-dimensional trans-thoracic echocardiographic assessment of aortic stenosis and regurgitation. *Cardiol Clin* **25**:327–234.

3. Ge S, Warner JG, Jr., Abraham TP, *et al.* (1998) Three-dimensional surface area of the aortic valve orifice by three-dimensional echocardiography: clinical validation of a novel index for assessment of aortic stenosis. *Am Heart J* **136**:1042–1050.

4. Kasprzak JD, Salustri A, Roelandt JR, & Ten Cate FJ (1998) Three-dimensional echocardiography of the aortic valve: feasibility, clinical potential, and limitations. *Echocardiography* **15**:127–138.

5. Goland S, Trento A, Iida K, *et al.* (2007) Assessment of aortic stenosis by three-dimensional echocardiography: an accurate and novel approach. *Heart* **93**:801–807.

6. Williams DE, Sahn DJ, & Friedman WF (1976) Cross-sectional echocardiographic localization of sites of left ventricular outflow tract obstruction. *Am J Cardiol* **37**:250–255.

7. Chang S, Clements S, & Chang J (1977) Aortic stenosis: echocardiographic cusp separation and surgical description of aortic valve in 22 patients. *Am J Cardiol* **39**:499–504.

8. Lesbre JP, Scheuble C, Kalisa A, Lalau JD, & Andrejak MT (1983) [Echocardiography in the diagnosis of severe aortic valve stenosis in adults]. *Arch Mal Coeur Vaiss* **76**:1–12.

9. DeMaria AN, Bommer W, Joye J, Lee G, Bouteller J, & Mason DT (1980) Value and limitations of cross-sectional echocardiography of the aortic valve in the diagnosis and quantification of valvular aortic stenosis. *Circulation* **62**:304–312.

10. Godley RW, Green D, Dillon JC, Rogers EW, Feigenbaum H, & Weyman AE (1981) Reliability of two-dimensional echocardiography in assessing the severity of valvular aortic stenosis. *Chest* **79**:657–662.

11. Okura H, Yoshida K, Hozumi T, Akasaka T, & Yoshikawa J (1997) Planimetry and transthoracic two-dimensional echocardiography in noninvasive assessment of aortic valve area in patients with valvular aortic stenosis. *J Am Coll Cardiol* **30**:753–759.

12. Weyman AE, Feigebaum H, Dillon JC, & Chang S (1975) Cross-sectional echocardiography in assessing the severity of valvular aortic stenosis. *Circulation* **52**:828–834.

13. Cormier B, Iung B, Porte JM, Barbant S, & Vahanian A (1996) Value of multiplane transesophageal echocardiography in determining aortic valve area in aortic stenosis. *Am J Cardiol* **77**:882–885.

14. Tribouilloy C, Shen WF, Peltier M, Mirode A, Rey JL, & Lesbre JP (1994) Quantitation of aortic valve area in aortic stenosis with multiplane transesophageal echocardiography: comparison with monoplane transesophageal approach. *Am Heart J* **128**:526–532.

15. Hoffmann R, Flachskampf FA, & Hanrath P (1993) Planimetry of orifice area in aortic stenosis using multiplane transesophageal echocardiography. *J Am Coll Cardiol* **22**:529–534.

16. Kim CJ, Berglund H, Nishioka T, Luo H, & Siegel RJ (1996) Correspondence of aortic valve area determination from transesophageal echocardiography, transthoracic echocardiography, and cardiac catheterization. *Am Heart J* **132**:1163–1172.

17. Stoddard MF, Arce J, Liddell NE, Peters G, Dillon S, & Kupersmith J (1991) Two-dimensional transesophageal echocardiographic determination of aortic valve area in adults with aortic stenosis. *Am Heart J* **122**:1415–1422.

18. Bernard Y, Meneveau N, Vuillemenot A, *et al.* (1997) Planimetry of aortic valve area using multiplane transoesophageal echocardiography is not a reliable method for assessing severity of aortic stenosis. *Heart* **78**:68–73.

19. Blot-Souletie N, Hebrard A, Acar P, Carrie D, & Puel J (2007) Comparison of accuracy of aortic valve area assessment in aortic stenosis by real time three-dimensional echocardiography in biplane mode versus two-dimensional transthoracic and transesophageal echocardiography. *Echocardiography* **24**:1065–1072.

20. Garcia D & Kadem L (2006) What do you mean by aortic valve area: geometric orifice area, effective orifice area, or Gorlin area? *J Heart Valve Dis* **15**:601–608.

21. Kadem L, Rieu R, Dumesnil JG, Durand LG, & Pibarot P (2006) Flow-dependent changes in Doppler-derived aortic valve effective orifice area are real and not due to artifact. *J Am Coll Cardiol* **47**:131–137.

22. Donal E, Novaro GM, Deserrano D, *et al.* (2005) Planimetric assessment of anatomic valve area overestimates effective orifice area in bicuspid aortic stenosis. *J Am Soc Echocardiogr* **18**:1392–1398.

23. Otto CM (2006) Valvular aortic stenosis: disease severity and timing of intervention. *J Am Coll Cardiol* **47**:2141–2151.

24. Currie PJ, Seward JB, Reeder GS, *et al.* (1985) Continuous-wave Doppler echocardiographic assessment of severity of calcific aortic stenosis: a simultaneous Doppler-catheter correlative study in 100 adult patients. *Circulation* **71**:1162–1169.

25. Berger M, Berdoff RL, Gallerstein PE, & Goldberg E (1984) Evaluation of aortic stenosis by continuous wave Doppler ultrasound. *J Am Coll Cardiol* **3**:150–156.

26. Kosturakis D, Allen HD, Goldberg SJ, Sahn DJ, & Valdes-Cruz LM (1984) Noninvasive quantification of stenotic semilunar valve areas by Doppler echocardiography. *J Am Coll Cardiol* **3**:1256–1262.

27. Simpson IA, Houston AB, Sheldon CD, Hutton I, & Lawrie TD (1985) Clinical value of Doppler echocardiography in the assessment of adults with aortic stenosis. *Br Heart J* **53**:636–639.

28. Pellikka PA, Nishimura RA, Bailey KR, & Tajik AJ (1990) The natural history of adults with asymptomatic, hemodynamically significant aortic stenosis. *J Am Coll Cardiol* **15**:1012–1017.

29. Bonow RO, Carabello BA, Kanu C, *et al.* (2006) ACC/AHA 2006 guidelines for the management of patients with valvular heart disease: a report of the American College of Cardiology/American Heart Association Task Force on Practice Guidelines (writing Committee to Revise the 1998 guidelines for the management of patients with valvular heart disease) developed in

collaboration with the Society of Cardiovascular Anesthesiologists endorsed by the Society for Cardiovascular Angiography and Interventions and the Society of Thoracic Surgeons. *J Am Coll Cardiol* **48**:e1–148.

30. Kadem L, Garcia D, Durand LG, Rieu R, Dumesnil JG, & Pibarot P (2006) Value and limitations of peak-to-peak gradient for evaluation of aortic stenosis. *J Heart Valve Dis* **15**:609–616.

31. Adele C, Vaitkus PT, & Tischler MD (1997) Evaluation of the significance of a transvalvular catheter on aortic valve gradient in aortic stenosis: a direct hemodynamic and Doppler echocardiographic study. *Am J Cardiol* **79**:513–516.

32. Laskey WK & Kussmaul WG (1994) Pressure recovery in aortic valve stenosis. *Circulation* **89**:116–121.

33. Voelker W, Reul H, Stelzer T, Schmidt A, & Karsch KR (1992) Pressure recovery in aortic stenosis: an in vitro study in a pulsatile flow model. *J Am Coll Cardiol* **20**:1585–1593.

34. Baumgartner H, Khan S, DeRobertis M, Czer L, & Maurer G (1990) Discrepancies between Doppler and catheter gradients in aortic prosthetic valves in vitro. A manifestation of localized gradients and pressure recovery. *Circulation* **82**:1467–1475.

35. Levine RA, Jimoh A, Cape EG, McMillan S, Yoganathan AP, & Weyman AE (1989) Pressure recovery distal to a stenosis: potential cause of gradient "overestimation" by Doppler echocardiography. *J Am Coll Cardiol* **13**:706–715.

36. Cape EG, Jones M, Yamada I, VanAuker MD, & Valdes-Cruz LM (1996) Turbulent/viscous interactions control Doppler/catheter pressure discrepancies in aortic stenosis. The role of the Reynolds number. *Circulation* **94**:2975–2981.

37. Niederberger J, Schima H, Maurer G, & Baumgartner H (1996) Importance of pressure recovery for the assessment of aortic stenosis by Doppler ultrasound. Role of aortic size, aortic valve area, and direction of the stenotic jet in vitro. *Circulation* **94**:1934–1940.

38. Rhodes KD, Stroml JA, Rahman MM, & VanAuker MD (2007) Prediction of pressure recovery location in aortic valve stenosis: an in-vitro validation study. *J Heart Valve Dis* **16**:489–494.

39. Garcia D, Dumesnil JG, Durand LG, Kadem L, & Pibarot P (2003) Discrepancies between catheter and Doppler estimates of valve effective orifice area can be predicted from the pressure recovery phenomenon: practical implications with regard to quantification of aortic stenosis severity. *J Am Coll Cardiol* **41**:435–442.

40. Razzolini R, Manica A, Tarantini G, Ramondo A, Napodano M, & Iliceto S (2007) Discrepancies between catheter and Doppler estimates of aortic stenosis: the role of pressure recovery evaluated "in vivo". *J Heart Valve Dis* **16**:225–229.

41. Isaaz K, Gaillard O, Cerisier A, *et al.* (2004) How important is the impact of pressure recovery on routine evaluation of aortic stenosis? A clinical study in 91 patients. *J Heart Valve Dis* **13**:347–356.

42. Zoghbi WA, Farmer KL, Soto JG, Nelson JG, & Quinones MA (1986) Accurate noninvasive quantification of stenotic aortic valve area by Doppler echocardiography. *Circulation* **73**:452–459.

43. Skjaerpe T, Hegrenaes L, & Hatle L (1985) Noninvasive estimation of valve area in patients with aortic stenosis by Doppler ultrasound and two-dimensional echocardiography. *Circulation* **72**:810–818.

44. Otto CM, Pearlman AS, Comess KA, Reamer RP, Janko CL, & Huntsman LL (1986) Determination of the stenotic aortic valve area in adults using Doppler echocardiography. *J Am Coll Cardiol* **7**:509–517.

45. Richards KL, Cannon SR, Miller JF, & Crawford MH (1986) Calculation of aortic valve area by Doppler echocardiography: a direct application of the continuity equation. *Circulation* **73**:964–969.

46. Dittmann H, Voelker W, Karsch KR, & Seipel L (1987) Influence of sampling site and flow area on cardiac output measurements by Doppler echocardiography. *J Am Coll Cardiol* **10**:818–823.

47. Oh JK, Taliercio CP, Holmes DR, Jr., *et al.* (1988) Prediction of the severity of aortic stenosis by Doppler aortic valve area determination: prospective Doppler-catheterization correlation in 100 patients. *J Am Coll Cardiol* **11**:1227–1234.

48. Teirstein P, Yeager M, Yock PG, & Popp RL (1986) Doppler echocardiographic measurement of aortic valve area in aortic stenosis: a noninvasive application of the Gorlin formula. *J Am Coll Cardiol* **8**:1059–1065.

49. Cannon SR, Richards KL, & Crawford M (1985) Hydraulic estimation of stenotic orifice area: a correction of the Gorlin formula. *Circulation* **71**:1170–1178.

50. Blackshear JL, Kapples EJ, Lane GE, & Safford RE (1992) Beat-by-beat aortic valve area measurements indicate constant orifice area in aortic stenosis: analysis of Doppler data with varying RR intervals. *J Am Soc Echocardiogr* **5**:414–420.

51. Casale PN, Palacios IF, Abascal VM, *et al.* (1992) Effects of dobutamine on Gorlin and continuity equation valve areas and valve resistance in valvular aortic stenosis. *Am J Cardiol* **70**:1175–1179.

52. Lee TM, Su SF, Chen MF, Liau CS, & Lee YT (1996) Effects of increasing flow rate on aortic stenotic indices: evidence from percutaneous transvenous balloon dilatation of the mitral valve in patients with combined aortic and mitral stenosis. *Heart* **76**:490–494.

53. Burwash IG, Pearlman AS, Kraft CD, Miyake-Hull C, Healy NL, & Otto CM (1994) Flow dependence of measures of aortic stenosis severity during exercise. *J Am Coll Cardiol* **24**:1342–1350.

54. Burwash IG, Thomas DD, Sadahiro M, *et al.* (1994) Dependence of Gorlin formula and continuity equation valve areas on transvalvular volume flow rate in valvular aortic stenosis. *Circulation* **89**:827–835.

55. Rask LP, Karp KH, & Eriksson NP (1996) Flow dependence of the aortic valve area in patients with aortic stenosis: assessment by application of the continuity equation. *J Am Soc Echocardiogr* **9**:295–299.

56. Myreng Y, Molstad P, Endresen K, & Ihlen H (1990) Reproducibility of echocardiographic estimates of the area of stenosed aortic valves using the continuity equation. *Int J Cardiol* **26**:349–354; discussion 355–359.

57. Gutierrez-Chico JL, Zamorano JL, Prieto-Moriche E, *et al.* (2008) Real-time three-dimensional echocardiography in aortic stenosis: a novel, simple, and reliable method to improve accuracy in area calculation. *Eur Heart J* **29**:1296–1306.

58. Doddamani S, Bello R, Friedman MA, *et al.* (2007) Demonstration of left ventricular outflow tract eccentricity by real time 3D echocardiography: implications for the determination of aortic valve area. *Echocardiography* **24**:860–866.

59. Gueret P, Meerbaum S, Zwehl W, *et al.* (1981) Two-dimensional echocardiographic assessment of left ventricular stroke volume:

experimental correlation with thermodilution and cineangiography in normal and ischemic states. *Cathet Cardiovasc Diagn* **7**:247–258.

60. Mercier JC, DiSessa TG, Jarmakani JM, *et al.* (1982) Two-dimensional echocardiographic assessment of left ventricular volumes and ejection fraction in children. *Circulation* **65**:962–969.

61. St John Sutton M, Otterstat JE, Plappert T, *et al.* (1998) Quantitation of left ventricular volumes and ejection fraction in post-infarction patients from biplane and single plane two-dimensional echocardiograms. A prospective longitudinal study of 371 patients. *Eur Heart J* **19**:808–816.

62. Wahr DW, Wang YS, & Schiller NB (1983) Left ventricular volumes determined by two-dimensional echocardiography in a normal adult population. *J Am Coll Cardiol* **1**:863–868.

63. Dumont Y & Arsenault M (2003) An alternative to standard continuity equation for the calculation of aortic valve area by echocardiography. *J Am Soc Echocardiogr* **16**:1309–1315.

64. Kim WY, Sogaard P, Egeblad H, Andersen NT, & Kristensen B (2001) Three-dimensional echocardiography with tissue harmonic imaging shows excellent reproducibility in assessment of left ventricular volumes. *J Am Soc Echocardiogr* **14**:612–617.

65. Kim WY, Sogaard P, Mortensen PT, *et al.* (2001) Three dimensional echocardiography documents haemodynamic improvement by biventricular pacing in patients with severe heart failure. *Heart* **85**:514–520.

66. Mannaerts HF, Van Der Heide JA, Kamp O, *et al.* (2003) Quantification of left ventricular volumes and ejection fraction using freehand transthoracic three-dimensional echocardiography: comparison with magnetic resonance imaging. *J Am Soc Echocardiogr* **16**:101–109.

67. Lange RA & Hillis LD (2006) Dobutamine stress echocardiography in patients with low-gradient aortic stenosis. *Circulation* **113**:1718–1720.

68. deFilippi CR, Willett DL, Brickner ME, *et al.* (1995) Usefulness of dobutamine echocardiography in distinguishing severe from nonsevere valvular aortic stenosis in patients with depressed left ventricular function and low transvalvular gradients. *Am J Cardiol* **75**:191–194.

69. Bermejo J & Yotti R (2007) Low-gradient aortic valve stenosis: value and limitations of dobutamine stress testing. *Heart* **93**:298–302.

70. Schwammenthal E, Vered Z, Moshkowitz Y, *et al.* (2001) Dobutamine echocardiography in patients with aortic stenosis and left ventricular dysfunction: predicting outcome as a function of management strategy. *Chest* **119**:1766–1777.

71. Monin JL, Quere JP, Monchi M, *et al.* (2003) Low-gradient aortic stenosis: operative risk stratification and predictors for long-term outcome: a multicenter study using dobutamine stress hemodynamics. *Circulation* **108**:319–324.

72. Wu WC, Ireland LA, & Sadaniantz A (2004) Evaluation of aortic valve disorders using stress echocardiography. *Echocardiography* **21**:459–466.

73. Chambers J (2006) Low "gradient", low flow aortic stenosis. *Heart* **92**:554–558.

74. Monin JL, Monchi M, Gest V, Duval-Moulin AM, Dubois-Rande JL, & Gueret P (2001) Aortic stenosis with severe left ventricular dysfunction and low transvalvular pressure gradients: risk stratification by low-dose dobutamine echocardiography. *J Am Coll Cardiol* **37**:2101–2107.

75. Blais C, Burwash IG, Mundigler G, *et al.* (2006) Projected valve area at normal flow rate improves the assessment of stenosis severity in patients with low-flow, low-gradient aortic stenosis: the multicenter TOPAS (Truly or Pseudo-Severe Aortic Stenosis) study. *Circulation* **113**:711–721.

76. Nishimura RA, Grantham JA, Connolly HM, Schaff HV, Higano ST, & Holmes DR, Jr. (2002) Low-output, low-gradient aortic stenosis in patients with depressed left ventricular systolic function: the clinical utility of the dobutamine challenge in the catheterization laboratory. *Circulation* **106**:809–813.

77. Quere JP, Monin JL, Levy F, *et al.* (2006) Influence of preoperative left ventricular contractile reserve on postoperative ejection fraction in low-gradient aortic stenosis. *Circulation* **113**:1738–1744.

78. Burwash IG, Hay KM, & Chan KL (2002) Hemodynamic stability of valve area, valve resistance, and stroke work loss in aortic stenosis: a comparative analysis. *J Am Soc Echocardiogr* **15**:814–822.

79. Blais C, Pibarot P, Dumesnil JG, Garcia D, Chen D, & Durand LG (2001) Comparison of valve resistance with effective orifice area regarding flow dependence. *Am J Cardiol* **88**:45–52.

80. Lin SS, Roger VL, Pascoe R, Seward JB, & Pellikka PA (1998) Dobutamine stress Doppler hemodynamics in patients with aortic stenosis: feasibility, safety, and surgical correlations. *Am Heart J* **136**:1010–1016.

81. Plonska E, Szyszka A, Kasprzak J, *et al.* (2001) [Side effects during dobutamine stress echocardiography in patients with aortic stenosis]. *Pol Merkur Lekarski* **11**:406–410.

82. Takeda S, Rimington H, & Chambers J (2001) Prediction of symptom-onset in aortic stenosis: a comparison of pressure drop/flow slope and haemodynamic measures at rest. *Int J Cardiol* **81**:131–137, discussion 138–139.

83. Bountioukos M, Kertai MD, Schinkel AF, *et al.* (2003) Safety of dobutamine stress echocardiography in patients with aortic stenosis. *J Heart Valve Dis* **12**:441–446.

84. Ennezat PV, Toussaint J, Marechaux S, *et al.* (2007) Low-level exercise echocardiography fails to elicit left ventricular contractile reserve in patients with aortic stenosis, reduced ejection fraction, and low transvalvular gradient. *Echocardiography* **24**:47–51.

85. Hoffer EP, Dewe W, Celentano C, & Pierard LA (1999) Low-level exercise echocardiography detects contractile reserve and predicts reversible dysfunction after acute myocardial infarction: comparison with low-dose dobutamine echocardiography. *J Am Coll Cardiol* **34**:989–997.

86. Otto CM, Pearlman AS, Kraft CD, Miyake-Hull CY, Burwash IG, & Gardner CJ (1992) Physiologic changes with maximal exercise in asymptomatic valvular aortic stenosis assessed by Doppler echocardiography. *J Am Coll Cardiol* **20**:1160–1167.

87. Das P, Rimington H, & Chambers J (2005) Exercise testing to stratify risk in aortic stenosis. *Eur Heart J* **26**:1309–1313.

88. Chambers J & Das P (2001) Treadmill exercise in apparently asymptomatic aortic stenosis. *Heart* **86**:361–362.

89. Lancellotti P, Lebois F, Simon M, Tombeux C, Chauvel C, & Pierard LA (2005) Prognostic importance of quantitative exercise Doppler echocardiography in asymptomatic valvular aortic stenosis. *Circulation* **112**(Suppl.):I377–I382.

90. Antonini-Canterin F, Faggiano P, Zanuttini D, & Ribichini F (1999) Is aortic valve resistance more clinically meaningful than valve area in aortic stenosis? *Heart* **82**:9–10.

91. Bermejo J, Garcia-Fernandez MA, Torrecilla EG, *et al.* (1996) Effects of dobutamine on Doppler echocardiographic indexes of aortic stenosis. *J Am Coll Cardiol* **28**:1206–1213.

92. Blitz LR & Herrmann HC (1996) Hemodynamic assessment of patients with low-flow, low-gradient valvular aortic stenosis. *Am J Cardiol* **78**:657–661.

93. Cannon JD Jr., Zile MR, Crawford FA, Jr., & Carabello BA (1992) Aortic valve resistance as an adjunct to the Gorlin formula in assessing the severity of aortic stenosis in symptomatic patients. *J Am Coll Cardiol* **20**:1517–1523.

94. Ho PP, Pauls GL, Lamberton DF, Portnoff JS, Pai RG, & Shah PM (1994) Doppler derived aortic valve resistance in aortic stenosis: its hemodynamic validation. *J Heart Valve Dis* **3**:283–287.

95. Mascherbauer J, Schima H, Rosenhek R, Czerny M, Maurer G, & Baumgartner H (2004) Value and limitations of aortic valve resistance with particular consideration of low flow-low gradient aortic stenosis: an in vitro study. *Eur Heart J* **25**:787–793.

96. Roger VL, Seward JB, Bailey KR, Oh JK, & Mullany CJ (1997) Aortic valve resistance in aortic stenosis: Doppler echocardiographic study and surgical correlation. *Am Heart J* **134**:924–929.

97. Voelker W, Reul H, Nienhaus G, *et al.* (1995) Comparison of valvular resistance, stroke work loss, and Gorlin valve area for quantification of aortic stenosis. An in vitro study in a pulsatile aortic flow model. *Circulation* **91**:1196–1204.

98. Rosenhek R, Binder T, Porenta G, *et al.* (2000) Predictors of outcome in severe, asymptomatic aortic stenosis. *N Engl J Med* **343**:611–617.

99. Bahler RC, Desser DR, Finkelhor RS, Brener SJ, & Youssefi M (1999) Factors leading to progression of valvular aortic stenosis. *Am J Cardiol* **84**:1044–1048.

100. Shavelle DM, Buljabasic N, Takasu J, *et al.* (2006) Validation of the severity index by cardiac catheterization and Doppler echocardiography in patients with aortic sclerosis and stenosis. *Cardiovasc Ultrasound* **4**:12.

101. Dwivedi G, Hickman M, & Senior R (2006) Accurate assessment of aortic stenosis with intravenous contrast. *Eur J Echocardiogr* **7**:65–67.

102. Smith LA, Cowell SJ, White AC, *et al.* (2004) Contrast agent increases Doppler velocities and improves reproducibility of aortic valve area measurements in patients with aortic stenosis. *J Am Soc Echocardiogr* **17**:247–252.

103. Hansen WH, Behrenbeck T, Spittell PC, Gilman G, & Seward JB (2005) Biphasic Doppler pattern of the descending thoracic aorta: a new echocardiographic finding in patients with aortic valve stenosis. *J Am Soc Echocardiogr* **18**:860–864.

104. Chambers J, Rajani R, Hankins M, & Cook R (2005) The peak to mean pressure decrease ratio: a new method of assessing aortic stenosis. *J Am Soc Echocardiogr* **18**:674–678.

105. Haghi D, Kaden JJ, & Suselbeck T (2007) Validation of the peak to mean pressure decrease ratio as a new method of assessing aortic stenosis using the Gorlin formula and the cardiovascular magnetic resonance-based hybrid method. *Echocardiography* **24**:335–339.

106. Haghi D, Papavassiliu T, Kalmar G, *et al.* (2005) A hybrid approach for quantification of aortic valve stenosis using cardiac magnetic resonance imaging and echocardiography. *J Cardiovasc Magn Reson* **7**:581–586.

107. Douglas PS, Khandheria B, Stainback RF, *et al.* (2007) ACCF/ASE/ACEP/ASNC/SCAI/SCCT/SCMR 2007 appropriateness criteria for transthoracic and transesophageal echocardiography: a report of the American College of Cardiology Foundation Quality Strategic Directions Committee Appropriateness Criteria Working Group, American Society of Echocardiography, American College of Emergency Physicians, American Society of Nuclear Cardiology, Society for Cardiovascular Angiography and Interventions, Society of Cardiovascular Computed Tomography, and the Society for Cardiovascular Magnetic Resonance. Endorsed by the American College of Chest Physicians and the Society of Critical Care Medicine. *J Am Soc Echocardiogr* **20**:787–805.

9   MRI of Aortic Stenosis

Daniel Thomas & Torsten Sommer

Department of Radiology, University of Bonn, Bonn, Germany

Introduction

Currently available magnetic resonance imaging (MRI) sequences offer a variety of approaches for the assessment of aortic valvular stenosis. Sophisticated vector-ECG and respiratory compensation techniques allow us to "freeze" cardiac motion and thus provide artifact-free imaging of the aortic valve throughout the cardiac cycle. The aortic valve and aortic valve area (AVA) can be imaged in any desired plane. Being a tomographic imaging technique, MRI is not limited by an acoustic window. Using turbo spin-echo sequences with blood suppression (BB-TSE) or fast gradient echo (GRE) sequences—of which the balanced steady-state free precession (b-SSFP) sequences have become the standard for cardiac applications—the anatomy of the left ventricular outflow tract and the aortic valve leaflets can be visualized clearly [1,2]. Furthermore, flow-sensitive imaging sequences, which allow for quantitative assessment of through-plane and in-plane blood flow, permit quantitative assessment of cross-plane transvalvular blood flow throughout the cardiac cycle as well as the in-plane depiction of the poststenotic jet area [3,4]. Thus, very much like echocardiography and invasive catheterization, aortic stenosis severity can be assessed by two distinct approaches. They are used in direct anatomic assessment of the valve leaflets and planimetry of the aortic valve area (echocardiography), as well as indirect assessment of stenosis severity by calculation of the functional aortic valve area using the continuity equation (echocardiography) [5] or Gorlin formula (invasive catheter angiography) [6]. However, unlike echocardiography, MRI does not suffer from limitations given by a poor acoustic window. Also, with echocardiography, anatomic assessment of the valve and valve area is often limited by heavy valvular calcification, whereas flow measurements may be limited by eccentric poststenotic jet morphology. In addition, reliable direct planimetry of the valve area using echo generally requires

a transesophageal echocardiographic approach, which is invasive and associated with significant patient discomfort. Assessment of aortic stenosis by invasive angiography is associated with a significant risk of cerebral embolism in addition to the general risk of invasive angiography [7]. As stated above, MRI using a multiparametric approach allows a comprehensive assessment of aortic valve stenosis within only one noninvasive examination. Practical and technical considerations, as well as the extensive research that has been performed, underscoring the suitability of MRI for imaging of the aortic valve, will be outlined and discussed in the following chapter.

Assessment of left ventricular outflow tract, valve anatomy, and stenotic jet

Magnetic resonance imaging protocol

A standard protocol for imaging of the outflow tract and valve anatomy, including the valve area, should comprise of the following MRI sequences:

• After acquisition of appropriate localizer images, a true four-chamber, two-chamber, short-axis, and left ventricular outflow tract (LVOT) cine sequence (b-SSFP; balanced steady-state free precession) is acquired.

• The LVOT should then be covered in a second, preferably coronal, plane. Using both planes transecting the aortic valve longitudinally will allow planning of subsequent cine (b-SSFP) and anatomic (BB-TSE; turbo spin-echo sequences with blood suppression) sequences orthogonal to the aortic valve.

• Optionally, three-dimensional (3-D) contrast-enhanced angiography of the aorta can be considered, allowing excellent assessment of the aortic root and ascending aorta.

Left ventricular outflow tract and aortic valve anatomy

The imaging protocol presented above allows for the assessment of typical morphologic findings associated with aortic stenosis [1,8–10]. In degenerative or rheumatoid disease, calcification or thickening of the valve leaflets can be seen (Figs. 9.1 and 9.2). Congenital abnormalities such as bicuspid

Cardiovascular Interventions in Clinical Practice. Edited by Jürgen Haase, Hans-Joachim Schäfers, Horst Sievert and Ron Waksman. © 2010 Blackwell Publishing.

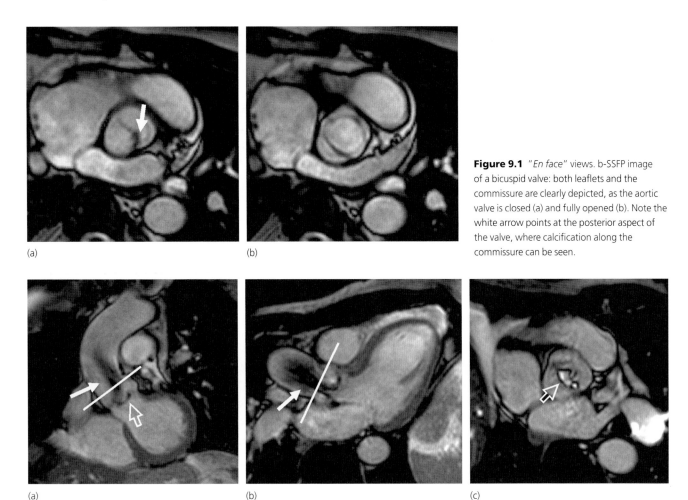

Figure 9.1 *"En face"* views. b-SSFP image of a bicuspid valve: both leaflets and the commissure are clearly depicted, as the aortic valve is closed (a) and fully opened (b). Note the white arrow points at the posterior aspect of the valve, where calcification along the commissure can be seen.

Figure 9.2 Coronal (a), LVOT (b), and *en face* (c) view of the aortic valve: The *"en face"* view (c) has been planned on images (a) and (b) (white line in a and b). The white closed arrow (a, b) points at the stenotic jet, which corresponds to a signal void due to spin dephasing. The jet emerges right distally to the opening of the heavily calcified valve (open arrow in a). The *en face* view demonstrates the reduced orifice of the aortic valve, where the commissures do not open sufficiently (open arrow in c). Planimetry of the orifice revealed an AVA of 1.2 cm², consistent with moderate stenosis.

valves can also be easily depicted (Fig. 9.1). It should be noted, however, that the temporal and spatial resolution of MRI is currently insufficient to visualize valvular vegetations on a routine basis, although visualization of vegetation has been reported [9]. Although simple valve morphology can be depicted using standard BB-TSE sequences, b-SSFP cine images will allow assessment of abnormal valve motion such as restricted valve mobility, doming, or altered pliability. An imaging protocol covering the LVOT and entire left ventricle will allow the exclusion of subvalvular (caused by, for example, hypertrophic obstructive cardiomyopathy; HOCM) or supravalvular aortic stenosis. Particularly in the case of subvalvular stenosis caused by HOCM, MRI will allow the visualization of high-velocity blood flow caused by obstruction of the outflow tract as well as an associated systolic anterior movement (SAM) phenomenon (of the mitral valve). In addition, MRI can be used to quantify the LVOT obstruction by planimetry in HOCM [11,12]. Assessment of aortic stenosis using MRI should not focus only on assessment of

degree of stenosis but should include determination of global left ventricular function (ejection fraction, volume) and mass [13,14]. Although the decision to undertake surgical intervention in aortic stenosis will depend primarily on clinical symptoms, following the American Heart Association and American College of Cardiology (AHA/ACC) guidelines, significant ventricular dysfunction is another cornerstone supporting the decision for surgery [15]. Use of a comprehensive imaging protocol allows the characterization of left ventricular concentric hypertrophy and dilation of the left atrium, which are associated with aortic stenosis. In the case of high-grade stenosis, the jet flow beyond the valve may exert shear forces on the ascending aorta, ultimately leading to aortic dilation. Such consequences of a stenotic valve can be depicted easily using coronal images as described above. However, if there is suspicion of an enlargement of the ascending aorta, standard contrast-enhanced 3-D magnetic resonance angiography will allow reliable assessment of the thoracic aorta [16].

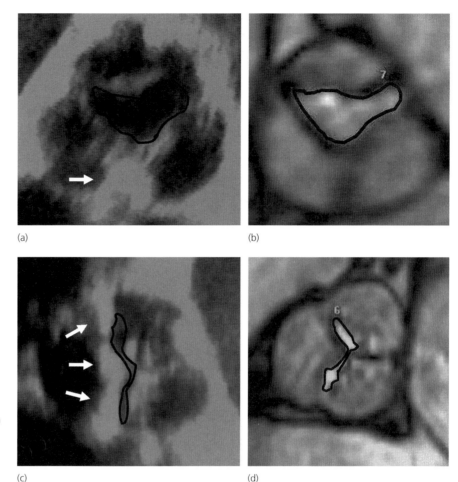

Figure 9.3 *En face* views of corresponding TEE and MRI studies (a and b and c and d): The valve orifice is clearly visualized by both TEE (a, c) and MRI (b, d). However, heavy valve calcification, which can be seen in both cases (arrows in a and c), renders clear delineation of the commissure difficult by TEE (c). Although the AVA was 1.5 cm² in the first patient (a, b) consistent with low-grade stenosis, it was 1.0 cm² in the second patient (c, d) with moderate stenosis.

Imaging of stenotic jet and area of signal loss

Turbulent flow and associated magnetic spin dephasing will lead to signal loss distal to a stenotic vessel on gradient-echo images [10,17,18]. According to the flow dynamics across a stenotic valve, a stable central jet core can be visualized with lateral zones of turbulence. In an experimental setting there is a correlation between the area of signal loss and the blood flow velocity/pressure gradient across the stenosis, and thus the degree of stenosis [18]. However, in a clinical setting there are a number of factors influencing the degree of signal loss and appearance of the jet. These are anatomic factors, such as the geometry of the AVA and the geometry of the LVOT, exerting direct effects on the jet direction and configuration through shear forces and higher orders of motion. On the other hand, the imaging sequence itself has a great influence on the appearance of the jet. Newer b-SSFP sequences are inherently less sensitive to flow disturbances than are conventional GRE sequences, and thus show smaller areas of signal loss than GRE sequences across the same stenosis [2,19]. Another factor with significant impact on appearance of the jet and area of signal loss is echo time, for which the simple rule is that the longer the echo time, the more spin dephasing will occur, and subsequently the larger the jet will

appear. That said, it becomes apparent that mere assessment of the jet and the area of signal loss cannot be used for reliable stenosis quantitation. However, in a routine clinical setting, in which imaging protocols and planning of imaging planes are standardized, the jet appearance can be used well for a first appraisal of a stenotic valve.

Direct assessment of aortic stenosis severity by measurement of the aortic valve area

In comparison with techniques indirectly measuring the valve area by calculation of the functional valve area, direct planimetry of the valve orifice is less dependent on cardiac output and function, which influences flow-dependent measures of the aortic valve area (e.g., Gorlin formula), and may influence noninvasive pressure measurements (e.g., the Bernoulli equation) [20–22]. For accurate planimetry of the AVA, three or more cine b-SSFP imaging slices should be acquired orthogonal to the aortic valve, such that valve area can be assessed at the narrowest location at end-systole and planimetry is not performed below or above the tips of the leaflets (Fig. 9.3). Alternatively, a standard GRE sequence can be used but the b-SSFP sequence-derived measurements have been shown to correlate more closely with TEE (mean difference b-SSFP versus TEE $0.15 \pm 0.13\,\text{cm}^2$, and GRE versus TEE $0.29 \pm 0.17\,\text{cm}^2$) [23]. Using the planimetry approach, very good correlation in the range of $r = 0.86–0.96\,\text{cm}^2$ and good agreement with mean differences in the range of $0.05–0.1\,\text{cm}^2$ between MRI and TEE have been found by various investigators [24–28]. Similarly, recent studies comparing MRI and multi-slice computed tomography for assessment of AVA with TEE found good agreement ($r = 0.98$) between all three techniques [29]. In comparison, correlation with TTE has been slightly less than with TEE direct planimetry [26,28]. Both MRI and TEE overestimate AVA compared with measures indirectly derived from the continuity equation with TEE or the Gorlin formula with invasive catheterization [24,25,27,28]. Over-estimation ranged from 15% to 30% in previously published studies. The reason for this discrepancy can be explained by the fact that planimetry directly measures anatomic orifice area, whereas the continuity equation and Gorlin formula calculate the effective functional valve area. It has been shown that the calculated effective orifice area depends on the geometric orifice area and the inflow shape of the stenosis [30]. In addition, the calculated AVA is obtained from data averaged over the cardiac cycle, whereas planimetry is performed at one time point during systole. Furthermore, standard AHA/ACC guidelines for grading of aortic stenosis by valve area are based on measurements of the effective valve area by transthoracic echocardiography (TTE) and TEE [15]. These facts have to be kept in mind for clinical decision-making based on planimetric-derived measures of AVA, and they must be considered when choosing an appropriate tool for follow-up of patients with aortic stenosis.

Indirect assessment of aortic stenosis severity by measurement of the functional valve area and estimating the pressure gradient

Magnetic resonance imaging protocol

Assessment of aortic stenosis following the above-mentioned imaging protocol will allow for planimetry of the AVA and assessment of the size of the area of signal loss/stenotic jet beyond the stenotic valve. However, for jet velocity mapping and for calculation of pressure gradients across the valve, as well as application of the continuity equation for assessment of valve area, two more imaging sequences are needed. A flow-sensitive GRE sequence in the LVOT and in a second oblique plane transecting the aortic valve should be acquired to assess the maximum flow velocity across the stenotic orifice. The planes of the flow-sensitive sequence must be strictly perpendicular and in-plane to the proximal stenotic jet (vena contracta), avoiding misangulation and misregistration. Otherwise, the measurements will underestimate the true flow velocity. Also, care must be taken to choose an appropriate velocity encoding (VENC) range, which covers the expected flow velocity across the valve, such that aliasing is avoided.

Measurement of the aortic pressure gradient using the modified Bernoulli equation

The degree of aortic stenosis can be graded by the pressure gradient across the valve. As previously stated, MRI allows accurate assessment of flow velocity in the jet originating from a stenotic valve. The maximum flow velocity should preferably be obtained from a combination of through-plane and in-plane velocity measurements through the aortic valve. Also, it is recommended that the valve orifice is covered with three or more parallel slices to ensure that the maximum velocity within the jet is covered. An appropriate VENC range would be in the order of 3–5 m/s, depending on the stenosis severity expected, and must be chosen to avoid aliasing in the flow measurements. As the maximum flow velocity has been determined, the pressure gradient across the valve can be calculated using the modified Bernoulli equation:

$$P_1 - P_2 = 4(V_2^2 - V_1^2)$$

where P_1 is the pressure proximal and P_2 the pressure distal to the obstruction, V_1 is the flow velocity proximal and V_2 the flow velocity distal to the obstruction. As V_1 rarely exceeds 1 m/s it can be neglected and the equation can further be simplified to:

$$\Delta P = 4 \times V_2^2$$

Studies comparing MRI-derived pressure gradients with manometer measurements *in vitro* [31] as well as invasive measurements *in vivo* [32] showed very close correlation across a wide range of pressure gradients ($r = 0.97$ for comparison with invasive pressure measurements across the aortic valve). Similarly, MRI-derived flow measurements agreed very well with those measured by Doppler (mean of differences 0.23 m/s $\pm$ 0.49 m/s) [18]. Although the pressure gradient across the valve is a good means for quantitation of the hemodynamic significance of stenosis severity, it must be considered that its determinants may vary substantially, given the varying aortic pressure and left ventricular function [21,33]. Particularly in patients with heart failure and reduced cardiac output, a stenosis still may be severe, but the mean gradient may be less than 50 mmHg.

Measurement of the aortic valve area using the continuity equation

Using TTE for measurement of the AVA generally implies the use of the continuity equation for calculation of the orifice area, rather than direct planimetry [5]. By means of the continuity equation, the AVA can be calculated as follows:

$$\text{AVA} = A_{\text{LVOT}} = (V_{\text{LVOT}}/V_{\text{AV}})$$

where A_{LVOT} is the area of the LVOT and V_{LVOT} and V_{AV} are maximum flow velocities recorded at the level of the stenotic valve or directly thereafter as well as at the level of the LVOT. Alternatively, the velocity–time integral (VTI) in the corresponding locations can be measured (LVOT$_{VTI}$/AV$_{VTI}$) and used for the calculation of AVA. An advantage over TTE is that with MRI the LVOT area can readily be planimetered on in-plane and cross-plane b-SSFP cine images [11,26,34]. The maximum flow velocities or VTI can directly be derived from the flow measurements performed in the imaging planes. Good correlation in the range of $r = 0.83$–0.98 as well as high intra- and interobserver variability between AVA measurements derived from the continuity equation using MRI and TTE has been reported [3,26,34]. The continuity equation offers an advantage over pressure measurements in that it is not influenced by a low cardiac output state; however, it requires the input of three variables and thus requires accurate measurements in order to exclude systemic errors.

Conclusion

Using MRI, the aortic valve area can be planimetered directly, just as with TEE. Also, MRI is noninvasive, with measurements less limited by valve calcification. The valve area can be determined by use of the continuity equation, just as with TTE. The area of the LVOT can be assessed more accurately and MRI is not limited by an acoustic window. Pressure gradients can indirectly be calculated by use of the Bernoulli equation, correlating well with invasive measurements obtained by cardiac catheterization. In addition, MRI provides accurate detailed information on myocardial function and changes in left ventricular geometry associated with stenosis. All these characteristics make MRI a unique tool for assessment of aortic stenosis, which may well be used as an alternative or adjunct to existing diagnostic imaging modalities.

References

1. Arai AE, Epstein FH, Bove KE, & Wolff SD (1999) Visualization of aortic valve leaflets using black blood MRI. *J Magn Reson Imaging* **10**:771–777.

2. Krombach GA, Kuhl H, Bucker A, *et al.* (2004) Cine MR imaging of heart valve dysfunction with segmented true fast imaging with steady state free precession. *J Magn Reson Imaging* **19**:59–67.

3. Caruthers SD, Lin SJ, Brown P, *et al.* (2003) Practical value of cardiac magnetic resonance imaging for clinical quantification of aortic valve stenosis: comparison with echocardiography. *Circulation* **108**:2236–2243.

4. Kilner PJ, Firmin DN, Rees RS, *et al.* (1991) Valve and great vessel stenosis: assessment with MR jet velocity mapping. *Radiology* **178**:229–235.

5. Skjaerpe T, Hegrenaes L, & Hatle L (1985) Noninvasive estimation of valve area in patients with aortic stenosis by Doppler ultrasound and two-dimensional echocardiography. *Circulation* **72**:810–818.

6. Gorlin R & Gorlin SG (1951) Hydraulic formula for calculation of the area of the stenotic mitral valve, other cardiac valves, and central circulatory shunts. I. *Am Heart J* **41**:1–29.

7. Omran H, Schmidt H, Hackenbroch M, *et al.* (2003) Silent and apparent cerebral embolism after retrograde catheterisation of the aortic valve in valvular stenosis: a prospective, randomised study. *Lancet* **361**(9365):1241–1246.

8. Globits S & Higgins CB (1995) Assessment of valvular heart disease by magnetic resonance imaging. *Am Heart J* **129**: 369–381.

9. Caduff JH, Hernandez RJ, & Ludomirsky A (1996) MR visualization of aortic valve vegetations. *J Comput Assist Tomogr* **20**: 613–615.

10. Duerinckx AJ & Higgins CB (1994) Valvular heart disease. *Radiol Clin North Am* **32**:613–630.

11. Schulz-Menger J, Strohm O, Waigand J, Uhlich F, Dietz R, & Friedrich MG (2000) The value of magnetic resonance imaging of the left ventricular outflow tract in patients with hypertrophic obstructive cardiomyopathy after septal artery embolization. *Circulation* **101**:1764–1766.

12. Schulz-Menger J, Abdel-Aty H, Busjahn A, *et al.* (2006) Left ventricular outflow tract planimetry by cardiovascular magnetic resonance differentiates obstructive from non-obstructive hypertrophic cardiomyopathy. *J Cardiovasc Magn Reson* **8**:741–746.

13. Sandstede JJ, Beer M, Hofmann S, *et al.* (2000) Changes in left and right ventricular cardiac function after valve replacement for aortic stenosis determined by cine MR imaging. *J Magn Reson Imaging* **12**:240–246.

14. Lamb HJ, Beyerbacht HP, de Roos A, *et al.* (2002) Left ventricular remodeling early after aortic valve replacement: differential effects on diastolic function in aortic valve stenosis and aortic regurgitation. *J Am Coll Cardiol* **40**:2182–2188.

15. Bonow RO, Carabello BA, Chatterjee K, *et al.* (2006) ACC/AHA 2006 guidelines for the management of patients with valvular heart disease: a report of the American College of Cardiology/ American Heart Association Task Force on Practice Guidelines (writing Committee to Revise the 1998 guidelines for the management of patients with valvular heart disease) developed in collaboration with the Society of Cardiovascular Anesthesiologists endorsed by the Society for Cardiovascular Angiography and Interventions and the Society of Thoracic Surgeons. *J Am Coll Cardiol* **48**:e1–148.

16. Leung DA & Debatin JF (1997) Three-dimensional contrast-enhanced magnetic resonance angiography of the thoracic vasculature. *Eur Radiol* **7**:981–989.

17. Keegan J, Gatehouse PD, John AS, Mohiaddin RH, & Firmin DN (2003) Breath-hold signal-loss sequence for the qualitative assessment of flow disturbances in cardiovascular MR. *J Magn Reson Imaging* **18**:496–501.

18. Kilner PJ, Manzara CC, Mohiaddin RH, *et al.* (1993) Magnetic resonance jet velocity mapping in mitral and aortic valve stenosis. *Circulation* **87**:1239–1248.

19. Barkhausen J, Ruehm SG, Goyen M, Buck T, Laub G, & Debatin JF (2001) MR evaluation of ventricular function: true fast imaging with steady-state precession versus fast low-angle shot cine MR imaging: feasibility study. *Radiology* **219**:264–269.

20. Danielsen R, Nordrehaug JE, & Vik-Mo H (1989) Factors affecting Doppler echocardiographic valve area assessment in aortic stenosis. *Am J Cardiol* **63**:1107–1111.

21. Burwash IG, Thomas DD, Sadahiro M, *et al.* (1994) Dependence of Gorlin formula and continuity equation valve areas on transvalvular volume flow rate in valvular aortic stenosis. *Circulation* **89**:827–835.

22. Cannon SR, Richards KL, & Crawford M (1985) Hydraulic estimation of stenotic orifice area: a correction of the Gorlin formula. *Circulation* **71**:1170–1178.

23. Schlosser T, Malyar N, Jochims M, *et al.* (2007) Quantification of aortic valve stenosis in MRI-comparison of steady-state free precession and fast low-angle shot sequences. *Eur Radiol* **17**:1284–1290.

24. Debl K, Djavidani B, Seitz J, *et al.* (2005) Planimetry of aortic valve area in aortic stenosis by magnetic resonance imaging. *Invest Radiol* **40**:631–636.

25. Malyar NM, Schlosser T, Barkhausen J, *et al.* (2008) Assessment of aortic valve area in aortic stenosis using cardiac magnetic resonance tomography: comparison with echocardiography. *Cardiology* **109**:126–134.

26. Pouleur AC, le Polain de Waroux JB, Pasquet A, Vancraeynest D, Vanoverschelde JL, & Gerber BL (2007) Planimetric and continuity equation assessment of aortic valve area: head to head comparison between cardiac magnetic resonance and echocardiography. *J Magn Reson Imaging* **26**:1436–1443.

27. Reant P, Lederlin M, Lafitte S, *et al.* (2006) Absolute assessment of aortic valve stenosis by planimetry using cardiovascular magnetic resonance imaging: comparison with transesophageal echocardiography, transthoracic echocardiography, and cardiac catheterisation. *Eur J Radiol* **59**:276–283.

28. Kupfahl C, Honold M, Meinhardt G, *et al.* (2004) Evaluation of aortic stenosis by cardiovascular magnetic resonance imaging: comparison with established routine clinical techniques. *Heart* **90**:893–901.

29. Pouleur AC, le Polain de Waroux JB, Pasquet A, Vanoverschelde JL, & Gerber BL (2007) Aortic valve area assessment: multidetector CT compared with cine MR imaging and transthoracic and transesophageal echocardiography. *Radiology* **244**:745–754.

30. Garcia D, Pibarot P, Landry C, *et al.* (2004) Estimation of aortic valve effective orifice area by Doppler echocardiography: effects of valve inflow shape and flow rate. *J Am Soc Echocardiogr* **17**:756–765.

31. Sondergaard L, Stahlberg F, Thomsen C, Stensgaard A, Lindvig K, & Henriksen O (1993) Accuracy and precision of MR velocity mapping in measurement of stenotic cross-sectional area, flow rate, and pressure gradient. *J Magn Reson Imaging* **3**:433–437.

32. Eichenberger AC, Jenni R, & von Schulthess GK (1993) Aortic valve pressure gradients in patients with aortic valve stenosis: quantification with velocity-encoded cine MR imaging. *AJR Am J Roentgenol* **160**:971–977.

33. Danielsen R, Nordrehaug JE, Stangeland L, & Vik-Mo H (1988) Limitations in assessing the severity of aortic stenosis by Doppler gradients. *Br Heart J* **59**:551–555.

34. Tanaka K, Makaryus AN, & Wolff SD (2007) Correlation of aortic valve area obtained by the velocity-encoded phase contrast continuity method to direct planimetry using cardiovascular magnetic resonance. *J Cardiovasc Magn Reson* **9**:799–805.

10 Surgical Replacement of the Aortic Valve

Anton Moritz & Mirko Doss

J.W. Goethe-University Frankfurt am Main, Germany

History

The first successful attempt to correct an aortic valve lesion with an artificial prosthesis was performed by Hufnagel in 1951 [1]. He implanted a caged ball prosthesis in the descending aorta, to correct an aortic valve insufficiency. The drawback of this procedure was that cardiac function, coronary circulation, and cerebral perfusion did not normalize after the operation.

The first successful aortic valve replacement was performed by Harken and colleagues in 1960 [2]. With the use of cardiopulmonary bypass, they were able to replace a stenotic aortic valve with a caged ball valve.

The first commercially available, and technically mature, mechanical prosthesis entered the market in the same year. It was designed by Edwards and first successfully implanted by Starr and Edwards in 1960 [3]. Use of the procedure subsequently spread worldwide, and numerous different mechanical valve designs were developed. However, as a result of widespread use, complications inherent in mechanical prostheses became evident. Systemic anticoagulation was necessary to avoid thromboembolism but was associated with the risk of severe bleeding complications. Thus, alternate valve substitutes were sought.

The first aortic homograft was implanted by Ross in 1962 [4]. Because of technical difficulties associated with the implantation of this valve substitute, most surgeons continued to prefer mechanical valves.

The first stent-mounted biological aortic valve prosthesis was implanted by Binet and colleagues in 1965 [5]. They used a formaldehyde-fixed porcine bioprosthesis that did not necessitate systemic anticoagulation of the patient. Unfortunately, clinical results with were not satisfactory, as the prosthesis degenerated after only a few years.

Ross introduced the use of a pulmonary autograft as an aortic valve substitute in 1967 [6]. The harvested pulmonary autograft was replaced by a homograft and the whole procedure became known as the Ross procedure.

Cardiovascular Interventions in Clinical Practice. Edited by Jürgen Haase, Hans-Joachim Schäfers, Horst Sievert and Ron Waksman. © 2010 Blackwell Publishing.

In 1967, glutaraldehyde fixation of porcine bioprostheses was introduced by Carpentier and colleagues [7]. A further innovation of the time was the introduction of bovine pericardial stented bioprostheses, by Ionescu and colleagues in 1971 [8]. Both prostheses were now fixed with glutaraldehyde and the early degeneration, reported for formaldehyde fixation, was no longer observed. To further improve durability of theses prostheses, zero-pressure fixation and anticalcification treatments were introduced.

However, calcification of biological tissues in the aortic position is also dependent on stresses acting upon such tissues during the movement of the leaflets. Furthermore, it became evident that the stented frame of bioprostheses caused a significant obstruction that occasionally led to elevated transvalvular gradients and incomplete regression of left ventricular hypertrophy. To overcome these problems, stentless bioprostheses were introduced by David and colleagues in 1988 [9]. During exercise in particular, a significant reduction in transvalvular gradients has been reported with these bioprostheses.

Pathophysiology

Aortic valve stenosis

In adults, the most common cause of aortic valve stenosis is calcific degeneration. This occurs in about 3% of the elderly population. During the cardiac cycle, shear stresses occur on the leaflets with every cardiac contraction, leading to calcium deposition in the collagen framework of the cusps. As the calcium load increases, the orifice progressively decreases in size and the valve becomes bulky and rigid in structure. The average decrease in effective orifice area is $0.1\,cm^2$ per year. This occurs fastest in degenerative stenosis. However, significant hemodynamic impairment does not occur until the effective orifice area is reduced to half the normal valve area of $3-4\,cm^2$. Beyond this point, left ventricular outflow obstruction rapidly increases. The distribution of calcification is not confined to the leaflets but may extend to the annulus, down the membranous septum, and over the ventricular surface of the anterior mitral valve leaflet.

The aortic valve usually has a tricuspid configuration. However, up to 2% of the population have congenitally bicuspid aortic valves. In the bicuspid aortic valve, shear stresses are greater and calcific degeneration of the leaflets occurs decades earlier. Particularly in patients with a bicuspid aortic valve, a turbulent flow in the ascending aorta occurs and may cause poststenotic dilation.

In patients with aortic valve stenosis resulting from rheumatic disease, fibrous thickening of the leaflets and fusion of one or more commissures typically occur. These changes also result in an increased rate of calcific changes in the cusps.

The permanent reduction in effective orifice area results in several structural changes. As a response to pressure overload, concentric hypertrophy of the left ventricle occurs. In contrast to eccentric hypertrophy, which occurs in aortic insufficiency, concentric hypertrophy maintains left ventricular volume. Myocytes become thicker as myofibrils increase in number. There is also an increase in interstitial collagen but not much fibrosis. Initially, hypertrophy allows the generation of high interventricular pressures, required to maintain cardiac output throughout the stenosis, without dysfunction (compensated aortic stenosis). This is explained by Laplace's law, which states that wall stress is directly proportional to chamber pressure and radius, and is inversely proportional to two times the wall thickness. Thus, concentric hypertrophy acts to normalize peak systolic wall stress (afterload).

Structural changes of the left ventricle in response to aortic valve stenosis cause several functional changes. In contrast to compensated aortic valve stenosis, in which systolic left ventricular function is preserved, decompensated aortic valve stenosis results in a decline in cardiac function. As hypertrophy cannot keep up with the degree of stenosis, ejection fraction, end-systolic volume, fractional shortening, and velocity of shortening decline. The pressure–volume loop shifts to the right. Concentric hypertrophy also reduces compliance of the left ventricle and thus diastolic function. Isotonic relaxation in diastole is dependent on normal compliance. However, with aortic valve stenosis end-diastolic pressure is increased, and rapid left ventricular filling, in the energy-dependent isovolumetric relaxation phase of diastole, is also impaired. These changes eventually lead to congestive cardiac failure.

Increased diastolic pressures reduce coronary blood flow in diastole, in which the major part of coronary perfusion normally occurs. Aortic valve stenosis also causes turbulent blood flow in the sinus of Valsalva, which has been shown to reduce coronary perfusion pressure, especially during systole. This is exacerbated by exercise-induced peripheral vasodilation. These changes contribute to a myocardial oxygen supply–demand mismatch in patients with aortic valve stenosis.

Aortic valve insufficiency

Aortic valve insufficiency can be caused by pathology of any component of the aortic root that prevents leaflet coaptation.

At annular level, annuloaortic ectasia caused by connective tissue disorders, such as cystic media necrosis and Marfan's disease, as well as isolated annular dilation, prevents coaptation of the normal aortic leaflets. At leaflet level, regurgitation can be caused by restricted mobility, as in calcific degeneration, rheumatic disease, and native valve endocarditis. Furthermore, regurgitation can be caused by pathologic mobility as in leaflet prolapse, or it can be caused by shortening of the free leaflet edges or perforation of leaflets with normal mobility. In patients with aortic valve insufficiency, several structural and functional changes occur: chronic aortic insufficiency, decompensated aortic insufficiency, and acute aortic insufficiency.

Chronic aortic insufficiency results in both volume and pressure overload. Volume overload results in eccentric hypertrophy and left ventricular dilation, whereas pressure overload results in concentric hypertrophy with the same increase in myofibrils and interstitial collagen as in aortic valve stenosis. In compensated aortic insufficiency, ventricular dilation results in a larger stroke volume, with all of the additional blood being ejected into the aorta. The resultant increase in pulse pressure causes systemic hypertension and a significant increase in left ventricular afterload.

In decompensated aortic insufficiency, left ventricular end-diastolic pressures and left atrial pressures increase further, leading to pulmonary hypertension and congestive cardiac failure. Eventually, as myocytes are stretched beyond their limit of effective contraction, left ventricular systolic function decreases and left ventricular end-systolic dilation progresses at a rate of about 7 mm per year.

Acute aortic insufficiency is most commonly caused by endocarditis, aortic dissection or thoracic trauma and constitutes a surgical emergency. There is no time for any of the adaptive changes to develop that characterize chronic aortic insufficiency. The sudden volume overload results in pulmonary edema as filling pressures increase in the noncompliant left ventricle. Reduced coronary blood flow, low cardiac output, and hypoxia lead to end-organ ischemia.

Indications

According to the American College of Cardiology and American Heart Association (ACC/AHA) practical guidelines for the management of patients with valvular heart disease, indications for aortic valve replacement can be summarized as follows [76]:

Aortic valve stenosis

High level of evidence based on individual randomized controlled trials with a narrow confidence interval
- Patients with severe aortic valve stenosis and any symptoms.

High level of evidence based on all or none randomized controlled trials
• Patients with severe aortic valve stenosis undergoing coronary artery bypass surgery (CABG), surgery of the ascending aorta, or surgery on another heart valve.
• Asymptomatic patients with severe aortic valve stenosis and systolic left ventricular ejection fraction of <50%.

Moderate level of evidence based on systematic reviews of cohort studies
• Asymptomatic patients with severe aortic valve stenosis and abnormal exercise testing, showing symptoms on exercise.

Moderate level of evidence based on systematic reviews of cohort studies displaying worrisome heterogeneity
• Asymptomatic patients with severe aortic valve stenosis and an abnormal exercise test showing a fall in blood pressure below the baseline.
• Patients with moderate aortic valve stenosis undergoing coronary artery bypass surgery, surgery of the ascending aorta, or surgery on another heart valve.
• Asymptomatic patients with severe aortic valve stenosis and moderate to severe calcification, and a rate of peak velocity progression >0.3 m/s per year.
• Aortic valve stenosis with a gradient below 40 mmHg and left ventricular dysfunction with contractile reserve.

Moderate level of evidence based on individual cohort study or low-quality randomized controlled trial
• Asymptomatic patients with severe aortic valve stenosis and abnormal exercise testing showing complex ventricular arrhythmias.
• Asymptomatic patients with severe aortic valve stenosis and excessive left ventricular hypertrophy (>1.5 mm), unless this is a result of hypertension.
• Aortic valve stenosis with a gradient below 40 mmHg and left ventricular dysfunction without contractile reserve.

Low level of evidence based on individual case–control study
• Aortic valve replacement is not useful for the prevention of sudden death in asymptomatic patients with severe aortic valve stenosis who have none of the findings listed above.

Aortic valve insufficiency

Patients with severe aortic valve insufficiency

High level of evidence based on individual randomized controlled trials with narrow confidence intervals
• Symptomatic patients showing dyspnea or angina.
• Asymptomatic patients with resting left ventricular ejection fraction of <50%.

High level of evidence based on all or none randomized controlled trials
• Patients undergoing CABG, surgery of the ascending aorta, or surgery on another heart valve.

Moderate level of evidence based on systematic reviews of cohort studies
• Asymptomatic patients with a resting left ventricular ejection fraction <50% with severe dilation (end-diastolic dimension <70 mm or end-systolic dimension <50 mm).

Patients with any level of severity of aortic valve insufficiency

High level of evidence based on all or none randomized controlled trials
Patients with aortic root disease due to Marfan's syndrome, with an aortic diameter >45 mm.

Moderate level of evidence based on systematic reviews of cohort studies
• Patients with aortic root disease with a bicuspid valve and an aortic diameter >50 mm.
• Patients with aortic root disease, with an aortic diameter >55 mm.

Technical aspects

Surgical implantation
Access to the heart is gained via a median sternotomy. The patient is fully heparinized, and cardiopulmonary bypass is established via aortic cannulation of the distal ascending aorta and the right atrial appendage, using a single two-stage venous cannula. In patients with an increased risk for aortic cannulation, such as those with a porcelain aorta undergoing redo surgery, right axillary artery cannulation may be a good alternative. Cardiopulmonary bypass is initiated and a vent catheter placed in the apex of the left ventricle or the right superior pulmonary vein.

For cardioplegia, a retrograde balloon-tipped catheter is placed in the coronary sinus. The aorta is clamped and an initial dose of retrograde cardioplegia is administered.

Access to the aortic valve is gained through a transverse aortotomy. Special care is taken to stay well away from the right and left coronary ostia and, in the case of stentless valve implantation, above the sinotubular junction, as the commissural posts of the prosthesis are attached in its close proximity, or to allow for a distal suture line. A transverse aortotomy is chosen over the hockey stick incision, in order not to disturb the geometry of the sinuses and thus allowing for exact orientation of the leaflets. The aortic valve is then inspected. It is important at this point to assess that the commissures are evenly located at 120° apart or if one sinus is proportionally larger than the others. This needs to be respected later when the prosthesis is implanted. Attention is also paid to coronary ostium abnormalities, calcifications of the aortic wall, and mismatches between annulus and sinotubular junction.

Excision of the native aortic valve and debridement of the aortic annulus is then carried out using scissors and rangeurs. Care is taken not to excise too much of the annular tissue. Radical debridement can lead to dehiscence of the aortoventricular continuity, damage of the anterior mitral leaflet, and perforation of the interventricular septum.

After excision of the native valve and decalcification of the annulus, the aortic root is meticulously cleaned, removing calcium and flushing with a saline solution. The annulus is then sized. Although it is desirable to implant a large valve size, care must be taken not to choose a prosthesis that is to large for the patient's aortic root. A valve that is too large can cause coronary obstruction, strut perforation of the aortic wall, and, if forced in place, aortic dissection. Most bioprostheses then require rinsing in saline solution for three 2-min intervals. During this time, 12–16 interrupted, mattressed, pledgeted 2–0 Ethibond sutures are placed circumferentially from below the annulus. Special care is taken when placing sutures below the right commissure to noncoronary commissure to prevent third-degree heart block by not taking exceedingly deep bites in this region. The sutures are then passed through the sewing ring of the prosthesis. The valves are implanted in the supra-annular position, with the stent positioned so as not to interfere with the coronary ostia. The valve is then lowered into the aortic root and the sutures tied. The first sutures to be tied are the ones below the left and right coronary ostium, making sure that the sewing ring of the valve sits low enough so as not to obstruct the coronary ostia. The suture at the lowest point in the noncoronary sinus is then tied, thus already anchoring the valve in the desired plane before the remaining sutures are subsequently tied. The coronary ostia are then inspected for patency and the aortic root is flushed with a saline solution to remove any debris. The aortotomy is then closed with a horizontal mattress suture and a second running suture using 4–0 Prolene.

Minimally invasive aortic valve replacement

Patients are placed in a supine position. A limited median skin incision (7–9 cm) is made from just beneath the sternal angle to the fourth intercostal space. The soft tissue is dissected and a flap is raised to allow access to the sternal notch. The sternum is opened from the sternal angle to the fourth or fifth intercostal space. The sternal incision is extended into the left fourth or fifth intercostal space. Care is taken not to damage the left internal thoracic artery. A standard arterial cannula and a 28F, straight, two-stage venous cannula are placed directly into the ascending aorta and the right atrial appendage after the pericardium is opened and tacked to the drapes under tension with stay sutures. In our experience, this maneuver elevates the heart anteriorly and results in good

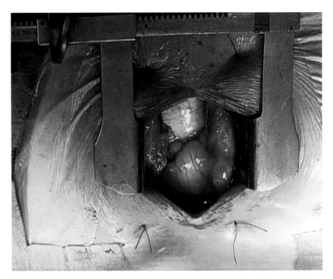

Figure 10.1 Partial upper sternotomy giving excellent exposition of the aorta, right atrium and right ventricle.

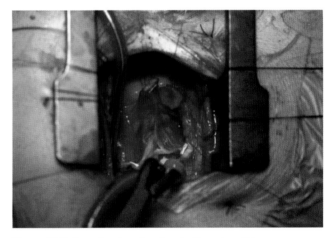

Figure 10.2 Operative view of aortic valve through partial upper sternotomy. Even complex aortic valve procedures are possible through this limited incision.

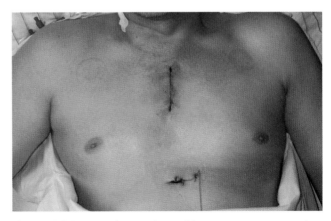

Figure 10.3 Postoperative scar after partial upper sternotomy, measuring 8 cm.

exposure of the aorta and the right atrium. Cardiopulmonary bypass is initiated. The field is flooded with carbon dioxide to aid de-airing of the heart. A cold swab is placed on the anterior surface of the right ventricle for added myocardial protection. After occluding the aorta with a standard aortic cross-clamp, cardioplegia is delivered only antegrade, using an aortic root cannula, and after aortotomy by selective coronary intubation. All subsequent steps of the procedure equal those of routine aortic valve replacement via a median sternotomy. For closure of the chest, a pericardial chest tube is inserted through a subxiphoid skin incision. The sternotomy is closed with stainless-steel wires, and the soft tissue is closed with running absorbable sutures (Figs. 10.1–10.3).

Results

Evaluation of operative risk

In patients undergoing aortic valve procedures, the European system for cardiac operative risk evaluation (EuroSCORE) model has been shown to be predictive of early mortality [10], postoperative complications [11], prolonged length of stay [11], and long-term mortality [12]. The use of EuroSCORE in predicting operative mortality for high-risk patients undergoing isolated aortic valve replacement (AVR) has yet to be validated. Although the logistic EuroSCORE model has been shown to be a better predictor of mortality than the additive EuroSCORE in high-risk populations [13,14], several studies have found that the logistic EuroSCORE model may overestimate the mortality of such patients undergoing valve procedures [15,16]. This is particularly true for patients aged 80 years and older [17]. On the other hand, it is evident that the logistic EuroSCORE may underestimate the actual risk of mortality in patients younger than 80 years, as several preoperative comorbidities, including coronary artery disease, presence of mitral valve insufficiency, hepatic disease, malignancies, cardiovascular risk factors (smoking history, hypertension, hyperlipidemia), and radiation of the chest, are not reflected [18]. Currently, there is no uniformly accepted and validated risk stratification model specifically designed for aortic valve surgery. However, the EuroSCORE estimate of operative risk complies with data presented in recent clinical series, and thus provides a reliable indication of patients' postoperative course [18,19].

Early survival

Elective aortic valve replacement can be performed with a perioperative mortality rate between 2% and 5%. According to the large databases (The Society of Thoracic Surgeons [STS] database and the German National Registry), this figure has not changed in the last 10 years. The perioperative mortality in octogenarians undergoing elective isolated aortic valve replacement is higher, at 8–14% [20–26]. In reoperations on the aortic valve, the perioperative mortality is also significantly increased and ranges between 6% and 15% [27]. In patients undergoing concomitant coronary artery bypass grafting, the perioperative risk is increased to 6–9% [28,29].

In isolated aortic valve replacement certain preoperative risk factors and intraoperative variables have been identified to mitigate in-hospital mortality. Perioperative factors include left ventricular hypertrophy, congestive heart failure status, age, and renal insufficiency. Intraoperative variables include concomitant coronary artery bypass surgery, redo surgery, coexisting ascending aortic aneurysm needing surgery, and the length of aortic cross-clamp time. The causes of perioperative mortality after isolated aortic valve replacement in >50% of patients are cardiac in nature. The primary causes are cardiac failure and myocardial infarction. Further common causes of perioperative mortality are thromboembolism, malignant arrhythmias, infection, and bleeding complications [30,31].

Late survival

Long-term survival after aortic valve replacement has been inferior to bypass surgery, despite being a curative operation. The 10- to 15-year survival rates show a wide range [32–42], even with the use of the same type of prosthesis (Table 10.1). Much research has been performed in an attempt to identify and design an ideal prosthesis and to improve long-term survival rates. However, it has become evident that patient-related risk factors, rather than the type of valve substitute, most significantly influence late survival. Significant risk factors for late mortality after aortic valve replacement include the age of the patient at time of implant, left ventricular impairment at time of implant, residual left ventricular hypertrophy, and concomitant coronary artery disease [35,36,39]. Further comorbidities, such as renal disease, chronic lung disease, diabetes, and pulmonary and systemic hypertension, have been documented to lower long-term survival [36].

The older the patient at the time of operation, the lower the long-term survival. Older patients are more likely to have clinically significant comorbidities that adversely affect survival. It has been reported that, among patients undergoing aortic valve replacement, 10-year survival was 27% ± 8% in those with renal disease, 30% ± 6% in those with chronic lung disease, 35% ± 6% in those with an ejection fraction <40%, 35% ± 5% in those with concomitant coronary artery disease [43]. These data indicate that patient characteristics at the time of operation are a major determinant of late mortality after aortic valve replacement.

Regression of left ventricular hypertrophy

Evidence from hypertensive patient populations and unoperated patient cohorts with aortic valve stenosis suggests that poor long-term results may be related to the incomplete regression of left ventricular hypertrophy [46,47].

Table 10.1 Long-term mortality after aortic valve replacement.

Prosthesis	10-year mortality (%)	15-year mortality (%)
Bioprostheses		
Carpentier-Edwards stented aortic valve	40.6 ± 2.1	70.7 ± 1.5
Perimount	29 ± 7	60.7 ± 3.1
Hancock	48 ± 2	64%
Hancock II	39 ± 2	53 ± 3
Mechanical valves		
St. Jude	42 ± 5	—
Medtronic Hall	36	55
Bjork-Shiley	30	46
Starr Edwards	40.4	55

Stented bioprosthetic valve substitutes are commonly employed in the elderly. The incidence of structural valve deterioration in a group of patients 65 years old and above was reported to be 6% at 15 years postoperatively [44]. The obstructive nature of the stent and sewing ring, or patient–prosthesis mismatch, have been held accountable for persistently elevated transvalvular gradients. In the late 1980s, stentless bioprostheses were introduced to circumvent these problems by offering a maximal orifice area for flow and eliminating the valvular sewing ring and stent. Thus, stentless valves seem to be the optimal choice for patients eligible for biological aortic valve replacement.

Significant postoperative regression of hypertrophy and improvement in left ventricular function is achieved in most patients following insertion of prostheses. However, residual left ventricular hypertrophy is common after AVR and impairs left ventricular diastolic function, which can lead to late congestive cardiac failure. Jamieson and colleagues [45] reported on a cohort of patients in whom incomplete regression of left ventricular hypertrophy significantly reduced 10-year survival. Unresolved left ventricular hypertrophy not only increases mortality, but also compromises quality of life and increases morbidity [46]. Michel and colleagues [47] found an increased incidence and severity of ventricular arrhythmias in patients with left ventricular hypertrophy after aortic valve replacement. Persistent hypertrophy may be a result of the obstructive nature of the valve itself, host-related factors, or patient–prosthesis mismatch. Valve-related left ventricular pressure increase is an important reason for incomplete regression of cellular hypertrophy and the development of increased interstitial fibrosis postoperatively [48].

Thus, one could argue that, to achieve an optimal postoperative result, the prosthesis chosen should combine the minimum obstructiveness with the best hemodynamic performance. Such prostheses would be expected to result in faster and more complete regression of left ventricular hyper-

trophy. Based on valve performance and its effects on regression of left ventricular hypertrophy, the current study was designed to provide some rationale to select the optimal valve substitute for patients in a certain age group.

The beneficial effects of a less obstructive valve (pulmonary autografts, stentless valves) have often been demonstrated [49–52]. However, there have been no randomized trials of pulmonary autografts and only four of stentless valves, comparing their performance with more obstructive valves (stented bioprosthesis, mechanical valves).

At the University of Frankfurt, a total of 120 patients with isolated aortic valve stenosis were included in a prospective randomized trial [53]. They were allocated to three groups according to their age. Group 1 patients (age < 60 years) were randomly assigned to receive a pulmonary autograft (n = 20) or a mechanical prosthesis [Edwards Mira (Edwards Lifesciences, Irvine, CA); n = 20]. Group 2 patients (age 60–75 years) received a stentless bioprosthesis [Carpentier-Edwards Prima Plus (Edwards Lifesciences, Irvine, CA); n = 20] or a mechanical prosthesis [Edwards Mira (Edwards Lifesciences, Irvine, CA); n = 20]. Group 3 patients (age > 75 years) received a stentless bioprosthesis (Carpentier-Edwards Prima Plus; n = 20) or a stented bioprosthesis (Carpentier-Edwards Perimount; n = 20).

The authors found that pulmonary autografts had significantly lower transvalvular gradients than the mechanical valves (pulmonary autografts 4.8 mmHg and mechanical valves 16.2 mmHg), however, left ventricular mass regression was similar in both groups at 6 and 12 months, despite the superior hemodynamic performance of the pulmonary autografts. Significant regression of left ventricular hypertrophy has been reported in literature after aortic valve replacement with both substitutes [52,54–56]. The 12-month postoperative follow-up period also seems to be sufficient to assess the regression of left ventricular hypertrophy. Several authors have reported that there is no difference in left ventricular mass regression between 1 year and 3 years of follow-up

Table 10.2 Comparative hydrodynamic evaluation of bioprosthetic heart valves [61].

Prosthesis	Mean transvalvular gradient (mmHg)	Effective orifice area (cm²)
Carpentier-Edwards stented aortic valve	8	1.52
Perimount stented pericardial	4.9	2.12
Mosaic stented porcine	10.8	1.5
Hancock II stented porcine	11	1.49
Mitroflow stented pericardial	6.3	1.53
Toronto stentless porcine	5.1	2.12
Prima Plus stentless porcine	6.2	2.0

In vitro transvalvular gradients and effective orifice areas measured at 5 L/min cardiac output in 25-mm prostheses.

[51,56,57]. Walter and colleagues [58] reported a significant difference in the rate of left ventricular mass regression in patients with peak transvalvular pressure gradients of 16.7 mmHg compared with 21 mmHg in a randomized cohort of 180 patients.

The authors also report on a randomized comparison of stentless against stented bioprostheses. They found no difference in transvalvular gradients and also no difference in the rate and completeness of left ventricular regression [59]. A number of nonrandomized studies have also been published, especially comparing stentless with stented bioprosthesis. Jin *et al.* [55] evaluated the regression of a left ventricular mass in a large number of patients who had undergone AVR, with different types of valve substitutes used. They found that the reduction in left ventricular mass was greater in patients who received stentless valves or homografts than in patients who received a stented bioprosthesis or mechanical valve. They also found that complete left ventricular mass regression was achieved 6 months postoperatively in patients with stentless valves, whereas, in patients who received stented or mechanical valves, regression remained incomplete after 12 months [51]. De Paulis [48] and colleagues compared stented, stentless, and mechanical valves, and, although stentless valves resulted in a significantly lower peak systolic gradient, there was no significant difference in the rate and completeness of left ventricular mass regression after 12 months.

Cohen *et al.* [56] also conducted a prospective randomized trial. Ninety-nine patients were randomly assigned to stentless or stented valves. Interestingly, they reported no difference in the rate and completeness of left ventricular mass regression and also no statistically significant difference in hemodynamic performance between these valves.

Structural valve deterioration

Mechanical valves in the aortic position have an extremely low rate of structural valve deterioration regardless of patient age. However, this is not true of bioprostheses, the rate of deterioration of which is related to the age of the patient at the time of operation [60]. In patients aged 16–39 years, structural valve deterioration is 60% at 10 years' follow-up and >90% at 16 years. In patients aged >70 years, structural valve deterioration is <15% at 15 years' follow-up [37]. The rate of structural valve deterioration in patients with porcine biological prostheses and homografts is higher than in patients with Carpentier-Edwards pericardial bioprostheses [60]. This finding is partly explained by the older age of the patients in the pericardial group at the time of operation. In *in vitro* studies, gradients are lower and effective orifice areas are larger in patients with pericardial valves than in patients with several other prosthetic heart valves (Table 10.2) [61]. These findings indicate that the pericardial aortic valve may be the bioprosthesis of choice in elderly patients. The rate of structural valve deterioration is not significantly different for Hancock and Carpentier-Edwards porcine valves [62]. The rate of structural valve deterioration of newer porcine stented and stentless valves at 9 years is within the expected range of valve deterioration observed in earlier stented porcine valves. The data suggest that all porcine valves have similar rates of structural valve deterioration.

Minimally invasive aortic valve replacement

The large number of recent reports on minimally invasive techniques for cardiac operations underscores the explosion of interest in less invasive surgical approaches [63–68]. The benefits of minimally invasive heart valve surgery may be realized after a relatively short learning curve by surgeons. With experience, cardiopulmonary bypass and aortic cross-clamp times approach those achieved with median sternotomy. Aortic valve operations can be performed safely through smaller incisions.

The partial upper sternotomy for aortic valve replacement has several advantages over other approaches. Cardiopulmonary bypass is accomplished easily via central cannulation. The internal mammary arteries are preserved, and good exposure of the ascending aorta is achieved. If necessary, conversion to full median sternotomy is easily performed. Visualization of the aortic valve is excellent. There are few contraindications to this approach, and some surgeons have reported successful aortic valve reoperations with this incision. However, concomitant coronary artery disease cannot be treated via this approach.

Recent data demonstrate that minimally invasive heart valve surgery results in tangible benefits. Several studies demonstrate substantial reductions in blood loss and transfusion requirements using smaller incisions. The smaller incision and reduced surgical trauma may result in earlier extubation, shorter intensive care unit stays, and shorter hospital stays. These factors, in turn, may decrease hospital costs and charges by 10–20%. Although most of these data come from retrospective studies, Machler et al. [69] confirmed several of these findings in a large prospective study of patients undergoing aortic valve surgery.

Complications after aortic valve replacement

To approve a prosthetic heart valve, the Food and Drug Administration (FDA) requires studies with more than 800 valve-years of follow-up. The incidence of complications should be <2% per valve-year, to conform with optimal performance characteristics determined by the FDA [70,71], which were calculated to allow an alpha error of 5% ($P<0.05$) and a beta error of 20% (power 80%) (Table 10.3).

The available literature suggests that there is no significant difference in complication rates among the various mechanical valves and also among the various bioprostheses with regards to the incidence of anticoagulation-related hemorrhage, valve thrombosis, endocarditis, and paravalvular leaks [60,72–74]. However, use of mechanical valves is associated with an increased risk of thromboembolism compared with bioprostheses.

The most common complication after aortic valve replacement is anticoagulation-related hemorrhage. The incidence ranges up to 2.5% per patient-year [75–77]. The second most

common complication after aortic valve replacement is thromboembolism. The incidence ranges up to 2.3% per patient-year. Fifty percent of patients experience thromboembolic complications manifested as strokes [75–77]. Paravalvular leaks are surgeon-related complications, which vary according to experience between centers. A rate of <0.1% per patient-year is considered an acceptable rate [78].

Endocarditis is a rare complication after aortic valve replacement. Freedom from endocarditis after heart valve replacement is 97% after 20 years [77,79]. Early onset of endocarditis (less than 60 days postoperatively) occurs in 60% of these patients. Valve thrombosis is also rare after aortic valve replacement. The incidence is <0.3% per patient-year [77,79].

These data confirm that FDA-approved prosthetic heart valves are associated with low complication rates, and that higher complication rates are, like mortality rates after aortic valve replacement, related to factors other than the type of heart valve. Thus, the lowest rates of thromboembolism can be expected in young patients in sinus rhythm, with normal ejection fraction, who do not smoke, without peripheral vascular disease, diabetes, or hypertension, and without clotting disorders.

Summary

After the introduction of prosthetic heart valves in the 1960s, aortic valve replacement became established as the treatment of choice for all aortic valve pathologies. With regards to morbidity and mortality rates, it has become evident that clinical outcomes are significantly dependent on patient-related factors. Thus, baseline demographic data and comorbid conditions of the patients at the time of surgery have moved into focus when comparing outcomes of different types of aortic valve surgery procedures and prostheses.

The EuroSCORE remains a valid tool to estimate perioperative risk in patients undergoing aortic valve replacement. However, operative risk tends to be overestimated in the elderly and underestimated in young patients.

Current stentless bioprostheses provide no advantage of over stented bioprostheses or mechanical valves in terms of hemodynamics and regression of left ventricular hypertrophy.

Anticoagulation-related complications remain a major drawback of mechanical valves. Structural valve deterioration of bioprostheses is dependent on the tissue and not on the design of the valves. Porcine stented valves degenerate at the same rate as stentless porcine valves.

Minimally invasive aortic valve surgery can be performed safely with reproducible results. Apart from cosmetic considerations, it leads to improved postoperative thorax stability, thus improving respiratory function and reducing blood loss and hospital stay. Thus, it provides patients with a high perioperative risk an excellent alternative to conventional surgery.

Table 10.3 FDA objective performance criteria for prosthetic heart valves.

Complications	% per valve-year
Thromboembolism	2.5
Valve thrombosis	0.2
All hemorrhage	1.4
Severe hemorrhage	0.9
All paravalvular leaks	1.2
Severe paravalvular leaks	0.6
Endocarditis	1.2

References

1. Hufnagel CA (1951) Aortic plastic valvular prosthesis. *Bull Georgetown Univ Med Cent* **4**:128–134.

2. Harken DE, Soroff HS, Taylor WJ, Lefermine AA, Guipa SS, & Lunzer S (1960) Partial and complete prostheses in aortic insufficiency. *J Thorac Surg* **36**:563–570.

3. Starr A & Edwards ML (1960) Mitral replacement: the shielded ball valve prosthesis. *J Thorac Cardiovasc Surg* **40**:744–762.

4. Ross DN (1962) Homograft replacement of the aortic valve. *Lancet* **2**:487.

5. Binet JP, Duran CG, Carpentier A, & Langlois J (1965) Heterologous aortic valve transplantation. *Lancet* **2**:1275.

6. Ross DN (1967) Replacement of aortic and mitral valve with a pulmonary autograft. *Lancet* **2**:956.

7. Carpentier A, Lemaigre G, Robert L, Carpentier S, & Dubost C (1969) Biological factors affecting long-term results of valvular heterografts. *J Thorac Cardiovasc Surg* **58**:467.

8. Ionescu MI, Pakrashi BC, Holden MP, Mary DH, & Wooler GH (1993) Results of aortic valve replacement with frame supported fascia lata and pericardial grafts. *J Thorac Cardiovasc Surg* **105**:154.

9. David TE, Pollick C, & Bos J (1990) Aortic valve replacement with stentless porcine aortic bioprosthesis. *J Thorac Cardiovasc Surg* **99**:113–118.

10. Roques F, Nashef SA, & Michel P (2001) Risk factors for early mortality after valve surgery in Europe in the 1990s: lessons from the EuroSCORE pilot program. *J Heart Valve Dis* **10**:572–577; discussion 577–578.

11. Toumpoulis IK, Anagnostopoulos CE, DeRose JJ, & Swistel DG (2005) Does EuroSCORE predict length of stay and specific postoperative complications after coronary artery bypass grafting? *Int J Cardiol* **105**:19–25.

12. Toumpoulis IK, Anagnostopoulos CE, Toumpoulis SK, DeRose JJ Jr., & Swistel DG (2005) EuroSCORE predicts long-term mortality after heart valve surgery. *Ann Thorac Surg* **79**:1902–1908.

13. Michel P, Roques F, & Nashef SA (2003) Logistic or additive EuroSCORE for high-risk patients? *Eur J Cardiothorac Surg* **23**:684–687; discussion 687.

14. Sergeant P, de Worm E, & Meyns B (2001) Single centre, single domain validation of the EuroSCORE on a consecutive sample of primary and repeat CABG. *Eur J Cardiothorac Surg* **20**:1176–1182.

15. Collart F, Feier H, Kerbaul F, et al. (2005) Valvular surgery in octogenarians: operative risks factors, evaluation of Euroscore and long term results. *Eur J Cardiothorac Surg* **27**:276–280.

16. Collart F, Feier H, Kerbaul F, et al. (2005) Primary valvular surgery in octogenarians: perioperative outcome. *J Heart Valve Dis* **14**:238–242; discussion 242.

17. Grossi EA, Schwartz CF, Yu PJ, et al. (2008) High-risk aortic valve replacement: are the outcomes as bad as predicted? *Ann Thorac Surg* **85**:102–106; discussion 107.

18. Walther T, Simon P, Dewey T, et al. (2007) Transapical minimally invasive aortic valve implantation: multicenter experience. *Circulation* **116**(11 Suppl.):I240–245.

19. Walther T, Falk V, Borger MA, et al. (2007) Minimally invasive transapical beating heart aortic valve implantation—proof of concept. *Eur J Cardiothorac Surg* **31**:9–15.

20. Melby SJ, Zierer A, Kaiser SP, et al. (2007) Aortic valve replacement in octogenarians: risk factors for early and late mortality. *Ann Thorac Surg* **83**:1651–1656; discussion 1656–1657.

21. Sundt TM, Bailey MS, Moon MR, et al. (2000) Quality of life after aortic valve replacement at the age of >80 years. *Circulation* **102**(19 Suppl. 3):III70–74.

22. Roberts WC, Ko JM, Garner WL, et al. (2007) Valve structure and survival in octogenarians having aortic valve replacement for aortic stenosis (+/– aortic regurgitation) with versus without coronary artery bypass grafting at a single US medical center 1993 to 2005. *Am J Cardiol* **100**:489–495.

23. Bose AK, Aitchison JD, & Dark JH (2007) Aortic valve replacement in octogenarians. *J Cardiothorac Surg* **2**:33.

24. Urso S, Sadaba R, Greco E, et al. (2007) One-hundred aortic valve replacements in octogenarians: outcomes and risk factors for early mortality. *J Heart Valve Dis* **16**:139–144.

25. Kolh P, Kerzmann A, Honore C, Comte L, & Limet R (2007) Aortic valve surgery in octogenarians: predictive factors for operative and long-term results. *Eur J Cardiothorac Surg* **31**:600–606.

26. Alexander KP, Anstrom KJ, Muhlbaier LH, et al. (2000) Outcomes of cardiac surgery in patients ≥ 80 years: results from the National Cardiovascular Network. *J Am Coll Cardiol* **35**:731–738.

27. Cohn LH (1994) Aortic valve prostheses. *Cardiol Rev* **2**:219.

28. Jin XY & Pepper JR (2002) Do stentless valves make a difference? *Eur J Cardiothorac Surg* **22**:95–100.

29. Westaby S, Jonson A, Payne N, et al. (2001) Does the use of a stentless bioprosthesis increase surgical risk? *Semin Thorac Cardiovasc Surg* **13**:143–147.

30. Jamieson WRE, Munro AI, Burr LH, Germann E, Miyagishima RT, & Ling H (1995) Influence of coronary artery bypass and age on clinical performance after aortic and mitral valve replacement with biological and mechanical prostheses. *Circulation* **92**:101–106.

31. Lytle BW, Cosgrove PM, & Taylor PC (1989) Primary isolated aortic valve replacement: early and late results. *J Thorac Cardiovasc Surg* **97**:675.

32. Orszulak TA, Schaff HV, & Puga FJ (1997) Event status of the Starr-Edwards aortic valve to 20 years: a benchmark for comparison. *Ann Thorac Surg* **63**:620–626.

33. Lindblom D (1988) Long-term clinical results after aortic valve replacement with the Bjork–Shiley prosthesis. *J Thorac Cardiovasc Surg* **95**:658–667.

34. Lund O, Nielson SL, Arildsen H, Ilkjaer LB, & Pilegard HK (2000) Standard aortic St. Jude valve at 18 years: performance profile and determinants of outcome. *Ann Thorac Surg* **69**:1459–1465.

35. Butchart EG, Li HH, Payne N, Buchan K, & Grunkemeier GL (2001) Twenty years' experience with the Medtronic hall valve. *J Thorac Cardiovasc Surg* **121**:1090–1100.

36. Petersheim DS, Chen Y-Y, & Cheruvu S (1999) outcome after biological versus mechanical aortic valve replacement in 841 patients. *J Thorac Cardiovasc Surg* **117**:890–897.

37. Yun KL, Miller DC, & Moore KA (1995) Durability of the Hancock MO bioprosthesis compared with the standard aortic valve bioprosthesis. *Ann Thorac Surg* **60**:S221–228.

38. Jamieson WRE, Burr LH, Munro AI, Tyres FO, & Miyagishima RT (1995) Carpentier-Edwards supra-annular porcine bioprosthesis: clinical performance to twelve years. *Ann Thorac Surg* **60**:S235–240.

39. Cohn LH, Collins JJ Jr, Rizzo RJ, Adams DH, Cooper GS, & Avanki SF (1998) Twenty year follow-up of the Hancock modified orifice porcine aortic valve. *Ann Thorac Surg* **66**:S30–34.

40. Khan SS, Chaux A, & Blanche C (1998) A twenty-year experience with the Hancock porcine xenograft in the elderly. *Ann Thorac Surg* **66**:S35–39.

41. Frater RWM, Furlong P, & Cosgrove DM (1998) Long-term durability and patient functional status of the Carpentier-Edwards Perimount pericardial bioprosthesis in the aortic position. *J Heart Valve Dis* **7**:48–53.

42. David TE, Ivanor J, Armstrong S, Feindel CM, & Cohen G (2001) Late results of heart valve replacement with the Hancock II bioprosthesis. *J Thorac Cardiovasc Surg* **121**:268–278.

43. Grunkemeier GL, Li H-H, & Starr A (1999) Heart valve replacement: a statistical review of 35 years results. *J Heart Valve Dis* **8**:466–471.

44. Hammermeister K, Sethi GK, Henderson WG, Grover FL, Oprian C, & Rahimtoola SH (2000) Outcomes 15 years after valve replacement with a mechanical versus a bioprosthetic valve: final report of the Veterans Affairs randomized trial. *J Am Coll Cardiol* **36**:1152–1158.

45. Jamieson WR, Burr LH, Tyers GF, Munro AI (1994) Carpentier-Edwards standard and supra-annular porcine bioprostheses: 10 year comparison of structural valve deterioration. *J Heart Valve Dis* **3**:59–65.

46. Rossi A, Tomaino M, Golia G, Anselmi M, Fuca G, & Zardini P (2000) Echocardiographic prediction of clinical outcome in medically treated patients with aortic stenosis. *Am Heart J* **140**:766–771.

47. Levy D (1991) Clinical significance of left ventricular hypertrophy: insights from the Framingham Study. *J Cardiovasc Pharmacol* **17**(Suppl. 2):S1–6.

48. Casabona R, De Paulis R, Zattera GF, *et al.* (1992) Stentless porcine and pericardial valve in aortic position. *Ann Thorac Surg* **54**:681–684; discussion 685.

49. Bikkina M, Larson MG, & Levy D (1993) Asymptomatic ventricular arrhythmias and mortality risk in subjects with left ventricular hypertrophy. *J Am Coll Cardiol* **22**:1111–1116.

50. Sen S & Tarazi RC (1983) Regression of myocardial hypertrophy and influence of adrenergic system. *Am J Physiol* **244**:H97–101.

51. Kurnik PB, Innerfield M, Wachspress JD, Eldredge WJ, & Waxman HL (1990) Left ventricular mass regression after aortic valve replacement measured by ultrafast computed tomography. *Am Heart J* **120**:919–927.

52. Ghali JK, Liao Y, Simmons B, Castaner A, Cao G, & Cooper RS (1992) The prognostic role of left ventricular hypertrophy in patients with or without coronary artery disease. *Ann Intern Med* **117**:831–836.

53. Doss M, Wood JP, Martens S, Wimmer-Greinecker G, & Moritz A (2005) Do pulmonary autografts provide better outcomes than mechanical valves? A prospective randomized trial. *Ann Thorac Surg* **80**:2194–2198.

54. Pibarot P, Dumesnil JG, Jobin J, Cartier P, Honos G, & Durand LG (1999) Hemodynamic and physical performance during maximal exercise in patients with an aortic bioprosthetic valve: comparison of stentless versus stented bioprostheses. *J Am Coll Cardiol* **34**:1609–1617.

55. Jin XY, Zhang ZM, Gibson DG, Yacoub MH, & Pepper JR (1996) Effects of valve substitute on changes in left ventricular function and hypertrophy after aortic valve replacement. *Ann Thorac Surg* **62**:683–690.

56. Cohen G, Christakis GT, Joyner CD, *et al.* (2002) Are stentless valves hemodynamically superior to stented valves? A prospective randomized trial. *Ann Thorac Surg* **73**:767–775; discussion 775–778.

57. Monrad ES, Hess OM, Murakami T, Nonogi H, Corin WJ, & Krayenbuehl HP (1988) Time course of regression of left ventricular hypertrophy after aortic valve replacement. *Circulation* **77**:1345–1355.

58. Walther T, Falk V, Langebartels G, *et al.* (1999) Prospectively randomized evaluation of stentless versus conventional biological aortic valves: impact on early regression of left ventricular hypertrophy. *Circulation* **100**(19 Suppl.):II6–10.

59. Doss M, Martens S, Wood JP, *et al.* (2003) Performance of stentless versus stented aortic valve bioprostheses in the elderly patient: a prospective randomized trial. *Eur J Cardiothorac Surg* **23**:299–304.

60. Grunkemeier GL, Li H-H, Naftel DC, Starr A, & Rahimtoola SH (2000) Long-term performance of heart valve prosthesis. *Curr Probl Cardiol* **25**:73–156.

61. Marquez S, Hon RT, & Yogonathan AP (2001) Comparative hydrodynamic evaluation of bioprosthetic heart valves. *J Heart Valve Dis* **10**:802–811.

62. David TE, Feindel CM, Scully HE, Bos J, & Rakowski H (1998) Aortic valve replacement with stentless porcine aortic valves: a ten-year experience. *J Heart Valve Dis* **7**:250–254.

63. Dogan, S, Dzemali O, Wimmer-Greinecker O, *et al.* (2003) Minimally invasive versus conventional aortic valve replacement: a prospective randomized trial. *J Heart Valve Dis* **12**:76–80.

64. Cohn LH, Adams DH, Couper GS, & Bichell DP (1997) Minimally invasive aortic valve replacement. *Semin Thorac Cardiovasc Surg* **9**:331–336.

65. Cosgrove DM 3rd & Sabik JF (1996) Minimally invasive approach for aortic valve operations. *Ann Thorac Surg* **62**:596–597.

66. Boehm J, Libera P, Will A, Martinoff S, & Wildhirt SM (2007) Partial median "I" sternotomy: minimally invasive alternate approach for aortic valve replacement. *Ann Thorac Surg* **84**:1053–1055.

67. Chang YS, Lin PJ, Chang CH, Chu JJ, & Tan PP (1999) "I" ministernotomy for aortic valve replacement. *Ann Thorac Surg* **68**:40–45.

68. Tabata M, Umakanthan R, Cohn LH, *et al.* (2008) Early and late outcomes of 1000 minimally invasive aortic valve operations. *Eur J Cardiothorac Surg* **33**:537–541.

69. Machler IIE, Bergmann P, & Anelli-Monti M (1999) Minimally invasive versus conventional aortic valve operations: a prospective study in 120 patients. *Ann Thorac Surg* **67**:1001–1005.

70. Johnson DM & Sapirstein W (1994) FDA's requirements for in vivo performance data for prosthetic heart valves. *J Heart Valve Dis* **3**:350–355.

71. Grunkemeier GL & Anderson WN Jr. (1998) Clinical evaluation and analysis of heart valve substitute. *J Heart Valve Dis* **7**:163–169.

72. Rahimtoola SH (1988) Lessons learned about the determinants of the results of valve surgery. *Circulation* **78**:1505–1507.

73. Bonow RO, Carabello B, de Leon AC Jr., *et al.* (2006) ACC/AHA Guidelines for the management of patients with valvular heart disease. *J Am Coll Cardiol* **48**:e1–148.

74. Butchart EG, Lewis PA, Bethel JA, & Brekenridge IM (1991) Adjusting anticoagulation to prosthesis thrombogenicity and patient risk factors: recommendations for the Medtronic hall valve. *Circulation* **84**(Suppl.):III 61–69.

75. Oxenham H, Bloomfield P, Wheatley DJ, *et al.* (2003) Twenty-year comparison of a Bjork-Shiley mechanical heart valve with porcine bioprostheses. *Heart* **89**:697.

76. Khan SS, Trento A, DeRobertis M, *et al.* (2001) Twenty-year comparison of tissue and mechanical valve replacement. *J Thorac Cardiovasc Surg* **122**:257.

77. Emery RW, Krogh CC, Arom DV, *et al.* (2005) The St. Jude Medical cardiac valve prosthesis: A 25-year experience with single valve replacement. *Ann Thorac Surg* **79**:776.

78. Schaff HV, Carrel TP, Jamieson WRE, *et al.* (2002) Paravalvular leak and other events in silzone-coated mechanical heart valves: a report from AVERT. *Ann Thorac Surg* **73**:785.

79. Ikonomidis JS, Kratz JM, Crumbley AJ, *et al.* (2003) Twenty-year experience with the St Jude Medical mechanical valve prosthesis. *J Thorac Cardiovasc Surg* **126**:2002–2031.

11 Percutaneous Implantation of Aortic Valve Prostheses

Robert H. Boone & John G. Webb

St. Paul's Hospital, University of British Columbia, Vancouver, British Columbia, Canada

Historical background

Calcific aortic stenosis, the prevalence of which increases with increasing age, is the most frequent expression of valvular heart disease in the Western world, and is the leading indication for valve replacement. For patients aged 55–64, 65–74, and ≥75 years, the prevalence of moderate or severe aortic stenosis is 0.6%, 1.4%, and up to 4.6%, respectively [1]. Surgical aortic valve replacement (AVR) is currently the preferred treatment strategy for symptomatic patients but, in the presence of comorbidities and advanced age, operative risks are increased and often considered prohibitive.

Given the risk of morbidity and mortality of surgical AVR, patients, or their physicians, may hesitate when considering surgical options. It is difficult to know how large this untreated population may be, but a 3-month survey of European hospitals in 2001 found that 9.8% of patients with aortic stenosis and indications for surgery were not offered intervention [2]. The study subsequently looked at elderly patients (age >75 years) with aortic stenosis and found that 33% were not offered intervention [2]. Others have reported that this rate may be as high as 40–60% [3,4]. Despite 1-, 5-, and 10-year medical therapy survival rates of 60%, 30%, and 18%, respectively, patient refusal of surgical therapy is a consistent reason for conservative treatment [5].

The search for a less invasive treatment option for patients with severe aortic stenosis was pioneered by Andersen *et al.* [6] in 1992 when they developed a balloon-expandable aortic valve that could be implanted within a porcine model. Subsequently, the feasibility of percutaneous prosthetic valve delivery was demonstrated by others [7–11], and in 2000 Bonhoeffer *et al.* [12] described the first successfully implanted catheter-based stent valve in a pulmonary conduit. Transcatheter aortic valve implantation (TAVI) was first performed using an antegrade approach via the femoral vein by Cribier

et al. in 2002 [13]. Subsequently, we described the development of a retrograde approach via the femoral artery [14], and an off-pump transapical approach via a minithoractomy [15,16].

Morphology and pathophysiology

Acquired aortic stenosis may occur as a result of calcific degeneration of a trileaflet valve, calcific degeneration of a bicuspid valve, or rheumatic valve disease. The atherosclerotic process may play a role in the pathogenesis of degenerative calcific aortic stenosis, with early lesions showing similar features including lipid accumulation, inflammatory cell infiltration, and calcification. Myofibroblasts have been implicated in the process of calcium deposition over many years [17]. Once calcified, leaflet mobility is reduced, transvalvular pressure gradients increase, left ventricular outflow becomes obstructed, and systolic pressure overload occurs. In response to higher pressure, the left ventricular wall thickens to maintain chamber size, wall stress, and ejection fraction [18]. This process is both beneficial and detrimental. The hypertrophied myocardium becomes increasingly vulnerable to ischemia given the lower coronary flow per gram of tissue and lack of vasodilatory reserve [19–21]. The tendency toward ischemic insult must be considered during TAVI, for which transient left ventricular outflow obstruction and rapid pacing are procedurally required.

For adults with aortic stenosis, the natural history is that of a prolonged latent period, during which morbidity and mortality are very low. With the continued active deposition of calcium, there is continued increase in the transvalvular gradient with eventual development of the cardinal symptoms of aortic stenosis: heart failure, angina, and syncope. The rate of progression from mild to severe aortic stenosis is variable but, once moderate aortic stenosis is present, aortic valve area (AVA) decreases, on average, at a rate of $0.1 \, cm^2$/year [22]. Although the rate of change can be predicted, it is the transition to a symptomatic state that marks a dramatic change in the natural history of the disease. Once symptomatic, the average survival is 2–3 years [23–25] and the risk of

Cardiovascular Interventions in Clinical Practice. Edited by Jürgen Haase, Hans-Joachim Schäfers, Horst Sievert and Ron Waksman. © 2010 Blackwell Publishing.

Table 11.1 ACC/AHA recommended indications for AVR in patients with aortic stenosis [27].

Indication	Class[a]	Level of evidence[b]
Severe aortic stenosis[c] and symptoms	I	B
Severe aortic stenosis, undergoing CABG	I	C
Severe aortic stenosis, undergoing aortic or other valve surgery	I	C
Severe aortic stenosis and EF <50%	I	C
Moderate aortic stenosis[d], undergoing CABG, aortic or other valve surgery	IIa	B
Asymptomatic, severe aortic stenosis, and abnormal exercise response[e]	IIb	C
Asymptomatic, severe aortic stenosis, and features suggesting rapid progression[f] or potential delay of surgery at the time of symptom onset	IIb	C
Mild aortic stenosis, undergoing CABG, and features suggesting rapid progression[f]	IIb	C
Asymptomatic, extremely severe aortic stenosis,[g] and expected operative mortality <1%	IIb	C
Asymptomatic, no findings listed above	III	B

ACC, American College of Cardiology; AHA, American Heart Association, AVR: aortic valve replacement; CABG, coronary artery bypass grafting; EF, ejection fraction; AVA, aortic valve area.

[a]Class I: conditions for which there is evidence for and/or general agreement that the procedure or treatment is beneficial, useful, and effective. Class II: conditions for which there is conflicting evidence and/or a divergence of opinion about the usefulness/efficacy of a procedure or treatment: IIa—weight of evidence/opinion is in favor of usefulness/efficacy; IIb—usefulness/efficacy is less well established by evidence/opinion. Class III: conditions for which there is evidence and/or general agreement that the procedure/treatment is not useful/effective and in some cases may be harmful.

[b]A, Data derived from multiple randomized clinical trials; B, data derived from a single randomized trial or nonrandomized studies; C, only consensus opinion of experts, case studies, or standard of are.

[c]Severe aortic stenosis: AVA <1 cm², AVA index <0.6 cm²/m², mean gradient >40 mmHg, and/or jet velocity >4 m/s [27].

[d]Moderate aortic stenosis: AVA 1.5–1 cm², mean gradient 25–40 mmHg, and/or jet velocity 3–4 m/s [27].

[e]Development of symptoms or asymptomatic hypotension.

[f]Age, calcification, and CAD.

[g]AVA <0.6 cm², mean gradient >60 mmHg, and jet velocity >5 m/s.

sudden death increases. Thus, it is with the development of symptoms that AVR must be contemplated [26].

Indications

Surgical AVR offers survival and symptom benefits in patients with severe aortic stenosis, and can be performed with a low risk, providing a durable result in most patient groups. The current Valvular Heart Disease Guidelines provided by the American College of Cardiology (ACC)/American Heart Association (AHA) give a class I recommendation of surgical AVR for patients with severe aortic stenosis in combination with symptoms, left ventricular ejection fraction (LVEF) <50%, or concomitant aortic, heart valve, or coronary bypass surgery [27]. Table 11.1 summarizes these guidelines. However, a large number of patients with severe aortic stenosis felt to be at excessive risk for perioperative morbidity and mortality, and are often deemed nonsurgical. It is this group to whom TAVI has been applied, and therefore an under-

standing of surgical risk is fundamental to the process of TAVI selection.

The risk of surgical AVR is best estimated by large databases providing retrospective analysis of surgical outcomes. The Society of Thoracic Surgeons (STS) database provides such a registry, and reports the average perioperative mortality as 3–4% for isolated AVR (1998–2005) and 5–7% for AVR plus coronary artery bypass grafts (CABGs) [28]. Other large registries report mortalities of 5–15% for isolated AVR, with higher rates in the presence of comorbidities or the need for additional cardiac procedures [29–36]. Beyond mortality, morbidity is a significant risk with surgical AVR, and often a prime patient concern. In the case of very elderly patients, postoperative stay is often longer than 2 weeks, a majority are discharged to nursing care or rehabilitation facilities, and the need for rehospitalizations can be as high as 20% [37,38].

Currently, TAVI procedures are being performed in an elderly cohort of "high-risk" or nonsurgical patients with symptomatic severe aortic stenosis. Quantitative risk estimates of 30-day mortality for surgical AVR can be obtained from risk calculators

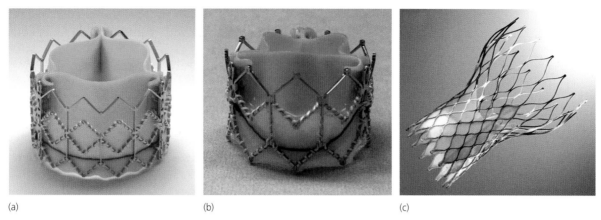

(a)   (b)   (c)

Figure 11.1 Currently available transcatheter aortic valves: (a) Edwards Lifesciences Sapien™ valve, (b) Edwards Lifesciences next-generation cobalt–chromium valve, (c) CoreValve Revalving™ valve.

generated by the European System for Cardiac Operative Risk Evaluation (EuroSCORE) [39,40] and the STS database [41]. Ambler *et al.* [42] developed an alternative risk model specifically for patients undergoing valve surgery using the database of the Society of Cardiothoracic Surgeons of Great Britain and Ireland (SCTS), but it remains less well utilized. All groups have facilitated risk calculations by providing on-line calculators: euroscore.org/calc.html, 66.89.112.110/STSWeb RiskCalc/, and www.ucl.ac.uk/stats/research/riskmodel/.

Eligibility for TAVI has been commonly defined, in part, by an objective assessment of individual risk using the above-listed databases [43]. Published case series have typically seen average EuroSCOREs of >20 [44,45]. Furthermore, the inclusion criteria for ongoing randomized trials include an objective risk measurement, with the threshold for the PARTNER (Placement of Aortic Transcatheter Valves) Trial set at an STS score >10 (or for those with STS <10, patients can be included if there is agreement by two senior cardiac surgeons that the risk of severe irreversible morbidity and/or mortality is >50%).

Not all patients with symptomatic severe aortic stenosis are eligible for TAVI. It is important to emphasize that surgical AVR is currently the treatment of choice for most patients with severe aortic stenosis, and at present TAVI should be considered only in patients felt to be at a high risk of morbidity or mortality with surgical AVR. Other factors that might preclude TAVI include (1) duration or quality of life being severely limited by comorbidities that are unlikely to be affected by relief of severe aortic stenosis, (2) an aortic annulus that is either too large or too small for the available prosthesis (i.e., the current Edwards Sapien™ is unsuitable for patients in whom the diameter of the aortic annulus at the level of the leaflet attachment is <18 or >26 mm as assessed by transesophageal echocardiography), and (3) for transarterial approaches, severe iliofemoral arterial disease. Recent papers have emphasized accurate measurements of aortic annular dimensions in patient selection to minimize the likelihood of postimplant significant aortic insufficiency [46].

Technical aspects

Balloon expandable aortic valve

Valve

The currently available Sapien™ prosthesis (Edwards Lifesciences LLC, Irvine, CA, USA) is a balloon-expandable valve consisting of three bovine pericardial leaflets hand-sewn to a stainless-steel, tubular, slotted, balloon-expandable stent (Fig. 11.1). The bottom portion of the stent is covered with a fabric sealing cuff, designed to facilitate a seal with the aortic annulus and prevent paravalvular leak. The bovine pericardium is processed with the same Thermafix™ (Edwards Lifesciences, lrvine, CA) anticalcification treatment utilized in the Carpentier-Edwards Perimount Magna™ (Edwards Lifesciences, lrvine, CA) surgical valves. Leaflet stress is low, and coaptation is maximized by a leaflet geometry that is similar to that of surgical heart valves, resulting in a naturally open-valve design. Currently, the valve is available in 23 and 26 mm diameters, with heights of 14.5 and 16 mm, respectively. The Sapien valve replaces the Cribier-Edwards equine stainless-steel stent valve that was used for the early published experience with balloon-expandable valves.

The valve is symmetrically compressed onto a valvuloplasty balloon using a specialized manual crimping tool. The balloon is custom manufactured by Edwards Lifesciences LLC (Irvine, CA, USA) and is 30 mm long. Before crimping, the balloon is accurately sized by preinflation within a sizing device. The balloon diameters are measured by injection of precise volumes of dilute contrast. A final balloon diameter of 22 mm is used for the 23-mm valve, and 25 mm for the 26-mm valve.

The evolution in Edwards Lifesciences transcatheter heart valve technology has been the development of valves whose struts are constructed from a cobalt–chromium alloy (Fig. 11.1). This has allowed the struts to be thinner without loss of structural strength or effective orifice area, and allows for a lower crimped profile. Crush force resistance, radial stiffness, fatigue, and corrosion resistance are similar to those of the stainless-steel Sapien valve. Initial implants used a delivery system 2F smaller in diameter than would have been required with the Sapien valve [47]. It is anticipated that with modification of the delivery system the new 23- and 26-mm valves will utilize 18F and 19F delivery systems, respectively. Furthermore, 20- and 29-mm valves can be produced with this new technology.

Access: Transvenous

Initial TAVI procedures were performed using an antegrade transvenous approach. Following percutaneous puncture of the femoral vein, atrial trans-septal puncture was performed to gain access to the left heart. A wire was then passed from the femoral vein through the trans-septal puncture and left heart, where it could be snared from the femoral artery to complete a full wire loop from venous to arterial systems and provide support for catheter and prosthesis introduction. The valve stent prosthesis was crimped on a valvuloplasty balloon and introduced from the femoral vein, across the dilated trans-septal puncture, into the left atrium and across the mitral valve to allow "antegrade" introduction to the aortic position. This procedure established the feasibility of TAVI [13], but was complex and difficult to replicate, and results were variable [48].

Access: Transarterial

The initial retrograde transarterial TAVI procedures employed a similar valve stent crimped on standard valvuloplasty balloons but, although they were successful, they were technically challenging [49,50]. The procedure was refined and made more reproducible with the development of a steerable guiding catheter (Flex Catheter, Edwards Lifesciences LLC), which has been further refined to the currently available RetroFlex™ II catheter (Edwards Lifesciences, Irvine, CA), as discussed below [14].

The RetroFlex™ II delivery catheter requires a 22F (7.3 mm) sheath for the 23-mm valve and a 24F (8 mm) sheath for the 26-mm valve. Given the large sheath size, and the fact that these procedures have generally been performed in elderly patients with a high prevalence of vascular disease, the potential for vascular complications is high. Our current practice is to obtain both traditional and computed tomography angiograms and of the descending aorta, iliac, and femoral systems. Common femoral and iliac size, tortuosity, and calcification (particularly circumferential) must all be considered in making decisions about the suitability for a transarterial (femoral) TAVI. We currently exclude patients in whom the vessel diameter is <7 mm, and are concerned when we see circumferential calcification within the iliofemoral system. Abdominal aortic aneurysm has not been problematic in our experience.

There have been a variety of approaches to arterial access and closure, with some centers using surgical cut-down and closure for arterial access. It has been our practice to use fluoroscopically guided percutaneous puncture of the common femoral artery at the level of the femoral head. Following placement of a 7F arterial sheath, we have been using one or two Prostar® XL perclose devices (Abbott Vascular, Inc., Redwood City, CA, USA) to place sutures before the introduction of larger sheaths for balloon valvuloplasty and TAVI. With experience, this has permitted arterial closure without the need for surgical intervention in most cases. Successful percutaneous closure necessitates accurate puncture of the anterior wall of the common femoral artery, which may be facilitated by ultrasound guidance. In the opposite groin, we place a 7F venous sheath for placement of a transvenous pacemaker, and a second 7F arterial sheath for placement of a pigtail catheter, which is advanced to the ascending aorta to help with prosthesis positioning at the time of implantation.

Following arterial access, we utilize standard techniques to place a catheter across the aortic valve. Most often this is accomplished by the use of a straight wire with an Amplatz Left I diagnostic catheter (Boston Scientific Corporation, Natick, MA). Subsequently, an exaggerated J is manually formed at the end of a of standard J-tipped 0.035-inch Amplatz extra support exchange wire. The wire is placed in the left ventricle and the catheter withdrawn. Once the wire is across the native valve, obsessive care must be exercised to ensure the wire is not withdrawn until after the prosthesis is placed.

It is important to choose an imaging angle at which all three leaflets of the native aortic valve are easily appreciated. We usually start in the anteroposterior view; however, the plane of the aortic valve is typically best seen with slight left anterior oblique (LAO) with or without cranial angulation or right anterior oblique (RAO) with or without caudal angulation. Prosthesis positioning depends upon an accurate understanding of the native aortic annulus, and having a view perpendicular to the annulus will greatly improve the likelihood of a successful procedure.

Balloon valvuloplasty is performed under rapid burst ventricular pacing with fluoroscopic guidance. We generally use 50 mm by 20 mm (or 22 mm) Z-Med II valvuloplasty balloons (NuMed, Inc., Hopkinton, NY, USA) to stretch the native valve enough to allow the TAVI prosthesis/stent balloon to cross the stenotic orifice. A single effective balloon dilation is often sufficient. We give standard doses of intravenous heparin before the valvuloplasty and maintain an activated clotting time of >250 s for the duration of the procedure. Following balloon valvuloplasty, the femoral artery is progressively dilated using a series of hydrophilic dilators followed by introduction of the larger delivery sheath under fluoroscopic guidance.

Delivery catheter and positioning

The RetroFlex II delivery catheter consists of three components incorporated in coaxial fashion: (1) a retractable nosecone catheter, (2) a balloon catheter (upon which the prosthesis is crimped), and (3) a deflectable steering catheter (Fig. 11.2). The catheter is advanced over the wire through the hemostatic

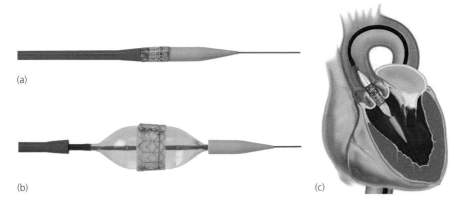

(a)

(b)

(c)

Figure 11.2 The Edwards Lifesciences RetroFlex II™ catheter: (a) photograph of the catheter assembled before introduction, (b) photograph of the catheter with nose-cone advanced and balloon exposed to allow for prosthesis deployment, and (c) diagrammatic representation of the device in position with nose-cone advanced, flexion catheter withdrawn and prosthesis placed with the aortic annulus.

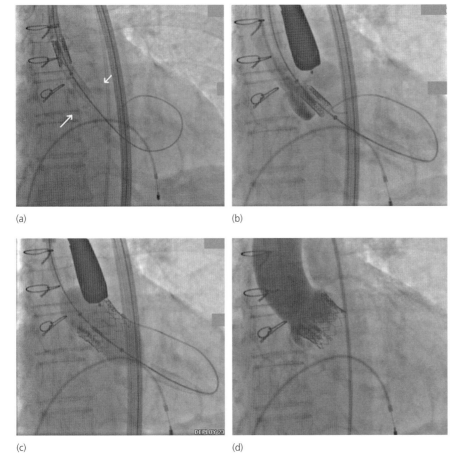

(a)

(b)

(c)

(d)

Figure 11.3 Implantation of a Sapien™ valve using the RetroFlex II system: (a) steerable delivery catheter with nosecone and prosthesis crimped on delivery balloon approaching calcified stenotic aortic valve; (b) delivery catheter withdrawn, nosecone advanced, and prosthesis in position within aortic annulus; (c) balloon inflation; (d) valve fully expanded with no aortic insufficiency.

valves of the sheath and into the descending thoracic aorta. As the catheter is advanced toward the aortic arch, a control knob on the catheter hub is rotated to deflect the delivery catheter over the arch in an atraumatic fashion and approach the native stenotic valve in a coaxial direction. The nosecone helps with atraumatic delivery of the prosthesis/balloon through the stenotic native valve and into the ventricle. The delivery catheter is then retracted while keeping the prosthesis/balloon in the ventricle and the nosecone is advanced to expose the distal end of the balloon. The whole system is then retracted to position the prosthesis within the native valve. The prosthesis is typically positioned so that approximately half of the prosthesis is ventricular to the insertion plane of the native valve leaflets. When the prosthesis is correctly positioned, rapid burst ventricular pacing is initiated and the deployment balloon is manually inflated with dilute contrast to achieve the predetermined size (Fig. 11.3). Following rapid inflation and deflation, the balloon is readvanced into the ventricle, the nosecone retracted onto the distal end of the balloon, and the system atraumatically withdrawn through the newly implanted valve. Finally, the delivery catheter, balloon, and nosecone are approximated in the descending aorta and removed through the delivery sheath. Following withdrawal of the large sheath and percutaneous closure of the arteriotomy, we routinely image the site of insertion by selective femoral angiogram, performed from the contralateral femoral artery.

Imaging and sizing

All our procedures are performed with fluoroscopic and transesophageal echocardiographic guidance. With the currently available prostheses, we require the diameter of the aortic annulus to be ≥18 mm and ≤26 mm. We routinely screen for this using transthoracic echocardiography (TTE), but in instances of annular dimensions >24 mm or <18 mm on TTE, a preprocedure transesophageal echocardiogram (TEE) is obtained. TEE measurements are routinely larger than TTE measurements. The average difference is 1.36 mm, but we have seen differences as large as 4 mm [51]. At the time of the procedure, decisions about prosthesis size are made based upon TEE imaging. We use a 23-mm prosthesis if the annulus is ≥18 mm and <22 mm and a 26-mm prosthesis if the annulus is >21 mm and ≤26 mm. We also find the input from experienced echocardiographers helpful with positioning and the assessment of postprocedure aortic insufficiency, and, in the case of complications, real-time echocardiography often complements fluoroscopy. Although some groups advocate balloon sizing to accurately choose prosthesis size [52], we continue to size based on TEE annular measurements.

Other procedural issues

Burst rapid pacing of the right ventricle is utilized to minimize transvalvular flow at the time of balloon valvuloplasty and during deployment of the prosthesis [53]. Under continuous pressure monitoring we test the pace at rates between 160 and 220 bpm to ensure that cardiac output can be transiently halted. Transient arrest of transvalvular flow is fundamental for accurate prosthesis deployment. The primary operator instructs either a trained registered nurse or the anesthesiologist as to the initiation and cessation of rapid pacing.

We have performed the majority of our operations using general anesthesia. There are several advantages of this, including patient comfort for vascular access, patient comfort with a TEE probe in place, and allowing the TAVI operator to concentrate on the procedural details while another physician can concentrate on patient physiology and hemodynamic stability. However, general anesthesia may have disadvantages in terms of hypotension and respiratory compromise in certain patients. It appears that both approaches will be valid in the future.

Often patients have some hemodynamic instability with the procedure, and transient hypotension is common when intervening in patients with critical aortic stenosis. Hypotension is a particular concern owing to the possibility of reduced coronary perfusion and progressive myocardial dysfunction.

We suggest that hypotension should be treated initially with vasopressors, such as phenylephrine or norepinephrine, and volume as required. Inotropic and chronotropic medications are problematic as they may worsen myocardial ischemia and myocardial dysfunction in the presence of untreated aortic stenosis. In our centre we have elected to provide pre-TAVI coronary revascularization if significant stenosis subtend a large myocardial territory. However, the indications for pre-procedure coronary revascularization is an area of ongoing active research. For the most part, TAVI procedures have been performed in the cardiac catheterization laboratory, but more recently various groups have perceived potential advantages to a hybrid cardiac catheterization/cardiac operating room setting with the potential for surgical and cardiopulmonary support when needed.

Preprocedure medical therapy includes bolus dosing with clopidogrel (300 mg) on the day before the procedure with maintenance for 3 months. All patients should be on chronic aspirin therapy (81 mg daily). We give a bolus dose of antibiotics on call to the procedure, and recommend that patients are referred for dental assessment before valve implantation if there are concerns around the need for dental procedures following valve implantation. Recommendations surrounding endocarditis prophylaxis are the same as with any surgical bioprosthetic valve [54].

Access: Transapical

Direct puncture of the left ventricular apex permits fluoroscopically guided antegrade wire advancement across the aortic valve. TAVI procedures can then be performed in a manner similar to the transfemoral retrograde approach. This "transapical" technique was initially developed to facilitate testing of transcatheter valves [11], and has been refined to become a clinical procedure in recent years [15,16,55–57]. In this procedure, the left ventricle is exposed through anterolateral minithoracotomy, which permits needle puncture of the left ventricular apex. A standard arterial sheath (7F) is then advanced over a wire into the left ventricular cavity. Fluoroscopy is used to advance an extra support wire through the stenotic aortic valve into the descending aorta. Balloon valvuloplasty is generally performed. Subsequently, a large access sheath is placed and the prosthesis is crimped onto a balloon catheter. The balloon/prosthesis is positioned under fluoroscopic and echocardiographic guidance and deployed with rapid burst ventricular pacing, as described above. The apex is surgically closed with pledgeted sutures, and a chest tube is placed. This approach has been widely adopted with demonstrated reproducibility [56,58,59]. Currently, it is our practice to employ a transfemoral approach for routine procedures, as our results have been more favorable to date. However, the transapical approach may be advantageous in cases limited by iliofemoral arterial disease, and the smaller distance between the prosthesis and site of arterial access may facilitate accurate positioning. Nevertheless, it appears likely that, as procedures and equipment evolve, the transarterial and transapical approaches will be complementary.

Self-expanding aortic valve

The CoreValve ReValving™ System (CoreValve, Inc., Irvine, CA, USA) utilizes a self-expanding, rather than balloon-expandable, prosthesis. The valve is constructed of a laser-cut nitinol alloy frame to which is sutured porcine pericardial leaflets and a sealing cuff. With cooling in ice water the frame is malleable and can be constrained inside a sheath. With retraction of the restraining sheath, the nitinol stent alloy expands to its predetermined shape, forming a rigid tubular frame with a trileaflet pericardial tissue valve (Fig. 11.1).

The CoreValve device measures 50 mm in axial length. The frame incorporates three distinct areas of radial force. The lower portion implants within the subannular region with high radial force. The middle supra-annular portion is tapered and contains the valve leaflets. The tapered portion is not intended to be apposed to the aorta or coronary sinuses so as to allow unobstructed blood flow to the coronary ostia through the stent struts. The upper portion of the frame is flared and anchors the prosthesis against the ascending aorta, providing longitudinal stability [60]. The valve is currently available in two sizes depending on the diameter of the ascending aorta and the aortic annulus. Initially, the delivery system was 24F, but subsequently evolved to 21F with a more recent 18F iteration [44,60].

As with all other current TAVI procedures, balloon valvuloplasty is typically performed before valve implantation. Initially, the CoreValve procedure was performed with femoral–femoral cardiopulmonary support and bilateral femoral surgical cut-downs. With reduction in the diameter of the delivery system and other technical improvements, cardiopulmonary support is no longer utilized and percutaneous closure has become the norm.

Results

The success of TAVI procedures can be considered by procedure type and duration of follow-up. Most authors report procedural success and 30-day mortality/majority cardiac events (MACE). As time moves on, follow-up will be extended, but, currently, the largest reported series have followed patients out to 1 year, with the longest follow-up of over 4 years reported in only a few patients.

Balloon-expandable transcatheter valves

Between 2002 and early 2008, over 1000 patients received a balloon-expandable transcatheter valve. Early experience with 59 patients undergoing surgery using an antegrade/transvenous approach was followed by 628 patients using a retrograde/transarterial approach and 457 patients using a transapical approach.

Transvenous approach

Cribier and colleagues demonstrated initial success of TAVI utilizing a transvenous technique with puncture of the femoral vein and interatrial septum to permit antegrade access to the left heart and aortic valve [61,62]. They published the results of their first 36 patients in 2006, and showed that valve implantation was successful in 75%, with failures secondary to embolization of the stent valve, hemodynamic instability, and inability to cross the native aortic valve [49]. Postprocedure hemodynamics confirmed excellent valve function with a significant decrease in gradient and increase in valve area, but the occurrence of moderate to severe paravalvular aortic insufficiency in 63% of patients was a major concern. There was a high rate of procedure-related in-hospital complications (26%) with worrisome procedural mortality rates. Nevertheless, extended follow-up has demonstrated sustained normal bioprosthetic valve function for over 4 years in two late survivors, providing proof that TAVI could be performed with a durable result. However, it was apparent that the transvenous antegrade approach was technically complex and not generalizable [63].

Transarterial approach

Early experience with the retrograde transarterial approach was limited by technical difficulties, which included issues of arterial access with large sheaths and catheters, difficulty with passage of large-diameter prostheses around the aortic arch, problems with retrograde crossing of severely stenotic calcified valves, and problematic positioning and deployment. Subsequently, a reproducible retrograde transarterial approach was developed and described by our group in 2006 [14]. TAVI was performed in 18 elderly high-risk patients (logistic EuroSCORE 26%) with success in 14 and a 30-day mortality of 11.1%, demonstrating the feasibility of this approach. Reproducibility and improving outcomes were subsequently demonstrated in a larger 50-patient cohort study [45]. Valve implantation was successful in 86% of patients, and 30-day mortality was 12% (logistic EuroSCORE estimate of 28%). With experience, procedural success increased from 76% in the first 25 patients to 96% after the first 25 patients, and 30-day mortality fell from 16% to 8%. In a subsequent report of the newer RetroFlex II delivery system, procedural success in the initial 25 patients was 100%, with no 30-day mortality [47].

We published further reports of an 85-patient series [64] and most recently a 168-patient series of 113 transfemoral and 55 transapical patients [65]. There have been significant improvements in valve area, left ventricular ejection fraction, mitral regurgitation and functional class, with improvements maintained at 1 year [66] (Fig. 11.4). None of the patients had moderate or severe aortic insufficiency, and although mild paravalvular aortic regurgitation was common, it remained stable, with no clinical consequences at 1 year. Thirty-day mortality has continued to fall to an overall rate of 11.3% (transfemoral 8% vs. transapical 18.2% ($P = 0.07$)), and evidence of

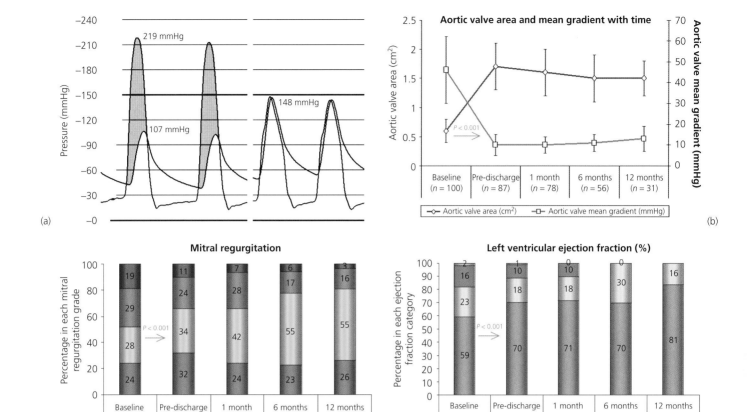

Figure 11.4 Hemodynamic and functional outcome of 100 elderly patients treated with Edwards Lifesciences bovine pericardial balloon-expandable aortic valve: (a) immediate hemodynamic results before and after valve implantation showing preprocedure simultaneous left ventricular and femoral artery mean gradient of 108 mmHg converted to postprocedure mean gradient of 3 mmHg; (b) graphic representation showing sustained improvement in aortic valve area and mean gradient out to 1 year of follow-up; (c) graph showing improvement in mitral regurgitation over time as evidenced by increasing proportion of patients with no or mild mitral regurgitation over time; (d) graph showing change in left ventricular ejection fraction over time.

a learning curve continued, with mortality falling from 14.3% to 8.3% between the first and second half of the series. [From 12.3% to 3.6% ($P = 0.16$) in transfemoral patients and from 25% to 11.1% ($P = 0.30$) in transapical patients.] Functional class improved over the year following the procedure ($P < 0.001$). Survival at 1 year was 74%, with the bulk of late re-admissions and mortality occurring as a function of comorbidities rather than procedure or valve-related events. The 1-year survival of 74% compares favourably with the reported 1-year survivals of 51% and 66% in elderly patients with aortic stenosis who were not considered to be surgical candidates or who declined surgery, respectively [67].

Importantly, this favourable experience has been confirmed in the 55-patient US multicenter REVIVAL II (randomization of endovascular implantation of valves trial) study where 30-day mortality was 7.4% (logistic EuroSCORE 33.1%, STS 12.8%) [68]. In September 2007, the SAPIEN™ valve received CE mark in the European community and as of May 2009 there have been over 2500 SAPIEN™ implants worldwide. The

Edwards Lifesciences SOURCE registry contains data on over 1000 implants, and confirms the structural and hemodynamic integrity of the valve with follow-up to 1 year, and the transfemoral ($n = 459$ patients) 30-day mortality was 6.3% with 93.3% of the cohort having a logistic EuroScore of >20% (mean 33.3%). One-year survival was approximately 75% (Edwards Lifesciences LLC., unpublished data).

Experience from the Canadian Registry of EndoVascular Implantation of Valves in Europe (REVIVE II), REVIVAL II, and other as yet unpublished registries has provided the impetus for the development of a randomized clinical trial: the PARTNER Trial is a prospective, randomized, controlled, multicenter, noninferiority pivotal trial evaluating the safety and effectiveness of the Edwards Sapien transcatheter heart valve in a stratified population of 600 patients with symptomatic severe aortic stenosis. The study population consists of two cohorts: (1) high-risk surgery patients (operative mortality estimated at >15% and STS ≥10) randomized to either TAVI or surgical aortic valve replacement and (2) inoperable patients (surgical consensus that the probability of death or serious, irreversible morbidity exceeds 50%) randomized to medical therapy or TAVI. The primary outcome is 1-year mortality, and enrolment is largely completed.

Transapical approach

Early experience with TAVI was limited to transfemoral approaches. Animal models utilized direct balloon catheter implantation of experimental prosthesis via the left ventricular apex [11], and was subsequently trialed extensively in animals [55]. The first human applications utilized a median sternotomy with cardiopulmonary bypass, but this has been supplanted by the current approach of intercostal thoracotomy without cardiopulmonary bypass [15,16,56,57,69].

The transapical approach avoids problems related to arterial access, and the short distance from the left ventricular apex to the aortic valve may facilitate antegrade crossing and prosthesis positioning. However, disadvantages include the need for a general anesthetic, thoracotomy, chest tube, and apical repair, and the possibility of injury to the mitral apparatus. Experience with this procedure is growing. As of early 2008, 457 procedures had been performed in a variety of centers in Canada, Europe, and the USA. The largest experience from four centers in Europe and North America was recently published and highlights the success of this approach. Fifty-nine patients with average logistic EuroScore of $26.8 \pm 13.5\%$ underwent transapical TAVR. Thirty-day mortality was 13.6%, and actuarial survival was $75.7 \pm 5.9\%$ at a follow-up interval of 110 ± 77 days (range 1 to 255 days) [56]. A slightly larger series of 61 patients showed 6- and 12-month survival of $74.4 \pm 6.6\%$ and $70.5 \pm 7.3\%$, respectively [69]. This procedural success was recently replicated by Walther *et al.* [70], where procedural success was 92.8% in a cohort of 168 patients. Thirty-day and 6-month mortality was 16% and 30%, respectively.

Self expanding aortic valves

The CoreValve Revalving™ (Corevalve Inc., Irvine, CA) procedures were initially performed in India with apparent procedural success but less favorable clinical outcomes. The first published reports from Germany in 2005 [71] and 2006 [60] demonstrated the reproducibility of the procedure. Valve implantation was successful in 88% of 25 patients. Mean transvalvular gradients were significantly reduced, but major in-hospital adverse events occurred in 32%. In-hospital mortality was 20% in this high-risk group with a median logistic EuroSCORE of 11%. A more recent report describes 86 operations performed using the newer 21F and 18F systems [44]. The group had a mean age of 81.3 ± 5.2 (21F) and 83.4 ± 6.7 years (18Fr), and a mean logistic EuroSCORE of $23.4\% \pm 13.5\%$ (21Fr) and $19.1\% \pm 11.1\%$ (18F). Valve implantation was successful in 88% of patients, with a marked reduction in mean transvalvular gradient and no change in aortic regurgitation grade. Periprocedural stroke and tamponade were concerns, but intraprocedural mortality was 6%, and overall

30-day mortality was 12%, which was a significant improvement over the earlier case series. The most recent series, of 1243 patients, shows 30-day mortality has decreased to 6.7% (Logistic EUROscore $22.9 \pm 4.1\%$), and postprocedure pacemaker implant was required in 12% [72]. Importantly, the 18Fr system has allowed transition to a percutaneous approach under local anesthesia without hemodynamic support [44].

Long-term outcome and complications

Valve function

Evaluation of transcatheter valves show excellent valve function post implantation (Fig. 11.4). In comparison with surgical prostheses, transcatheter valve orifice areas are typically larger owing to the absence of sewing rings and the ability to implant oversized prosthesis following balloon dilation. Follow-up echocardiographic data commonly show gradients of $<10\,\mathrm{mmHg}$ and effective orifice areas of $>1.5\,\mathrm{cm}^2$ for both currently available prostheses [67,69,73].

Paravalvular leak following TAVI is common. However, although initial experience often documented severe paravalvular regurgitation [8,60], most current series have found such leaks to be mild to moderate and generally well tolerated when procedures have been performed with routine oversizing and careful attention to positioning [14,44,45,51]. Clinically important hemolysis has not been observed [14,45,74].

There are few clinical data upon which to make conclusive statements about valve durability. *In vitro* valve testing with the Cribier-Edwards Sapien, and CoreValve devices predict durability similar to that seen with surgical bioprostheses. Structural valve deterioration has not been reported, but follow-up in a reasonable number of patients is limited to 2 years, with a few patients followed to 4 years. Nevertheless, *in vivo* valve failure must be expected eventually, and it remains to be determined if this will occur significantly before that expected with a surgical bioprosthesis. Importantly, early experience with implantation of transcatheter valves within failed surgically implanted bioprostheses sets the scene for a "valve-in-valve" procedure that may be, at least in a limited sense, repeatable when percutaneous valves do fail [75–77].

Complications of percutaneous valves

The manipulation of large catheters through the vasculature raises the possibility of arterial dissection or perforation. Although these complications still occur, their incidence has been reduced by careful screening, particularly of the femoral artery, experience, the advent of new technology, and the possibility of a transapical approach [49,78]. Cardiogenic shock and myocardial ischemia may occur in any procedure in patients with severe aortic stenosis. Coronary revascularization may help to mitigate against this possibility, but a consensus as to what lesions require revascularization before TAVI is an ongoing area of research. The potential for coronary obstruction by displacement of a bulky native leaflet over the coronary ostium is of particular concern to TAVI procedures. Although this has been reported [62], the frequency of such occurrence is unknown and a better understanding of methods of screening for this complication requires further investigation. The risk of atrioventricular block and pacemaker dependence is of concern, given the anatomical proximity of the aortic annulus to the bundle of His/Purkinje system. Initial reports of heart block with balloon-expandable valves suggests a risk similar to that associated with surgical AVR [79]. Initial reports suggest that this risk may be higher with the CoreValve device, presumably because the area of contact with the interventricular septum is larger. Finally, stroke is a primary concern of both physicians and patients given the possibility of embolization of aortic atheroma, friable material from a calcified aortic valve, catheter induced thrombus, or air. Despite this risk, our experience with over 200 transcatheter procedures is of a stroke rate of 4%, although the rate of undetected embolic events may be higher. Walther and colleagues [69] report a stroke rate of 0% in their series of transapical procedures, and the largest multicenter 86-patient CoreValve series reported stroke rates of 10% [44]. Despite this range of events, it is likely that stroke risk will decrease with experience and the development of less traumatic delivery systems. Our group recently published a review paper highlighting the complications of multicenters utilizing different systems and techniques in an effort to prevent others from having similar problems and highlight management strategies [80].

Learning curve

Transcatheter aortic valve implantation is a complex procedure being performed in elderly patients with multiple comorbidities and severe aortic stenosis. Technical errors are not well tolerated and mortality may ensue. Nevertheless, the procedure has proven reproducibility across multiple centers, and outcomes will continue to improve with improvements in equipment, techniques and experience [44,45]. Consequently, cautious dissemination appears prudent. Formal educational programs, virtual simulators, and proctoring have been utilized and appear helpful. Regional centers of expertise may be desirable to optimize outcomes.

Conclusion

Severe aortic stenosis is a mechanical problem that cannot be treated medically, but requires a mechanical solution for durable long-term results. Surgical aortic valve replacement continues to be the treatment of choice for patients at low operative risk, but many patients at high operative risk do not receive definitive therapy. Transcatheter aortic valve implantation is a feasible and reproducible therapeutic option for patients with symptomatic severe aortic stenosis and high surgical risk. Despite appropriate initial skepticism, this approach is gaining rapid acceptance. A variety of devices and implan-

tation techniques have been developed, and technologic improvements continue to increase procedural ease and success. Early and longer-term outcome data from a variety of international registries suggest that TAVI is a reasonable therapeutic option for patients with comorbidities in whom the risk of morbidity and mortality with open heart surgery is unacceptable. Although implications of this therapy are still not fully known, clinical trials are ongoing. We suspect that TAVI within native or prosthetic valves will become a viable therapeutic option applicable beyond those currently considered nonsurgical candidates.

Conflict of interest disclosure

Dr. Webb is a consultant to Edwards Lifesciences, LLB.

References

1. Nkomo VT, Gardin JM, Skelton TN, *et al.* (2006) Burden of valvular heart diseases: a population-based study. *Lancet* **368**:1005–1011.
2. Iung B, Cachier A, Baron G, *et al.* (2005) Decision-making in elderly patients with severe aortic stenosis: why are so many denied surgery? *Eur Heart J* **26**:2714–2720.
3. Bouma BJ, van Den Brink RB, van Der Meulen JH, *et al.* (1999) To operate or not on elderly patients with aortic stenosis: the decision and its consequences. *Heart* **82**:143–148.
4. Varadarajan P, Kapoor N, Bansal RC, *et al.* (2006) Clinical profile and natural history of 453 nonsurgically managed patients with severe aortic stenosis. *Ann Thorac Surg* **82**:2111–2115.
5. Pai RG, Kapoor N, Bansal RC, *et al.* (2006) Malignant natural history of asymptomatic severe aortic stenosis: benefit of aortic valve replacement. *Ann Thorac Surg* **82**:2116–2122.
6. Andersen HR, Knudsen LL, & Hasenkam JM (1992) Transluminal implantation of artificial heart valves. Description of a new expandable aortic valve and initial results with implantation by catheter technique in closed chest pigs. *Eur Heart J* **13**:704–708.
7. Boudjemline Y, Agnoletti G, Bonnet D, *et al.* (2004) Percutaneous pulmonary valve replacement in a large right ventricular outflow tract: an experimental study. *J Am Coll Cardiol* **43**:1082–1087.
8. Cribier A, Eltchaninoff H, Bash A, *et al.* (2001) Trans-catheter implantation of balloon-expandable prosthetic heart valves. Early results in an animal model. *Circulation* **104**(Suppl. 2):I552.
9. Lutter G, Kuklinski D, Berg G, *et al.* (2002) Percutaneous aortic valve replacement: an experimental study. I. Studies on implantation. *J Thorac Cardiovasc Surg* **123**:768–776.
10. Sochman J, Peregrin JH, Pavcnik D, *et al.* (2000) Percutaneous transcatheter aortic disc valve prosthesis implantation: a feasibility study. *Cardiovasc Intervent Radiol* **23**:384–388.
11. Webb JG, Munt B, Makkar RR, *et al.* (2004) Percutaneous stent-mounted valve for treatment of aortic or pulmonary valve disease. *Catheter Cardiovas Interv* **63**:89–93.
12. Bonhoeffer P, Boudjemline Y, Saliba Z, *et al.* (2000) Percutaneous replacement of pulmonary valve in a right-ventricle to pulmonary-artery prosthetic conduit with valve dysfunction. *Lancet* **356**:1403–1405.

13. Cribier A, Eltchaninoff H, Bash A, *et al.* (2002) Percutaneous transcatheter implantation of an aortic valve prosthesis for calcific aortic stenosis: first human case description. *Circulation* **106**:3006–3008.

14. Webb JG, Chandavimol M, Thompson CR, *et al.* (2006) Percutaneous aortic valve implantation retrograde from the femoral artery. *Circulation* **113**:842–850.

15. Ye J, Cheung A, Lichtenstein SV, *et al.* (2007) Six-month outcome of transapical transcatheter aortic valve implantation in the initial seven patients. *Eur J Cardiothorac Surg* **31**:16–21.

16. Lichtenstein SV, Cheung A, Ye J, *et al.* (2006) Transapical transcatheter aortic valve implantation in humans: initial clinical experience. *Circulation* **114**:591–596.

17. Freeman RV & Otto CM (2005) Spectrum of calcific aortic valve disease: pathogenesis, disease progression, and treatment strategies. *Circulation* **111**:3316–3326.

18. Gunther S & Grossman W (1979) Determinants of ventricular function in pressure-overload hypertrophy in man. *Circulation* **59**:679–688.

19. Bache RJ, Vrobel TR, Ring WS, *et al.* (1981) Regional myocardial blood flow during exercise in dogs with chronic left ventricular hypertrophy. *Circ Res* **48**:76–87.

20. Gaasch WH, Zile MR, Hoshino PK, *et al.* (1990) Tolerance of the hypertrophic heart to ischemia. Studies in compensated and failing dog hearts with pressure overload hypertrophy. *Circulation* **81**:1644–1653.

21. Marcus ML, Doty DB, Hiratzka LF, *et al.* (1982) Decreased coronary reserve: a mechanism for angina pectoris in patients with aortic stenosis and normal coronary arteries. *N Engl J Med* **307**:1362–1366.

22. Rosenhek R, Binder T, Porenta G, *et al.* (2000) Predictors of outcome in severe, asymptomatic aortic stenosis. *N Engl J Med* **343**:611–617.

23. Pellikka PA, Sarano ME, Nishimura RA, *et al.* (2005) Outcome of 622 adults with asymptomatic, hemodynamically significant aortic stenosis during prolonged follow-up [see comment]. *Circulation* **111**:3290–3295.

24. Ross J Jr. & Braunwald E (1968) Aortic stenosis. *Circulation* **38**(1 Suppl.):61–67.

25. Turina J, Hess O, Sepulcri F, *et al.* (1987) Spontaneous course of aortic valve disease. *Eur Heart J* **8**:471–483.

26. Otto CM (2006) Valvular aortic stenosis: disease severity and timing of intervention. *J Am Coll Cardiol* **47**:2141–2151.

27. Bonow RO, Carabello BA, Kanu C, *et al.* (2006) ACC/AHA 2006 guidelines for the management of patients with valvular heart disease: a report of the American College of Cardiology/American Heart Association Task Force on Practice Guidelines (writing committee to revise the 1998 Guidelines for the Management of Patients With Valvular Heart Disease): developed in collaboration with the Society of Cardiovascular Anesthesiologists: endorsed by the Society for Cardiovascular Angiography and Interventions and the Society of Thoracic Surgeons. *Circulation* **114**:e84–231.

28. Society of Thoracic Surgeons National Cardiac Surgery Database. 2006 Executive Summary. http://www.sts.org/documents/pdf/STS-ExecutiveSummarySpring2006.pdf (accessed August 28, 2007).

29. Alexander KP, Anstrom KJ, Muhlbaier LH, *et al.* (2000) Outcomes of cardiac surgery in patients ≥ 80 years: results from the National Cardiovascular Network. *J Am Coll Cardiol Mar* **35**:731–738.

30. Asimakopoulos G, Edwards MB, & Taylor KM (1997) Aortic valve replacement in patients 80 years of age and older: survival and cause of death based on 1100 cases: collective results from the UK Heart Valve Registry. *Circulation* **96**:3403–3408.

31. Dalrymple-Hay MJ, Alzetani A, Aboel-Nazar S, *et al.* (1999) Cardiac surgery in the elderly. *Eur J Cardiothorac Surg* **15**:61–66.

32. Kolh P, Kerzmann A, Honore C, *et al.* (2007) Aortic valve surgery in octogenarians: predictive factors for operative and long-term results. *Eur J Cardiothorac Surg* **31**:600–606.

33. Kolh P, Kerzmann A, Lahaye L, *et al.* (2001) Cardiac surgery in octogenarians; peri-operative outcome and long-term results. *Eur Heart J* **22**:1235–1243.

34. Langanay T, De Latour B, Ligier K, *et al.* (2004) Surgery for aortic stenosis in octogenarians: influence of coronary disease and other comorbidities on hospital mortality. *J Heart Valve Dis* **13**:545–552; discussion 52–3.

35. Suttie SA, Jamieson WRE, Burr LH, *et al.* (2006) Elderly valve replacement with bioprostheses and mechanical prostheses. Comparison by composites of complications. *J Cardiovasc Surg* **47**:191–199.

36. Vahanian A, Baumgartner H, Bax J, *et al.* (2007) Guidelines on the management of valvular heart disease: The Task Force on the Management of Valvular Heart Disease of the European Society of Cardiology. *Eur Heart J* **28**:230–268.

37. Goodney PP, Stukel TA, Lucas FL, *et al.* (2003) Hospital volume, length of stay, and readmission rates in high-risk surgery [see comment]. *Ann Surg* **238**:161–167.

38. Hara H, Pedersen WR, Ladich E, *et al.* (2007) Percutaneous balloon aortic valvuloplasty revisited: time for a renaissance? *Circulation* **115**(12):e334–338.

39. Nashef SA, Roques F, Michel P, *et al.* (1999) European system for cardiac operative risk evaluation (EuroSCORE). *Eur J Cardiothorac Surg* **16**:9–13.

40. Nashef SAM, Roques F, Hammill BG, *et al.* (2002) Validation of European System for Cardiac Operative Risk Evaluation (EuroSCORE) in North American cardiac surgery. *Eur J Cardiothorac Surg* **22**:101–105.

41. Shroyer ALW, Coombs LP, Peterson ED, *et al.* (2003) The Society of Thoracic Surgeons: 30-day operative mortality and morbidity risk models. *Ann Thorac Surg* **75**:1856–1864; discussion 64–65.

42. Ambler G, Omar RZ, Royston P, *et al.* (2005) Generic, simple risk stratification model for heart valve surgery. *Circulation* **112**:224–231.

43. Vassiliades TA Jr., Block PC, Cohn LH, *et al.* (2005) The clinical development of percutaneous heart valve technology: a position statement of the Society of Thoracic Surgeons (STS), the American Association for Thoracic Surgery (AATS), and the Society for Cardiovascular Angiography and Interventions (SCAI) Endorsed by the American College of Cardiology Foundation (ACCF) and the American Heart Association (AHA). *J Am Coll Cardiol* **45**:1554–1560.

44. Grube E, Schuler G, Buellesfeld L, *et al.* (2007) Percutaneous aortic valve replacement for severe aortic stenosis in high-risk patients using the second- and current third-generation self-expanding CoreValve prosthesis: device success and 30-day clinical outcome. *J Am Coll Cardiol* **50**:69–76.

45. Webb J, Pasupati S, Humphries K, *et al.* (2007) Percutaneous transarterial aortic valve replacement in selected high-risk patients with aortic stenosis. *Circulation* **116**:755–763.

46. Detaint D, Lepage L, Himbert D, *et al.* (2009) Determinants of significant paravalvular regurgitation after transcatheter aortic

valve implantation: impact of device and annulus discongruence. *J Am Coll Cardiol* **2**:821–827.

47. Webb JG, Altwegg L, Masson JB, *et al.* (2009) A new transcatheter aortic valve and percutaneous valve delivery system. *J Am Coll Cardiol* **53**:1855–1888.

48. Cribier A, Eltchaninoff H, Tron C, *et al.* (2006) Treatment of calcific aortic stenosis with the percutaneous heart valve: mid-term follow-up from the initial feasibility studies: the French experience. *J Am Coll Cardiol* **47**:1214–1223.

49. Cribier A, Eltchaninoff H, Tron C, *et al.* (2006) Percutaneous implantation of aortic valve prosthesis in patients with calcific aortic stenosis: technical advances, clinical results and future strategies. *J Intervent Cardiol* **19**:S87–S96.

50. Hanzel GS, Harrity PJ, Schreiber TL, *et al.* (2005) Retrograde percutaneous aortic valve implantation for critical aortic stenosis. *Catheter Cardiovasc Interv* **64**:322–326.

51. Moss RR, Ivens E, Pasupati S, *et al.* (2008) Role of echocardiography in percutaneous aortic valve implantation. *J Am Coll Cardiol Imaging* **1**:15–24.

52. Babaliaros VC, Liff D, Chen EP, *et al.* (2008) Can balloon aortic valvuloplasty help determine appropriate transcatheter aortic valve size? *J Am Coll Cardiol* **1**:580–586.

53. Webb JG, Pasupati S, Achtem L, *et al.* (2006) Rapid pacing to facilitate transcatheter prosthetic heart valve implantation. *Catheter Cardiovasc Interv* **68**:199–204.

54. Wilson W, Taubert KA, Gewitz M, *et al.* (2007) Prevention of infective endocarditis: guidelines from the American Heart Association. *Circulation* **116**:1736–1754.

55. Walther T, Dewey T, Wimmer-Greinecker G, *et al.* (2006) Transapical approach for sutureless stent-fixed aortic valve implantation: experimental results. *Eur J Cardiothorac Surg* **29**:703–708.

56. Walther T, Simon P, Dewey T, *et al.* (2007) Transapical minimally invasive aortic valve implantation: multicenter experience. *Circulation* 116(Suppl. I):I240-I5.

57. Ye J, Cheung A, Lichtenstein SV, *et al.* (2006) Transapical aortic valve implantation in humans. *J Thorac Cardiovasc Surg* **131**:1194–1196.

58. Antunes MJ (2007) Off-pump aortic valve replacement with catheter-mounted valved stents. Is the future already here? *Eur J Cardiothorac Surg* **31**:1–3.

59. Huber CH & von Segesser LK (2006) Direct access valve replacement (DAVR)—are we entering a new era in cardiac surgery? *Eur J Cardiothorac Surg* **29**:380–385.

60. Grube E, Laborde JC, Gerckens U, *et al.* (2006) Percutaneous implantation of the CoreValve self-expanding valve prosthesis in high-risk patients with aortic valve disease: the Siegburg first-in-man study. *Circulation* **114**:1616–1624.

61. Cribier A, Eltchaninoff H, Tron C, *et al.* (2004) Early experience with percutaneous transcatheter implantation of heart valve prosthesis for the treatment of end-stage inoperable patients with calcific aortic stenosis. *J Am Coll Cardiol* **43**:698–703.

62. Eltchaninoff H, Tron C, & Cribier A (2003) Percutaneous implantation of aortic valve prosthesis in patients with calcific aortic stenosis: technical aspects. *J Intervent Cardiol* **16**:515–521.

63. Sakata Y, Syed Z, Salinger MH, *et al.* (2005) Percutaneous balloon aortic valvuloplasty: antegrade transseptal vs. conventional retrograde transarterial approach. *Catheter Cardiovasc Intervent* **64**:314–321.

64. Pasupati S, Humphries K, Altwegg L, *et al.* (2007) Transarterial percutaneous aortic valve [PAV] insertion: Canadian single-centre experience. *Am J Cardiol* **100**(Suppl.):56L.

65. Webb JG, Altwegg L, Boone RH, *et al.* (2009) Transcatheter aortic valve implantation. Impact on clinical and valve-related outcomes. *Circulation* **119**:3009–3016.

66. Pasupati S, Humphries K, AlAli A, *et al.* (2007) Balloon expandable aortic valve [BEAV] implantation. The first 100 Canadian patients. *Circulation* **116**(Suppl. II):357b. Abstract 1700.

67. Kojodjojo P, Gohil N, Barker D, *et al.* (2008) Outcomes of elderly patients aged 80 and over with symptomatic, severe aortic stenosis: impact of patient's choice of refusing aortic valve replacement on survival. *Q J Med* **101**:567–573.

68. Kodali S, O'Neill WO, Moses J, *et al.* (2007) Six month to one year clinical outcomes following retrograde percutaneous aortic valve replacement in high risk patients: a report from the REVIVAL-II trial. *Am J Cardiol* **100**(Suppl. 1):56L.

69. Walther T, Falk V, Borger MA, *et al.* (2007) Transapical aortic valve implantation at one year. *Circulation* **116**(Suppl. II):543. (AHA Meeting Abstracts: Abstract 2466).

70. Walther T (2008) Transapical aortic valve implantation: Traverse Feasibility Study. *Transcatheter Cardiovascular Therapeutics*, Washington, DC.

71. Grube E, Laborde JC, Zickmann B, *et al.* (2005) First report on a human percutaneous transluminal implantation of a self-expanding valve prosthesis for interventional treatment of aortic valve stenosis. *Catheter Cardiovasc Intervent* **66**:465–469.

72. Laborde JC (2008) Transcatheter aortic valve implantation with the CoreValve ReValving device. *Transcatheter Cardiovascular Therapeutics*, Washington, DC.

73. Borger MA, Walther T, Kempfert J, *et al.* (2007) Transapical aortic valve implantation in high risk surgical patients: medium term results. *Am J Cardiol* **100**;8(Suppl. 1):56L.

74. Murphy C, Pasupati S, Naiman S, *et al.* (2007) Hemolysis after transcatheter balloon expandable aortic valve insertion. *Can J Cardiol* **23**:78.

75. Walther T, Kempfert J, Borger MA, *et al.* (2008) Human minimally invasive off-pump valve-in-a-valve implantation. *Ann Thoracic Surgery* **85**:1072–1073.

76. Webb JG (2007) Transcatheter valve in valve implants for failed prosthetic valves. *Catheter Cardiovasc Intervent* **70**:765–766.

77. Wenaweser P, Buellesfeld L, Gerckens U, *et al.* (2007) Percutaneous aortic valve replacement for severe aortic regurgitation in degenerated bioprosthesis: the first valve in valve procedure using the CoreValve Revalving system [see comment]. *Catheter Cardiovasc Intervent* **70**:760–764.

78. Webb JG (2008) Complications of percutaneous aortic valve implantation. In: Hijazi Z, Feldman T, Cheatham J, & Sievert H, eds. *Complications in Percutaneous Interventions for Congenital & Structural heart Disease*. London: Informa.

79. Sinhal A, Altwegg L, Pasupati S, *et al.* (2008) Atrioventricular block after transcatheter balloon expandable aortic valve implantation. *J Am Coll Cardiol Cardiovasc Intervent* (in press).

80. Masson JB, Kovac J, Schuler G, *et al.* (2009) Transcatheter aortic valve implantation: review of the nature, management, and avoidance of procedural complications. *JACC Cardiovasc Interv* **2**:811–820.

12   Pathology of Aortic Insufficiency

Philipp A. Schnabel[1], Artur Lichtenberg[2], Esther Herpel[1], Arne Warth[1] & Nikolaus Gassler[3]

[1]Institute of Pathology, University Clinics Heidelberg, Germany
[2]Clinic for Cardiovascular Surgery, University of Düsseldorf, Düsseldorf, Germany
[3]Institute of Pathology, RWTH Aachen University, Germany

Definition

Aortic insufficiency (AI) is a pathologic condition characterized by the backflow of blood from the ascending aorta into the left ventricle [1]. AI is caused by diseases of the a aortic valve and/or of the aortic root [2] and may be acute or chronic.

Frequency

Pure AI represents the second most frequent reason for aortic valve surgery [2,3]. In the surgical literature, up to 20% of all aortic valve surgeries are performed because of pure AI. However, aortic stenosis is by far the most common reason for aortic surgery (see Chapter 7). In addition, a considerable percentage of patients have combined aortic stenosis and AI [4,5]. In the era of Doppler echocardiography, many cases of mild AI have been identified in the general population (up to 8.5% of women and up to 13% of men).

Etiology

In more than 50% of cases, AI is caused by dilation of the aortic root (annuloaortic ectasia) [2,3]. This dilation of the aortic root is often idiopathic, and sometimes it is associated with arterial hypertension and aging.

The second most frequent cause of AI is a congenital bicuspid (i.e., bicommissural) aortic valve, which may be associated with dilation of the aortic root [2,6–15]. Moreover, AI may be due to or associated with other congenital heart diseases, for example ventricular septal defect, subvalvular aortic stenosis, dysplasia of valve cusps without fusion of commissures, absence of valve leaflets, or even, rarely, the presence of additional aortic valve leaflets [16–22].

Causes of acute acquired AI include aortic dissection [23,24], spontaneous rupture of fenestrated cusps [25–28], trauma [29–31], complications following different interventions [32–35], endocarditis [36–40], systemic diseases (such as rheumatic fever) [41–43], connective tissue syndromes, and Turner's syndrome, leading to aortic dissection [44–46]. In pregnancy, aortic dissection with or without aneurysms and/or aortic dilation may also occur in the absence of Marfan's syndrome, Ehlers–Danlos syndrome, or other connective tissue syndromes [47–49]. Very rarely, acute aortic valve insufficiency can be due to isolated giant cell inflammation of the aortic leaflets [50]. Acute aortic insufficiency may also be caused by giant cell arteritis [51].

Chronic dilation of the aortic root may, on the one hand, be due to connective tissue syndromes in various collagen vascular diseases such as Marfan's syndrome [45], Ehlers–Danlos syndrome, or other diseases leading to destruction of elastic laminae [52], but rarely in Turner's syndrome [53]. On the other hand, chronic dilation of the aortic root may be due to inflammatory diseases of the aortic root, as found in syphilis, Reiter's disease [52], giant cell arteritis (Horton's disease/arteritis temporalis) [52,54,55], Behçet's disease [56], ankylosing spondylitis [57,58], Takayasu's arteritis [59], and very rarely in Crohn's disease [60].

Chronic AI due to aortic valvular diseases in addition to congenital malformations may be caused by postinflammatory alterations, following infectious or noninfectious endocarditis, chronic rheumatic disease [3,52,61], systemic lupus erythematosus (endocarditis Libman–Sachs), and rarely in Fabry's disease [62] or Kawasaki's disease [63].

Moreover, AI may be associated with certain medications (e.g., serotonin uptake inhibitors, dexfenfluramine isotopes or analogs, dopamine agonists), but the literature in this field is controversial [64–69].

The main causes of acute or chronic AI in relation to alterations of the aortic root and/or aortic valve (cusps) are summarized in Table 12.1.

Anatomy and physiology of the aortic valve and the aortic root

Gross and microscopic anatomy of the aortic valve are described in Chapter 7.

Cardiovascular Interventions in Clinical Practice. Edited by Jürgen Haase, Hans-Joachim Schäfers, Horst Sievert and Ron Waksman. © 2010 Blackwell Publishing.

Table 12.1 Causes of aortic insufficiency (AI) in relation to aortic cusp and/or aortic root pathology.

Causes of AI	Pathology	
	Predominantly valvular disease	Predominantly aortic root disease
Acute AI		
Acute endocarditis	+++	(+)
Aortic dissection	(+)	+++
Trauma	++	++
Rupture of fenestrated cusps	+++	(+)
Chronic AI		
Annuloaortic ectasia	(+)	+++
Congenital bicuspid aortic valve	+++	++
Rheumatic heart disease	+++	+
Vasculitis	(+)	+++

In the context of AI, it is of great importance to realize that the aortic valve cannot be viewed as an isolated structure [2,70]: the aortic valve, anatomically, is a part of the aortic root and, physiologically, is a functional unit together with the aortic root. Anatomically, the cranial borders of the aortic valve are marked by the commissures and the sinotubular transition; the caudal border is marked by the aortoventricular transition [71]. The three cusps of the aortic valve are attached by fibrous strands to the aortic root. The size of the aortic ring is determined by the sinotubular diameter, the aortoventricular transition, and the width of the sinus. During the cardiac cycle, the aortic root undergoes complex movements that precede and support the opening and the closing of the aortic valve, which is an active process and not only passively driven by the pressure gradient between left ventricle and aorta [2,70]. Thus, AI is caused by functional disturbances of the aortic root (e.g., by increased rigidity with age or dilation/aneurysm), as well as by morphologic alterations of the cusps, or both.

Pathophysiology

In AI the incomplete closure of the aortic valve permits backflow of blood from the aorta into the left ventricle. In this situation the aorta is acting like a compression chamber. There is a steep drop in diastolic pressure in the ascending aorta. The regurgitation of blood leads to increased left ventricular blood volume, which causes volume hypertrophy. In contrast to pressure hypertrophy (e.g., in aortic stenosis; see Chapter 7), in volume hypertrophy ventricular dilation develops earlier (excentric dilation). Moreover, the diastolic reflux of blood to the left ventricle can reduce blood influx into the coronary arteries. This reduced coronary flow deteriorates the relative coronary insufficiency, which is due to left

ventricular hypertrophy. This results in myocardial ischemia and fibrosis.

In AI cardiac failure occurs much earlier than in aortic stenosis. Clinically the patients show lung edema with the symptoms of severe dyspnea, which can develop dramatically in acute AI.

In a rat model of acute severe AI significant macroscopic and microscopic abnormalities were present soon after induction of AI [72]: considerable hypertrophy, perivascular fibrosis and extracellular matrix remodeling were found after only 14 days. In a rabbit model of chronic AI caused heart failure and myocyte degeneration (necrosis) and fibrosis [73]. Autophagy has been identified as a mechanism for cell death in degenerative aortic valve disease in addition to atherosclerosis, heart failure and regions around myocardial infarcts [74].

Gross and histologic pathology of aortic insufficiency

Main features of gross and microscopic pathology of the aortic valve are given in Chapter 07 and discussed in detail regarding congenital versus acquired aortic valve disease, endothelial damage, inflammation, lipid accumulation, extracellular matrix remodeling, and loss of flexibility, calcification/ossification, as well as neovascularization. Some special macroscopic and microscopic features of AI are shown in (Figs. 12.1, 12.2, and 12.3).

Dilation and/or aneurysms can best be demonstrated macroscopically or echocardiographically. Figure 12.1a shows an aortic aneurysm *in situ*, and Figure 12.1b shows the surgical reconstruction of the aortic valve. The aorta is severely dilated owing to so-called mucoid degeneration of the media, with loss of elastic lamellae. In a mouse model of mucopolysaccharidosis I, aortic dilation is probably due to degradation of elastin by matrix metalloproteinase (MMP)-12 and/or

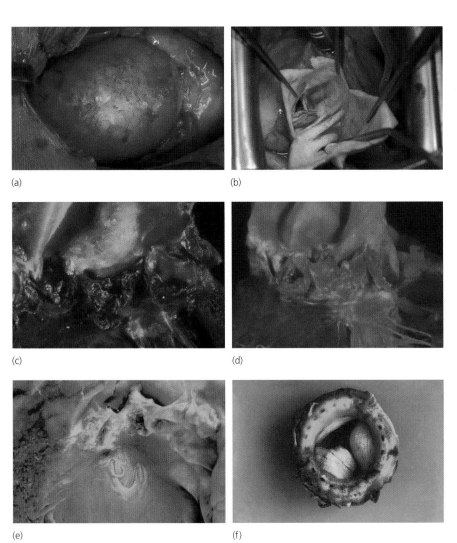

(a)

(b)

(c)

(d)

(e)

(f)

Figure 12.1 Aortic insufficiency I. (a) Aortic aneurysm *in situ* in a 45-year-old man. (b) Surgical reconstruction of the aortic valve in the same patient. (c) Macroscopic view of acute bacterial endocarditis in a severely calcified aortic valve: autopsy specimen from a 56-year-old man. (d and e) Postinflammatory alterations of insufficient aortic valves. (d) Predominance of fibrotic changes in an autopsy specimen from a 52-year-old woman. (e) Calcification and a lesion in the parietal endocardium due to aortic insufficiency with a regurgitation jet ("Zahn's sign of valve insufficiency") in a autopsy specimen from a 64-year-old man. (f) Insufficient "historical unphysiologic" aortic valve bioprosthesis, from which one of the cusps manufactured from fascia lata is completely lost, in a specimen from a 43-year-old woman.

cathepsin S [75]. The detailed mechanisms of elastin degradation in aortic dilation or aneurysm in association with different manifestations of AI in humans remain to be determined. Valve-preserving aortic root reconstruction can be done with an

in-hospital and 30-day mortality rate of 3.7% compared with 4.0% for a composite valve conduit reconstruction [76].

Figure 12.1c shows the macroscopic view of an acute bacterial endocarditis in a severely calcified aortic valve.

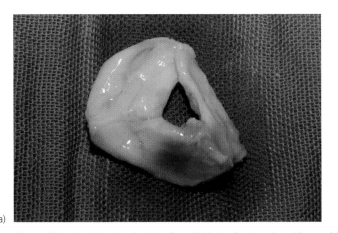

(a)

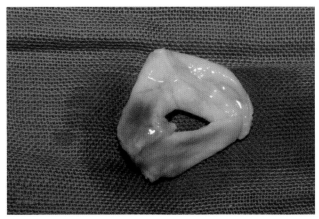

(b)

Figure 12.2 Combined aortic vitium (a and b) Excised aortic valve with a combined aortic stenosis and aortic insufficiency: postinflammatory, as indicated by the fused commissures. Specimen from a 53-year-old woman.

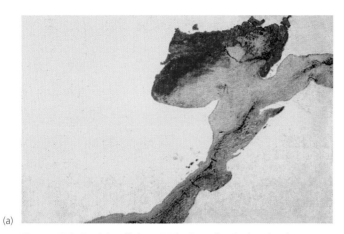

(a)

(b)

Figure 12.3 Aortic insufficiency II. Histology of excised aortic valves. (a) Parts of an aortic cusp showing abacterial thrombotic endocarditis (endocarditis Libman–Sachs) from a 31-year-old woman with systemic lupus erythematosus (hematoxylin and eosin, original magnification ×5). (b) Severe dystrophic calcification without any signs of inflammation, from a 45-year old man (hematoxylin and eosin, original magnification ×5).

Calcification may lead to aortic stenosis, AI, or both [77]. However, detailed investigations of the calcification process suggest that the cause and mechanism of calcification differ between rheumatic valvular disease, degenerative aortic valve disease, and congenitally bicuspid aortic valves [77]. In Figure 12.1d and e, postinflammatory alterations of insufficient aortic valves are obvious: in Figure 12.1d with predominance of fibrotic changes, and in Figure 12.1e with calcification and a lesion in the parietal endocardium due to AI with a regurgitation jet ("Zahn's sign of valve insufficiency"). Figure 12.1f depicts an insufficient, "historical unphysiologic" aortic valve bioprosthesis, a prosthesis in which one of the cusps, manufactured from fascia lata, is completely lost.

In Figure 12.2a and b, an excised aortic valve with a combined aortic stenosis and AI is also postinflammatory, as indicated by the fused commissures.

Figure 12.3a and b shows histologic features of excised aortic valves. Figure 12.3a presents parts of an aortic cusp with an abacterial thrombotic endocarditis (endocarditis Libman–Sachs) in a patient with systemic lupus erythematosus. Figure 12.3b shows severe dystrophic calcification without any signs of inflammation.

Similar to the mitral valve (see Chapter 21), but more rarely, "mucinous infiltration" of "dystrophic" aortic valves may occur [78], resembling "myxomatous/myxoid degeneration" of the mitral valve [79]. Lad *et al.* [79] concluded that patients with combined mitral regurgitation due to myxomatous degeneration and bicuspid aortic valve disease requiring operations often have a large, prolapsing anterior leaflet of the mitral valve and dilated aortic annulus with AI due to cusp prolapse. Myxomatous degeneration of the "floppy" aortic valve [80] may be associated with cystic media necrosis of the aortic root, and in very few cases with a "floppy mitral valve" (see Chapter 21).

In Figure 12.4a and b, typical histopathologic features of severe cardiomyocyte hypertrophy in chronic AI are presented. With both magnifications, myocytes are enlarged in diameter

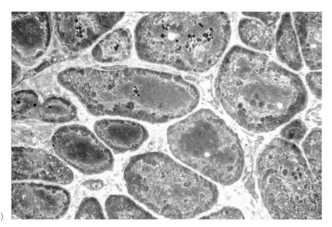

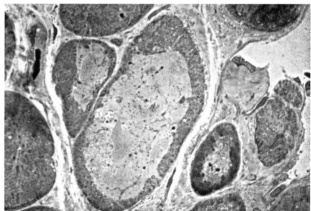

(a)

(b)

Figure 12.4 Left ventricular hypertrophy. (a, b) Histopathology of severe cardiomyocyte hypertrophy in chronic aortic insufficiency from a 48-year-old man. Myocytes are enlarged in diameter and reveal extended central vacuolization due to loss of myofibrils (semithin section, Di St. Agnese, original magnification: a, ×10, b, ×20).

and reveal extended central vacuolization due to loss of myofibrils (see above: Pathophysiology).

Treatment

In acute AI, surgical therapy is the only life-saving option [81]. In asymptomatic patients with severe chronic AI and normal left ventricular function, vasodilators may prolong the compensated phase of chronic AI [81,82], but proof that vasodilators modify the time of aortic surgery is limited [81,83]. In patients without symptoms and without left ventricular enlargement, the time-point for surgery remains debatable [82,83]. But after enlargement of the left ventricle, symptoms and/or functional parameters can indicate surgical therapy. Decline in ejection fraction, increase in echocardiographic diameters, a left ventricular dysfunction, the presence of pulmonary hypertension, or atrial fibrillation are parameters for this decision [82,83]. Annuloaortic ectasia requires surgery when the diameter reaches 50–55 mm [84]. In cases with unique valve lesions, indications for surgery include major radiographic cardiomegaly (cardiothoracic ratio >0.58), evidence of major left ventricular dilation by echocardiography (end-diastolic diameter >70 mm, end-systolic diameter >50 mm), and alterations of systolic function (ejection fraction <0.50 or 0.55) [84]. The preoperative indexed end-systolic left ventricular diameter improves the prediction of unfavorable outcomes [85]. As there are new methods for reconstructive surgery of AI with regard to the recent knowledge about the anatomy and physiology of the aortic valve and the aortic root, depending on the individual medical history [70,86–91] and pathology of each patient, the indications for the various treatment strategies are still "in progress" [2,78,92–99]. The long-term results of reconstructive surgical techniques in comparison with aortic valve replacement remain to be determined.

Acknowledgments

Ms. S. Berger is highly acknowledged for assistance in preparing the manuscript, and Mr. John J. Moyers for preparing the figures. This chapter is dedicated to Hilde Schnabel, who was very brave with her rheumatic valvular disease.

References

1. Bekeredjian R & Grayburn PA (2005) Valvular heart disease: aortic regurgitation. *Circulation* **112**:125–134.

2. Schaefers HJ & Boehm M (2004) Ursachen und Behandlungsstrategien der Aortenklappeninsuffizienz. *Dtsch Arztebl* **101**:A2475–2479.

3. Dare AJ, Veinot JP, Edwards WD, Tazelaar HD, & Schaff HV (1993) New observations on the etiology of aortic valve disease: a surgical pathologic study of 236 cases from 1990. *Hum Pathol* **24**:1330–1338.

4. Subramanian R, Olson LJ, & Edwards WD (1985) Surgical pathology of combined aortic stenosis and insufficiency: a study of 213 cases. *Mayo Clin Proc* **60**:247–254.

5. Chuangsuwanich T, Warnnissorn M, Leksrisakul P, Laksanabunsong P, Thongcharoen P, & Sahasakui Y (2004) Pathology and etiology of 110 consecutively removed aortic valves. *Med Assoc Thai* **87**:921–934.

6. Bauer M (2005) *Bikuspide Aortenklappe und Dilation der Aorta ascendens*. Berlin: Med Habilschr.

7. Bauer M, Bauer U, Siniawski H, & Hetzer R (2007) Differences in clinical manifestations in patients with bicuspid and tricuspid aortic valves undergoing surgery of the aortic valve and/or ascending aorta. *Thorac Cardiov Surg* **55**:485–490.

8. Butany J, Vaideeswar P, Dixit V, Lad V, Vegas A, & David TE (2009) Ascending aortic aneurysms in unicommissural aortic valve disease. *Cardiovasc Pathol* **18**:11–18.

9. Cecconi M, Nistri S, Quarti A, Manfrin M, Colonna PL, Molini E, & Perna GP (2006) Aortic dilation in patients with bicuspid aortic valve. *J Cardiovasc Med (Hagerstown)* **7**:11–20.

10. Host NB (2008) Bicuspid aortic valve. Do we take it sufficiently seriously? *Ugeskr Laeger* **16**:2242–2245.

11. Olson LJ, Subramanian R, & Edwards WD (1984) Surgical pathology of pure aortic insufficiency: a study of 225 cases. *Mayo Clin Proc* **59**:835–841.

12. Russo CF, Cannata A, Lanfranconi M, Vitali E, Garatti A, & Bonacina E (2008) Is aortic wall degeneration related to bicuspid aortic valve anatomy in patients with valvular disease? *J Thorac Cardiovasc Surg* **136**:937–942.

13. Sabet HY, Edwards WD, Tazelaar HD, & Daly RC (1999) Congenitally bicuspid aortic valves: a surgical pathology study of 542 cases (1991 through 1996) and a literature review of 2,715 additional cases. *Mayo Cin Proc* **74**:14–26.

14. Sadee AS, Becker AE, Verheul HA, Bouma B, & Hedemaker G (1992) Aortic valve regurgitation and the congenitally bicuspid aortic valve: a clinico-pathological correlation. *Br Heart J* **67**:439–441.

15. Yener N, Oktar GL, Erer D, Yardimci MM, & Yener A (2002) Bicuspid aortic valve. *Ann Thorac Cardiovasc Surg* **8**:264–267.

16. Nadas AS, Thilenius OG, Lafarge CG, & Hauck AJ (1964) Ventricular septal defect with aortic regurgitation—Medical and pathological aspects. *Circulation* **29**:862–873.

17. Vaideeswar P & Deshpande JR (2003) Congenital aortic regurgitation due to aortic valvar fenestration with associated aortic dissection. *J Postgrad Med* **49**:369.

18. Di Pino A, Gitto P, Silvia A, & Bianca I (2008) Congenital quadricuspid aortic valve in children. *Cardiol Young* **18**:324–327.

19. Godefroid O, Colles P, Vercauteren S, Louagie Y, & Marchandise B (2006) Quadricuspid aortic valve: a rare etiology of aortic regurgitation. *Eur J Echocardiogr* **7**:168–170.

20. Kawanishi Y, Tanaka H, Nakagiri K, Yamashita T, Okada K, & Okita Y (2008) Congenital quadricuspid aortic valve associated with severe regurgitation. *Asian Cardiovasc Thorac Ann* **16**:e40–e41.

21. Seki A, Sasaki M, Masumoto H, Kajiyama M, & Asaoka M (1996) Quadricuspid aortic valve: report of a case associated with severe aortic regurgitation. *Kyobu Geka* **49**:1027–1031.

22. Timperley J, Milner R, Marshall AJ, & Gilbert TJ (2002) Quadricuspid aortic valves. *Clin Cardiol* **25**:548–552.

23. Butany J, El Demellawy D, Collins MJ, *et al.* (2005) Ascending aortic aneurysm with dissection and aortic insufficiency. *J Card Surg* **20**: 85–89.

24. Golzari M & Riebman JB (2004) The four seasons of ruptured sinus of valsalva aneurysms: case presentations and review. *Heart Surg Forum* **7**:E577–E583.

25. Akiyama K, Ohsawa S, Hirota J, & Takiguchi M (1998) Massive aortic regurgitation by spontaneous rupture of a fibrous strand in a fenestrated aortic valve. *J Heart Valve Dis* **7**:521–523.

26. Blaszyk H, Witkiewicz AJ, & Edwards WD (1999) Acute aortic regurgitation due to spontaneous rupture of a fenestrated cusp: report in 65-year-old man and review of seven additional cases. *Cardiovasc Pathol* **8**:213–216.

27. Bourgault C, Couture C, Martineau A, Dagenais F, Poirier P, & Sénéchal M (Nov. 2007) Incidental mobile aortic valve lesion: a case of aortic valve fenestration. *J Heart Valve Dis* **16**:692–694.

28. Ide H, Ino T, Yamada S, & Terada Y (1991) Spontaneous aortic cusp rupture. *Nippon Kyobu Geka Gakkai Zasshi* **39**:1816–1820.

29. Imamamki M, Shimakura T, Kurihara H, Maeda T, & Sugawara Y (1996) Surgical treatment of traumatic rupture of the aortic valve. *Nippon Kyobu Geka Gakkai Zasshi* **44**:2050–2053.

30. Kaljusto ML, Vengen OA, & Tønnessen T (2008) Traumatic aortic valve rupture after a high-speed motor vehicle. *J Heart Valve Dis* **17**:586–588.

31. Mullenix PS, Parsa CJ, Mackensen GB, Jollis JG, Harrison JK, & Hughes GC (2008) Pannus-related prosthetic valve dysfunction and life-threatening aortic regurgitation. *J Heart Valve Dis* **17**:666–669.

32. Nascimento J, Lemos C, Marques AM, Antunes MJ, & Gonsalves A (1996) Traumatic aortic valve insufficiency *Rev Port Cardiol* **15**:147–152.

33. Lee AP, Walley VM, Ascah KJ, Veinot JP, Davies RA, & Keon WJ (1996) A fenestrated aortic valve contributing to iatrogenic aortic insufficiency post mitral valve replacement. *Cardiovasc Pathol* **5**:81–83.

34. Kervan U, Bardakci H, Altintas G, Tufekcioglu O, & Birincioglu CL (2008) A case of intraventricular septum dissection presenting with aneurysmal dilation through the outflow track of the left ventricle. *J Card Surg* **23**:173–176.

35. Momeni M, Van Caenegem O, & Van Dyck MJ (2005) Aortic regurgitation after left ventricular assist device placement. *J Cardiothorac Vasc Anesth* **19**:409–410.

36. Fayad G, Modine T, Mokhtari S, *et al.* (2003) Pasteurella multocida aortic valve endocarditis: case report and literature review. *J Heart Valve Dis* **12**:261–263.

37. Franz M, Bahrmann P, Berndt A, *et al.* (2008) Surgical therapy of infective endocarditis. General aspects and case report. *Med Klin (Munich)* **103**:349–355.

38. Hisata Y, Hazama S, Izumi K, & Eishi K (2008) Triple-valve treatment for prosthetic valve endocarditis occurring 20 years after implantation of a Carpentier–Edwards pericardial bioprosthesis in the aortic valve. *Gen Thorac Cardiovasc Surg* **56**:595–598.

39. Lim YT, Lim MC, Choo MH, & Gamini K (1994) Severe aortic regurgitation due to *Neisseria mucosa* endocarditis. *Singapore Med J* **35**:650–652.

40. Raval AN, Menkis AH, & Boughner DR (2002) Mitral valve aneurysm associated with aortic valve endocarditis and regurgitation. *Heart Surg For* **5**, 298–299.

41. Chand EM, Freant LJ, & Rubin JW (1999) Aortic valve rheumatoid nodules producing clinical aortic regurgitation and a review of the literature. *Cardiovasc Pathol* **8**:333–338.

42. Feldman T (1996) Rheumatic heart disease *Curr Opin Cardiol* **11**:126–130.

43. Minematsu N, Yoshikai M, Kamohara K, & Tomimitsu S (2004) Aortic valve regurgitation associated with rheumatoid arthritis; report of a case. *Kyobu Geka* **57**:391–394.

44. Bondy CA (2008) Aortic dissection in Turner syndrome. *Curr Opin Cardiol* **23**:519–526.

45. Carrel T (1997) Cardiovascular surgery in Marfan syndrome. A review with case examples. *Schweiz Med Wochenschr* **127**:992–1006.

46. Shaker WH, Refaat AA, Hakamei MA, & Ibrahim MF (2008) Acute type A aortic dissection at seven weeks of gestation in a Marfan patient: case report. *J Card Surg* **23**:569–570.

47. Horstkotte D, Fassbender D, & Piper C (2003) Congenital heart disease and acquired valvular lesions in pregnancy. *Herz* **28**:227–239.

48. Williams GM, Gott VL, Brawley RK, Schauble JF, & Labs JD (1988) Aortic disease associated with pregnancy. *J Vasc Surg* **8**:470–475.

49. Snir E, Levinsky L, Salomon J, Findler M, Levy MJ, & Vidne BA (1988) Dissecting aortic aneurysm in pregnant women without Marfan disease. *Surg Gynecol Obstet* **167**:463–465.

50. Niclauss L, Letovanec I, Chassot PG, Gersbach PA, & von Segesser LK (2008) Acute aortic valve insufficiency and cardiogenic shock due to an isolated giant cell inflammation of the aortic valve leaflets: case report and review of the literature. *J Heart Valve Dis* **17**:343–347.

51. Tandon R & Fahy R (2006) Giant cell arteritis in a patient with acute aortic insufficiency with thyrotoxicosis. *Clin Rheumatol* **25**:254–257.

52. Guiney TE, Davies MJ, Parker DJ, Leech GJ, & Leatham A (1987) The etiology and course of isolated severe aortic regurgitation: a clinical, pathological, and echocardiographic study. *Br Heart J* **58**:358–368.

53. Sachdev V, Matura LA, Sidenko S, *et al.* (2008) Aortic valve disease in Turner syndrome. *J Am Coll Cardiol* **51**:1904–1909.

54. Costello JM & Nicholson WJ (1990) Severe aortic regurgitation as a late complication of temporal arteritis. *Chest* **98**:875–877.

55. Le Tourneau T, Millaire A, Asseman P, De Groote P, Théry C, & Ducloux G (1996) Aortitis in Horton disease. Review of the literature *Ann Med Interne (Paris)* **147**:361–368.

56. Lee I, Park S, Hwang I, *et al.* (2008) Cardiac Behçet disease presenting as aortic valvulitis/aortitis or right heart inflammatory mass: a clinicopathologic study of 12 cases. *Am J Surg Pathol* **32**:390–398.

57. Palazzi C, D'Angelo S, Lubrano E, & Olivieri I (2008) Aortic involvement in ankylosing spondylitis. *Clin Exp Rheumatol* **26**(Suppl. 49):S131–S134.

58. Gregersen PK, Gallerstein P, Jaffe W, & Enlow RW (1982) Valvular heart disease associated with juvenile onset ankylosing spondylitis: a case report and review of the literature. *Bull Hosp It Dis Orthop Inst* **42**:103–114.

59. Matsuura K, Ogino H, Kobayashi J, *et al.* (2005) Surgical treatment of aortic regurgitation due to Takayasu arteritis—Long-term morbidity and mortality. *Circulation* **112**:3707–3712.

60. Wäckerlin A, Zünd G, Maggiorini M, Jenni R, Turina M, & Follath F (1997) Aortic valve insufficiency in Crohn disease. *Schweiz Med Wochenschr* **127**:935–939.

61. Hlavaty L & Vander Heide R (1998) Causes of isolated aortic insufficiency in an urban population in the 1990s. A review of 56 surgical pathology cases. *Cardiovasc Pathol* **7**:313–319.

62. Choi S, Seo H, Park M, *et al.* (2009) Fabry disease with aortic regurgitation. *Ann Thorac Surg* **87**:625–628.

63. Sotelo N & González LA (2007) Kawasaki disease: a rare pediatric pathology in Mexico. Twenty cases report form the Hospital Infantil del Estado de Sonora. *Arch Cardiol Mex* **77**:299–307.

64. Antonini A & Poewe W (2007) Fibrotic heart-valve reaction to dopamine-agonist treatment in Parkinson's disease. *Lancet Neurol* **6**:826–829.

65. Boutet K, Frachon I, Jobic Y, *et al.* (2009) Fenfluramine-like cardiovascular side-effects of benfluorex. *Eur Resp J* **33**:684–688.

66. Coalo A, Marek J, Goth MI, *et al.* (2008) No greater incidence or worsening of cardiac valve regurgitation with somatostatin analog treatment of acromegaly. *J Clin Endocrinol Metab* **93**:2243–2248.

67. Kars M, Delgado V, Holman ER, *et al.* (2008) Aortic valve calcification and mild tricuspid regurgitation but no clinical heart disease after 8 years of dopamine agonist therapy for prolactinoma. *J Clin Endocrinol Metab* **93**:3348–3356.

68. Kars M, Pereira AM, Bax JJ, & Romijn JA (2008) Cabergoline and cardiac valve disease in prolactinoma patients: additional studies during long-term treatment are required. *Eu J Enocrinol* **159**:363–367.

69. Lancellotti P, Livadariu E, Markov. M, *et al.* (2008) Cabergoline and the risk of valvular lesions in endocrine disease. *Eur J Endocrinol* **159**:1–5.

70. Bechtel JF, Erasmi AW, Misfeld M, & Sievers HH (2006) Reconstructive surgery of the aortic valve: the Ross, David and Yacoub procedures. *Herz* **31**:413–422.

71. Anderson RH (2000) Clinical anatomy of the aortic root. *Heart* **84**:670–673.

72. Lachance D, Plante E, Roussel E, Drolet MC, Couet J, & Arsenault M (2008) Early left ventricular remodeling in acute severe aortic regurgitation: insights from an animal model. *J Heart Valve Dis* **17**:300–308.

73. Liu S-K, Magid NR, Fox PR, Goldfine SM, & Borer JS (1998) Fibrosis, myocyte degeneration and heart failure in chronic experimental aortic regurgitation. *Cardiology* **90**:101–109.

74. Mistiaen WP, Somer P, Knaapen MW, & Kockx MM (2006) Autophagy as mechanism for cell death in degenerative aortic valve disease. *Autophagy* **2**:221–223.

75. Ma X, Tittiger M, Knutsen RH, *et al.* (2008) Upregulation of elastase proteins results in aortic dilation in mucopolysaccharidosis in mice. *Mol Genet Metab* **94**:298–304.

76. Zehr KJ, Orszulak TA, Mullany CJ, *et al.* (2004) Surgery for aneurysms of the aortic root: a 30-year-experience. *Circulation* **110**:1364–1371.

77. Togashi M, Tamura K, Masuda Y, & Fukuda Y (2008) Comparative study of calcified changes in aortic valvular diseases. *J Nippon Med Sch* **75**:138–145.

78. Michel PL, Hanania G, Chomette G, *et al.* (1991) Insuffisance aortique dystrophique: influence de la dilation de l'aorte ascendante sur l'evolution secondaire. *Arch Mal Coeur Vaiss* **84**:477–482.

79. Lad V, David TE, & Vegas A (2009) Mitral regurgitation due to myxomatous degeneration combined with bicuspid aortic valve disease is often due to prolapse of the anterior leaflet of the mitral valve *Ann Thorac Surg* **87**:79–82.

80. Bellitti R, Caruso A, Festa M, *et al.* (1985) Prolapse of the "floppy" aortic valve as a cause of aortic regurgitation. A clinico-morphologic study. *Int J Cardiol* **9**:399–410.

81. Scheuble A & Vahanian A (2005) Aortic insufficiency: defining the role of pharmacotherapy. *Am J Cardiovasc Drugs* **5**:113–120.

82. Goldbarg SH & Halperin JL (2008) Aortic regurgitation: disease progression and management. *Nat Clin Pract Cardiovasc Med* **5**:269–279.

83. de Gevigney G, Groupe de travail sur les valvulopathies de la Scociete francaise de cardiologie (2007) The best of valvular heart disease in 2006. *Arch Mal Coeur Vaiss* **100**(Spec No 1): 19–28.

84. Acar J, Michel PL, & de Gevigney G (2000) When is surgery needed for minimally symptomatic or asymptomatic acquired valvulopathy? *Presse Med* **29(34)**:1867–1875.

85. Sambola A, Tornos P, Ferreira-Gonzalez I, & Evangelista A (2008) Prognostic value of preoperative indexed end-systolic left ventricle diameter in the outcome after surgery in patients with chronic aortic regurgitation. *Am Heart J* **155**:1114–1120.

86. Böhm JO, Hemmer W, Rein JG, *et al.* (2009) A single-institution experience with the Ross operation over 11 years. *Ann Thorac Surg* **87**:514–520.

87. Hanke T, Charitos EI, Stierle U, *et al.* (2009) Factors associated with the development of aortic valve regurgitation over time after two different techniques of valve-sparing aortic root surgery. *J Thorac Cardiovasc Surg* **137**:314–319.

88. Mutsuga M, Tamaki S, Yokoyama Y, *et al.* (2008) Surgical treatment for aortic root dilation and aortic regurgitation after arterial switch operation. *Kyobu Geka* **61**:1043–1047.

89. Nagy Z & Watterson KG (2008) Ross procedure versus mechanical aortic valve replacement in young adults. *Magy Seb* **61**(Suppl.):23–27.

90. Roos-Hesselink JW, Schoelzel BE, Heijdra RJ, *et al.* (2003) Aortic valve and aortic arch pathology after coarctation repair. *Heart* **89**:1074–1077.

91. Schwartz ML, Gauvreau K, del Nido P, Mayer JE, & Colan SD (2004) Long-term predictors of aortic root dilation and aortic regurgitation after arterial switch operation. *Circulation* **110**(Suppl. 1):II128–II132.

92. Boodhwani M, de Kerchove L, Glineur D, *et al.* (2009) Repair-orientated classification of aortic insufficiency: impact on surgical techniques and clinical outcomes. *J Thorac Cardiovasc Surg* **137**:286–294.

93. Hicks GL & Massey HT (2002) Update on indications for surgery in aortic insufficiency. *Curr Opin Cardiol* **17**:172–178.

94. Kawazoe K, Izumoto H, Satoh Y, Eishi K, & Ishibashi K (2001) Annuloaortic repair in the treatment of aortic regurgitation and aortic root pathology. *Surg Today* **31**:27–31.

95. McDonald ML, Smedira NG, Blackstone EH, *et al.* (2000) Reduced survival in women after valve surgery for aortic regurgitation: effect of aortic enlargement and late aortic rupture. *J Thorac Cardiovasc Surg* **119**:1205–1215.

96. Misfeld M, Bechtel M, & Sievers HH (2007) Types of reconstructive surgery of the aortic valve. *J Cardiovasc Surg (Torino)* **48**:781–790.

97. Pettersson GB, Crucean AC, Savage R, *et al.* (2008) Toward predictable repair of regurgitant aortic valves: a systematic morphology-directed approach to bicommissural repair. *J Am Coll Cardiol* **52**:40–49.

98. Urbanski PP & Frank S (2008) New vascular graft for simplification of the aortic valve reimplantation technique. *Interact Cardiovasc Thorac Surg* **7**:552–554.

99. Van Son JAM, Battellini R, Mierzwa M, Walther T, Autschbach R, & Mohr FW (1999) Aortic root reconstruction with preservation of native aortic valve and sinuses in aortic root dilation with aortic regurgitation. *J Thorac Cardiovasc Surg* **117**:1151–1156.

13 Echocardiography of Aortic Insufficiency

Martin G. Keane & Susan E. Wiegers

University of Pennsylvania School of Medicine, Philadelphia, PA, USA

Epidemiology of aortic insufficiency

Insufficiency of the aortic valve is a relatively common abnormality, with an overall prevalence of 4.9% in the Framingham offspring population [1]. However, in healthy young individuals, even trace aortic insufficiency is rare, typically found in <1% [2]. The prevalence of insufficiency increases with age [2–4]. Mild degrees of aortic insufficiency are present in up to 10–14% of middle-aged and elderly patients [1,5,6]. In patients with acute aortic insufficiency, there is high morbidity and mortality from the sudden and often severe left ventricular volume overload which results from acute systolic heart failure, pulmonary edema, and hemodynamic collapse [7]. Rapid diagnosis of the underlying cause of acute insufficiency in the emergency department or intensive care unit is essential for appropriate emergent intervention.

Chronic aortic insufficiency of varying degree is typically asymptomatic initially, but is equally detrimental in terms of long-term morbidity and mortality [8,9]. Chronic aortic regurgitation results in long-term volume overload of the left ventricle, which is accompanied by compensatory cavity dilation and hypertrophy of the left ventricular myocardium [10]. As a result of these compensatory responses, patients with chronic insufficiency of the aortic valve remain asymptomatic for many years. Mortality is not appreciably increased in asymptomatic patients with aortic insufficiency compared with the general population [8,9,11], but such patients do have elevated cardiac event rates—including a need for surgical valve replacement—and onset of congestive heart failure [12]. Ongoing ventricular remodeling, however, ultimately results in progressive systolic and diastolic dysfunction and the late onset of congestive symptoms [7,10]. Once symptomatic, a patient frequently has advanced degrees of ventricular failure, and may benefit minimally from surgical replacement of the aortic valve [8]. Of key importance, therefore, is the use of intermittent noninvasive ventricular evaluation in the asymptomatic patient with significant aortic insufficiency to allow intervention before significant deterioration of ventricular function occurs.

Pathophysiology of aortic insufficiency

Primary valve abnormalities

The structure of the aortic valve is complex, and has been described in detail in Chapter 12. The typical normal aortic valve consists of three "semilunar" cusps that are suspended by extensions of tissue upward into the sinuses of Valsalva, forming the commissures. During diastole the edges of these cup-like leaflets are drawn together tightly to prevent the backwards flow of blood into the left ventricle after systolic ejection. Anomalies of leaflet structure, destruction of all or part of a leaflet, or excessive thickening or calcification of any one of the cusps leads to interruption of the tight coaptation during diastole. Even the nonspecific thickening of the cusps that occurs with age may cause mild degrees of insufficiency [13].

The most common primary valvular abnormalities are listed in Table 13.1. Unlike aortic stenosis, which has the common final pathway of restricted aortic valve motion and reduced systolic orifice, the causes of aortic regurgitation involve multiple structures and must be assessed echocardiographically for a complete diagnosis. Congenital abnormalities of aortic valve structure include unicuspid, bicuspid, and quadricuspid leaflet morphologies, and are found in approximately 2–3% of the adult population [14]. The bicuspid aortic valve is the most common congenital cause of premature aortic valve stenosis and insufficiency in the third and fourth decades. Acquired valve abnormalities that lead to aortic insufficiency include valve thickening and calcific degeneration in later decades, often resulting in combined aortic stenosis and insufficiency. Thickening and leaflet retraction that occur from rheumatic valvulitis commonly result in aortic insufficiency through mechanical malcoaptation. Rheumatic distortion of valve leaflet morphology was once a common cause of aortic valve insufficiency, but is seen more rarely in developed countries today. Destruction or distortion of valve leaflets by endocarditis or malcoaptation due to large vegetations

Cardiovascular Interventions in Clinical Practice. Edited by Jürgen Haase, Hans-Joachim Schäfers, Horst Sievert and Ron Waksman. © 2010 Blackwell Publishing.

Table 13.1 Causes of aortic regurgitation.

Primary valve abnormalities
Congenital (bicuspid aortic valve, subaortic stenosis)
Endocarditis
Degenerative
Traumatic
Rheumatic

Primary root abnormalities
Dilated aortic root
    Syndromic (Marfan, Loeys–Dietz, Ehlers–Danlos)
    Familial aortic aneurysm
    Hypertension
    Vasculitis
Aortic dissection

frequently causes valve insufficiency. Traumatic tearing of aortic valve leaflets is a rare, albeit acute, cause of typically severe aortic insufficiency.

Aortic root abnormalities and secondary aortic valve insufficiency

The structure and proper function of the aortic valve depend intimately on the surrounding aortic root and proximal ascending aorta [15]. The leaflets of the aortic valve are intricately three-dimensional, with the commissures "suspended" from the sinuses of Valsalva in a complex fashion. Forming the base of the valve, the junction between the left ventricular outflow tract and the aorta constitutes the aortic annulus. Although the annulus consists primarily of fibrous tissue, the posterior aspect of the annulus is ventricular myocardium [16]. Any disruption to the annulus, the sinuses of Valsalva, or the proximal ascending aorta just distal to the sinotubular junction may compromise normal aortic leaflet function and coaptation. Common causes of paravalvular disruption are noted in Table 13.1. Dilation of the aortic root or proximal aneurysm formation are the most common causes of secondary aortic insufficiency [17], and is commonly seen in Marfan's syndrome, Ehlers–Danlos syndrome, and with the aortopathy associated with bicuspid aortic valve disease [18–20]. Leaflet malcoaptation from proximal aortic dilation results in insufficiency at the center of the valve and in severe dilation, along all of the commissures. In addition to dilation, mechanical tearing of the intimal layer from the elastic support of the media during aortic dissection or from trauma undermines the suspensory portions of the commissures, and can result in varying degrees of aortic leaflet prolapse and aortic insufficiency [21]. The degree of insufficiency correlates with the extent of disruption of the commissural supports defined by the percentage of the annulus that is dissected [22].

Finally, destruction of subvalvular components of the valve destabilizes the annulus and causes insufficiency by annular

dilation as well as interruption of leaflet morphology. Common causes of subvalvular disruption include abscess formation from endocarditis, and occasionally trauma or dissection [23,24]. Subvalvular membranes in congenital subvalvular stenosis obstruct flow and cause excess turbulence immediately below the valve. The high-velocity turbulent jet striking the ventricular side of the aortic valve causes endothelial damage and progressive thickening, and may lead to prolapse. A subaortic membrane is invariably associated with some degree of aortic insufficiency in the patients with congenital subvalvular stenosis. [25]. Another example of congenital subvalvular pathology is the perimembranous ventricular septal defect, in which the associated high-velocity jet may disrupt valve architecture and result in prolapse of the right coronary cusp [26,27].

Echocardiographic evaluation of aortic insufficiency

Two-dimensional echocardiography is the primary noninvasive modality used in clinical practice for anatomic assessment of the aortic valve and surrounding tissue. Doppler echocardiography, however, represents a noninvasive and accurate technique for determination of severity of insufficiency that is more applicable to a wide variety of clinical situations [28].

Two-dimensional echocardiography of the aortic valve has been described in detail in Chapter 8. Special considerations in the anatomic assessment of the insufficient aortic valve include careful visualization of valve morphology in the parasternal short-axis view. Any focal or diffuse thickening or calcification of a trileaflet aortic valve should be evaluated and localized. The presence of vegetations or abscesses can also be detected. It is also important to discern the presence of congenital abnormalities, such as bicuspid or unicuspid valves. The bicuspid valve is best identified in its open position during systole, with an ellipsoid systolic orifice (Fig. 13.1b). A ridge of tissue (or raphe) may be present at the site of the fused commissure, mimicking the appearance of a trileaflet valve when the valve is closed in diastole. Unicuspid valves are rare, and usually present with severe stenosis in early childhood or infancy. Care must be taken to image the entire root area scanning through multiple short-axis planes to define the single commissural connection to the aortic wall of the unicuspid valve.

The parasternal long-axis view contributes additional information about valvular structure and the mechanisms of valve insufficiency. This view also allows additional assessment of the severity of leaflet calcification and thickening. Systolic doming of the valve leaflets indicates the presence of rheumatic disease or a congenitally abnormal valve. Disruption of coaptation, valve prolapse, and the presence of vegetations are usually best seen in this view. As described below, color flow Doppler imaging demonstrates aortic insufficiency in the left

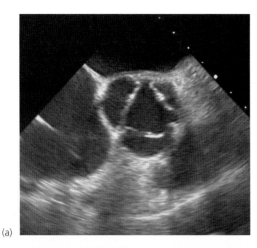

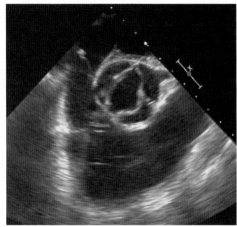

(a)

(b)

Figure 13.1 (a) Transesophageal echocardiogram of the aortic valve in systole from the midesophageal position, imaging angle 60°. The leaflets open along the commissures. The noncoronary cusp is identified by its relationship to the interatrial septum which transects it. The right coronary cusp is the most anterior leaflet and so is imaged at the bottom of the screen. (b) Transesophageal echocardiogram in a similar position as (a) in a patient with a bicuspid valve. The orifice is an ellipsoid, due to the fusion of the commissure between what would have been the right and left coronary cusps. The left main coronary ostium is visualized to the right of the image arising from the aortic root.

ventricular outflow tract arising from the level of the aortic valve leaflets in diastole. The left ventricular outflow tract dimension, which is essential for semiquantitative assessment of insufficiency, is measured immediately below the attachment of the cusps in this view. Para-annular abnormalities such as abscesses can sometimes be seen in transthoracic studies, but transesophageal imaging is more sensitive for detection of abscess.

The parasternal long-axis view is also essential for measuring the dimensions of the aortic root, sinotubular junction, and proximal portions of the ascending aorta (Fig.13.2). The larger diameter at the level of the sinuses of Valsalva is evident, as is the relative narrowing of the root at the sinotubular junction. Only the most proximal portion of the ascending aorta may

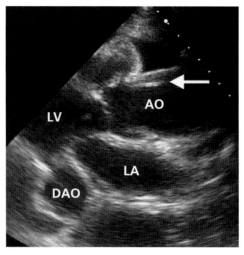

Figure 13.2 Parasternal long axis of the ascending aorta. The transducer has been moved cranially one interspace to image the aorta. The dimensions of the aorta can be measured from the two-dimensional image. This patient has an intramural hematoma (arrow) extending to the right coronary ostium that required emergency surgery. AO, ascending aorta; DAO, descending thoracic aorta; LA, left atrium; LV, left ventricle.

be imaged on the standard parasternal long-axis view, but abnormalities of these proximal portions are those most likely to undermine the aortic valve structure and create insufficiency. Additionally, the transducer may be moved to a higher inter-costal interspace to image the proximal ascending aorta more completely. According to the American Society of Echo-cardiography Standards, measurements should be made per-pendicular to the long axis of the aorta and are made from leading edge to leading edge [29]. There are standard normal values of aortic dimension published [30], but "normal" aortic size does increase with larger overall body size [31]. Assessment of abnormal dilation or aneurysm should take body size into account via indexing, but use of static aortic root measurements is still common clinically and in the literature.

The aortic valve and root morphology is typically poorly visualized in the apical five-chamber view and the apical long axis. However, these views are optimal for Doppler assessment of insufficiency, as the ultrasound beam is parallel to the blood flow. A short-axis view of the aortic valve can also be obtained from the subcostal view, which may be helpful when the parasternal images are suboptimal.

Transesophageal imaging of the aortic valve can be utilized when more detailed evaluation of valve structure and abnor-malities is warranted. The short axis of the aortic valve in midesophageal view allows rapid assessment of the competency of the valve commissures, and the structure of the sinuses of Valsalva is best seen in this view (Fig. 13.1a). The midesopha-geal long-axis view of the valve and root (approximately 120° imaging angle) offers the best assessment of the out-flow tract, annulus, sinuses, and sinotubular junction. The modified four-chamber view from the transverse plane in the midesophageal position visualizes the left ventricular outflow tract. This is particularly important because vegetations of the aortic valve are generally attached to the ventricular surface of the aortic valve and may be seen in the modified four-chamber view prolapsing into the outflow tract. Transgastric imaging does not afford adequate assessment of the valve but does allow for the Doppler interrogation of the aortic valve gradients and aortic insufficiency [32].

Color Doppler semi quantitative assessment

A number of echocardiographic measures for assessment of aortic insufficiency exist, and this fact demonstrates that none is able to stand alone in the quantitative assessment of the degree of insufficiency. The philosophy of the various techniques may be summarized as an effort to assess either the regurgitant volume or the effective regurgitant orifice area of the insufficient valve. The assessment of the severity by echocardiography typically entails incorporation of a number of different techniques in a cumulative fashion. Data from each technique are interpreted in concert with the others, with a careful recognition of the technical limitations of each, to provide an overall assessment.

Aortic insufficiency is most easily detected via color Doppler as a high-velocity turbulent jet, arising at the level of the aortic valve cusps and extending into the left ventricular outflow tract for a variable distance. The color Doppler signal is best demonstrated in the parasternal or apical long-axis or in the apical five-chamber view. Parasternal or subcostal short-axis views of the aortic valve with color Doppler may also detect the diastolic jet and pinpoint the origin with regard to the aortic valve architecture. In the oldest quantitation system, the degree of insufficiency is graded by the extent of the regurgitant jet in the left ventricle [33]. Trace insufficiency is visible only immediately below the valve. Grade I jets are present only in the proximal left ventricular outflow tract, and grade II jets extend to the tips of the mitral valve leaflets. Grade III and IV jets extend to the papillary muscle tips and beyond, respectively. A number of factors affect the extent of the visible color Doppler regurgitant jet other than the actual regurgitant volume. Variation in left ventricular compliance and aortic diastolic pressure can limit or facilitate the flow of regurgitation toward the apex, and therefore shorten or lengthen the color Doppler trail. Furthermore, this technique is significantly affected by the settings of the ultrasound machine, including color gain, Nyquist limit, pulse repetition frequency, and the transmission frequency [34–37]. To minimize this variability, a number of other measurements have been proposed.

A more reliable color Doppler technique estimates the size of the regurgitant orifice of the insufficient valve [33]. The height of the regurgitant jet as measured in the left ventricular outflow tract from the parasternal long axis or the trans-

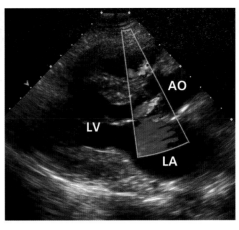

Figure 13.3 Parasternal long-axis view in diastole of a patient with mild aortic insufficiency. The high velocity and turbulent jet arises at the level of the aortic valve leaflets and extends into the outflow tract. AO, ascending aorta; LA, left atrium; LV, left ventricle.

esophageal long-axis view is measured at a point just below the bottoms of the valve cusps (Fig. 13.3). The jet height compared with the overall diameter of the left ventricular outflow tract (LVOT) is expressed as a ratio. This ratio of jet height to LVOT width correlates well with the degree of insufficiency as assessed by aortography, itself a qualitative assessment [33]. A ratio of <25% is consistent with mild aortic regurgitation. Moderate aortic regurgitation has a ratio between 25% and 40%, and a ratio of >40% is consistent with severe aortic insufficiency. Markedly eccentric jets may lead to an underestimation of the width [38]. This measurement may also be made accurately in transesophageal views, but should not be utilized in the apical transthoracic views, in which the jet of insufficiency is in the far field and cannot be measured reliably. The width of the jet must be measured directly below the aortic valve leaflets because of dispersion of the jet as it travels down the outflow tract.

Measurement of the jet height is easy and most accurate in cases of centrally directed aortic insufficiency, in which the jet flows freely from a roughly circular and symmetrical regurgitant orifice. When there is prolapse of aortic valve leaflets or more complex valve damage, the regurgitant orifice may have complex anatomy or the jet may be directed eccentrically. In these cases, use of the jet height in a single plane is not representative of the actual size of the regurgitant jet, and can either over- or underestimate the severity of aortic valve insufficiency, depending on the orientation of the lesion. Eccentric jets, furthermore, spread laterally across the walls of the LVOT and appear thin and ribbon-like in the transverse visualization of the parasternal long-axis view. This eccentricity, therefore, results in significant underestimation of the degree of insufficiency. Despite these limitations, this "method of Perry" is easy to perform with accuracy, and has served as a very useful color Doppler measure of aortic insufficiency in general clinical practice [33,39,40].

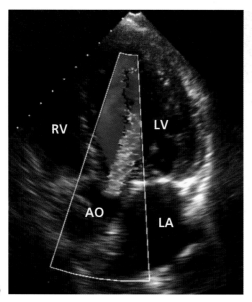

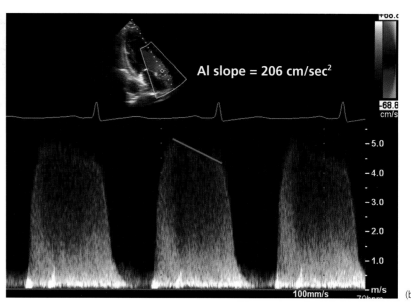

(a)

(b)

Figure 13.4 (a) Apical five-chamber view in diastole. The turbulent jet of moderate aortic insufficiency extends into the left ventricle (LV) well past the mitral valve leaflets. The jet is parallel to the ultrasound beam from this position, allowing for Doppler interrogation of the velocity. Of particular note is the proximal acceleration of the jet (PISA) in the aortic root (AO).

(b) Spectral display of continuous wave Doppler from the apical long-axis position from a different patient. The deceleration slope of the spectral envelope is 206 cm/s² consistent with mild to moderate aortic insufficiency. LA, left atrium; RV, right ventricle.

The short-axis view of the aortic valve with color Doppler imaging may also be utilized; an analogous comparison of the aortic insufficiency jet area to the short axis of the LVOT area estimates the size of the regurgitant orifice [33]. These measurements must be made at the level of the commissural coaptation, and has demonstrated acceptable reproducibility and reliability [38]. The short-axis view of insufficiency also allows better assessment of complex or asymmetric jets, as well as visualization of the origin of highly eccentric jets that are difficult to assess in parasternal long-axis views. Positioning of the transducer higher or lower than the commissures, however, can respectively under- or overestimate the jet [41].

Assessment of vena contracta

An alternative estimation of the regurgitant orifice of an insufficient aortic valve entails the measurement of the vena contracta in the parasternal long-axis view. The vena contracta represents the origin of the jet of insufficiency within the aortic valve itself. It is measured using color Doppler at a more proximal location than the jet width/LVOT width location [42]. Although less affected by eccentricity of the jet, the vena contracta may still underestimate severity of aortic insufficiency in cases of asymmetric regurgitant orifices. Furthermore, measurements of small color Doppler jets, such as the vena contracta, are limited by the anteroposterior linear resolution of color Doppler, which may introduce uncertainty in the measurement of very small differences in vena contracta size [43].

Estimation of the effective regurgitant orifice area of the insufficient aortic valve may be calculated from the measured diameter of the vena contracta. This estimation assumes a circular diameter of the regurgitant orifice, and the effective regurgitant orifice (ERO) = $\pi \times$ (vena contracta width/2)². Although the severity of aortic insufficiency measured by this method correlates with invasive regurgitant orifice, measurements in animal studies and in humans, the presence of significant measurement uncertainty of the vena contracta width is magnified by squaring in the ERO calculation [42,44,45].

Other semiquantitative Doppler techniques

Continuous-wave Doppler can be used in the apical five-chamber or apical long axis to measure the velocity of aortic insufficiency. The deceleration slope of the spectral envelope of the aortic insufficiency jet correlates with the change in pressure gradient between the aorta and left ventricle over the course of diastole (Fig. 13.4). A steeper deceleration slope indicates more rapid equilibration between the two chambers and so more severe insufficiency [46,47]. A slope of less than 200 cm/s² is considered an indication of mild aortic insufficiency, and a slope greater than 350 cm/s² as an indication of severe insufficiency [39,48–50].

The slope of the diastolic aortic spectral Doppler is also affected by left ventricular compliance. In patients with left ventricular hypertrophy or other abnormalities of relaxation, there is an exaggerated rapid rise in left ventricular diastolic pressure and concomitant increase in the slope of aortic–left ventricle equilibration. This leads to a steep deceleration slope and overestimation of the severity of insufficiency [51]. This technique is also not applicable to acute aortic regurgitation, in which ventricular compliance is severely compromised by sudden onset of large regurgitant volumes [52].

Pulse-wave Doppler can be used to detect reversal of diastolic flow in the descending thoracic or abdominal aorta, which is an indication of aortic insufficiency [53]. Special care must be taken, however, to place the pulse-wave volume in a the region well beyond the left subclavian artery, so that flow into the left subclavian is not misinterpreted as aortic flow reversal. When diastolic flow reversal is limited to the early portion of diastole, more moderate degrees of aortic insufficiency are suggested [54]. Flow reversal that continues throughout diastole is consistent with severe aortic regurgitation, particularly if end-diastolic velocity exceeds 32 cm/s [54]. The presence of surgical atrioventricular fistulas in the left arm may also be responsible for false-positive detection of descending aortic flow reversal. Knowledge of pertinent clinical history of the patient is therefore crucial for accurate interpretation.

Volumetric quantitative techniques

The Doppler techniques described above, for the large part, attempt to semiquantitatively estimate the severity of aortic valve insufficiency by approximating the size of the regurgitant orifice. Other techniques more directly address estimation of actual regurgitant volume or regurgitant fraction through the insufficient valve. Although these techniques are more quantitative than the Doppler methods described previously, they too suffer from measurement inaccuracies and geometric assumptions that may not pertain in the *in vivo* state. However, they both represent important additional assessment tools for aortic insufficiency.

Quantitation of regurgitant volume

The regurgitant volume is equal to the difference between the forward flow in systole across the aortic valve (which includes both forward systemic flow and the additional flow that later regurgitates across the insufficient valve) and the flow in diastole across the mitral valve (which represents forward systemic flow only) [12]. Pulse-wave Doppler can be utilized to quantify these volumes of flow across mitral and aortic valves. The regurgitant fraction is given by the equation:

$$\text{Regurgitant fraction} = SV_{AO} - SV_{MV}/SV_{AO}$$

where SV_{AO} is the stroke volume across the aortic valve and SV_{MV} is the stroke volume across the mitral valve.

Although simple in theory, and ideally fully quantitative, this volumetric technique is more difficult to perform accurately in practice. Calculation of forward aortic stroke volume is relative easy to measure in clinical practice, and the geometric assumptions of the circular nature of the outflow tract are

accurate. Unfortunately, calculation of the mitral stroke volume is far less reliable. Pulse-wave Doppler measurement of the flow through the mitral orifice is performed in the apical views, and is accurate. Estimation of the mitral inflow orifice, however, is more limited owing to the complex nature of the mitral annular apparatus, which is not circular. Furthermore, the shape and size of the mitral annulus change significantly over the course of diastole. Thus, this volumetric technique is limited by underlying assumptions of geometry and dynamic valvular changes throughout the cardiac cycle. Systolic flow in the pulmonary artery may be used in place of the mitral valve stroke volume if mitral insufficiency is present, and may suffer less from dynamic changes in geometry over systole.

Proximal isovelocity surface area

The proximal isovelocity surface area (PISA) method has been used to calculate both the regurgitant volumes and the effective regurgitant orifice area. Flow toward a small orifice accelerates such that, at any given radius from the center of the orifice, the velocity of the jet is uniform across the hemisphere formed by the radius [55]. Thus, the flow across the orifice is equal to the flow across the isovelocity hemispheres. The flow rate across the surface area of the hemisphere is calculated by the equation:

$$RF = 2\pi r^2 \times v_r$$

where RF is the flow rate in cm^3/s, r is the radius from the center of the orifice, and v_r is the velocity of the flow at radius r. The concept of continuity of flow, in which flow through the isovelocity hemisphere must be equal to the flow through the insufficient aortic valve, allows calculation of effective regurgitant orifice area (EROA) = RF/v_{max}, where v_{max} is the maximum velocity of the aortic regurgitant jet in diastole measured by continuous-wave Doppler. Mild insufficiency is associated with an effective regurgitant orifice of 0.1 cm^2 or less using the proximal convergence method [42]. Estimated regurgitant orifice measurements between 0.1 and 0.3 cm^2 denote moderate insufficiency, and areas larger than 0.3 cm^2 are consistent with severe insufficiency [42].

Values obtained from the flow convergence method correlate with effective regurgitant orifice areas measured invasively [56]. The PISA method is feasible in most patients [57]. Apical imaging of the aortic flow results in artifacts and difficulty in alignment, reducing the utility of the method for aortic insufficiency [58]. Imaging from the high right parasternal edge in the right lateral decubitus position may allow better visualization and alignment of eccentric flow convergence surfaces with the ultrasound beam [43]. Regurgitant volume per beat may be calculated by multiplying the effective regurgitant orifice area by the velocity–time integral of the continuous-wave Doppler envelope [59]. Similarly, the regurgitant fraction may be computed as the ratio of regurgitant volume to the left ventricular stroke volume. A regurgitant fraction of <20% correlates with mild aortic insufficiency and of greater than 55% with severe insufficiency [38].

New echo frontiers

Newer echo techniques, including three dimensional (3-D) echocardiography and intracardiac echocardiography, offer new frontiers for the assessment of the anatomy of the insufficient aortic valve and for the quantitation of the severity of insufficiency. Three-dimensional transthoracic imaging offers more robust visualization of the entire aortic and root structure in real time [60]. Initial limitations to resolution and "stitching artifact" introduced by multibeat acquisition of different sectors improve with each new generation of 3-D technology. Three-dimensional echocardiographic imaging allows multiple slices at varying "nontraditional" angles, and facilitates measurements such as direct tracing of the regurgitant vena contracta—including those with complex geometry that would be less accurately measured using two-dimensional assumptions. Vena contracta measurements attained in this way correlate well with actual findings at surgery [61].

Evaluation of secondary left ventricular changes

Ventricular adaptation to the chronic volume load of severe aortic insufficiency leads to eccentric hypertrophy of the left ventricle. The ventricle frequently dilates in a globular fashion with the minor axis approaching the length of the major axis. The ventricular geometry may be visualized by left ventriculography and by magnetic resonance imaging, but echocardiography is the dominant clinical method, primarily because of the ease of application and the ability to perform serial studies. Radionuclide angiography has also been used to measure left ventricular ejection fraction but gives no information on valvular morphology.

Patients may remain asymptomatic despite severe chronic aortic insufficiency. The initial normalization of the wall stress, provided by left ventricular remodeling, eventually fails and the left ventricular function declines. Contractile function may not improve after relief of the volume load by valve replacement. The fall in ejection fraction may occur despite an absence of symptoms even in patients who are not sedentary. Symptoms associated with aortic insufficiency are associated with a poor prognosis and some patients will not have recovery of left ventricular systolic function after valve replacement. A physical examination is sensitive for the diagnosis of chronic severe aortic insufficiency but not for more mild degrees [62]. Echocardiography remains the only efficient method for detection of aortic insufficiency and for serial examinations. Similarly, echocardiography is the ideal tool for assessment of left ventricular remodeling and the development of systolic dysfunction.

Patients with severe, chronic insufficiency require frequent assessment of the left ventricular size and function to identify the appropriate timing of surgery and avoid irreversible ventricular dysfunction. Medical therapy with afterload reduction is indicated for asymptomatic patients with chronic severe aortic insufficiency and normal left ventricular systolic function [7,12]. Afterload reduction reduces the remodeling associated with chronic severe aortic insufficiency and may result in decreased left ventricular volumes and regurgitant fraction in some patients [63–65]. Others have not found a change in left ventricular volumes with chronic afterload reduction; however, a decrease in left ventricle mass may be seen [66].

Monitoring of left ventricular size and function is indicated in patients with chronic severe aortic insufficiency, even if the patient is asymptomatic. Echocardiograms at an interval of 2–3 months will establish the stability of the left ventricular function and size. Subsequently, asymptomatic patients should have echocardiograms performed at least at yearly intervals. Those patients with more severe aortic insufficiency and those with bicuspid valves tend to have faster rates of progression of insufficiency and larger ventricular volumes [67]. The size of the aortic root and ascending aorta should also be assessed during these examinations. Radionuclide angiography can be performed if the patient has inadequate echocardiographic windows or if the change in left ventricular systolic dysfunction identified on echocardiography is equivocal. The onset of symptoms should precipitate immediate evaluation with assessment of left ventricular systolic function and size. Serial testing is not recommended for patients with mild degrees of aortic insufficiency or moderate insufficiency, and normal left ventricular dimensions and systolic function.

Acute aortic insufficiency is very poorly tolerated if the regurgitant fraction is significant. The ventricle does not have time to remodel to accommodate the sudden increase in volume and its ability to increase ejection fraction is limited. The patient may present in cardiogenic shock and the murmur of aortic insufficiency may be quiet owing to the low pressure gradient between the left ventricle and the aorta or may be obscured by respiratory noise. Acute severe aortic insufficiency may be difficult to diagnose by echocardiography. With severe aortic insufficiency resulting from acute flail of one or two leaflets, the pressure in the left ventricle and the proximal aorta may equilibrate rapidly after ventricular contraction has ceased. The color flow jet may encompass the entire outflow tract and occur only in early diastole. The color flow may be difficult to visualize. Other echocardiographic signs of severe decompensated aortic insufficiency include early closure of the mitral valve in the absence of first-degree atrioventricular block. Diastolic opening of the aortic valve has also been described [68]. However, in some patients, the only echocardiographic sign may be the movement of the aortic cusps demonstrating a complete flail of a leaflet. Acute severe aortic insufficiency requires emergency surgical intervention if the patient is to survive.

Conclusion

Echocardiography is a reliable method to diagnose aortic insufficiency and to assess its severity. The lack of a true invasive gold standard for aortic insufficiency has led to a number of echocardiographic parameters that should ideally all be assessed in a given patient. Furthermore, serial assessment of asymptomatic patients with severe chronic aortic insufficiency is indicated to identify those patients who require surgical intervention.

References

1. Singh JP, Evans JC, Levy D, *et al.* (1999) Prevalence and clinical determinants of mitral, tricuspid and aortic regurgitation. The Framingham Heart Study. *Am J Cardiol* **83**:897–902.

2. Nkomo VT, Gardin JM, Skelton TN, Gottdiener JS, Scott CG, & Enriquez-Sarano M (2006) Burden of valvular heart diseases: a population-based study. *Lancet* **368**:1005–1011.

3. Kim M, Roman MJ, Cavallini MC, Schwartz JE, Pickering TG, & Devereux RB (1996) Effect of hypertension on aortic root size and prevalence of aortic regurgitation. *Hypertension* **28**:47–52.

4. Vasan RS, Larson MG, Levy D, *et al.* (1995) Determinants of echocardiographic aortic root size. *Circulation* **91**:734–740.

5. Lavie CJ, Hebert K, & Cassidy M (1993) Prevalence and severity of Doppler-detected valvular regurgitation and estimation of right-sided cardiac pressures in patients with normal two-dimensional echocardiograms. *Chest* **103**:226–231.

6. Lebowitz NE, Bella JN, Roman MJ, *et al.* (2000) Prevalence and correlates of aortic regurgitation in American Indians: the Strong Heart Study. *J Am Coll Cardiol* **36**:461–477.

7. Maurer G (2006) Aortic regurgitation. *Heart* **92**:994–1000.

8. Bonow RO, Lakatos E, Maron BJ, & Epstein SE (1991) Serial long-term assessment of the natural history of asymptomatic patients with chronic aortic regurgitation and normal left ventricular systolic function. *Circulation* **84**:1625–1635.

9. Borer JS, Hochreiter C, Herrold EM, *et al.* (1998) Prediction of indication for valve replacement among asymptomatic or minimally symptomatic patients with chronic aortic regurgitation and normal left ventricular performance. *Circulation* **97**:525–534.

10. Bekeredjian R & Grayburn PA (2005) Valvular heart disease: aortic regurgitation. *Circulation* **112**:125–134.

11. Dujardin KS, Enriquez-Sarano M, Schaff HV, Bailey KR, Seward JB, & Tajik AJ (1999) Mortality and morbidity of aortic regurgitation in clinical practice: a long-term follow up study. *Circulation* **99**:1851–1857.

12. Enriquez-Sarano M & Tajik AJ (2004) Aortic regurgitation. *N Engl J Med* **351**:1539–1546.

13. Margonato A, Cianflone D, Carlino M, Conversano A, Nitti C, & Chierchia S (1989) Frequency and significance of aortic valve thickening in older asymptomatic patients and its relation to aortic regurgitation. *Am J Cardiol* **64**:1061–1062.

14. Roberts WC & Ko JM (2005) Frequency by decades of unicuspid, bicuspid and tricuspid aortic valves in adults having isolated aortic valve replacement for aortic stenosis, with or without associated aortic regurgitation. *Circulation* **111**:920–925.

15. Dagum P, Green GR, Nistal FJ, *et al.* (1999) Deformational dynamics of the aortic root: modes and physiologic determinants. *Circulation* **100**(19 Suppl.):II54–62.

16. Anderson R, Devine WA, Ho SY, Smith A, & McKay R (1991) The myth of the aortic annulus: the anatomy of the subaortic outflow tract. *Ann Thorac Surg* **59**:640–646.

17. Roman MJ, Devereux RB, Niles NW, *et al.* (1987) Aortic root dilatation as a cause of isolated, severe aortic regurgitation: prevalence, clinical and echocardiographic patterns, and relation to left ventricular hypertrophy and function. *Ann Int Med* **106**:800–807.

18. Keane MG & Pyeritz RE (2008) Medical management of Marfan syndrome. *Circulation* **117**:2802–2813.

19. Keane MG, Wiegers SE, Plappert T, Pochettino A, Bavaria JE, & Sutton MG (2000) Bicuspid aortic valves are associated with aortic dilatation out of proportion to underlying valvular disease. *Circulation* **102**:35–39.

20. Nistri S, Sorbo MD, Marin M, Palisi M, Scognamiglio R, & Thiene G (1999) Aortic root dilatation in young men with normally functioning bicuspid aortic valves. *Heart* **82**:19–22.

21. Kai H, Koyanagi S, & Takeshita A (1992) Aortic valve prolapse with aortic regurgitation assessed by Doppler color-flow echocardiography. *Am Heart J* **124**:1297–1304.

22. Keane MG, Wiegers SE, Yang E, Ferrari VA, St John Sutton MG, & Bavaria JE (2000) Aortic regurgitation in Type A dissection: structural determinants and the role of valvular resuspension. *Am J Cardiol* **85**:604–610.

23. Movsowitz HD, Levine RA, Hilgenberg AD, & Isselbacher EM (2000) Transesophageal echocardiographic description of the mechanisms of aortic regurgitation in acute type A aortic dissection: implications for aortic valve repair. *J Am Coll Cardiol* **36**:884–890.

24. Rambaud G, Francois B, Cornu E, Allot V, & Vignon P (1999) Diagnosis and management of traumatic aortic regurgitation associated with laceration of the aortic isthmus. *J Trauma-Inj Infect Crit Care* **46**:717–720.

25. Erentug V, Bozbuga N, Kirali K, *et al.* (2005) Surgical treatment of subaortic obstruction in adolescent and adults: long-term follow-up. *J Card Surg* **20**:16–21.

26. Leung MP, Chau KT, Chiu C, Yung TC, & Mok CK (1996) Intraoperative TEE assessment of ventricular septal defect with aortic regurgitation. *Ann Thorac Surg* **61**:854–860.

27. Tohyama K, Satomi G, & Momma K (1997) Aortic valve prolapse and aortic regurgitation associated with subpulmonic ventricular septal defect. *Am J Cardiol* **79**:1285–1289.

28. Jacob R & Stewart WJ (2007) A practical approach to the quantification of valvular regurgitation. *Curr Cardiol Rep* **9**:105–111.

29. Roman MJ, Devereux RB, Kramer-Fox R, & O'Loughlin J (1989) Two-dimensional echocardiographic aortic root dimensions in normal children and adults. *Am J Cardiol* **64**:507–512.

30. Lang RM, Bierig M, Devereux RB, *et al.* (2005) Recommendations for chamber quantification: a report from the American Society of Echocardiography's Guidelines and Standards Committee and the Chamber Quantification Writing Group, developed in conjunction with the European Association of Echocardiography, a branch of the European Society of Cardiology. *J Am Soc Echocardiogr* **18**:1440–1463.

31. Kinoshita N, Mimura J, Obayashi C, Katsukawa F, Onishi S, & Yamazaki H (2000) Aortic root dilatation among young competitive athletes: echocardiographic screening of 1929 athletes between 15 and 34 years of age. *Am Heart J* **139**:723–728.

32. Stoddard MF, Hammons RT, & Longaker RA (1996) Doppler transesophageal echocardiographic determination of aortic valve area in adults with aortic stenosis. *Am Heart J* **132**:337–342.

33. Perry GJ, *et al.* (1987) Evaluation of aortic insufficiency by Doppler color flow mapping. *J Am Coll Cardiol* **9**:952–959.

34. Smith MD, Grayburn PA, Spain MG, & DeMaria AN (1988) Observer variability in the quantitation of Doppler color flow jet areas for mitral and aortic regurgitation. *J Am Coll Cardiol* **11**:579–584.

35. Smith MD, Kwan O, & Spain MG (1992) Temporal variability of color Doppler jet areas in patients with mitral and aortic regurgitation. *Am Heart J* **123**:953–960.

36. Spain MG & Smith MD (1990) Effect of isometric exercise on mitral and aortic regurgitation as assessed by color Doppler flow imaging. *Am J Cardiol* **65**:78–83.

37. Wong M, Matsumura M, Suzuki K, & Omoto R (1987) Technical and biologic sources of variability in the mapping of aortic, mitral and tricuspid color flow jets. *Am J Cardiol* **69**:847–851.

38. Evangelista A, delCastillo HG, & Calvo F (2000) Strategy for optimal aortic regurgitation quantification by Doppler echocardiography: agreement among different methods. *Am Heart J* **139**:773–781.

39. Dolan MS, Castello R, St Vrain JA, Aguirre F, & Labovitz AJ (1995) Quantitation of aortic regurgitation by Doppler echocardiography: a practical approach. *Am Heart J* **129**:1014–1020.

40. Zarauza J, Ares M, Vilchez FG, *et al.* (1998) An integrated approach to the quantification of aortic regurgitation by Doppler echocardiography. *Am Heart J* **136**:1030–1041.

41. Taylor A, Eichhorn EJ, Brickner ME, Eberhart RC, & Grayburn PA (1990) Aortic valve morphology: an important in vitro determinant of proximal regurgitant jet width by color Doppler flow mapping. *J Am Coll Cardiol* **16**:405–412.

42. Tribouilloy CM, Enriquez-Sarano M, Bailey KR, Seward JB, & Tajik AJ (2000) Assessment of severity of aortic regurgitation using the width of the vena contracta: a clinical color Doppler imaging study. *Circulation* **102**:558–564.

43. Shiota T, Jones M, Agler DA, *et al.* (1999) New echocardiographic windows for quantitative determination of aortic regurgitation volume using color Doppler flow convergence and vena contracta. *Am J Cardiol* **83**:1064–1068.

44. Ishii K, Jones M, Shiota T, *et al.* (1997) Quantifying aortic regurgitation by using the color Doppler-imaged vena contracta. *Circulation* **96**:2009–2015.

45. Yeung A, Plappert T, & St. John Sutton MG (1992) Calculation of aortic regurgitation orifice area by Doppler echocardiography: an application of the continuity equation. *Br Heart J* **68**:236–240.

46. Grayburn PA, Smith MD, Handshoe R, Friedman BJ, & DeMaria AN (1986) Detection of aortic insufficiency by standard echocardiography, pulsed Doppler echocardiography and auscultation. *Ann Int Med* **104**:599–605.

47. Masuyama T, Kitabatake A, Kodama K, Uematsu M, Nakatani S, & Kamada T (1989) Semiquantitative evaluation of aortic regurgitation by Doppler echocardiography: effects of associated mitral stenosis. *Am Heart J* **117**:133–139.

48. Beyer R, Ramirez M, Josephson MA, & Shah PM (1987) Correlation of continuous wave Doppler assessment of chronic aortic regurgitation with hemodynamics and angiography. *Am J Cardiol* **60**:852–856.

49. Labovitz AJ, Ferrara RP, Kern MJ, Bryg RJ, Mrosek DG, & Williams GA (1986) Quantitative evaluation of aortic insufficiency by continuous wave Doppler echocardiography. *J Am Coll Cardiol* **8**:1341–1347.

50. Vanoverschelde J, Taymans-Robert AR, Raphael DA, & Cosyns JR (1989) Influence of transmitral filling dynamics on continuous wave Doppler assessment of aortic regurgitation by half-time methods. *Am J Cardiol* **64**:614–619.

51. deMarchi SF, Windecker S, Aeschbacher BC, & Seiler C (1999) Influence of left ventricular relaxation on the pressure half time of aortic regurgitation. *Heart* **82**:607–613.

52. Griffin BP, Flachskampf FA, Siu S, Weyman AE, & Thomas JD (1991) The effect of regurgitant orifice size, chamber compliance and systemic vascular resistance on aortic regurgitant velocity slope and pressure half-time. *Am Heart J* **122**:1049–1056.

53. Touche T, Prasquier R, Nitenberg A, de Zuttere D, & Gourgon R (1985) Assessment and follow up of patient with aortic regurgitation by an updated Doppler echocardiographic measurement of the regurgitant fraction in the aortic arch. *Circulation* **72**:819–824.

54. Reimold SC, Maier SE, Aggarwal K, *et al.* (1996) Aortic flow velocity patterns in chronic aortic regurgitation: implications for Doppler echocardiography. *J Am Soc Echocardiogr* **9**:675–683.

55. Bargaggia GS, Tronconi L, Sahn DJ, *et al.* (1991) A new method for quantitation of mitral regurgitation based on color flow Doppler imaging of flow convergence proximal to regurgitant orifice. *Circulation* **84**:1481–1489.

56. Shiota T, Jones M, Yamada I, *et al.* (1996) Effective regurgitant orifice area by the color Doppler flow convergence method for evaluating the severity of chronic aortic regurgitation. *Circulation* **93**:594–602.

57. Tribouilloy CM, Enriquez-Sarano M, Fett SL, Bailey KR, Seward JB, & Tajik AJ (1998) Application of the proximal flow convergence method to calculate the effective regurgitant orifice area in aortic regurgitation. *J Am Coll Cardiol* **32**:1032–1039.

58. Yamachika S, Reid CL, Savani D, *et al.* (1997) Usefulness of color Doppler proximal isovelocity surface area method in quantitating valvular regurgitation. *J Am Soc Echocardiogr* **10**:159–168.

59. Quinones M, Otto CM, Stoddard M, Waggoner A, & Zoghbi WA (2002) Recommendations for quantification of Doppler echocardiography: a report from the Doppler Quantification Task Force of the Nomenclature and Standards Committee of the American Society of Echocardiography. *J Am Soc Echocardiogr* **15**:167–181.

60. Mallavarapu RK & Nanda NC (2007) Three-dimensional transthoracic echocardiographic assessment of aortic stenosis and regurgitation. *Cardiol Clin* **25**:327–334.

61. Fang L, Hsiung MC, Miller AP, *et al.* (2005) Assessment of aortic regurgitation by live three-dimensional transthoracic echocardiographic measurements of vena contracta area: usefulness and validation. *Echocardiography* **22**:775–781.

62. Aronow W & Kronzon I (1989) Correlation of prevalence and severity of aortic regurgitation detected by pulsed Doppler echocardiography with the murmur of aortic regurgitation in

elderly patients in a long-term health care facility. *Am J Cardiol* **63**:128–129.

63. Lin M, Chiang HT, Lin SL, *et al.* (1994) Vasodilator therapy in chronic asymptomatic aortic regurgitation: enalapril versus hydralazine therapy. *J Am Coll Cardiol* **24**:1046–1053.

64. Scognamiglio R, Fasoli G, Ponchia A, & Dalla-Volta S (1990) Long-term nifedipine unloading therapy in asymptomatic patient with chronic severe aortic regurgitation. *J Am Coll Cardiol* **16**:424–429.

65. Scognamiglio R, Rahmitoola S, & Fasoli G (1994) Nifedipine in asymptomatic patients with severe aortic regurgitation and normal left ventricular function. *N Engl J Med* **331**:689–694.

66. Sondergaard L, Aldershvile J, & Hildebrandt P (2000) Vasodilation with felodipine in chronic asymptomatic aortic regurgitation. *Am Heart J* **139**:667–674.

67. Padial LR, Oliver A, Vivaldi M, *et al.* (1997) Doppler echocardiographic assessment of progression of aortic regurgitation. *Am J Cardiol* **80**:306–314.

68. Meyer T, Sareli P, Pocock WA, Dean H, Epstein M, & Barlow J (1987) Echocardiographic and hemodynamic correlates of diastolic closure of the mitral valve and diastolic opening of the aortic valve in severe aortic regurgitation. *Am J Cardiol* **59**:1144–1148.

14   MRI of Aortic Insufficiency

Joachim Lotz

Hanover Medical School, Hannover, Germany

Introduction

Using magnetic resonance imaging (MRI) for the diagnosis of aortic insufficiency seems to be disproportionate at first glance. Echocardiography is routinely used to evaluate valvular function, morphology, and associated ventricular function. Imaging can be done in real time and arrhythmias have to be severe to really render echocardiography impossible. Several qualitative and quantitative techniques are usually combined to quantify the amount of valvular insufficiency (see Chapter 13); however, echocardiography has its limitations. Quantitative measurements of aortic insufficiency in echocardiography have relevant intrinsic limitations [1] such that the values obtained should be viewed with caution and only in the context of the qualitative signs of severity.

There are advantages for using MRI in certain situations: MRI is not dependent on acoustic windows. Aortic insufficiency can be assessed quantitatively with flow measurements. Ventricular volumes and function as well as ventricular mass are quantified using a three-dimensional (3-D) approach, and thereby MRI is insensitive to errors induced by akinetic or dyskinetic wall segments. Involvement of the ascending aorta can be assessed by either 3-D or two-dimensional (2-D) approaches, both of which are robust and easy to use. MRI, however, does have its drawbacks. Imaging with high spatial and temporal resolution requires nonreal-time imaging. This makes MRI sensitive to arrhythmias. MRI still is not recommended for patients with cardiac pacemakers or any metallic implant in neural tissues (cochlear implants, brainstem implants) or intraocular and intracerebral metallic foreign bodies.

Complete evaluation of aortic valve insufficiency includes assessment of the aortic valve, ventricular function, and volumes, as well as the evaluation of the aortic bulb and ascending aorta.

Cardiovascular Interventions in Clinical Practice. Edited by Jürgen Haase, Hans-Joachim Schäfers, Horst Sievert and Ron Waksman. © 2010 Blackwell Publishing.

Grading of aortic insufficiency

Grading of aortic insufficiency in MRI is usually done by quantitation of the regurgitated volume of the incompetent valve. Qualitative approaches have been used initially but most techniques have been dismissed for the grading of aortic insufficiency. They are, however, used to characterize the morphologic alterations of the valve and to visualize the presence of an aortic valve insufficiency.

Quantitative grading—flow measurement

Quantitation of aortic insufficiency in MRI is usually carried out with phase-contrast flow measurements: a moving particle induces a phase shift in the MRI signal. This phase shift can be manipulated to be linear to the velocity of the moving particle, thus enabling a quantitative flow measurement [2]. A phase-contrast flow measurement yields two data sets. The magnitude images resemble normal cine images with detailed anatomy of the vessel and its environment (Fig. 14.1a). The second data set includes the velocity images that are unique to phase contrast techniques. Every voxel in these images encodes the velocity at this position as a grayscale from black (flow away from the observer) to white (flow toward the observer) (Fig. 14.1b). Specific software is necessary to extract the quantitative flow information, resulting in time-resolved data on maximum and minimum flow velocities, mean flow volume, forward as well as reverse flow volumes, and area of the vessel during cardiac cycle. Phase-contrast flow measurements are usually performed either in suspended respiration or during free breathing. Both techniques interpolate the data from a number of heartbeats to calculate the flow dynamics of one cardiac cycle. Time resolution of flow measurements vary between 30 ms and approximately 150 ms, depending on the technique used. As with Doppler echocardiography, the range of velocities to be assessed has to be defined before the flow measurement. If this encoding velocity is too low, aliasing of velocity information occurs and the scan has to be repeated with an increased encoding velocity to yield a valid measurement.

To quantify the regurgitated fraction of an aortic valve, a flow measurement is prescribed approximately 2 cm

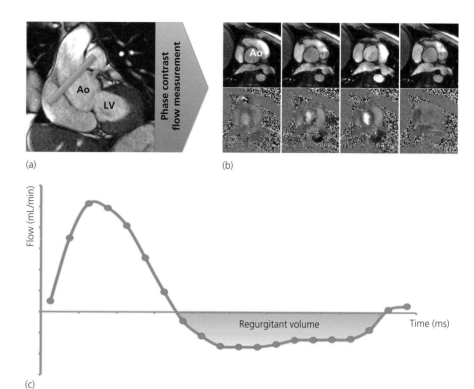

(a)

(b)

Figure 14.1 Phase-contrast flow measurement for aortic insufficiency. (a) Imaging plane at the sinotubular junction, perpendicular to the aortic wall. (b) Phase contrast flow measurements yield a time-resolved data set with magnitude images (above) and velocity images (below). (c) Dedicated software can extrude velocity information for the whole area of the aorta to yield a flow volume curve over the whole cardiac cycle, including calculation of regurgitant volume and regurgitant fraction of aortic valve insufficiency.

(c)

above the aortic valve, perpendicular to the aorta (Fig. 14.1a). Analysis of this measurement yields a volume–flow curve in which forward and reverse flow can easily be seen. Most dedicated software tools for MR flow analysis are able to automatically calculate the regurgitated flow–volume, insufficiency fraction, and effective cardiac output from these data (Fig. 14.1c).

Although the technique of flow measurement in MRI is quite robust, there are some pitfalls for this technique when applied to aortic insufficiency. Owing to the compliance of the aorta, the regurgitated volume gets smaller with increasing distance to the aortic valve. It has been estimated that the fraction of regurgitation can be underestimated by more than 20% if flow measurement is taken not at the aortic valve but more distally at the level of the pulmonary artery bifurcation, or just proximal to the origin of the brachiocephalic trunk [3]. Flow measurements should therefore be taken in the vicinity of the aortic valve. Measurements within the aortic valve, however, are subject to errors induced by turbulent and accelerating flow; the plane of the aortic valve moves 6–9 mm during the cardiac cycle [4]. As the imaging plane in MRI is usually fixed during the data acquisition, movement of the aortic valve through the imaging plane can occur; this may invalidate the measurement. Thus, an imaging plane 2 cm distal to the aortic valve, just in or above the sinotubular junction [5], is usually chosen for the evaluation of aortic insufficiency. In this position, flow to the coronary arteries during diastole is included in the regurgitated volume as a systematic, but acceptable, error.

There is no accepted standard to translate the fraction of regurgitation into a three- or four-point scale grading of aortic insufficiency. All published reports that compare echocardiography with MRI for aortic insufficiency describe a good correlation between the two modalities [5–7]. The intervals of regurgitated volumes or fractions mapped to the degree of aortic insufficiency cannot be compared between the studies. The discrepancies can be explained by differences in the techniques used in echocardiography as well as differences in techniques used in MRI. Therefore, the translation of quantitative fraction of regurgitation into the qualitative grading of aortic insufficiency has to be defined for each institution based on their (always identical) technique used in MRI as well as echocardiography. The main point of a written report of an MRI evaluation of aortic insufficiency should be a qualitative grading in combination with the quantitative number of the fraction of regurgitation. We also prefer to add a line about the MRI technique used for the flow measurement in the final report (Table 14.1).

Qualitative magnetic resonance imaging of aortic insufficiency

Attempts have been made to circumvent the need for dedicated software for the quantitation of aortic insufficiency. Initial approaches tried to use the length and width of the regurgitant jet on MR cine images to quantify valvular insufficiencies. This approach was dismissed because many parameters of the MRI technique have significant effects on the dimensions of the jet. Nevertheless, these techniques are still used to detect a valvular

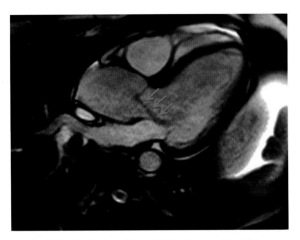

Figure 14.2 Aortic valve insufficiency in cine images. Cine MR images can visualize aortic valve insufficiency jets as seen in this example of mild aortic insufficiency (proven by echocardiography).

jet of insufficiency, irrespective of its severity (Fig. 14.2). Mild aortic insufficiency, in particular, can be seen on these images, even though it might be below the threshold of detection by quantitative MR flow measurements. These sequences also help to define the origin of the insufficiency and the morphologic alterations of the aortic valve per se, including the differentiation of bicuspid and tricuspid valve anatomy. Calcifications of the valve leaflets are seen as signal voids but usually do not interfere with the interpretation of the images [8,9].

Morphologic information can be used to further support results from flow measurements. Debl *et al.* [10] published an approach to use planimetry of the maximum insufficiency area of the aortic valve during diastole. The area correlated well with findings in echocardiography and invasive measurements

for moderate and severe aortic valve insufficiencies. Gradient echo cine sequences may be useful in the detection of insufficiency jets or a paravalvular leakage [11] in all types of valve replacements, including aortic valve stent grafts. This is not true for aortic stent grafts and nonbiologic valve replacements with supporting structures made out of steel because steel will destroy the MR signal within the valve and the adjacent structures (Fig. 14.3).

Evaluation of the aortic bulb and ascending aorta

In addition to imaging planes that run parallel to the aortic valve, perpendicularly oriented cine imaging planes can be used to assess the aortic bulb and parts of the aortic leaflets (Fig. 14.4). From these images, exact values to assess the dilation of the aortic root and proximal ascending aorta can be inferred. Especially in patients with contraindication to contrast media, these 2-D imaging techniques can be used instead of contrast-based 3-D MR angiography.

For complete assessment of the ascending aorta and aortic arch, a contrast-based 3-D MR angiogram is the fastest and most effective imaging technique (see Chapter 9).

Quantification of ventricular function and volumes

In addition to the characterization of the aortic valve itself, a complete workup of aortic insufficiency includes ventricular volumes and function as well as left ventricular mass. These parameters are the most important ones in the follow-up of a known high-grade aortic insufficiency [12].

For the estimation of left ventricular function and volumes, a stack of short-axis cine images is acquired from the ventricular apex to the level of the atria. Dedicated software is used for segmentation of the endocardial and epicardial border in

Table 14.1 Translation of quantitative regurgitation into grading of aortic valve insufficiency.

	Grading of aortic insufficiency		
	I (mild)	II (moderate)	III (severe)
Fraction of diastolic aortic regurgitation	<15%	16–30%	>30%

Translation of regurgitation volume into a grading scale for aortic valve regurgitation as used by the authors and supported by the publication of Ley *et al.* [5]. The thresholds for the different gradings are strongly dependent on the position and temporal resolution of flow measurement in the ascending aorta. The written report of the quantitative grading of aortic insufficiency should therefore include technical information as shown in this example.

Example of flow report
Aortic valve flow measurements
Forward volume   75 mL/heart beat
Regurgitant volume   18 mL/heart beat
Effective forward volume   55 mL/heart beat
Insufficiency fraction   24%

Severity of aortic insufficiency: moderate (grade II/III)
Technique: Phase contrast flow measurement; temp. resolution: 110 ms; slice position: sinotubular junction; suspended respiration; heart rate: 69 bpm

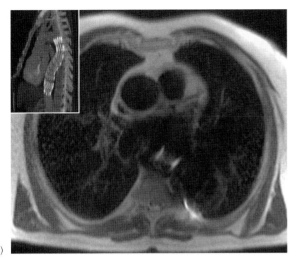

(a)

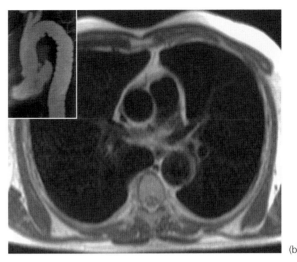

(b)

Figure 14.3 Effects of steel-supported stent graft on MRI. Steel implants significantly impede MRI. (a) Patient with an aortic stent graft with supporting springs made out of steel. No diagnostic information can be retrieved from the image. Inset shows sagittal image from CT-exam of the

same patient. (b) Patient with an aortic stent graft with supporting springs made out of nitinol. The supporting structures can be clearly delineated but do not cause artifacts in transverse images as well as MR-angiography (inset).

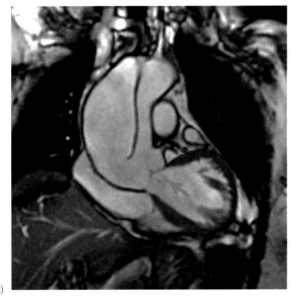

(a)

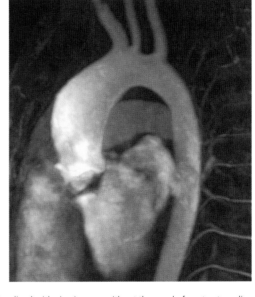

(b)

Figure 14.4 Evaluation of aortic root with MRI. Patient with mild aortic insufficiency and chronic type A aortic dissection. (a) The relationship of aortic valve leaflets, origin of coronary arteries, dimension of sinus of Valsalva and—in this case—the proximal end of the aortic dissection can be

visualized with cine images without the need of contrast media application. (b) For the complete evaluation of the ascending aorta, a 3-D MR angiogram using a gadolinium-based contrast agent is more efficient than cine images in terms of overview, time effectiveness, and patient comfort.

systole and diastole of this 3-D data set of the left ventricle. The data derived from this method of segmentation include end-diastolic and end-systolic volume, left ventricular output, ejection fraction, and all variables derived therefrom. The high reproducibility and high accuracy of this method have made MRI the reference standard in the estimation of left ventricular function and volumes [13]. This technique can be used even in low-output ventricles with ejection fractions below 20%. Large akinetic areas or ventricular wall aneurysms can be correctly included into the calculation of ventricular

volumes. Reliable normal ranges for ventricular volumes and volume indices have been compiled and stratified by sex and age [14,15]. It is common practice to supply the end-diastolic diameter in addition to the volumetric values of the left ventricle in order to keep the compatibility with the American Heart Association criteria for operative correction of aortic insufficiency and to make it easier to compare MRI data with echocardiography-derived data. The end-diastolic diameter of the left ventricle is usually measured on a midventricular slice of the short axis where both papillary muscles can be seen.

The difference of stroke volumes of the left and right ventricle was used in early reports to quantify aortic insufficiencies. This technique has not gained wide acceptance because the reliable volumetric segmentation of the right ventricle is technically demanding owing to the extensive trabecular network. In experienced hands this technique might yield accurate results; in general, it is regarded to be less reliable than flow measurements. Furthermore, any other concomitant valvular insufficiency of the right or left ventricle invalidates this approach.

Conclusion

Magnetic resonance imaging can be used to evaluate all aspects of aortic valve insufficiency, including insufficiency fraction, ventricular volumes, and aortic root dilation. It is the most reliable source for the evaluation of left ventricular volumes, function, and myocardial mass. For grading of aortic insufficiency, it is the responsibility of the local MRI team to translate the quantitative data of regurgitated flow volumes into a three-point scale of aortic insufficiency.

Magnetic resonance imaging might be used in the initial diagnosis, as well as the long-term follow-up, before and after aortic valve replacement. However, it remains the second-line imaging modality after transthoracic and transesophageal echocardiography.

References

1. Maurer G (2006) Aortic regurgitation. *Heart* **92**:994–1000.
2. Lotz J, Meier C, Leppert A, & Galanski M (2002) Cardiovascular flow measurement with phase-contrast MR imaging: basic facts and implementation. *Radiographics* **22**:651–671.
3. Chatzimavroudis GP, Walker PG, Oshinski JN, Franch RH, Pettigrew RI, & Yoganathan AP (1997) Slice location dependence of aortic regurgitation measurements with MR phase velocity mapping. *Magn Reson Med* **37**:545–551.
4. Kozerke S, Scheidegger MB, Pedersen EM, & Boesiger P (1999) Heart motion adapted cine phase-contrast flow measurements through the aortic valve. *Magn Reson Med* **42**:970–978.
5. Ley S, Eichhorn J, Ley-Zaporozhan J, *et al.* (2007) Evaluation of aortic regurgitation in congenital heart disease: value of MR imaging in comparison to echocardiography. *Pediatr Radiol* **37**:426–436.
6. Gelfand EV, Hughes S, Hauser TH, *et al.* (2006) Severity of mitral and aortic regurgitation as assessed by cardiovascular magnetic resonance: optimizing correlation with Doppler echocardiography. *J Cardiovasc Magn Reson* **8**:503–507.
7. Engels G, Reynen K, Muller E, Wilke N, & Bachmann K (1993) [Quantitative evaluation of aortic valve insufficiency in magnetic resonance tomography]. *Z Kardiol* **82**:345–351.
8. Debl K, Djavidani B, Seitz J, *et al.* (2005) Planimetry of aortic valve area in aortic stenosis by magnetic resonance imaging. *Invest Radiol* **40**:631–636.
9. Friedrich MG, Schulz-Menger J, Poetsch T, Pilz B, Uhlich F, & Dietz R (2002) Quantification of valvular aortic stenosis by magnetic resonance imaging. *Am Heart J* **144**:329–334.
10. Debl K, Djavidani B, Buchner S, *et al.* (2008) Assessment of the anatomic regurgitant orifice in aortic regurgitation: a clinical magnetic resonance imaging study. *Heart* **94**:e8.
11. Pflaumer A, Schwaiger M, Hess J, Lange R, & Stern H (2005) Quantification of periprosthetic valve leakage with multiple regurgitation jets by magnetic resonance imaging. *Pediatr Cardiol* **26**:593–594.
12. ACC/AHA (2006) Guidelines for the Management of Patients With Valvular Heart Disease: a report of the American College of Cardiology/American Heart Association Task Force on Practice Guidelines (Writing Committee to Revise the (1998) Guidelines for the Management of Patients With Valvular Heart Disease): developed in collaboration with the Society of Cardiovascular Anesthesiologists: endorsed by the Society for Cardiovascular Angiography and Interventions and the Society of Thoracic Surgeons. *Circulation* **114**:e84–231.
13. Grothues F, Smith GC, Moon JC, *et al.* (2002) Comparison of interstudy reproducibility of cardiovascular magnetic resonance with two-dimensional echocardiography in normal subjects and in patients with heart failure or left ventricular hypertrophy. *Am J Cardiol* **90**:29–34.
14. Sandstede J, Lipke C, Beer M, *et al.* (2000) Age- and gender-specific differences in left and right ventricular cardiac function and mass determined by cine magnetic resonance imaging. *Eur Radiol* **10**:438–442.
15. Lorenz CH, Walker ES, Morgan VL, Klein SS, & Graham TP Jr. (1999) Normal human right and left ventricular mass, systolic function, and gender differences by cine magnetic resonance imaging. *J Cardiovasc Magn Reson* **1**:7–21.

15 Surgical Reconstruction of the Aortic Valve

Diana Aicher & Hans-Joachim Schäfers

University Hospitals of Saarland, Homburg, Germany

Historical background

The first attempts at reconstructive surgery of the aortic valve were undertaken in the early days of cardiac surgery. The development of extracorporeal circulation opened up a window of new treatment options for congenital heart disease [1]. The technology was soon applied also to the surgical treatment of diseases of the heart valves.

The first operations to reconstruct the aortic valve were performed in the late 1950s and early 1960s. Based on animal experiments, Hurwitt *et al.* [2] proposed a repair approach for the insufficient aortic valve, in which one sinus and cusp of the aortic valve were excised and the valve effectively "bicuspidized." Shortening of the free cusp margin was used for aortic insufficiency by Spencer and Trusler as early as 1973 [3]. Cabrol *et al.* [4] published a technique of root plication for the insufficient aortic valve in 1961, and Ross [5] used pericardium for replacement or extension of cusp tissue [5].

Limited information is available on the functional results of this operation and the long-term durability. Although some of these techniques continued to be used occasionally over the subsequent decades, aortic valve surgery was revolutionized by the first heart valve replacement [6]. The new mechanical valves were applicable to all aortic diseases, and their insertion proved to be very reproducible. Research subsequently focused on design improvements of mechanical valve substitutes. Later, homografts, the autograft concept, and also xenograft heart valves were introduced in order to provide a reproducible substitute without the need of long-term anticoagulation and its disadvantages [7]. In particular, biologic xenografts were enthusiastically used in the 1970s because of their availability and ease of implantation.

In the 1980s it became evident that the durability of biologic heart valves was less than anticipated [8]. At the same time, the limited but continued activity in mitral repair demonstrated that reconstructive heart valve surgery could provide a stable

Cardiovascular Interventions in Clinical Practice. Edited by Jürgen Haase, Hans-Joachim Schäfers, Horst Sievert and Ron Waksman. © 2010 Blackwell Publishing.

long-term solution without the need for anticoagulation and with a low incidence of valve-related complications [9]. These observations led to increased activity in mitral valve repair and stimulated the development of new reconstructive approaches to the insufficient aortic valve.

Frater [10] first described correction of aortic dilation by adjustment of the intercommissural distance at the sinus rim level—the so-called sinotubular junction (STJ) remodeling. David and Feindel [11] and Sarsam and Yacoub [12] developed and proposed two different reconstructive operations for patients with insufficient aortic valves resulting from dilation of the aortic root. Cosgrove and co-workers [13] showed that cusp deformation (i.e., prolapse) could be reproducibly treated by reconstructive surgery. Attempts were also made to correct congenital malformation of the aortic valve [14]. Positive and very encouraging results published by some groups [14–16] led to increased enthusiasm in aortic valve reconstruction. Currently, an increasing number of surgeons worldwide engage in activities to discover optimal indications and repair techniques for the insufficient aortic valve.

Morphology and pathophysiology

To understand the pathophysiology of aortic insufficiency it is important to carefully analyze the anatomy and physiology of a normally functioning aortic valve. Anatomically, the aortic valve is part of the aortic root, which is defined by the commissures and the sinotubular junction cranially, and the basal ring caudally [17,18]. The annulus of the aortic valve is a coronet-shaped structure formed by the semilunar attachment of the fibrous parts of the cusps. Aortic ring size is primarily determined by the sinotubular and aortoventricular diameter, and to a lesser extent the diameter of the sinuses (Fig. 15.1).

It has been demonstrated that aortic root diameters show a positive correlation with body size [19], but the normal geometric relationship of aortic root and cusps is still poorly understood. Swanson and Clark [20], who examined silicone rubber molds of pressurized normal human aortic roots, found a constant ratio of the base radius (aortoventricular diameter) to the commissure radius of 1, and a ratio of the

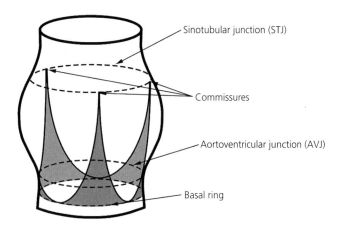

Figure 15.1 Aortic ring parameters.

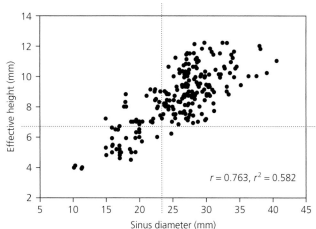

$r = 0.763, r^2 = 0.582$

Figure 15.2 Correlation of the effective height with sinus diameter in healthy adults and infants.

sinus height to the commissure radius of 1.2. Thubrikar *et al.* [18] carried out similar measurements in dogs and obtained ratios of 1.2 and 1.4, respectively, suggesting that the geometry of canine and human aortic valves is similar. Kunzelman *et al.* [21] found a relatively constant relationship between root diameter and cusp dimensions. Because the measurements were performed under nonpressurized conditions, they are not transferable to normal conditions with the aortic root and cusps under pressure.

To obtain data that can be used for decision-making in aortic valve repair, we have performed echocardiographic studies in healthy individuals. We have been able to confirm previous reports regarding standard diameters of aortoventricular and sinotubular junction in adults [22]. Most importantly, we have found a constant geometric configuration typical of the normal aortic valve with respect to height difference of central coaptation of cusp margins and their aortic insertion. This height difference—the effective height—correlates with root dimensions (aortoventricular diameter, sinus, sinotubular junction) and body size in the normal aortic valve (Fig. 15.2).

Functionally, the aortic valve is not a passive structure in which components move as a result of blood flow, but it has been demonstrated that the aortic valve and the aortic root are subjected to dynamic changes during the cardiac cycle [21,22]. Although the cusps are the most dynamic part of the aortic valve, the motions of other parts of the valve, such as the commissures and the annulus, are also important. Expansion of the aortic root starts during isovolumic contraction, first at the base and then at the commissures, followed by the sinotubular junction and the ascending aorta, and reaching its maximum expansion during the first third of ejection [23]. Thus, significant aortic root expansion (37.7% ± 2.7% of volume increase) occurs before ejection and initiates a stressless aortic cusp separation [24]. The pre-ejectional expansion of the aortic root is a result of commissural and annular base expansion related to volume redistribution in the left ventricular outflow tract via the interleaflet triangles [25,26]. The cusp movement during systole can be expressed in four phases: (1) a rapid

opening phase, (2) a phase of very little movement, (3) a slow closure phase, and (4) a rapid closure phase [24,27]. Based on these findings, it is only reasonable to regard the aortic root and valve as a functional unit. It is also evident that any geometric and functional disturbance of the unit will inhibit the natural process of valve closure and can thus lead to aortic insufficiency.

Causes of aortic insufficiency

The most common reason for aortic insufficiency is dilation of the aortic root. Over 60% of aortic insufficiency is caused by dilation of the ascending aorta or aortic root [28,29]. Aortic root diameter has been shown to increase with increasing age [19]. Atherosclerotic dilation due to hypertension, which is observed with increasing prevalence beyond the age of 60 years, involves mostly the distal segment of the aortic root, i.e., at the level of the sinuses and the sinotubular junction [30]. Congenital connective tissue disease, such as Marfan's syndrome, also leads to dilation of the aortic root, which involves mostly the sinotubular, sinus, and aortoventricular diameter in the first to the fourth decades of life [31].

Bicuspid anatomy of the aortic valve is also associated with dilation of the proximal aorta. Aortic aneurysm has been observed in up to 50% of individuals with bicuspid aortic valves irrespective of the hemodynamic performance of the valve [32,33]. The degree of dilation has been found to be inversely correlated with endothelial nitric oxide synthase (eNOS) expression in bicuspid aortic valves, with different patterns in normotensive or hypertensive patients [34]. A separate root pathology that leads to impaired closure of the aortic valve is aortic dissection. The dissecting process—regardless of the presence of pre-existing root dilation—commonly involves at least one and in most instances both commissures of the noncoronary aortic cusp. Consequently, this cusp loses its hinge points and is deformed during diastole, leading to aortic insufficiency of a variable degree.

The second component that may be responsible for aortic insufficiency—either alone or in combination with root dilation—is pathology of the aortic cusps. The most frequent form is a cusp prolapse, resulting from stretching of the cusp tissue, and most often seen on the fused cusp in bicuspid anatomy or as myxomatous degeneration in tricuspid aortic valves [35]. The prolapse may also be due to congenital cusp fenestrations in tricuspid, and less frequently in bicuspid, aortic valves [36,37]. These fenestrations are located in the paracommissural areas of the cusps and do not directly lead to aortic insufficiency because they are limited to the coaptation zone. They do, however, represent an area of reduced mechanical stability of the cusp because the free margin is only string-like and not supported by adjacent cusp tissue. Elongation of these marginal strands or their rupture will lead to deformation of the cusp, which can occur acutely in the presence of rupture. Quadricuspid aortic valves develop aortic insufficiency, mostly resulting from the restriction of cusp motion by the additional commissure. Unicuspid valves exhibit a combined geometric problem of cusp fusion and inadequate commissural height [38].

Currently, there is only limited information regarding the prevalence of cusp prolapse. This is because the rapid motion of the aortic cusps is difficult to follow with the time resolution of current echocardiography equipment. As a consequence, direct echocardiographic evidence of prolapse is difficult to provide, and most often the eccentricity of the regurgitant jet is a more reliable indicator of cusp deformation [39,40]. The difficulty of diagnosis is increased by the fact that, as yet, there are no clear and accepted criteria for the definition of prolapse. Prolapse is mostly defined as the bulging of cusp tissue into the left ventricular outflow tract [35]. Taking the geometry of the aortic valve into consideration, it is probably better defined as an insufficient height of a free cusp margin relative to the other margins. Prolapse may also coexist with root dilation, and it may be induced by reduction of root diameters, particularly at the sinotubular level.

Aortic insufficiency can also occur as a result of cusp retraction in rheumatic aortic valve disease, in which the usually thickened and retracted cusps fail to coapt adequately, despite preserved mobility. Restricted mobility of the cusp can also be caused by limited calcification—often seen in the fused cusp of a bicuspid aortic valve. Aortic insufficiency resulting from infective endocarditis can be induced by a broad spectrum of defects—starting with limited perforation of a cusp, to complete destruction of a cusp, to destruction of the aortic root. Acute aortic insufficiency is a rare complication of blunt chest traumas as a result of the rupture of a cusp or a commissure.

Technical aspects

Although repair of the insufficient mitral valve has long become a routine procedure, the development of similar concepts for the aortic valve is lagging behind. This is, at least in part, due to technical aspects that differ between mitral valve and aortic valve surgery, and make intraoperative assessment of valve geometry and judgment of surgical technical maneuvers difficult.

The majority of insufficient aortic valves are of normal, tricuspid geometry. This automatically implies the presence of three coaptation lines, compared with only one coaptation line of an axial symmetric valve, such as the mitral valve. Any manipulation on one cusp will automatically have an effect on at least two coaptation zones. Moreover, the aortic valve is always seen from its outflow side, unlike the mitral valve, which is seen from its inflow side. Most importantly, the surgeon always sees the valve under cardioplegic arrest. Under these conditions the aortic root is collapsed and the geometry of the root and aortic valve is completely different from normal, pressurized conditions. Finally, knowledge of the normal geometry of the aortic valve and root and the geometric prerequisites of an ideal repair result is still limited. The majority of these procedures are currently performed by surgeons who have developed a sufficient degree of (subjective) judgment needed to deal with the complex geometry.

To make aortic valve repair more reproducible, some groups, including ours, have developed specific technical solutions for these problems. Commissural stay sutures put under tension are used by the more active groups so as to mimic root geometry under pressurized conditions. Alternatively, the use of endoscopy has been proposed for the use of crystalloid cardioplegia [41]. As yet, no standardized assessment of cusp geometry is accepted. Although El Khoury *et al.* [62] suggest establishing the height of the cusp margin sufficiently high in the wide portion of the sinuses, we have taken a more analytic approach. Based on echocardiographic studies in normal patients, we have found a typical height difference between cusp margin and the nadir of these sinuses or aortic insertion, essentially the effective height (Fig. 15.3a). Based on our own observations in normal aortic valves in adults, we aim at an effective height of 9–10 mm. This has been reproducible and helpful in assessing pre-existing cusp pathology and the effect of cusp repair (Fig. 15.3b).

Operative techniques

Root procedures

Aortic dilation can be treated by sinotubular junction (STJ) remodeling [10] or subvalvular annuloplasty [4]—techniques that do not require root replacement—with subsequent reimplantation of the coronaries. Both techniques have a limited effect on the pre-existing size of the root, but they can aid in restoring aortic valve competence. Root remodeling [12] or reimplantation of the aortic valve within a vascular graft [11] are the techniques that involve root replacement and thus allow for the complete elimination of dilated aortic wall in the root.

Sinotubular remodeling consists simply of anastomosing a vascular graft to the aortic root at sinotubular level with a

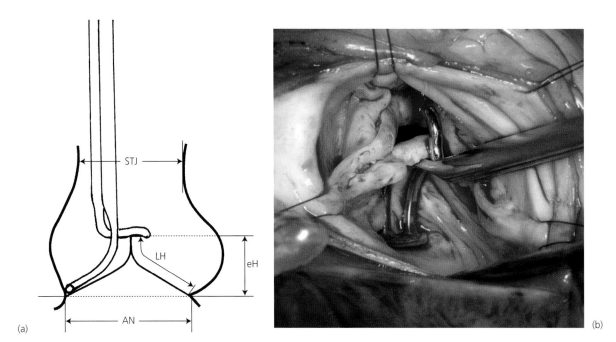

Figure 15.3 (a) Definition of the effective height. (b) Caliper for intraoperative measurement of the effective height.

continuous suture. It is probably the most appropriate option for patients with aortic aneurysm that involves primarily the ascending aorta and has only limited extension into the aortic root. Graft size is best chosen after holding the aortic commissures in a position that results in good cusp coaptation. Alternatively, the graft is chosen according to the size of the aortoventricular junction, an approach we prefer. In suturing, care must be taken not to distort the circumferential orientation of the aortic commissures, as this will lead to alterations of cusp geometry and function.

A subvalvular annuloplasty is commonly performed, as published initially by Cabrol *et al.* [4]. Although its exact geometric and functional role has still to be defined, it is probably helpful as an additional technical maneuver to cusp repair if there is borderline dilation of the root (aortoventricular diameter 26–30 mm) or borderline cusp tissue (geometric height < 20 mm). Horizontal mattress sutures buttressed with Teflon felt are placed through the annulus on each side of a commissure and tied. This reduces the circumference of the annulus and increases cusp coaptation without interfering with cusp motion. The amount of plication depends on the level at which the sutures are placed, i.e., a more caudal placement will lead to more plication. The plication may be used on selected or all commissures.

The two techniques used most frequently for more extensive root dilation are root remodeling [12] and reimplantation of the aortic valve within a graft [11]. Although prognostic data are not available, root replacement appears to be necessary in the presence of sinus diameters > 50 mm (transesophageal echocardiography; TEE), and it is probably advisable for sinus diameters > 40–45 mm. The relative importance of remodeling

versus reimplantation has been the subject of controversial discussion [43–46]. Remodeling, as the less invasive procedure, appears justified in cases of root dilation that do not involve the aortoventricular junction. It has been shown to result in almost normal cusp motion in both systole and diastole [47]. Reimplantation, on the other hand, definitely also stabilizes the aortic root at aortoventricular level, and is currently the only option that does so. The advantage of this technique is the support of the valve by the Dacron® graft (Intervascular; Datascope Intervascular GmbH, Bensheim, Germany), which is thought to enhance competence and prevent future dilation. There is concern, however, that the cusps can touch the graft and, consequently, degenerate. Moreover the absence of distensibility and the sinuses of Valsalva has been shown to result in abnormal cusp motion [48].

For aortic root remodeling, the dilated aortic tissue is excised close to the cusp insertion lines, leaving a limited rim of aortic wall for subsequent suturing (Fig. 15.4). A Dacron graft is chosen with a diameter close to that of the native aortoventricular junction, and three tongues are created so that the resected sinus wall can be replaced (Fig. 15.5). The graft is then sutured into the remnants of the aortic root, with the suture line closely following the cusp insertion lines (Fig. 15.6). Care is taken to create new commissures of adequate height. The result is a re-constructed root that is of normal configuration and still has some of its physiologic distensibility in the cardiac cycle. Near-normal cusp motion has been reported with this technique [47].

Aortic valve reimplantation, introduced by David and Feindel [11], allows not only for normalization of sinus and sinotubular junction, but also for stabilization of the aortoventricular junction. Resection of aortic wall is similar

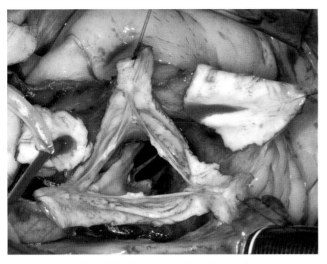

Figure 15.4 Excising of the dilated aortic tissue close to the cusp insertion lines, leaving a limited rim of aortic wall for subsequent suturing for root remodeling.

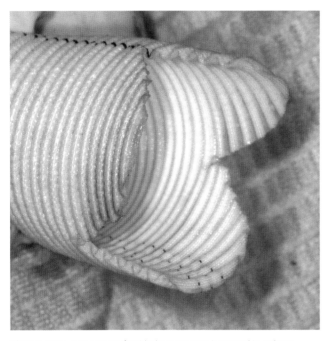

Figure 15.5 A Dacron graft with three tongues is created in order to replace the resected sinus wall.

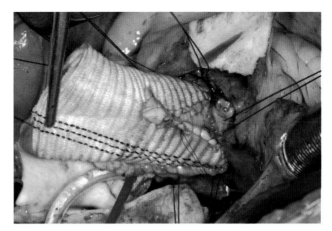

Figure 15.6 The suture line closely follows the cusp insertion lines.

as for root remodeling. In addition, the aortic valve is mobilized to the level of the basal ring/aortoventricular junction. Sutures are then placed through the root remnants at the lowest points of dissection, and these sutures are then passed through the end of a vascular graft, which is thus anchored to the left ventricular outflow tract. The commissures of the aortic valve are fixed at adequate height and circumferential orientation in the graft in order to create a geometry of the aortic valve that is close to normal. Finally, the remnants of aortic wall are fixed inside the graft by a continuous suture.

Initially both valve-sparing techniques were designed for patients with normal aortic cusps in whom regurgitation was either limited or solely a result of aortic dilation. As cusp prolapse may be present in conjunction with aortic dilation, a combined approach appears necessary for a relevant proportion of patients. We have previously shown not only that the combination of cusp and root repair for these individuals is feasible, but that valve stability actually improved and was more successful than isolated root repair [49]. Most importantly, the combined approach has allowed extension of reconstructive surgery for a large proportion of patients with aortic insufficiency, regardless of its preoperative severity.

As published by Langer *et al.* [50], we developed our own approach to the root according to the degree of dilation. No surgical procedure on the root is undertaken if dimensions appeared preserved (sinotubular diameter ≤27 mm, aorto-ventricular diameter ≤27 mm). In the presence of mild dilation (sinotubular diameter ≤32 mm, aortoventricular diameter ≤29 mm) subcommissural plication is performed. If dilation is more pronounced at the level of sinotubular junction and in the sinuses (sinotubular diameter >32 mm, sinus diameter >40–45 mm), root remodeling is chosen to restore near-normal root dimension [12]. In the presence of more severe root dilation at the level of the aortoventricular junction (≥30 mm) or the presence of Marfan's syndrome, the aortic valve is reimplanted within a vascular graft [11].

Cusp procedures

The primary goal of cusp repair is to correct distorted geometry and thereby normalize coaptation. The most common cusp alteration is prolapse, followed by restriction and congenital malformation. Cusp prolapse can be treated by central plication of the free margin [51], paracommissural plication [5], or triangular resection of redundant cusp tissue [9]. The triangular resection technique was proposed by Carpentier for tricuspid valves and later used by others for the correction of cusp prolapse in bicuspid and tricuspid aortic valves [13]. The technical variants have specific characteristics. Paracommissural

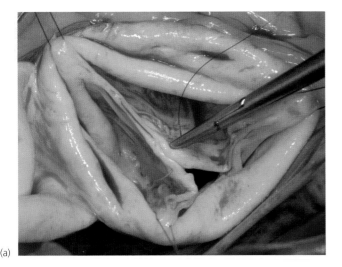

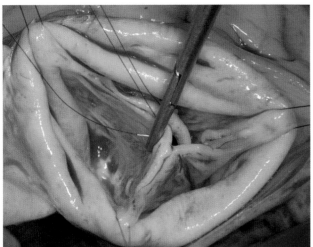

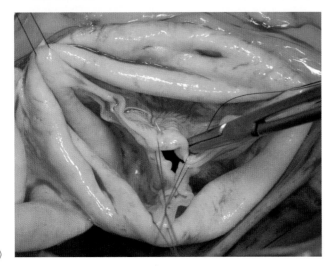

Figure 15.7 Stay sutures in the middle of the free cusp margins facilitate the assessment of cusp length.

plication corrects tissue redundancy in a high-stress zone of the free margin, and can thus be expected to be associated with an elevated risk of suture dehiscence. In fact, late results of this technique have supported this assumption [52]. By comparison, plication in the central part of the free cusp margin places sutures in an area of low stress [53]. Early in our experience we used paracommissural sutures, only to be facing recurrence of regurgitation from suture dehiscence. Over the past 11 years we have consistently preferred central plication, and the proportion of patients requiring reoperation for suture dehiscence has been small. Interestingly, we have primarily seen the need for reoperation as a result of a prolapse undercorrected at the time of initial surgery, and suture dehiscence was only seen in bicuspid valves, with an assumedly higher stress load on the margin of the fused cusp. Triangular resection intuitively appears as a more complex procedure, in which suture dehiscence can result in severe aortic insufficiency. We have therefore employed this technique with reservation, even though midterm stability has been as good as that of central free-margin plication [54].

Assessment of cusp geometry is of paramount importance for successful cusp repair. This is most reproducibly achieved with the use of stay sutures on the free cusp margins (Fig. 15.7). The measurement of effective height has been a helpful tool in the past years [55]. We preferably perform plication of the central portion of the free margin using single 5–0 or 6–0 Prolene sutures for correction of prolapse. Depending on the extent of prolapse, one to five plication stitches are placed in a stepwise fashion until an adequate cusp configuration is achieved. In the presence of marked tissue redundancy (>10 mm) or dense fibrosis/calcification, we choose a triangular resection of the diseased cusp tissue, readapting the remaining tissue by interrupted stitches (6–0 Prolene). If the resulting tissue defect after triangular resection is too large to allow for direct readaption, we insert a pericardial patch.

Other cusp pathologies have posed a bigger challenge to repair. Cusp retraction may be corrected by augmentation of the affected cusp with pericardial tissue [56,57]. We have found, however, that restriction not only involves the geometric height of the cusp, but also results in shortening of cusp tissue between the commissures, i.e., in its length. Restoration of normal cusp geometry has been difficult in these instances. More unusual congenital anomalies, such as unicuspid or quadricuspid anatomy, require specific maneuvers that not only address the direct mechanism of regurgitation, but also create a design with better a prognosis for durability. The conversion of quadricuspid anatomy to a tricuspid design with or without cusp augmentation has been a reproducible approach [58]. Bicuspidization of the unicuspid valve is a relatively young concept that has allowed reconstructive surgery in most patients with this variant. Using pericardial tissue a bicuspid valve with two commissures of normal height can be created, and the hemodynamic function has been equivalent to normally functioning bicuspid aortic valves [38].

Indications

Current indications for aortic valve repair are essentially those accepted for aortic valve replacement [59]. Current guidelines have not included earlier operative treatment, as in mitral valve surgery, except for the possibility of surgical treatment of aortic aneurysm at smaller aortic dimensions if valve preservation is possible by surgeons experienced in valve repair [59].

Symptomatic acute aortic insufficiency is an unequivocal indication for urgent intervention. In chronic severe aortic insufficiency, the onset of symptoms is accepted as an indication for surgery (class IB), also in asymptomatic patients with severe aortic insufficiency and impaired left ventricular function at rest (resting ejection fraction $\leq 50\%$) (class IB). Surgery is also suggested in patients with severe aortic insufficiency undergoing coronary artery bypass grafting, surgery of the ascending aorta or another valve (class IC). Similarly, surgery should also be considered in asymptomatic patients with severe aortic insufficiency with a resting left ventricular ejection fraction $> 50\%$ but severe left ventricular dilation (left ventricular end-diastolic diameter $> 70\,mm$ and/or left ventricular end-systolic diameter $> 50\,mm$ [or $> 25\,mm/m^2$ body surface area]) (class IC). A rapid increase in ventricular parameters on serial testing is another reason to consider surgery. Aortic root dilation $\geq 55\,mm$ should be a surgical indication, irrespective of the degree of aortic insufficiency (class IIaC). In patients with Marfan's syndrome (class IC) or bicuspid aortic valves (class IIaC), even lower degrees of root dilation (≥ 45 and $\geq 50\,mm$, respectively) have been proposed as indications for surgery, especially when there is a rapid increase in aortic diameter between serial measurements (5 mm per year) or family history of aortic dissection. Lower thresholds of aortic diameters can also be considered for indicating surgery if valve repair can be performed by experienced surgeons [59].

Results

Repair results have mostly focused on single techniques rather than repair as therapy for aortic insufficiency. In addition, few series report which proportion of patients with aortic insufficiency underwent repair rather than replacement. Minakata *et al.* [60] reported on 160 patients who were treated using aortic valve repair techniques and operated on over a 15-year period, constituting 13% of all individuals treated for aortic insufficiency during the same period. We established standardized techniques and then consistently tried to treat the unit of root and valve by a combined approach. This has allowed an increasing rate of repair in aortic insufficiency, reaching 90% of all procedures for aortic insufficiency in the last 4 years.

Root remodeling resulted in variable success rates with respect to valve stability. Yacoub *et al.* [61] reported in their series of 158 patients a freedom from reoperation at 1, 5, and 10 years of 97%, 89%, and 89%, respectively. El Khoury *et al.* [62] found good early results with the remodeling technique, with only one reoperation out of 45 patients at a follow-up of 30 months; the reason for reoperation was cusp repair failure. Luciani *et al.* [63] showed early restoration of valve competence after remodeling, but in a high proportion of patients (37%) recurrence of severe aortic insufficiency with the need for reoperation was described within the first 2 years after operation. Annuloaortic ectasia was identified as one of the risk factors for reoperation. Similar results were reported by Leyh *et al.* [45], who found a high failure rate of aortic root remodeling in patients with acute type A dissection with a rate of reoperation of 37% within 2 years. The reason for recurrent aortic insufficiency in all cases was prolapsing cusps. In 350 patients treated using remodeling techniques, we found a good long-term valve stability with a freedom from aortic insufficiency $\geq II$ of 89% of patients after 5 years and 88% after 10 years. Freedom from reoperation at 5 years and 10 years was 96% and 95%, respectively. Eleven patients had to be reoperated. The most common cause was cusp prolapse, in seven patients. Other reasons were rupture of a Trusler stitch ($n = 1$), endocarditis ($n = 1$), degeneration ($n = 1$), and suture dehiscence ($n = 1$). Out of 49 patients with acute dissection type A treated using remodeling techniques, only one patient had to be reoperated because of cup prolapse 11 months after the initial repair.

Numerous modifications of the reimplantation technique have been developed [64–67], and several series have resulted in good valve stability [44,68,69]. The level of cusp coaptation within the graft has been identified as a risk factor for the development of aortic insufficiency after reimplantation [46]. The less physiologic motion pattern of the cusps has not yet been proven to result in impairment of valve function up to 10 years postoperatively [47]. In patients with Marfan's syndrome, remodeling and reimplantation provide similar results with regard to valve stability [70,71]. We have treated 29 patients by reimplantation of the aortic valve, 12 with Marfan's syndrome. Freedom from reoperation at 5 and 10 years was 92% and 85%, respectively.

Many different techniques for isolated aortic valve repair are described with limited comparability, and mostly in small series. Cosgrove *et al.* [13] repaired cusp prolapse preferably in insufficient bicuspid aortic valves. Casselman *et al.* [72] published midterm follow-up data of this series with a freedom from reoperation of 95%, 87%, and 84% at 1, 5, and 7 years, respectively, in 94 patients; residual aortic insufficiency was identified as a risk factor for reoperation. Trusler *et al.* [52] published their late results of aortic valve repair in 70 patients with aortic insufficiency associated with ventricular septal defect. Freedom from reoperation was 85% after 10 and 15 years. The biggest series was published by Minakata *et al.* [60] from the Mayo Clinic. They found a freedom from reoperation of 89% and 85% after 5 and 7 years, respectively.

All publications show a low hospital mortality: Casselman *et al.* 0%; Trusler *et al.* 0%, Minakata *et al.* 0.6%. This is in

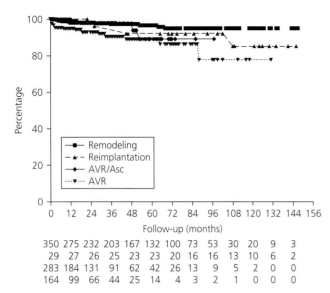

Figure 15.8 Freedom from reoperation for the different repair techniques.

agreement with our results, with one death out of 156 patients (0.6%) after isolated aortic valve repair. Hospital mortality for all patients was 2.8% (23/826) and depended largely on the age and comorbidity of the patient. Mortality of emergency operations for acute dissection has been as low as 7.6%.

Data about long-term valve-related complications after aortic valve repair are very limited. Casselman *et al.* [72] found no episode of thromboembolism or endocarditis in their series after a follow-up of 5 years. Trusler *et al.* [52] reported about three cases of endocarditis. No information about thromboembolic events was given. Minakata *et al.* [60] reported rates of freedom from stroke, bleeding, and endocarditis at 5 years of 98%, 94%, and 100%, respectively.

In our own patients, postoperative morbidity has been low; there was no postoperative aortoventricular block. There were 10 episodes of thromboembolism early postoperatively in conjunction with intermittent atrial fibrillation, with a linearized rate of 0.3% per patient-year. Mean systolic gradients were low, in both tricuspid (6.9 ± 5.7 mmHg) and bicuspid (10.6 ± 7.7 mmHg) aortic valves. Postoperative endocarditis of the reconstructed aortic valve (<60 days) was seen in two patients. Both could be stabilized by antibiotic treatment. They underwent reoperation for recurrent insufficiency within the first postoperative year and both recovered without problems. Another two patients developed endocarditis later after the operation (19 months/5 years). Both were treated by valve replacement and recovered well. The resulting linearized incidence of endocarditis was 0.15% per patient per year.

In our patients, aortic valve function remained stable in the vast majority throughout the follow-up period. Reoperation was necessary for recurrent insufficiency in 41 patients. Reasons for reoperation were active or healed endocarditis (*n* = 4), cusp retraction (*n* = 3), secondary aortic root dilation

(*n* = 2), suture line dehiscence after complex cusp repair (*n* = 8), progressive cusp prolapse (*n* = 23), and recurrent root dissection (*n* = 1). At reoperation the valve was replaced in 24 patients; valve and root were replaced with a composite graft in two. In 17 instances the aortic valve was re-repaired.

Freedom from reoperation at 5 years is 96% after remodeling, 92% after reimplantation, and 89% after isolated valve repair (Fig. 15.8). With increasing experience and improved understanding of optimal aortic valve configuration, we have been able to re-repair a relevant proportion of the failing aortic valves. Freedom from valve replacement at 5 and 10 years is thus 96% and 94%. Freedom from all valve-related complications is 92% after 5 years and 88% after 10 years.

Conclusion

Although the first reconstructive operations for the aortic valve were performed in the late 1950s, aortic valve repair remained an operation utilized for few selected patients. The realization that heart valve prostheses carry a relevant risk of valve-related complications stimulated the development of new reconstructive approaches for aortic insufficiency.

It is now known that aortic insufficiency is the result of dysfunction of the unit of aortic valve and root. Repair of the aortic valve has to address the functional unit of the root and cusps. Aortic dilation can be treated by STJ remodeling or subvalvular annuloplasty. Root remodeling or reimplantation of the aortic valve within a vascular graft are the techniques that involve root replacement, and thus allow for the complete elimination of dilated aortic wall in the root. The most common cusp alteration due to degeneration is cusp prolapse; it can be treated by central plication, paracommissural plication or triangular resection. Other cusp pathologies, such as restriction, congenital fenestration, or endocarditic lesions, may be corrected by the use of pericardial patches.

Root remodeling and aortoventricular reimplantation have been used with variable success rates with respect to valve stability. Also, for isolated aortic valve repair different techniques have been able to restore aortic valve function. Morbidity and valve-related complications are low.

Aortic valve repair is a new alternative to valve replacement. The stability is similar to mitral reconstruction and the incidence of valve-related complications is low.

In view of the current results, aortic valve reconstruction is a good option not only for a selected subgroup, but for all patients in whom aortic valve pathology allows reconstruction with a predictable functional result.

References

1. Kirklin JW, Donald DE, Harshbarger HG, *et al.* (1956) Studies in extracorporeal circulation. I. Applicability of Gibbon-type

pump-oxygenator to human intracardiac surgery: 40 cases. *Ann Surg* **144**:2–8.

2. Hurwitt ES, Hoffert PW, & Rosenblatt A (1960) Plication of the aortic ring in the correction of aortic insufficiency. *J Thorac Cardiovasc Surg* **39**:654–662.

3. Trusler GA, Moes CA, & Kidd BS (1973) Repair of ventricular septal defect with aortic insufficiency. *J Thorac Cardiovasc Surg* **66**:394–403.

4. Cabrol C, Cabrol A, Guiraudon G, & Bertrand M (1966) Le traitement de l'insuffisance aortique par'annuloplastie aortique. *Arch Mal Coeur Vaiss* **59**:1305–1322.

5. Ross DN (1963) Surgical reconstruction of the aortic valve. *Lancet* **1**:571–574.

6. Hufnagel CA, Harvey WP, Rabil PJ, & McDermott TF (1954) Surgical correction of aortic insufficiency. *Surgery* **35**:673–683.

7. Ross DN (1962) Homograft replacement of the aortic valve. *Lancet* **2**:487.

8. Bortolotti U, Milano A, Thiene G, *et al.* (1987) Early mechanical failures of the Hancock pericardial xenograft. *J Thorac Cardiovasc Surg* **94**:200–207.

9. Carpentier A (1983) Cardiac valve surgery—the "French correction". *J Thorac Cardiovasc Surg* **86**:323–337.

10. Frater RW (1986) Aortic valve insufficiency due to aortic dilatation: correction by sinus rim adjustment. *Circulation* **74**(3 Pt 2):I136–I142.

11. David TE & Feindel CM (1992) An aortic valve-sparing operation for patients with aortic incompetence and aneurysm of the ascending aorta. *J Thorac Cardiovasc Surg* **103**:617–621.

12. Sarsam MA & Yacoub M (1993) Remodeling of the aortic valve annulus. *J Thorac Cardiovasc Surg* **105**:435–438.

13. Cosgrove DM, Rosenkranz ER, Hendren WG, Bartlett JC, & Stewart WJ (1991) Valvuloplasty for aortic insufficiency. *J Thorac Cardiovasc Surg* **102**:571–576.

14. Tolan MJ, Daubeney PE, Slavik Z, Keeton BR, Salmon AP, & Monro JL (1997) Aortic valve repair of congenital stenosis with bovine pericardium. *Ann Thorac Surg* **63**:465–469.

15. Kalangos A, Beghetti M, Baldovinos A, Vala D, Bichel T, Mermillod B, *et al.* (1999) Aortic valve repair by cusp extension with the use of fresh autologous pericardium in children with rheumatic aortic insufficiency. *J Thorac Cardiovasc Surg* **118**:225–236.

16. Alsoufi B, Karamlou T, Bradley T, *et al.* (2006) Short and midterm results of aortic valve cusp extension in the treatment of children with congenital aortic valve disease. *Ann Thorac Surg* **82**:1292–1299.

17. Anderson RH (2000) Clinical anatomy of the aortic root. *Heart* **84**:670–673.

18. Thubrikar M, Piepgrass WC, Shaner TW, & Nolan SP (1981) The design of the normal aortic valve. *Am J Physiol* **241**:H795–H801.

19. Roman MJ, Devereux RB, Niles NW, *et al.* (1987) Aortic root dilatation as a cause of isolated, severe aortic regurgitation. Prevalence, clinical and echocardiographic patterns, and relation to left ventricular hypertrophy and function. *Ann Intern Med* **106**:800–807.

20. Swanson M & Clark RE (1974) Dimensions and geometric relationships of the human aortic valve as a function of pressure. *Circ Res* **35**:871–882.

21. Kunzelman KS, Grande KJ, David TE, Cochran RP, & Verrier ED (1994) Aortic root and valve relationships. Impact on surgical repair. *J Thorac Cardiovasc Surg* **107**:162–170.

22. Vasan RS, Larson MG, & Levy D (1995) Determinants of echocardiographic aortic root size. The Framingham Heart Study. *Circulation* **91**:734–740.

23. Dagum P, Green GR, Nistal FJ, Daughters GT, Timek TA, Foppiano LE, *et al.* (1999) Deformational dynamics of the aortic root: modes and physiologic determinants. *Circulation* **100**(19 Suppl.): II54–II62.

24. Lansac E, Lim HS, Shomura Y, *et al.* (2002) A four-dimensional study of the aortic root dynamics. *Eur J Cardiothorac Surg* **22**:497–503.

25. Erasmi A, Sievers HH, Scharfschwerdt M, Eckel T, & Misfeld M (2005) In vitro hydrodynamics, cusp-bending deformation, and root distensibility for different types of aortic valve-sparing operations: remodeling, sinus prosthesis, and reimplantation. *J Thorac Cardiovasc Surg* **130**:1044–1049.

26. Rodriguez F, Green GR, Dagum P, *et al.* (2006) Left ventricular volume shifts and aortic root expansion during isovolumic contraction. *J Heart Valve Dis* **15**:465–473.

27. Grande-Allen KJ, Cochran RP, Reinhall PG & Kunzelman KS (2000) Re-creation of sinuses is important for sparing the aortic valve: a finite element study. *J Thorac Cardiovasc Surg* **119**(4 Pt 1):753–763.

28. Devereux RB & Roman MJ (1999) Aortic disease in Marfan's syndrome. *N Engl J Med* **340**:1358–1359.

29. Muluk SC, Gertler JP, Brewster DC, *et al.* (1994) Presentation and patterns of aortic aneurysms in young patients. *J Vasc Surg* **20**:880–886.

30. Kim M, Roman MJ, Cavallini MC, Schwartz JE, Pickering TG, & Devereux RB (1996) Effect of hypertension on aortic root size and prevalence of aortic regurgitation. *Hypertension* **28**:47–52.

31. Marsalese DL, Moodie DS, Lytle BW, *et al.* (1990) Cystic medial necrosis of the aorta in patients without Marfan's syndrome: surgical outcome and long-term follow-up. *J Am Coll Cardiol* **16**:68–73.

32. Nistri S, Sorbo MD, Marin M, Palisi M, Scognamiglio R, & Thiene G (1999) Aortic root dilatation in young men with normally functioning bicuspid aortic valves. *Heart* **82**:19–22.

33. Nkomo VT, Enriquez-Sarano M, Ammash NM, *et al.* (2003) Bicuspid aortic valve associated with aortic dilatation: a community-based study. *Arterioscler Thromb Vasc Biol* **23**:351–356.

34. Aicher D, Urbich C, Zeiher A, Dimmeler S, & Schafers HJ (2007) Endothelial nitric oxide synthase in bicuspid aortic valve disease. *Ann Thorac Surg* **83**:1290–1294.

35. Shapiro LM, Thwaites B, Westgate C, & Donaldson R (1985) Prevalence and clinical significance of aortic valve prolapse. *Br Heart J* **54**:179–183.

36. Akiyama K, Hirota J, Taniyasu N, Maisawa K, Kobayashi Y, & Tsuda M (2004) Pathogenetic significance of myxomatous degeneration in fenestration-related massive aortic regurgitation. *Circ J* **68**:439–443.

37. Symbas PN, Walter PF, Hurst JW, & Schlant RC (1969) Fenestration of aortic cusps causing aortic regurgitation. *J Thorac Cardiovasc Surg* **57**:464–470.

38. Schafers HJ, Aicher D, Riodionycheva S, *et al.* (2008) Bicuspidization of the unicuspid aortic valve: a new reconstructive approach. *Ann Thorac Surg* **85**:2012–2018.

39. Kai H, Koyanagi S, & Takeshita A (1992) Aortic valve prolapse with aortic regurgitation assessed by Doppler color-flow echocardiography. *Am Heart J* **124**:1297–1304.

40. Cohen GI, Duffy CI, Klein AL, Miller DP, Cosgrove DM, & Stewart WJ (1996) Color Doppler and two-dimensional echocardiographic determination of the mechanism of aortic regurgitation with surgical correlation. *J Am Soc Echocardiogr* **9**:508–515.

41. Ohtsubo S, Itoh T, Natsuaki M, *et al.* (2000) Successful valve-sparing in aortic root reconstruction under endoscopic guidance. *Eur J Cardiothorac Surg* **17**:420–425.

42. Jeanmart H, de Kerchove L, Glineur D, *et al.* (2007) Aortic valve repair: the functional approach to leaflet prolapse and valve-sparing surgery. *Ann Thorac Surg* **83**:S746–S751.

43. Burkhart HM, Zehr KJ, Schaff HV, Daly RC, Dearani JA, & Orszulak TA (2003) Valve-preserving aortic root reconstruction: a comparison of techniques. *J Heart Valve Dis* **12**:62–67.

44. David TE, Feindel CM, Webb GD, Colman JM, Armstrong S, & Maganti M (2006) Long-term results of aortic valve-sparing operations for aortic root aneurysm. *J Thorac Cardiovasc Surg* **132**:347–354.

45. Leyh RG, Fischer S, Kallenbach K, *et al.* (2002) High failure rate after valve-sparing aortic root replacement using the "remodeling technique" in acute type A aortic dissection. *Circulation* **106**(12 Suppl. 1):I229–I233.

46. Pethig K, Milz A, Hagl C, Harringer W, & Haverich A (2002) Aortic valve reimplantation in ascending aortic aneurysm: risk factors for early valve failure. *Ann Thorac Surg* **73**(1):29–33.

47. Leyh RG, Schmidtke C, Sievers HH, Yacoub MH (1999) Opening and closing characteristics of the aortic valve after different types of valve-preserving surgery. *Circulation* **100**:2153–2160.

48. Fries R, Graeter T, Aicher D, *et al.* (2006) In vitro comparison of aortic valve movement after valve-preserving aortic replacement. *J Thorac Cardiovasc Surg* **132**:32–37.

49. Langer F, Graeter T, Nikoloudakis N, Aicher D, Wendler O, & Schafers HJ (2001) Valve-preserving aortic replacement: does the additional repair of leaflet prolapse adversely affect the results? *J Thorac Cardiovasc Surg* **122**:270–277.

50. Langer F, Aicher D, Kissinger A, *et al.* (2004) Aortic valve repair using a differentiated surgical strategy. *Circulation* **110**(11 Suppl. 1): II67–II73.

51. Spencer FC, Bahnson HT, & Neill CA (1962) The treatment of aortic regurgitation associated with a ventricular septal defect. *J Thorac Cardiovasc Surg* **43**:222–233.

52. Trusler GA, Williams WG, Smallhorn JF, & Freedom RM (1992) Late results after repair of aortic insufficiency associated with ventricular septal defect. *J Thorac Cardiovasc Surg* **103**:276–281.

53. Beck A, Thubrikar MJ, & Robicsek F (2001) Stress analysis of the aortic valve with and without the sinuses of valsalva. *J Heart Valve Dis* **10**:1–11.

54. Aicher D, Langer F, Adam O, Tscholl D, Lausberg H, & Schafers HJ (2007) Cusp repair in aortic valve reconstruction: does the technique affect stability? *J Thorac Cardiovasc Surg* **134**:1533–1538.

55. Schafers HJ, Bierbach B, & Aicher D (2006) A new approach to the assessment of aortic cusp geometry. *J Thorac Cardiovasc Surg* **132**:436–438.

56. Grinda JM, Latremouille C, Berrebi AJ, *et al.* (2002) Aortic cusp extension valvuloplasty for rheumatic aortic valve disease: midterm results. *Ann Thorac Surg* **74**:438–443.

57. Al Halees Z, Al Shahid M, Al Sanei A, Sallehuddin A, & Duran C (2005) Up to 16 years follow-up of aortic valve reconstruction with pericardium: a stentless readily available cheap valve? *Eur J Cardiothorac Surg* **28**:200–205.

58. Schmidt KI, Jeserich M, Aicher D, & Schafers HJ (2008) Tricuspidization of the quadricuspid aortic valve. *Ann Thorac Surg* **85**:1087–1089.

59. Vahanian A, Baumgartner H, Bax J, *et al.* (2007) Guidelines on the management of valvular heart disease: The Task Force on the Management of Valvular Heart Disease of the European Society of Cardiology. *Eur Heart J* **28**:230–268.

60. Minakata K, Schaff HV, Zehr KJ, *et al.* (2004) Is repair of aortic valve regurgitation a safe alternative to valve replacement? *J Thorac Cardiovasc Surg* **127**:645–653.

61. Yacoub M, Gehle P, Chandrasekaran V, Birks E, Child A, & Radley-Smith R (1998) Late results of a valve-preserving operation in patients with aneurysms of the ascending aorta and root. *J Thorac Cardiovasc Surg* **115**:1080–1084.

62. El Khoury GA, Underwood MJ, Glineur D, Derouck D, & Dion RA (2000) Reconstruction of the ascending aorta and aortic root: experience in 45 consecutive patients. *Ann Thorac Surg* **70**: 1246–1250.

63. Luciani GB, Casali G, Tomezzoli A, & Mazzucco A (1999) Recurrence of aortic insufficiency after aortic root remodeling with valve preservation. *Ann Thorac Surg* **67**:1849–1852.

64. David TE (1997) Aortic root aneurysms: remodeling or composite replacement? *Ann Thorac Surg* **64**:1564–1568.

65. Hopkins RA (2003) Aortic valve leaflet sparing and salvage surgery: evolution of techniques for aortic root reconstruction. *Eur J Cardiothorac Surg* **24**:886–897.

66. David TE (2002) Aortic valve sparing operations. *Ann Thorac Surg* **73**:1029–1030.

67. Svensson LG (2003) Sizing for modified David's reimplantation procedure. *Ann Thorac Surg* **76**:1751–1753.

68. Kallenbach K, Karck M, Pak D, *et al.* (2005) Decade of aortic valve sparing reimplantation: are we pushing the limits too far? *Circulation* **112**(9 Suppl.):I253–I259.

69. Harringer W, Pethig K, Hagl C, Wahlers T, Cremer J, & Haverich A (1999) Replacement of ascending aorta with aortic valve reimplantation: midterm results. *Eur J Cardiothorac Surg* **15**:803–807.

70. de Oliveira NC, David TE, Ivanov J, *et al.* (2003) Results of surgery for aortic root aneurysm in patients with Marfan syndrome. *J Thorac Cardiovasc Surg* **125**:789–796.

71. Birks EJ, Webb C, Child A, Radley-Smith R, & Yacoub MH (1999) Early and long-term results of a valve-sparing operation for Marfan syndrome. *Circulation* **100**(19 Suppl.):II29–II35.

72. Casselman FP, Gillinov AM, Akhrass R, Kasirajan V, Blackstone EH, & Cosgrove DM (1999) Intermediate-term durability of bicuspid aortic valve repair for prolapsing leaflet. *Eur J Cardiothorac Surg* **15**:302–308.

16   Pathology of Mitral Stenosis

Arne Warth, Esther Herpel & Philipp A. Schnabel

Institute of Pathology, University Clinics Heidelberg, Heidelberg, Germany

Definition

Mitral stenosis is mainly caused by inflammation (predominantly rheumatic fever), which leads to fibrosis and scarring with a reduced mitral valve orifice area.

Epidemiology

Mitral valve stenosis is one of the most frequent acquired heart valve pathologies worldwide and is found more often in women than in men [1]. In Western countries, the incidence of mitral stenosis has decreased over the past decades owing to the use of antibiotics, such as penicillin [2]. Mitral stenosis is frequently found in combination with mitral valve regurgitation and occasionally with aortic valve stenosis or insufficiency, which causes left ventricular dysfunction. The 10-year survival for New York Heart Association (NYHA) grade I and II patients is about 85%, and for NYHA III patients about 40%. The 5-year survival for NYHA grade IV patients is only 15%. The main causes of death are lung edema and right heart failure [1,3], arterial and lung embolism [4], and endocarditis [1,3].

Etiology

By far the most common cause of mitral stenosis is rheumatic fever, or, more precisely, the resulting endocarditis [1]. About 90% of all patients with rheumatic heart disease show an involvement of the mitral valve. However, rheumatic fever is evident in only 50–70% of all patients' histories. Further causes such as endocarditis due to bacterial infections or congenital mitral stenosis are rare. Patients with congenital mitral stenosis may have further cardiac abnormalities, including bicuspid aortic valve and coarctation of the aorta. Other rare etiologies for mitral stenosis include annular calcification,

Table 16.1 Causes and frequency of mitral stenosis.

Causes	Frequency
Endocarditis due to rheumatic fever	+++
Bacterial endocarditis	+
Congenital	(+)
Endomyocardial fibrosis	(+)
Systemic immunologic diseases: rheumatoid arthritis, lupus erythematosus, antiphospholipid syndrome, systemic vasculitides	(+)

+++, very frequent; +, sometimes; (+), rare.

systemic lupus erythematosus, carcinoid heart disease, endomyocardial fibrosis, and rheumatoid arthritis (Table 16.1) [1].

The symptoms of mitral stenosis become evident after an asymptomatic latent period of up to 40 years, with a mean interval of 16.3 years from the initial episode of rheumatic fever [1–5]. Data concerning the onset of symptoms in patients with nonrheumatic mitral stenosis are limited. However, a study of patients with mitral stenosis due to endocarditis revealed that these patients became symptomatic about 5 years after the initial event [1].

Anatomy and physiology of the mitral valve

The mitral valve arises from the annulus fibrosus, which surrounds the ostia atrioventricularia. The leaflets (cusps) are attached to the annulus fibrosus but also extend into the ventricular lumen. There, the free edges of the usually two leaflets are irregularly shaped. The number of effective leaflets in the atrioventricular valves is more often augmented than decreased owing to deep indentations of the leaflets. Each leaflet is linked with the ventricular papillary muscles or, in some instances, directly with the ventricular wall by the chordae tendineae, which are ramified and differ in thickness. The thinner chordae are attached to the free edges of the leaflets, and the chordae of median thickness are attached to

Cardiovascular Interventions in Clinical Practice. Edited by Jürgen Haase, Hans-Joachim Schäfers, Horst Sievert and Ron Waksman. © 2010 Blackwell Publishing.

the surface of the ventricular surface of the leaflets, only a few millimeters away, distant to the free edge. The thickest chordae are fixed to the ventricular surface of the leaflets near their origin from the annulus fibrosus. The atrial surface of the leaflets is smooth and bright; however, the ventricular surface is irregularly shaped and interweaved with bundles of chordae tendineae, which are fixed there. Each leaflet receives chordae from more than one papillary muscle, and each papillary muscle delivers chordae tendineae to more than one leaflet.

Owing to the special functional requirements, the anatomy of the mitral valve is far more complex and thus more susceptible to dysfunction than the aortic valve (compare Chapters 7 and 12) [1]. This is because the "normal" mitral valve apparatus has to comply with a high diastolic flow, especially in high cardiac output, a situation that is worsened by a relatively short diastole in the presence of high heart rates [1]. Thus, complete closure of the mitral valve is necessary to protect the lungs from high backpressure during ventricular systole. The circumference, shape, and location of the mitral valve are subjected to continuous changes during the cardiac cycle. Under these conditions, a broad coaptation of the closing portions of the leaflets and a firm fixation of the leaflets in the closed position by the subvalvular apparatus are prerequisites for mitral valve competence.

Pathophysiology

Mitral stenosis following rheumatic fever is the result of postinflammatory, slowly progressing degenerative changes of the mitral valve and the chordae tendineae due to a cross-reactivity between the streptococcal antigen and the valve tissue. Fibrosis and annular calcifications lead to thickening and immobility of the valve leaflets, as well as fusion of leaflet commissures and shortening of the chordae tendineae. Progression of the disease is slow in asymptomatic patients, but becomes more rapid after the onset of symptoms. The normal cross-sectional valve orifice area varies between 4 and 6 cm^2. Hemodynamically relevant changes occur when more than 50% of the valve orifice is degeneratively stenosed, resulting in increased pressure gradients between the left atrium and left ventricle and impaired left ventricular filling. An orifice area of <1 cm^2 is considered to represent critical mitral stenosis. Significantly increased transmitral pressure gradients result in dilation of the left atrium (Fig. 16.1). This dilation significantly contributes to atrial fibrillation [6], with the risk of thrombus formation and consequent arterial embolism [7], as well as pulmonary hypertension with hypertrophy of the pulmonary artery muscular layer and organic obliterative changes in the pulmonary vascular bed [8]. In later disease stages this leads to pressure exposure of the right ventricle, dilation of the right heart, and right-sided heart failure. The increased pulmonary blood pressure results in an

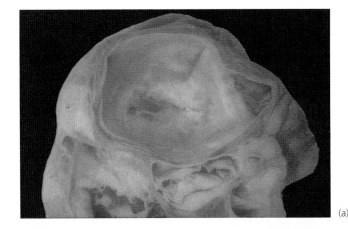
(a)

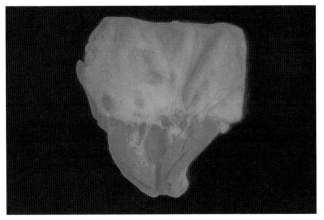
(b)

Figure 16.1 Mitral valve with severe mitral stenosis ("buttonhole stenosis"): autopsy specimen from a 36-year-old woman (courtesy of W. Doerr). (a) View of the significantly reduced mitral orifice area from the enlarged left atrium. (b) View of the left-sided heart with an extremely enlarged left atrium and an almost "atrophic" left ventricle.

adaptation mechanism, with increased pulmonary lymph flow, decreased permeability of the alveolar capillary membranes, and reactive constriction of the pulmonary vessels. This leads to reduced blood flow and a gradual reduction in hydrostatic pressure to prevent the risk of lung edema, which occurs at left atrial or pulmonary capillary pressures >25–30 mmHg at rest, or in combination with exercise, fever, anemia, tachycardia, or pregnancy. When the capacity of the described counter-mechanisms is exhausted, the symptoms of chronic lung congestion become evident. These include dyspnea, orthopnea, and, especially nocturnal cough.

Hemodynamic changes and the clinical appearance depend on the grade of valve obstruction, transmitral blood flow, heart rhythm, and heart frequency, as well as secondary changes in the pulmonary vessels. The classic symptom of mitral stenosis is dyspnea due to blood backpressure into the lungs [3]. Dyspnea often becomes symptomatic during exercise, with an increase in heart rate per minute. In severe stenoses, dyspnea even at rest is possible. Further symptoms are chest pain and hemoptysis due to diffuse alveolar hemorrhage [8], especially at night. In some cases, the patient's sputum includes hemosiderin-laden macrophages with dense, iron-positive intracellular inclusions. Chronic mitral stenosis is characterized by the so-called facies mitralis, or "mitral face.". This describes red to blue cheeks in combination with peripheral cyanosis and signs of right heart insufficiency. In some cases, the diagnosis of mitral stenosis comes after the diagnosis of tachyarrhythmia absoluta with atrial fibrillation.

Histopathology and clinical consequences

For histology/histopathology of the mitral valve we refer to Chapter 21 (see also Chapters 7 and 12 for histopathologic alterations of the aortic valve). A main histopathologic feature of mitral stenosis is fibrosis (i.e., augmentation of mainly collagen fibers, sometimes also elastic fibers), whereas calcification plays a minor role in mitral stenosis (for details see Chapter 21). Fibrosis can also rarely be seen in the parietal endocardium, where it is usually associated with hypereosinophilia [9]. Fibrosis occurs in the myocardium, especially in the left atrium, together with myocyte hypertrophy as a consequence of increased left atrial volume and pressure due to long-lasting mitral stenosis. The reasons for and consequences of myocardial fibrosis differ between heart diseases [10]. Endomyocardial fibrosis (e.g., in hypereosinophilia [Loeffler's syndrome] or carcinoid heart disease) may lead to ventricular failure [11]. Myocardial fibrosis and hypertrophy (e.g., as a consequence of aortic stenosis or insufficiency) is discussed in Chapters 7 and 12.

In the case of mitral stenosis, however, rheumatic fever, bacterial infections, annular calcification, systemic lupus erythematosus, carcinoid heart disease, endomyocardial fibrosis, and rheumatoid arthritis, besides rare congenital cases, have been identified as causal factors (see Table 16.1) [1].

Rheumatic fever
Rheumatic fever classically occurs in children between 4 and 9 years, 2–3 weeks after infection of the upper airways with streptococcal bacteria. Today the disease is quite rare owing to the existence of antibiotics [2]. The main symptoms of the disease include migratory arthritis of the large joints, carditis, central nervous system symptoms, erythema marginatum, fever, elongated PQ intervals, and elevated serum parameters of inflammation [12]. The involvement of the heart is characterized by a more or less distinct pancarditis, including myocarditis, endocarditis, and pericarditis. The most severe long-term consequence of the disease is therefore mitral stenosis [13].

Bacterial endocarditis
Although rare, infective endocarditis continues to be associated with significant morbidity and mortality, despite recent advances in its management, and remains a serious and challenging condition requiring a multidisciplinary approach. Surgery is essential in at least 50% of cases [5,14].

Endomyocardial fibrosis
Endomyocardial fibrosis is an idiopathic disorder with clinical parallels to rheumatic heart diseases, indicating an auto-aggressive pathogenesis [9]. The disease is characterized by fibrosis of the myocardium and fibrotic thickening and hyalinization of the endocardium with focal lymphocytic infiltrations, most commonly located in the left ventricular apex and the dorsal mitral valve leaflet. This may lead to parietal thrombus formations and concomitant pericarditis [10].

Carcinoid heart disease
Carcinoid heart disease is characterized by subendocardial cellular proliferations and endocardial thickening due to hormones (serotonin, bradykinin) that are secreted by gastrointestinal neuroendocrine tumors. Pathogenetically, these hormones are suggested to stimulate fibroblast proliferation and endocardial endothelial dysfunction [11]. However, as the hormones pass the right side of the heart before reaching the left endocardium, the disease is much more common in the right side of the heart [1].

Systemic immunologic disorders
Inflammatory rheumatic diseases, such as rheumatoid arthritis, lupus erythematosus, antiphospholipid syndrome, or systemic vasculitides, potentially involve organs and structures beyond the musculoskeletal system, and all structures of the heart may be affected [12,13,15–20]. Less than 10% of rheumatoid arthritis-affected patients have clinical signs of a cardiac involvement, but up to 30% are affected by clinically inapparent pericardial effusions. Myocarditis or endocarditis is caused by granulomatous infiltrates ("rheumatic nodules" or "Aschoff nodules"), which can typically be seen as a histomorphologic correlate of the disease [13].

Although involvement of the kidneys or the central nervous system means much more severe complications of systemic lupus erythematosus, cardiac involvement is very common and has manifold characteristics [16,21]. Pericarditis is evident in up to half of all patients with systemic lupus erythematosus, with resulting constrictive pericarditis in the long term [13], and some patients additionally develop an aseptic, so-called Libman–Sacks endocarditis [21,22] (see Fig. 12.3a).

Both the aortic and the mitral valve are affected in about 50% of all cases with a high association to antiphospholipid syndrome [13].

Among the systemic vasculitides, the antineutrophil cytoplasmic antibody-associated diseases (Morbus Wegener, microscopic polyangiitis, Churg–Strauss syndrome) as well as a large cell Takayasu arteritis are the most common ones that may affect the heart with peri- and myocarditis [13] (see Chapter 12).

Annular calcification

The etiology of annular calcification is unclear. The disease is characterized by dystrophic calcifications of the mitral annulus, normally without degenerative changes of the mitral valve leaflets. Thus, the disease classically leads to mitral valve regurgitation rather than to mitral stenosis (see Chapter 21) [15].

Treatment

Today, medical treatment is mainly reserved for early or mild cases of mitral stenosis, and especially for the treatment of atrial fibrillation and prevention of systemic embolization [5]. The natural history of mitral stenosis is well known from the literature [1–4,23]. The choice of percutaneous mitral balloon valvotomy, surgical valvotomy, commissurotomy, or valve replacement depends on the severity and the extent of the disease, the presence of comorbidity, the patient's age and situation (e.g., pregnancy), and the pathologic anatomy [5].

Acknowledgments

Mr. John J. Moyers is gratefully acknowledged for assistance in preparing the figures.

References

1. Horstkotte D, Niehues R, & Strauer BE (1991) Pathomorphological aspects, etiology and natural history of acquired mitral valve stenosis. *Eur Heart J* **1**(Suppl. B):55–60.

2. Gordis L (1991) The virtual disappearance of rheumatic fever in the United States: lessons in the rise and fall of disease. T. Duckett Jones memorial lecture. *Circulation* **72**:1155–1162.

3. Rowe JC, Bland EF, Sprague HB, & White PD (1960) The course of mitral stenosis without surgery: ten- and twenty-year perspectives. *Ann Intern Med* **52**:741–749.

4. Selzer A & Cohn KE (1972) Natural history of mitral stenosis: a review. *Circulation* **45**:878–890.

5. Bonow RO, Carabello BA, Chatterjee K, *et al.* (2006) ACC/AHA 2006 guidelines for the management of patients with valvular heart disease: a report of the American College of Cardiology/ American Heart Association Task Force on Practice Guidelines (writing Committee to Revise the 1998 guidelines for the management of patients with valvular heart disease) developed in collaboration with the Society of Cardiovascular Anesthesiologists endorsed by the Society for Cardiovascular Angiography and Interventions and the Society of Thoracic Surgeons. *J Am Coll Cardiol* **48**:e1–148.

6. Diker E, Aydogdu S, Ozdemir M, *et al.* (1996) Prevalence and predictors atrial fibrillation in rheumatic valvular heart disease. *Am J Cardiol* **77**:96–98.

7. Chiang CW, Lo SK, Ko YS, Cheng NJ, Lin PJ, & Chang CH (1998) Predictors of systemic embolism in patients with mitral stenosis. A prospective study. *Ann Intern Med* **128**:885–889.

8. Woolley K & Stark P (1999) Pulmonary parenchymal manifestations of mitral valve disease. *Radiographics* **19**:965–972.

9. Andy JJ (2001) Etiology of endomyocardial fibrosis (EMF). *West Afr J Med* **20**:199–207.

10. Maisch B & Rupp H (2006) [Myocardial fibrosis: a cardiopathophysiologic Janus head]. *Herz* **31**:260–268.

11. Andries LJ, Kaluza G, De Keulenaer GW, Mebazaa A, Brutsaert DL, & Sys SU (1996) Endocardial endothelial dysfunction and heart failure. *J Card Fail* **2**(Suppl.):S195–202.

12. Specker C (2006) [Cardiac manifestations of rheumatic diseases]. *Med Klin* (*Munich*) **101**(Suppl. 1):40–43.

13. Specker C (2007) [The heart in rheumatic diseases]. *Internist* (*Berl*) **48**:284–289.

14. Zakkar M, Chan KM, Amirak E, Herrey A, & Punjabi PP (2009) Infective endocarditis of the mitral valve: optimal management. *Prog Cardiovasc Dis* **51**:472–474.

15. Boudoulas H (2003) Etiology of valvular heart disease. *Expert Rev Cardiovasc Ther* **1**:523–532.

16. Goodsona NJ & Solomon DH (2006) The cardiovascular manifestations of rheumatic diseases. *Curr Opin Rheumatol* **18**:135–140.

17. Roberts WC (1983) Morphologic features of the normal and abnormal mitral valve. *Am J Cardiol* **51**:1005–1028.

18. Hanson TP, Edwards BS, & Edwards JE (1985) Pathology of surgically excised mitral valves. One hundred consecutive cases. *Arch Pathol Lab Med* **109**:823–828.

19. Iung B, Baron G, & Butchart EG, *et al.* (2003) A prospective survey of patients with valvular heart disease in Europe: The Euro Heart Survey on Valvular Heart Disease. *Eur Heart J* **24**:1231–1243.

20. Leong SW, Soor GS, Butany J, Henry J, Thangaroopan M, & Leask RL (2006) Morphological findings in 192 surgically excised native mitral valves. *Can J Cardiol* **22**:1055–1061.

21. Moder KG, Miller TD, & Tazelaar HD (1999) Cardiac involvement in systemic lupus erythematodes. *Mayo Clin Proc* **74**: 275–284.

22. Moyssakis I, Tektonidou MG, Vasilliou VA, Samarkos M, Votteas V, & Moutsopoulos HM (2007) Libman–Sacks endocarditis in systemic lupus erythematosus: prevalence, associations, and evolution. *Am J Med* **120**:636–642.

23. Olesen KH (1962) The natural history of 271 patients with mitral stenosis under medical treatment. *Heart* **23**:349–357.

17   Echocardiography of Mitral Stenosis

Wolfgang Fehske

St. Vinzenz-Hospital, Köln, Germany

Introduction

The anterior leaflet of the mitral valve is the most prominent reflector when the heart is investigated by ultrasound. This was discovered when the first experimental investigations were performed in humans [1]. Rheumatic mitral valve stenosis was the most frequent acquired heart valve disease during the very early stages of the new diagnostic method. Consequently, the first important clinical application of echocardiography became its contribution to the diagnosis of this specific valve disorder. With the developing ultrasound technologies, the diagnostic capabilities of echocardiography increased and, since the introduction of Doppler echocardiography, the comprehensive ultrasound examination is referred to as the standard diagnostic tool for the investigation of patients with mitral valve stenosis [2,3].

Pathophysiology of mitral stenosis

The severity of a mitral valve stenosis is mainly classified by the residual morphologic opening area (see Table 17.1), resulting in a more or less important pressure drop at the valve level. Pressure losses and opening areas are inversely correlated.

If heart rate and stroke volume were fixed, one could directly calculate the opening area from the mean pressure difference and vice versa. Consequently, under standard conditions ("normal" heart rate and "normal" stroke volume), the severity of mitral valve stenosis could also be classified by using the mean pressure differences (see Table 17.1). But there is a large interindividual variability in how the overall hemodynamic situation is adapted to the stenotic mitral valve.

One cornerstone within the broad spectrum of pathophysiologic possibilities is the development of cardiac output, which is either maintained over a long period of time or reduced, probably early in the course of the disease [4]. It can be assumed that

the age of the patients at the primary rheumatic carditis is important for the different developments [5]. At one end of the spectrum are young adults with severely reduced opening areas who remain asymptomatic for a long period of time [6]. They remain in sinus rhythm and maintain a normal cardiac output, with the capacity to even moderately increase it under stress conditions. In these patients, a high pressure loss across the mitral valve is mandatory, and consequently they also have a high systolic pulmonary pressure, which occasionally may exceed the systemic arterial pressure [7]. Symptoms in these patients may exclusively develop from exertional angina pectoris without an underlying coronary artery stenosis. Angina is caused by the increased wall stress induced by the pressure load to the right ventricle [8]. At the other end of the spectrum are older patients with a reduced cardiac output [9]. Even with a moderate to severe degree of mitral stenosis, they show only a relative low pressure loss across the valve, and under resting conditions one measures at most slightly elevated systolic pulmonary pressures. These patients typically develop symptoms of early onset of atrial fibrillation, peripheral arterial emboli, or exertional dyspnea with pulmonary congestion and/or edema. There is an ongoing debate as to why these patients suffer from pulmonary edema whereas patient groups in whom with cardiac output is maintained and who have chronically high blood pressures within the left atrium and the pulmonary veins are generally protected against pulmonary edema [3,10]. One major difference might be that in the latter group there is change in the permeability of the pulmonary microvascular structure. However, the whole complex pathophysiology of elevated systolic pulmonary blood pressure, reduced global pulmonary arterial vessel diameter, increased pulmonary vascular resistance, and reduced compliance of the left atrium and the pulmonary veins is part of an adaptational process in all patients with mitral valve stenosis. Finally, even those patients with reduced cardiac output and relatively low pressure losses across the mitral valve will develop pulmonary hypertension as a consequence of a secondary vasoconstriction of the pulmonary arterioles and partial obstruction of the pulmonary veins. Other than the independent effects of chronic hypoxia on the pulmonary vascular bed in these patients, the main cause of the elevating

Cardiovascular Interventions in Clinical Practice. Edited by Jürgen Haase, Hans-Joachim Schäfers, Horst Sievert and Ron Waksman. © 2010 Blackwell Publishing.

Table 17.1 Classification of severity of mitral valve stenosis according to the AHA/ACC guidelines for the management of patients with valvular heart disease [5].

Mitral valve stenosis: classification of severity	Opening area (cm²)	Mean pressure drop (mmHg)	Systolic pulmonary pressure (mmHg)
Normal	4.0–5.0	<1	<30
Mild	>1.5	<5	<30
Moderate	1.0–1.5	5–10	30–50
Severe	<1.0	>10	>50

ACC, American College of Cardiology; AHA, American Heart Association.

pulmonary vascular resistance in all patients with mitral stenosis is most likely chronic distension of the pulmonary veins (pulmonary venous hypertension). The exact trigger mechanisms and the neural and/or biochemical mediation within this process are not completely understood, and it is unclear to what extent the hemodynamic and morphologic adaptations are reversible after relief of the initial mitral stenosis [11].

Depending on the course of the disease, the first symptoms in patients with mitral stenosis are the onset of atrial fibrillation with enlarged left atria, peripheral emboli, or, less frequently, angina pectoris. Common to all patient groups is a gradual decrease in exercise tolerance, normally more than 10 years after the rheumatic disease has affected the heart. In the course of the untreated disease, further pulmonary [12] and cardiac symptoms will mainly arise from sequelae of pulmonary hypertension characterized by right heart congestion, primarily induced by chronic pressure overload and secondarily by volume overload as a consequence of increasing severity of tricuspid regurgitation.

After many years with no symptoms, the more rapid progression of the disease in the so-called "Third World" populations with younger patients is mainly attributed to recurrent rheumatic infections, but in older patients living in North America or in Europe the slower progression is mainly a consequence of secondary degenerative changes of the mitral valve or possibly of constantly increasing pulmonary resistance, even with no additional morphologic changes in the valve itself [10,13,14].

The overall course of the disease is also determined by the degree of a concomitant mitral insufficiency and/or additional rheumatic involvement of either the aortic and/or tricuspid valves, which must be diagnosed and treated separately. Finally, specific attention should be paid to the systolic and diastolic function of the left ventricle, which has generally been affected by the acute rheumatic cardiac disease. The normally small ventricle with a more or less healed myocardium has, once the stenosis of the mitral valve is removed, to take over the relative circulatory volume load that previously acted to "protect" the ventricle during the course of the disease. To preview the left ventricular outcome after successful

valvotomy or surgical treatment of mitral valve stenosis is a fundamental challenge of the echocardiographic examination in each of theses patients.

An improved understanding of the pathophysiologic changes, combined with cardiac surgery better conditions and the introduction of percutaneous mitral balloon valvotomy (PMBV), has led to a worldwide decrease in the numbers of patients with mitral valve stenosis [15]. Currently, patients are diagnosed and fundamentally treated much earlier than 20 years ago, when only severely symptomatic patients were categorized as suitable candidates for replacement of the mitral valve, or for closed or open commissurotomy. The international guidelines for the management of patients with heart valve diseases reflect these changes.

Echocardiographic parameters used within the guidelines

Two sets of international guidelines have recently been presented [2,3]. The European guidelines do not substantially differ from the American guidelines regarding the treatment of mitral valve stenosis, although the latter provide more pathophysiologic background. Both writing committees have carefully reviewed the current literature. Thus, we will refer mainly to the texts of the guidelines in respect of the basic considerations—why and when indications for a PMBV or surgical procedures are given—and will only add specific aspects, and a few newer references, for the subsequent echocardiographic section.

Both guidelines ascertain that echocardiography is the standard method to establish the qualitative and quantitative diagnosis in patients with mitral valve stenosis. A comprehensive echocardiographic examination should allow the extraction of the key parameters, which form the basis for all decisions in treatment:
- specific morphologic changes of the valve leaflets and the subvalvular apparatus;
- mitral valve area (MVA);
- systolic pulmonary artery pressure (SAP).

Although the American guidelines subdivide symptomatic patients into those with New York Heart Association (NYHA) class II and those with NYHA class III or IV classifications, the European guidelines differentiate only between symptomatic and asymptomatic patients in general. The latter recommend either PMBV, surgery, or conservative treatment only for patients with at least moderate degrees of stenoses (MVA <1.5 cm^2), whereas the American guidelines additionally include symptomatic patients with mild forms of stenosis (>1.5 cm^2). With the exception of one class IIaC indication for PMBV in asymptomatic patients with a resting pulmonary pressure >50 mmHg, the European guidelines do not specifically mention pressure measurements. The American guidelines incoporate all the parameters given in Table 17.1. They also include the category "severe pulmonary hypertension" for patients with systolic pulmonary pressures of >60–80 mmHg, who are considered to be suitable surgical treatment if symptoms are mild and conditions are unfavorable for PMBV.

Both guidelines differentiate between patients with conditions appropriate for PMBV and those with unfavorable conditions. This division is mainly based on the results of a scoring system that takes account of morphologic and motion aspects of the valve, the patient's age, and any concomitant mitral insufficiency (degree >2+). The scoring system is described in more detail in the European guidelines (see below), but in both cases assignment to the categories "appropriate" or "inappropriate" for PMBV is left to the individual physician.

In patients with questionable symptoms and a moderate or severe stenosis, or in symptomatic patients with only a mild stenosis, both guidelines recommend stress echocardiography (see below), but only the American guidelines provide threshold values for the indication for PMBV or a surgical intervention (systolic pulmonary pressure >60 mmHg, pulmonary wedge pressure ≥25 mmHg, mitral valve gradient >15 mmHg).

To understand and apply the concepts of diagnosis and treatment of patients with mitral stenosis, the guidelines should be consulted directly [2,3].

The echocardiographic examination

A standardized transthoracic echocardiographic examination (TTE) should include a basic set of loops, Doppler spectra, and motion modes (M-modes), which are registered from the parasternal, apical, and subcostal acoustic windows [16,17]. In patients with mitral valve stenosis it should always be possible to establish the correct diagnosis with all the important qualitative and quantitative parameters from the digital records of such a *standard examination* alone. An *extended examination* may be necessary if additional questions have to be answered or in the case of application of new echocardiographic methods and/or parameters aimed at improving morphologic or hemodynamic diagnostic potential.

As well as looking at the three key parameters highlighted in the guidelines (see above), we will focus on all the important cardiac aspects that are related to the disease and which should be diagnosed by echocardiography. For each of the specific questions we primarily refer to the possibilities of the *standard examination* before referring to the complementary part of the *extended examination*. The quantitative parameters that should be measured in a standard examination are especially important for patients with a mitral valve stenosis (Table 17.2).

Left ventricle

Standard examination

The size and the global and regional function of the left ventricle can be comprehensively diagnosed by standard techniques, mainly based on the evaluation of two-dimensional (2-D) imaging loops [18]. The diastolic and systolic left ventricular volumes should be measured and the resulting ejection fraction should be calculated. Reference values for classifying left ventricular volumes and function should be extracted from the national or international recommendations [16,18]. If there is no important concomitant mitral and/or aortic insufficiency, then in patients with mitral valve stenosis, in general, the left ventricle is small and contracts normally and the walls are of normal thickness. A reduced ejection fraction (<50%) suggests a negative prognosis [19–21]. However, even when the ejection fraction is normal, the sequelae of the original rheumatic carditis may be suspected when the typical features of diastolic dysfunction [22] are observed [23]. All other causes of a reduced left ventricular systolic or diastolic function (e.g., scars after myocardial infarctions or different stages of a hypertensive heart disease) can be detected or excluded by the standard investigation [18].

Cardiac output

The quantitation of stroke volume (SV) and cardiac output (CO = heart rate × SV) is of particular importance in patients with mitral valve stenosis (see above). If there is no aortic valve disease, the easiest and most popular approach to calculate cardiac output is to combine the cross-section of the left ventricular outflow tract (LVOT) with the corresponding pulsed Doppler velocity–time integral (VTI) as registered within the apical five-chamber view. The LVOT diameter (D) is taken from the parasternal long-axis view, with the calculated cross-section being $LVOT_{area} = (D/2)^2 × \pi$. One major reason for calculating stroke volume values arises from the integration of these results to any of the numerous applications of the continuity equation [24–26]. In the case of all types of arrhythmias, average measurements should be inserted instead of maximal or minimal values.

Extended examination

Tissue velocity imaging (TVI) with additional evaluation of deformation parameters has also been used in patients

Table 17.2 Proposed parameters to be measured within a standard echocardiographic examination of patients with a mitral valve stenosis.

	Parameter	Window	Imaging plane	Echocardiography method	Calculation
1.	End-diastolic LV volume	Apical	biplane: 2- and 4-chamber views alternatively: monoplane long axis or 4-chamber view	2-D	Method of disks
2.	End-systolic LV volume	Apical	See 1	2-D	Method of disks
3.	LV ejection fraction				$1-2/1 \times 100$
4.	IVS diastolic	Parasternal, alternatively with anatomical M-mode any long axis plane	Preferably short axis—papillary muscle level	Standard M-mode (alt. anatomical M-mode)	
5.	LV posterior wall	See 4	See 4	See 4	
6.	LA diameter (see 4)	See 4	(Preferably short axis) aorta/LA level	See 4	
7.	LV end-systolic diameter	See 4	See 4	See 4	
8.	RV end-diastolic diameter	See 4	See 4	See 4	
9.	LA volume	Apical	Four-chamber view	2-D	Method of disks end-systolic frame
10.	Systolic pulmonary artery pressure (SAP)	Mainly apical, alternative windows (small angle between TI jet and Doppler cursor)	Four-chamber view, or two-chamber view RV	Continuous wave	$4 \times TIV^2_{max}$ plus central venous pressure
LV output					
11a.	LVOT area	Parasternal	Long axis	2-D	(LVOT diameter/2)$^2 \times \pi$
11b.	Stroke volume	Apical	Five-chamber view	Pulsed Doppler	$VTI_{LVOT} \times$ LVOT area
11c.	Cardiac output				SV $\times$ heart rate
12.	Mean pressure drop mitral valve	Apical	Long axis	Continuous wave alternatively pulsed Doppler	Mean value of instantaneous pressure differences ($4 \times V^2_{max}$)
13.	Tricuspid annulus diameter	Apical	Four-chamber view	2-D	
14.	TAPSE (tricuspid annular plane systolic excursion)	Apical	Four-chamber view	M-Mode	Difference in relative height to apex of lateral tricuspid annulus
15.	Opening area by planimetry	Parasternal	Short-axis mitral valve	2-D	
16.	Opening area with mitral valve PHT[a]	Apical	Long axis	Continuous wave	220/PHT

For further explanation see text of the article. Reference values for the MVA, mean pressure drop, and systolic pulmonary pressure are extracted from the *ACC/AHA 2006 guidelines for the management of patients with valvular heart disease* [5] and are separately shown in Table 17.1. For all other reference values the standard recommendations for echocardiographic examinations should be used [19,21].

LA, left atrium; LV, left ventricle; RV, right ventricle; SV, stroke volume; TI, tricuspid insufficiency.

[a]The method for determining the pressure halftime from the diastolic mitral valve-Doppler spectrum is described within the text.

with mitral valve stenosis [27–29]. In our experience, however, the application of TVI methods does not add significant new information to the recognition of the left ventricular function in patients with mitral valve stenosis.

Left atrium

Standard examination

The characteristic changes in the left atrium in patients with mitral valve stenosis are part of the different pathophysiologic

Table 17.3 The Wilkins score system for categorizing morphology and mobility of a stenosed mitral valve [48].

Grade	Mobility	Subvalvular thickening	Thickening	Calcification
1	Highly mobile valve with only leaflet tips restricted	Minimal thickening just below the mitral leaflets	Leaflets near normal in thickness (4–5 mm)	A single area of increased echocardiography brightness
2	Leaflet mid and base portions have normal mobility	Thickening of chordal structures extending up to one-third of the chordal length	Mid leaflets normal, considerable thickening of margins (5–8 mm)	Scattered areas of brightness confined to leaflet margins
3	Valve continues to move forward in diastole, mainly from the base	Thickening extending to the distal third of the chords	Thickening extending through the entire leaflet (5–8 mm)	Brightness extending into the mid portion of the leaflets
4	No or minimal forward movement of the leaflets in diastole	Extensive thickening and shortening of all chordal structures extending down to the papillary muscles	Considerable thickening of all leaflet tissue (greater than 8–10 mm)	Extensive brightness throughout much of the leaflet tissue

developments. The size of the left atrium should be measured and categorized, preferably from the four-chamber view, using the method of disks [18], although the conventional diameter derived from an M-mode recording is widely accepted as a single characteristic parameter for the size of the left atrium [16]. Normal values and subdivisions into different categories of left atrial enlargement should be extracted from the standard recommendations [16,18].

In rare instances, left atrial thrombi can be detected by the transthoracic examination. However, if left atrial thrombi have to be excluded as part of the therapeutic strategy, a transesophageal echocardiographic examination must always be added.

Extended examination

For the assessment of the risk of cerebral or peripheral emboli in patients with mitral valve stenosis, transesophageal echocardiography (TEE) is the method of choice to prove or exclude left atrial thrombi, which are mostly located within the left atrial appendage (LAA) [30,31]. A standard transesophageal echocardiographic investigation should always visualize the LAA in at least two orthogonal planes, and a pulsed spectral Doppler interrogation of the flow should be included [32]. Dense spontaneous echo contrast is categorized with similar prognostic importance as to the risk of peripheral embolization [2]. LAA function analysis as determined by TVI techniques has been proposed as a follow-up parameter specifically for the characterization of the risk of formation of new left atrial thrombi, and has shown a significant recovery of LAA function after PMBV [33–37].

Tissue velocity imaging of the mitral ring has also been used to predict the probability of LAA thrombi and spontaneous echo contrast [36,38], but the method is not accepted as a substitute for TEE.

Morphology and functional anatomy of the mitral valve with special focus on the predictable outcome of balloon valvotomy

Standard examination

Two-dimensional echocardiography in standard imaging planes should always enable the exclusion of functional causes of left ventricular inflow obstruction other than rheumatic mitral valve stenosis. Examples of other pathologic conditions are large left atrial myxoma, congenital anomalies such as cor triatriatum, or a parachute mitral valve [39]. Patients with exclusively severe degenerative changes in their mitral valves should be strictly separated from patients with a primarily rheumatic mitral valve stenosis [40,41]. In these patients, the restriction of the MVA in general is not severe and the therapeutic options regarding PMBV or surgical valve-sparing procedures cannot be applied in the same way.

Two-dimensional transthoracic echocardiography (TTE) enables the visualization of most morphologic changes in mitral valve stenosis. The valve should be investigated from all acoustic windows using all standard imaging planes, with particular focus given to the long-axis and commissural two-chamber views from the apical window and the short- and long-axis imaging planes from the parasternal window. Various scoring systems can be used to categorize and semiquantitatively analyze changes in the underlying morphology and the functional anatomy in individual patients. The commonly used Wilkins score [42] is described in Table 17.3. This score represents the earliest attempt to categorize the morphologic and functional characteristics as detected by echocardiography in patients with mitral valve stenosis. It evaluates four separate parameters: *leaflet mobility*, *leaflet thickening*, *subvalvular thickening*, and *calcification*. These are categorized according to a four-grade scale of increasing severity. The result is a semiquantitative description of the valve pathology using a single numerical value. The score has mainly been used to differentiate patients with morphology seemingly appropriate for PMBV from those with an assumedly unfavorable outcome. A score of <8 is generally taken as the cut-off point for predicting a good result [43]. Of the four parameters, the thickness and the mobility of the anterior mitral leaflet are reported to be most important, and the morphology and motion of the posterior leaflet and the degree of commissural calcification are less important, for predicting the outcome after PMBV [44,45].

The Wilkins score represents an international standard [46], and recently its clinical value was confirmed when, in a series of 518 patients who were followed for 0.5–16.5 years after PMBV, a sophisticated Cox regression multiparameter analysis revealed that an echographic cut-off value of >8 in combination with the postprocedure mitral valve area (higher is better) and preprocedure functional class (lower is better) was associated with restenosis whereas the combination of Wilkins score of <8 and patient's age at intervention (the younger the better) proved to be highly significant predictors of event-free survival [47].

Additional scoring systems have been proposed to predict significant postprocedural mitral insufficiency [48] or to characterize more specifically the feasibility of splitting the anterolateral and the posteromedial commissures by scoring the severity of noncalcified fusions by TEE [49]. The European guidelines add another proposal classifying three groups of combined anatomical changes for predicting the outcome of PMBV [50].

We apply the Wilkins score in all patients with mitral valve stenosis, but its decision-making value is low if a PMBV is to be performed. In a patient who meets the general indications for PMBV in the American guidelines, we abstain from PMBV only in the presence of contraindications such as pre-existing MI ≥2+ or atrial thrombi: we would not abstain from the procedure if the Wilkins score alone indicated an unfavorable outcome. In the result is unsatisfactory, a surgical procedure should subsequently be performed.

Extended examination

Transesophageal echocardiography
Morphologic analysis of the mitral valve should always be possible within a standard TTE investigation. Little further information will be added during a subsequent TEE examination.

Three-dimensional echocardiography
Three-dimensional (3-D) echocardiographic techniques have mainly been applied in patients with mitral valve stenosis to measure the mitral valve opening area (see below) [51,52]. New parameters are proposed for distinguishing between a more conical or a more funnel-like geometry and a flat supravalvular inflow region. The first results need further evaluation and confirmation by other groups, in terms of

selection of appropriate candidates for PMBV, before they should be applied [53]. 3-D echocardiography has also been used to analyze the morphology of the commissures but provided no additional value compared with 2-D echocardiography alone [54].

Opening area

Soon after the first description of 2-D planimetry in 1975 [55], the method became the standard diagnostic tool for the quantitative evaluation of this key parameter in patients with mitral valve stenosis. With the introduction of Doppler echocardiography, the pressure half-time (PHT) method and the continuity equation were added to the echocardiographic armamentarium [56], and later, following the application of the flow convergence or proximal isovelocity surface area (PISA) principle for measurements of retrograde flow values in mitral insufficiency [24], this method was additionally proposed for estimating the size of the stenotic area in patients with mitral valve stenosis [26]. These methods are all currently available. Their relative importance and applicability have been systematically compared [57], and it was found that, compared with 2-D planimetry of a pathologic specimen, the PHT and PISA methods provide a reliable measurement of the size of the anatomic orifice. The flow area method using the continuity equation provided a less reliable correlation. Based on these data it is surprising that the American guidelines refer only to the PHT method for measuring the MVA [2], with the European guidelines establishing 2-D planimetry as the reference method [3]. As both reference methods are fast and easy to use they should be part of the *standard examination*, but application of the continuity equation and/or the PISA method is more time-consuming and thus these methods are part of the *extended examination* as well as the newly proposed 3-D approach.

Standard examination

Two-dimensional imaging
Planimetry of the stenotic mitral valve area should always be performed within the parasternal short-axis view. Standard gain settings should be used to avoid a too small planimetry caused by blooming. These rules were already been established in the first description of the method [55].

Recently, a mitral leaflet separation index (distance between mitral leaflets) was proposed as a parameter of mitral valve stenosis severity. It was found to be useful, but it cannot replace planimetry [58]. A standard approach for assessing MVA by parasternal 2-D imaging is shown in Figure 17.1.

Pressure half-time
The PHT method can be applied in almost all patients with mitral valve stenosis because the continuous-wave Doppler mitral valve inflow signal is very strong. The method is based on the original observation that the speed of the diastolic

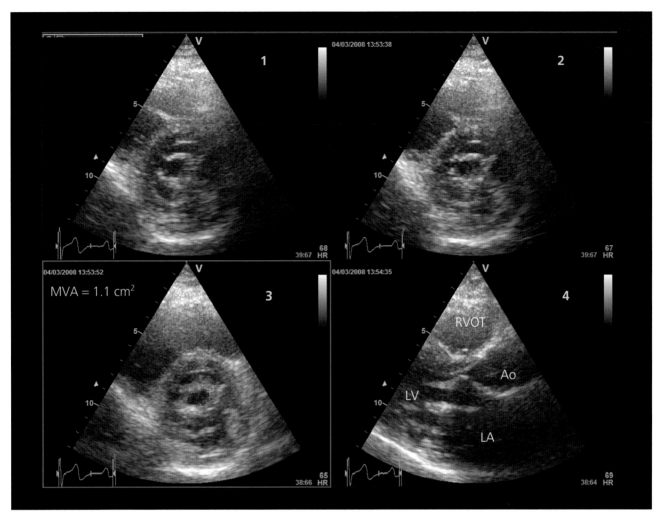

Figure 17.1 Standard approach to delineate the *narrowest* opening of the mitral valve. Sequential loops are recorded within a parasternal short-axis position to find out the optimal image, which in this case is seen in the loop (image 3). Image 1 is the corresponding long-axis aspect from the same parasternal window position. LA, left atrium; LV, left ventricle; Ao, aorta; RVOT, right ventricular outflow tract.

velocity decay is characteristic of the severity of mitral valve stenosis. As for the catheter technique, a reference value of 220 ms was taken to establish the simple to use standard formula, which can currently be used with any echocardiographic system: $MVA_{PHT} = 220/PHT$. The method of defining the PHT was first described, after the introduction of continuous-wave Doppler, in clinical echocardiography [56,59]: the half-time of the diastolic decrease in pressure loss (PHT) is recorded by measuring the time–distance between the maximum mitral valve velocity and the velocity of that numerical value divided by the square root of 2, which corresponds to half of the initial pressure loss. This parameter should ideally be independent of stroke volume and should be applicable in patients with atrial fibrillation.

The application, with all its technical specifications and limitations, has been reviewed several times [60]. One major concern refers to the unknown changes in the diastolic properties of the left ventricle, and it has been suggested that the method should not be applied in patients older than 65 years [61], in patients with tachycardia, and in patients with significant aortic insufficiency [62–64]; however, in hypertensive patients the degree of mitral valve stenosis will be underestimated using this method [40].

Finally, there has been a highly sophisticated debate on the potential disadvantages of the PHT method based on a theoretical background and *in vitro* investigations regarding the net atrioventricular compliance as the driving force for the mainly passive volume shift between left atrium and left ventricle during early diastole [65,66]. It was shown that if a severely stenosed valve is missed by the PHT method, this is most probably due to a reduced net atrioventricular compliance. A simplified method for calculating the net atrioventricular compliance is proposed: $C_n = 1270 \times (MV_{area}/\text{E-wave downslope})$ [66], where C_n is the net compliance (measured in mL/mmHg, MV_{area} is measured in cm^2, and E-wave downslope is measured in cm/s^2. This equation, however, assumes an unrestricted compliance of the left ventricle, which is clearly not the case in all patients. Recently, it was proposed that the calculated net atrioventricular compliance should be used as a prognostic indicator of the need for mitral valve replacement or PMBV [67]. Because a simple stress test has an even higher clinical significance, we recommend that this parameter is not used routinely. In general, the calculation of the net atrioventricular compliance should at most be part of an extended investigation.

Despite the restrictions of the PHT method, it is still reasonable to apply it. In the majority of patients, it allows one basic parameter for quantitation of the severity of mitral valve stenosis to be dteermined very easily.

Extended investigation

Proximal isovelocity surface area
The basic principle of quantifying the MVA in patients with mitral valve stenosis using the PISA method is derived from its application in mitral insufficiency. However, some specific adaptations have been described for mitral valve stenosis area calculation [26]. Numerous reports have been published on the reliability of this method under various conditions, such as atrial fibrillation, concomitant aortic insufficiency, and severely calcified valves with high Wilkins scores [68–71]. Simplifying modifications have also been proposed [72,73]. However, the method has not achieved great popularity, probably because it requires too many assumptions.

Continuity equation
Although the PISA method is based on the same hemodynamica principle, in echocardiography the term "continuity equation" is normally used for the calculation of the areas of stenosed aortic valves [25]. The same principle can be applied for the determination of MVAs in patients with mitral valve stenosis [74–79]. The calculation is simple, $MVA = SV/VTI_{MS}$, where SV is the stroke volume, preferably measured within the LVOT (see above), and VTI_{MS} is the mitral valve stenosis velocity–time integral. Restrictions to the application exist only if there is either a concomitant significant mitral insufficiency or aortic valve disease.

Transesophageal echocardiography
For determination of the MVA, TEE adds little information to conventional transthoracic examination. Only occasionally is one able with a short-axis transgastric view to visualize the opening of the stenotic mitral valve as considerable restrictions prevent the imaging plane being adapted to the smallest MVA.

Three-dimensional echocardiography
Since the introduction of real-time 3-D echocardiography for transthoracic and transesophageal imaging, several investigators have shown that the method is able to visualize the stenotic valve area—as the whole mitral valve apparatus—

embedded within the complete volume data set [80–85]. The ideal imaging plane, which reveals the narrowest opening, can be systematically reconstructed, even when there is no parasternal acoustic window for registration of the standard 2-D loops [40,83,84]. As in 2-D imaging, the morphologic information can additionally be combined with Doppler color flow data [40]. With the exception of one paper revealing only weak correlations between MVAs measured with 3-D compared with conventional echocardiographic methods [53], all other authors report excellent results with the same correlations [52,80,83,85,86]. Our own experience with the application of 3-D echocardiography leads us to be less enthusiastic; the quality of 3-D images is always worse than that of standard 2-D parasternal images, and the former should not replace the latter if the parasternal window is accessible. 3-D imaging from the parasternal window for MVA determination does not add to the information that an experienced investigator can extract from the 2-D examination alone [53]. A comparison of apical 3-D images and parasternal 2-D images of a pre- and postinterventional MVA is shown in Figure 17.2.

The "gold standard"
The recent description of the 3-D technique for measuring the MVA by planimetry within reconstructed planes from a 3-D voxel data set has again raised the question of which method should be regarded as the "gold standard" [51]. An editorial comment asserted an equal rank for 2-D planimetry and the Gorlin formula (the value of the 3-D methods had yet to be documented) [87]. We agree, in principle, but suggest that the Gorlin formula—combining pressure and cardiac output measurements—should not be the reference method for measuring the anatomically defined MVA in patients with rheumatic mitral valve stenosis. This is particularly true in the case of patients with atrial fibrillation.

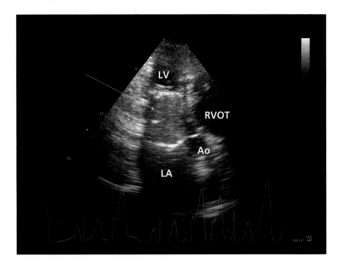

Figure 17.2 Echocardiographic guidance of mitral valvuloplasty. The Inoue balloon is visualized in the correct position inflated for valvuloplasty. Arrow points to the balloon. LA, left atrium; LV, left ventricle; Ao, aorta; RVOT, right ventricular outflow tract.

Pressure loss across the mitral valve

Standard investigation

Since the introduction of continuous-wave Doppler into routine echocardiography, the application of the simplified Bernoulli equation ($\Delta p \approx 4 \times v_{\max}^2$, where Δp is the hydrodynamic pressure difference and $v_{\max}$ is the maximal instantaneous velocity along the blood flow through the stenosis) has proved to be reliable and robust. Today, Doppler estimation of pressure differences across stenosed mitral valves is considered the standard reference method [88,89].

The diastolic mean pressure drop (Δp mean) should be calculated by outlining the mitral valve stenosis–continuous wave spectra throughout diastole. The reference values for the pressure loss measurements are listed in Table 17.1. In patients with atrial fibrillation, an appropriate number of heart cycles should be averaged.

Extended examination

Concerning the mean pressure drop, there is no need for additional measurements as the calculation of that parameter is already part of the standard examination.

Mitral valve resistance

The ratio of mitral valve mean pressure drop and flow has been proposed as a significant predictor of severity of the disease, and the parameter was reported to be a predictor of individual exercise capacity as well as of the systolic pulmonary pressures under maximal stress conditions [90]. However, because it contains exactly the same information as is used for the calculation of the effective orifice area by the continuity equation (see above), we do not integrate the calculation of mitral valve resistance (MVR) in the investigation protocol in mitral valve stenosis.

Pulmonary artery pressure

The pressure and—later within the course of the disease—the volume load to the right ventricle are the consequences of the increased resistance to the left ventricular inflow by the stenotic mitral valve. The differentiation between precapillary increase in pulmonary resistance and postcapillary pressure increase due to predominant elevation of left atrial and lung vein pressures is not possible by means of any of the echocardiographic parameters. However, the SAP can reliably be measured and should be part of any standard echocardiographic investigation.

Standard investigation

As well as a number of indirect signs of pressure overload of the right ventricle, such as systolic flattening of the IVS, right ventricular dilation, and hypertrophy [18,91], the most important parameter to be determined during the standard investigation is the SAP. It is estimated by applying the simplified Bernoulli equation to the maximal velocity within the continuous-wave Doppler spectrum, derived from a tricuspid insufficiency jet

[92,93]. The central venous pressure—or the right atrial pressure—must be added to the pressure difference as extracted from the tricuspid insufficiency velocity. In nearly 90% of all investigations a trained user will be able to detect a tricuspid insufficiency jet, and measurements can even be performed with very tiny insufficiency jets. The right atrial pressure cannot directly be measured by echocardiography. However, it is generally estimated from the size and respiratory variation of the inferior vena cava [91]. At our institution, we do not give a numerical value for the estimated right atrial pressure, but within the echocardiography reports we indicate if there are signs of no, moderate, or severe right atrial congestion, which means that to obtain the true SAP we should add the corresponding values of 0–20 mmHg, or even more, to the peak pressure difference calculated from the tricuspid insufficiency.

If the SAP cannot be measured from the standard echocardiographic investigation, one major parameter for decision-making in patients with mitral valve stenosis is missed, and completion of the diagnosis by invasive means should always be discussed [2,3].

Extended examination

From the end-diastolic velocity measurements in the pulmonary insufficiency jet, the diastolic pulmonary artery pressure can be estimated [91].

Numerous proposals have been published for calculating the total pulmonary vascular resistance. These are mostly prone to unpredictable influences of heart rate, respiratory variations, and Doppler signal quality. We do not routinely use these parameters in patients with mitral valve stenosis. For more details, we recommend referring to articles reviewing the current literature [91].

Right ventricular function

The systolic and diastolic function of the right ventricle is very important for the clinical course of the patients with mitral valve stenosis. It is possible to visualize most parts of the right ventricle and the right atrium by TTE. However, until now, no parameter that comprehensively characterizes the overall right ventricular function and functional reserve has been described. The subdivision into standard and extended investigational parts is relatively arbitrary.

The increasing pressure load to the right ventricle leads to an increasing chamber size, and finally to dilation of the atrioventricular ring, with consequent increas in the severity of tricuspid insufficiency.

Standard investigation

The size of the right ventricle can be estimated from a standard M-mode registration or from an apical four-chamber view. Reference values for the systolic and diastolic diameters of the right ventricular outflow tract (RVOT; M-mode), as well as for the areas of tricuspid insufficiency and right atrial and fractional right ventricular area changes, are given within the official recommendations for chamber quantitation [18] and within a recently published review paper [94]. International recommendations for diagnosing and quantifying a tricuspid insufficiency should be applied [95], and the semiquantitative parameters should be used within any standard investigation.

A single parameter for dynamic functional analysis of the tricuspid insufficiency is widely used and should be integrated into the standard investigation: the tricuspid annular plane systolic excursion can easily be measured from the apical four-chamber view at the lateral tricuspid ring. A value of less than 1.5 cm has been described as being associated with poor prognosis [96]. However, the reliability of this parameter to exclusively reflect right ventricular function has been questioned [94,97].

Extended examination

Numerous attempts to use new echocardiographic facilities to characterize right ventricular function have been described: parameters derived from tissue velocity imaging, speckle tracking, 3-D registrations, and time interval measurements all have insufficient clinical significance [94,97–101].

Stress echocardiography

Following the guidelines [2,3], a stress test should be performed in asymptomatic patients with mild or moderate to severe stenosis in whom the resting systolic pulmonary arterial pressure (PAP) is less than 50 mmHg, and in any symptomatic patient with only mild stenosis. In general, interventional or operative treatment is indicated when the mean pressure drop increases by more than 15 mmHg and/or PAP increases to >60 mmHg.

A physical stress echocardiographic examination with the patient in a left lateral decubital position is ideal [75,102,103], although the results and their interpretation differ slightly between authors. We strongly recommend that—whenever possible—a physical stress test should be performed. Dobutamine stress testing is associated with unpredictable pharmacologic effects that do not really simulate the conditions under which the threshold values for active treatment in patients with mitral valve stenosis were defined within the guidelines.

A typical stress echocardiographic investigation of a patient with a moderate to severe mitral valve stenosis is shown in Figure 17.3.

Specific conditions in patients with mitral valve stenosis

Some specific conditions should be considered within this chapter on the echocardiographic examination of patients with mitral valve stenosis.

Concomitant mitral insufficiency

If there is a significant concomitant MI, PMBV should not be performed. The recognition and semiquantitative description should follow the international recommendations, which

have also been integrated into the guidelines for heart valve disease [95].

Concomitant aortic valve diseases

Concomitant aortic insufficiency will always shorten the PHT in patients with mitral valve stenosis, and consequently will underscore the severity of the stenosis. A central question is aimed at the progression of aortic insufficiency after treating mitral valve stenosis. This question has been extensively discussed in the literature, and it is generally reported that mild aortic insufficiency present at the time of mitral valve intervention progresses very slowly and rarely necessitates reintervention [104–106]. The rare combination of mitral valve stenosis and severe aortic stenosis should be diagnosed separately, and indications for operation should be observed for each single valve lesion.

Pregnancy

As blood volume is significantly increased during a normal pregnancy, and this is associated with a corresponding increase in cardiac output with an additional increase in heart rate in the range 10–20 beats/min, the hemodynamic conditions for a given degree of mitral valve stenosis are dramatically worsened. This development peaks at 20–24 weeks of gestation, and it is reversed only 6 weeks after delivery [107]. One should always be aware of this physiologic situation in an asymptomatic nonpregnant young woman who presents with only moderate mitral valve stenosis. There are a number of reports of how to treat symptomatic pregnant women, and PMBV has been reported to give excellent results for maternal and fetal outcome, provided the preinterventional status is better than a NYHA III classification [107–110]. Interestingly, PMBV has been reported to be performed without any radiation under either complete TTE guidance [111,112] or, in an exceptional case, under the guidance of intracardiac echocardiography [113].

Guidance of percutaneous mitral balloon valvulotomy

Currently, in most institutions, PMBV is performed in the catheterization laboratory. The whole procedure is generally guided by 2-D TTE, and is particularly helpful in controlling the puncture site of the interatrial septum, and the position of the balloon inside the valve before inflating, and for the analysis of the final procedural results. A TEE investigation is necessary only if TTE image quality is unacceptable [114]. The use of intracardiac echocardiography (ICE) has been reported to be an attractive alternative, as the image quality is excellent and any sedation necessary for TEE can be avoided [115]. Intracardiac echocardiographic catheters are expensive and can be reused only a few times, and, with the available 2-D approach, the intracardiac orientation is worse than with a parallel investigation with TEE [116]. The application of transthoracic 3-D technology for guidance of PMBV has been

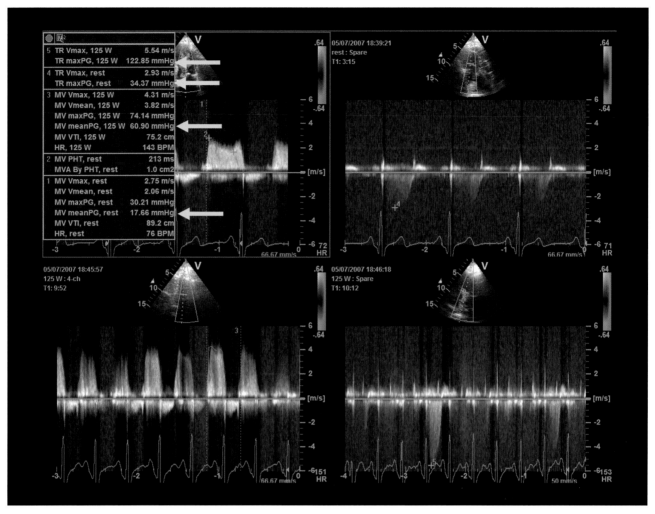

Figure 17.3 Standard Doppler measurements in a patient with a moderate to severe mitral valve stenosis under resting (two upper spectra) and under stress conditions of 125-W bicycle stress (lower row). On the left side the continuous wave spectra from the mitral valve inflow are seen, and on the right side the corresponding spectra from the tricuspid insufficiency is seen. Using the simplified Bernoulli equation, it can be read from the summary report of the echocardiographic system that the mean pressure drop increased from 17 to 61 mmHg, and the systolic pulmonary artery pressure increased from 34 to 123 mmHg. The measurement of the MVA by the PHT method is useful only under resting conditions (1.0 cm²). The relevant measurement values are indicated by the arrows. HR, heart rate; MV, mitral valve; TR, tricuspid insufflation.

reported to be even more effective than that of 2-D echocardiography, with both approaches (TEE or TTE) [52]. Until now, it has not been clear if the 3-D concept, in general, will partly or completely replace the 2-D concept. The handling of the 3-D software for adjusting the imaging projections and the image quality itself are still arguments for keeping 2-D echocardiography as standard.

Since the first description of echocardiography guidance of PMBV, it has become known that the application of the PHT method is not useful for assessing the morphologic and hemodynamic results of the procedure [76,117–119]. It has been explained extensively by several authors that this is due to the diastolic properties of the left ventricle and the net chamber compliance, which are substantially changed during PMBV. If possible, parasternal planimetry should be used instead. In addition to the determination of the widened MVA, the major goals of the postprocedural echocardiographic control are to review the morphologic changes induced by the valvulotomy and to detect and categorize a new or increased mitral insufficiency.

A typical image of an apical long-axis investigation during PMBV is shown in Figure 17.4.

Follow-up investigations

The time interval between two subsequent investigations for detecting possible changes in patients with mitral valve stenosis should depend on the expected natural course of the untreated disease or the expected changes after PMBV and MVR, respectively. In individual patients, the rate of mitral valve narrowing is variable and cannot be predicted by the initial

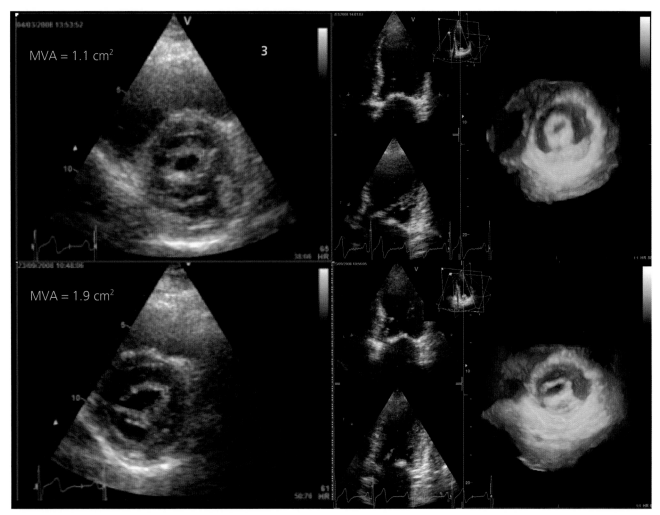

Figure 17.4 Pre- and postinterventional two-dimensional and transthoracic three-dimensional aspects of a mitral valve stenosis. On the left side, the planimetry is shown before and after valvuloplasty, a significant increase from 1.1 to 1.9 cm^2 is documented. On the right side, surface-rendered three-dimensional images qualitatively show that both commissures have been significantly dilated.

analysis. Right heart disease can progress independently from mitral valve narrowing [13]. For all patient groups with moderate to severe forms of mitral valve stenosis, we propose a 6- to 12-month interval between standard examinations. In larger series of follow-up investigations a trend is reported that, in patients with milder forms of mitral valve stenosis and in those with concomitant aortic insufficiency, a faster increase in the severity of the disease is detected [13,14]. The first episode of atrial fibrillation is normally combined with some degree of clinical deterioration and will directly lead to an echocardiographic reinvestigation.

Several follow-up series of patients after valvulotomy have been published, mainly with the aim of finding out parameters that predict the individual postinterventional prognosis [44,120,121]. In general, prognosis is shown to be reduced in patients older than 55 years of age [5] with low flow, low gradient, and low ejection fraction, and severe mitral valve stenosis [121]. Significant restenosis should always be ruled out, but it may be observed, specifically in patients with a significant postinterventional mitral insufficiency [122]. Our own experience with younger symptomatic patients treated with PMBV corresponds to the early reports in literature of a progressive improvement in pulmonary vascular resistance, even several months after the intervention [123].

References

1. Edler I (1955) The diagnostic use of ultrasound in heart disease. *Med Scand* **308**(Suppl.): 32.
2. Bonow R, Carabello B, Kanu C, *et al.* (2006) ACC/AHA 2006 guidelines for the management of patients with valvular heart disease: a report of the American College of Cardiology/American Heart Association Task Force on Practice Guidelines (writing committee to revise the 1998 Guidelines for the Management of Patients With Valvular Heart Disease): developed in

collaboration with the Society of Cardiovascular Anesthesiologists: endorsed by the Society for Cardiovascular Angiography and Interventions and the Society of Thoracic Surgeons. *Circulation* **114**:e84–231.

3. Vahanian A, Baumgartner H, Bax J, *et al.* (2007) Guidelines on the management of valvular heart disease: The Task Force on the Management of Valvular Heart Disease of the European Society of Cardiology. *Eur Heart J* **28**:230–268.

4. Hugenholtz PG, Ryan TJ, Stein SW, & Belmann WH (1962) The spectrum of pure mitral stenosis: hemodynamic studies in relation to clinical disability. *Am J Cardiol* **10**:773–784.

5. Shaw TR, Sutaria N, & Prendergast B (2003) Clinical and haemodynamic profiles of young, middle aged, and elderly patients with mitral stenosis undergoing mitral balloon valvotomy. *Heart* **89**:1430–1436.

6. Selzer A & Cohn KE (1972) Natural history of mitral stenosis: a review. *Circulation* **45**:878–890.

7. Bahl V, Chandra S, Talwar K, Kaul U, Sharma S, & Wasir H (1995) Balloon mitral valvotomy in patients with systemic and suprasystemic pulmonary artery pressures. *Cathet Cardiovasc Diagn* **36**:211–215.

8. Friedensohn A, Stryjer D, & Schlesinger Z (1983) Myocardial ischemia in mitral stenosis with normal coronary arteries. *Heart Lung* **12**:653–655.

9. Carroll JD & Feldman T (1993) Percutaneous mitral balloon valvotomy and the new demographics of mitral stenosis. *JAMA* **270**:1731–1736.

10. Otto C & Bonow R (2008) Valvular heart disease–mitral stenosis. In: Libby P, Bonow R, Mann D, & Zipes D (eds). *Braunwald's Heart Disease*, 8th edn. Philadelphia: Saunders Elsevier, pp. 1646–1656.

11. Rich S & McLaughlin V (2008) Pulmonary hypertension. In: Libby P, Bonow R, Mann D, & Zipes D (eds). *Braunwald's Heart Disease*, 8th edn. Philadelphia: Saunders Elsevier, p. 1903.

12. Jebavy P, Hurych J, & Widimsky J (1978) Influence of pulmonary hypertension on pulmonary diffusing capacity in patients with mitral stenosis. *Respiration* **35**:1–7.

13. Sagie A, Freitas N, Padial L, *et al.* (1996) Doppler echocardiographic assessment of long-term progression of mitral stenosis in 103 patients: valve area and right heart disease. *J Am Coll Cardiol* **28**:472–479.

14. Gordon SP, Douglas PS, Come PC, & Manning WJ (1992) Two-dimensional and Doppler echocardiographic determinants of the natural history of mitral valve narrowing in patients with rheumatic mitral stenosis: implications for follow-up. *J Am Coll Cardiol* **19**:968–973.

15. Iung B, Baron G, Butchart E, *et al.* (2003) A prospective survey of patients with valvular heart disease in Europe: The Euro Heart Survey on Valvular Heart Disease. *Eur Heart J* **24**:1231–1243.

16. Voelker W (2004) [A structured report data set for documentation of echocardiographic studies—Update (2004)]. *Z Kardiol* **93**:987–1004.

17. Evangelista A, Flachskampf F, Lancellotti P, *et al.* (2008) European Association of Echocardiography recommendations for standardization of performance, digital storage and reporting of echocardiographic studies. *Eur J Echocardiogr* **9**:438–448.

18. Lang R, Bierig M, Devereux R, *et al.* (2006) Recommendations for chamber quantification. *Eur J Echocardiogr* **7**:79–108.

19. Sanchez P, Rodriguez-Alemparte M, Inglessis I, & Palacios I (2005) The impact of age in the immediate and long-term outcomes of percutaneous mitral balloon valvuloplasty. *J Interv Cardiol* **18**:217–225.

20. Ramondo A, Napodano M, Fraccaro C, Razzolini R, Tarantini G, & Iliceto S (2006) Relation of patient age to outcome of percutaneous mitral valvuloplasty. *Am J Cardiol* **98**:1493–1500.

21. Iung B & Vahanian A (2002) The long-term outcome of balloon valvuloplasty for mitral stenosis. *Curr Cardiol Rep* **4**:118–124.

22. Kasner M, Westermann D, Steendijk P, *et al.* (2007) Utility of Doppler echocardiography and tissue Doppler imaging in the estimation of diastolic function in heart failure with normal ejection fraction: a comparative Doppler-conductance catheterization study. *Circulation* **116**:637–647.

23. Surdacki A, Legutko J, Turek P, Dudek D, Zmudka K, & Dubiel J (1996) Determinants of depressed left ventricular ejection fraction in pure mitral stenosis with preserved sinus rhythm. *J Heart Valve Dis* **5**:1–9.

24. Bargiggia GS, Tronconi L, Sahn DJ, *et al.* (1991) A new method for quantitation of mitral regurgitation based on color flow Doppler imaging of flow convergence proximal to regurgitant orifice. *Circulation* **84**:1481–1489.

25. Skjaerpe T, Hegrenaes L, & Hatle L (1985) Noninvasive estimation of valve area in patients with aortic stenosis by Doppler ultrasound and two-dimensional echocardiography. *Circulation* **72**:810–818.

26. Rodriguez L, Thomas JD, Monterroso V, *et al.* (1993) Validation of the proximal flow convergence method. Calculation of orifice area in patients with mitral stenosis. *Circulation* **88**:1157–1165.

27. Sengupta P, Mohan J, Mehta V, *et al.* (2004) Effects of percutaneous mitral commissurotomy on longitudinal left ventricular dynamics in mitral stenosis: quantitative assessment by tissue velocity imaging. *J Am Soc Echocardiogr* **17**:824–818.

28. Ozdemir K, Altunkeser B, Gok H, Icli A, & Temizhan A (2002) Analysis of the myocardial velocities in patients with mitral stenosis. *J Am Soc Echocardiogr* **15**:1472–1478.

29. Dogan S, Aydin M, Gursurer M, Dursun A, Onuk T, & Madak H (2006) Prediction of subclinical left ventricular dysfunction with strain rate imaging in patients with mild to moderate rheumatic mitral stenosis. *J Am Soc Echocardiogr* **19**:243–248.

30. Berger M (2004) Natural history of mitral stenosis and echocardiographic criteria and pitfalls in selecting patients for balloon valvuloplasty. *Adv Cardiol* **41**:87–94.

31. Silaruks S, Thinkhamrop B, Tantikosum W, Wongvipaporn C, Tatsanavivat P, & Klungboonkrong V (2002) A prognostic model for predicting the disappearance of left atrial thrombi among candidates for percutaneous transvenous mitral commissurotomy. *J Am Coll Cardiol* **39**:886–891.

32. Flachskampf FA, Decoodt P, Fraser AG, Daniel WG, & Roelandt JR (2001) Guidelines from the Working Group. Recommendations for performing transesophageal echocardiography. *Eur J Echocardiogr* **2**:8–21.

33. Topsakal R, Eryol N, Ozdogru I, *et al.* (2004) Color Doppler tissue imaging to evaluate left atrial appendage function in patients with mitral stenosis in sinus rhythm. *Echocardiography* **21**:235–240.

34. Karakaya O, Turkmen M, Bitigen A, *et al.* (2006) Effect of percutaneous mitral balloon valvuloplasty on left atrial appendage function: a Doppler tissue study. *J Am Soc Echocardiogr* **19**:434–437.

35. Gurlertop Y, Yilmaz M, Acikel M, *et al.* (2004) Tissue Doppler properties of the left atrial appendage in patients with mitral valve disease. *Echocardiography* **21**:319–324.

36. Cayly M, Kanadasi M, Demir M, & Acarturk E (2006) Mitral annular systolic velocity reflects the left atrial appendage function in mitral stenosis. *Echocardiography* **23**:546–552.

37. Bauer F, Verdonck A, Schuster I, *et al.* (2005) Left atrial appendage function analyzed by tissue Doppler imaging in mitral stenosis: effect of afterload reduction after mitral valve commissurotomy. *J Am Soc Echocardiogr* **18**:934–939.

38. Cayli M, Acarturk E, Kanadasi M, & Demir M (2007) Annular systolic velocity predicts the presence of spontaneous echo contrast in mitral stenosis patients with sinus rhythm. *Clin Cardiol* **30**:459–463.

39. Sosland R, Vacek J, & Gorton M (2007) Congenital mitral stenosis: a rare presentation and novel approach to management. *J Thorac Cardiovasc Surg* **133**:572–573.

40. Chu J, Levine R, Chua S, *et al.* (2008) Assessing mitral valve area and orifice geometry in calcific mitral stenosis: a new solution by real-time three-dimensional echocardiography. *J Am Soc Echocardiogr* **21**:1006–1009.

41. Akram M, Chan T, McAuliffe S, & Chenzbraun A (2009) Non-rheumatic annular mitral stenosis: prevalence and characteristics. *Eur J Echocardiogr* **10**:103–105.

42. Wilkins G, Weyman A, Abascal V, Block P, & Palacios I (1988) Percutaneous balloon dilatation of the mitral valve: an analysis of echocardiographic variables related to outcome and the mechanism of dilatation. *Br Heart J* **60**:299–308.

43. Abascal V, Wilkins G, O'Shea J, *et al.* (1990) Prediction of successful outcome in 130 patients undergoing percutaneous balloon mitral valvotomy. *Circulation* **82**:448–456.

44. Reid C, Chandraratna P, Kawanishi D, Kotlewski A, & Rahimtoola S (1989) Influence of mitral valve morphology on double-balloon catheter balloon valvuloplasty in patients with mitral stenosis. Analysis of factors predicting immediate and 3-month results. *Circulation* **80**:515–524.

45. Turgeman Y, Atar S, Feldman A, *et al.* (2005) "Frozen" posterior mitral leaflet in rheumatic mitral stenosis: incidence and impact on outcome of balloon mitral commissurotomy. *J Heart Valve Dis* **14**:282–285.

46. Fawzy M, Shoukri M, Hassan W, Nambiar V, Stefadouros M, & Canver C (2007) The impact of mitral valve morphology on the long-term outcome of mitral balloon valvuloplasty. *Catheter Cardiovasc Interv* **69**:40–46.

47. Fawzy M, Fadel B, Al-Sergani H, *et al.* (2007) Long-term results (up to 16.5 years) of mitral balloon valvuloplasty in a series of 518 patients and predictors of long-term outcome. *J Interv Cardiol* **20**:66–72.

48. Padial L, Abascal V, Moreno P, Weyman A, Levine R, & Palacios I (1999) Echocardiography can predict the development of severe mitral regurgitation after percutaneous mitral valvuloplasty by the Inoue technique. *Am J Cardiol* **83**:1210–1213.

49. Sutaria N, Shaw T, Prendergast B, & Northridge D (2006) Transoesophageal echocardiographic assessment of mitral valve commissural morphology predicts outcome after balloon mitral valvotomy. *Heart* **92**:52–57.

50. Iung B, Cormier B, Ducimetiere P, *et al.* (1996) Immediate results of percutaneous mitral commissurotomy. A predictive model on a series of 1514 patients. *Circulation* **94**:2124–2130.

51. Perez DIL, Casanova C, Almeria C, *et al.* (2007) Which method should be the reference method to evaluate the severity of rheumatic mitral stenosis? Gorlin's method versus 3D-echo. *Eur J Echocardiogr* **8**:470–473.

52. Zamorano J, Perez dIL, Sugeng L, *et al.* (2004) Non-invasive assessment of mitral valve area during percutaneous balloon mitral valvuloplasty: role of real-time 3D echocardiography. *Eur Heart J* **25**:2086–2091.

53. Valocik G, Kamp O, Mannaerts H, & Visser C (2007) New quantitative three-dimensional echocardiographic indices of mitral valve stenosis: new 3D indices of mitral stenosis. *Int J Cardiovasc Imaging* **23**:707–716.

54. Messika-Zeitoun D, Brochet E, Holmin C, *et al.* (2007) Three-dimensional evaluation of the mitral valve area and commissural opening before and after percutaneous mitral commissurotomy in patients with mitral stenosis. *Eur Heart J* **28**:72–79.

55. Henry W, Griffith J, Michaelis L, McIntosh C, Morrow A, & Epstein S (1975) Measurement of mitral orifice area in patients with mitral valve disease by real-time, two-dimensional echocardiography. *Circulation* **51**:827–831.

56. Hatle L (1984) Noninvasive assessment of valve lesions with Doppler ultrasound. *Herz* **9**:213–221.

57. Faletra F, Pezzano A, Fusco R, *et al.* (1996) Measurement of mitral valve area in mitral stenosis: four echocardiographic methods compared with direct measurement of anatomic orifices. *J Am Coll Cardiol* **28**:1190–1197.

58. Holmin C, Messika-Zeitoun D, Mezalek A, *et al.* (2007) Mitral leaflet separation index: a new method for the evaluation of the severity of mitral stenosis? Usefulness before and after percutaneous mitral commissurotomy. *J Am Soc Echocardiogr* **20**:1119–1124.

59. Hatle L, Angelsen B, & Tromsdal A (1979) Noninvasive assessment of atrioventricular pressure half-time by Doppler ultrasound. *Circulation* **60**:1096–1104.

60. Hatle L (1990) Doppler echocardiographic evaluation of mitral stenosis. *Cardiol Clin* **8**:233–247.

61. Abascal V, Moreno P, Rodriguez L, *et al.* (1996) Comparison of the usefulness of Doppler pressure half-time in mitral stenosis in patients <65 and > or =65 years of age. *Am J Cardiol* **78**:1390–1393.

62. Smith M, Wisenbaugh T, Grayburn P, Gurley J, Spain M, & De MA (1991) Value and limitations of Doppler pressure half-time in quantifying mitral stenosis: a comparison with micromanometer catheter recordings. *Am Heart J* **121**(2 Pt 1):480–488.

63. Moro E, Nicolosi G, Zanuttini D, Cervesato E, & Roelandt J (1988) Influence of aortic regurgitation on the assessment of the pressure half-time and derived mitral-valve area in patients with mitral stenosis. *Eur Heart J* **9**:1010–1017.

64. Flachskampf F, Weyman A, Gillam L, Liu C, Abascal V, & Thomas J (1990) Aortic regurgitation shortens Doppler pressure half-time in mitral stenosis: clinical evidence, in vitro simulation and theoretic analysis. *J Am Coll Cardiol* **16**:396–404.

65. Schwammenthal E, Vered Z, Agranat O, Kaplinsky E, Rabinowitz B, & Feinberg MS (2000) Impact of atrioventricular compliance on pulmonary artery pressure in mitral stenosis: an exercise echocardiographic study. *Circulation* **102**:2378–2384.

66. Flachskampf FA, Weyman AE, Guerrero JL, & Thomas JD (1992) Calculation of atrioventricular compliance from the mitral flow profile: analytic and in vitro study. *J Am Coll Cardiol* **19**:998–1004.

67. Kim H, Kim Y, Hwang S, *et al.* (2008) Hemodynamic and prognostic implications of net atrioventricular compliance in patients with mitral stenosis. *J Am Soc Echocardiogr* **21**:482–486.

68. Bennis A, Drighil A, & Tribouilloy C, Chraibi N (2002) Clinical application in routine practice of the proximal flow convergence method to calculate the mitral surface area in mitral valve stenosis. *Int J Cardiovasc Imaging* **18**:443–451.

69. Sunil RT, Krishnan M, Koshy C, *et al.* (2005) Comparison of proximal isovelocity surface area method and pressure half time method for evaluation of mitral valve area in patients undergoing balloon mitral valvotomy. *Echocardiography* **22**:707–712.

70. Messika-Zeitoun D, Meizels A, Cachier A, *et al.* (2005) Echocardiographic evaluation of the mitral valve area before and after percutaneous mitral commissurotomy: the pressure half-time method revisited. *J Am Soc Echocardiogr* **18**:1409–1414.

71. Lee T, Tseng C, Chiao C, *et al.* (2004) Clinical applicability for the assessment of the valvular mitral stenosis severity with Doppler echocardiography and the proximal isovelocity surface area (PISA) method. *Echocardiography* **21**:1–6.

72. Uzun M & Yokusoglu M (2007) The PISA method simplified. *Eur J Echocardiogr* **8**:1–2; author reply 3.

73. Messika-Zeitoun D, Cachier A, Brochet E, Cormier B, Iung B, & Vahanian A (2007) Evaluation of mitral valve area by the proximal isovelocity surface area method in mitral stenosis: could it be simplified? *Eur J Echocardiogr* **8**:116–121.

74. Dahan M, Paillole C, Martin D, & Gourgon R (1993) Determinants of stroke volume response to exercise in patients with mitral stenosis: a Doppler echocardiographic study. *J Am Coll Cardiol* **21**:384–389.

75. Eren M, Arikan E, Gorgulu S, *et al.* (2002) Relationship between resting parameters of the mitral valve and exercise capacity in patients with mitral stenosis: can the diastolic filling period predict exercise capacity? *J Heart Valve Dis* **11**:191–198.

76. Klarich K, Rihal C, & Nishimura R (1996) Variability between methods of calculating mitral valve area: simultaneous Doppler echocardiographic and cardiac catheterization studies conducted before and after percutaneous mitral valvuloplasty. *J Am Soc Echocardiogr* **9**:684–690.

77. Mohan J, Chawla R, & Arora R (1996) Methodological variation and agreement in assessing mitral valve orifice area by echo-Doppler methods in mitral stenosis. *Indian Heart J* **48**:653–657.

78. Nakatani S, Masuyama T, Kodama K, Kitabatake A, Fujii K, & Kamada T (1988) Value and limitations of Doppler echocardiography in the quantification of stenotic mitral valve area: comparison of the pressure half-time and the continuity equation methods. *Circulation* **77**:78–85.

79. Voelker W, Berner A, Regele B, *et al.* (1993) Effect of exercise on valvular resistance in patients with mitral stenosis. *J Am Coll Cardiol* **22**:777–782.

80. Binder T, Rosenhek R, Porenta G, Maurer G, & Baumgartner H (2000) Improved assessment of mitral valve stenosis by volumetric real-time three-dimensional echocardiography. *J Am Coll Cardiol* **36**:1355–1361.

81. Langerveld J, Valocik G, Plokker H, *et al.* (2003) Additional value of three-dimensional transesophageal echocardiography for patients with mitral valve stenosis undergoing balloon valvuloplasty. *J Am Soc Echocardiogr* **16**:841–849.

82. Singh V, Nanda N, Agrawal G, *et al.* (2003) Live three-dimensional echocardiographic assessment of mitral stenosis. *Echocardiography* **20**:743–750.

83. Zamorano J, Cordeiro P, Sugeng L, *et al.* (2004) Real-time three-dimensional echocardiography for rheumatic mitral valve stenosis evaluation: an accurate and novel approach. *J Am Coll Cardiol* **43**:2091–2096.

84. Sebag I, Morgan J, Handschumacher M, *et al.* (2005) Usefulness of three-dimensionally guided assessment of mitral stenosis using matrix-array ultrasound. *Am J Cardiol* **96**:1151–1156.

85. de Agustin J, Nanda N, Gill E, de IL, & Zamorano J (2007) The use of three-dimensional echocardiography for the evaluation of and treatment of mitral stenosis. *Cardiol Clin* **25**:311–318.

86. Poutanen T, Tikanoja T, Sairanen H, & Jokinen E (2006) Normal mitral and aortic valve areas assessed by three- and two-dimensional echocardiography in 168 children and young adults. *Pediatr Cardiol* **27**:217–225.

87. Flachskampf F & Klinghammer L (2008) Determination of stenotic mitral valve area: new, old, and gold standards. *Eur J Echocardiogr* **9**:321.

88. Nishimura R, Rihal C, Tajik A, & Holmes D (1994) Accurate measurement of the transmitral gradient in patients with mitral stenosis: a simultaneous catheterization and Doppler echocardiographic study. *J Am Coll Cardiol* **24**:152–158.

89. David D, Lang R, Marcus R, *et al.* (1991) Doppler echocardiographic estimation of transmitral pressure gradients and correlations with micromanometer gradients in mitral stenosis. *Am J Cardiol* **67**:1161–1164.

90. Izgi C, Ozdemir N, Cevik C, *et al.* (2007) Mitral valve resistance as a determinant of resting and stress pulmonary artery pressure in patients with mitral stenosis: a dobutamine stress study. *J Am Soc Echocardiogr* **20**:1160–1166.

91. Lee KS, Abbas AE, Khandheria BK, & Lester SJ (2007) Echocardiographic assessment of right heart hemodynamic parameters. *J Am Soc Echocardiogr* **20**:773–782.

92. Skjaerpe T & Hatle L (1986) Noninvasive estimation of systolic pressure in the right ventricle in patients with tricuspid regurgitation. *Eur Heart J* **7**:704–710.

93. Hatle L (1984) Maximal blood flow velocities—haemodynamic data obtained noninvasively with CW Doppler. *Ultrasound Med Biol* **10**:225–237.

94. Lindqvist P, Calcutteea A, & Henein M (2008) Echocardiography in the assessment of right heart function. *Eur J Echocardiogr* **9**:225–234.

95. Zoghbi WA, Enriquez-Sarano M, Foster E, *et al.* (2003) Recommendations for evaluation of the severity of native valvular regurgitation with two-dimensional and Doppler echocardiography. *J Am Soc Echocardiogr* **16**:777–802.

96. Samad BA, Alam M, & Jensen-Urstad K (2002) Prognostic impact of right ventricular involvement as assessed by tricuspid annular motion in patients with acute myocardial infarction. *Am J Cardiol* **90**:778–781.

97. Kjaergaard J, Petersen C, Kjaer A, Schaadt B, Oh J, & Hassager C (2006) Evaluation of right ventricular volume and function by 2D and 3D echocardiography compared to MRI. *Eur J Echocardiogr* **7**:430–438.

98. Wang A, Krasuski R, Warner J, *et al.* (2002) Serial echocardiographic evaluation of restenosis after successful percutaneous mitral commissurotomy. *J Am Coll Cardiol* **39**:328–334.

99. Lamia B, Teboul J, Monnet X, Richard C, & Chemla D (2007) Relationship between the tricuspid annular plane systolic excursion and right and left ventricular function in critically ill patients. *Intensive Care Med* **33**:2143–2149.

100. Meluzin J, Spinarova L, Hude P, *et al.* (2005) Prognostic importance of various echocardiographic right ventricular functional parameters in patients with symptomatic heart failure. *J Am Soc Echocardiogr* **18**:435–444.

101. Lanzarini L, Fontana A, Campana C, & Klersy C (2005) Two simple echo-Doppler measurements can accurately identify pulmonary hypertension in the large majority of patients with chronic heart failure. *J Heart Lung Transplant* **24**:745–754.

102. Rayburn B & Fortuin N (1996) Severely symptomatic mitral stenosis with a low gradient: a case for low-technology medicine. *Am Heart J* **132**:628–632.

103. Lev E, Sagie A, Vaturi M, Sela N, Battler A, & Shapira Y (2004) Value of exercise echocardiography in rheumatic mitral stenosis with and without significant mitral regurgitation. *Am J Cardiol* **93**:1060–1063.

104. Choudhary S, Talwar S, Juneja R, & Kumar A (2001) Fate of mild aortic valve disease after mitral valve intervention. *J Thorac Cardiovasc Surg* **122**:583–586.

105. Chen C, Cheng T, Chen J, Zhou Y, Mei J, & Ma T (1993) Percutaneous balloon mitral valvuloplasty for mitral stenosis with and without associated aortic regurgitation. *Am Heart J* **125**:128–137.

106. Sanchez-Ledesma M, Cruz-Gonzalez I, Sanchez P, *et al.* (2008) Impact of concomitant aortic regurgitation on percutaneous mitral valvuloplasty: immediate results, short-term, and long-term outcome. *Am Heart J* **156**:361–366.

107. Reimold S & Rutherford J (2003) Clinical practice. Valvular heart disease in pregnancy. *N Engl J Med* **349**:52–59.

108. Desai D, Adanlawo M, Naidoo D, Moodley J, & Kleinschmidt I (2000) Mitral stenosis in pregnancy: a four-year experience at King Edward VIII Hospital, Durban, South Africa. *BJOG* **107**:953–958.

109. Esteves C, Munoz J, Braga S, *et al.* (2006) Immediate and long-term follow-up of percutaneous balloon mitral valvuloplasty in pregnant patients with rheumatic mitral stenosis. *Am J Cardiol* **98**:812–816.

110. Sivadasanpillai H, Srinivasan A, Sivasubramoniam S, *et al.* (2005) Long-term outcome of patients undergoing balloon mitral valvotomy in pregnancy. *Am J Cardiol* **95**:1504–1506.

111. Chiang C, Hsu L, Chu P, Ho W, Lo H, & Chang C (2003) Feasibility of simplifying balloon mitral valvuloplasty by obviating left-sided cardiac catheterization using on-line guidance with transesophageal echocardiography. *Chest* **123**:1957–1963.

112. Trehan V, Mukhopadhyay S, Nigam A, *et al.* (2005) Mitral valvuloplasty by inoue balloon under transthoracic echocardiographic guidance. *J Am Soc Echocardiogr* **18**:964–969.

113. Yap S, de JP, Ligthart J, Serruys P, & Roos-Hesselink J (2006) Percutaneous triple-valve balloon valvulotomy in a pregnant woman using intracardiac echocardiography: case report. *J Heart Valve Dis* **15**:459–464.

114. Feldman T (2004) Intraprocedure guidance for percutaneous mitral valve interventions: TTE, TEE, ICE, or X-ray? *Catheter Cardiovasc Interv* **63**:395–396.

115. Green N, Hansgen A, & Carroll J (2004) Initial clinical experience with intracardiac echocardiography in guiding balloon mitral valvuloplasty: technique, safety, utility, and limitations. *Catheter Cardiovasc Interv* **63**:385–394.

116. Chiang C, Huang H, & Ko Y (2007) Echocardiography-guided balloon mitral valvotomy: transesophageal echocardiography versus intracardiac echocardiography. *J Heart Valve Dis* **16**:596–601.

117. Thomas J, Wilkins G, Choong C, *et al.* (1988) Inaccuracy of mitral pressure half-time immediately after percutaneous mitral valvotomy. Dependence on transmitral gradient and left atrial and ventricular compliance. *Circulation* **78**:980–993.

118. Reid CL & Rahimtoola SH (1991) The role of echocardiography/Doppler in catheter balloon treatment of adults with aortic and mitral stenosis. *Circulation* **84**(3 Suppl.):I240–249.

119. Abascal VM, Wilkins GT, Choong CY, *et al.* (1988) Echocardiographic evaluation of mitral valve structure and function in patients followed for at least 6 months after percutaneous balloon mitral valvuloplasty. *J Am Coll Cardiol* **12**:606–615.

120. Iung B, Garbarz E, Michaud P, *et al.* (1999) Late results of percutaneous mitral commissurotomy in a series of 1024 patients. Analysis of late clinical deterioration: frequency, anatomic findings, and predictive factors. *Circulation* **99**:3272–3278.

121. Turgeman Y, Atar S, Suleiman K, Bloch L, & Rosenfeld T (2003) Percutaneous balloon mitral valvuloplasty in patients with severe mitral stenosis and low transmitral diastolic pressure gradient. *Int J Cardiovasc Intervent* **5**:200–205.

122. Chmielak Z, Ruzyllo W, Demkow M, *et al.* (2002) Late results of percutaneous balloon mitral commissurotomy in patients with restenosis after surgical commissurotomy compared to patients with "de-novo" stenosis. *J Heart Valve Dis* **11**:509–516.

123. Levine M, Weinstein J, Diver D, *et al.* (1989) Progressive improvement in pulmonary vascular resistance after percutaneous mitral valvuloplasty. *Circulation* **79**:1061–1067.

18   MRI of Mitral Stenosis

Matthias Gutberlet

University Leipzig, Leipzig Heart Center, Leipzig, Germany

Introduction

General requirements for an imaging modality to assess valvular disease are as follows:
- visualization of anatomic structures (valve thickness, number of leaflets, occurrence of calcifications and the presence of endocarditic vegetations);
- assessment of valvular function (gradation of the severity of valvular stenosis and the ability of a sufficient coaptation of the leaflets);
- assessment of the effect of valvular dysfunction on ventricular size, geometry, muscle mass and ventricular function.

Visualization of valve morphology

Echocardiography, and especially transesophageal echocardiography, is still the method of choice for the visualization of mitral valve morphology. Nevertheless, rough valve morphology is usually already assessable with standard electrocardiography (ECG)-gated magnetic resonance (MR) sequences such as "black blood" spin-echo sequences, especially of the atrioventricular valves. Nevertheless, the best imaging sequence with magnetic resonance for the visualization of valve morphology and function is SSFP sequences, which are called true FISP, FIESTA or balanced FFE on scanners from different vendors [1,2].

These sequences allow not only the assessment of valve morphology, but also a functional evaluation, because the movement of the valve can be visualized by so-called cine MRI. Turbulence or increased blood flow could additionally enhance the assessment as a result of signal void caused by spin dephasing at the leaflet edges.

The best visualization of the mitral valve can be achieved in the two-chamber long-axis view, the four-chamber view, the left ventricular outflow tract (LVOT) view (Fig. 18.1a and b), and in short-axis slices parallel to the orientation of the

Cardiovascular Interventions in Clinical Practice. Edited by Jürgen Haase, Hans-Joachim Schäfers, Horst Sievert and Ron Waksman. © 2010 Blackwell Publishing.

atrioventricular valve itself (Fig. 18.1c and d). Owing to the in-plane motion of the valve itself, a stack of several parallel slices should be acquired to cover the mitral valve during the whole cardiac cycle, and to ensure that the maximal orifice area during diastole can be planimetered (Fig. 18.1a) sufficiently.

Assessment of ventricular function

Cine MRI using SSFP sequences is the gold standard for the noninvasive assessment of left and especially right ventricular volumes, muscle mass, and function. As a result, biventricular stroke volumes and ejection fraction can be calculated simultaneously. As a consequence of mitral stenosis, left atrial enlargement, pulmonary congestion, right ventricular dysfunction, and pulmonary valve incompetence occur, which can be easily assessed using MRI.

Flow measurements

Cine MRI, especially when using simple gradient-echo sequences (GREs) allows for a qualitative assessment of valvular stenosis owing to a signal void due to dephasing as a result of increased blood velocity or turbulences caused by a stenosis (Fig. 18.1a and b). These sequences can be used only to detect an area of a stenosis, but not for quantitation because the amount of dephasing depends not only on the peak velocity, but also on the echo time of the sequence and is therefore very variable [3]. Shorter echo times lead to a more pronounced signal void, whereas sequences with a longer echo time, especially high-grade stenosis, produce only a low signal void. Furthermore, signal loss is less marked on the usually used SSFP sequences.

A similar approach to Doppler echocardiography, in which the semiquantitative description of the length and width of a jet can be used to assess the severity of a valvular incompetence, is therefore not possible. To quantify the degree of a mitral valve stenosis, measurements analogous to Doppler echocardiography flow measurements can be used. Phase velocity mapping is the magnetic resonance technique usually used to quantify blood flow in patients with valvular heart disease. This technique enables the measurement of peak and mean velocity

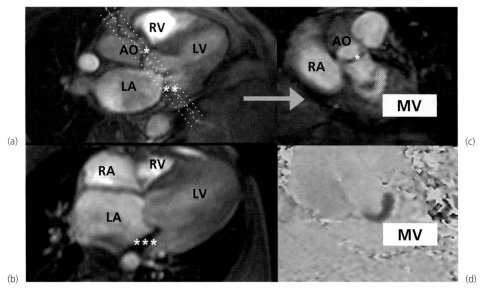

Figure 18.1 (a) Cine MRI gradient-echo sequence in the left ventricular outflow tract (LVOT) view during diastole demonstrates a thickened and calcified aortic valve (*), as well as a thickened and calcified mitral valve with decreased mobility (**) indicated by a "doming" of the mitral valve during diastole. The left atrium (LA) is enlarged. The mitral valve stenosis was graded as a high-grade mitral valve stenosis. Additionally, the lines (------) for the image plane planning for the short-axis views (c, d) are indicated. This acquisition should contain several slices orientated perpendicular to the LVOT and/or four-chamber view acquisitions, and orientated parallel to the mitral valve (MV).

(b) The 4-chamber view acquisition during systole with a remarkable flow void below the mitral valve (***) indicating a mitral valve insufficiency. (c) Modulus image of the flow sensitive gradient-echo sequence in short-axis orientation through the mitral valve during diastole demonstrates the severely reduced mitral valve orifice area (red area), which can also be assessed even more easily in the corresponding flow or phase image. The moon-shaped dark area represents in-plane flow through the severely reduced mitral valve orifice area. The signal intensity indicates the increased flow velocity. AO, aorta; LV, left ventricle; RA, right atrium; RV, right ventricle.

over a stenosis as well as the measurement of flow volume. Hemodynamic relevance occurs when the mitral valve orifice area is below 2.5 cm^2 [4]. This causes a diastolic transmitral gradient, which can be assessed by measuring the peak velocity across the mitral valve. Peak velocity measurements over the mitral valve are usually performed in the short-axis view, directly distally of the leaflets (Fig. 18.1c and d).

The flow measurements can be performed in-plane (perpendicular to the mitral valve) or through-plane (parallel to the mitral valve). Through-plane magnetic resonance flow measurements are usually more accurate than in-plane measurements [4]. In general, magnetic resonance flow measurements correlate well with flow measurements obtained using Doppler echocardiography [5]. As with Doppler echocardiography, the expected peak velocity, the so-called "encoded velocity" (V_{enc}), has to be adjusted in advance to avoid aliasing [6]. Like in echocardiography, the resulting flow curves can be used to calculate the mitral pressure half time (PHT). The PHT can be used to make an estimate of the mitral valve area by using the following formula:

$$\text{Valve area (cm}^2) = 220\,\text{PHT (ms)}$$

Measuring the pulmonary vein flow can also be used to evaluate the severity of mitral valve stenosis [7]. In severe mitral valve stenosis, pulmonary vein flow can be reversed. Usually the segmentation of the mitral valve orifice area is performed on the SSFP images parallel to the mitral valve. The modulus or phase images of the flow-sensitive GRE can also be used to measure the valve orifice area (Fig. 18.1c and d). Owing to the high inflow contrast, the edges can usually be visualized with high image quality.

References

1. Sondergaard l, Lindvig K, Hildebrandt P, *et al.* (1993) Valve area and cardiac output in aortic stenosis. *Am Heart J* **127**:1156–1164.
2. Friedrich MG, Schulz-Menger J, Poetsch T, *et al.* (2002) Quantification of valvular aortic stenosis by magnetic resonance imaging. *Am Heart J* **144**:329–334.
3. Kilner PJ, Firmin DN, Rees RSO, *et al.* (1991) Valve and great vessel stenosis: assessment with MR jet velocity mapping. *Radiology* **178**:229–235.
4. Taylor AM & Bogaert J (2005) Valvular Heart Disease. In: Bogaert J, Dymarkowski S, & Taylor AM (eds). *Clinical Cardiac MRI*. Springer Verlag: Berlin, Heidelberg, New York, pp. 353–379.
5. Heidenreich PA, Steffens JC, Fujita N, *et al.* (1995) The evaluation of mitral stenosis with velocity-encoded cine MRI. *Am J Cardiol* **75**:365–369.
6. Gutberlet M, Abdul-Khaliq H, Stobbe H, *et al.* (2001) Einsatz moderner Schnittbildverfahren in der Diagnostik von Herzklappenerkrankungen. *Z Kardiol* **90** (Suppl. 6):2–12.
7. Mohiaddin RH, Amanuma M, Kilner PJ, *et al.* (1991) MR phase-shift velocity mapping of mitral and pulmonary venous flow. *J Comput Assist Tomogr* **15**:237–243.

19   Catheter-based Mitral Valvuloplasty

Prafulla G. Kerkar & Milind S. Phadke

Seth GS Medical College and KEM Hospital, Mumbai, India

Historical background

Mitral stenosis is not only one of the most distressing forms of heart disease, but when advanced resists all treatment by medications. On looking at the contracted mitral orifice in a severe case of this disease the wish unconsciously arises that one could divide the constriction as easily during life as one can after death The risk which such an operation would entail naturally makes one shrink from it [1].

Based on this concept put forth by Lauder Brunton, after initial unsuccessful attempts in the 1920s [2], Harken *et al.* [3] performed the first successful surgical commissurotomy in 1948. The surgical technique evolved from using the finger, to using a knife, to eventually using the Tubb's [4] dilator to split the fused commissures. It was only logical that a cardiac surgeon, Kanji Inoue, was to use the balloon catheter, introduced percutaneously, to perform the first successful catheter-based mitral valvuloplasty (CBMV) in June 1982 [5]. Since then, various catheter-based techniques [6–13] have been used to perform CBMV, which has become established as a procedure of choice for symptomatic, severe, pliable rheumatic mitral stenosis.

Morphology and pathophysiology

Rheumatic involvement is overwhelmingly the most common cause of mitral stenosis, and the mitral valve is most often involved in rheumatic heart disease [14]. Mitral stenosis occurs as a progressive delayed sequel of mitral valvulitis as a result of acute rheumatic fever. The normal mitral valve area (MVA) is 4–6 cm². In severe mitral stenosis (MVA $\leq 1.0\,cm^2$), there is thickening of the cusps, fusion of the commissures, and shortening and fusion of the chordae tendineae [15]. In more advanced forms, there may be calcification of the leaflets and commissures. These features are well visualized by conventional

two-dimensional (2-D) echocardiography, and can be graded by the Wilkins score [16]. This score includes four variables, each of which is graded on a scale of 0 to 4. The variables include leaflet thickening, leaflet mobility, subvalvular thickening, and extent and severity of calcification. The maximum possible score is 16. The mechanism of increase in the mitral valve area with CBMV is a splitting of one or both commissures, in a manner similar to surgical commissurotomy [17,18]. An additional mechanism may involve fracture of the calcific nodular deposits on the valve [19].

The hemodynamic hallmark of severe mitral stenosis is the presence of a significant diastolic gradient (Fig. 19.1) between the left atrium and the left ventricle. This leads to elevated left atrial pressures and pulmonary venous hypertension. The latter causes most of the symptoms in severe mitral stenosis (dyspnea, orthopnea, paroxysmal nocturnal dyspnea, pulmonary edema, cough, and hemoptysis) and, if unrelieved, can eventually lead to pulmonary arterial hypertension.

Indications

The American College of Cardiology and American Heart Association (ACC/AHA) guidelines suggest that CBMV be performed only by skilled operators at institutions with extensive experience in performing the technique [20]. The European Society of Cardiology (ESC) guidelines (Table 19.1) recommend that intervention should be performed only in patients with clinically significant mitral stenosis (MVA < 1.5 cm² or < 1.7–1.8 cm², particularly in unusually large patients) [21]. Symptomatic patients with favorable valve anatomy should undergo CBMV. Also, CBMV is the procedure of choice in patients who are poor surgical candidates owing to comorbid factors. Indications for patients with unfavorable characteristics are debatable because of the unpredictable results of CBMV in this heterogeneous group. In general, the relative experience of the interventional cardiologist and the cardiac surgeon should be taken into account. For patients with unfavorable characteristics, our policy is to perform a CBMV with the surgical team on standby (especially in younger patients in the hope of postponing valve replacement). Owing to the inherent risks of the procedure (particularly the occurrence of unpredictable mitral

Cardiovascular Interventions in Clinical Practice. Edited by Jürgen Haase, Hans-Joachim Schäfers, Horst Sievert and Ron Waksman. © 2010 Blackwell Publishing.

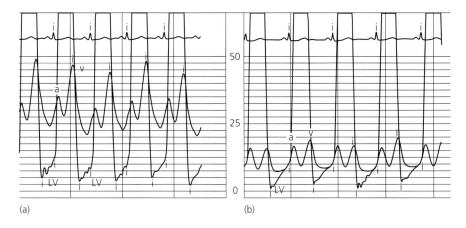

(a)　　　　　　　　　　　　　　(b)

Figure 19.1 Simultaneous pre-CBMV (a) and post-CBMV (b) pressure recordings of the left atrium and left ventricle showing a significant drop in transmitral gradient.

Table 19.1 Indications for percutaneous mitral commissurotomy in patients with a mitral valve area < 1.5 cm² (modified from reference 21, with permission from the publisher).

Indications	Class
Symptomatic patients with favorable characteristics[a] for percutaneous mitral commissurotomy	IB
Symptomatic patients with contraindication or high risk for surgery	IC
As initial treatment in symptomatic patients with unfavorable anatomy but otherwise favorable clinical characteristics[a]	IIaC
Asymptomatic patients with favorable characteristics and high thromboembolic risk or high risk of hemodynamic decompensation	
Previous history of embolism	IIaC
Dense spontaneous contrast in the left atrium	IIaC
Recent or paroxysmal atrial fibrillation	IIaC
Systolic pulmonary pressure greater than 50 mm at rest	IIaC
Need of major noncardiac surgery	IIaC
Desire for pregnancy	IIaC

[a]Favorable characteristics for percutaneous mitral commissurotomy can be defined as absence of several of the following: *clinical characteristics* (old age, history of commissurotomy, NYHA class IV, atrial fibrillation, and severe pulmonary hypertension) and *anatomical characteristics* (echo score >8, Cormier score 3 [calcification of mitral valve of any extent as assessed by fluoroscopy], very small mitral valve area, and severe tricuspid insufficiency).

insufficiency), truly asymptomatic patients are not subjected to CBMV, unless there is evidence of hemodynamic decompensation, increased risk of thromboembolism, or a desire for pregnancy (Table 19.1).

The presence of left atrial thrombus, coexisting moderate (3+) or severe (4+) mitral insufficiency, severe or bicommissural calcification, and concomitant severe aortic valve disease, severe combined tricuspid stenosis and insufficiency, or coronary artery disease requiring surgery are considered

contraindications for CBMV [21]. When the thrombus is located in the left atrial appendage and not in the cavity, and if intervention is not urgent (or if surgery is contraindicated), it is our policy to anticoagulate the patient for a period ranging from 3 to 6 months for complete resolution of the thrombus (documented on transesophageal echocardiography, TEE) after which CBMV can be safely performed. It has been shown that anticoagulation can cause regression of thrombi (especially smaller ones) in a significant proportion of patients [22].

Technique

Preprocedure evaluation

All patients should undergo a detailed clinical, roentgenographic, electrocardiographic, and echocardiographic examination. Valve area is calculated by both planimetry and Doppler PHT methods. Valve suitability is assessed by the Wilkins score [16]. A score of up to 8 is considered ideal for CBMV, although the procedure may be performed in patients with higher scores. In addition, commissural calcification and thickening, being important predictors of postprocedural acute mitral insufficiency, should be specifically looked for [23]. TEE is performed only in patients with atrial fibrillation, in those with recent cerebral symptoms, or in those with suspicion of left atrial thrombus on transthoracic echocardiography (TTE).

Procedure

Access

Right femoral vein access is preferred over access to the left because it is easier to perform the trans-septal puncture (TSP) and subsequent steps by this route. Although the procedure itself is performed through the venous route, an arterial access is additionally taken, primarily for monitoring the intra-arterial pressure, and for positioning a pigtail catheter in the root of the aorta for guidance during the TSP.

Trans-septal puncture

The TSP can be technically challenging, but is one of the most crucial steps in the procedure. An appropriately executed TSP at a precise site is critical not only for the safety of the procedure to avoid cardiac perforation, but also for ensuring easy passage of the balloon across the stenosed mitral valve. The site of puncture on the interatrial septum is located in the small region of the fossa ovalis, which tends to enlarge and become displaced with mitral valve disease. The equipment required consists of a standard Brockenbrough needle, a 7F or 8F Mullins sheath and a dilator. Although biplane fluoroscopy could be advantageous for a TSP, single plane fluoroscopy is sufficient for most skilled operators. We perform the TSP using the anteroposterior and lateral views, although others have suggested additional and alternative fluoroscopic angulations [24–28].

Landmarks for the puncture site

The target puncture site is usually located at the intersection of a horizontal line crossing the center of the mitral annulus (M-line) and a vertical line assumed to divide the interatrial septum into anterior and posterior halves [28]. However, this is only an approximation, and the site often has to be appropriately modified in individual cases according to the morphology. In patients in whom the left atrium is large, the puncture site is often lower than usual, whereas in those with small left atria or with associated aortic valve disease, a higher site is preferred.

The horizontal and vertical lines were initially described by Inoue using recirculation right atrial angiography [29]. However, the *angiographic* method is usually reserved only for difficult circumstances, such as patients with kyphoscoliosis or when the atrial silhouettes are not well visualized. In the more commonly utilized *fluoroscopic* method, a pigtail catheter is positioned in the noncoronary sinus of Valsalva, touching the aortic valve, which is taken to be the anterior septal limit in the frontal view [28]. The medial left atrial silhouette, usually very well discernible in mitral stenosis, is considered to be the posterior septal limit. The vertical line bisects the anterior and posterior septal limits so determined. The horizontal line, passing through the center of the mitral annulus, is ideally determined from a diastolic freeze frame of the left ventriculogram [28]. However, for practical purposes, we assume it to be about half a vertebral body to one vertebral body lower than the pigtail tip.

Technique of trans-septal puncture

The right femoral vein is punctured and a 0.032-inch guidewire is positioned in the mid-portion of the superior vena cava (SVC). The groin puncture site is well dilated to create a friction-free passage for the trans-septal catheter to facilitate tactile–visual perception of the left atrial pulsations before TSP. The Mullins trans-septal introducer set is then advanced to the SVC and the guidewire removed. The dilator is aspirated, flushed, and made air free. While continuously flushing, the Brockenbrough needle is advanced through the dilator under fluoroscopic guidance, allowing it to freely rotate within the dilator. If resistance is encountered, the needle is withdrawn and gently rotated to look anteriorly, or the assembly may be advanced as a whole. The needle is then attached by a 6-inch flexible connecting tube to a bivalve to enable continuous pressure monitoring and contrast injection. At all times, care should be taken to keep the unit air free. Moreover, it is important to ensure that the sharp tip of this needle remains 2–3 mm inside the tip of the dilator. For this, the index finger could be made into a "stopcock" by placing it at all times between the hub of the dilator and the metallic arrow of the needle [27]. High-resolution fluoroscopy is essential to visualize the tip of the needle and the tip of the dilator. Under anteroposterior fluoroscopy guidance and right atrial pressure monitoring, the entire assembly is withdrawn gradually. During this initial descent from the SVC to the right atrium, the needle is oriented at 3 o'clock and then rotated clockwise from 3 o'clock to 4 o'clock to 5 or 6 o'clock during subsequent withdrawal. Three leftward deflections of the unit are noted during descent—the first as the catheter enters the right atrium, the second gradual one over the ascending aortic bulge, and the third deflection as the catheter tip clears the limbic ledge and engages the fossa ovalis [24]. Catheter tip position is then checked in the lateral fluoroscopic view. Before TSP, the catheter tip is pointed upwards and slightly posteriorly.

To confirm the site of puncture, a number of methods are suggested. The most reliable one is to tent the expected site of the fossa ovalis with the assembly and feel for the transmitted left atrial pulsations. If there is any doubt about the site, the septal flush or stain method is used [27]. In the *septal flush* technique the needle is disengaged from the fossa by pointing it slightly anteriorly, and contrast is flushed continuously in the cavity to outline the right atrial margin of the septum (Fig. 19.2a). In the *septal stain* method, originally described by Mullins [30] as the "tag", about 0.5 mL of undiluted contrast is injected against resistance after intentionally engaging the septum (Fig. 19.2b). The septal flush and septal stain proceeds in the lateral projection, which serves to confirm the appropriate posterior direction of the needle–catheter assembly [28]. Viewed in the lateral projection, the upper part of the septum is vertical (Fig. 19.2b) and the lower part is more or less horizontal (Fig. 19.2a), depending on left atrial enlargement. It is best to avoid TSP in the upper vertical part of the septum because (1) the engagement of the septum is difficult here as the catheter–needle assembly tends to slide upwards (Fig. 19.2b) and (2) there is a risk of dissection of the septum. Once the site is identified, after engaging the septum or tenting it with the dilator, the needle is advanced out of the dilator and a "popping" sensation is usually experienced as the needle enters the left atrium. Left atrial entry is confirmed by the pressure recording, contrast injection, or oximetry of the left atrial blood. Further steps are undertaken *only* after confirming left atrial entry.

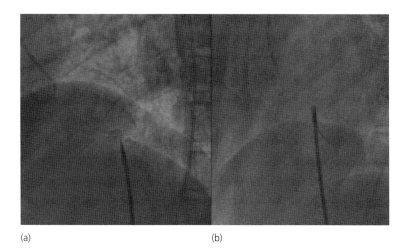

(a)   (b)

Figure 19.2 Lateral fluoroscopic view showing the septal flush and septal stain methods. (a) The needle is disengaged from the septum and undiluted contrast is injected into the right atrial cavity to outline the interatrial septum (in this instance the lower horizontal part). In the septal stain method (b), undiluted contrast agent is injected against resistance after engaging the septum. The needle has slid up to stain the upper vertical part of the septum.

The needle and the trans-septal set are then advanced together as a unit, and a second "give" is often appreciated as the dilator traverses the septum. After advancing the dilator a short distance into the left atrium, the needle and the assembly are rotated anteriorly to the 3 o'clock position—to avoid any posterior left atrial wall puncture, and also because there is more space anteriorly. The needle is simultaneously withdrawn into the dilator. After stepping on the needle and the dilator, the Mullins sheath is then advanced about 4–5 cm into the left atrium. Since the radiopacity of the Mullins sheath is suboptimal [31], the degree of advancement of the tip of the sheath over the dilator can be made out from the scale (in centimeters) at the proximal end of the dilator. Resistance is often encountered at the septum during advancement of the sheath over the dilator, and it is imperative that the operator does not let go of the needle and the dilator during this step, to prevent inadvertent left atrial perforation with the needle or the dilator. The dilator and needle are then removed. The sheath is allowed to back bleed and to be flushed, and the left atrial pressure is recorded. The patient receives the full dose of heparin 100 units/kg at this stage. The pigtail catheter is advanced into the left ventricle, and the left atrial and ventricular pressures are recorded simultaneously to assess the transmitral gradient. For the Inoue technique, the Mullins sheath can be dispensed with, and only the dilator and the needle are used for the TSP.

Choosing an optimal puncture site is a matter of judgment and experience. Care must be taken not to puncture the septum medial to the "midline", as the needle can injure important structures such as the aorta, tricuspid valve, and the coronary sinus [28]. Also, such medial punctures would be too close to the mitral valve, making crossing of the mitral valve with the bulky balloons more difficult. Owing to distorted anatomy of the fossa, the septum, and the atria in diseased states, the puncture site may not always be on the fossa ovalis. In general, the sites that are posterior and more lateral (as seen in the anteroposterior fluoroscopy) are more suitable for easy access to the stenotic mitral valve with the balloon. Lower puncture sites are preferred for the double-balloon technique and higher

ones for the Inoue technique [24]. Although a posterior low puncture is desirable for easy access to the mitral valve, it is fraught with the risk of an "atrial stitch" (accidental entry into the left atrium extrapericardially without traversing the septum) causing cardiac tamponade [27,32]. With a low anterior puncture close to the mitral valve, it may be extremely difficult to enter the mitral valve. In such instances the reverse "loop" technique can be used [33].

Because of the expanding indications of TSP, there has been a resurgence of interest in the development of technology that can make the procedure easier and safer [34]. These technologies include better imaging of the fossa ovalis with intracardiac echocardiography [35–37], three-dimensional (3-D) echocardiography, special infrared-emitting catheters [34] and the use of radiofrequency [38] or excimer laser energy [39] for safer TSP.

Techniques of catheter-based mitral valvuloplasty

The retrograde or transarterial route or the transvenous or antegrade route [40] can be used to perform CBMV.

The advantage of the retrograde or transarterial route—with or without trans-septal catheterization [8,9]—is that it minimizes or even eliminates the possible hazards associated with a trans-septal puncture. However, there remains the risk of potential peripheral arterial damage as a result of the bulky balloons. The retrograde non-trans-septal technique obviates the need for trans-septal catheterization, but can often be technically more demanding. Moreover, it carries the risk of potential damage to the subvalvular mitral valve apparatus and pulmonary vein perforation. The retrograde route is therefore not widely used. Nonetheless, it may sometimes be the only feasible alternative in patients with venous obstruction [41].

The transvenous or antegrade route is the most widely used route [42,43]. It is performed through the femoral vein; rarely, the jugular vein may be used [13]. The transvenous route mandates trans-septal heart catheterization skills. Through this route, balloon dilation of the mitral valve may be performed by an *over-the-wire* technique, utilizing a single

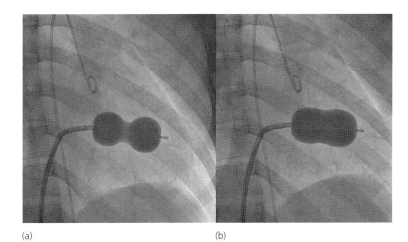

Figure 19.3 The Inoue technique. Partial inflation (a) and full inflation (b) of the Inoue balloon across the mitral valve in right anterior oblique (30°) projection.

(a)   (b)

large balloon over one wire (single balloon technique) [6], two balloons over a single wire (multitrack technique) [11], or two balloons over two wires (the double balloon technique, DBT) [7]. In the Inoue technique [5], a single rubber balloon is used *without a wire* across the mitral valve. Instead of the balloon, a metallic commissurotomy can also be used [12] by the transvenous route. The two main balloon dilation methods are the Inoue technique and the DBT described below.

Inoue technique of catheter-based mitral valvuloplasty

The first CBMV was performed by the Inoue technique [5], which is currently the most widely used method. The Inoue balloon, a most ingeniously designed device, is made of nylon and rubber micromesh and is self-positioning and pressure expandable [43]. It has three parts with a sequential inflation profile, and is available in sizes from 20 to 30 mm.

After gaining left atrial access, the spring guidewire is passed into the left atrium. Over this wire the 14F dilator is advanced to dilate the groin as well as the TSP site. The slenderized balloon catheter is then passed into the left atrium and the spring guidewire is removed along with the stainless-steel slenderizer. The central port of the balloon is flushed and 1–2 mL of diluted contrast is injected into the balloon port to make the balloon into a flotation catheter. The J-shaped stylet is then passed into the balloon and rotated counterclockwise to make the balloon coaxial with the mitral valve (appreciated by the to and fro bobbing motion of the balloon). Stepping on the stylet, the balloon is floated into the left ventricle during diastole. The diluted contrast is then injected into the balloon port, when the balloon inflates sequentially as a result of its unique design. Initially, the distal half of the balloon inflates when it is pulled back from the apex of the left ventricle on to the constricted mitral valve. The proximal half then inflates so that the balloon's shape now resembles a dumbbell (Fig. 19.3a). Finally, the central waist inflates at full inflation (Fig. 19.3b). Balloon size is chosen according to the height of the patient as per the Inoue formula—"maximal balloon size

in mm is equal to height in cm divided by 10 plus 10." Thus, the balloon size for a patient with a height of 150 cm would be 25 mm ([150/10)] + 10 = 25). The inflation is generally commenced with a balloon size 4 mm smaller than the maximal permissible balloon diameter, and then increased in increments of 2 mm each based on the drop in mitral valve gradients, appearance of or increase in audible mitral insufficiency, and the bedside echocardiographic findings.

Double-balloon technique

This technique was first introduced by Al Zaibag and coworkers [7] in 1986. After left atrial access with the Mullins sheath, a right coronary catheter or a balloon-tipped catheter is passed into the left ventricle, often with the help of a preshaped hard end of a regular guidewire [10]. Through this, an exchange-length (260 cm) guidewire with a preformed distal loop is placed at the left ventricular apex. The Mullins sheath is then advanced into the left ventricle and the catheter removed, taking care to maintain the position of the guidewire at the left ventricular apex. A second exchange-length guidewire with a preformed distal loop is then placed through the Mullins sheath in the left ventricular apex, following which the sheath is removed. Over one of these two wires, the septum is dilated with a 6–8 mm peripheral angioplasty balloon. The mitral valve is then sequentially dilated with a single balloon followed by two balloons (each balloon 4 cm long and varying between 15 and 20 mm in diameter, as required) (Fig. 19.4).

Comparison of the Inoue and double-balloon techniques

These techniques differ as regards the shape and compliance characteristics of the dilating balloons, and in the ability to perform a stepwise dilation. There are a few randomized studies [44–46] comparing the two techniques. In general, the Inoue technique is less cumbersome, requires shorter procedure and fluoroscopy times (relevant for use with pregnant patients), and needs fewer skilled personnel. Moreover, the Inoue balloon is easier to position and maintain across the mitral valve.

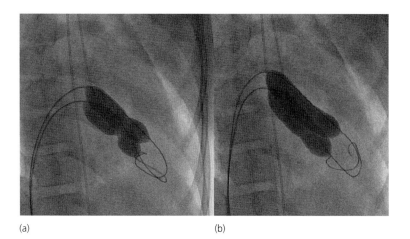

(a)   (b)

Figure 19.4 The double-balloon technique: Two over-the-wire balloons are inflated across the mitral valve in right anterior oblique (30°). (a) Partially inflated balloons with a waist at the site of stenosis. (b) Full inflation with disappearance of the waist.

Although, theoretically, there could be a higher possibility of bicommissural splitting with the DBT (owing to alignment of the two balloons in the elliptical mitral valve orifice), both techniques have been found to be equally efficacious and safe [44]. With the Inoue technique, the risk of left ventricular perforation is almost nonexistent because no guidewires are introduced into this chamber. Moreover, if stepwise dilation is undertaken, the risk of severe mitral insufficiency could be lower [45–50]. The occurrence of atrial level shunts at the puncture site is similar. However, the risk of balloon rupture (and consequent embolism) is lower with the Inoue technique, though not rare [51]. The chief disadvantage of the Inoue balloon is its high cost.

The metallic commissurotome

The metallic commissurotome was first introduced by Cribier and coworkers [12,52]. In this over-the-wire technique, a metallic commissurotome, similar to the Tubb's dilator used by surgeons, is utilized instead of the balloon to dilate the mitral valve. The dilator is reusable and can be screwed onto the distal end of the catheter. The septum is dilated with an 18F dilator and a stiff guidewire is used to track this bulky device. Though the efficacy is similar to the Inoue balloon [53], the probability of left ventricular perforation and tamponade is significantly higher. Moreover, this method is technically demanding and requires more skilled personnel when compared with the Inoue technique. The greatest advantage is the reusability of the metallic head, and therefore a potential for cost savings [54,55]—often an important consideration in developing countries. In our own unpublished experience, we were able to use a single metallic dilator in over 35 cases. Another advantage of the commissurotomy is that it splits calcified commissures better [55].

Assessment of immediate results in the catheterization laboratory

The immediate results can be assessed in the catheterization laboratory by clinical, hemodynamic and echocardiographic parameters. A decrease in the length of the mid-diastolic murmur of mitral stenosis and the appearance of a new pansystolic murmur of mitral insufficiency on auscultation are reliable clinical clues to the procedural success and occurrence of mitral insufficiency, respectively. Hemodynamically, a decrease in the mean mitral valve gradient and mean left atrial pressure suggests successful CBMV (Fig. 19.1). An increase in the v-wave indicates development of acute mitral insufficiency. Calculation of valve area by hemodynamic measurements is subject to fallacies. Transthoracic echocardiography in the catheterization laboratory is cumbersome. Though used routinely in many centers, we utilize it only (1) in doubtful situations to assess commissural splitting, before resorting to further dilation with a larger balloon size, (2) during a suspected complication, e.g., to rule out hemopericardium as a cause of hypotension, (3) during CBMV in patients with unsuitable morphology, or (4) during CBMV in patients who are pregnant. TEE and intracardiac echocardiography have been used to guide TSP because of their vastly superior imaging of the atrial septum [35–37].

There is much debate about the gold standard for measuring the mitral valve area following CBMV. Pressure half time is exquisitely dependent on the compliances of the left atrium and the left ventricle, as well as on the initial pressure gradient, and the former show marked variation in the postprocedure period [56]. Therefore, the PHT method is often inaccurate for measurement of the MVA for several days following a CBMV. A recent study found that the proximal isovelocity surface area (PISA) method for estimation of MVA correlated well with 2-D planimetry after CBMV [57].

We use the following end-points for CBMV in our laboratory: (1) a 50% drop in the mean transmitral gradient, (2) a significant increase in the v-wave in left atrial pressure, (3) maximal permissible size of the balloon used for dilation, (4) complete opening of at least one of the commissures on echocardiography, or (5) appearance of new mitral insufficiency clinically or increment in grade of mitral insufficiency on color Doppler echocardiography.

Results

Immediate outcomes

The acute hemodynamic results and symptom relief following CBMV are excellent in many large series in a broad spectrum of patients and in various clinical settings [58–64], making it one of the most gratifying procedures in the field of interventional cardiology. The usual criteria for procedural success include a postprocedural MVA of >1.5 cm^2 or a doubling of the pre-procedural MVA, with postprocedure mitral insufficiency of less than grade III. On average, the MVA is expected to double after a CBMV.

Our experience

Since our first case in 1990, more than 4000 CBMV procedures have been performed at our institute. We retrospectively analyzed the immediate outcomes of 1085 patients undergoing CBMV during the 3-year period from January 2005 to December 2007. The mean age was 28.7 ± 5.8 years, and 79% were females. Overall, 239 patients (22%) were under 20 years of age (juvenile mitral stenosis) and 786 (65%) were classified as New York Heart Association (NYHA) class III or IV. Atrial fibrillation was present in 93 patients (8.6%). A high Wilkins score (≥8) was seen in 32.5% of patients. Compared with Western series [65,66], our patient population undergoing CBMV was much younger. The technical success rate was 98.9%. In 12 patients (1.1%) there were technical failures—for reasons including inability to perform the TSP or cross the valve, thrombosis of the access veins, and abandonment of the procedure due to pericardial puncture or the development of cardiac tamponade. In the remaining 1073 patients, procedural success as defined above was achieved in 970 patients (90.4%). There was an increase in the MVA from 0.78 ± 0.26 cm^2 to 1.64 ± 0.31 cm^2, with a fall in the mean transmitral gradient from 19.2 ± 4.2 mmHg to 6.3 ± 1.9 mmHg. The pulmonary artery systolic pressures declined from 59.3 ± 27.1 mmHg to 41.3 ± 17.5 mmHg as assessed on color Doppler echocardiography. Following CBMV, 92% of patients were categorized as NYHA class II or less. There were two deaths, one due to cardiac tamponade and one due to acute severe mitral insufficiency with cardiogenic shock. Acute severe mitral insufficiency was seen in 41 (3.8%). Of these, 27 required emergency surgery (within 24 hours), and the rest were operated at an elective date.

The immediate results of CBMV are similar to those of open or closed surgical mitral valvotomy [67,68]. An echocardiographic score of greater than 8, severe subvalvular involvement, and significant (especially commissural) calcification are predictive of a suboptimal result after CBMV [16,69,70]. Other variables that can predict immediate results include the patient's age [58,71–73], functional class [71,74], the presence of atrial fibrillation [75], and a history of previous surgical commissurotomy [71,72].

Complications

Since its introduction, over the past two decades, CBMV has continued to remain a safe procedure, particularly with careful patient selection on the basis of the echocardiographic morphology of the valve. Nevertheless, it is important to realize that there is a definite learning curve [76], and that complications are often more common in the early phase of the operator's career.

Death

Mortality following CBMV is usually 1–3% [59,69,64,77–78]. The common causes of death include cardiac tamponade, acute severe mitral insufficiency, and cerebrovascular events. Emergency CBMV carries a significantly increased risk of mortality [79] (see below).

Acute mitral insufficiency

Although mitral insufficiency of some degree can occur in up to 15% of patients following a CBMV [80], it is usually mild. The incidence of acute severe mitral insufficiency, a potentially catastrophic complication, is between 3% and 8% [81–83]. Acute mitral insufficiency generally results from a noncommissural tear—the valve leaflets or the chordae are usually involved, as seen in surgical [82,84] and autopsy [85] findings. Commissural calcification [86] and balloon overinflation are associated with increased risk of this complication. The large regurgitant volume delivered to a relatively noncompliant left atrium causes a precipitous rise in the left atrial pressure and v-waves, resulting in acute pulmonary edema. Cardiac output may also be impaired, as the acuteness of the mitral insufficiency does not allow the left ventricle to use its compensatory mechanism of preload reserve for pumping the excess volume [87]. Bedside 2-D echo/color Doppler is extremely useful in visualizing the site of the tear and quantifying the grade of mitral insufficiency. In hemodynamically unstable patients, prompt surgery with mitral valve repair/replacement is recommended. While preparing for surgery, the patient is usually stabilized using intravenous diuretics, inotropes, and intra-aortic balloon pump (IABP) support in severe cases. Anesthetic agents that increase the afterload should preferably be avoided. Semi-emergent surgery may be chosen in patients who are hemodynamically stable.

Cardiac tamponade

The incidence of cardiac tamponade, another potentially fatal complication, is usually <1% [84,88]. The operator's experience and increasing patient age have been identified as factors predicting an increased risk of tamponade [89]. During the TSP, tamponade can occur owing to trauma to the right and left atria, the coronary sinus, or the aortic root. In the double balloon technique, it may result from left ventricular perforation by the guidewires or the balloons. Tamponade is suspected when there is an unexplained drop in the arterial pressure or an increase in the size of the cardiac silhouette, with lack of pulsations on fluoroscopy. Immediate bedside 2-D echocardiography will demonstrate the presence of fluid in the pericardial cavity. Management consists of immediate pericardiocentesis, rapid infusion of crystalloids and/or packed cells, and rapidly shifting the patient for surgical correction. If the tamponade is noticed on withdrawing the septal dilator, the dilator should be reinserted across the TSP site and left *in situ* to prevent further accumulation of blood in the pericardium. Prevention of tamponade requires a good knowledge of the fluoroscopic anatomy of the interatrial septum and adjacent structures, a sound puncture technique, and gentle manipulation of the assembly while entering the left atrium and crossing the mitral valve.

Atrial septal defect

Although an echocardiographic incidence of 20–24% [90–93] has been described for residual ASDs with left-to-right shunting at the TSP site, most defects close spontaneously, and hemodynamically significant shunts are uncommon [94–96]. Rarely, in the presence of severe pulmonary hypertension, right-to-left shunting can occur at the site of the defect and may occasionally cause cyanosis [97,98] or paradoxical embolism [99].

Systemic embolism

The most important embolic complication is the occurrence of cerebral emboli. Although microembolism to the brain (detectable with MRI) is not uncommon [100], clinically significant cerebral emboli are rare (0.5–1%) [80,88]. Shaw *et al.* [101] found a higher incidence (5%) of systemic emboli in elderly patients (age ≥70 years). Atrial fibrillation and the presence of left atrial thrombi before the procedure may be important predictors of this complication.

Long-term results

Follow-up data of up to 17 years are now available [102]. Overall, the clinical outcomes are quite satisfactory [44,103–106]. Iung *et al.* [107], in a study of 1024 consecutive patients, found the 10-year survival rate to be 85%, with freedom from reoperation in 61% and a good functional status (NYHA class I and II) in 56%. Fawzy *et al.* [102], in a study of 520 patients, found that actuarial freedom from restenosis at 10, 15, and 17 years was $73 \pm 2\%$, $43 \pm 4\%$, and $23 \pm 6\%$, respectively. Event-free survival (death, redo MBV, mitral valve replacement, NYHA class III or IV) at 10, 15, and 17 years was $82 \pm 2\%$, $45 \pm 5\%$, and $31 \pm 6\%$, respectively. Predictors of unfavorable long-term results include higher preprocedure valve scores, older age, a higher NYHA class before valvuloplasty, history of previous commissurotomy, severe tricuspid insufficiency, cardiomegaly, and high pulmonary vascular resistances. Atrial fibrillation, suboptimal postprocedure results, and the presence of more than grade II mitral insufficiency also predict poor late results [43,71,105,108,109].

The pulmonary artery pressures show a significant reduction following CBMV. This fall is often seen immediately post procedure, and continues at follow-up. Even patients with severe pulmonary hypertension can show near-normalization of the pulmonary artery systolic pressures at long-term follow-up [110,111], although some may continue to have elevated pressure and pulmonary vascular resistance [112], despite adequate relief of mitral stenosis. Significant reductions in the left atrial size [113], left atrial hypercoagulability [114], and the incidence of systemic embolism [115] have been documented following CBMV.

Catheter-based mitral valvuloplasty in special situations

Pregnancy

Prophylactic CBMV is offered to women with severe mitral stenosis who want to get pregnant in the hope of preventing the expected clinical worsening in the second trimester and peripartum [118–120], and to reduce the need for pharmacologic and procedural intervention during pregnancy [118]. However, the decision to undertake CBMV in pregnant patients with moderate mitral stenosis should be based on the clinical judgment, taking into account the functional class, severity of mitral stenosis, and the morphology of the valve. In patients with moderate mitral stenosis of unfavorable morphology who are asymptomatic or mildly symptomatic, medical therapy may be preferable to a CBMV. This is because CBMV may be complicated by significant mitral insufficiency which may necessitate mitral valve replacement before pregnancy, with its attendant hazards of anticoagulation.

Pregnant patients often present with an exacerbation of symptoms of mitral stenosis in the second trimester as a result of the hemodynamic burden imposed by the physiologic circulatory changes of pregnancy. Some may be first detected to have severe mitral stenosis during gestation. In symptomatic patients with severe mitral stenosis, CBMV is usually electively done in the second trimester, at about 24–26 weeks gestational age. It should be done with adequate shielding of the abdomen and pelvis, limiting fluoroscopic time to the minimum. In a high-volume institute like ours, the average fluoroscopy time is usually less than 10 min [119]. Radiation exposure can be reduced by using echocardiography in the catheterization laboratory to assess the results. The Inoue technique is preferred over the double-balloon technique to reduce procedure and fluoroscopy time [120]. Though the reported maternal and fetal outcomes have been variable, they are satisfactory [121,122] in most large series. Long-term follow-up of the children has shown normal growth and development in the majority [123–125], suggesting that the amount of radiation delivered during a CBMV may be tolerated by the fetus.

It is debatable whether CBMV should be performed prophylactically in asymptomatic or mildly symptomatic women with moderate or severe mitral stenosis during pregnancy [126] because of variable maternal and fetal outcomes reported in literature [116,117,127–129]. On the basis of available information, therefore, it seems reasonable to limit CBMV during pregnancy to symptomatic patients with severe mitral stenosis who do not respond to medical therapy or who cannot be provided with close and expert follow-up during pregnancy, labor, and delivery [126].

Mitral restenosis

Mitral restenosis following CBMV is usually uncommon within 3 years, and the incidence progressively increases with time [130,131]. Following surgical valvotomy, a repeat surgical procedure may be needed in 10–30% of patients after 5–15 years [132–134]. Restenosis is usually defined as MVA smaller than 1.5 cm², with a loss ≥50% of the gain achieved with valve dilation [135]. Repeat CBMV is useful in patients with mitral restenosis following previous surgical commissurotomy or CBMV, although technical difficulties may sometimes be encountered. In a study of 614 consecutive patients undergoing CBMV at our institute, Gupta *et al.* [136] identified 84 patients (13.7%) with mitral restenosis following previous surgical mitral valvotomy and compared them with 530 patients who had not undergone previous surgery. The success rates (more than 90% in both groups), final mitral valve area, mean transmitral gradient, and mean pulmonary artery pressure were similar. There were no significant differences in mortality or the occurrence of postprocedural acute mitral insufficiency. The beneficial acute outcome was found to be sustained at intermediate-term follow-up. In another study, Fawzy *et al.* [137] found a satisfactory, though inferior, 10-year event-free survival rate (54 ± 7% vs. 80 ± 3%, *P* < 0.005) among patients with mitral restenosis following previous surgical commissurotomy or CBMV compared with *de novo* mitral stenosis patients. More than 50% patients remained improved at 10 years, thus enabling the operation or reoperation to be deferred. Although CBMV gives good immediate results in mitral restenosis, the long-term outcomes are generally considered to be inferior to those of surgical therapy [138,139].

Juvenile mitral stenosis

Catheter-based mitral valvuloplasty is the procedure of choice in patients below 20 years of age unless the valve is unsuitable for the procedure. The threshold for advising valve replacement for this group should obviously be high, considering the problems with long-term anticoagulation. A number of studies have shown that CBMV gives excellent results in children and adolescents [140–142]. The long-term results are similar to those in adults [143,144]. The use of a metallic commissurotomy as an alternative to the Inoue balloon catheter has also been studied in patients with juvenile mitral stenosis, and has shown similar procedural success and complication rates in the immediate and intermediate-term follow-up [54].

Mitral stenosis in the elderly

Older patients are often not suitable for CBMV, as they tend to have severe subvalvular involvement and or extensive calcification. However, palliative CBMV may be attempted in those individuals who are poor surgical candidates because of other comorbid conditions and have relatively less severe subvalvular involvement or calcification. Several studies in patients aged 70 years or older have shown CBMV to be a useful palliative measure in high-risk surgical candidates [145,146]. The outcomes are generally less favorable than in younger patients, with an increased risk of complications [101].

Emergent catheter-based mitral valvuloplasty

In developing countries, owing to socioeconomic constraints, many patients do not undergo elective relief of mitral stenosis and present in an advanced critically ill state with pulmonary edema, cardiogenic shock, or even cardiac arrest. In such patients, the surgical mortality is very high, and emergent CBMV can be considered as a life-saving treatment option. A study [79] from our institute of 40 such patients (mean age 40 ± 13 years) undergoing emergent CBMV found that these patients were significantly older and that the incidence of atrial fibrillation, valve scores, and pulmonary artery systolic pressure were significantly higher, and mitral valve area significantly lower, than in patients who underwent elective CBMV. Mitral insufficiency occurred in 15%, and the mortality was 35%. Stepwise logistic regression analysis identified a mitral valvuloplasty score ≥ 8, pulmonary artery systolic pressure (PASP) ≥ 65 mmHg, and cardiac output ≤ 3.15 L/min as significant predictors of a fatal outcome. Follow-up of 1–16 months was available in 20 out of the 26 survivors, of whom 15 were asymptomatic. The gain in mitral valve area and the decrease in transmitral gradient and PASP obtained immediately after CBMV persisted during the follow-up period.

Double-valve balloon valvuloplasty

Aortic stenosis and tricuspid stenosis can coexist with rheumatic mitral stenosis, and there have been several reports of successful concurrent catheter-based valvuloplasty of the stenosed aortic or tricuspid valve during CBMV [147–149]. The sequence of dilation of the stenosed valves in this situation can be problematic. Usually, the distal stenosis is addressed first. During concomitant aortic valvuloplasty and CBMV, the TSP is performed first so that heparin can be given before crossing the stenosed aortic valve. We prefer to then dilate the aortic valve by over-the-wire balloon technique followed by CBMV with the Inoue technique. Others have performed concurrent anterograde CBMV and aortic valvuloplasty using the Inoue balloon with safe and effective outcomes [149,150]. The occurrence of severe mitral insufficiency during CBMV in the face of unrelieved severe aortic stenosis may not be well tolerated. In the presence of combined mitral stenosis and tricuspid stenosis, CBMV is usually performed first. Both valves can be dilated by the Inoue technique with good results

[148]. The immediate results are often rewarding, and some investigators have also been able to demonstrate a sustained benefit on long-term follow-up [151]. Concurrent mitral–aortic and mitral–tricuspid balloon valvuloplasty has been performed through the jugular route as well [152].

Conclusion

Catheter-based mitral valvuloplasty is safe and effective for a wide range of patients with mitral stenosis, and remains the treatment of choice in most patients with rheumatic mitral stenosis with suitable valve morphology. With a growing body of evidence now demonstrating sustained long-term results, and given the significant global disease burden and expanding indications for trans-septal puncture, the importance of training interventional cardiologists to perform this procedure cannot be overemphasized.

Acknowledgments

The authors are grateful to Dr. Rahul R. Gupta, Registrar in Cardiology, for his assistance in collection and analysis of our data, and to our faculty doctors, P. Nathani, P. Nyayadhish, C. Lanjewar, and A. Nabar, for their invaluable role in the conduct of mitral valvuloplasty procedures.

References

1. Brunton L (1902) Preliminary note on the possibility of treating mitral stenosis by surgical methods. *Lancet* **1**:352.
2. Bland EF (1952) Surgery for mitral stenosis. *Circulation* **5**:290–299.
3. Harken DE, Ellis LB, Ware PF, *et al.* (1948) The surgical treatment of mitral stenosis. *N Engl J Med* **239**:801–809.
4. Westaby S & Bosher C (1998) Development of Surgery in Valvular heart Disease. In: Westaby S & Bosher C (ed.). *Landmarks in Cardiac Surgery*. Oxford: Oxford University Press, p. 180.
5. Inoue K, Owaki T, Nakamura T, *et al.* (1984) Clinical application of transvenous mitral commissurotomy by a new balloon catheter. *J Thorac Cardiovasc Surg* **87**:394–402.
6. Lock JE, Khalilullah M, Shrivastava S, *et al.* (1985) Percutaneous catheter commissurotomy in rheumatic mitral stenosis. *N Engl J Med* **313**:1515–1518.
7. Al Zaibag M, Ribeiro PA, Al Kasab S, *et al.* (1986) Percutaneous double-balloon mitral valvotomy for rheumatic mitral valve stenosis. *Lancet* **1**:757–761.
8. Babic UU, Pejcic P, Djurisic Z, *et al.* (1986) Percutaneous transarterial balloon valvuloplasty for mitral valve stenosis. *Am J Cardiol* **57**:1101–1104.
9. Stefanidis C, Stratos C, Pitsavos C, *et al.* (1992) Retrograde non-transseptal balloon mitral valvuloplasty: immediate and long-term follow up. *Circulation* **85**:1760–1767.
10. Kerkar P, Lokhandwala Y, & Vora A (1994) A simple technique to cross mitral valve during percutaneous balloon mitral valvuloplasty. *Cathet Cardiovasc Diagn* **31**:161–162.
11. Bonhoeffer P, Piechaud JF, Sidi D, *et al.* (1995) Mitral dilatation with the Multi-Track system: an alternative approach. *Cathet Cardiovasc Diagn* **36**:189–193.
12. Cribier A, Lath PC, & Letac B (1997) Percutaneous mitral valvotomy with a metal dilator. *Lancet* **349**:1667.
13. Joseph G, George OK, Mandalay A, *et al.* (2002) Transjugular approach to balloon mitral valvuloplasty helps overcome impediments caused by anatomical alterations. *Cathet Cardiovasc Intervent* **57**:353–362.
14. Bland EF & Jones TD (1951) Rheumatic fever and rheumatic heart disease *Circulation* **4**:836.
15. Roberts WC & Perloff JK (1972) Mitral valvular disease. *Ann Intern Med* **77**:939.
16. Wilkins GT, Weyman AE, Abascal LM, Block PC, & Palacios IF (1988) Percutaneous balloon dilatation of the mitral valve: an analysis of echocardiographic variables related to outcome and the mechanism of dilatation. *Br Heart J* **60**: 299–308.
17. Kaplan JD, Isner JM, Karas RH, *et al.* (1987) In vitro analysis of balloon valvuloplasty of stenotic mitral valves. *Am J Cardiol* **59**:318–323.
18. Block PC, Palacios IL, Jacobs ML, *et al.* (1987) Mechanism of percutaneous mitral valvotomy. *Am J Cardiol* **59**:178–179.
19. Reifart N, Nowak B, Baykut D, *et al.* (1990) Experimental balloon valvuloplasty of fibrotic and calcific mitral valves. *Circulation* **81**:1005–1011.
20. Bonow RO, Carabello BA, Kanu C, *et al.* (2006) ACC/AHA 2006 guidelines for the management of patients with valvular heart disease: a report of the American College of Cardiology/American Heart Association Task Force on Practice Guidelines (writing committee to revise the 1998 Guidelines for the Management of Patients With Valvular Heart Disease): developed in collaboration with the Society of Cardiovascular Anesthesiologists: endorsed by the Society for Cardiovascular Angiography and Interventions and the Society of Thoracic Surgeons. *Circulation* **114**:e84–231.
21. Vahanian A, Baumgartner H, Bax J, *et al.* (2007) Guidelines on the management of valvular heart disease: The Task Force on the Management of Valvular Heart Disease of the European Society of Cardiology. *Eur Heart J* **28**:230–268.
22. Silaruks S, Thinkhamrop B, Kiatchoosakun S, *et al.* (2004) Resolution of left atrial thrombus after 6 months of anti-coagulation in candidates for percutaneous transvenous mitral commissurotomy. *Ann Intern Med* **140**:101–105.
23. Padial LR, Abascal VM, Moreno PR, *et al.* (1999) Echocardio-graphy can predict the development of severe mitral regurgitation after percutaneous mitral valvulotomy by the Inoue technique. *Am J Cardiol* **83**:1210–1213.
24. Clugston R, Lau FY, & Ruis C (1992) Transseptal catheterization update 1992. *Cathet Cardiovasc Diagn* **26**:266–274.
25. Rocha P, Berland j, Rigaud M, *et al.* (1991) Fluoroscopic guidance in transseptal catheterization in percutaneous mitral balloon valvotomy *Cathet Cardiovasc Diagn* **23**:172–176.
26. Doorey A & Goldenburg EM (1991) Transseptal catheterization in adults: enhanced efficacy and safety in low volume operators using a non-standard technique. *Cathet Cardiovasc Diagn* **24**:166–172.
27. Hung JS (1992) Atrial septal puncture technique in percutaneous transvenous mitral commissurotomy: mitral valvuloplasty

using the Inoue balloon catheter technique. *Cathet Cardiovasc Diagn* **26**:275–284.

28. Hung J & Lau K (2006) Trans-septal access in Inoue-balloon mitral valvuloplasty. *Indian Heart J* **58**:463–465.

29. Inoue K, Lau KW, & Jung KS (2002) Percutaneous transvenous mitral commissurotomy. In: Grech ED & Ramsdale DR. *Practical Interventional Cardiology*, 2nd edn. London, UK: Martin Dunitz Ltd, p. 373.

30. Mullins CE (1983) Transseptal left heart catheterization: experience with a new technique in 520 pediatric and adult patients. *Pediatr Cardiol* **4**:239–246.

31. Dalvi B, Vora A, & Kerkar P (1992) Radio-opaque tipped Mullins sheath. *Cathet Cardiovasc Diagn* **27**:244–245.

32. Kerkar PG, Vora AM, Sivaraman A, *et al.* (1994) Balloon mitral commissurotomy complicated by fatal pericardial tamponade due to "Atrial Stitch". *J Inv Cardiol* **6**:17–20.

33. Hung JS & Lau KW (1996) Pitfalls and tips in Inoue balloon mitral commissurotomy. *Cathet Cardiovasc Diagn* **37**:188–199.

34. Babaliaros VC, Green JT, Lerakis S, *et al.* (2008) Emerging applications for transseptal left heart catheterization: old techniques for new procedures. *J Am Coll Cardiol* **51**:2116–2122.

35. Green NE, Hansgen AR, & Carroll JD (2004) Initial clinical experience with intracardiac echocardiography (ICE) in guiding balloon mitral valvuloplasty: technique, safety, utility & limitations. *Catheter Cardiovasc Interv* **63**:385–394.

36. Cafri C, de la Guardia B, Barasch E, *et al.* (2000) Transseptal puncture guided by intracardiac echocardiography during percutaneous transvenous mitral commissurotomy in patients with distorted anatomy of the fossa ovalis *Catheter Cardiovasc Interv* **50**:463–467.

37. Cheng A & Calkins H (2007) A conservative approach to performing transseptal punctures without the use of intracardiac echocardiography: stepwise approach with real-time video clips. *J Cardiovasc Electrophysiol* **18**:686–689.

38. Sherman W, Lee P, Hartley A, & Love B (2005) Transatrial septal catheterization using a new radiofrequency probe *Catheter Cardiovasc Interv* **66**:14–17.

39. Elagha AA, Kim AH, Kocaturk O, & Lederman RJ (2007) Blunt atrial transseptal puncture using excimer laser in swine. *Catheter Cardiovasc Interv* **70**:585–590.

40. Vahanian A, Iung B, & Cormier B (2003). Mitral Valvuloplasty. In Topol EJ (ed.). *Textbook of Interventional Cardiology*. 4th edn. Philadelphia: Saunders, Elsevier, pp. 921–940.

41. Vora A, Kerkar P, Kulkarni H, *et al.* (1995) Percutaneous balloon mitral valvuloplasty by the retrograde (babic) technique in a patient with inferior vena cava stenosis. *Cathet Cardiovasc Diagn* **36**:291–292.

42. Holmes D (1992) Trans-septal catheterization 1992: it is here to stay. *Catheter Cardiovasc Diagn* **26**:264–265.

43. Himbert D, Brochet E, Iung B, *et al.* (2008) State-of-the-art nonvascular interventions: mitral valvuloplasty. *J Invasive Cardiol* **20**:e114–119.

44. Kang DS, Park SW, Song JK, *et al.* (2000) Long-term clinical and echocardiographic outcome of percutaneous mitral valvuloplasty: randomized comparison of Inoue and double-balloon techniques. *J Am Coll Cardiol* **35**:169–175.

45. Chen CR, Huang ZD, Lo ZX, *et al.* (1990) Comparison of single rubber-nylon balloon and double polyethylene balloon valvulo-plasty in 94 patients with rheumatic mitral stenosis. *Am Heart J* **119**:102–111.

46. Bassand JP, Schiele F, Bernard Y, *et al.* (1991) the double balloon and Inoue techniques in percutaneous mitral valvulo-plasty: comparative results in a series of 232 cases. *J Am Coll Cardiol* **18**:982–989.

47. Riberio PA, Fawzy ME, Arafat MA, *et al.* (1991) Comparison of mitral valve area results of balloon mitral valvotomy using the Inoue and double balloon techniques. *Am J Cardiol* **68**:687–688.

48. Fernandez Ortiz A, Macaya C, Afonso F, *et al.* (1992) Mono versus double-balloon technique for commissural splitting after percutaneous mitral valvotomy. *Am J Cardiol* **69**:1100–1101.

49. Ruiz CE, Zhang HP, Macaya C, *et al.* (1992) Comparison of Inoue single balloon versus double balloon technique for percutaneous mitral valvotomy. *Am Heart J* **123**:942–947.

50. Rihal CS & Holmes DR (1994) Percutaneous balloon mitral valvuloplasty: issues involved in comparing techniques. *Catheter Cardiovasc Diagn* **2**:35–41.

51. Kerkar PG, Vora AM, & Sethi JP (1994) Unusual tear in Inoue balloon during percutaneous balloon mitral valvuloplasty in a patient with calcific mitral stenosis. *Cathet Cardiovasc Diagn* **31**:127–129.

52. Cribier A, Eltchanikoff M, Carloff R, *et al.* (2000) Percutaneous mechanical mitral commissurotomy with the metallic valvulo-tome: detailed technical aspects and overview of the results of the multicenter registry on 882 patients. *J Int Cardiol* **13**:255–262.

53. Bhat A, Harikrishnan S, Tharakan JM, *et al.* (2002) Comparison of percutaneous transmitral commissurotomy with Inoue balloon technique and metallic commissurotomy: immediate and short-term follow-up results of a randomized study. *Am Heart J* **144**:1074–1080.

54. Harikrishnan S, Nair K, Tharakan JM, *et al.* (2006) Percutaneous mitral commissurotomy in juvenile mitral stenosis—comparison of long term results of Inoue balloon technique and metallic commissurotomy. *Catheter Cardiovasc Interv* **67**:453–459.

55. Zaki AM, Kasem HH, Bakhoum S, *et al.* (2002) Comparison of early results of percutaneous metallic mitral commissurotome with Inoue balloon technique in patients with high mitral echocardiographic scores. *Cathet Cardiovasc Interv* **57**:312–317.

56. Thomas JD, Wilkins GT, Choong CY, *et al.* (1988) Inaccuracy of mitral pressure half-time immediately after percutaneous mitral valvotomy—dependence on transmitral gradient and left atrial and left ventricular compliance. *Circulation* **78**:980–993.

57. Sunil Roy TN, Krishnan MN, Koshy C, *et al.* (2005) Comparison of proximal isovelocity surface area method and pressure half time method for evaluation of mitral valve area in patients undergoing balloon mitral valvotomy. *Echocardiography* **22**:707–712.

58. Iung B, Cormier B, Ducimetiere P, *et al.* (1996) Immediate results of percutaneous mitral commissurotomy. A predictive model on a series of 1514 patients. *Circulation* **94**:2124–2130.

59. Arora R, Singh Kalra G, Ramachandra Murty GS, *et al.* (1994) Percutaneous transatrial mitral commissurotomy: immediate and intermediate results. *J Am Coll Cardiol* **23**:1327–1332.

60. Chen CR & Cheng TO (1995) Percutaneous balloon mitral valvuloplasty by the Inoue technique: a multicenter study of 4832 patients in China. *Am Heart J* **129**:1197–1202.

61. Neumayer U, Schmidt HK, Fassbender D, *et al.* (2002) Early (three-month) results of percutaneous mitral valvotomy with the Inoue balloon in 1123 consecutive patients comparing various age groups. *Am J Cardiol* **90**:190–193.

62. Tuzcu EM, Block PC, Griffin BP, *et al.* (1992) Immediate and long-term outcome of percutaneous mitral valvotomy in patients 65 years and older. *Circulation* **85**:963–971.

63. Mishra S, Narang R, Sharma M, *et al.* (2001) Percutaneous transseptal mitral commissurotomy in pregnant women with critical mitral stenosis. *Indian Heart J* **53**:192–196.

64. Iung B, Nicoud-Houel A, Fondard O, *et al.* (2004) Temporal trends in percutaneous mitral commissurotomy over a 15-year period. *Eur Heart J* **25**:702–708.

65. Palacios IF (1994) Percutaneous mitral balloon valvotomy for patients with mitral stenosis. *Curr Opin Cardiol* **9**:164–175.

66. Feldman T (1994) Hemodynamic results, clinical outcome, and complications of Inoue balloon mitral valvotomy. *Cathet Cardiovasc Diagn* **2**:2–7.

67. Turi ZG, Reyes VP, Raju BS, *et al.* (1991) Percutaneous balloon versus surgical closed commissurotomy for mitral stenosis. A prospective, randomized trial. *Circulation* **83**:1179–1185.

68. Reyes BP, Raju BS, Wynne J, *et al.* (1994) Percutaneous balloon valvuloplasty compared with open surgical commissurotomy for mitral stenosis. *N Engl J Med* **331**:961.

69. Fatkin D, Roy, Morgan J, *et al.* (1993) Percutaneous balloon mitral valvotomy with the Inoue single balloon catheter: commissural morphology as a determinant of outcome. *J Am Coll Cardiol* **21**:390–397.

70. Reid CL, Otto CM, & Davis KB (1992) Influence of mitral valve morphology on mitral balloon commissurotomy: immediate and six-month results from the NHLBI Balloon Valotomy Registry. *Am Heart J* **124**:657–665.

71. Palacios IF, Tuzcu ME, Weyman AE, *et al.* (1995) Clinical follow-up of patients undergoing percutaneous mitral balloon valvotomy. *Circulation* **91**:671–676.

72. Herrmann HC, Ramaswamy K, Isner JM, *et al.* (1992) Factors influencing immediate results, complications, and short-term follow-up status after Inoue balloon mitral valvotomy: a North-American multicenter study. *Am Heart J* **124**:160–166.

73. Valentini P, Vegni FE, & Nihoyannopoulos P (2002) Age, a predictive factor for the reduction in the mean transmitral pressure gradient after percutaneous balloon mitral valvotomy. *Ital Heart J* **3**:462–466.

74. Dean LS, Mickel M, Bonan R, *et al.* (1996) Four-year follow-up of patients undergoing percutaneous balloon mitral commissurotomy. A report from the National Heart, Lung and Blood Institute Balloon Valvuloplasty Registry. *J Am Coll Cardiol* **28**:145.

75. Leon MN, Harrell LC, Simosa HF, *et al.* (1999) Mitral balloon valvotomy for patients with mitral stenosis in atrial fibrillation: immediate and long-term results. *J Am Coll Cardiol* **34**:1145–1152.

76. Sanchez PL, Harrell LC, Salas RE, *et al.* (2001) Learning curve of the Inoue technique of percutaneous mitral balloon valvuloplasty. *Am J Cardiol* **88**:662–667.

77. Iung B, Cormier B, Ducimetiere P, *et al.* (1996) Immediate results of percutaneous mitral commissurotomy. *Circulation* **94**:2124–2130.

78. The National Heart, Lung, and Blood Institute Balloon Valvuloplasty Registry. (1992) Complications and mortality of percutaneous balloon mitral commissurotomy. *Circulation* **85**:2014–2024.

79. Lokhandwala Y, Banker D, Vora M, *et al.* (1998) Emergent balloon mitral valvotomy in patients presenting with cardiac arrest, cardiogenic shock or refractory pulmonary edema. *J Am Coll Cardiol* (1998) **32**:154–158.

80. Fawzy M (2007) Percutaneous mitral balloon valvotomy. *Catheter Cardiovasc Interv* **69**:313–321.

81. Kaul UA, Singh S, Kalra GS, *et al.* (2000) Mitral regurgitation following percutaneous transvenous mitral commissurotomy: a single-center experience. *J Heart Valve Dis* **9**:262–266; discussion 266–268.

82. Hernandez R, Macaya C, Banuelos C, *et al.* (1992) Predictors, mechanisms and outcome of severe mitral regurgitation complicating percutaneous mitral valvotomy with the Inoue balloon. *Am J Cardiol* **70**:1169–1174.

83. Hermann HC, Lima JA, Feldman T, *et al.* (1993) Mechanisms and outcome of severe mitral regurgitation after Inoue balloon valvuloplasty. *J Am Coll Cardiol* **22**:783–789.

84. Varma PK, Theodore S, Neema PK, *et al.* (2005) Emergency surgery after percutaneous transmitral commissurotomy: operative versus echocardiographic findings, mechanisms of complications, and outcomes. *J Thorac Cardiovasc Surg* **130**:772–776.

85. Deshpande J, Vaideeswar P, Sivaraman J, *et al.* (1995) Balloon mitral valvotomy: an autopsy study. *Int J Cardiol* **52**:67–76.

86. Cannan C, Nishimura R, Reeder G, *et al.* (1997) Echocardiographic assessment of commissural calcium: a simple predictor of outcome after percutaneous mitral balloon valvotomy. *J Am Coll Cardiol* **29**:175–180.

87. Tempe D, Gupta B, Banerjee A, *et al.* (2004) Surgical interventions in patients undergoing percutaneous balloon mitral valvotomy: a retrospective analysis of anesthetic considerations. *Ann Cardiac Anesth* **7**:129–136.

88. Zeng Z, Fang Y, & Fu H (1999) Clinical analysis of percutaneous balloon mitral valvotomy in 1063 patients. *Hua Xi Yi Ke Da Xue Xue Bao* **30**:85–87.

89. Joseph G, Chandy ST, & Krishnaswami S (1997) Mechanisms of cardiac perforation leading to tamponade in balloon mitral valvuloplasty. *Catheter Cardiovasc Diagn* **42**:138–146.

90. Palacios IF, Block PC, Wilkins GT *et al.* (1989) Follow-up of patients undergoing percutaneous mitral balloon valvotomy. *Circulation* **79**:573–579.

91. O'Shea JP, Abascal VM, & Marshall JE (1988) Long term persistence of atrial septal defect following percutaneous mitral valvuloplasty a doppler-echocardiographic follow-up study. *Circulation* **78**(Suppl. 2):2–1. Abstract.

92. Yoshida K, Yoshikawa J, Akasaka T, *et al.* (1989) Assessment of left-to-right atrial shunting after percutaneous mitral valvuloplasty by transoesophageal color doppler flow-mapping. *Circulation* **80**:1521–1526.

93. Fawzy ME, Fadel B, Al Sergani H, *et al.* (2007) Long-term results (up to 16.5 years) of mitral balloon valvuloplasty in a series of 518 patients and predictors of long-term outcome. *J Interv Cardiol* **20**:66–72.

94. Harrison JK, Wilson JS, Hearne SE, & Bashore TM (1994) Complications related to percutaneous transvenous mitral commissurotomy. *Cathet Cardiovasc Diagn* (Suppl. 2):52–60.

95. Carroll JD & Feldman T (1993) Percutaneous mitral balloon valvotomy and the new demographics of mitral stenosis. *JAMA* **270**:1731–1736.

96. Cequier A, Bonan R, Serra A, *et al.* (1990) Left to right atrial shunting after percutaneous mitral valvuloplasty. *Circulation* **81**:1190–1197.

97. Goldberg N, Roman CF, & Cha SD (1989) Right to left interatrial shunting following balloon mitral valvuloplasty. *Cathet Cardiovasc Diagn* **16**:133–135.

98. Nakao M, Ch'ng JK, & Sin YK (2008) Acquired right-to-left shunt through an atrial septal perforation with cyanosis after percutaneous transvenous mitral commissurotomy. *J Thorac Cardiovasc Surg* **135**:690–691.

99. Harikrishnan S, Titus T, Tharakan JN (2005) Septal defects after percutaneous mitral valvotomy—all are not innocent. *J Am Soc Echocardiogr* **18**:183–184.

100. Rocha P, Quanadli S, Strumza P, *et al.* (1999) Brain "embolism" detected by magnetic resonance imaging during percutaneous mitral balloon commissurotomy. *Cardiovasc Intervent Radiol* **22**:268–273.

101. Shaw TR, Sutaria N, Prendergast GB (2003) Clinical and haemodynamic profiles of young, middle aged, and elderly patients with mitral stenosis undergoing mitral balloon valvotomy. *Heart* **89**:1430–1436.

102. Fawzy ME, Shoukri M, Al Buraiki J, *et al.* (2007) Seventeen years' clinical and echocardiographic follow up of mitral balloon valvuloplasty in 520 patients, and predictors of long-term outcome. *J Heart Valve Dis* **16**:454–460.

103. Orrange SE, Kawanishi DT, Lopez BM, *et al.* (1997) Actuarial outcome after catheter balloon commissurotomy in patients with mitral stenosis. *Circulation* **95**:382–389.

104. Pan M, Medina A, Suarez de Lezo J, *et al.* (1993) Factors determining late success after mitral balloon valvulotomy. *Am J Cardiol* **71**:1181–1185.

105. Ben-Fahrat M, Betbout F, Gamra H, *et al.* (2001) Predictors of long-term event-free survival and of freedom from restenosis after percutaneous balloon mitral commissurotomy *Am Heart J* **142**:1072–1079.

106. Joseph PK, Bhat A, Francis B, *et al.* (1997) Percutaneous transvenous mitral commissurotomy using an Inoue balloon in children with rheumatic mitral stenosis. *Int J Cardiol* **62**:19–22.

107. Iung B, Garbarz E, Michaud P, *et al.* (1999) Late results of percutaneous mitral valvotomy in a series of 1024 patients: frequency, anatomic findings, and predictive factors. *Circulation* **99**:3272–3278.

108. Kohen DJ, Kuntz RE, Gordon SP *et al.* (1992) Predictors of long-term outcome after percutaneous balloon mitral valvuloplasty. *N Engl J Med* **327**:1329–1335.

109. Fawzy ME, Shoukry M, Hassan WH, *et al.* (2007) The impact of mitral valve morphology on the long-term outcome of mitral balloon valvuloplasty. *Catheter Cardiovasc Interv* **69**:40–46.

110. Umesan CV, Kapur A, Sinha N, *et al.* (2000) Effect of Inoue balloon mitral valvotomy on severe pulmonary arterial hypertension in 315 patients with rheumatic mitral stenosis: immediate and long-term results. *J Heart Valve Dis* **9**:609–615.

111. Fawzy ME, Hassan W, Stefadouros M, *et al.* (2004) Prevalence and fate of severe pulmonary hypertension in 559 consecutive patients with severe rheumatic mitral stenosis undergoing mitral balloon valvotomy. *J Heart Valve Dis* **13**:942–947; discussion 947–948.

112. Bahl VK, Chandra S, Talwar KK, *et al.* (1995) Balloon mitral valvotomy in patients with systemic and suprasystemic pulmonary artery pressures. *Cathet Cardiovasc Diagn* **36**:211–215.

113. Stefadouros MA, Fawzi ME, & Malik S (1999) The long-term effect of successful mitral balloon valvotomy on left atrial size. *J Heart Valve Dis* **8**:543–550.

114. Peverill RE, Harper RW, Harris G, *et al.* (1995) Amelioration of regional left atrial hypercoagulability by balloon mitral valvuloplasty in patients with mitral stenosis. *Circulation* **92**(Suppl. 1):1–21.

115. Chiang C-W, Lo S-K, Ko Y-S, Cheng N-J, Lin PJ, & Chang C-H (1998) Predictors of systemic embolism in patients with mitral stenosis: a prospective study. *Ann Int Med* **128**:885–889.

116. Hameed A, Karaalp IS, Tummala PP, *et al.* (2001) The effect of valvular heart disease on maternal and fetal outcome of pregnancy. *J Am Coll Cardiol* **37**:893–899.

117. Silversides CK, Colman JM, Sermer M, & Siu SC (2003) Cardiac risk in pregnant women with rheumatic mitral stenosis. *Am J Cardiol* **91**:1382–1385.

118. Bhatla N, Lal S, Behera G, *et al.* (2003) Cardiac disease in pregnancy. *Int J Gynaecol Obstet* **82**:153–159.

119. Gupta A, Lokhandwala YY, Satoskar PR, *et al.* (1998) Balloon mitral valvotomy in pregnancy: maternal and fetal outcomes. *J Am Coll Cardiol* **187**:409–415.

120. Cheng TO (2002) Percutaneous mitral valvuloplasty by the Inoue balloon technique is the ideal procedure for treatment of significant mitral stenosis in pregnant women. *Cathet Cardiovasc Interv* Nov;**57**(3):323–4.

121. Mishra S, Narang R, Sharma M, *et al.* (2001) Percutaneous transseptal mitral commissurotomy in pregnant women with critical mitral stenosis. *Indian Heart J* **53**:192–196.

122. Sivadasanpillai H, Srinivasan A, Sivasubramoniam S, *et al.* (2005) Long-term outcome of patients undergoing balloon mitral valvotomy in pregnancy. *Am J Cardiol* **95**:1504–1506.

123. Manquione JM, Lourenco RM, dos Santos ES, *et al.* (2000) Long-term follow-up of pregnant women after percutaneous mitral valvuloplasty. *Catheter Cardiovasc Interv* **50**:413–417.

124. Esteves CA, Munoz JS, Braga S, *et al.* (2006) Immediate and long-term follow up of percutaneous balloon mitral valvuloplasty in pregnant patients with rheumatic mitral stenosis. *Am J Cardiol* **98**:812–816.

125. Kinsara AJ, Ismai O, & Fawzi ME (2002) Effect of balloon mitral valvoplasty during pregnancy on childhood development. *Cardiology* **97**:155–158.

126. Elkayam U & Bitar F (2005) Valvular heart disease and pregnancy part I: native valves. *J Am Coll Cardiol* **46**:223–230.

127. Kramer MS, Demissie K, Yang H, Platt RW, Sauvé R, & Liston R (2000) The contribution of mild and moderate preterm birth to infant mortality. Fetal and Infant Health Study Group of the Canadian Perinatal Surveillance System. *JAMA* **284**:843–849.

128. Barker DJ & Osmond C (1989) Growth in utero, blood pressure in childhood and adult life, and mortality from cardiovascular disease. *BMJ* **298**:564–567.

129. Ben Farhat M, Gamra H, Betbout F, *et al.* (1997) Percutaneous balloon mitral commissurotomy during pregnancy. *Heart* **77**:564–567.

130. Guerios E, Bueno R, Nercolini D, *et al.* (2005) Mitral stenosis and percutaneous mitral valvuloplasty (Part 1). *J Invasive Cardiol* **17**:382–386.

131. Hernandez R, Banuelos C, Alfonso F, *et al.* (1999) Long-term clinical and echocardiographic follow-up after percutaneous mitral valvuloplasty with the Inoue balloon. *Circulation* **99**: 1580–1586.

132. John S, Perianayagam WJ, Abraham K, *et al.* (1978) Restenosis of the mitral valve: surgical considerations and results of operation. *Ann Thorac Surg* **25**:316–321.

133. Gross RI, Cunningham JN Jr, Snively SL, *et al.* (1981) Long-term results of open radical mitral commissurotomy: ten year follow-up study of 202 patients. *Am J Cardiol* **47**:821–825.

134. Harken DE, Black H, Taylor WJ, *et al.* (1961) Reoperation for mitral stenosis. A discussion of post-operative deterioration and methods of improving initial and secondary operation. *Circulation* **23**:7–12.

135. Turi ZG (1998) Restenosis after mitral valvuloplasty. A proxy for short-term palliation versus long-term cure. *Cathet Cardiovasc Diagn* **143**:42.

136. Gupta S, Vora A, Lokhandwala Y, Kerkar P, Kulkarni H, & Dalvi B (1996) Percutaneous mitral valvotomy in mitral restenosis. *Eur Heart J* **17**:1560–1564.

137. Fawzy ME, Hassan W, Shoukri M, *et al.* (2005) Immediate and long-term results of mitral balloon valvotomy for restenosis following previous surgical or balloon mitral commissurotomy. *Am J Cardiol* **96**:971–975.

138. Kim JB, Ha JW, Kim JS, *et al.* (2007) Comparison of long-term outcome after mitral valve replacement or repeated balloon mitral valvotomy in patients with restenosis after previous balloon valvotomy. *Am J Cardiol* **99**:1571–1574.

139. Pathan AZ, Mahdi MA, & Leon MN (1999) Is redo percutaneous mitral balloon valvuloplasty (PMV) indicated in patients with post-PMV mitral restenosis? *J Am Coll Cardiol* **34**:49–54.

140. Kinsara AJ, Fawzy ME, & Sivnandan V (2002) Immediate and midterm outcome of balloon mitral valvotomy in children and adolescents. *Can J Cardiol* **18**:967–971.

141. Krishnamoorthy KM & Tharakan JA (2003) Balloon mitral valvulotomy in children aged ≤ 12 years. *J Heart Valve Dis* **12**:461–468.

142. Zaki A, Salama M, El Masry M, *et al.* (1999) Five-year follow-up after percutaneous balloon mitral valvuloplasty in children and adolescents. *Am J Cardiol* **83**:735–739.

143. Fawzy M, Stefadourus M, Hegazy H, *et al.* (2005) Long term clinical and echocardiographic results of mitral balloon valvotomy in children and adolescents. *Heart* **91**:743–748.

144. Sinha N, Kapur A, Kumar AS, *et al.* (1997) Immediate and follow up results of Inoue balloon mitral valvotomy in juvenile rheumatic mitral stenosis. *J Heart Valve Dis* **6**:599–603.

145. Sutaria N, Elder AT, & Shaw TR (2000) Long term outcome of percutaneous mitral balloon valvotomy in patients aged 70 and over. *Heart* **83**:433–438.

146. Sutaria N, Elder AT, & Shaw TR (2000) Mitral balloon valvotomy for the treatment of mitral stenosis in octogenarians. *J Am Geriatr Soc* **48**:971–974.

147. Sharma S, Loya YS, & Desai D (1997) Percutaneous double-valve balloon valvotomy for multivalve stenosis: immediate results and intermediate-term follow-up. *Am Heart J* **133**:64–70.

148. Sharma S, Loya YS, & Daxini BV (1991) Concurrent double balloon valvotomy for combined rheumatic mitral and tricuspid stenosis. *Cathet Cardiovasc Diagn* **23**:42–46.

149. Krishnan MN, Syamkumar MD, Sajeev CG, *et al.* (2007) Snare-assisted anterograde balloon mitral and aortic valvotomy using Inoue balloon catheter. *Int J Cardiol* **114**:e9–11.

150. Bahl K, Chandra S, Goswami KC, *et al.* (1998) Combined mitral and aortic valvuloplasty by antegrade transseptal approach using Inoue balloon catheter. *Int J Cardiol* **63**:313–315.

151. Sancaktar O, Kumbasar SD, & Semiz E (1998) Late results of combined percutaneous balloon valvuloplasty of mitral and tricuspid valves. *Cathet Cardiovasc Diagn* **45**:246–250.

152. Joseph G, Rajendiran G, Rajpal KA, *et al.* (2000) Trans-jugular approach to concurrent mitral-aortic and mitral-tricuspid balloon valvuloplasty. *Catheter Cardiovasc Interv* **49**:335–341.

20 Surgical Management of Mitral Stenosis

Kevin L. Greason & Hartzell V. Schaff

Mayo Clinic, Rochester, MN, USA

Introduction

Mitral stenosis causes obstruction to left ventricle inflow at the level of the mitral valve leaflets and subvalvular apparatus, and results from a structural abnormality of the mitral valve complex that prevents proper opening during diastolic filling of the left ventricle [1]. A study in the surgical management of mitral stenosis is almost entirely a study of rheumatic mitral valve disease. Isolated mitral stenosis occurs in 40% of all patients presenting with rheumatic heart disease. The ratio of women to men presenting with isolated mitral stenosis is 2:1. Acquired causes of mitral obstruction, other than rheumatic heart disease, are rare and include left atrial myxoma, ball valve thrombosis, mucopolysaccharidosis, and severe mitral annular calcification [2].

Mitral valve anatomy

The mitral valve complex includes the orifice, annulus, anterior and posterior leaflets and the subvalvular apparatus that consists of chordae tendineae and papillary muscles. The left atrium is relatively unrelated to the form and function of the mitral valve complex, but it is greatly affected by valve function. The left ventricle is an important subunit of the mitral valve apparatus; ventricular dysfunction producing tethering of the chordae can directly affect leaflet motion/coaptation and may cause significant mitral insufficiency, and removal of the subvalvular structures during valve replacement may lead to some degree of ventricular dysfunction.

The mitral valve annulus consists of fibrocollagenous elements of varying consistency [3]. The annulus is strongest at the inner aspects of the left and right fibrous trigones. Spanning the zone between the trigones, the central part of the anterior mitral leaflet is the fibrous subaortic curtain, which descends from the adjacent halves of the left coronary and noncoronary

Cardiovascular Interventions in Clinical Practice. Edited by Jürgen Haase, Hans-Joachim Schäfers, Horst Sievert and Ron Waksman. © 2010 Blackwell Publishing.

cusp regions of the aortic valve annulus. The posterior annulus is made up of a more tenuous sheet of deformable fibroelastic connective tissue.

The leaflets are defined by the anterolateral and posteromedial commissures; two indentations on the posterior leaflet divide this structure into three anatomically individualized scallops. The scallops of the posterior leaflet are identified as P1 (anterolateral scallop), P2 (middle scallop), and P3 (posteromedial scallop). The three corresponding segments of the anterior leaflet are A1 (lateral segment), A2 (middle segment), and A3 (medial segment) [4].

There are generally two papillary muscles that vary considerably in their formation, from long and finger-like to short and stubby; occasionally, their tips are bifid. The muscles are named based on their point of origin from the free wall of the left ventricle: anterolateral and posteromedial. Chordae tendineae arise most commonly from the tip and margin of the apical third of each muscle, but occasionally they emerge near the base. The chordae from each muscle diverge and are inserted into corresponding points on both leaflets of the mitral valve.

The anterolateral and posteromedial chordae tendineae mostly arise near the tips of their corresponding papillary muscle as a single stem branching almost immediately into radiating strands like the struts of a fan and insert into the leaflets. Chordae of the mitral complex can be subdivided into commissural, leaflet, rough zone, cleft, and basal types depending on their area of insertion. In the majority of hearts, the chordae support the entire free edges of the leaflets.

The mean circumference of the mitral valve orifice averages 9–10 cm in adults and is slightly smaller in women than in men. The orifice is a dynamic structure whose area can reduce by as much as 40% during systole. The orifice changes from the circular profile characteristic of diastole to a D-shaped concentric form at the height of systole. The annular attachment of the anterior leaflet provides the concavity of the crescent, and the attachment of the posterior leaflet, although remaining convex, contracts toward the former.

Important anatomic relationships exist between the mitral valve and other structures that put them at risk during surgical manipulation of the mitral valve (Fig. 20.1). The anterior leaflet is in direct continuity with the aortic valve, specifically

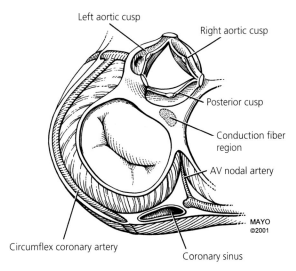

Figure 20.1 Anatomical relationship of mitral valve to other cardiac structures. (Modified from Burkhart and Zehr [5], with permission).

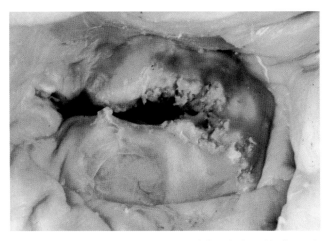

Figure 20.2 Rheumatic mitral valve. Note calcified, thickened leaflets with commissural fusion resulting in stenosis.

portions of the left and noncoronary aortic valve cusps. The conduction bundle is susceptible to damage in the area of the right fibrous trigone. Vascular structures vulnerable to damage include the circumflex coronary artery, which courses parallel to the posterior annulus on the left, and the coronary sinus, which is superficial to the posterior annulus on the right. In a left dominant coronary artery system, the circumflex coronary artery is at risk for damage along the entire length of the posterior annulus [5].

Pathophysiology of mitral stenosis

A normal mitral valve opens to an area of 4–6 cm^2. Significant symptoms resulting from mitral valve stenosis generally occur when the valve area is <2–2.5 cm^2. The narrowing of the valve orifice results in a diastolic transmitral pressure gradient. Blood can flow from the left atrium to the left ventricle only if propelled by a pressure gradient. The diastolic pressure gradient is the fundamental expression of mitral stenosis and results in elevation of left atrial pressure, which is reflected back into the pulmonary venous circulation resulting in pulmonary congestion [1,2].

For any given orifice size, the transmitral gradient is a function of the square of the transvalvular flow rate. Thus, if there is an increase in transmitral flow or a decrease in the diastolic filling, symptoms may develop secondary to elevation of left atrial pressure, even when a given mitral valve area under ordinary circumstances may not be associated with symptoms. A mitral valve area of >2.5 cm^2 is usually not associated with symptoms at rest (mild mitral stenosis). Exercise, emotional stress, infection, pregnancy, or atrial fibrillation with increased ventricular rate may precipitate symptoms, however, by increasing the flow rate and decreasing the diastolic filling period [1,2].

As the orifice area decreases further, the left atrial pressure rises with a concomitant progression of symptoms. As the severity of stenosis increases, cardiac output becomes subnormal at rest and fails to increase during exercise. Once the valve area becomes less than 1 cm^2, severe mitral stenosis is present and nearly all patients have some degree of activity limitation. Pulmonary artery hypertension frequently complicates mitral stenosis. With increasing pulmonary hypertension, an increase in right ventricular end-diastolic volume and pressure as well as secondary tricuspid insufficiency may ensue, which may ultimately result in heart failure and systemic venous congestion. Further reduced forward output occurs with increasing pulmonary vascular resistance.

The natural history of rheumatic mitral stenosis was characterized in the 1950s and 1960s. The classic progression was 10 years from the occurrence of rheumatic fever to the onset of symptoms in women in their second and third decades of life. Ten years later symptoms would become disabling as a result of severe heart failure and/or pulmonary hypertension. In North America and Europe, this classic history of mitral stenosis has been replaced by a milder delayed course owing to the decline in rheumatic fever. The mean age at presentation is now in the fifth and sixth decades of life. Women still predominate, however, making up two-thirds of all patients with rheumatic mitral stenosis. Serial hemodynamic and Doppler echocardiographic studies have reported annual loss of mitral valve area, ranging from 0.09 to 0.32 cm^2 [1,2,6].

Pathology of rheumatic mitral stenosis

Rheumatic fever results in characteristic changes in the mitral valve, including thickening of the leaflets, fusion of the commissures, and chordal shortening and fusion (Fig. 20.2). With acute rheumatic fever, there is inflammation and edema of the leaflets, with small fibrin–platelet thrombi along the leaflet contact zones. Subsequent scarring leads to the characteristic valve deformity with obliteration of the normal leaflet architecture

Table 20.1 Severity of mitral stenosis [2].

	Mild	Moderate	Severe
Mean gradient (mmHg)	<5	5–10	>10
Pulmonary artery systolic pressure (mmHg)	<30	30–50	>50
Valve area (cm^2)	>1.5	1.0–1.5	<1.0

These are accepted criteria when heart rate is between 60 and 90 beats/min.

by fibrosis, neovascularization, and increased collagen and tissue cellularity. Superimposed calcification results in further dysfunction [6].

Diagnostic evaluation

Echocardiography is indicated in patients for the diagnosis of mitral stenosis, assessment of hemodynamic severity (mean gradient, mitral valve area, and pulmonary artery pressure), assessment of concomitant valvular lesions, and assessment of valve morphology (to determine suitability for percutaneous mitral valve balloon valvotomy). Echocardiography confirms the diagnosis and identification of acquired causes of mitral stenosis that require further therapy. The severity of stenosis is based on mean transvalvular gradient, resting pulmonary artery pressures, and calculated valve area (Table 20.1) [2].

Additional indications for echocardiography include re-evaluation of patients with known mitral stenosis and changing symptoms or signs. Echocardiography should be performed for assessment of the hemodynamic response of the mean gradient and pulmonary artery pressure by exercise Doppler echocardiography in patients with mitral stenosis when there is discrepancy between resting Doppler echocardiography

findings, clinical findings, symptoms and/or signs. Transesophageal echocardiography is indicated to assess the presence or absence of left atrial thrombus and to further evaluate the severity of mitral insufficiency in patients considered for mitral valve intervention [2].

An echocardiographic score has been developed to describe the morphology of the mitral valve complex. Commonly used scores evaluate four factors: leaflet mobility, degree of subvalvular fusion, leaflet thickness, and leaflet calcification (Table 20.2). Each factor is given a score of 1–4, with 1 being least involved and 4 being most involved. The sum of the four factors is the total score (minimum score, 4; maximum score, 16). This scoring grade predicts the acute and intermediate term outcome of percutaneous mitral valve balloon valvotomy. Patients with a total score of ≤8 often achieve excellent immediate results with a low incidence of complications. Patients with a score >10 have less optimal results and a higher risk of complications to include restenosis [1,2].

Cardiac catheterization for hemodynamic evaluation is no longer necessary for all patients and, at our clinic, is reserved for patients in whom further information is required after a comprehensive two-dimensional and Doppler echocardiography assessment. Reasonable indications include a discrepancy between noninvasive tests and clinical findings regarding the severity of mitral stenosis, the presence of doubt as to the severity of pulmonary arterial hypertension when out of proportion to the severity of the mitral stenosis as determined by noninvasive testing, and assessment of the hemodynamic response of pulmonary artery and left atrial pressures to exercise when clinical symptoms and resting hemodynamics are discordant [1,2].

Indications for intervention

Percutaneous mitral valve balloon valvotomy is indicated and is effective for symptomatic patients (New York Heart

Table 20.2 Echocardiographic score for percutaneous mitral valve balloon valvotomy [2].

Score	Leaflet mobility	Subvalvular thickening	Leaflet thickening	Leaflet calcification
1	Highly mobile valve with only leaflet tips restricted	Minimal thickening just below the mitral leaflets	Leaflets near normal in thickness (4–5 mm)	A single area of increased echocardiography brightness
2	Leaflet mid and base portions have normal mobility	Thickening of chordal structures extending up to one-third of the chordal length	Mid leaflets normal, considerable thickening of margins (5–8 mm)	Scattered areas of brightness confined to leaflet margins
3	Valve continues to move forward in diastole, mainly from the base	Thickening extending to the distal third of the chords	Thickening extending through the entire leaflet (5–8 mm)	Brightness extending into the mid portion of the leaflets
4	No or minimal forward movement of the leaflets in diastole	Extensive thickening and shortening of all chordal structures extending down to the papillary muscles	Considerable thickening of all leaflet tissue (more than 8–10 mm)	Extensive brightness throughout much of the leaflet tissue

Association [NYHA] functional class II, III, or IV) with moderate or severe mitral stenosis and valve morphology favorable for percutaneous mitral valve balloon valvotomy; it can be safely performed in pregnant patients. It is also effective for asymptomatic patients with moderate or severe mitral stenosis and favorable valve morphology who have severe pulmonary hypertension (pulmonary artery systolic pressure of >50 mmHg at rest or >60 mmHg with exercise), although it is controversial as to whether these patients with severe pulmonary hypertension should be referred directly for mitral valve replacement to prevent right ventricular failure. Percutaneous mitral valve balloon valvotomy should not be performed in patients with moderate or worse mitral insufficiency or left atrial thrombus [2].

Mitral valve operation is indicated in patients with symptomatic (NYHA functional class III or IV) moderate, or severe mitral stenosis when (1) percutaneous mitral valve balloon valvotomy is unavailable, (2) percutaneous mitral valve balloon valvotomy is contraindicated because of left atrial thrombus, despite anticoagulation, or because concomitant moderate or worse mitral insufficiency is present, or (3) the valve morphology is not favorable for percutaneous mitral valve balloon valvotomy in a patient with acceptable operative risk. Operation is also reasonable for patients with severe mitral stenosis and severe pulmonary hypertension, with NYHA functional class I or II symptoms, who are not considered candidates for percutaneous mitral valve balloon valvotomy. Mitral valve repair may be considered for asymptomatic patients with moderate or worse mitral stenosis who have had recurrent embolic events while receiving adequate anticoagulation and who have valve morphology favorable for repair [2].

Surgical technique

Mitral valve exposure

Our standard approach to the mitral valve is via median sternotomy, although alternate incisions and robotic assistance are used in selected cases [5]. Sternotomy allows complete access to all the cardiac chambers and great vessels. Cannulation for cardiopulmonary bypass, managing aortic valve insufficiency, monitoring the left ventricle for distention, and evacuating air are all easier when using the midline approach. In addition, median sternotomy allows for other cardiac procedures, such as coronary artery revascularization and arrhythmia operation, if necessary.

After median sternotomy is performed, cardiopulmonary bypass is instituted with cannulation of the aorta and right atrium. A single two-stage venous atrial cannula provides satisfactory venous return for most patients. If the left atrium is small or if blood return from the superior vena cava to the single cannula is obstructed during atrial retraction, separate cannulae for the cavae should be used. Typically, this includes

a right-angle superior vena cava cannula and a straight or right-angle inferior vena cava cannula. Dual venous cannulation is also advantageous during reoperations on the mitral valve; after isolation of the right atrium, incision across the atrial septum gives excellent exposure to the mitral valve.

Other maneuvers that may improve mitral valve exposure include lifting up on the right pericardial sutures, avoiding traction sutures on the left, and mobilizing the superior and inferior venae cavae. In patients with pericardial adhesions (e.g., reoperations) freeing the apex of the heart from adhesions and/or opening the left pleural space allows the apex of the heart to fall posteriorly, and thus improves exposure of the mitral valve.

Occasionally, a right anterolateral thoracotomy is preferred for mitral valve surgery. Short inframammary incisions are useful in women who have concerns about the cosmetic appearance of the midline incision; and the approach is also useful in selected patients with previous median sternotomy and anatomic considerations that make repeat median sternotomy risky. Typical patients include those with patent arterial coronary bypass grafts, especially if they cross the midline, and patients with other potential hazards, such as previous sternotomy and an enlarged right ventricle. There is also increasing experience in using minimally invasive techniques (video assisted, robotic) to repair the mitral valve. Exposure in such instances is a variation of the right anterolateral thoracotomy approach.

For the right anterolateral thoracotomy approach, the patient is positioned at a 30° tilt, right side up, and the patient's right arm is positioned overhead. The chest is entered through the fifth interspace via an incision made from just right of the sternum to the anterior axillary line. One-lung ventilation is preferred. Pulling the diaphragm down with stay sutures, brought through the inferior intercostal spaces and tagged on traction enhances exposure of the atria. The nonventilated lung is retracted posteriorly, and cardiopulmonary bypass cannulae (two venous, one arterial) are placed. Peripheral cannulation using the femoral artery and femoral vein facilitates these smaller incisions. Vacuum assist is a helpful adjunct for venous drainage in this setting.

Atriotomy

After cardiopulmonary bypass is established at normothermia or mild hypothermia, the aortic cross-clamp is applied and cold blood cardioplegia is administered, producing complete cardiac arrest [5]. In most patients, the mitral valve is exposed with an incision in the left atrium just posterior to the interatrial groove. Before making the atriotomy, the interatrial groove can be developed several centimeters with sharp dissection. The incision begins on the anterolateral left atrium near the junction of the right superior pulmonary vein and left atrium, posterior to Waterston's groove. It continues inferiorly between the right inferior pulmonary vein and the inferior vena cava. By developing the interatrial

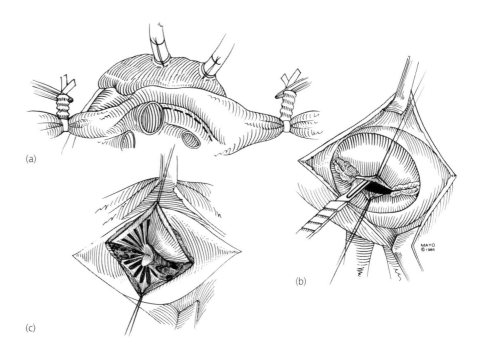

Figure 20.3 Technique of open commissurotomy.

plane, the left atrial incision can be made approximately 2–4 cm from the right pulmonary veins, giving closer exposure of the mitral valve.

Other atrial incisions may be useful in circumstances in which exposure is poor, as sometimes occurs in patients with a large anteroposterior chest diameter, patients with marked concentric left ventricular hypertrophy, and in some patients undergoing reoperation. For example, a simple trans-septal incision provides excellent exposure of the mitral valve and is favored when a right atriotomy is necessary for treatment of concomitant tricuspid valve disease. This approach is also useful in patients who have had multiple previous operations; with repeated left atriotomies the tissue may be stiff and fibrotic, making retraction and valve exposure difficult.

In rare situations, it may be impossible to adequately expose the mitral valve through a standard left atriotomy, and the surgeon may use additional incisions, such as the biatrial transseptal incision as described by Brawley [7] or other modifications of the original Dubost technique. Additionally, the extended vertical transatrial septal approach as described by Guiraudon *et al.* [8] opens both atria widely, giving excellent mitral valve exposure, even in the setting of a small left atrium.

Mitral valve examination

After the heart has been arrested and the atriotomy has been performed, the left atrial appendage is examined for thrombi and the mitral valve is inspected. Thrombi are removed and the ostium of the left atrial appendage is usually oversewn. The entire mitral valve complex must be carefully examined to confirm the mechanism of the mitral stenosis and to assess the feasibility of reconstruction. Important features to be noted include leaflet pliability, thickness, induration and

retraction, chordal thickening, degree of mitral insufficiency, and site and extent of any calcification [9].

Mitral valve repair

Exploration for possible valve repair is indicated in a selected group of patients with relatively preserved and pliable anterior leaflet and subvalvular apparatus. Open mitral commissurotomy is the preferred technique and begins at the anterolateral commissure [10]. A blunt-ended, long-handled hook is placed beneath each leaflet on either side of the anterolateral commissure and gentle traction is applied. The anterior hook is pulled anteroinferiorly, and the posterior hook is pulled posteroinferiorly. This displays and spreads out the region of the anterolateral commissure. Alternatively, a 3–0 Prolene suture can be placed in the mid portion of the anterior and posterior leaflets to serve as retraction sutures. The commissure is identified carefully and the surgeon should note the underlying chordal anatomy. In some patients, the commissure can be opened with gentle blunt dissection, and in other patients the commissure is recreated by a sharp incision with a knife (Fig. 20.3).

An important step in surgical commissurotomy is incision and mobilization of fused chordae; the incision in the fused chordae can be carried through the papillary muscle to further increase mobility of the leaflets. When incising the commissure, care is taken to maintain a distance of about 3–4 mm from the annulus. Otherwise, if the commissure is incised too close to the annulus, there is risk of producing a flail anterior leaflet and subsequent postoperative eccentric mitral insufficiency.

Following successful treatment of the anterolateral commissure, a similar procedure is repeated on the posteromedial commissure. After release of the fused commissural and sub-valvular components, the pliability of the mitral leaflets may be improved by leaflet thinning. It is important to check for regurgitation after commissurotomy, and in some patients, commissural plication may be necessary to shorten the posterior annulus and increase the area of leaflet coaptation to prevent eccentric mitral insufficiency.

Annular dilation can result in repair failure. The simple means to avoid this, as described by Carpentier (quoted by Yau *et al.* [11]), is to use a prosthetic ring to reinforce the annulus. It is important to use a large prosthetic ring in rheumatic valvular disease to compensate for the increased rigidity of the leaflets and to reduce the incidence of recurrent stenosis. The ring is secured to the annulus with interrupted 2–0 Ethibond sutures. In rare cases, leaflet extension of the anterior, posterior, or both leaflets using glutaraldehyde-treated autologous pericardium may be necessary.

Completion transesophageal echocardiography

It is important for the echocardiographer and surgeon to be familiar with the characteristics of the repaired valve that may increase the likelihood of residual insufficiency or repair failure. Residual mitral insufficiency greater than grade I or mild must be addressed surgically during the same operation by a either a re-repair or replacement. Although the exact location of mitral insufficiency may not be as important to identify before the first attempt at repair, it is very helpful to determine which segment is causing a residual leak post repair, using transesophageal echocardiography before repeat surgical exploration. If the first repair was felt to be satisfactory by visual examination, the transesophageal echocardiogram may be the only guide to aid the surgeon attempting a re-repair of the mitral valve [12].

Mitral valve replacement

When mitral valve replacement is necessary, consideration should be given to preservation of the subvalvular apparatus [5]. We usually excise the anterior leaflet but preserve the posterior leaflet and its subvalvular apparatus if they are not involved by infection or extensive calcification. However, in many patients the posterior leaflet is so thickened and abnormal that it cannot be preserved because the tissue interferes with an adequate-sized prosthesis or may interfere with the prosthetic valve function. In such instances, we would resect the portions of the posterior leaflet and subvalvular apparatus. Preservation of chordae helps maintain ventricular geometry and function of the papillary muscles. The intact posterior chordae reduce longitudinal tension on the posterior left ventricular free wall and reduce the risk of atrioventricular groove disruption [13].

To anchor the prosthetic valve, we use 2–0 Ethibond mattress sutures with the pledgets situated on the ventricular side. If a tissue valve is placed and the mitral orifice is large, the leaflet tissues are simply pinned up toward the annulus. If a mechanical valve is being placed, it may be difficult to tether the leaflet tissue and chordae safely out of the way of the valvular mechanism. In this situation, resection of the leaflet and subvalvular apparatus may be indicated. In contrast to the situation with degenerative mitral valve disease, it is rarely possible to preserve the anterior leaflet during valve replacement for rheumatic mitral valve stenosis. One technique proposed for preservation of the leaflet involves detaching a rim of approximately 5 mm of leaflet tissue from the anterior annulus. The incision is carried to each commissure, freeing the anterior leaflet from the annulus. Two 1- to 2-cm pods of leaflet are retained that contain the chordae to each of the papillary muscles. The pods are secured to the annulus at the 2–3 and 9–10 o'clock positions with the corresponding pledgetted valve sutures [14].

Calcified annulus

Valve replacement in the face of a heavily calcified mitral annulus presents a special challenge. Aggressive debridement of calcification is risky, with possible complications including circumflex coronary artery damage and atrioventricular disruption. Fortunately, the calcification is posterior to the trigones in 98% of patients and rarely involves the leaflets (6%) or extensively the ventricular myocardium or papillary muscles (20%). Usually, the anterior annulus is spared [15]. In only a minority of cases will the calcium be so extensive as to require radical debridement. In our practice, as well as at other clinics, most surgeons avoid extensive debridement unless absolutely necessary [14].

With mild to moderate annular calcification, we remove the anterior leaflet, leaving a 5-mm rim of tissue for suture placement and leaving the posterior calcified annulus intact. The sutures can usually be placed in the usual fashion, taking generous tissue bites and avoiding the calcium as much as possible. The sutures being placed with the pledgets on the ventricular side allow direct tissue–sewing ring apposition. It is helpful to choose a valve with a generous sewing cuff that prevents leakage between crevices of calcium.

If calcification is more severe and sutures can not be placed through the annulus, one option is to anchor the prosthesis directly to the leaflets themselves; one may have to downsize the prosthesis a size or two to obtain a good fit. Another option involves seating the prosthesis in a supra-annular position by placing mattress sutures within the left atrium, just above the calcified annulus. Pledgetted sutures placed from the atrial to the ventricular side are best for this technique.

Rarely, heavy circumferential leaflet and annular calcification precludes safe suture placement, and the only option may be to debride the calcium. Caution must be carried out during this portion of the procedure to avoid injury to the circumflex coronary artery and atrioventricular connection (Fig. 20.1). If debridement is extensive and puts the patient at risk of atrioventricular disruption, pericardial reconstruction of the annular defect with pledgetted sutures is indicated. Horizontal mattress sutures can be passed through the pericardium creating a new portion of the annulus to anchor the valve prosthesis [5].

Management of the left atrial appendage

Because of the risk of thrombosis formation and systemic embolization, the left atrial appendage should be excluded from the circulation by ligation or oversewing of the orifice. This is advisable for all patients who are in atrial fibrillation and for most patients having mitral valve replacement for rheumatic heart disease. The major exception would be patients with very friable tissue who might be at risk of bleeding.

Management of associated atrial fibrillation

Atrial remodeling in mitral stenosis is characterized by left atrial enlargement, loss of myocardium, and scarring, which produces widespread conduction abnormalities and is associated with a heightened inducibility of atrial fibrillation. Indeed, atrial fibrillation is present in 30–50% of patients who require mitral valve surgery, and the risk of ischemic stroke is increased sixfold in patients with atrial fibrillation compared with the normal population. Loss of atrial contraction with the onset of atrial fibrillation often precipitates symptoms in patients with rheumatic mitral valve stenosis.

Consideration should be given to performing the Cox maze procedure or one of its modifications in patients with rheumatic mitral valve disease undergoing valve repair or replacement. Maintenance of sinus rhythm may improve functional capacity, and recent studies suggest that risk of development of late tricuspid valve regurgitation after mitral valve surgery is reduced when sinus rhythm is maintained [16].

It is important to recognize, however, that success in restoring sinus rhythm in patients with rheumatic heart disease and atrial fibrillation (60–70%) is lower than that observed in patients who have had Cox maze procedures for lone atrial fibrillation or for atrial fibrillation associated with degenerative mitral valve disease (80–90%). An additional factor is that most patients having valve replacement for rheumatic heart disease will receive mechanical prostheses and require long-term anticoagulation with coumadin. Therefore, if there is concern that the additional time and manipulation of surgical ablation of atrial fibrillation at the time of mitral valve surgery might increase the hazard of operation, it may be advisable to simply replace or repair the valve and obliterate the left atrial appendage.

Management of associated tricuspid valve disease

Rheumatic involvement of the tricuspid valve leaflets and chordae may aggravate right heart failure in patients with rheumatic mitral valve disease. Scarring of the tricuspid valve (organic tricuspid valve disease) usually produces both stenosis and insufficiency because of the fixed small orifice, and when this is present in patients undergoing mitral valve surgery the tricuspid valve should be replaced with a mechanical or biologic prosthesis. Methods of repair have been described, but results are much less satisfactory than with pure insufficiency of the mitral valve, and there is risk of ongoing scarring and subsequent valve malfunction.

A more common problem is central tricuspid valve insufficiency, with normal leaflets and variable degrees of annular dilation and pulmonary artery hypertension. Tricuspid valve leakage in such circumstances is termed functional (or secondary) regurgitation, but this may be a misnomer because the rheumatic process can cause dilation of the tricuspid valve annulus without significant pulmonary hypertension. Clinical experience and longitudinal studies have shown that valve replacement for severe mitral valve stenosis does not always lead to regression of pulmonary artery hypertension or to reduction in tricuspid valve annulus enlargement. Indeed, some surgeons advise that concomitant tricuspid valve repair be undertaken when the diameter of the tricuspid valve annulus is ≥70 mm, regardless of the degree of valve leakage [17].

An additional complicating factor is that tricuspid valve regurgitation often appears less severe when using transesophageal echocardiography during general anesthesia than with the degree assessed by transthoracic study preoperatively. It is our practice, therefore, to perform tricuspid valve annuloplasty in all patients with moderate or greater tricuspid valve insufficiency who undergo operation for rheumatic mitral valve disease. Further, we would consider tricuspid annuloplasty in patients with any degree of tricuspid valve leakage when there is clinical evidence of right heart failure (hepatic congestion, peripheral edema, etc.) or when the annulus is greatly dilated.

Results

The immediate results of percutaneous mitral valve balloon valvotomy are similar to those of open mitral commissurotomy. The mean valve area usually doubles (from $1–2 \, cm^2$), with a 50–60% reduction in transmitral gradient. Overall, the procedure is successful in 80–95% of patients, which is defined as a mitral valve area greater than $1.5 \, cm^2$ and a decrease in left atrial pressure to < 18 mmHg in the absence of complications. The most common acute complications include severe mitral insufficiency, which occurs in 2–10%, and a residual atrial septal defect, which occurs in 5–12%. Less frequent complications include perforation of the left ventricle (0.5–4%), embolic events (0.5–3%), and myocardial infarction (0.3–0.5%). The mortality rate ranges from 1% to 2% [2].

Event-free survival (freedom from death, repeat valvotomy, or mitral valve operation) after percutaneous mitral valve balloon valvotomy is 50–65% at 3–7 years, with an event-free survival of 80–90% in patients with favorable mitral valve pathology. More than 90% of patients free of events remain in NYHA functional class I or II after percutaneous mitral valve balloon valvotomy. Patients with valvular calcification, thickened fibrotic leaflets with decreased mobility, and subvalvular fusion have a higher incidence of acute complications and a higher rate of recurrent stenosis on follow-up. In many cases, mitral valve operation is preferable for patients with severe calcification and deformity.

Mitral valve repair is possible in less than one-fourth of patients operated on for rheumatic mitral disease [10,12]. Repair techniques include open commissurotomy (with or without annuloplasty) in isolated mitral stenosis or more complex repairs in patients with mixed stenosis and insufficiency. Early results are excellent with operative mortality rates of <1% and overall 5- and 10-year survival of 97% and 88%, respectively. As with percutaneous mitral valve balloon valvotomy, however, restenosis may occur late after operation, and freedom from reoperation at 10 years ranges from 72% to 87%. Further, 5- and 10-year freedom from thromboembolic complications are both reported at 93% with an annualized rate of 0.5% per patient-year.

Most patients having operation for rheumatic mitral disease undergo valve replacement. Significant valvular calcification, thickened fibrotic leaflets with decreased mobility, and subvalvular fusion often preclude an attempt at valve repair. Operative mortality at the Mayo Clinic is 1% for elective mitral valve replacement in patients younger than 75 years [5]. In a series of over 573 mitral valve operations for rheumatic disease, Yau *et al.* [11] reported that overall 5- and 10-year survival is not significantly different between bioprosthetic (83% and 70%, respectively) and mechanical valves (88% and 73%, respectively). As expected, 5- and 10-year freedom from reoperation rates are significantly lower with bioprosthetic (94% and 69%, respectively) than with mechanical valves (96% and 95%, respectively). Conversely, 5- and 10-year freedom from thromboembolic complications rates are higher with bioprosthetic (94% and 93%, respectively) than with mechanical valves (89% and 72%, respectively). There is, however, no significant difference in late valve-related morbidity (5- and 10-year freedom reoperation, endocarditis, or thromboembolic event) comparing mechanical and bioprosthesis valves [12].

The decision for repair versus replacement in rheumatic mitral disease is difficult in some patients. In Yau *et al.*'s series [11], better late cardiac survival was independently predicted by valve repair rather than by replacement. However, freedom from reoperation was greatest, and freedom from thromboembolic complications rate was lowest, after mechanical valve replacement [12]. Importantly, 23 patients in their series (16%) underwent reoperation after initial valve repair with no operative deaths, thus somewhat minimizing the effect of reoperation on the long-term outcome of patients treated with initial valve repair. We believe that rheumatic mitral valves should be repaired when pathologic findings are favorable because this late survival is the best and freedom from thromboembolic complications is excellent. But young patients undergoing open commissurotomy should be informed of the probable need for late valve replacement.

References

1. Bruce CJ & Nishimura RA (1998) Clinical assessment and management of mitral stenosis. *Cardiol Clin* **16**:375–403.
2. Bonow RO, Carabello BA, Chatterjee K, *et al.* (2006) ACC/AHA 2006 guidelines for the management of patients with valvular heart disease: a report of the American College of Cardiology/American Heart Association Task Force on Practice Guidelines (Writing Committee to Develop Guidelines for the Management of Patients With Valvular Heart Disease). *Circulation* **114**:e84–e231.
3. Shah P (2005) Heart and great vessels. In: Standring S, Ellis H, Healy JC, *et al.* (eds). *Gray's Anatomy*: *The Anatomical Basis of Clinical Practice*, 39th edn. Edinburgh: Elsevier, pp. 1006–1008.
4. Filsoufi F & Carpentier A (2007) Principles of reconstructive surgery in degenerative mitral valve disease. *Semin Thorac Cardiovasc Surg* **19**:103–110.
5. Burkhart HM & Zehr KJ 2004) Mitral valve replacement. In: Yang SC & Cameron DE (eds). *Current Therapy in Thoracic and Cardiovascular Surgery*. Philadelphia: Mosby Publishing, pp. 623–626.
6. Otto CM & Bonow R (2008) Valvular heart disease. In: Braunwald E (ed.). *Braunwald's Heart Disease*: *A Textbook of Cardiovascular Medicine*. Philadelphia: Saunders, Elsevier, pp. 1646–1657.
7. Brawley RF (1980) Improved exposure of the mitral valve in patients with a small left atrium. *Ann Thorac Surg* **29**:179–181.
8. Guiraudon GM, Ofiesh JG, & Kaushik R (1991) Extended vertical transatrial septal approach to the mitral valve. *Ann Thorac Surg* **52**:1058–1060.
9. Ghosh PK, Choudhary A, Agarwal SK *et al.* (1997) Role of an operative score in mitral reconstruction in dominantly stenotic lesions. *Eur J Cardiothorac Surg* **11**:274–279.
10. Choudhary SK, Dhareshwar J, Govil A *et al.* (2003) Open mitral commissurotomy in the current era: indications, technique, and results. *Ann Thorac Surg* **75**:41–46.
11. Yau Tm, Farag El-Ghoneimi YA, Armstong S *et al.* (2000) Mitral valve repair and replacement for rheumatic disease. *J Thorac Cardiovasc Surg* **119**:53–61.
12. Suri RM & Orszulak TA (2005) Triangular resection for repair of mitral regurgitation due to degenerative disease. *Oper Tech Thorac Cardiovasc Surg* **10**:194–199.
13. Glower DD (2000) Mitral valve implantation. *Oper Tech Thorac Cardiovasc Surg* **5**:242–250.
14. Smedira NG (2003) Mitral valve replacement with a calcified annulus. *Oper Tech Thorac Cardiovasc Surg* **8**:2–13.
15. Carpentier AF, Pellerin M, Fuzellier JF, *et al.* (1996) Extensive calcification of the mitral valve annulus: pathology and surgical management. *J Thorac Cardiovasc Surg* **111**:718–730.
16. Stulak JM, Schaff HV, Dearani JA, *et al.* (2008) Restoration of sinus rhythm by the Maze procedure halts progression of tricuspid regurgitation after mitral surgery. *Ann Thorac Surg* **86**:40–44.
17. Dreyfus GD, Corbi PJ, Chan KM, *et al.* (2005) Secondary tricuspid regurgitation or dilatation: which should be the criteria for surgical repair? *Ann Thorac Surg* **79**:127–132.

21   Pathology of Mitral Insufficiency

Esther Herpel[1], Arne Warth[1], Artur Lichtenberg[2] & Philipp A. Schnabel[1]

[1]Institute of Pathology, University Clinics Heidelberg, Germany
[2]Clinic for Cardiovascular Surgery, University of Düsseldorf, Düsseldorf, Germany

Definition

Mitral insufficiency is characterized by an inability of the mitral valve to close completely. Acute mitral insufficiency is distinguished from chronic mitral insufficiency according to the time course [1].

Epidemiology

Mitral insufficiency is the second most frequent reason for valve surgery and is one of the most frequent acquired heart valve pathologies worldwide [2–6].

Etiology

Mitral insufficiency may be secondary to abnormalities of the valve leaflets, mitral annulus, papillary muscles, and their adjacent musculature. Chronic rheumatoid heart disease, leading to mitral valve retraction and/or shortening of chordae tendineae, accounts for about one-third of cases of severe mitral insufficiency, and occurs more frequently in males [7–9]. Further common causes that may affect these structures are degenerative diseases such as mitral valve prolapse, which leads to elongated chordae tendineae, rupture of chordae tendineae with a "flail leaflet," annular dilation, as in Marfan's syndrome, and calcification.

Ischemic mitral regurgitation is another cause of mitral regurgitation, and leads to reduced movement as a result of eccentric papillary muscle tension. It is caused by coronary heart disease, acute myocardial infarction or scarring of the myocardium after infarction, and left ventricular impairment and dilation. An extremely dramatic event leading to acute mitral regurgitation is the rupture of a papillary muscle as a result of acute myocardial infarction [10].

Cardiovascular Interventions in Clinical Practice. Edited by Jürgen Haase, Hans-Joachim Schäfers, Horst Sievert and Ron Waksman. © 2010 Blackwell Publishing.

Infrequent etiologies for mitral valve insufficiency are systemic lupus erythematosus (endocarditis Libman–Sacks), hypertrophic obstructive cardiomyopathy, trauma, a mitral valve cleft or an insufficient valvular prosthesis, and ankylosing spondylitis [11–15]. Congenital mitral insufficiency is less frequent, and in 10% the etiology is unclear [2]. Extreme calcifications are predominantly reported in elderly women.

Table 21.1 summarizes the causes of mitral insufficiency in relation to mitral leaflet, subvalvular apparatus, and myocardial pathology/dysfunction.

Anatomy and physiology of the mitral valve

"Normal" anatomy and physiology are described in Chapter 16. The competence and functional integrity of the mitral valve depend on the following anatomic structures: (1) posterior left atrial wall, (2) annulus fibrosus, (3) leaflets/valve cups, (4) chordae tendineae, (5) papillary muscle, and (6) left ventricular wall [16]. If any of these anatomic structures is affected by acquired or congenital disorders, the finely coordinated mechanism upholding functional integrity is deranged and leads to abnormal function [7,17]. The normal mean perimeter of the mitral valve is about 8.2–9.9 cm. Perimeters longer than 12 cm suggest mitral valve insufficiency.

Pathophysiology

The exact mechanical alterations leading to the development of ischemic mitral insufficiency are not well defined [1,17]. In experimental studies, ischemic mitral insufficiency was attributed to global changes in the left ventricle geometry [18–20]. More recently, *in vitro* [21] and animal studies [22–25] have suggested that the pathogenesis is more complex, related to alterations in spatial relationships between the left ventricle and the mitral valve apparatus. In human studies, mitral annulus enlargement, increased mitral tenting area, and loss of systolic mitral annular contraction [23–25] have been proposed as possible mechanisms. However, restrictions in imaging and analysis of mitral insufficiency degree, mitral

Table 21.1 Causes of mitral insufficiency (MI) in relation to mitral leaflet, subvalvular apparatus, and myocardial pathology/dysfunction.

Causes of MI	Predominantly		
	Leaflets	Subvalvular apparatus	Myocardium
Acute MI			
Myocardial infarction	–	+/++	+++
Rupture of chordae tendineae	–	+++	–
Acute endocarditis	+++	+	(+)
Heart failure	–	(+)	+++
Chronic MI			
Rheumatic heart disease	++	++	–
Degenerative MI	++/+++	+/++	–
Calcifying MI	+/++	++/+++	(+)
Ischemic MI	–	+	++
Floppy mitral valve	++/+++	++	–
Systemic immunologic disorder	++/+++	++	+

deformation, and global and local left ventricle remodeling have limited these studies.

The insufficient mitral orifice may be considered to lie in parallel with the aortic orifice, and, thus, resistance to left ventricular emptying is reduced in patients with mitral insufficiency. Consequently, the left ventricle is decompressed into the left atrium during ejection. Accompanying the reduction in left ventricular size is a rapid decline in the left ventricular wall tension. This leads to a progressive reduction in left ventricular afterload, allowing a greater proportion of left ventricular contractile activity to be expended in shortening. The initial compensation of mitral insufficiency consists of more complete systolic emptying of the left ventricle. A progressive increase in the left ventricular end-diastolic volume occurs as the severity of the regurgitation increases and the function of the ventricle deteriorates. Left ventricular end-diastolic pressure may be slightly elevated. However, in chronic mitral insufficiency, there is often an increase in left ventricular compliance so that the ventricular volume may be increased with little elevation in the end-diastolic pressure gradient. If this end-diastolic pressure gradient persists throughout diastole, in the presence of an associated mitral stenosis of significant degree, a brief early diastolic gradient may occur in patients with pure regurgitation (mitral insufficiency) as a result of the torrential flow of blood across a normal-sized mitral orifice.

Patients with severe mitral insufficiency may be divided into four subgroups, depending on the compliance (i.e., the pressure–volume relationship of the left atrium and pulmonary venous bed and the regurgitation fraction of stroke volume).

The first group comprises patients with acute mitral insufficiency resulting from infarction, rupture of chordae tendineae, or papillary muscle rupture. These patients show little enlarge-

ment of the left atrium but left atrial pressure is markedly increased and regurgitation fraction is more than 50% of the stroke volume. Compliance is normal or reduced.

The second group consists of patients with chronic or long-term severe mitral insufficiency. The regurgitation fraction is about 30–50%. of the stroke volume. The left atrium is massively enlarged and shows thinning of the walls. Left atrial pressure and pulmonary vascular resistance are normal or only slightly elevated.

The third group of patients show hemodynamic features, such as a regurgitation fraction of 15–30% of stroke volume. There is a moderate increase in compliance. The patient's left atrium shows variable degrees of enlargement with significant elevation of left atrial pressure. Sooner or later the hemodynamic parameters deteriorate and these patients must be recategorized into the second group.

The fourth group shows a very mild form of mitral insufficiency, with only mild hemodynamic features. The regurgitation fraction is less than 15% of stroke volume.

Histopathology and clinical consequences

The anatomic elements of the mitral apparatus are given above (under Anatomy and physiology of the mitral valve) and in Chapter 16.

The macroscopic and histopathologic alterations of large series of surgically excised mitral valves have been described [7–9,26]. The most important findings in mitral insufficiency are rheumatic heart disease, degenerative mitral insufficiency, calcifying mitral insufficiency (annular calcification), ischemic mitral insufficiency (specifically in floppy mitral valve disease), and systemic immunologic disorders.

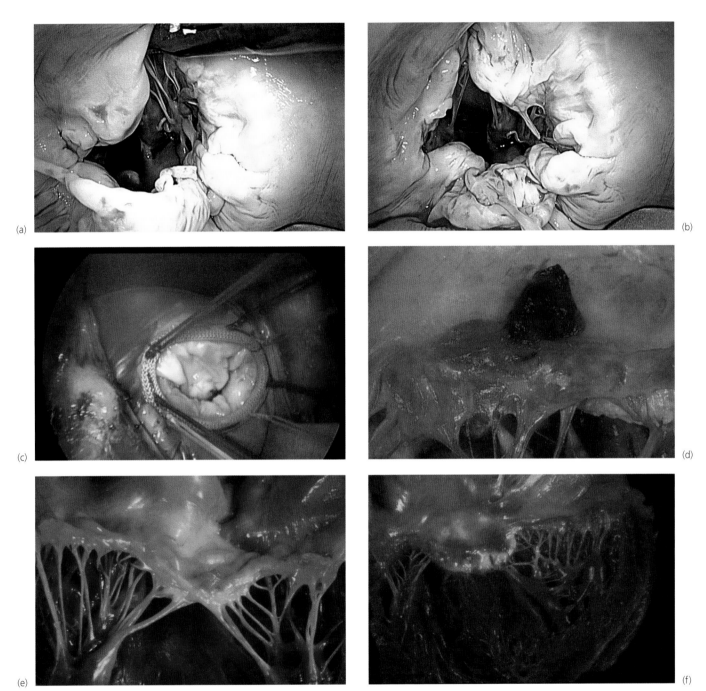

Figure 21.1 Mitral insufficiency. (a–c) Surgical reconstruction of a floppy mitral valve in a 53-year-old woman: (a) view on the bulged mitral leaflets and the large mitral orifice area from the left atrium, (b) view on the bulged mitral leaflets, an enlarged mitral orifice, and a torn chordae tendineae, (c) sufficient closure of the reconstructed mitral valve after insertion of a Carpentier ring. (d) Part of a mitral valve with a thrombus on the atrial surface post rheumatic endocarditis: autopsy specimen from a 45-year-old man. (e) Part of a mitral valve showing a small "nodule" on the atrial surface after abacterial Libman–Sacks endocarditis due to systemic lupus erythematodes: autopsy specimen from a 36-year-old woman. (f) View on a degenerated mitral valve and the dilated left ventricle autopsy in a 56-year-old man.

Rheumatic heart disease

Rheumatic heart disease leads to valve cups that macroscopically show rigidity, deformity, and retraction. There is also commissural fusion and shortening, retraction, and fusion of the chordae tendineae. The histologic alterations

have been described by different groups [7–9,27] and are considered further in Chapters 7, 12, and 16. Figure 21.1d shows a thrombus on the atrial surface after rheumatic endocarditis in an autopsy specimen from a 45-year-old man.

Degenerative mitral insufficiency

Degenerative alterations of the mitral valve are described and discussed in Chapter 16, and of the aortic valve in Chapters 7 and 12. As already discussed in these chapters, there are microscopic and clinical findings that suggest similarities with atheroinflammatory conditions [28] and, moreover, sometimes also with amyloid depositions.

Figure 21.1f shows a degenerated mitral valve with slight localized "bulging" of the thickened leaflets near the free margin in direction of the left atrium and the dilated left ventricle in an autopsy case from a 56-year-old man.

Calcifying mitral insufficiency (annular calcification)

The etiology of annular calcification is unclear. The disease is characterized by dystrophic calcifications of the mitral annulus, normally without degenerative changes of the mitral valve leaflets. Thus, the disease classically leads to mitral insufficiency and not to mitral stenosis [29] (see also Chapter 16).

Mitral annular calcification, if sufficiently extensive, prevents systolic contraction of the atrioventricular annulus. The dense calcification of the entire submittal region in its most severe form is a rigid curved bar or ring of calcium that encircles the mitral orifice, and calcific spurs may project into the adjacent left ventricular myocardium. The calcification may involve the basal portion of the valve leaflets and causes distortion of the posterior mitral valve leaflet with limitation of motion. The base of the posterior cusp is pushed up toward the atria, often stimulating a degree of mitral prolapse. This may result in insufficient leaflet area for coaptation, leading to regurgitation and congestive failure if untreated. Mitral insufficiency can be severe if found with ruptured chordae tendineae or with severely elongated chordae billowing into the atrium [30].

Ischemic mitral insufficiency

Ischemic mitral insufficiency was introduced above (under Etiology) and discussed (under Pathophysiology). Ischemic mitral insufficiency has been intensively investigated experimentally in different species and clinically in humans [31–48].

Floppy mitral valve disease

Macroscopically, the longitudinal diameter and the transverse diameter of one leaflet or both leaflets are extended, and they bulge out into the atrium like an opened parachute (Fig. 21.1a–c). The hindmost leaflet is commonly affected. Focally, there is a streaky fibrosis found in the parietal endocardium directly behind the leaflets. The chordae tendineae are mainly thickened, sometimes thinned, roughed up or frayed, and sometimes elongated. The leaflets appear jelly-like, thickened, and show interchordal bumps and bulges with a smooth surface on the atrial surface ("mitral prolapse"). The commissures are maintained, and they are never fused. Moreover, the valve tissue is never calcified [26].

Histologically, there are abundant acid mucopolysaccharides within the thickened valve, showing a strong reaction to the periodic acid–Schiff staining and Alcian-blue staining. The mucoid material is predominantly located in the spongiosa and sometimes penetrates the fibrosa, which is sometimes deleted by the mucoid material. Within the atrial part of the valve there are strong deposits of fibrosis due to dysfunction of the remodeling of the extracellular matrix [26,49].

Systemic immunologic disorders

Inflammatory rheumatoid diseases, such as rheumatoid arthritis, lupus erythematosus, antiphospholipid syndrome or systemic vasculitides, potentially involve organs and structures beyond the musculoskeletal system, including the heart, in which all structures/tissues may be affected [50,51]. In systemic lupus erythematosus, the so-called Libman–Sacks endocarditis may also lead to mitral stenosis [52], in addition to other valvular manifestations (see Chapters 12 and 16). Figure 21.1e reveals a small "nodule" on the atrial surface after abacterial Libman–Sacks endocarditis due to systemic lupus erythematosus in an autopsy specimen from a 36-year-old woman.

Treatment

Medical treatment today is mainly preserved for early, slight, or inoperable cases of mitral insufficiency [13]. The natural history of mitral insufficiency is well known from the literature [1,6,13]. Depending on the severity, extent and type of underlying disease, comorbidities, age, the special situation of the patient, and the pathologic anatomy, surgical reconstruction (Fig. 21.1a–c), interventional repair, or valve replacement may be performed.

Acknowledgments

Mr. John J. Moyers is gratefully acknowledged for assistance in preparing the figures.

References

1. Braunwald E, Zipes DP, & Libby P (2001) Valvular heart disease. In: Braunwald E, Zipes DP, Libby P (eds). *Heart Disease: A Textbook of Cardiovascular Medicine*, 6th edn. Philadelphia, PA: WB Saunders Co., pp. 1653–1660.
2. Luxereau PR, Dorent R, De Gevigney G, Bruneaval P, Chomette G, & Delahaye G (1991) Etiology of surgically treated mitral regurgitation. *Eur Heart J* **12**(Suppl. B):2–4.
3. Iung B, Baron G, Butchart EG, *et al.* (2003) A prospective survey of patients with valvular heart disease in Europe: The Euro Heart Survey on Valvular Heart Disease. *Eur Heart J* **24**:1231–1243.
4. Martinez-Selles M, Garcia-Fernandez MA, Moreno M, Larios E, García-Robles JA, & Pinto A (2006) [Influence of gender on the etiology of mitral regurgitation]. *Rev Esp Cardiol* **59**:1335–1338.

5. Iung B, Baron G, Tornos P, Gohlke-Bärwolf C, Butchart EG, & Vahanian A (2007) Valvular heart disease in the community: a European experience. *Curr Probl Cardiol* **32**:609–61.

6. Mirabel M, Iung B, Baron G, *et al.* (2007) What are the characteristics of patients with severe, symptomatic, mitral regurgitation who are denied surgery? *Eur Heart J* **28**:1358–1365.

7. Roberts WC (1983) Morphologic features of the normal and abnormal mitral valve. *Am J Cardiol* **51**:1005–1028.

8. Hanson TP, Edwards BS, & Edwards JE (1985) Pathology of surgically excised mitral valves. One hundred consecutive cases. *Arch Pathol Lab Med* **109**:823–828.

9. Leong SW, Soor GS, Butany J, Henry J, Thangaroopan M, & Leask RL (2006) Morphological findings in 192 surgically excised native mitral valves. *Can J Cardiol* **22**:1055–1061.

10. Flachskampf FA & Daniel WG (2006). [Mitral regurgitation]. *Internist (Berl)* **47**:275–283.

11. Rowe JC, Bland EF, Sprague HB, & White PD (1960) The course of mitral stenosis without surgery: ten- and twenty-year perspectives. *Ann Intern Med* **52**:741–749.

12. Gordis L (1985) The virtual disappearance of rheumatic fever in the United States: lessons in the rise and fall of disease. T. Duckett Jones memorial lecture. *Circulation* **72**:1155–1162.

13. Bonow RO, Carabello BA, Chatterjee K, *et al.* (2006) ACC/AHA 2006 guidelines for the management of patients with valvular heart disease: a report of the American College of Cardiology/American Heart Association Task Force on Practice Guidelines (writing Committee to Revise the 1998 guidelines for the management of patients with valvular heart disease) developed in collaboration with the Society of Cardiovascular Anesthesiologists endorsed by the Society for Cardiovascular Angiography and Interventions and the Society of Thoracic Surgeons. *J Am Coll Cardiol* **48**:e1–148.

14. Borghetti V, Nardi S, Bovelli D, *et al.* (2007) [Mitral regurgitation and left ventricular dysfunction: pathophysiology and surgical therapy]. *G Ital Cardiol (Rome)* **8**:498–507.

15. Brueck M, Bandorski D, & Kramer W (2007) [Flail mitral valve leaflet as incidental finding]. *Med Klin (Munich)* **102**:931–933.

16. Perloff J K & Roberts WC (1972) The mitral apparatus. Functional anatomy of mitral regurgitation. *Circulation* **46**:227–239.

17. Crawford MH, DiMarco JP, & Paulus WJ (2004) *Cardiology*, 2nd edn. London: Mosby, pp 1039–1083.

18. Blumlein S, Bouchard A, Schiller MB *et al.* (1986) Quantitation of mitral regurgitation by Doppler echocardiography. *Circulation* **74**:306–314.

19. Rokey R, Sterling LL, Zoghbi WA, *et al.* (1986) Determination of regurgitant fraction in isolated mitral or aortic regurgitation by pulsed Doppler two-dimensional echocardiography. *J Am Coll Cardiol* **7**:1273–1278.

20. Lamas G, Mitchell GF, Flaker GC, *et al.* (1997) Clinical significance of mitral regurgitation after acute myocardial infarction. Survival and Ventricular Enlargement Investigators. *Circulation* **96**:827–833.

21. He S, Fontaine, AA *et al.* (1997) Integrated mechanism for functional mitral regurgitation: leaflet restriction versus coapting force: in vitro studies. *Circulation* **96**:1826–1834.

22. Komeda M, Glasson JR, Bolger AF, *et al.* (1997) Geometric determinants of ischemic mitral regurgitation. *Circulation* **96**(Suppl.):II-128–133.

23. Gorman RC, McCaughan JS, Ratcliffe MB, *et al.* (1995) Pathogenesis of acute ischemic mitral regurgitation in three dimensions. *J Thorac Cardiovasc Surg* **109**:684–693.

24. Guy TS, Moainie SL, Gorman JH 3rd, *et al.* (2004) Prevention of ischemic mitral regurgitation does not influence the outcome of remodeling after posterolateral myocardial infarction. *J Am Coll Cardiol* **43**:377–383.

25. Enomoto Y, Gorman JH 3rd *et al.* (2005) Surgical treatment of ischemic mitral regurgitation might not influence ventricular remodeling. *J Thorac Cardiovasc Surg* **129**:504–511.

26. Turri M, Thiene G, Bortolotti U, Mazzucco A, & Gallucci V (1989) Surgical pathology of disease of the mitral valve, with special reference to lesions promoting valvar incompetence. *Int J Cardiol* **22**:213–219.

27. Hutchison SJ, Tak T, Mummaneni M, *et al.* (1995) Morphological characteristics of the regurgitant rheumatic mitral valve. *Can J Cardiol* **11**:765–769.

28. Kristen AV, Schnabel PA, Winter B, *et al.* (2009) High prevalence of amyloid in 150 surgically removed heart valves—a comparison of histological and clinical data reveals a correlation to athero-inflammatory conditions. *Cardiovasc Pathol* (Epub ahead of print).

29. Boudoulas H (2003) Etiology of valvular heart disease. *Expert Rev Cardiovasc Ther* **1**:523–532.

30. Ng CK, Punzengruber C, Pachinger O, *et al.* (2000) Valve repair in mitral regurgitation complicated by severe annulus calcification. *Ann Thorac Surg* **70**:53–58.

31. Cochran RP, Kunzelman KS, Chuong CJ, Sacks MS, & Eberhart RC (1991) Nondestructive analysis of mitral valve collagen fiber orientation. *ASAIO Trans* **37**:M447–448.

32. Kunzelman KS & Cochran RP (1992) Stress/strain characteristics of porcine mitral valve tissue: parallel versus perpendicular collagen orientation. *J Card Surg* **7**:71–78.

33. Kunzelman KS, Cochran RP, Murphree SS, Ring WS, Verrier ED, & Eberhart RC (1993) Differential collagen distribution in the mitral valve and its influence on biomechanical behaviour. *J Heart Valve Dis* **2**:236–244.

34. Kunzelman KS, Reimink MS, Verrier ED, & Cochran RP (1996) Replacement of mitral valve posterior chordae tendineae with expanded polytetrafluoroethylene suture: a finite element study. *J Card Surg* **11**:136–145; discussion 146.

35. Kunzelman KS, Reimink MS, & Cochran RP (1997) Annular dilatation increases stress in the mitral valve and delays coaptation: a finite element computer model. *Cardiovasc Surg* **5**:427–434.

36. Quick DW, Kunzelman KS, Kneebone JM, & Cochrane RP (1997) Collagen synthesis is upregulated in mitral valves subjected to altered stress. *Asaio J* **43**:181–186.

37. Kunzelman KS, Quick DW, & Cochran RP (1998) Altered collagen concentration in mitral valve leaflets: biochemical and finite element analysis. *Ann Thorac Surg* **66**(Suppl.):S198–205.

38. Otsuji Y, Handschumacher MD, Kisanuki A, Tei C, & Levine RA (1998) Functional mitral regurgitation. *Cardiologia* **43**:1011–1016.

39. Otsuji Y, Handschumacher MD, Liel-Cohen N, *et al.* (2001) Mechanism of ischemic mitral regurgitation with segmental left ventricular dysfunction: three-dimensional echocardiographic studies in models of acute and chronic progressive regurgitation. *J Am Coll Cardiol* **37**:641–648.

40. Otsuji Y, Kumanohoso T, Yoshifuku S, *et al.* (2002) Isolated annular dilation does not usually cause important functional

mitral regurgitation: comparison between patients with lone atrial fibrillation and those with idiopathic or ischemic cardiomyopathy. *J Am Coll Cardiol* **39**:1651–1656.

41. Sedransk KL, Grande-Allen KJ, & Vesely I (2002) Failure mechanics of mitral valve chordae tendineae. *J Heart Valve Dis* **11**:644–650.

42. Einstein DR, Kunzelman KS, Reinhall PG, Nicosia MA, & Cochran RP (2005) The relationship of normal and abnormal microstructural proliferation to the mitral valve closure sound. *J Biomech Eng* **127**:134–147.

43. Grande-Allen KJ, Barber JE, Klatka KM *et al.* (2005) Mitral valve stiffening in end-stage heart failure: evidence of an organic contribution to functional mitral regurgitation. *J Thorac Cardiovasc Surg* **130**:783–790.

44. Grande-Allen KJ, Borowski AG, Troughton AW, *et al.* (2005) Apparently normal mitral valves in patients with heart failure demonstrate biochemical and structural derangements: an extracellular matrix and echocardiographic study. *J Am Coll Cardiol* **45**:54–61.

45. Kuwahara E, Otsuji Y, Iguro Y, *et al.* (2006) Mechanism of recurrent/persistent ischemic/functional mitral regurgitation in the chronic phase after surgical annuloplasty: importance of augmented posterior leaflet tethering. *Circulation* **114**(Suppl.): I529–1534.

46. Ueno T, Sakata R, Iguro Y, Nagata T, Otsuji Y, & Tei C (2006) New surgical approach to reduce tethering in ischemic mitral regurgitation by relocation of separate heads of the posterior papillary muscle. *Ann Thorac Surg* **81**:2324–2325.

47. Kunzelman KS, Einstein DR, & Cochran RP (2007) Fluid-structure interaction models of the mitral valve: function in normal and pathological states. *Philos Trans R Soc Lond B Biol Sci* **362**:1393–1406.

48. Blevins TL, Peterson SB, Lee EL, *et al.* (2008). Mitral valvular interstitial cells demonstrate regional, adhesional, and synthetic heterogeneity. *Cells Tissues Organs* **187**:113–122.

49. Tamura K, Fukuda Y, Ishizaki M, Masuda Y, Yamanaka N, & Ferrans VJ (1995). Abnormalities in elastic fibers and other connective-tissue components of floppy mitral valve. *Am Heart J* **129**:1149–1158.

50. Specker C (2006) [Cardiac manifestations of rheumatic diseases]. *Med Klin* (Munich) **101**(Suppl. 1):40–43.

51. Specker C (2007) [The heart in rheumatic diseases]. *Internist* (*Berl*) **48**:284–289.

52. Moyssakis I, Tektonidou MG, Vassiliou VA, Samarkos M, Votteas V, & Moutsopoulos HM (2007) Libman-Sacks endocarditis in systemic lupus erythematosus: prevalence, associations, and evolution. *Am J Med* **120**:636–642.

22 Echocardiography of Mitral Insufficiency

Juan Luis Gutiérrez-Chico[1], Pedro Marcos-Alberca[2] & José Luis Zamorano[2]

[1]Vigo University Hospital, Spain
[2]Hospital Clinico San Carlos, Madrid, Spain

Introduction

Echocardiography has become the cornerstone for the diagnosis of mitral insufficiency: it can be used to confirm the diagnosis and to grade its severity, it gives important clues to the etiology of the disease, and it enables evaluation of the repercussion on left ventricle, left atrium, and pulmonary system. Accurate interpretation of echocardiograms requires an intimate knowledge of mitral valve anatomy and of the pathophysiologic mechanisms leading to mitral insufficiency.

Conventional transthoracic study

Motion modulation

Motion modulation (M-mode) today plays only a modest role in the evaluation of mitral insufficiency.

Anteroposterior motion of the aortic root

The left atrium lies between the rigid spinal column posteriorly and the aortic root anteriorly, so that an increase in left atrial volume displaces the aortic root anteriorly. Because mitral insufficiency results in increased left atrial volume in systole followed by an abrupt decrease in diastole, anteroposterior motion of the aortic root will appear exaggerated in M-mode.

Mitral prolapse

M-mode was previously a useful tool for the diagnosis of mitral prolapse, but the advent of two-dimensional (2-D), transesophageal (TEE), and three-dimensional (3-D) technology has enabled visualization of the spatial complexity of mitral prolapse, surpassing the modest M-mode capabilities. M-mode may be still very useful in the diagnosis of *chordal rupture* in some cases in which the 2-D image is dubious (Fig. 22.1).

Cardiovascular Interventions in Clinical Practice. Edited by Jürgen Haase, Hans-Joachim Schäfers, Horst Sievert and Ron Waksman. © 2010 Blackwell Publishing.

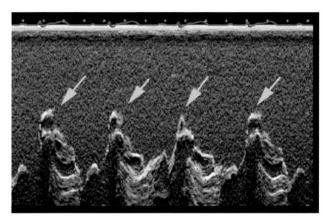

Figure 22.1 M-mode showing chordal rupture in the mitral apparatus (arrows).

Two-dimensional echocardiography study

The principal aim of transthoracic 2-D study in mitral insufficiency should be to discover the *etiology* and to assess its functional and structural *repercussion* (mainly in the left ventricle and left atrium).

Etiology

A superior systolic displacement of the mitral leaflets ≥2 mm above the annular plane into the left atrium in the parasternal long-axis view is required for the diagnosis of *mitral prolapse* using 2-D echocardiography [1–5]. This simple and objective criterion was adopted after Levine's studies [6–8] of the 3-D structure of the mitral valve, and helped enormously to augment the specificity of the diagnosis and to dissipate the confusion about mitral prolapse. However, its sensitivity is poor as only prolapses involving central scallops (A2, P2) will fulfill this criterion [9]. If the leaflet thickness is ≥5 mm in maximal diastasis, mitral prolapse is considered "classic," presumably associated with myxomatous degeneration and valve redundancy (dilated annulus, longer leaflets). Several studies have suggested that "classic prolapse" is associated with a poorer prognosis than "nonclassic prolapse," although mitral insufficiency severity could be the main predictor of complications [10], rather than leaflet thickness itself.

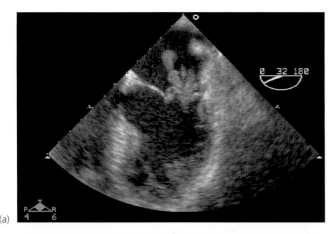

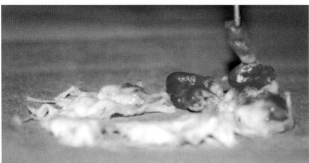

Figure 22.2 Infective endocarditis of the posterior leaflet.
(a) Transesophageal study showing vegetations and (b) macroscopic
appearance of the surgical piece excised.

A segmental contractility defect in the left ventricle points
to an *ischemic* origin of the regurgitation. Mechanic complications in the setting of an ST-elevation myocardial infarction
are also easily recognizable in 2-D studies.

Endocarditis results in mitral insufficiency as a result of leaflet
destruction, perforation, or deformity. Mobile oscillating vegetations attached to the valve (Fig. 22.2), or cardiac abscesses, in
a specific clinical setting, are Duke's major diagnostic criteria
for the diagnosis of endocarditis. In many cases, however, echocardiographic images will be just "consistent with infectious
endocarditis": echocardiography is then a minor criterion,
and needs to be contrasted with other clinical–microbiologic
variables to establish the diagnosis.

Commissural fusion, thickening of the leaflet tips, coexisting
mitral stenosis of any degree with diastolic doming, or typical
affectation of other cardiac valves are features pointing to
rheumatic mitral valve.

Age-related *degenerative* changes affect both the mitral
annulus and leaflets. Mitral annular calcification appears as
an area of increased echogenicity on the annulus immediately
adjacent to the attachment point of the posterior leaflet.
Acoustic shadowing, due to the presence of calcium, is seen.
In short-axis views, the annular calcium usually involves the
entire U-shaped posterior annulus. The region of anterior mitral
leaflet–aortic root continuity is involved rarely. Irregular areas
of thickening and increased echogenicity can also be observed
in the leaflets. Degenerative changes may render the mitral
valve incompetent, or favor chordal rupture and subsequent
acute severe mitral insufficiency.

Chordal disruption or *elongation* may occur in mitral prolapse, age-related degeneration or ischemic cardiomyopathy.
When chordal rupture is present, a flail segment of the leaflet
protrudes into the left atrium. Current harmonic 2-D technology permits the visualization of waving ruptured chordae
at the tip of flail segments in most cases; if there is any
doubt, M-mode can be helpful. 3-D technologies, contrary to
popular belief, are scarcely sensitive enough to detect chordal
ruptures.

Papillary muscle rupture can occur as a mechanical complication of myocardial infarction. As each papillary muscle
attaches to both leaflets, when the entire papillary muscle is
ruptured, 2-D imaging shows a mobile mass, attached to flail
segments of anterior and posterior leaflets; however, color
Doppler shows free mitral insufficiency (Fig. 22.3). Partial
rupture is the rupture of one "head" of the papillary muscle
(seen only in posterolateral muscle rupture) or a partial
disconnection of the base of the muscle.

As a general rule, the best way to increase sensitivity and
specificity in 2-D imaging for the etiologic diagnosis of mitral
insufficiency is looking at the screen with one eye and looking
to the clinical history with the other.

Repercussion of the regurgitation
Current guidelines admit indication of mitral valve repair
or replacement for those patients with severe mitral insufficiency and a left ventricular ejection fraction of ≤60% or
end-systolic diameter ≥40 mm [1]. If the left ventricle is
severely impaired, the surgical risk rises dramatically, and
thus surgical intervention is discouraged for those patients
with left ventricular ejection fractions of <30% or end-systolic
diameters of >55 mm [1].

Left atrial enlargement must be reported with anteroposterior
and superoinferior diameters; it is an independent predictor
of comorbidity [10].

Doppler study
The main focus of the 2-D Doppler study will be the assessment of the *severity* of mitral insufficiency.

Continuous Doppler
The continuous-wave Doppler spectral recording of mitral
insufficiency shows a rapid rise in velocity during isovolumic
contraction to a maximum of 5–6 m/s. The velocity stays
high throughout systole, paralleling the rise and fall of left
ventricular pressure (given a normal left atrial pressure).
During isovolumic relaxation, the velocity rapidly returns to
baseline.

The intensity of the mitral regurgitant signal, in comparison
with antegrade flow, is related to mitral insufficiency severity.

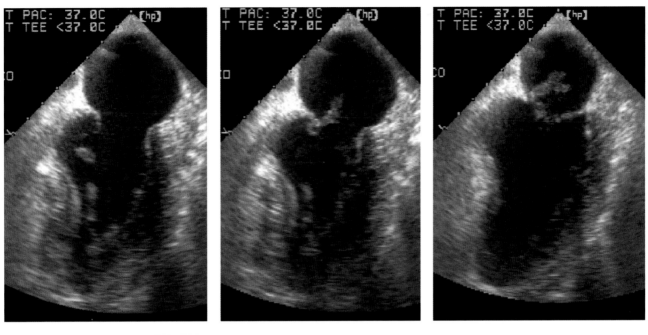

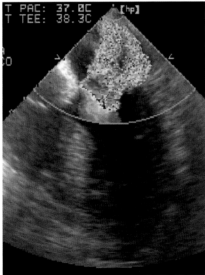

Figure 22.3 Rupture of the posteromedial papillary muscle after myocardial infarction. Color Doppler shows massive acute mitral insufficiency.

Thus, a dense continuous Doppler signal during regurgitant flow, as intense as the signal of antegrade flow throughout systole, strongly suggests severe mitral insufficiency.

In acute mitral insufficiency, the low compliance of the left atrium favors a late systolic pressure increase, (corresponding to the v-wave of the pressure curve). Continuous Doppler will reflect this "v-wave" as a high initial velocity followed by a more rapid fall in mid and late systole (Fig. 22.4), showing a typically asymmetric curve.

Pulsed Doppler

Pulsed-wave Doppler recording offers an objective method to quantify the regurgitant volume (the volumetric method), as well as useful indirect markers of severity.

Volumetric method

The continuity equation can be employed to calculate the mitral regurgitant volume and the effective regurgitant orifice (ERO). Regurgitant volume (RV) can be obtained subtracting the net forward stroke volume ($SV_{forward}$) measured in the left ventricular outflow tract (LVOT) from the total stroke volume (SV_{total}), measured in the inflow mitral annulus.

$$RV = SV_{total} - SV_{forward}$$

Assuming a circular shape of the LVOT, its cross-sectional area can be calculated by the formula:

$$Area = \pi r^2$$

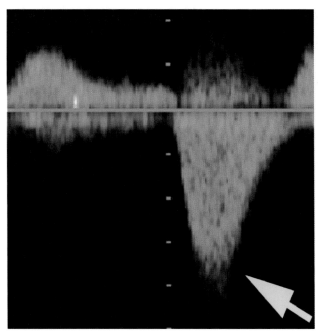

Figure 22.4 Continuous-wave Doppler pattern of "v-wave" (arrow) in a patient with acute severe mitral insufficiency.

Because we measured directly the LVOT diameter, instead of the radius, in the parasternal long-axis view, the formula appears as follows:

$$\text{LVOT}_{area} = \pi(\text{LVOT}_{diameter}/2)^2$$

We can calculate then the net forward stroke volume from this area plus the time–velocity integral in the LVOT (TVI_{LVOT}):

$$\text{SV}_{forward} = \text{LVOT}_{area} \times \text{TVI}_{LVOT}$$

$$\text{SV}_{forward} = \pi(\text{LVOT}_{diameter}/2)^2 \times \text{TVI}_{LVOT}$$

Assuming an elliptical shape of the mitral annulus, its cross-sectional area can be calculated by the formula

$$\text{Mitral area} = \pi(D_1 \times D_2)/4$$

where D_1 and D_2 are mitral annular diameters measured in two orthogonal views. We can calculate then the total stroke volume (SV_{total}) from this area plus the time–velocity integral in the mitral inflow pulsed Doppler recording ($\text{TVI}_{mi\,inflow}$):

$$\text{SV}_{total} = \text{mitral area} \times \text{TVI}_{mi\,inflow}$$

$$\text{SV}_{total} = \pi([D_1 \times D_2]/4) \times \text{TVI}_{mi\,inflow}$$

Once we have calculated $\text{SV}_{forward}$ and SV_{total}, we can calculate the regurgitant volume:

$$\text{RV} = \text{SV}_{total} - \text{SV}_{forward}$$

$$\text{RV} = \pi([D_1 \times D_2]/4) \times \text{TVI}_{mi\,inflow} - \pi(\text{LVOT}_{diameter}/2)^2 \times \text{TVI}_{LVOT}$$

Derived from the regurgitant volume, we can calculate the regurgitant fraction (RF) and the effective regurgitant orifice:

$$\text{RF} = \text{RV}/\text{SV}_{total}$$

$$\text{ERO} = \text{RV}/\text{TVI}_{mi\,inflow}$$

Potential pitfalls

The 2-D pulsed Doppler volumetric method tends to *overestimate* the severity of mitral insufficiency [11] for several reasons: improper positioning of the Doppler sample volume can result in overestimation of the $\text{TVI}_{mi\,inflow}$ because of the increase in velocity from the annulus to the tip of the leaflets [12]—meticulous positioning of the sample volume at the level of the annulus, where D_1 and D_2 are measured, is mandatory to avoid this bias; TVI_{LVOT} can be underestimated if the ultrasound beam and the direction of blood flow are not parallel; and inaccuracy in the measurement of mitral diameters is common—small errors in diameters mean large errors in cross-sectional area. These potential sources of error may contribute to reported regurgitant fractions of up to 20% in normal subjects [13]. In current clinical practice this method is seldom employed because of the advantages of color Doppler quantitative methods (see below).

Indirect markers of regurgitation severity

Pulmonary vein systolic flow reversal

When severe mitral insufficiency is present, pulsed Doppler echocardiography shows a negative reversal pulmonary vein systolic (PVs) wave (Fig. 22.5). This sign predicts a large effective regurgitant orifice (ERO) of >0.3 cm² [14]. Blunted PVs (rather than reversal) is much less predictive, being found in a wide spectrum of severity, from mild to severe. False-negatives occur when the left atrium is severely enlarged and compliant so that all the excess volume is contained in the left atrium without displacement into the pulmonary veins. False-positive results occur when an eccentric jet is directed into a pulmonary vein, causing flow reversal even when regurgitation is not severe. To optimize the sensitivity of the pulmonary vein systolic flow reversal, it is important to sample both right and left pulmonary veins because the direction of the jet can influence the pulmonary vein's flow pattern [15].

Peak E-wave velocity

The volume overload represented by the regurgitant volume in the left atrium increases the atrioventricular pressure gradient at early systole, thus increasing the peak E-wave velocity [16]. A peak E-wave velocity of >1.2 m/s has a modest positive predictive value (75%) for severe mitral insufficiency

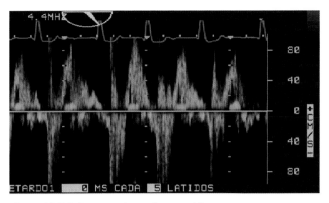

Figure 22.5 Pulmonary vein systolic reversal flow.

[17]. Moreover, a high peak E-wave velocity can also be found in patients with severe aortic regurgitation, or in other clinical settings, and its diagnostic value in acute mitral insufficiency is uncertain. Therefore, it should never be used in isolation to judge regurgitant severity.

Color Doppler

Doppler color flow mapping provides real-time visualization of regurgitant flow signals. Although Doppler color flow images are derived from autocorrelation techniques that provide mathematical estimates of mean velocities along each scan line, this technique is most commonly applied qualitatively to assess the presence and spatial distribution of the flow disturbance due to valvular regurgitation.

Color Doppler mapping for semiquantitative grading of severity

Depth of jet penetration into the left atrium [18] and maximal jet area have been correlated with angiographic severity of mitral insufficiency. Improved correlation has been observed when the mitral regurgitant jet area is corrected for left atrial area [19]. Thus, a mitral regurgitant jet reaching the posterior wall of the left atrium, or whose color flow area is ≥ 40% of the left atrial size, is considered very suggestive of severe mitral insufficiency.

Although these criteria based on color flow mapping correlate well with the semiquantitative grade of severity, they correlate poorly with quantitative measures of regurgitant volume or fraction ($r = 0.55$; $r = 0.62$, respectively) [20]. This lack of correlation is related to several geometric, physiologic, and instrumental factors.

Geometric factors

Regurgitant jet area depends on the geometry and direction of the jet [21]. Doppler color flow mapping of free regurgitant jets that are unbounded by surrounding structures may lead to overestimation of severity owing to entrainment of adjacent fluid by the high-velocity jet [22]. In contrast, the area of an eccentric jet is only 40% of the area of a free jet with the same regurgitant fraction [21].

Physiologic factors

Color Doppler jet area varies enormously depending on loading conditions and hemodynamic state. For example, acute severe mitral insufficiency may be underestimated by color Doppler mapping because of increased heart rate, decreased systemic blood pressure, and a rapid rise in pressure in the noncompliant left atrium [23].

Instrumental factors

Color Doppler area also depends on the echocardiographic approach, transducer frequency, gain settings, and several instrumental parameters. For instance, the same regurgitant jet appears more severe on transesophageal echocardiography than on transthoracic echocardiography. Color Doppler area is subject to great inter/intraobserver variability, as well as day-to-day variability.

On this basis, evaluation of mitral insufficiency severity should not be based merely on the measurement of color Doppler area or penetration into the left atrium. The abundant limitations of this approach, together with the current development and simple application of more accurate quantitative methods, such as PISA or vena contracta, make the mere semiquantitative estimation based on color Doppler areas hardly justifiable today.

Proximal isovelocity surface area method

When blood in the left ventricle converges toward the mitral regurgitant orifice, blood flow velocity increases and forms a series of concentric isovelocity layers. Flow reaches its maximal velocity at the level of the regurgitant orifice. When this phenomenon is observed with color Doppler, a clear hemisphere in the ventricular face of the valve can be seen, defining the area in which the flow velocity equals the Nyquist limit. This phenomenon is the basis of the proximal isovelocity surface area (PISA) method. Compared with the turbulent flow downstream, this laminar and more predictable flow pattern in the proximal flow convergence region offers interesting advantages for quantitation of the regurgitation severity. In theory, PISA is less dependent on the geometrical, physiohemodynamic, and instrumental factors that influence the spatial extent of the regurgitant jet in the receiving chamber, and is much less influenced by other concomitant valvular lesions. In practice, the method has been validated *in vitro* [24] and in clinical studies [25], demonstrating higher accuracy than any other noninvasive methods for quantitation of the severity of mitral insufficiency [26].

The first step of the method consists of calculating the instantaneous volume flow rate at the level of the hemisphere. The image and color Doppler parameters must be properly adjusted: zooming in on the mitral valve and shifting the color Doppler zero line in the same direction as the regurgitant flow (downward in transthoracic, upward in transesophageal study) to obtain a larger hemisphere are useful tips (Fig. 22.6). We then freeze the image and search for the frame in which

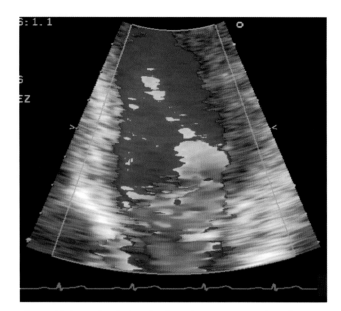

Figure 22.6 PISA hemisphere in a (transthoracic/transesophageal) echocardiographic study of a patient with mitral insufficiency. Notice the zoom over the area and the shift of the zero level.

an optimal PISA radius (r) can be measured, from the mitral leaflets to the aliasing limit. As the area of a sphere surface is $4\pi r^2$, the area of the surface of our hemisphere (PISA) will be:

$$PISA = 2\pi r^2$$

where r is the radius that we have measured in the aliasing hemisphere. The instantaneous volume flow rate is then:

$$\text{Flow rate} = PISA \times \text{aliasing velocity} = 2\pi r^2 \times \text{aliasing velocity}$$

The second step consists then of the application of the instantaneous continuity principle for the flow rate. The flow rate at the PISA is equal to the flow rate across the ERO:

$$\text{Flow rate}_{PISA} = \text{flow rate}_{ERO}$$

$$2\pi r^2 \times \text{aliasing velocity} = ERO \times \text{peak mitral regurgitation velocity}$$

$$ERO = (2\pi r^2 \times \text{aliasing velocity})/ \text{(peak mitral regurgitation velocity)}$$

Once ERO has been calculated, mitral regurgitant volume can also be obtained:

$$RV = ERO \times \text{mitral regurgitation TVI}$$

Technical considerations

The flow convergence layers flatten progressively as they approach the regurgitant orifice [27]. Moreover, the hemi-

spheric assumption of the method can be accepted only if the Nyquist velocity is much less than the orifice velocity. These physical considerations have several implications:
• PISA radius measurements performed close to the regurgitant orifice will systematically underestimate the regurgitation severity.
• They underscore the importance of shifting the color Doppler zero line toward the regurgitant flow direction. It allows a large PISA hemisphere, at the maximal affordable difference between the Nyquist and regurgitant flow velocities. This optimizes the accuracy of the method.
• The PISA method is not valid for patients with very mild mitral insufficiency, because they do not have a visible proximal acceleration zone at the Nyquist range.

Theoretically, PISA should be independent of orifice shape, and of the presence of single or multiple orifices. It has been suggested that the method can be consistently applied with irregular or multiple orifices [24], given that the measurement are obtained far enough from the regurgitant orifice. The application and validity of PISA in this particular clinical setting is still controversial. In the case of a geometrical constrain avoiding formation of a full PISA hemisphere, an angle correction should be added to the formula:

$$ERO = (2\pi r^2 \times \text{aliasing velocity})/ \text{(peak mitral regurgitation velocity)} \times (\alpha/180)$$

Simplifications of the proximal isovelocity surface area method

If aliasing velocity is 40 cm/s, and the mitral insufficiency velocity is assumed to be 500 cm/s.

$$ERO = (6.28 \times r^2 \times 40)/500 = (251 \times r^2)/500 = r^2/2$$

If aliasing velocity is 30 cm/s, and the mitral insufficiency velocity is assumed to be 500 cm/s, ERO becomes 0.38 cm^2 when the PISA radius is 1 cm. Hence, a PISA radius of ≥1 cm indicates severe mitral insufficiency. The relationship between TVI and peak velocity of mitral insufficiency has been shown to be relatively constant [28]:

$$MR\ TVI/MR\ \text{peak velocity} = 1/3.25$$

Therefore, mitral regurgitant volume can be calculated as follows:

$$RV = (2\pi r^2 \times \text{aliasing velocity})/ \text{peak mitral regurgitation velocity} \times MR$$

$$TVI = (6.28 r^2 \times \text{aliasing velocity})/3.25 = 2r^2 \times \text{aliasing velocity}$$

Vena contracta

The vena contracta width (VCW) is defined as the narrowest diameter of regurgitant flow immediately downstream from the flow convergence region. It is a transition area between

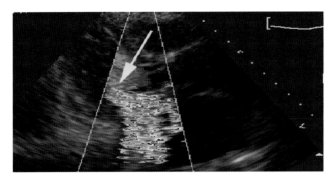

Figure 22.7 Vena contracta in a patient with severe mitral insufficiency. Transesophageal study. Notice the zoom and small sector angle to maximize the accuracy of the measurement.

the laminar flow of the proximal convergence region and the turbulent flow of the proximal jet (Fig. 22.7). It is not a direct measurement of regurgitant orifice diameter; in fact, it is smaller than the anatomic orifice by a factor of 0.8 (coefficient of contraction).

Similar to PISA, it is not so affected by geometric or physio-hemodynamic factors, and remains accurate in the presence of eccentric jets. VCW is more accurate and predictive of the severity of mitral insufficiency than color Doppler jet area, penetration, left atrial size, or pulmonary venous flow. Its feasibility ranges between 92% and 97% of patients, and highest accuracy is reached when measured by multiplane TEE, compared with single-plane TEE or transthoracic echocardiography. Thus, it has been proposed as a simple yet accurate method for intraoperative assessment of mitral insufficiency.

A VCW of ≥5 mm suggests severe mitral insufficiency; whereas a VCW of <3 mm suggests mild mitral insufficiency. Between 3 and 5 mm there is an intermediate region of uncertainty, where the method is not so predictive, and further quantitation methods should be employed. The ERO can be estimated from the VCW, assuming that VCW represents the diameter of the ERO:

$$ERO = \pi r^2 = \pi(VCW/2)^2$$

Although independent from geometric and hemodynamic conditions, VCW is critically dependent on appropriate instrumental adjusting. It requires optimized axial resolution, a smaller sector angle, high frame rate, and a zoom to obtain an accurate and reproducible measurement.

Beyond the mitral valve

In addition to the capital role played by the Doppler study in the assessment of the severity of mitral insufficiency, it must be also employed to estimate the pulmonary systolic pressure (PSP) from the right ventricle–right atrium peak gradient, given the presence of any degree of tricuspid regurgitation that makes this calculation possible.

Echocardiographic criteria for severe mitral insufficiency

The following criteria are diagnostic of definite severe mitral insufficiency:
- 2-D echocardiographic evidence of disruption of the mitral valve apparatus (papillary muscle rupture, flail mitral leaflet…)
- ERO ≥0.4 cm^2
- mitral regurgitant volume ≥60 mL
- regurgitation fraction ≥55%
- pulmonary vein systolic flow reversal
- mitral insufficiency color flow jet reaching the posterior wall of the left atrium (with a high aliasing velocity of color map).

The following criteria are suggestive of severe mitral insufficiency:
- color flow area ≥40% of left atrial size
- eccentric mitral insufficiency jet reaching the posterior wall of the left atrium
- dense continuous-wave Doppler signal
- increased E velocity (≥1.2 m/s for native valve; 2 m/s for prosthesis)
- dilated left ventricle or left atrium (≥5.5 cm).

Transthoracic protocol for the patient with mitral insufficiency

- 2-D echocardiography:
  - etiology of mitral insufficiency
  - repercussion of mitral insufficiency:
    - left atrial dilation
    - left ventricle:
        dilation (end-systolic diameter)
        systolic function
- Severity of mitral insufficiency:
  - continuous Doppler signal density
  - pulmonary vein systolic flow reversal
  - PISA
  - eventually other quantitative methods: vena contracta, volumetric method.

After performing all these calculations, the echocardiographer should define regurgitation severity as mild, moderate, or severe, avoiding annoying "confidence intervals" (mild–moderate, moderate–severe, …), particularly those involving the term "severe," as they do not help the clinician in the decision-making process. In the case of discrepancies, the experienced echocardiographer should know which method is the most reliable, and which one could be biased in every particular case.
- Estimation of pulmonary systolic pressure.

Transesophageal study

Mitral insufficiency is the valvular heart disease that most often requires transesophageal evaluation. It is frequently difficult to assess the mechanism, the cause, and the magnitude of mitral insufficiency with a transthoracic approach because the mitral valve is quite distant from the chest wall, the acoustic window is often of suboptimal quality, and the mitral regurgitant jet is directed away from the transducer. TEE overcomes all these limitations: the acoustic beam is generated in the esophagus, a few millimeters behind the left atrium, and therefore the transducer frequency can be higher, the echo attenuation is minimal, and the image quality is optimal. Furthermore, the regurgitant jet is directed against the transducer, forming a very precise Doppler signal.

In the evaluation of critically ill patients, TEE is very useful, which is the usual scenario in which acute mitral insufficiency is found.

Severity of mitral insufficiency will be most accurately evaluated using TEE. Pulmonary vein systolic flow reversal, PISA, and vena contracta can be easily and quickly measured with TEE. Planimetry of the color Doppler jet area is often performed, notwithstanding its limitations. The regurgitation area by TEE uses to be significantly larger than by transthoracic echo. If the transthoracic study is not conclusive about the regurgitation severity, TEE is mandatory.

Current guidelines for the management of patients with valvular heart disease admit the indication (IIa) of surgery in those asymptomatic patients with severe mitral insufficiency, left ventricular ejection fraction >60%, end-systolic diameter <40 mm, in whom the likelihood of successful repair is estimated as >90% [1]. Although transthoracic 2-D study can predict the repair likelihood in a large proportion of patients [29], TEE evaluation is often required. If the cause of the regurgitation is mitral prolapse, TEE is the only echocardiographic method properly validated to perform a systematic segmental analysis [30–37]. TEE also provides detailed information about eventual chordal ruptures and the state of subvalvular apparatus. Transthoracic real-time 3-D echocardiography also has outstanding proven accuracy in segmental analysis [38,39], but TEE is still superior in the depiction of chordal and subvalvular apparatus.

Intraoperative TEE is normally performed immediately before cardioplegia and on-pump connection, with the aim of informing the surgeon about the functional anatomy of the valve, and to reconfirm the regurgitant severity under the loading conditions of general anesthesia, serving as a baseline for later comparison. After concluding the intervention, restoring cardiac beat, and weaning from cardiopulmonary bypass, TEE is repeated with the aim of evaluating the functional result of the repair. Persistence of more than mild residual mitral insufficiency after repair is an independent predictor of complications and poor outcomes; thus. the surgeon should consider the possibility of repairing again or replacing the valve. Intraoperative TEE must be performed under normal hemodynamic conditions; hypotension secondary to the on-pump status can lead to underestimation of the magnitude of the residual mitral insufficiency. Other complications of valve repair, such as dynamic LVOT obstruction or functional mitral stenosis, as well as left ventricular systolic functions must be also assessed.

Three-dimensional study

Transthoracic real-time three-dimensional echocardiography

Real-time 3-D echocardiography (RT 3-D) offers a detailed 3-D view of the mitral valve, which is particularly useful in the evaluation of mitral stenosis [40], postvalvotomy patients [41], or mitral prolapse [38,39].

Interesting geometric differences have been found by RT 3-D echocardiography in the valvular apparatus between

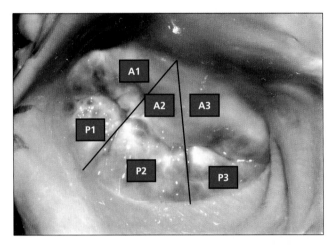

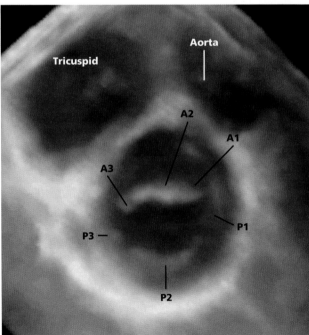

Figure 22.8 Carpentier's nomenclature for the mitral scallops (surgical view above, echocardiographic view below). Scallops of the anterior leaflet are named A, and scallops of the posterior leaflet are named P. Scallops are numbered as 1, 2 or 3, starting from the left atrial appendage (anterolateral commissure).

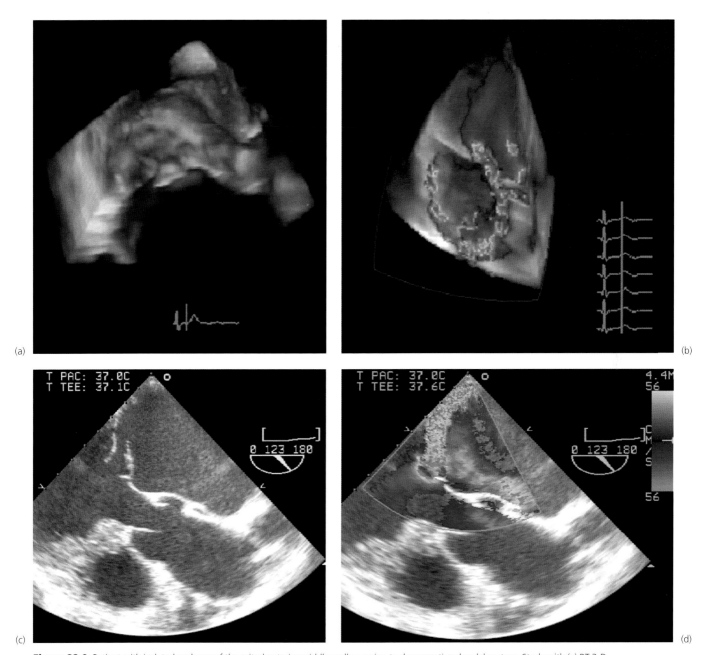

(a)

(b)

(c)

(d)

Figure 22.9 Patient with isolated prolapse of the mitral anterior middle scallop owing to degenerative chordal rupture. Study with (a) RT 3-D echocardiography, (b) 3-D colour-Doppler, (c) TEE, and (d) colour Doppler TEE.

ischemic and secondary to dilated cardiomyopathy mitral insufficiency [42]. These findings, although important for physiopathologic and investigational points of view, have limited clinical applicability. In mitral prolapse, RT 3-D echocardiography has proven high accuracy in performing a transthoracic segmental analysis (Fig. 22.8) and in predicting the likelihood of repair [38,39]. However, it is time-consuming, and TEE is superior in detecting chordal rupture or in the assessment of regurgitation severity. This is the reason why many echocardiographers still prefer TEE to decide the likeli-

hood of repair of a patient with mitral prolapse and significant mitral insufficiency.

Although 2-D colour-Doppler analysis of the regurgitant jets indicates the *leaflet* predominantly affected, analysis with RT 3-D colour-Doppler indicates the *scallops* predominantly affected in a mitral prolapse [43]. This analysis is complex and time-consuming but offers interesting possibilities for the future (Fig. 22.9).

For the evaluation and follow-up of patients after surgical mitral valve repair, RT 3-D is the tool of choice. The *en face* 3-D

Table 22.1 Differential features between chronic and acute mitral insufficiency.

	Chronic	Acute
Etiology	Myxomatous degeneration	Endocarditis
	Dilated cardiomyopathy	Chordal rupture
		Papillary muscle rupture
Left ventricle size	Dilated	Normal
Left ventricle systolic function	Initially hyperdynamic	Hyperdynamic
	Normal or depressed in later stages	
Left atrial size	Dilated	Normal
Continuous-wave Doppler	High velocity throughout systole	Late systolic velocity decline (v-wave)

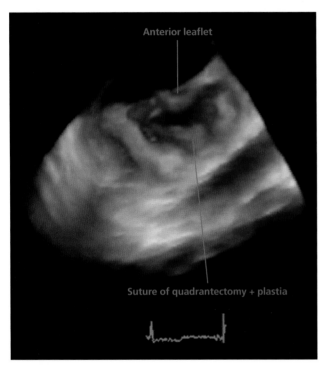

Figure 22.10 Real-time 3-D echocardiography of a patient with prolapse of the posterior middle scallop after mitral valve repair. Notice the hyperrefringence of the annulus, the suture of the quadrantectomy plus sliding plastia, and the reattachment of chordae.

views of the repaired valve give a simple, quick, and detailed depiction of the morphologic result (Fig. 22.10), whereas 2-D imaging would require longer studies, multiple views, and more experienced interpretation.

Transesophageal three-dimensional echocardiography

Rotational 3-D transesophageal reconstruction has been an interesting tool to evaluate the mitral anatomy [44,45]. It consists of a sequential acquisition of 2-D transesophageal planes, obtained with a multiplane probe rotating every 2–3°. These planes are processed by specific software to obtain a dynamic 3-D reconstruction of the cardiac structures. It renders

high-quality images, detailed depiction of cardiac structures, and dynamic 3-D functional anatomy, in contrast with the static view of the valve in the surgical inspection and with the limitations of 2-D study. The main disadvantage is complexity.

The recent appearance of RT 3-D TEE permits an easy acquisition of real-time dynamic 3-D images. The image quality is higher than any with other echocardiographic method, and allows every kind of spatial approach to the valve. The cropping tools provide high-quality and precisely defined 2-D planes of the desired structures at the desired level. There is no evidence yet of its diagnostic value, but it is easy to predict that RT 3-D TEE will soon become the gold standard for precise evaluation of multiple mitral problems, such as mitral prolapse or intraoperative monitoring of mitral valve repair.

Challenging issues

Acute versus chronic mitral insufficiency

The clinical presentation of an acute mitral insufficiency has nothing to do with chronic mitral insufficiency, even if the latter occurs in decompensated heart failure. Regardless of this, it is interesting to know some echocardiographic features in which they differ (Table 22.1).

Ischemic mitral insufficiency: will it improve with revascularization?

The indication for mitral valve operation in the patient who undergoes coronary artery bypass graft (CABG) with mild to moderate mitral insufficiency is still unclear, but there are data to indicate benefit of mitral valve repair in such patients [46–49]. CABG alone may improve left ventricular function and reduce ischemic mitral insufficiency in selected patients, especially those with transient severe mitral insufficiency resulting from ischemia. Low-dose dobutamine echocardiography may be helpful to identify those patients in whom mitral insufficiency will improve after revascularization [50]; if regurgitation severity becomes reduced during low-dose dobutamine echocardiography, it may be possible to avoid the intervention on the valve during CABG revascularization.

References

1. Bonow RO, Carabello BA, Chatterjee K, *et al.* (2006) ACC/AHA 2006 Guidelines for the Management of Patients With Valvular Heart Disease: A Report of the American College of Cardiology/American Heart Association Task Force on Practice Guidelines (Writing Committee to Revise the 1998 Guidelines for the Management of Patients With Valvular Heart Disease) Developed in Collaboration With the Society of Cardiovascular Anesthesiologists Endorsed by the Society for Cardiovascular Angiography and Interventions and the Society of Thoracic Surgeons. *J Am Coll Cardiol* **48**:e1–148.

2. Cheitlin MD, Armstrong WF, Aurigemma GP, *et al.* (2003) ACC/AHA/ASE 2003 Guideline Update for the Clinical Application of Echocardiography: summary article. A report of the American College of Cardiology/American Heart Association Task Force on Practice Guidelines (ACC/AHA/ASE Committee to Update the 1997 Guidelines for the Clinical Application of Echocardiography). *J Am Soc Echocardiogr* **16**:1091–1110.

3. Otto CM (2007) *The Practice of Clinical Echocardiography*, 3rd edn. Philadelphia, PA: Saunders.

4. Otto CM (2004) *Textbook of Clinical Echocardiography*, 3rd edn. Philadelphia, PA: Saunders.

5. Oh JK, Seward JB, & Tajik AJ (2006) *The Echo Manual*, 3rd edn. Philadelphia, PA: Lippincott Williams & Wilkins.

6. Levine RA, Triulzi MO, Harrigan P, & Weyman AE (1987) The relationship of mitral annular shape to the diagnosis of mitral valve prolapse. *Circulation* **75**:756–767.

7. Levine RA, Stathogiannis E, Newell JB, Harrigan P, & Weyman AE (1988) Reconsideration of echocardiographic standards for mitral valve prolapse: lack of association between leaflet displacement isolated to the apical four chamber view and independent echocardiographic evidence of abnormality. *J Am Coll Cardiol* **11**:1010–1019.

8. Levine RA, Handschumacher MD, Sanfilippo AJ, *et al.* (1989) Three-dimensional echocardiographic reconstruction of the mitral valve, with implications for the diagnosis of mitral valve prolapse. *Circulation* **80**:589–598.

9. Gutiérrez-Chico J (2008) *Usefulness of Real-Time Three-Dimensional Transthoracic Echocardiography for Segmental Analysis in Mitral Prolapse*. PhD Thesis, Universidad Complutense de Madrid, Madris.

10. Avierinos JF, Gersh BJ, Melton LJ III, *et al.* (2002) Natural history of asymptomatic mitral valve prolapse in the community. *Circulation* **106**:1355–1361.

11. Enriquez-Sarano M, Bailey KR, Seward JB, Tajik AJ, Krohn MJ, & Mays JM (1993) Quantitative Doppler assessment of valvular regurgitation. *Circulation* **87**:841–848.

12. Samstad SO, Rossvoll O, Torp HG, Skjaerpe T, & Hatle L (1992) Cross-sectional early mitral flow-velocity profiles from color Doppler in patients with mitral valve disease. *Circulation* **86**:748–755.

13. Rokey R, Sterling LL, Zoghbi WA, *et al.* (1986) Determination of regurgitant fraction in isolated mitral or aortic regurgitation by pulsed Doppler two-dimensional echocardiography. *J Am Coll Cardiol* **7**:1273–1278.

14. Pu M, Griffin BP, Vandervoort PM, *et al.* (1999) The value of assessing pulmonary venous flow velocity for predicting severity of mitral regurgitation: a quantitative assessment integrating left ventricular function. *J Am Soc Echocardiogr* **12**:736–743.

15. Yoshida K, Yoshikawa J, Yamaura Y, *et al.* (1990) Value of acceleration flows and regurgitant jet direction by color Doppler flow mapping in the evaluation of mitral valve prolapse. *Circulation* **81**:879–885.

16. Appleton CP, Hatle LK, Nellessen U, Schnittger I, & Popp RL (1990) Flow velocity acceleration in the left ventricle: a useful Doppler echocardiographic sign of hemodynamically significant mitral regurgitation. *J Am Soc Echocardiogr* **3**:35–45.

17. Thomas L, Foster E, & Schiller NB (1998) Peak mitral inflow velocity predicts mitral regurgitation severity. *J Am Coll Cardiol* **31**:174–179.

18. Miyatake K, Izumi S, Okamoto M, *et al.* (1986) Semiquantitative grading of severity of mitral regurgitation by real-time two-dimensional Doppler flow imaging technique. *J Am Coll Cardiol* **7**:82–88.

19. Helmcke F, Nanda NC, Hsiung MC, *et al.* (1987) Color Doppler assessment of mitral regurgitation with orthogonal planes. *Circulation* **75**:175–183.

20. Spain MG, Smith MD, Grayburn PA, Harlamert EA, & DeMaria AN (1989) Quantitative assessment of mitral regurgitation by Doppler color flow imaging: angiographic and hemodynamic correlations. *J Am Coll Cardiol* **13**:585–590.

21. Chen CG, Thomas JD, Anconina J, *et al.* (1991) Impact of impinging wall jet on color Doppler quantification of mitral regurgitation. *Circulation* **84**:712–720.

22. McCully RB, Enriquez-Sarano M, Tajik AJ, & Seward JB (1994) Overestimation of severity of ischemic/functional mitral regurgitation by color Doppler jet area. *Am J Cardiol* **74**:790–793.

23. Cape EG, Yoganathan AP, & Levine RA (1993) Increased heart rate can cause underestimation of regurgitant jet size by Doppler color flow mapping. *J Am Coll Cardiol* **21**:1029–1037.

24. Recusani F, Bargiggia GS, Yoganathan AP, *et al.* (1991) A new method for quantification of regurgitant flow rate using color Doppler flow imaging of the flow convergence region proximal to a discrete orifice. An in vitro study. *Circulation* **83**:594–604.

25. Rivera JM, Vandervoort PM, Thoreau DH, Levine RA, Weyman AE, & Thomas JD (1992) Quantification of mitral regurgitation with the proximal flow convergence method: a clinical study. *Am Heart J* **124**:1289–1296.

26. Flachskampf FA, Frieske R, Engelhard B, *et al.* (1998) Comparison of transesophageal Doppler methods with angiography for evaluation of the severity of mitral regurgitation. *J Am Soc Echocardiogr* **11**:882–892.

27. Vandervoort PM, Thoreau DH, Rivera JM, Levine RA, Weyman AE, & Thomas JD (1993) Automated flow rate calculations based on digital analysis of flow convergence proximal to regurgitant orifices. *J Am Coll Cardiol* **22**:535–541.

28. Rossi A, Dujardin KS, Bailey KR, Seward JB, & Enriquez-Sarano M (1998) Rapid estimation of regurgitant volume by the proximal isovelocity surface area method in mitral regurgitation: Can continuous-wave Doppler echocardiography be omitted? *J Am Soc Echocardiogr* **11**:138–148.

29. Monin JL, Dehant P, Roiron C, *et al.* (2005) Functional assessment of mitral regurgitation by transthoracic echocardiography using standardized imaging planes diagnostic accuracy and outcome implications. *J Am Coll Cardiol* **46**:302–309.

30. Zamorano J, Erbel R, Mackowski T, Alfonso F, & Meyer J (1992) Usefulness of transesophageal echocardiography for diagnosis of mitral valve prolapse. *Am J Cardiol* **69**:419–422.

31. Caldarera I, Van Herwerden LA, Taams MA, Bos E, & Roelandt JR (1995) Multiplane transoesophageal echocardiography and morphology of regurgitant mitral valves in surgical repair. *Eur Heart J* **16**:999–1006.

32. Langholz D, Mackin WJ, Wallis DE, Jacobs WR, Scanlon PJ, & Louie EK (1998) Transesophageal echocardiographic assessment of systolic mitral leaflet displacement among patients with mitral valve prolapse. *Am Heart J* **135**:197–206.

33. Foster GP, Isselbacher EM, Rose GA, Torchiana DF, Akins CW, & Picard MH (1998) Accurate localization of mitral regurgitant defects using multiplane transesophageal echocardiography. *Ann Thorac Surg* **65**:1025–1031.

34. Grewal KS, Malkowski MJ, Kramer CM, Dianzumba S, & Reichek N (1998) Multiplane transesophageal echocardiographic identification of the involved scallop in patients with flail mitral valve leaflet: intraoperative correlation. *J Am Soc Echocardiogr* **11**:966–971.

35. Lambert AS, Miller JP, Merrick SH, *et al.* (1999) Improved evaluation of the location and mechanism of mitral valve regurgitation with a systematic transesophageal echocardiography examination. *Anesth Analg* **88**:1205.

36. Omran AS, Woo A, David TE, Feindel CM, Rakowski H, & Siu SC (2002) Intraoperative transesophageal echocardiography accurately predicts mitral valve anatomy and suitability for repair. *J Am Soc Echocardiogr* **15**:950–957.

37. Agricola E, Oppizzi M, De Bonis M, *et al.* (2003) Multiplane transesophageal echocardiography performed according to the guidelines of the American Society of Echocardiography in patients with mitral valve prolapse, flail, and endocarditis: diagnostic accuracy in the identification of mitral regurgitant defects by correlation with surgical findings. *J Am Soc Echocardiogr* **16**:61–66.

38. Gutierrez-Chico JL, Zamorano Gomez JL, Rodrigo-Lopez JL, *et al.* (2008) Accuracy of real-time 3-dimensional echocardiography in the assessment of mitral prolapse. Is transesophageal echocardiography still mandatory? *Am Heart J* **155**:694–698.

39. Pepi M, Tamborini G, Maltagliati A, *et al.* (2006) Head-to-head comparison of two- and three-dimensional transthoracic and transesophageal echocardiography in the localization of mitral valve prolapse. *J Am Coll Cardiol* **48**:2524–2530.

40. Zamorano J, Cordeiro P, Sugeng L, *et al.* (2004) Real-time three-dimensional echocardiography for rheumatic mitral valve stenosis evaluation: an accurate and novel approach. *J Am Coll Cardiol* **43**:2091–2096.

41. Zamorano J, Perez de Isla L, Sugeng L, *et al.* (2004) Non-invasive assessment of mitral valve area during percutaneous balloon mitral valvuloplasty: role of real-time 3D echocardiography. *Eur Heart J* **25**:2086–2091.

42. Kwan J, Shiota T, Agler DA, *et al.* (2003) Geometric differences of the mitral apparatus between ischemic and dilated cardiomyopathy with significant mitral regurgitation: real-time three-dimensional echocardiography study. *Circulation* **107**:1135–1140.

43. Gutierrez-Chico JL, Zamorano JL, Bover Freire R, Perez de Isla L, Almeria Valera C, & Macaya C (2005) Analysis with real-time 3D-echo of mitral regurgitant jets gives important information for segmental analysis in mitral prolapse. *Eur Heart J* **26**:691. Abstract.

44. Pai RG, Tanimoto M, Jintapakorn W, Azevedo J, Pandian NG, & Shah PM (1995) Volume-rendered three-dimensional dynamic anatomy of the mitral annulus using a transesophageal echocardiographic technique. *J Heart Valve Dis* **4**:623–627.

45. Salustri A, Becker AE, van Herwerden L, Vletter WB, Ten Cate FJ, & Roelandt JRTC (1996) Three-dimensional echocardiography of normal and pathologic mitral valve: a comparison with two-dimensional transesophageal echocardiography. *J Am Coll Cardiol* **27**:1502–1510.

46. Harris KM, Sundt TM III, Aeppli D, Sharma R, & Barzilai B (2002) Can late survival of patients with moderate ischemic mitral regurgitation be impacted by intervention on the valve? *Ann Thorac Surg* **74**:1468–1475.

47. Prifti E, Bonacchi M, Frati G, *et al.* (2001) Should mild-to-moderate and moderate ischemic mitral regurgitation be corrected in patients with impaired left ventricular function undergoing simultaneous coronary revascularization? *J Card Surg* **16**:473–483.

48. Lam BK, Gillinov AM, Blackstone EH, *et al.* (2005) Importance of moderate ischemic mitral regurgitation. *Ann Thorac Surg* **79**:462–470.

49. Schroder JN, Williams ML, Hata JA, *et al.* (2005) Impact of mitral valve regurgitation evaluated by intraoperative transesophageal echocardiography on long-term outcomes after coronary artery bypass grafting. *Circulation* **112**:I293–I298.

50. Roshanali F, Mandegar MH, Yousefnia MA, Alaeddini F, & Wann S (2006) Low-dose dobutamine stress echocardiography to predict reversibility of mitral regurgitation with CABG. *Echocardiography* **23**:31–37.

23   MRI of Mitral Insufficiency

Matthias Gutberlet

University Leipzig, Leipzig Heart Center, Leipzig, Germany

Introduction

General requirements for an imaging modality to assess valvular disease are as follows:

- visualization of anatomic structures (valve thickness, number of leaflets, occurrence of calcifications and the presence of endocarditic vegetations);
- assessment of valvular function (gradation of the severity of valvular stenosis and the ability of a sufficient coaptation of the leaflets);
- assessment of the effect of valvular dysfunction on ventricular size, geometry, muscle mass, and ventricular function.

Visualization of valve morphology

As for the visualization of mitral valve stenosis, the best imaging sequence with magnetic resonance for the visualization of valve morphology and function is SSFP sequences [1,2]. These sequences allow not only for the assessment of valve morphology, but also for a functional evaluation because the movement of the valve can be visualized by the so-called cine MRI. Turbulence or increased blood flow could additionally enhance the assessment as a result of signal void caused by spin dephasing at the leaflet edges.

When imaging patients with mitral valve insufficiency, it is important to also visualize the left atrium and atrial appendage to assess left atrial size and to exclude the presence of atrial thrombi. The best visualization of the mitral valve can be achieved in the two-chamber long-axis view, four-chamber view, left ventricular outflow tract (LVOT) view, and in short-axis slices parallel to the orientation of the atrioventricular valve (Fig. 23.1). Owing to the in-plane motion of the valve itself, a stack of several parallel slices (Fig. 23.1a) should be

Cardiovascular Interventions in Clinical Practice. Edited by Jürgen Haase, Hans-Joachim Schäfers, Horst Sievert and Ron Waksman. © 2010 Blackwell Publishing.

acquired to cover the mitral valve during the whole cardiac cycle and to ensure that the maximal regurgitant area during systole can be planimetered (Fig. 23.1d).

Furthermore, MRI can also be used to assess potential reasons for mitral valve insufficiency, i.e., in myocardial infarction (Fig. 23.2c and d) or hypertrophic cardiomyopathy [3].

Assessment of ventricular function

Cine-MRI using SSFP sequences is the "gold standard" for the noninvasive assessment of left and especially right ventricular volumes, muscle mass, and function [4]. This is especially important because chronic mitral valve insufficiency has hemodynamic consequences, i.e., left ventricular dilatation and, eventually, left ventricular failure. It is well known that surgical repair of mitral valve incompetence is less successful if the left ventricular ejection fraction is lower than 60% [5]. Therefore, MRI is an ideal method to monitor the effects of mitral valve insufficiency.

Three different methods are available for the quantification of mitral valve insufficiency by MRI. If only an isolated mitral valve insufficiency has to be quantified, simple volumetric measurements of the right and left ventricular stroke volumes are sufficient to quantify mitral regurgitation [6]. The difference between left ventricular stroke volume (LVSV, mL/beat) and right ventricular stroke volume (RVSV, mL/beat) represents the regurgitant volume (eqn 23.1), from which the regurgitant fraction (%) (eqn 232) can be calculated [7].

$$\text{Regurgitant volume (mL/beat)} = \text{LVSV} - \text{RVSV} \qquad (23.1)$$

$$\text{Regurgitant fraction (\%)} = (\text{regurgitant volume} \times 100)/\text{LVSV} \qquad (23.2)$$

If other valve disease is present [6], the mitral valve regurgitant volume can be calculated by a combination of volumetry of the LVSV and magnetic resonance flow measurements, using the technique of phase-shift velocity mapping in the aorta (eqn 23.3).

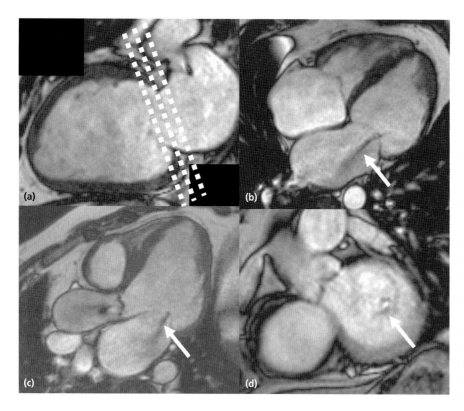

Figure 23.1 Steady-state free precession sequences from a 57-year-old man with a mild mitral insufficiency following myocardial infarction (occluded circumflex artery). (a) A two-chamber long-axis view. Dotted lines demonstrate the planning for the visualization of the mitral valve in two-chamber short-axis view. (b) A four-chamber view during systole demonstrates a holosystolic insufficiency jet (white arrow). (c) Additionally acquired images of the LVOT revealed an aortic valve stenosis with thickened aortic cusps. Again a holosystolic insufficiency jet (white arrow) is obvious owing to spin dephasing at areas of turbulent or increased flow. (d) The result of the short-axis view planning in (a) is shown. During systole a small orifice remains open (white arrow) indicating mild mitral valve insufficiency.

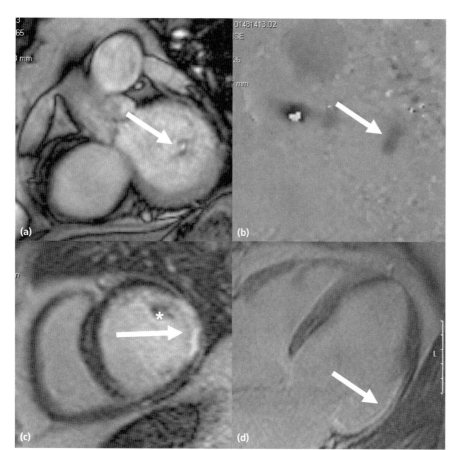

Figure 23.2 The same 57-year-old man as in Figure 23.1. (a) The modulus image of the flow-sensitive GRE sequence in short-axis orientation through the mitral valve during systole demonstrates a mild remaining open orifice (white arrow). (b) The phase image demonstrates retrograde flow (white arrow). "Late enhancement" images in (c) short-axis and (d) four-chamber view reveal an almost transmural scar at the lateral wall (white arrow) of the left ventricle. The origin of the anterior papillary muscle (*) is surrounded by scar tissue (bright signal).

Flow measurements

Cine-MRI, especially when using simple gradient echo (GRE) sequences, allows for a qualitative assessment of valvular insufficiency resulting from signal void as a result of dephasing due to increased blood velocity or turbulences caused by the regurgitant flow (Fig. 23.1). This sequence can be used only to detect an area of valvular insufficiency; it cannot be used to quantify as dephasing depends not only on the peak velocity, but also on the echo time of the sequence, and is therefore very variable. As already mentioned in Chapter 18 in respect of mitral valve stenosis, a shorter echo time leads to a more pronounced signal void, whereas sequences with a longer echo time, especially for high-grade stenosis, produce only a low signal void. Furthermore, signal loss is less marked with the commonly used SSFP sequences [8]. A similar approach to color Doppler echocardiography, in which the semiquantitative description of the length and width of a jet can be used to assess the severity of a valvular insufficiency, is therefore not possible.

Measuring the pulmonary vein flow can also be used to evaluate the severity of mitral valve stenosis [6]. As with severe mitral valve stenosis, pulmonary vein flow can be reversed in severe mitral valve insufficiency. Usually, the segmentation of the mitral valve orifice area is performed on the SSFP images parallel to the mitral valve (Fig. 23.1a and d). The modulus or phase images of the flow-sensitive gradient echo sequence can also be used to measure the mitral valve regurgitant area (Fig. 23.2b). Owing to the high inflow contrast, the edges can usually be visualized with high image quality.

As already mentioned (Fig. 23.2), absolute flow quantification (mL/s) is possible with MRI and can be used to quantify mitral valve insufficiency, even if additional valvular disease is present. Two methods can be used. The first one is a combination of the results of volumetric MRI measurements and flow quantification, using the following equation (eqn 23.3) to calculate the regurgitant volume:

Regurgitant volume (mL/beat) = LVSV − aortic forward flow (23.3)

The second method for mitral valve insufficiency quantification, using phase-shift velocity mapping, relies only on the flow measurement using the difference of the aortic outflow representing the ventricular outflow and the ventricular inflow (mL/beat) (eqn 23.4) [9]. The outflow measurement is usually performed in the ascending aorta, perpendicular to the vessel course and distal to the aortic valve and the origin of the coronary arteries. The inflow measurement is usually performed at the mitral valve annulus during diastole.

Regurgitant volume (mL/beat) =
left ventricular inflow − aortic forward flow (23.4)

Both methods showed good correlation to the semiquantification with Doppler echocardiography.

References

1. Sondergaard L, Lindvig K, Hildebrandt P, *et al.* (1993) Valve area and cardiac output in aortic stenosis. *Am Heart J* **127**:1156–1164.
2. Friedrich MG, Schulz-Menger J, Poetsch T, *et al.* (2002) Quantification of valvular aortic stenosis by magnetic resonance imaging. *Am Heart J* **144**:329–334.
3. Gutberlet M, Fröhlich M, Mehl S, *et al.* (2005) Myocardial viability assessment in patients with highly impaired left ventricular function: comparison of delayed enhancement, dobutamine stress MRI, end-diastolic wall thickness, and Tl201-SPECT with functional recovery after revascularization. *Eur Radiol* **15**:872–880.
3. Gutberlet M, Abdul-Khaliq H, Grothoff H, *et al.* (2003) Vergleich der transthorakalen 3D-Echokardiographie mit der MRT zur Bestimmung linksventrikulärer Volumina bei Patienten mit pathologischer Ventrikelgeometrie aufgrund angeborener Herzfehler. *Fortschr Röntgenstr* **175**:942–951.
5. Enriquez-Sarano M, Tajik A, Schaff H, *et al.* (1994) Echocardiographic prediction of survival after surgical correction of organic mitral regurgitation. *Circulation* **90**:830–837.
6. Taylor AM & Bogaert J (2005) *Valvular heart disease*. In: Bogaert J, Dymarkowski S, & Taylor AM (eds). *Clinical Cardiac MRI*. Berlin: Springer, pp. 353–379.
7. Hundley WG, Li HF, Willard JE, *et al.* (1995) Magnetic resonance imaging assessment of the severity of mitral regurgitation. *Circulation* **92**:1151–1158.
8. Kilner PJ, Firmin DN, Rees RSO, *et al.* (1991) Valve and great vessel stenosis: assessment with MR jet velocity mapping. *Radiology* **178**:229–235.
9. Fujita N, Chazoullieres AF, Hartiala JJ, *et al.* (1994) Quantification of mitral regurgitation by velocity encoded cine nuclear magnetic resonance imaging. *J Am Coll Cardiol* **23**:951–958.

24 Surgical Management of Mitral Insufficiency

Kevin L. Greason & Hartzell V. Schaff

Mayo Clinic, Rochester, MN, USA

Introduction

The common causes of mitral valve insufficiency include degenerative mitral valve disease, rheumatic heart disease, infective endocarditis, certain drugs, and collagen vascular diseases. Additionally, mitral insufficiency can result from ventricular enlargement, as occurs in dilated cardiomyopathy and in patients with left ventricular dysfunction resulting from coronary artery disease. In some cases, such as ruptured chordae tendineae, ruptured papillary muscle, or infective endocarditis, mitral insufficiency can be acute and severe. More often, mitral insufficiency worsens gradually over a prolonged period of time [1]. The most common etiology of mitral insufficiency in developed countries is degenerative mitral valve disease, and in most surgical practices pure mitral regurgitation now accounts for approximately 75% of patients requiring surgery [2].

The evolution in the surgical management of mitral insufficiency that has occurred over the past 20 years is largely attributable to advances in three areas:

1 There have been significant improvements in operative techniques that have led to predictable and durable results after valve repair.

2 Because of the decline in rheumatic heart disease in the USA, almost 80% of patients undergoing mitral valve operations today have pure insufficiency rather than valve stenosis or mixed insufficiency and stenosis.

3 A better understanding of the natural history of mitral insufficiency coupled with improved echocardiography techniques allows stratification of patients and selection of optimal treatment strategies [3].

Mitral valve anatomy

The mitral valve complex includes the orifice, annulus, anterior and posterior leaflets, and the subvalvular apparatus, which includes the chordae tendineae and papillary muscles. The left atrium is relatively unrelated to the form and function of the mitral valve complex. The left ventricle is an important subunit of the mitral valve apparatus, however, and ventricular dysfunction producing tethering of the chordae can directly affect leaflet motion/coaptation and may cause significant mitral insufficiency.

The mitral valve annulus is not a simple circumferential fibrous ring [4]. It consists of fibrocollagenous elements as well as muscle fibers allowing the annulus to contract during systole. The annulus is strongest at the inner aspects of the left and right fibrous trigones. Spanning the zone between the trigones, the central part of the anterior mitral leaflet is the fibrous subaortic curtain, which descends from the adjacent halves of the left coronary and noncoronary cusp regions of the aortic valve annulus. The posterior annulus is made up of a more tenuous sheet of deformable fibroelastic connective tissue.

Anatomists have proposed that the mitral valve leaflets consist of a continuous veil inserted around the entire circumference of the mitral orifice. Classically, the veil has been divided into the anterior (one-third orifice circumference) and posterior (two-thirds orifice circumference) leaflets that are divided by the anterolateral and posteromedial commissures. From a surgical standpoint, the valve is separated into six segments. Two indentations on the posterior leaflet divide this structure into three anatomically individualized scallops. The three scallops of the posterior leaflet are identified as P1 (anterolateral scallop), P2 (middle scallop), and P3 (posteromedial scallop). The three corresponding segments of the anterior leaflet are A1 (lateral segment), A2 (middle segment) and A3 (medial segment) [2].

There are generally two papillary muscles, which vary considerably in their formation, from long and finger-like to short and stubby; occasionally their tips are bifid. The muscles are named based on their point of origin from the free wall of the left ventricle: anterolateral and posteromedial. Chordae tendineae arise most commonly from the tip and margin of the apical third of each muscle, but occasionally they emerge near the base. The chordae from each muscle diverge and are inserted into corresponding points on both leaflets of the mitral valve.

Cardiovascular Interventions in Clinical Practice. Edited by Jürgen Haase, Hans-Joachim Schäfers, Horst Sievert and Ron Waksman. © 2010 Blackwell Publishing.

The anterolateral and posteromedial chordae tendineae mostly arise near the tips of their corresponding papillary muscle as a single stem branching almost immediately into radiating strands, like the struts of a fan, and insert into the leaflets. Chordae of the mitral complex can be subdivided into commissural, leaflet, rough zone, cleft, and basal types depending on their area of insertion. In the majority of hearts, the chordae support the entire free edges of the leaflets.

The mean circumference of the mitral valve orifice averages 9–10 cm in adults, but is slightly smaller in women than in men. Because of the contractile function of the mitral annulus the valve orifice represents a dynamic structure, the area reducing by as much as 40% during systole. The orifice changes from the circular profile characteristic of diastole to a D-shaped concentric form at the height of systole. The annular attachment of the anterior leaflet provides the concavity of the crescent, and the attachment of the posterior leaflet, although remaining convex, contracts toward the former.

Important anatomic relationships exist between the mitral valve and other structures that put them at risk during surgical manipulation of the mitral valve. The anterior leaflet is in direct continuity with the aortic valve, specifically portions of the left and noncoronary aortic valve cusps. The conduction bundle is susceptible to damage in the area of the right fibrous trigone. Vascular structures vulnerable to damage include the circumflex coronary artery, which courses parallel to the posterior annulus on the left, and the coronary sinus, which is superficial to the posterior annulus on the right. In a left dominant coronary artery system, the circumflex coronary artery is at risk for damage along the entire length of the posterior annulus [5].

Pathophysiology of mitral insufficiency

Mitral valve insufficiency caused by degenerative mitral valve disease usually results from segmental leaflet prolapse owing to ruptured or elongated chordae tendineae; the posterior middle scallop (P2) is involved most commonly. Secondary effects include fibrosis of the leaflets with thinning and/or elongation of other chordae tendineae, resulting in more leaflet dysfunction and valvular insufficiency. The left ventricle compensates for the insufficiency with an increase in left ventricle end-diastolic volume that results in an increase in total stroke volume, which allows for maintenance of forward cardiac output [1]. With echocardiography, the increase in end-diastolic volume can be followed easily by the change in left ventricle end-diastolic diameter.

As regurgitant volume increases and the left ventricular size increases to maintain cardiac output, there is additional dilation of the left atrium and the mitral valve annulus. The anterior portion of the mitral valve annulus is in fibrous continuity with the aortic valve and dilates less in response to chronic valve insufficiency than the posterior portion of the annulus. With worsening valve leakage and annular dilation, the normal systolic reduction of the annular diameter does not occur, thus further increasing the regurgitant volume.

Ischemic mitral valve insufficiency results when ischemic injury of the inferior or posterolateral aspects of the left ventricle leads to displacement or tethering of the papillary muscles, valvular tenting, and loss of systolic annular contraction (Carpentier type IIIb). With enlargement of the ventricle and valve annulus, there is increased sphericity of these structures, with dilation in the septal–lateral dimension, or distance from the anterior annulus to the posterior annulus. Some believe the annulus dilates asymmetrically at the posteromedial scallop (P3) and commissure [6].

Echocardiography

Transthoracic echocardiography is indicated in all patients suspected of having mitral insufficiency for baseline evaluation of left ventricular size and function, right and left atrial size, pulmonary artery pressure, and severity of mitral insufficiency. Intraoperative transesophageal echocardiography is indicated to establish the anatomic basis for severe mitral insufficiency and to assess the results of operative intervention on the valve. Quantitative data that stratify the degree of mitral insufficiency include the regurgitant volume (mild <30, moderate 30–59, and severe >60 mL/beat) and the effective regurgitant orifice area (mild <20, moderate 20–39, and severe >40 mm^2) [1].

Indications for operation

In acute, severe mitral insufficiency, most commonly caused by chordal rupture, endocarditis with leaflet perforation, or myocardial infarction with papillary muscle rupture/displacement, a sudden volume overload overwhelms the unprepared left atrium and left ventricle, resulting in acute pulmonary congestion. In this phase of the disease the patient has both reduced forward output (often with hemodynamic compromise) and simultaneous respiratory failure owing to pulmonary venous hypertension. The left ventricle adapts first by increasing ejection fraction, becoming hyperdynamic, and later by dilating to accommodate a larger end-diastolic volume. In some patients, the acute volume overload cannot be tolerated in the short term, and this is especially true with papillary muscle rupture associated with myocardial infarction; in such patients, placement of an intra-aortic balloon pump and urgent valve operation will be necessary [1].

Patients with chronic mitral valve insufficiency may have degenerative valve disease, rheumatic valve disease, or valve leakage owing to ischemic heart disease. Patients with chronic ischemic mitral insufficiency characteristically have an anatomically normal mitral valve. Insufficiency results when posterolateral scar leads to tethering of the mitral apparatus as described previously. New evidence suggests that even a moderate amount of mitral insufficiency in patients undergoing coronary artery revascularization may not resolve after coronary artery bypass alone, and may be associated with reduced long-term survival [6]. Patients with at least moderate or greater ischemic mitral insufficiency may benefit from concomitant mitral valve operation at the time of coronary artery revascularization.

Chronic mitral insufficiency from a primary mitral valve abnormality tends to progress over time with an increase in left ventricular volume overload due to an increase in the effective regurgitant orifice area. Such patients have a high likelihood of developing heart failure symptoms or left ventricle dysfunction. In 1996, Ling and colleagues [7] reported the late outcome of 229 patients with flail mitral valve leaflets, a condition which is uniformly associated with severe valve leakage. During follow-up, which extended to 10 years, 45 patients (20%) died under medical management, and 31 deaths (69%) were due to cardiac causes. Furthermore, congestive heart failure was observed in more than 60% of the patients 10 years after diagnosis; both the presence of symptoms (even the New York Heart Association [NYHA] class I and II) and degree of left ventricle dysfunction impacted late survival [7]. This study suggested that the natural history of severe mitral valve insufficiency is not benign, as previously thought, and that earlier operation might improve patient survival.

Operation is indicated in symptomatic patients with severe mitral insufficiency to improve exercise capacity and quality of life. Survival rates in symptomatic patients with severe valve leakage, particularly those with impaired ventricular function, are poor. Correction of mitral insufficiency should be performed in patients before left ventricular decompensation (ejection fraction <60% or left ventricle end diastolic diameter >45 mm) [5]. Operation should also be considered if patients develop atrial fibrillation or pulmonary hypertension (pulmonary artery systolic pressure >50 mmHg at rest) [1].

Prognosis and management of asymptomatic patients with mitral insufficiency has been controversial. Recent data suggest that with severe mitral insufficiency even patients who are completely asymptomatic are at risk for cardiac complications, including premature death. Enriquez-Sarano and coworkers [8] studied 456 asymptomatic patients with various degrees of organic mitral insufficiency. In this group, the estimated 5-year risk of death was 22% and the risk of any cardiac event (death from cardiac causes, heart failure, or new atrial fibrillation) was 33%. Outcome was linked directly to severity of mitral insufficiency.

In Enriquez-Sarano's study, effective regurgitant orifice area was an important independent determinant of survival in the asymptomatic patients (Fig. 24.1). Indeed, the predictive power of the effective regurgitant orifice area superseded all other qualitative and quantitative measures of mitral valve

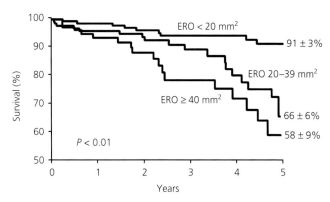

Figure 24.1 Overall survival (Kaplan–Meier estimates) among patients with asymptomatic mitral insufficiency under medical management, and stratified according to the effective regurgitant orifice area (modified from Schaff and coworkers [3] and Sarano and coworkers [8]).

leakage. Those patients with an orifice of at least 40 mm² had an increased risk of late death (both cardiac and overall deaths) and cardiac events (all $P < 0.01$). These data clearly show that patients with a regurgitant orifice of at least 40 mm² have a poor outcome with medical management alone and should be considered for valve repair. As discussed below, early repair of severe mitral regurgitation appears to improve late survival, and we advise operation before the development of symptoms or left ventricle dysfunction in patients with severe mitral insufficiency who have repairable valves.

Surgical technique

Mitral valve exposure

Our standard approach to the mitral valve is via median sternotomy, although alternate incisions and robotic assistance are used in selected cases [5]. Sternotomy allows complete access to all the cardiac chambers and great vessels. Cannulation for cardiopulmonary bypass, managing aortic valve insufficiency, monitoring the left ventricle for distension, and evacuating air are all easier when using the midline approach. In addition, median sternotomy allows for other cardiac procedures, such as coronary artery revascularization and arrhythmia operation, if necessary.

After median sternotomy is performed, cardiopulmonary bypass is instituted with cannulation of the aorta and right atrium. A single two-stage venous atrial cannula provides satisfactory venous return for most patients. If the left atrium is small or if blood return from the superior vena cava to the single cannula is obstructed during atrial retraction, separate cannulae for the cavae should be used. Typically, this includes a right-angle superior vena cava cannula and a straight or right-angle inferior vena cava cannula.

Other maneuvers that may improve mitral valve exposure include lifting up on the right pericardial sutures, avoiding traction sutures on the left, and mobilizing the superior and inferior venae cavae. In patients with pericardial adhesions (e.g., reoperations), freeing the apex of the heart from adhesions and/or opening the left pleural space allows the apex of the heart to fall posteriorly and thus improves exposure of the mitral valve.

Occasionally, a right anterolateral thoracotomy is preferred for mitral valve surgery, such as in a patient with previous median sternotomy and anatomic considerations that make repeat median sternotomy risky. Typical patients include those with patent arterial coronary bypass grafts, especially if they cross the midline, and patients with other potential hazards, such as an enlarged right ventricle. Female patients may prefer anterolateral thoracotomy for cosmetic reasons. There is also increasing experience in using minimally invasive techniques (video assisted, robotic) to repair the mitral valve. Exposure in such instances is a variation of the right anterolateral thoracotomy approach.

For the right anterolateral thoracotomy approach, the patient is positioned at a 30° tilt, right side up, and the patient's right arm is positioned overhead. The chest is entered through the fifth interspace via an incision made from just right of the sternum to the anterior axillary line. One-lung ventilation is preferred. Pulling the diaphragm down with stay sutures brought through the inferior intercostal spaces and tagged on traction enhances exposure of the atria. The nonventilated lung is retracted posteriorly, and cardiopulmonary bypass cannulae (two venous, one arterial) are placed. The aortic cannula may be difficult to insert from this exposure, necessitating use of the femoral artery for arterial cannulation. Additionally, venous drainage via a femoral venous long cannula passed into the right atrium can usually provide adequate flow. Vacuum assistance is a helpful adjunct for venous drainage in this setting.

Atriotomy

After cardiopulmonary bypass is established at normothermia or mild hypothermia, the aortic cross-clamp is applied and cold blood cardioplegia is instituted, producing complete cardiac arrest [5]. In most patients, the mitral valve is exposed with an incision in the left atrium just posterior to the interatrial groove. Before making the atriotomy, the interatrial groove can be developed several centimeters with sharp dissection. The incision begins on the anterolateral left atrium near the junction of the right superior pulmonary vein and left atrium, posterior to Waterston's groove. It continues inferiorly between the right inferior pulmonary vein and the inferior vena cava. By developing the interatrial plane, the left atrial incision can be made approximately 2–4 cm from the right pulmonary veins, giving closer exposure of the mitral valve.

Other atrial incisions may be useful in circumstances in which exposure is poor, as sometimes occurs in patients with a large anteroposterior chest diameter, patients with marked concentric left ventricular hypertrophy, and in some patients undergoing reoperation. For example, a simple trans-septal incision provides excellent exposure of the mitral valve and is favored when a right atriotomy is necessary for treatment of concomitant tricuspid valve disease. This approach is also useful in patients who have had multiple previous operations; with repeated left atriotomies the tissue may be stiff and fibrotic, making retraction and valve exposure difficult.

In rare situations, it may be impossible to adequately expose the mitral valve through a standard left atriotomy, and the surgeon may use additional incisions, such as the biatrial trans-septal incision as described by Brawley [9], or other modifications of the original Dubost technique. Additionally, the extended vertical transatrial septal approach, as described by Guiraudon *et al.* [10], opens both atria widely, giving excellent mitral valve exposure, even in the setting of a small left atrium.

Mitral valve examination

After the heart has been arrested and the atriotomy has been performed, the entire mitral valve complex must be examined carefully to confirm the mechanism of mitral insufficiency, to assess the feasibility of reconstruction, and to plan the exact operative strategy. The mitral annulus is examined to assess the severity of dilation, presence and extent of calcification, and severity and extent of leaflet prolapse according to segmental valve analysis. The anterolateral scallop of the posterior leaflet (P1) is often intact and can serve as a reference point. Applying traction to the free edge of other valvular segments and comparing them with the P1 segment determines the severity and extent of leaflet prolapse [2].

Mitral valve repair

The goals of reconstructive surgery are preservation or restoration of normal leaflet motion, creation of a large surface of coaptation, and stabilization of the entire annulus with a remodeling annuloplasty. Current surgical techniques allow surgeons to perform reconstructive surgery in almost all patients with degenerative mitral disease. Provided that these guidelines are followed, a durable repair can be expected in approximately 98% of patients with a mortality of <1% [11].

Not all regurgitant mitral valves are repairable, however. Significant postinflammatory changes, calcification, extensive bileaflet involvement, and severe ischemic valve tethering increase the complexity of valve repair and decrease the likelihood of a durable result. In such instances it is best to proceed directly to mitral valve replacement.

Posterior leaflet repair

The most common finding with leaflet prolapse is ruptured or elongated chordae tendineae to the middle scallop (P2) of the posterior leaflet. In such cases, the prolapsing segment is resected in a triangular fashion with the base of the triangle at

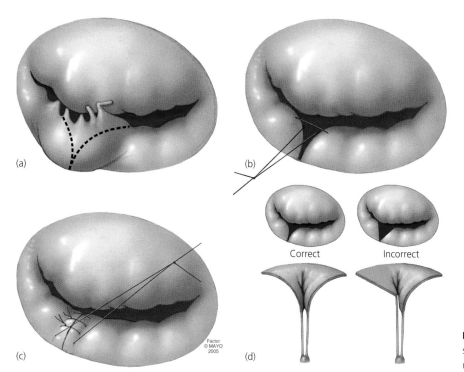

(a)

(b)

Correct   Incorrect

(c)   (d)

Factor
© MAYO
2005

Figure 24.2 Triangular resection prolapsed segment posterior leaflet mitral valve with repair (modified from Suri and Orszulak [12]).

the leading edge and the apex toward the annulus (Fig. 24.2). The defect is repaired in two layers with 4–0 Prolene sutures (Ethicon Inc., A Johnson & Johnson Company, Somerville, NJ, USA). We believe triangular resection has several advantages over quadrangular resection. The triangular repair is simple and eliminates the need for annular plication sutures and sliding plasty of the normal posterior leaflet. By eliminating plication of the posterior annulus, there is less risk of circumflex coronary artery kinking [12].

Anterior leaflet repair

Often, anterior leaflet prolapse is diffuse, extending over a long portion of the free edge of the valve. In such cases, annuloplasty alone is sufficient to restore coaptation with the posterior leaflet and to eliminate insufficiency [13]. When there is segmental prolapse of the anterior leaflet, as occurs with chordal rupture, we favor repair using artificial chordae tendineae. In this technique, both needles of a pledgetted double-armed 4–0 Gore-Tex™ suture (Gore-Tex™, W.L. Gore™ & Associates, Flagstaff, AZ, USA) are passed through the appropriate papillary muscle that gave rise to the abnormal chordae, with the sutures exiting the fibrous tip; the suture is not tied. Each suture is then passed twice through the leading edge of the prolapsing mitral leaflet segment near its center. The suture is then tied carefully so as to restore the free edge of the anterior leaflet to the plane of the valve annulus; multiple knots are required to prevent slippage [12].

Plication or limited resection of a prolapsing segment of the anterior leaflet can be used, but resection should be limited

to only one-third the distance between the leading edge of the valve leaflet and the annulus to prevent tethering. We rarely use triangular resection for anterior leaflet pathology, but the technique is used by other centers [14].

Bileaflet repair

It is important to note that, in many cases, bileaflet prolapse can be corrected by annuloplasty alone. When there are identifiable areas of both anterior and posterior leaflets that require repair, we often combine the above two techniques. The order of performance, however, is of importance. To gain the best exposure of the papillary muscle for placement of the artificial chordae, it is best to complete the posterior triangular resection first but without repairing the resultant defect. Next, the artificial chordae sutures are placed through the papillary muscle and prolapsing anterior leaflet as previously described; but, the sutures are not tied. The posterior leaflet triangular resection is then repaired. Finally, the artificial chordae are adjusted to length and tied as previously described [12].

Posterior annuloplasty

Annuloplasty is an integral part of mitral valve repair. Our preference is to place a standard partial 63-mm-long flexible annuloplasty ring or band along the posterior annulus between the right and left fibrous trigones (Fig. 24.3). The ring is secured to the annulus with 7–9 interrupted 2–0 Ethibond sutures (Ethicon Inc., A Johnson & Johnson Company, Somerville, NJ, USA). We use the same ring for most mitral valve repairs in

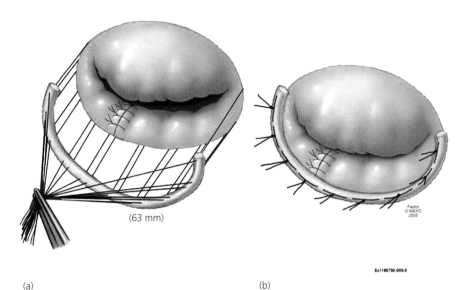

(63 mm)

Figure 24.3 Partial ring posterior annuloplasty. Flexible 63-mm annuloplasty ring or band placed between the right and left fibrous trigones (modified from Suri and Orszulak [12]).

(a)

(b)

the treatment of mitral insufficiency caused by degenerative mitral disease [12].

In repair of mitral valve insufficiency resulting from cardiomyopathy (dilated or ischemic), an "undersized" (restrictive) annuloplasty band is used (approximately 55 mm in length). Undersizing the annuloplasty is important, regardless of the method used. Some surgeons favor complete ring annuloplasty for repair of ischemic mitral valve insufficiency and cite the high rate of recurrent or residual insufficiency as a failure of annular remodeling with partial flexible rings. In addition, there are newly designed rings that, compared with conventional symmetric annuloplasty rings, have tailored reduction of the anteroposterior dimension; these asymmetric three-dimensional devices are intended to reduce middle-to-medial (P2–P3) curvature and increase coaptation of the tethered P2 and P3 segments [15]. Additional experience and follow-up will be necessary to determine whether or not these specially designed rings will prevent recurrence of ischemic mitral insufficiency.

Completion transesophageal echocardiography

It is important for the echocardiographer and surgeon to be familiar with the characteristics of the repaired valve that may increase the likelihood of residual insufficiency or repair failure. Residual mild mitral insufficiency or greater than grade I should be addressed surgically during the same operation by either a re-repair or replacement. Although the exact location of mitral insufficiency may not be as important to identify before the first attempt at repair, it is very helpful to determine which segment is causing a residual leak post repair, using transesophageal echocardiography before repeat surgical exploration. If the first repair was felt to be satisfactory by visual examination, the transesophageal echocardiogram may be the only guide to aid the surgeon attempting a re-repair of the mitral valve [12].

Mitral valve replacement

When mitral valve replacement is necessary, consideration should be given to preservation of the subvalvular apparatus [5]. We usually excise the anterior leaflet but preserve the posterior leaflet and its subvalvular apparatus, if not involved by infection or extensive calcification. An issue is whether saving thickened leaflets and chordae results in placement of a significantly smaller valve. If an adequately sized prosthesis cannot be placed, we would resect the portions of the posterior leaflet and subvalvular apparatus as necessary. Preservation of chordae helps to maintain ventricular geometry and function of the papillary muscles. The intact posterior chordae reduce longitudinal tension on the posterior left ventricular free wall and reduce the risk of atrioventricular groove disruption [16].

Our practice is to place 2–0 Ethibond sutures with the pledgets situated on the ventricular side. If a tissue valve is placed and the mitral orifice is large, the leaflet tissues are simply pinned up toward the annulus. If a mechanical valve is being placed, it may be difficult to tether the leaflet tissue and chordae safely out of the way of the valvular mechanism. In this situation, resection of the leaflet and subvalvular apparatus may be indicated.

Some surgeons make a point to preserve the anterior leaflet during valve replacement. It has been our experience that, if the anterior leaflet is pliable enough to persevere, then often the valve in repairable. Regardless, if the anterior leaflet is preserved, the surgeon must be sure that the preserved leaflet tissue does not impinge on the prosthesis or protrude into the left ventricular outflow tract, creating obstruction. One technique involves detaching a rim of approximately 5 mm of leaflet tissue from the anterior annulus. The incision is carried to each commissure, freeing the anterior leaflet from the annulus. Two 1- to 2-cm pods of leaflet are retained that contain the chordae to each of the papillary muscles. The pods are secured to the annulus at the 2 to 3 and 9 to 10 o'clock positions with the corresponding pledgetted valve sutures [17].

Calcified annulus

Valve replacement in the face of a heavily calcified mitral annulus presents a challenge. Aggressive debridement of calcification is risky, with possible complications including circumflex coronary artery damage and atrioventricular disruption. Fortunately, the calcification is posterior to the trigones in 98% of patients, and rarely involves the leaflets (6%), or extensively the ventricular myocardium or papillary muscles (20%). Usually the anterior annulus is spared [18]. In only a minority of cases will the calcium be so extensive as to require radical debridement. In our practice, as well as at other clinics, most surgeons avoid extensive debridement unless it is absolutely necessary [17].

With mild to moderate annular calcification, we remove the anterior leaflet, leaving a 5-mm rim of tissue for suture placement, and leaving the posterior calcified annulus intact. The sutures can usually be placed in the normal fashion, taking generous tissue bites and avoiding the calcium as much as possible. The sutures being placed with the pledgets on the ventricular side allow direct tissue-to-sewing ring apposition. It is helpful to choose a valve with a generous sewing cuff that prevents leakage between crevices of calcium. If calcification is more severe and sutures cannot be placed through the annulus, one option is to anchor the prosthesis directly to the leaflets themselves; one may have to downsize the prosthesis a size or two to obtain a good fit. Another option involves seating the prosthesis in a supra-annular position by placing mattress sutures within the left atrium, just above the calcified annulus. Pledgetted sutures placed from the atrial to the ventricular side are best for this technique.

Rarely, heavy circumferential leaflet and annular calcification precludes safe suture placement and the only option may be to debride the calcium. Caution must be carried out during this portion of the procedure to avoid injury to the circumflex coronary artery and atrioventricular connection. If debridement is extensive and puts the patient at risk of atrioventricular disruption, pericardial reconstruction of the annular defect with pledgetted sutures is indicated. Horizontal mattress sutures can be passed through the pericardium creating a new portion of the annulus to anchor the valve prosthesis [5].

Results

Operative mortality at the Mayo Clinic is 1% for elective mitral valve repair and replacement in patients younger than 75 years [5,12]. The availability of reproducible valve repair as an alternative to prosthetic replacement has dramatically influenced the indications for surgical intervention. With successful valve repair, patients who maintain sinus rhythm can resume full activities without the need for chronic anti-

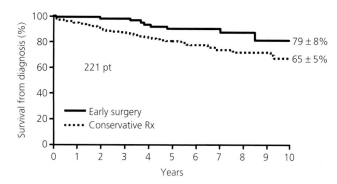

Figure 24.4 Overall survival from time of diagnosis in patients with mitral insufficiency due to flail leaflets according to the management strategy selected at baseline. Survival was significantly better in patients who underwent early surgery than in those who received conservative management (Rx) (modified from Schaff and coworkers [3] and Ling and coworkers [7]).

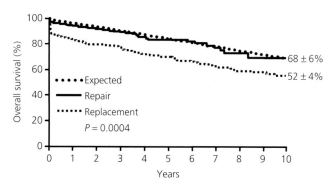

Figure 24.5 Overall survival of patients having valve repair or valve replacement for severe mitral insufficiency. Note the statistically significant difference between the groups ($P = 0.004$) and the similarity of survival of patients who had valve repair compared with the expected survival rate (modified from Schaff and coworkers [3] and Enriquez-Sarano and coworkers [11]).

coagulation. In addition to less morbidity, valve repair seems to improve patient survival more than prosthetic replacement. Earlier valve repair for mitral insufficiency should improve patient survival compared with previous strategies waiting for the development of symptoms before surgical referral (Fig. 24.4).

We previously evaluated 409 patient having correction of organic mitral insufficiency in the 1980s and found that, after valve repair, overall survival at 10 years was 68% ± 6% compared with 52% ± 4% for patients undergoing valve replacement ($P = 0.0004$); similarly, operative mortality was significantly reduced ($P = 0.002$) and late survival was significantly improved with repair compared with replacement (Fig. 24.5). Ejection fraction decreased significantly after operation in both groups, but was higher after valve repair ($P = 0.001$). Most importantly, multivariate analysis demonstrated an independent positive effect of valve repair on overall

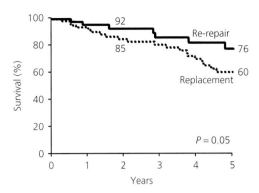

Figure 24.6 Late survival (>30 days or discharge from the hospital) after mitral valve re-repair or replacement at reoperation for recurrent mitral insufficiency. The late survival associated with mitral valve re-repair is greater than that seen after mitral valve replacement; mortality hazard ratio for re-repair, 0.49; P = 0.05 versus valve replacement (modified from Schaff and coworkers [3] and Suri and coworkers [22]).

survival (hazard ration, 0.39; P = 0.026), late survival (hazard ration, 0.44; P = 0.001), and postoperative ejection fraction (P = 0.001) [3].

There are likely several mechanisms whereby overall survival is improved with mitral valve repair compared with replacement. Operative mortality is lower with repair because of elimination of device-related complications, such as ventricular rupture, thrombus formation, and mechanical malfunction. With valve repair, the chordal apparatus is preserved, and studies in patients having valve replacement show that the preservation of mitral valve attachments preserves ventricular geometry and systolic function [19–21]. Also, the rate of late complications is much lower for valve repair than for prosthetic replacement. The survival advantage of repair over replacement extends to patients who undergo reoperation for late failure of initial repair (Fig. 24.6) [22]. Valve repair significantly improves postoperative outcome in patients with mitral insufficiency, and should be the preferred mode of surgical correction. The low operative mortality is an incentive for early surgery before ventricular dysfunction occurs.

Operative techniques in the surgical management of mitral insufficiency have evolved over the past 20 years and have predictable and durable results after valve repair. In current practice at our clinic, more than 90–95% of patients with pure mitral insufficiency as a result degenerative diseases have valvuloplasty rather than prosthetic replacement. With simplified methods of leaflet repair and annuloplasty, the risk of reoperation after correction of posterior leaflet prolapse is approximately 0.5% per year, and rates of reintervention after repair of the anterior or bileaflet prolapse are similarly low (1.6% and 0.9% per year, respectively). Furthermore, the durability of mitral repair for all leaflet prolapse subsets in the current era is similar to that after mitral valve replacement (0.74% per year overall) [23].

References

1. Bonow RO, Carabello BA, Chatterjee K, *et al.* (2006) ACC/AHA 2006 guidelines for the management of patients with valvular heart disease: a report of the American College of Cardiology/American Heart Association Task Force on Practice Guidelines (Writing Committee to Develop Guidelines for the Management of Patients with Valvular Heart Disease). *Circulation* **114**:e84–e231.

2. Filsoufi F & Carpentier A (2007) Principles of reconstructive surgery in degenerative mitral valve disease. *Semin Thorac Cardiovasc Surg* **19**:103–110.

3. Schaff HV, Suri RM, & Enriquez-Sarano M (2007) Indications for surgery in degenerative mitral valve disease. *Semin Thorac Cardiovasc Surg* **19**:97–102.

4. Shah P (2005) Heart and great vessels. In: Standring S, Ellis H, Healy JC, *et al.* (eds.). *Gray's Anatomy. The Anatomical Basis of Clinical Practice*, 39th edn. Edinburgh: Elsevier, pp. 1006–1008.

5. Burkhart HM & Zehr KJ (2004) Mitral valve replacement. In: Yang SC & Cameron DE (eds.). *Current Therapy in Thoracic and Cardiovascular Surgery*. Philadelphia: Mosby Publishing, pp. 623–626.

6. McGee EC & McCarthy PM (2005) Correction of ischemic mitral regurgitation. *Oper Tech Thorac Cardiovasc Surg* **10**:101–112.

7. Ling LH, Enriquez-Sarano M, Seward JB, *et al.* (1996) Clinical outcome of mitral regurgitation due to flail leaflet. *N Engl J Med* **335**:1417–1423.

8. Enriquez-Sarano M, Avierinos JF, Messika-Zeitoun D, *et al.* (2005) Quantitative determinants of the outcome of asymptomatic mitral regurgitation. *N Engl J Med* **352**:875–883.

9. Brawley RF (1980) Improved exposure of the mitral valve in patients with a small left atrium. *Ann Thorac Surg* **29**:179–181.

10. Guiraudon GM, Ofiesh JG, & Kaushik R (1991) Extended vertical transatrial septal approach to the mitral valve. *Ann Thorac Surg* **52**:1058–1060.

11. Enriquez-Sarano M, Orszulak TA, Schaff HV, *et al.* (1997) Mitral regurgitation: a new clinical perspective. *Mayo Clin Proc* **72**:1034–1043.

12. Suri RM & Orszulak TA (2005) Triangular resection for repair of mitral regurgitation due to degenerative disease. *Oper Tech Thorac Cardiovasc Surg* **10**:194–199.

13. Phillips MR, Daly RC, Schaff HV *et al.* (2000) Repair of anterior leaflet mitral valve prolapse: chordal replacement versus chordal shortening. *Ann Thorac Surg* **69**:25–29.

14. Seitelberger R, Bialy J, Gottardi R, *et al.* (2004) Triangular plication of the anterior mitral leaflet: a new operative technique. *Ann Thorac Surg* **78**:e36–37.

15. Daimon M, Fukuda S, Adams DH, *et al.* (2006) Mitral valve repair with Carpentier-McCarthy-Adams IMR ETlogix annuloplasty ring for ischemic mitral regurgitation: early echocardiographic results from a multi-center study. *Circulation* **114**:I588–593.

16. Glower DD (2000) Mitral valve implantation. *Oper Tech Thorac Cardiovasc Surg* **5**:242–250.

17. Smedira NG (2003) Mitral valve replacement with a calcified annulus. *Oper Tech Thorac Cardiovasc Surg* **8**:2–13.

18. Carpentier AF, Pellerin M, Fuzellier JF, *et al.* (1996) Extensive calcification of the mitral valve annulus: pathology and surgical management. *J Thorac Cardiovasc Surg* **111**:718–730.

19. Kouris N, Ikonomidis I, Kontogianni D, *et al.* (2005) Mitral valve repair versus replacement for isolated non-ischemic mitral regurgitation in patients with preoperative left ventricle dysfunction. A long-term follow-up echocardiography study. *Eur J Echocardiogr* **6**:435–442.

20. Lillehie CW (1995) New ideas and their acceptance as it has related to preservation of chordae tendinae and certain other discoveries. *J Heart Valve Dis* **4**(Suppl. 2):S106–114.

21. Reardon MJ, & David TE (1999) Mitral valve replacement with preservation of the subvalvular apparatus. *Curr Opin Cardiol* **14**:104–110.

22. Suri RM, Schaff HV, Dearani JA, *et al.* (2006) Recurrent mitral regurgitation after repair: should the mitral valve be re-repaired? *J Thoracic Cardiovasc Surg* **132**:1390–1397.

23. Suri RM, Schaff HV, Dearani JA, *et al.* (2006) Survival advantage and improved durability of mitral repair for leaflet prolapse subsets in the current era. *Ann Thorac Surg* **82**:819–826.

25 Perspectives on Percutaneous Mitral Valve Repair

Frederick St. Goar, Saibal Kar & Ted Feldman
Cardiovascular Institute, Mt View, CA, USA

Introduction

The mitral valve, so named because of its resemblance to a bishop's mitre, is characterized by systolic coaptation of the anterior and posterior leaflet scallops, and is designed to minimize leaflet, annular, and chordal strain. Optimal function of the valve requires synchrony of multiple components including leaflets, annulus, chordae tendineae, papillary muscles, and left ventricular muscle. Clinically significant mitral insufficiency is due to ineffective coaptation and is a common finding in heart failure. Patients with mild mitral insufficiency may remain asymptomatic for many years. However, moderate to severe mitral insufficiency produces either gradual or, at times, acute ventricular dilation and contractile dysfunction [1].

Mitral insufficiency is heterogeneous in its pathology. It is termed degenerative when it is caused by valve leaflet and chordal abnormalities and functional when it is the result of ventricular dysfunction. In patients with symptomatic moderate to severe or severe mitral insufficiency, surgical intervention is the recommended therapy. Surgery is also recommended for asymptomatic patients with severe mitral insufficiency who have evidence of left ventricular dysfunction, and/or atrial fibrillation or pulmonary hypertension [2].

The preferred surgical therapy for mitral insufficiency is mitral valve repair [3,4]. Patients undergoing mitral repair have consistently demonstrated improved short- and long-term outcomes compared with patients who receive a mitral valve prosthesis [5]. For functional mitral insufficiency, the most common surgical intervention is annuloplasty [6]. An annuloplasty, typically using a complete undersized ring, provides correction of annular dilation, an increase in leaflet coaptation, and reduction of chordal tension, and helps prevent future annular dilation. Although surgical intervention in patients suffering from functional mitral insufficiency is a therapeutic option, the beneficial impact, especially in patients with reduced left ventricular function resulting from an ischemic etiology,

Cardiovascular Interventions in Clinical Practice. Edited by Jürgen Haase, Hans-Joachim Schäfers, Horst Sievert and Ron Waksman. © 2010 Blackwell Publishing.

remains controversial owing to limited durability or the progression of the ischemic disease process [7,8]. In addition, patients with functional mitral insufficiency are often not suitable surgical candidates because of the presence of left ventricle dysfunction, comorbidities, and significant coronary artery disease. The frequently unacceptable morbidity associated with open heart surgery presently keeps many patients with clinically significant mitral insufficiency from receiving mitral surgery. A variety of new percutaneous, transcatheter mitral valve therapies are being developed with the goal of expanding the pool of patients who might dramatically benefit from a less traumatic approach to a reduction in mitral insufficiency.

Percutaneous annuloplasty

Approach

Percutaneous approaches to annular remodeling include coronary sinus-based annuloplasty, direct intracavitary annuloplasty, and other novel cinching devices. Thus far, published results have primarily focused on coronary sinus-based annular remodeling. The coronary sinus and great coronary vein course near the atrioventricular groove in proximity to the mitral annulus. Preclinical data demonstrate that placement of a device in the coronary sinus can alter mitral annular geometry and reduce mitral insufficiency in animal models [9–12]. Challenges related to implementing this approach include identification of patients with an appropriate anatomic relationship of the mitral annulus, coronary sinus, and great cardiac vein. In addition, the coronary sinus crosses over a circumflex coronary branch in as many as two-thirds of patients, making distortion and occlusion of the circumflex coronary artery a potential problem [13].

Device technologies

A number of technologies using percutaneous approaches to annular remodeling are currently being investigated in preclinical animal studies and clinical trials. The Carillon™ Mitral Contour System from Cardiac Dimensions (Kirkland, WA, USA) consists of a nitinol shaping ribbon with distal and proximal anchors (Fig. 25.1). Once the device is positioned in

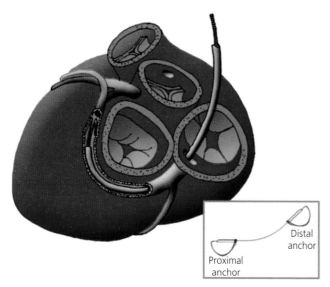

Figure 25.1 CARILLON™ device (Cardiac Dimensions, Kirkland, WA, USA). Two self expandable anchors connected by a ribbon.

the coronary sinus, tension is applied to the ribbon to reduce the mitral annular diameter. The treatment effect can be adjusted under echocardiographic guidance. Application of this device in an ovine rapid-pacing model of heart failure and variable degrees of mitral insufficiency demonstrated reduction of mitral insufficiency, increase in cardiac output, and reduction in pulmonary capillary wedge pressure [9]. Further study revealed that this treatment effect was maintained for 4 weeks and led to improvements in plasma norepinephrine and brain natriuretic peptide levels [10]. Evaluation in a canine model of heart failure confirmed similar beneficial effects on mitral insufficiency and hemodynamic indices. Preserved patency of the coronary sinus after chronic implantation was also demonstrated, and highlighted the importance of considering the anatomy of the circumflex coronary artery in relation to the coronary sinus before device deployment [11]. At the 2008 American College of Cardiology (ACC) meeting, preliminary data from the Carillon Phase 1 pilot study, AMADEUS, were reported. In this trial the device was successfully deployed in 30 patients with functional mitral insufficiency. In 19 patients (63%) the mitral insufficiency improved by one grade. There was one 30-day death and two small non-Q-wave myocardial infarctions [12].

Another indirect annuloplasty device, the percutaneous transvenous mitral annuloplasty (PTMA) system from Viacor Inc. (Wilmington, MA, USA) includes a 7F multilumen catheter that is positioned in the coronary sinus. Preformed stainless-steel elements are inserted into the lumina of the catheter, exerting a graded and adjustable change in mitral annular geometry without cinching (Fig. 25.4). The system allows a diagnostic component, enabling complete withdrawal if the effect is not satisfactory. In addition, the hub of the multilumen catheter is implanted in a subcutaneous pocket, theoretically

enabling repeat access and modification of the treatment effect at any time after the initial device implantation. Preclinical studies with a single-lumen prototype in an ovine model of acute ischemic mitral insufficiency confirmed the feasibility of annular remodeling to reduce mitral insufficiency [13]. A subsequent study of the multilumen catheter in an ovine model of chronic ischemic mitral insufficiency confirmed that PTMA-based annular remodeling reduced chronic ischemic mitral insufficiency by reducing the mitral annular diameter and tenting area. In preclinical models, long-term implantation (up to 6 months) has been associated with maintained reduction in mitral annular diameter, patency of the coronary sinus, and no damage to surrounding structures (circumflex coronary artery, mitral valve).

The Viacor annuloplasty device has been utilized temporarily in 10 patients undergoing open heart surgery for treatment of functional mitral insufficiency. Under this protocol, investigators had approximately 1 hour to perform a diagnostic PTMA. Initial experience with a single-lumen prototype device in five patients confirmed the feasibility of alteration of mitral annular geometry from the coronary sinus. In the remaining five patients, the multilumen device was employed; successful delivery occurred in four patients, with reduction of mitral insufficiency by two grades in two patients and no treatment effect in one. Of note, in the patient with no treatment effect, surgical annuloplasty also failed to reduce mitral insufficiency, and the patient underwent mitral valve replacement. In the fifth patient, there was reduction in mitral insufficiency grade by PTMA, but alterations in systemic blood pressure during the procedure made assessment of treatment effect problematic. Based on this proof-of-concept study, a clinical trial was initiated outside the USA. In the first 20 patients of this study, only seven patients showed any benefit; the device is undergoing redesign [12].

The MONARC™ Percutaneous Mitral Annuloplasty System (Edwards Lifesciences LLC, Irvine, CA, USA) consists of a self-expanding nitinol implant with distal and proximal self-expanding stent anchors (Fig. 25.2). The bridging member between the anchors has shape-memory properties that result in shortening forces at body temperature. As the bridge section tenses and shortens, the anchors are drawn toward each other, displacing the posterior annulus anteriorly. The bridge has the configuration of a spring, held open by bioabsorbable material. The spring shortens over 3–6 weeks as the material dissolves. Thus, the efficacy of the implant is not immediately apparent and neither is the potential impact on the circumflex coronary artery lumen.

The early clinical experience with the first generation of this device, the Edwards Viking Percutaneous Mitral Annuloplasty System, in five patients was recently reported [14]. The device was introduced percutaneously through an internal jugular vein puncture and positioned successfully in the coronary sinus in four out of five patients suffering from chronic ischemic mitral insufficiency. In one patient, the device could

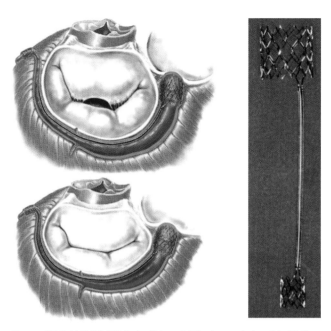

Figure 25.2 MONARC™ device (Edwards Lifesciences, Irvine, CA, USA). Two self-expandable nitinol stent-like anchors connected by a bridge.

not be advanced fully into the coronary sinus after two attempts, so it was not implanted. Coronary angiography was performed before the procedure and at 3 months. Baseline site-assessed mitral insufficiency was 3.0 ± 0.7, and three out of four patients with an implant had reduced severity of mitral insufficiency at discharge. Severity of mitral insufficiency was reduced to 1.6 ± 1.1 at the last postimplant visit in patients with an intact device. Separation of the bridge section of the device occurred in three out of four patients receiving an implant, and was detected 28–81 days after the procedure. There were no adverse events associated with bridge separation. The device was then redesigned as the Monarc™ and implanted in 59/69 additional patients. Mitral insufficiency was improved in 60% (19/31). Late bridge fractures occurred in several, and coronary compression was noted in three, with an acute mitral insufficiency resulting in death in one patient at 552 days [12]. These initial data confirm the feasibility but also the challenges of percutaneous, coronary sinus-based annular remodeling in humans, and demonstrate a potential beneficial effect on functional mitral insufficiency in selected patients.

Percutaneous annuloplasty: future directions

Patient selection is a key challenge with coronary sinus-based annular remodeling. It is likely that patients with certain specific anatomic configurations of the coronary sinus, great coronary vein, mitral valve, and left ventricle may be candidates for percutaneous, coronary-sinus based annuloplasty; however, clinical experience is necessary to identify and quantify these parameters and to identify appropriate patients. Preprocedural screening with noninvasive imaging modalities (e.g., multislice CTA) will be mandatory to avoid patients at

risk for circumflex coronary artery compression and the subsequent ischemia.

Once the profile of potential candidates is better understood and some of the technical challenges in device design are addressed, percutaneous annuloplasty as sole therapy will need to be compared with standard therapy as well as other percutaneous approaches. For patients with congestive heart failure and functional mitral insufficiency caused by left ventricular dysfunction, standard therapy is pharmacologic and, in some cases, includes cardiac resynchronization therapy. Few of these patients are currently referred for surgery because of the less than optimal outcomes. Therefore, trials of percutaneous annuloplasty are likely to be complex and will likely resemble randomized trial investigations of medical and device-based therapies for heart failure. Despite all the investigative hurdles and potential technical and clinical challenges, if a simple transvenous coronary sinus implant is able to safely and predictably reduce mitral insufficiency, it could become a very worthwhile therapy for many presently untreated patients.

A variety of other percutaneous annuloplasty systems are under development using a nonsinus approach. Percutaneous annular reconfiguration systems placed via the cavity of the left atrium or left ventricle include the Mitralign® Percutaneous Mitral Repair System (Mitralign Inc., Tewksbury, MA, USA), AccuCinch™ (Guided Delivery Systems, Santa Clara, CA, USA), and PS3 System™ (Ample Medical Inc., Foster City, CA, USA). These devices offer a compelling alternative approach that is more in line with the surgical paradigm. Although they may be more challenging to deliver than the sinoplasty systems, the fact that they avoid the issue of the coronary sinus–circumflex artery juxtaposition makes them intriguing technical alternatives. Finally, the i-Coapsys™ device (Myocor Inc., Maple Grove, MN, USA) is designed to alter ventricular and annular geometry by tensioning devices placed on the epicardial surface of the heart, and although there are interesting data from an off-pump beating heart surgical approach to placing this device, it remains to be seen whether it can be successfully placed using a transpericardial percutaneous approach. A phase I trial is planned in the USA for this approach.

Percutaneous edge-to-edge mitral repair

Surgical precedent

Degenerative mitral insufficiency (mitral prolapse and/or flail), which is the indication for over 75% of mitral valve surgical interventions, requires some form of leaflet and or chordal resection or reconstruction at the time of surgical repair. Although valve repair outcomes compare favorably with valve replacement, nationwide in the USA it is still performed only in fewer than half of the patients undergoing mitral valve surgery [15]. Valve replacement is selected based on anatomic factors, including leaflet pathology, annular calcification, comorbidities, and surgeon experience and

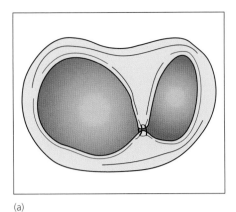

(a)

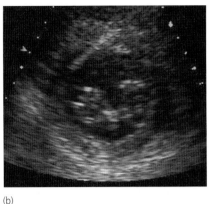

(b)

Figure 25.3 Edge-to-edge repair with suture apposing anterior and posterior leaflets, schematic and short axis transthoracic echocardiography image.

preference. Complex valvular pathology compromises the outcome of a repair [16]. To expand the number of potential candidates for repair, surgeons have developed novel repair techniques including chordal shortening and transposition, sliding leaflet repair, and the edge-to-edge technique [17].

A pioneering Italian cardiac surgeon, Ottavio Alfieri, first performed edge-to-edge repair of anterior leaflet prolapse in 1991. When operating on an atrial septal defect in a 29-year-old, he noted that she had a double-orifice mitral valve, a rare but well-described congenital defect [18]. Later that day, after performing mitral valve repair on a patient who had anterior leaflet prolapse, the surgeon initially obtained a suboptimal result. He processed what he had seen in the previous patient and insightfully elected to appose the middle scallops of the anterior and posterior leaflet with a stitch at the location of the remaining leak, creating an effectively functioning dual-orifice mitral valve (Fig. 25.3). This approach has now been successfully used to treat degenerative mitral insufficiency due to the prolapse of either one or both leaflets, as well as for functional insufficiency from ischemia or cardiomyopathy [19,20]. The edge-to-edge repair has received mixed reviews within the surgical community. It is worth noting that the technique, although routinely used by some, has most frequently served as a bail-out procedure when more conventional surgical approaches are suboptimal.

In a recent report from Alfieri's group [21], central double-orifice repair was performed in 260 patients followed for up to 7 years. The majority (81%) of the patients had degenerative etiology. At 5 years, survival was 94% and freedom from reoperation was 90%. Freedom from reoperation was lower (72% vs. 92%) in patients who did not undergo a concomitant annuloplasty procedure than in those who did; however, annuloplasty was not a multivariable predictor of freedom from reoperation [22]. In another report, Alfieri's group presented an intention-to-treat isolated edge-to-edge surgical repair patient. They showed a rate of freedom from reoperation of 90% and recurrent mitral insufficiency of >2+ at 5 years and almost 80% freedom from reoperation and recurrent mitral insufficiency of >2+ after 12 years [23]. These data sup-

port the notion that an isolated edge-to-edge mitral repair has the potential to be durable in selected patients. The clinical success and relative simplicity of this technique prompted interest in the development of a catheter-based, percutaneously delivered, edge-to-edge repair.

Development of percutaneous edge-to-edge repair

The first dedicated catheter based edge-to-edge repair system project was started in 1999 (Evalve, Inc., Menlo Park, CA, USA). The initial endeavor focused on reproducing the surgical paradigm of a suture-based approach. Various suture systems were tested in an isolated pig heart model, and in the process of these tests it became apparent that the leaflets needed to be stabilized first before being sutured. The model used for the development of the technology was created by removing the left atrium of a porcine heart and transecting primary chordae of the middle scallop of the posterior leaflet. With the heart immersed in a warm water bath, a tube was placed through the left ventricular apex and ventricular pressure varied to mimic the cardiac cycle and create physiologic mitral leaflet motion. It was discovered that the system that was developed to effectively stabilize the leaflets, a figure of 8 open loop introduced through the valve from the atrial side and then pulled up to catch the leaflets and produce leaflet coaptation (Fig. 25.4), also resolved the mitral insufficiency. This stabilization system eventually evolved, in an iterative fashion, in to what is now the Evalve MitraClip mitral repair system (Fig. 25.5).

The delivery system was refined for percutaneous endovascular placement in an acute porcine model. This included development of a steerable guide catheter, delivered transseptally into the left atrium via femoral vein access. A double orifice was created in 14 anesthetized normal adult pigs. Direct epicardial echocardiographic guidance was used to place the clip [24]. A double orifice was created in all 14 animals, sometimes requiring several grasps. There was no mitral insufficiency or echocardiographic evidence of mitral stenosis after clip deployment. In two animals, the clip released from the anterior leaflet, retrospectively determined to be related

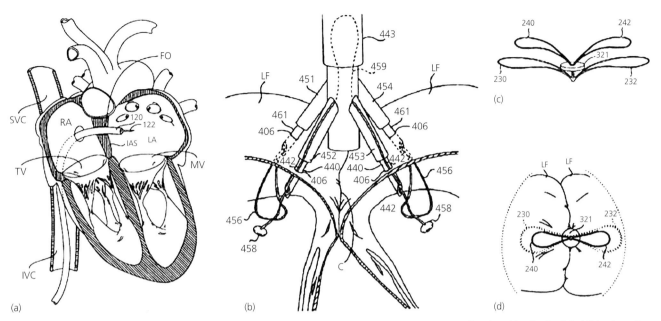

Figure 25.4 Evalve patent drawings. (a) Trans-septal approach of guide catheter. (b) Initial suture base concept abandoned for clip. (c, d) Stabilizing loops for atrial and ventricular sides of leaflets.

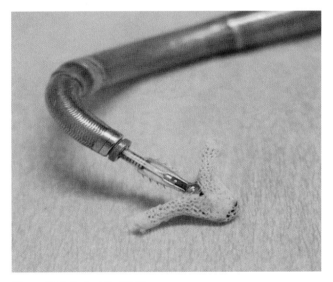

Figure 25.5 Evalve MitraClip™.

to an improper grasping technique with the clip not properly configured for grasping. Acute postmortem analysis confirmed a double orifice in the remaining 12 pigs, with clip deployment perpendicular to the line of coaptation.

Separate chronic animal studies were conducted to evaluate the healing response of the clip with extended follow-up [25]. At 4 weeks, the entire clip was encapsulated in a layer of tissue. There was evidence of tissue deposition and leaflet-to-leaflet healing. At 12 weeks, tissue encapsulation was further developed with leaflet-to-leaflet bridging between the arms of the clip. At 24 weeks, development of mature solid tissue bridging

was present. Scanning electron microscopy of three mitral valves (one each at 4 weeks, 12 weeks, and 24 weeks) showed complete tissue encapsulation of the clip with endothelial cells on the surface. In summary, the clip became well incorporated into the valve leaflets with no significant tissue growth beyond the sides of the clip or evidence of tissue necrosis between the clip arms. Privitera *et al.* [26] recently reported surgical pathologic findings of a patient who received isolated surgical edge-to-edge repair and then 4 years later underwent cardiac transplantation for progressive heart failure in spite of a competent nonstenotic mitral valve. The point of suture apposition of the anterior and posterior mitral leaflets was shown to be encapsulated with endothelial tissue surrounding a fibrous tissue bridge. The pathologic findings demonstrated at 6- and 12-month follow-up in the Evalve porcine model are remarkably similar to the pathology of the 4-year surgical result.

Percutaneous edge-to-edge repair with the MitraClip in humans is performed in the cardiac catheterization laboratory with a combination of echocardiographic and fluoroscopic guidance. Access to the left atrium is obtained via the femoral vein and a 24F guide catheter is placed across the intra-atrial septum using standard trans-septal techniques. A steerable clip delivery system is introduced through the guide and, using a series of iterative steps, positioned above the mitral leaflets at the location of the regurgitant jet. After the opened clip is passed through the leaflets, it is pulled back to grasp the free edges of the leaflets and then closed, resulting in a double-orifice valve (Fig. 25.6). The acute result is then evaluated with two-dimensional color-flow and pulsed Doppler imaging. If inadequate reduction in mitral insufficiency is obtained, the leaflets can be released and repositioned. In some cases, a

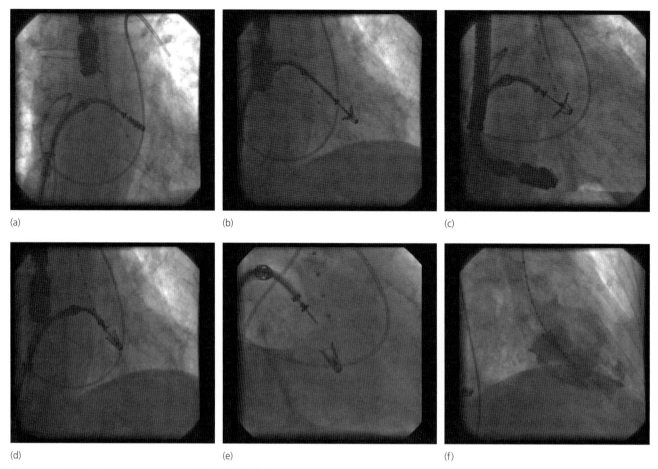

Figure 25.6 (a) Mitraclip™ advanced out guide catheter in left atrium. (b) Open clip advanced into left ventricle. (c) Clip pulled back to grasp leaflets. (d) Clip closed on leaflets. (e) Clip detached. (f) Left ventricular angiogram showing absence of residual mitral regurgitation.

single clip is not sufficient to adequately decrease the magnitude of mitral insufficiency. In this situation, a second clip can be placed adjacent to the first clip on the side of the residual jet. Repeat hemodynamic and echocardiographic assessments are then performed to verify the final results, at which point the delivery system is removed and groin hemostasis obtained with manual compression.

The procedure requires a dedicated team of physicians. Clear communication between the interventionalist and the echocardiographer providing the transesophageal echocardiographic guidance is imperative to achieve an optimal outcome [27]. The procedure is performed under general anesthesia and the anesthesiologist also plays a critical role. Although cardiologists are well versed in echocardiographic assessment of mitral insufficiency in the conscious unsedated patient, hemodynamics are altered in the anesthetized patient. Changes in blood pressure, afterload, and vascular tone need to be considered during the evaluation of procedural results in this setting. Working with an anesthesiologist who is versed in intraoperative echocardiographic interpretation facilitates assessment of an adequate result, in terms of the degree of reduction of mitral insufficiency.

Human studies

The first human implant of the Mitraclip was performed in June 2003. The first patient was a 48-year-old woman who suffered from anterior flail and severe symptomatic mitral insufficiency. Her mitral insufficiency was reduced to <2+. Two years after her procedure she was clinically stable and asymptomatic. Her mitral insufficiency grade remained at <2+ and, more importantly, her left ventricular volumes, which were abnormal before the procedure, had decreased and normalized [28]. Follow-up echocardiography performed in this patient 4 years post procedure demonstrated that the mitral insufficiency remained at <2+ per the echocardiography core laboratory.

The Mitraclip system has been successfully evaluated in a US phase I clinical trial (EVEREST I); the 6-month results have been published and the 12-month results have been reported [29,30]. The study population consisted of surgical candidates with moderate to severe or severe mitral insufficiency and clinical symptoms. Symptomatic patients were eligible if echocardiographic evidence of left ventricular dysfunction was present. American College of Cardiology/American Heart Association (ACC/AHA) guidelines for the criteria for surgical intervention were followed and patients were closely screened using American Society for Echocardiography methods for the assessment of mitral insufficiency severity [31,32]. An echocardiography core laboratory was used for the baseline and follow-up assessment of results. Echocardiographic anatomic inclusion criteria included specific leaflet morphologic findings, to determine if adequate tissue was available, and location of mitral insufficiency jet origin (from the central two-thirds of the line of coaptation), to determine if there was enough tissue coaptation for clip placement. The rigorous morphologic criteria effectively excluded patients with severe valve pathology and severe ventricular dilation. These criteria were developed with the help and insight of cardiovascular surgeons.

The primary end point for the EVEREST I trial was safety at 30 days. Safety was defined as freedom from death, myocardial infarction, cardiac tamponade, cardiac surgery for failed clip or device, clip detachment, permanent stroke, or septicemia. Secondary safety end points included hospital vascular complications, 30-day and 6-month bleeding, endocarditis, clip thrombosis, hemolysis, or mitral valve surgery, and the 6-month secondary safety end point was cardiac surgery for the failed clip or device.

The primary efficacy end point was reduction of mitral insufficiency to 2+ or less based on the fact that the ACC/AHA task force guidelines for valvular heart disease do not recommend valve surgery for 2+ mitral insufficiency or less. Secondary efficacy end points included successful implantation of the clip and implantation without major adverse events in the hospital. The 30-day, 6- and 12-month secondary efficacy end points included mitral insufficiency severity determined by echocardiography and mitral valve function, including transvalvular pressure gradient, mitral valve area, and cardiac output. New York Heart Association functional class was evaluated as a secondary efficacy end point.

A total of 107 patients (median age 71 years) were enrolled in the EVEREST I trial and the roll-in nonrandomized portion of the EVEREST II trial. Twenty-three patients (21%) suffered from pure functional mitral insufficiency and the rest had degenerative or combined degenerative and functional disease. Acute procedural success, which was defined as successful clip placement with reduction of mitral insufficiency severity to ≤2+, was achieved in 76% of patients. Ten of the 107 patients (9%) had a major adverse event, including a single death (unrelated to the clip), a single stroke with a neurologic deficit lasting more than 72 h that resolved within 30 days, nonelective cardiac surgery in two patients for trans-septal complications, and bleeding requiring transfusion ≥2 units in five patients. Partial clip detachment, defined as detachment of a single leaflet from the clip, occurred in 10 patients (9%). This occurred in three patients during clip placement, in one before hospital discharge, and in five patients between discharge and 30 days. Only one partial clip detachment occurred after 30 days. None of the partial clip detachments was associated with clinical events or the need

for urgent intervention. Overall, in-hospital mortality was <1%. Major adverse events within 30 days included partial clip detachment without embolization in 7% of patients, all of whom underwent successful elective valve surgery. A post-procedural stroke occurred in one patient. Symptoms totally resolved by 30 days. The average length of hospital stay was <2 days. When a clip was placed and the result was suboptimal and surgery was subsequently required, mitral repair using standard surgical techniques was possible as late as 18 months after the initial interventional procedure [33]. The fact that this percutaneous repair technique does not appear to impact the future surgical options for the treated patients is an important criterion for future clinical acceptance of this technique.

Durability data for this procedure, admittedly short term, now include, among patients discharged with a successful result, an actuarial 2-year freedom from death, mitral valve surgery, or recurrent mitral insufficiency of >2+ of 80%. Although these initial data are compelling, the strategy for application and indications for this procedure remain to be determined. To be deemed clinically successfully, this therapy will need to result in both an initial and a sustained mitral insufficiency reduction and, depending on the patient population, will need to compare favorably with surgical benchmarks. After surgical repair of degenerative disease, recurrence of mitral insufficiency has been reported with linearized recurrence rates of >2+ mitral insufficiency of 3.7% per year [34]. The EVERST II trial, which is currently enrolling, will report the results of Mitraclip therapy versus routine surgical therapy in 280 randomized in a 2:1 fashion.

As noted, both the Evalve feasibility study and the ongoing EVEREST II trial include patients with degenerative or functional mitral insufficiency who are candidates for mitral repair surgery and represent a broad patient population. At one end are younger patients in whom the longer-term results of mitral repair surgery are relatively well characterized. At the other end are elderly patients, often in their eighth decade of life, and sometimes with significant comorbidity, in whom surgery presents a higher risk. For this reason, a good number of these patients are not candidates for the randomized EVEREST II trial. These patients would benefit most from a percutaneous intervention. It is possible that, in this group, a lesser degree of efficacy in terms of mitral insufficiency reduction would be an acceptable outcome and a major clinical benefit, especially if the morbidity of the procedure is less than that of surgery. A group of high-risk surgical patients suffering from functional mitral regurgitation were evaluated with echocardiography 12 months after Mitraclip placement. Successful reduction in mitral regurgitation resulted in significant reduction in mitral annular diameter as well as left ventricular volumes [35].

The surgical approach for the treatment of functional mitral insufficiency (FMR) remains controversial. While untreated FMR has been associated with decreased survival, no clear long-term survival benefit has been demonstrated in patients with severely compromised left ventricular function undergoing surgery for FMR [36]. Although ring annuloplasty alone in FMR patients results in good freedom from reoperation, early reoccurrence of moderate to severe mitral insufficiency is frequent. McGee *et al.* [37] reported a 28% mitral insufficiency (>2+) reoccurrence rate as early as 6 months. The initial experience using the Mitraclip in patients with pure functional mitral insufficiency is still relatively small; however 23 patients had similar 12-month durability compared with the overall EVEREST I population [38].

Why might the edge-to-edge approach be an effective therapy in this patient population? It has been demonstrated in both animal and human explants that an edge-to-edge repair results in the formation of a tissue bridge between the anterior and posterior leaflets in the septal–lateral direction [25,26]. It is possible that the tissue bridge which develops around the clip may help support the annulus, limiting septal–lateral annular dilatation without impairing annular contractile function. Additionally, continuity created by the tissue bridge between the annulus, leaflets, chordae and papillary muscles may also help prevent dilation of the left ventricle. Maisano *et al.* reported 12-year outcomes with isolated surgical edge-to-edge repair without annuloplasty, with excellent results; the support from this tissue bridge might contribute to these good long-term outcomes [22].

In patients with severe heart failure and dilated cardiomyopathy, resynchronization therapy can result in reverse left ventricular remodeling and is associated with improved left ventricle function and favorable 1-year survival. Yu *et al.* [39] suggest that reverse left ventricular remodeling with a >9.5% reduction in left ventricular end-systolic volume is a predictor of lower long-term mortality and decreased heart failure events in patients with severe left ventricle dysfunction. Early reports from EVEREST I and EVEREST II roll-in showed that patients in whom mitral insufficiency was successfully reduced also exhibited measurable left ventricular reverse remodeling with changes in left ventricular end-systolic and end-diastolic volume and systolic and diastolic left ventricular internal diameter [38]. If these early results obtained in a small patient cohort can be replicated in a large study, decreasing mitral insufficiency from 3+ or greater to 2+ or less with a Mitraclip may have a dramatic impact on both the morbidity and mortality of patients suffering from functional mitral insufficiency.

Conclusions

The data from the initial MitraClip studies are encouraging and indicate that this first-class device can acutely decrease mitral insufficiency in the majority of patients in whom it is used. At 1 year's follow-up, a substantial portion of the patients treated successfully with the clip remained alive without the need for further surgery and with recurrent mitral insufficiency <2+. This patient population also demonstrateds significant improvement in symptoms that paralleled improved left ventricular remodeling, confirming that mitral insufficiency reduction resulted in clinical benefit. The Mitraclip is successful in reducing mitral insufficiency in patients with both degenerative and functional mitral insufficiency. Finally, in those patients in whom the device has been unsuccessful to date valve surgery options are uncompromised. Patients considered at high risk for surgery have also been treated successfully, suggesting that this new technology can satisfy an important unmet clinical need.

The significant interest in the development of percutaneous mitral valve repair therapies is sure to lead to a variety of effective technologies. As these technologies evolve there will be issues with operator techniques and device systems. Given the growing collaboration between the various cardiovascular subspecialties, including cardiac surgeons and cardiologists specializing in structural heart disease interventions, these issues are likely to be resolved. Significant questions also remain in terms of selecting the patients best served by the new percutaneous therapies, but data from rigorous, prospective, randomized clinical studies should help to provide answers. These new transcatheter mitral insufficiency therapeutics are showing compelling early promise and will undoubtedly extend a variety of treatment options to an expanding population of patients suffering from mitral valve disease.

Disclosure

Dr. St Goar is a founder and equity holder in Evalve. Drs. Feldman and Kar receive research support from Edwards Lifesciences and Evalve, Inc.

References

1. Enriquez-Sarano M, Nkomo V, Mohty D, Avierinos JF, Chaliki H (2002) Mitral regurgitation: predictors of outcome and natural history. *Adv Cardiol* **39**:133–143.

2. Bonow RO, Carabello B, de Leon AC Jr, *et al.* (1998) Guidelines for management of patients with valvular heart disease: executive summary. *Circulation* **98**:1949–1984.

3. Miller DC (2001) Ischemic mitral regurgitation redux–to repair or to replace? *J Thoracic Cardiovasc Surg* **122**:1059–1062.

4. Lawrie GM (1998) Mitral valve repair vs replacement: current recommendations and long-term results, *Cardiol Clin* **16**:437–448.

5. Enriquez-Sarano M, Schaff HV, & Orszulak TA (1995) Valve repair improves the outcome of surgery for mitral regurgitation: a multivariate analysis. *Circulation* **91**:1022–1028.

6. Calafiore AM, Gallina S, Di Mauro M, *et al.* (2001) Mitral valve procedure in dilate cardiomyopathy: repair or replacement. *Ann Thorac Surg* **71**:1146–1152.

7. Tahta SA, Oury JH, Maxwell JM, Hiro SP, & Duran CM (2002) Outcome after mitral valve repair for functional ischemic mitral regurgitation. *J Heart Valve Dis* **11**:11–18.

8. Hung J, Handschumacher MD, Rudski L, Chow CM, Guerrero JL, & Levine RA (1999) Persistence of ischemic mitral regurgitation despite annular ring reduction: mechanistic insights from 3D echocardiography. *Circulation* **100**:I-73.

9. Daimon M, Shiota T, Gillinov AM, *et al.* (2005) Percutaneous mitral valve repair for chronic ischemic mitral regurgitation: a real-time three-dimensional echocardiographic study in an ovine model. *Circulation* **111**:2183–2189.

10. Byrne MJ, Kaye DM, Mathis M, Reuter DG, Alferness CA, & Power JM (2004) Percutaneous mitral annular reduction provides continued benefit in an ovine model of dilated cardiomyopathy. *Circulation* **110**:3088–3092.

11. Lee MS, Shah AP, Dang N, *et al.* (2006) Coronary sinus is dilated and outwardly displaced in patients with mitral regurgitation: quantitative angiographic analysis. *Catheter Cardiovasc Interv* **67**:490–494.

12. Schofer J, Siminiak T, Haude M, *et al.* (2009) Percutaneous mitral valve annuloplasty for functional mitral regurgitation: results of the CARILLON Mitral Annuloplasty Device European Union study. *Circulation* **120**:326–333.

13. Liddicoat JR, Mac Neill BD, Gillinov AM, *et al.* (2003) Percutaneous mitral valve repair: a feasibility study in an ovine model of acute ischemic mitral regurgitation. *Catheter Cardiovasc Interv* **60**:410–416.

14. Webb J, Harnek J, Munt BI *et al.* (2006) Percutaneous transvenous mitral annuloplasty: initial human experience with device implantation in the coronary sinus. *Circulation* **113**:851–855.

15. Society of Thoracic Surgeons National Cardiac Surgery Database (2002) *Mitral Valve Repair and Replacement Patients: Incidence of Complications Summary.* Available at: www.sts.org

16. Fann JI, Ingels NB, & Miller C (1997) Pathophysiology of mitral valve disease and operative indications. In: Edmunds LH (ed.). *Cardiac Surgery in the Adult.* New York: McGraw-Hill, pp. 959–987.

17. Galloway AC, Grossi EA, Bizekis CE, *et al.* (2002) Evolving techniques for mitral valve reconstruction. *Ann Surg* **3**:288–294.

18. Trowitzsch E, Bano-Rodrijo A, Burger BM, *et al.* (1988) Two-dimensional echocardiographic findings in double orifice mitral valve. *J Am Coll Cardiol* **6**:383–387.

19. Umana JP, Salehizadeh B, DeRose JJ, *et al.* (1998) "Bow-tie" mitral valve repair: an adjuvant technique for ischemic mitral regurgitation. *Ann Thorac Surg* **66**:1640–1646.

20. Maisano F, Schreuder JJ, Oppizzi M, *et al.* (2000) The double orifice technique as a standardized approach to treat mitral regurgitation due to severe myxomatous disease: surgical technique. *Eur J Cardiothorac Surg* **17**:201–215.

21. Alfieri O, Maisano F, DeBonis M, *et al.* (2001) The edge-to-edge technique in mitral valve repair: a simple solution for complex problems. *J Thoracic Cardiovasc Surg* **122**:674–681.

22. Maisano F, Caldarola A, Blasio A, De Bonis M, La Canna G, & Alfieri O (2003) Midterm results of edge-to-edge mitral valve repair without annuloplasty. *J Thoracic Cardiovasc Surg* **126**:1987–1997.

23. Maisano F, Vigano G, Blasio A, Colombo A, Calabrese C, & Alfieri O (2006) Surgical isolated edge-to-edge mitral valve repair without annuloplasty: clinical proof of the principle for an endovascular approach. *Eur Interv* **2**:181–186.

24. St. Goar FG, Fann JI, Komtebedde J, *et al.* (2003) Endovascular edge-to-edge mitral valve repair: acute results in a porcine model. *Circulation* **108**:1990–1993.

25. Fann JI, St. Goar F, Komtebedde J, *et al.* (2003) Off pump edge-to-edge mitral valve technique using a mechanical clip in a chronic model. *Circulation* **108**:488–493.

26. Privitera S, Butany J, Cusimano RJ, *et al.* (2002) Alfieri mitral valve repair: clinical outcome and pathology. *Circulation* **106**:e173–174.

27. Silvestry FE, Rodriguez LL, Hermann HC, *et al.* (2007) echocardiographic guidance and assessment of percutaneous repair for mitral regurgitation with the Evalve MitraClip: lessons learned from EVEREST I. *J Am Soc Echocardiogr* **20**:1131–1140.

28. Condado JA, Acquatella H, Rodriguez, *et al.* (2006) Percutaneous edge-to-edge mitral valve repair: 2-year follow-up in the first human case. *Cath Cardiovasc Int* **67**:323–325.

29. Feldman T, Wasserman HS, Herrmann HC, *et al.* (2005) Percutaneous mitral valve repair using the edge-to-edge technique: six-month results of the EVEREST Phase 1 Clinical Trial. *J Am Coll Cardiol* **46**:2134–2140.

30. Feldman T, Kar S, Rinaldi M, *et al.* for the EVEREST Investigators (2009) Percutaneous mitral repair with the MitraClip system: safety and midterm durability in the initial EVEREST (Endovascular Valve Edge-to-Edge REpair Study) Cohort. *J Am Coll Cardid* **54**:686–694.

31. Bonow RO, Carabello BA, Cvaterjee K, *et al.* (2006) ACC/AHA 2006 guidelines for the management of patients with valvular heart disease: a report of the American College of Cardiology/American Heart Association Task Force on practice guidelines. *Circulation* **114**:450–457.

32. Zoghbi WA, Sarano ME, Foster E, *et al.* (2003) Recommendations for the evaluation of the severity of native valvular regurgitation with two-dimensional and Doppler echocardiography. *J Am Soc Echocardiogr* **16**:777–802.

33. Deng NC, Aboodi MS, Sakaguchi T, *et al.* (2005) Surgical revision after mitral valve repair with a clip. *Ann Thorac Surg* **80**:238–242.

34. Flameng W, Meuris B, Herijgers, *et al.* (2008) Durability of mitral valve repair in Barlow disease versus fibroelastic deficiency. *J Thorac Cardiovasc Surg* **135**:274–282.

35. Kar S, Whitlow P, Petersen W, *et al.* (2009) Successful MitraClip therapy results in favorable septo-lateral mitral annular diameter and left ventricular remodeling in high-risk surgical patients with functional MR. Presented TCT September 2009, San Francisco, CA, USA.

36. Bursi F, Enriquez-Sarano M, Jacobsen SJ, & Roger VL (2006) Mitral regurgitation after myocardial infarction: a review. *Am J Med* **119**:103–112.

37. McGee EC, Gillinov AM, Blackstone EH, *et al.* (2004) Recurrent mitral regurgitation after annuloplasty for functional ischemic mitral regurgitation. *J Thorac Cardiovasc Surg* **128**:916–924.

38. Hermiller J, Kar S, Fail P, *et al.* (2008) Percutaneous mitral repair with the MitraClip device for functional MR: acute success and one year durability in the initial EVEREST cohort. Late Breaking Clinical Trials presented at ACC, March 29–April 1 2008, Chicago, IL, USA.

39. Yu CK, Bleeker GB, Fung JWH, *et al.* (2005) Left ventricular reverse remodeling but not clinical improvement predicts long-term survival after cardiac resynchronization therapy. *Circulation* **112**:1580–1586.

2   Coronary Heart Disease

26   Pathology of Coronary Artery Disease

Paul Fefer[1], Jagdish Butany[2,3] & Bradley H. Strauss[1,2]

[1]Sunnybrook Research Institute, Toronto, Canada
[2]University of Toronto, Toronto, Canada
[3]University Health Network, Toronto, Canada

Anatomy of the coronary arteries

There is considerable interindividual variability in the relative size and position of the coronary arteries. Coronary anomalies will be discussed in the next section (Anomalies of the coronary arteries).

Left coronary artery

The left coronary artery (Fig. 26.1) supplies most of the left ventricular free walls and most of the ventricular septum. It also supplies most of the left atrium. The left main trunk originates from the left coronary aortic sinus and varies in length from a few millimeters to a few centimeters. It lies between the pulmonary trunk and the left atrial appendage before emerging into the atrioventricular groove. It then divides into two or three main branches: the left anterior descending artery (LAD), the left circumflex artery (LCx), and the ramus intermedius.

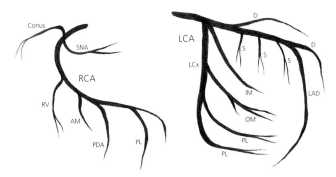

Figure 26.1 Schematic diagram of the left and right coronary arteries. AM, acute marginal branch; D, diagonal branch; IM, ramus intermedius branch; LAD, left anterior descending artery; LCA, left coronary artery; LCx, left circumflex artery; OM, obtuse marginal branch; PDA, posterior descending branch; PL, posterolateral branch; RCA, right coronary artery; RV, right ventricular branch; S, septal branch; SNA, sinus node artery.

Cardiovascular Interventions in Clinical Practice. Edited by Jürgen Haase, Hans-Joachim Schäfers, Horst Sievert and Ron Waksman. © 2010 Blackwell Publishing.

The LAD is usually the larger branch; it runs along the anterior interventricular groove down to the apex. In two-thirds of patients it turns round and runs a short distance in the posterior interventricular groove to meet the terminal portion of the posterior descending artery (PDA). The main branches coming off the LAD are the septal perforators, which supply the anterior two-thirds of the interventricular septum (small posterior septal branches supply the posterior third of the septum for a variable distance from the cardiac apex), and two to nine diagonal branches that cross the left ventricle's anterior aspect. Occasionally, one or two small right anterior ventricular branches arise from the LAD, and frequently a small left conus branch leaves the LAD from near its origin, anastomosing with the right ventricular conus branch.

The LCx is of similar caliber to the LAD. It originates at the left main bifurcation with the LAD, and courses left within the atrioventricular groove. In about 90% of patients, a large obtuse marginal branch (OM) arises from the LCx and ramifies over the rounded "obtuse" margin of the heart, supplying the lateral aspect of the left ventricle. Additional obtuse marginal branches supply the lateral and posterolateral territories of the left ventricle. In most cases it will terminate left of the crux (see Right coronary artery, below), but in approximately 8% it will reach the crux and form the PDA, which courses in the posterior interventricular groove and supplies the posterior one-third of the ventricular septum through the posterior septal perforators. This is termed "left dominance." In an additional 7% of hearts, there is a codominant system in which the posterior circulation of the heart is derived in roughly equal proportions from the LCx and the RCA. Additional branches arising from the LCx include the artery to the sinoatrial node in 35% of cases and a varying number of atrial branches.

The ramus intermedius branch arises at the angle between the LAD and LCx. It varies in caliber and length.

Right coronary artery

The right coronary artery (RCA) (Fig. 26.1) originates in the right coronary aortic sinus, courses anteriorly between the right atrial appendage and the pulmonary trunk and turns to

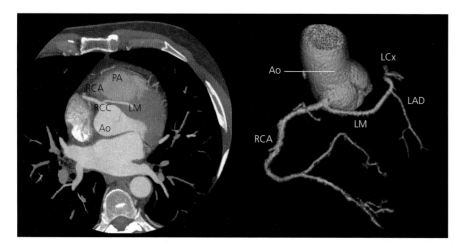

Figure 26.2 Computed tomographic angiography of anomalous origin of left coronary artery from right coronary cusp. LAD, left anterior descending artery; LCx, left circumflex artery; LM, left main stem artery; RCA, right coronary artery; RCC, right coronary cusp.

the right in the atrioventricular groove. In most cases it reaches the junction of the atrioventricular and interventricular grooves (the crux of the heart). In about 85% of individuals, it will give off the PDA and additional posterolateral branches. Usually the size of the right coronary system is inversely proportional to the size of the circumflex system. The first branch in about two-thirds of patients is the right conus artery, which supplies the right ventricular outflow tract and often anastomoses with the left conus artery originating from the LAD. In about one-third of patients, the conus artery originates as a separate artery with an independent origin in the right coronary cusp. Atrial branches originate from the proximal third of the RCA (the first segment). Two or three acute marginal branches usually originate from the mid-segment of the RCA, supplying the right ventricle. As the RCA approaches the crux, it produces one to three PDA branches (only one will actually run in the groove). The PDA is single in 70% and has parallel right coronary branches in 30% of individuals; it is replaced in about 10% by a left coronary branch from the LCx. A varying number of branches arise distal to the origin of the PDA at the crux. These form the posterolateral branches of the RCA and supply the posterolateral territory of the left ventricle.

The sinoatrial node is supplied by the RCA and LCx in 55% and 35% of cases, respectively. The atrioventricular node is supplied predominantly by the RCA, with only 10–20% of cases supplied by the LCx [1].

Intramyocardial coronary segments

The prevalence of intramuscular coronary arteries varies between 5% and 86% in autopsy series, and is reported between these extremes in angiographic series. Intramuscular segments were identified in 36 of 118 (30.5%) patients undergoing coronary CT angiography [2], in accordance with published pathologic series. The clinical significance of this finding has been debated, but the main relevance of this finding is in the potential for technical problems during coronary bypass surgery, including inadvertent perforation of the right ventricle.

Anomalies of the coronary arteries

It should be appreciated that there is much interindividual variation in the coronary artery anatomy. Coronary anomaly has been defined as a morphologic variant in <1% of the population [3]. Anomalies may be classified into those of origin and course, intrinsic coronary arterial anatomy, and coronary termination. For a full account of coronary anomalies, the interested reader is referred to further sources on this topic [4].

Anomalous origins of the coronary arteries are usually incidental findings without prognostic significance, although they can pose a diagnostic challenge in the catheterization laboratory. Some forms, however, are associated with symptoms (angina, infarction, syncope) and potentially catastrophic events (arrhythmias and sudden death). The exact prevalence of these disorders varies between different series (approximate frequencies in parenthesis have been taken from large series [3,4]).

Anomalous coronary origin from the opposite sinus (0.92% for anomalous RCA from the left sinus and 0.15% for anomalous LCA from the right sinus) is shown in Figure 26.2. The crucial factor determining the functional significance of these anomalies seems to depend on the course taken by the artery, rather than the anomalous origin itself. Specifically, a proximal arterial portion coursing between the aorta and pulmonary artery ("interarterial course") has been implicated in sudden death, especially in association with extreme physical exercise [5,6]. The cause of death is presumed to be related to myocardial ischemia. Correct identification of this anomaly is essential as surgical treatment is indicated in patients with myocardial ischemia. This anomaly can be identified by coronary angiography [7].

The following anomalies are not associated with adverse outcomes but can be challenging to demonstrate by selective coronary angiography using conventional (e.g., Judkins) catheters. These typically require additional fluoroscopy time, contrast agent, and catheters:

- separate ostia of the LAD and LCx (0.41%);
- origin of the LCx from the RCA or right sinus of Valsalva (0.37%)—LCx invariably follows a retroaortic route and passes posteriorly around the aortic root to its normal position;
- origin of the LAD from the right sinus of Valsalva or proximal RCA (rare).

Coronary artery fistulae are anomalies of coronary termination that may cause symptoms. Coronary artery fistulae may arise from both coronary arteries. Although fistulae may drain to any "cardiac venous structure" (vena cava, coronary sinus, pulmonary artery, or left atrium [8]), a majority will drain into the right side of the heart [9], and therefore cause a left-to-right intracardiac shunt. Chronic large-volume shunts through these fistulae may cause major aneurysmal enlargement of the proximal feeding artery, in addition to the receiving vessel or chamber. Owing to right heart dilation and pressure overload, or as a result of coronary steal, patients may experience breathlessness, chest pain, or arrhythmias. On rare occasions, vessel rupture, tamponade, or bacterial endocarditis may be the presenting findings. The use of modern imaging modalities, such as multidetector computed tomography (CT) angiography and cardiac magnetic resonance, allows for better visualization of coronary artery anomalies [10], enabling better risk stratification and planning of interventional treatment if indicated.

Atherosclerotic coronary artery disease

The most frequent underlying cause of coronary and vascular disease by far is atherosclerosis, a complex disease beginning in infancy. Thrombosis superimposed on atherosclerotic lesions is one of the major causes of morbidity and mortality worldwide. In this section we will elaborate on the development, classification, and biology of the atherosclerotic plaque.

Classification of coronary atherosclerosis

Our understanding of atherosclerotic heart disease is based predominantly on autopsy series, involving mainly young sudden death victims, and to a certain extent on angiographic data from living subjects. Thus, nonfatal clinical events are poorly represented in these series. Furthermore, reliable animal models of clinically significant atheroma are lacking. Therefore, there remains some debate as to the relative importance and clinical significance of the various pathologic findings. The American Heart Association (AHA) introduced a morphologic classification scheme for atherosclerotic lesions [11,12]. An attempt to simplify this classification (especially with regard to advanced atheroma) and integrate findings from later pathologic series was devised by Virmani *et al.* [13]. The following discussion integrates aspects of both classification schemes.

Much of what is known about the earliest lesions of atherosclerosis comes from animal studies. The AHA classification [14] divides atherosclerotic lesions into six classes: three pre-atheromatous (types I–III) and three atheromatous lesions (types IV–VI). Early histologic changes (type I lesion) are minimal and rarely visible to the unaided eye. Small, isolated groups of macrophages containing lipid droplets (foam cells) accumulate preferentially in regions of intimal thickening [15,16]. These intimal thickenings are present at constant locations from birth, do not obstruct the lumen, and represent an adaptation to local mechanical forces.

The fatty streak is present in AHA type II lesions. They have been found in autopsies of children dying of noncardiac causes. On gross inspection fatty streaks may be visible as yellow-colored streaks, patches, or spots on the intimal surface of the arteries. Microscopically, the lesions consist primarily of macrophage foam cells stratified in adjacent layers. Intimal smooth muscle cells also contain droplets. T lymphocytes are present but are less numerous than macrophages, and isolated mast cells are present. Most of the lipid in these lesions is intracellular, mainly found in macrophages, but a small quantity of extracellular lipid is also present. Some type II lesions will progress to more advanced atheromas (more likely at the so-called "atherosclerosis prone" areas with intimal thickening); however, most type II lesions will not progress and may even disappear. Whether a lesion will progress is largely determined by the mechanical forces that act on the vessel wall. In people whose plasma lipoproteins exceed certain thresholds, there is an increased influx and increased accumulation of lipid in these areas. Low shear stress increases the time of interaction between blood-borne particles (such as low-density lipoproteins, LDLs) and the vessel wall, leading to increased transendothelial diffusion of these particles [17]. In subjects with very high LDL levels (e.g., homozygous familial hypercholesterolemia), type II lesions rapidly develop into advanced lesions, even in arterial locations outside the progression-prone locations. Similarly, when serum cholesterol levels much higher than those usually found in human populations are induced in laboratory animals, resultant lesions are widely dispersed.

More advanced pre-atheromatous type III lesions form a morphologic and chemical bridge between the fatty streak and advanced atheromas. Its characteristic histologic features, in addition to the type II features described previously, are microscopically visible *extracellular* lipid droplets and particles, to the extent that pools of this material form among the layers of smooth muscle cells in the thickened intima. Electron microscopy reveals that the extracellular lipid droplets are either membrane bound or free. The lipid pool lies just below the layers of macrophage foam cells, replaces intercellular matrix proteoglycans and fibers, and drives smooth muscle cells apart. At this stage, a lipid core has not yet accumulated. Studies of many cases indicate that the lipid core forms by the

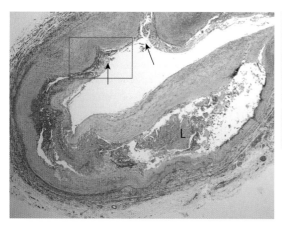
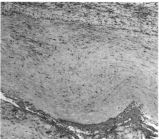

Figure 26.3 Movat stained section of coronary artery with plaque rupture. Extensive lipid (L) is present within the necrotic core. The two ends of the torn plaque are indicated by arrows. Inset shows fibrin clot.

increase and confluence of these separate extracellular lipid pools. Chemical analysis shows that these lesions contain more free cholesterol, fatty acid, sphingomyelin, lysolecithin, and triglyceride than type II lesions but less so than type IV lesions [18,19]. The difference in fatty acids between type II and advanced lesions may be explained by the massive overall increase in lipids and the change from intracellular to predominantly extracellular storage.

Advanced atheromatous lesions (AHA types IV–VI) are defined histologically by the accumulation of lipid, cells, and matrix components, including minerals. These lesions are associated with structural disorganization, repair, and thickening of the intima, as well as deformity of the arterial wall. These particular lesions may have variable effects on arterial narrowing and symptomatology and in some, but not all, cases, will be visible by angiography. The clinical significance of these lesions may be a result of arterial lumen narrowing or of superimposed complications, which may develop suddenly [20]. Broadly speaking, AHA type IV lesions are defined by the presence of the *lipid core*, which appears to develop from an increase in and the consequent confluence of small isolated pools of extracellular lipids that characterize AHA type III lesions [16]. These lesions initially are found in the same locations as adaptive intimal thickenings, and, at least initially, are eccentric. The tissue layer between the lipid core and the endothelial surface is still largely the intima that preceded lesion development. When this cover of the lipid core (the cap) later undergoes an increase in fibrous tissue (mainly collagen), the lesion is then labeled type V. These lesions usually encroach more on the vessel lumen than type IV lesions and can be multilayered with several lipid cores, separated by thick layers of fibrous connective tissue, stacked irregularly one above the other (*multilayered atheroma*). This may be explained at least in part by repeated disruptions of the lesion surface, hematomas, and thrombotic deposits. Both type IV and type V lesions may be the nidus for coronary thrombosis, owing to fissure, hematoma, and/or thrombus, and will then be defined as type VI lesions.

The later modification suggested by Virmani *et al.* [13] does not assume a linear progression of lesions, and instead suggests a classification based on morphologic description. The modification primarily focuses on advanced atheromatous lesions and replaces the AHA type IV, V, and VI lesions. The scheme is based on seven categories of lesion. These categories include intimal xanthoma, intimal thickening, pathologic thickening, fibrous cap atheroma, thin cap fibrous atheroma (TCFA), calcified nodule, and fibrocalcific plaque. We will expound on the TCFA and on complicated lesions. TCFA was added as a specific atheroma type not included in the AHA classification. The thickness of a "thin" fibrous cap has been defined as <65 μm. This definition was based on morphometric data from 41 ruptured plaques, in which 95% of the caps were <64 μm thick [20]. The TCFA is distinguished from the earlier "fibrous cap lesion" by the loss of smooth muscle cells, extracellular matrix, and inflammatory infiltrate; the necrotic core underlying the thin fibrous cap is usually large, hemorrhage and/or calcification is often present, and intraplaque vasa vasorum is abundant [22,23]. Lesions with thrombosis are classified as being affected principally by three distinct processes: rupture (Fig. 26.3), erosion (Fig. 26.4), and, less frequently, the calcified nodule. These lesions may coexist in any given coronary artery segment. Additional discussion of the processes is provided below (see Vulnerable plaque section, below).

Plaque biology

Stable plaque

The angiographic plaque morphology associated with chronic stable angina is similar to that of uncomplicated lesions described in postmortem studies [24]. These lesions tend to have a smooth outline and tapered shoulders, and appear symmetric or eccentric with a broad neck [25,26]. In contrast to small lipid-rich lesions that are prone to disruption, severely stenotic lesions tend to be fibrotic and stable [27]. Severe stenoses progress to total occlusion approximately

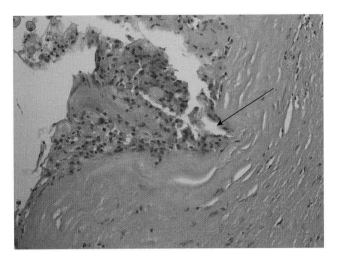

Figure 26.4 Hematoxylin and eosin stain of a coronary artery demonstrating plaque erosion at the surface of a coronary atherosclerotic plaque (arrow). Macrophages and thrombus are adherent to the torn edge.

three times more frequently than vessels with less severe stenoses [28], but less frequently lead to myocardial infarction (probably because of well-developed collateral vessels [29]).

Coronary angiography is the most widely utilized clinical tool for assessing severity of coronary stenoses. This is estimated by expressing the maximum stenotic diameter as a percentage of the adjacent, presumably normal, arterial diameter. Positive remodeling of the vessel will often leave the vessel lumen virtually unchanged until a lesion occupies more than 40% of the potential luminal area, as defined by the area within the internal elastic lamina [30], or until there has been an 80% increase in external arterial size [31]. In addition, percentage stenosis does not take into account additional factors of potential importance such as lesion length or geometry [32]. Despite the inaccuracies inherent in this system, percentage stenosis is clinically useful as a measure of obstruction to flow, particularly for stenoses below 50% or above 70%. Coronary flow reserve begins to decrease with stenoses >50% in diameter and decreases rapidly when the diameter exceeds 70%. Effort angina and rest angina occur when the diameter of stenosis exceeds 70% and 90%, respectively.

Natural history and mechanism of plaque progression

Generally, type II lesions appear in the coronary arteries around puberty [16], and slowly increase in size and number until about the age of 60 years [33]. In a histologic study of the proximal left coronary arteries of young people, 65% of those in the age group around puberty (age 12–14 years) had type I or II lesions, and an additional 8% also had more advanced lesions [16]. Because an increase in blood lipids is not associated with puberty, other factors must come into

play at puberty (e.g., rising blood pressure) [34]. Intermediate (type III) lesions may evolve soon after puberty and form the bridge between early and advanced lesions. Advanced (type IV) lesions are frequent from the third decade onwards, and type V and VI lesions begin to appear in middle-aged and older persons. These are often the predominant lesion types. Numerous mechanisms have been suggested to explain plaque progression: silent plaque rupture, intraplaque hemorrhage, and neovascularization.

Silent plaque rupture

Complicated plaques with overlying thrombosis that are not occlusive and fatal can contribute to lesion growth. The thrombus is overgrown by endothelial cells at the lumen and local production of cytokines and growth-regulatory molecules presumably stimulates changes in smooth muscle cell phenotypes with associated increases in proliferation, migration, and collagen synthesis, resulting in the organization of thrombotic deposits. Evidence for this mechanism was found in a study of 142 men who suffered sudden coronary death. The percentage of luminal area narrowing increased with increased numbers of healed sites of previous rupture, thus lending support to the notion that silent plaque rupture is a form of wound healing that results in lesion growth [35].

Intraplaque hemorrhage

Intraplaque hemorrhage is a common event in advanced coronary atherosclerotic lesions. In a postmortem study of 100 sudden cardiac death patients who were studied for the incidence of plaque hemorrhage in noninfarct-related segments, an association was found between plaque hemorrhage, an increase in the size of the necrotic core, and lesion instability in coronary plaques [36]. The proposed mechanism involves retention of erythrocyte membrane cholesterol and foam cells [37]. An animal model in rabbits provides evidence that acute hemorrhagic events promote the accumulation of free cholesterol and stimulate excessive influx of macrophages [36], and provide another explanation for episodic growth of atherosclerotic plaques.

Neovascularization

Neovascularization constitutes a key factor in the progression of atherosclerotic plaques by supplying them with lipoproteins, inflammatory cells, matrix proteases, and reactive oxygen species [38]. Low endothelial shear indirectly promotes intimal neovascularization by inducing compensatory intimal thickening, thus creating a state of relative ischemia with upregulation of vascular endothelial growth factor (VEGF) and other angiogenic growth factors [39].

Vulnerable plaque

Vulnerable plaque refers to a lesion that is likely to become unstable and prone to thrombosis, thus leading to either partial or complete vessel closure. This clinically culminates in an acute coronary syndrome, manifesting as unstable angina, non-ST elevation mycordial infarction (NSTEMI), ST elevation myocardial infarction (STEMI), or sudden cardiac death. Complicated AHA type IV or V lesions, in which disruptions of the lesion surface (hematoma, hemorrhage, or thrombotic deposits) have developed, are classified as type VI lesions. Although the complicated plaque is the nidus for coronary thrombosis, it must be stressed that, for thrombosis to occur, activation of the clotting system is needed. Various systemic factors contribute to this process, in part through activation of the clotting system (e.g., high plasma fibrinogen levels [40–42], high levels of LDL [43], smoking [44], and increased levels of type I plasminogen activator inhibitor and lipoprotein (a) [45,46]). Recognition of the precursor lesions of acute coronary syndrome has become a diagnostic target with the goal of identifying sites at high risk for coronary thrombosis. The hope is that early identification will enable intervention before acute coronary syndrome ensues, thus preventing irreversible myocardial damage or death.

Three different pathologies have been proposed for the vulnerable plaque. The most common cause of coronary thrombosis is plaque rupture (Fig. 26.3). TCFA, described above, closely resembles plaque rupture in morphology and is thus considered the precursor lesion of plaque rupture. It is characterized by a necrotic core with an overlying thin, ruptured cap infiltrated with macrophages. Smooth muscle cells within the cap are absent or few. The thickness of the fibrous cap near the rupture is $23 \pm 19\,\mu m$, with 95% of caps measuring $<65\,\mu m$ [21]. TCFAs differ from ruptured plaques by having a smaller necrotic core, less macrophage infiltration of the fibrous cap, less calcification, and less hemosiderin-laden macrophages [47]. A postmortem study examining luminal narrowings caused by various plaque types found that mean luminal narrowing was least in sections with thin cap atheroma (59.6%), intermediate for plaque hemorrhage (68.8%), and highest in plaque rupture (73.3%) or healed plaque rupture (72.8%). Over 50% of TCFAs occur in proximal portions of major coronary arteries (LAD, LCx, RCA). Another one-third are located in the mid-portion of these arteries, and the remainder in distal segments [48]. A similar distribution is found in ruptures and healed plaque ruptures. Monocyte infiltration of the thrombus correlates with the presence of occluding thrombus, and it is currently believed that circulating monocytes supply the tissue factor that propagates acute thrombi overlying unstable coronary plaques, and not plaque-derived macrophages as previously thought. Myeloperoxide (MPO)-staining monocytes and neutrophils have been demonstrated in the fibrous cap. Higher intraclot density of MPO-staining cells has been correlated with occlusive and long thrombi [47]. It was hypothesized that MPO, in addition to providing a prothrombotic milieu and increasing oxidized LDL, may be responsible for the disruption of the fibrous cap by production of hypochlorous acid [49]. The degree of lesion disruption determines the nature of the

ensuing clinical state. If only the endothelial surface of the lesion is disrupted, the thrombogenic stimulus is limited, and at most there is mural thrombus, without symptoms, and with possible subsequent lesion growth. If the disruption is deeper, as with fissuring, a transient thrombotic occlusion (i.e., lasting minutes) may take place and may even be repetitive [50], leading to unstable symptoms. If the disruption is very deep or ulceration exposes the lipid core, collagen, tissue factor and other elements, a relatively persistent thrombotic occlusion can ensue, resulting in acute STEMI [51]. This sequence of events has been supported by angiographic studies. Retrospective studies have shown that up to two-thirds of patients with unstable symptoms had rapid progression of previously relatively mild stenoses. Approximately 70% of lesions in patients with unstable angina had <50% diameter stenosis on a first angiogram [52].

Plaque erosion

The underlying plaque in this mechanism of acute coronary syndrome tends to be eccentric and calcified (Fig. 26.4) There is a lack of endothelium, and the media in these segments is intact and thicker, is rich in smooth muscle cells and extracellular matrix [53], and has few macrophages and lymphocytes. The most frequent location for plaque erosion and plaque rupture is the proximal LAD (66%), followed by the right coronary artery (18%) and the circumflex coronary artery (14%). Single-vessel disease (56%) is twice as frequent as double-vessel disease (26%). Erosions constitute about 40% of cases of thrombotic sudden coronary death [13,21,54,55]. The risk factors for erosion are poorly understood and are different from those for rupture. Plaque erosion is associated with smoking, especially in women. Patients are younger on average and have less severe narrowing at sites of thrombosis than patients suffering plaque rupture. Plaque erosion accounts for 80% of thrombi occurring in women under 50 years of age [47].

Calcified nodule

A calcified nodule is the least frequent lesion associated with coronary thrombosis. It consists of calcified plates without a necrotic core. The luminal region shows presence of breaks in the calcified plate, bone formation, and interspersed fibrin with a disrupted surface fibrous cap and overlying thrombus. It is more commonly seen in older male patients. It is thought to be more common in the carotid arteries and may be related to the frequent occurrence of plaque hemorrhage.

Coronary calcification

Calcification correlates highly with plaque burden. Radiographic coronary calcification is present in 46% of men and women under 40 years of age, 79% of men and women between 50 and 60 years old, and 100% of those over the age of 60. The extent of calcification shows a 10-year lag in women when compared with men, with equalization by the eighth decade [56]. There is a large variation in the degree of calcification of thin cap fibroatheromas, with no evidence of calcification in more than 50%. Likewise, plaque erosions show no calcification, but acute ruptures show speckled calcification. Calcified nodules, as their name suggests, carry the greatest amount of calcium but rarely trigger thrombosis and tend to occur in the RCA or LAD artery of older individuals [13].

Ectatic coronary arteries

The terms "coronary ectasia" and "aneurysm" have been used interchangeably. This is commonly defined as a diameter of an ectatic segment that is over 1.5 times larger than a healthy reference segment [57]; more than half are related to atherosclerosis. Other conditions associated with coronary ectasia include inflammatory and infectious conditions, such as syphilis, connective tissue disorders, and Kawasaki's disease [58]. Recent studies have documented an association of coronary ectasia with aneurysms in other vascular beds (e.g., abdominal and thoracic aorta). In an autopsy study, coronary arterial aneurysms were related to atherosclerosis in 38 of 52 patients. These patients were more often symptomatic and had increased heart weights, equal numbers of coronary arterial aneurysms in the right and left vessels, and the majority had single aneurysms with thrombi in the lumen. Patients with coronary arterial aneurysms secondary to inflammation were younger; the majority had a prodromal influenza-like syndrome and multiple coronary arterial aneurysms but the prevalence of ischemic heart disease was low. Various hypotheses have been put forth to explain the development of coronary ectasia. There is some evidence to suggest that chronic overstimulation of the endothelium by NO or NO donors may play a part [59,60]. Overexpression of metalloproteinases, enzymes involved in the proteolysis of the extracellular matrix proteins, may also contribute to ecstatic disease. Lamblin *et al.* [61] found a higher frequency of 5A/5A polymorphism of metalloproteinase-3 (MMP-3) in patients with ectatic coronary disease. Additionally, an association between coronary ectasia and elevated levels of inflammatory mediators [high-sensitivity C-reactive protein (hsCRP), interleukin 6 (IL-6), vascular cell adhesion molecule 1 (V-CAM-1), intercellular adhesion molecule (ICAM), and E-selectin] has been reported [58].

Chronic total occlusions

Chronic total occlusions (CTOs) are defined as arterial occlusions of at least 6 weeks' duration. They are reported in about 30% of coronary angiographic studies in patients with coronary artery disease. Surprisingly, there is a dearth of histopathologic data on this lesion type. Only two studies, involving a total of 71 patients, have been published [62,63]. It is generally assumed that a CTO forms on the basis of a ruptured atherosclerotic plaque [64]. The thrombus and lipid-rich cholesterol esters are gradually replaced by collagen, and

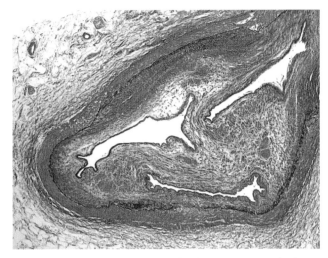

Figure 26.5 Movat stain of chronic total occlusion. Large recanalization channels are evident inside the occlusion.

in some cases calcification. In fact, approximately 50% of angiographic CTOs are not totally occluded when examined histologically [62]. Neovascularization manifested as microvessel formation within the occluded artery, or from the contralateral nonoccluded arteries, is a common angiographic and histologic feature (Fig. 26.5). Inflammatory cells (lymphocytes and macrophages) are commonly present in the intima of CTOs and likely play an active role in angiogenesis and atherosclerotic lesion progression [65]. So-called "soft plaques," comprising foam cells, loose fibrous tissue, and neovascular channels, are assumed to be more frequent in occlusions less than 1 year old. These lesions are easier to cross with an angioplasty guidewire than hard plaques, which are associated with increasing CTO age and increasing content of hard fibrous tissue and calcium.

Nonatherosclerotic coronary artery disease

Atherosclerosis remains the major cause of symptomatic coronary artery disease. However, acute coronary syndrome can rarely develop on the basis of nonatherosclerotic coronary artery disease. While a full discussion of this topic is beyond the scope of this chapter, a limited number of entities are discussed below.

Coronary artery dissection

Outside the setting of percutaneous coronary intervention, spontaneous dissection in atherosclerotic coronary disease is rare. In nonatherosclerotic coronary arteries, spontaneous coronary dissection is associated with connective tissue disease, especially Marfan's syndrome. The cardiac manifestations of this syndrome, related to a mutation in the fibrillin-1 gene, are related to weakening of the arterial media, and include aortic valve insufficiency, ascending aortic aneurysms, and mitral valve prolapse. The pathologic process is characterized by cystic medial necrosis, identified pathologically as fragmentation of elastic lamellae, apoptosis of medial smooth muscle and formation of proteoglycan-rich "mucoid pools." Coronary dissection in these patients usually results from retrograde extension of an aortic dissecting hematoma. Patients with bicuspid aortic valve are also at risk of developing cystic medial necrosis of the ascending aortic root and proximal coronary arteries, and subsequently are at increased risk for coronary dissection. Other extremely rare degenerative diseases associated with coronary artery dissection include Ehlers–Danlos disease type IV and heritable storage diseases [66].

Most spontaneous coronary dissections occur in women of reproductive age (75% of cases), of whom more than 30% are pregnant or peripartum [67]. Progesterone-dependent connective tissue changes are likely responsible for the association between dissection and pregnancy.

Coronary vasculitis

Coronary vasculitis is rare but varied in presentation. The most common form in children is Kawasaki's disease, a self-limiting type of vasculitis with acute onset. Although the full form includes involvement of skin, mucous membranes, and lymph nodes, the most important aspect of the disease is the development of coronary aneurysms in 15% of children. Most lesions remain asymptomatic. An infectious trigger is presumed [68]. Other vasculitides affecting the coronary arteries include polyarteritis nodosa (PAN), which involves the coronary arteries in 50% of patients, giant cell arteritis in older patients, and, rarely, isolated coronary vasculitis. Postinflammatory aneurysms can persist after the inflammatory process has resolved. Histopathology of the vessel wall is not fully diagnostic for specific vasculitides because various cellular patterns are common in different pathologic processes. The presence of adventitial infiltrates of B cells and dendritic cells, which closely resemble the mucosa associated lymphoid tissues, suggests that production of immunoglobulins occurs in the immediate proximity of the inflamed vessel [69].

Mediastinal radiation

Radiation therapy to the mediastinum is commonly used for treatment of several malignancies, particularly breast cancer and lymphoma. Significant coronary sclerosing intimal fibrosis is reported in up to 3% of patients. This occurs without an increase in intimal lipids. Usually there is accompanying adventitial fibrosis and bizarre-shaped fibroblasts.

Cocaine abuse

Cocaine and its derivatives specifically affect coronary arteries by inducing coronary spasm and thrombosis. Acute MI and sudden cardiac death can occur in the setting of normal coronary arteries, though more commonly cocaine abuse will precipitate coronary thrombosis at the site of an atherosclerotic stenosis. Atherosclerosis is accelerated in patients who abuse cocaine.

Conclusion

Coronary artery disease remains a major cause of morbidity and mortality worldwide. The study of coronary artery pathology has advanced our understanding of this complex disease process, and enabled us to develop novel therapies combating the disease at various stages of development. Cardiovascular interventions rely on a deep understanding of coronary anatomy and pathology. We have attempted to provide a useful outline of coronary anatomy and pathology for the cardiovascular interventionalist.

Disclosure

The authors declare they have no conflicts of interest relating to this manuscript.

References

1. Johnson D (2005) Thorax: heart and great vessels. In: Standrig S (ed.). *Gray's Anatomy*, 39th edn. Edinburgh: Elsevier Publishing. pp. 1014–1018.
2. Konen E, Goitein O, Sternik L, *et al.* (2007) The prevalence and anatomical patterns of intramuscular coronary arteries: a coronary computed tomography angiographic study. *J Am Coll Cardiol* **49**:587–593.
3. Angelini P (2007) Coronary artery anomalies: an entity in search of an identity. *Circulation* **115**:1296–1305.
4. Angelini P, Villason S, Chan AV, *et al.* (1999) Normal and anomalous coronary arteries in humans. In: Angelini P (ed.). *Coronary Artery Anomalies: A comprehensive Approach*. Philadelphia: Lippincott Williams & Wilkins, pp. 27–150.
5. Drory Y, Turetz Y, Hiss Y, *et al.* (1991) Sudden unexpected death in persons less than 40 years of age. *Am J Cardiol* **68**: 1388–1392.
6. Basso C, Maron BJ, & Thiene G (2000) Clinical profile of congenital coronary artery anomalies with origin from the wrong aortic sinus leading to sudden death in young competitive athletes. *J Am Coll Cardiol* **35**:1493–1501.
7. Bitar S & Kern MJ (2003) Angiographic data. In: Morton MJ (ed.). *The Cardiac Catheterization Handbook*, 4th edn. St. Louis: Mosby, pp. 253–262.
8. Armsby LR, Keane JF, Sherwood MC, *et al.* (2002) Management of coronary artery fistulae. Patient selection and results of transcatheter closure. *J Am Coll Cardiol* **39**:1026–1032.
9. Mavroudis C, Backer CL, Rocchini AP, *et al.* (1997) Coronary artery fistulas in infants and children: a surgical review and discussion of coil embolization. *Ann Thorac Surg* **63**:1235–1242.
10. Manghat NE, Morgan-Hughes GJ, Marshall AJ, *et al.* (2005) Multidetector row computed tomography: imaging congenital coronary artery anomalies in adults. *Heart* **91**:1515–1522.
11. Stary HC, Chandler AB, Glagov S, *et al.* (1994) A definition of initial, fatty streak, and intermediate lesions of atherosclerosis. A report from the Committee on Vascular Lesions of the Council

on Arteriosclerosis, American Heart Association. *Arterioscler Thromb* **14**:840–856.

12. Stary HC, Chandler AB, Dinsmore RE, *et al.* (1995) A definition of advanced types of atherosclerotic lesions and a histological classification of atherosclerosis. A report from the Committee on Vascular Lesions of the Council on Arteriosclerosis, American Heart Association. *Arterioscler Thromb Vasc Biol* **15**:1512–1531.

13. Virmani R, Kolodgie FD, Burke AP, *et al.* (2000) Lessons from sudden coronary death: a comprehensive morphological classification scheme for atherosclerotic lesions. *Arterioscler Thromb Vasc Biol* **20**:1262–1275.

14. Stary HC, Blankenhorn DH, Chandler AB, *et al.* (1992) A definition of the intima of human arteries and of its atherosclerosis-prone regions. A report from the Committee on Vascular Lesions of the Council on Arteriosclerosis, American Heart Association. *Circulation* **85**:391–405.

15. Stary HC (1987) Macrophages, macrophage foam cells, and eccentric intimal thickening in the coronary arteries of young children. *Atherosclerosis* **64**:91–108.

16. Stary HC (1989) Evolution and progression of atherosclerotic lesions in coronary arteries of children and young adults. *Arteriosclerosis* **9**, I19–32.

17. Glagov S, Zarins C, Giddens DP, *et al.* (1988) Hemodynamics and atherosclerosis. Insights and perspectives gained from studies of human arteries. *Arch Pathol Lab Med* **112**:1018–1031.

18. Katz SS, Shipley GG, Small DM (1976) Physical chemistry of the lipids of human atherosclerotic lesions. Demonstration of a lesion intermediate between fatty streaks and advanced plaques. *J Clin Invest* **58**:200–211.

19. Small DM (1988) George Lyman Duff memorial lecture. Progression and regression of atherosclerotic lesions. Insights from lipid physical biochemistry. *Arteriosclerosis* **8**:103–129.

20. Stary HC, Chandler AB, Dinsmore RE, *et al.* (1995) A definition of advanced types of atherosclerotic lesions and a histological classification of atherosclerosis. A report from the Committee on Vascular Lesions of the Council on Arteriosclerosis, American Heart Association. *Circulation* **92**:1355–1374.

21. Burke AP, Farb A, Malcom GT, *et al.* (1997) Coronary risk factors and plaque morphology in men with coronary disease who died suddenly. *N Engl J Med* **336**:1276–1282.

22. Burke AP, Farb A, Malcolm GT, *et al.* (1999) Plaque rupture and sudden death related to exertion in men with coronary artery disease. *JAMA* **281**:921–926.

23. Fishbein MC & Siegel RJ (1996) How big are coronary atherosclerotic plaques that rupture? *Circulation* **94**:2662–2666.

24. Levin DC & Fallon JT (1982) Significance of the angiographic morphology of localized coronary stenoses: histopathologic correlations. *Circulation* **66**:316–320.

25. Ambrose JA, Winters SL, Stern A, *et al.* (1985) Angiographic morphology and the pathogenesis of unstable angina pectoris. *J Am Coll Cardiol* **5**:609–616.

26. Ellis S, Alderman EL, Cain K, *et al.* (1989) Morphology of left anterior descending coronary territory lesions as a predictor of anterior myocardial infarction: a CASS Registry Study. *J Am Coll Cardiol* **13**:1481–1491.

27. Kragel AH, Gertz SD, & Roberts WC (1991) Morphologic comparison of frequency and types of acute lesions in the major epicardial coronary arteries in unstable angina pectoris, sudden

coronary death and acute myocardial infarction. *J Am Coll Cardiol* **18**:801–808.

28. Webster MSI, Chesebro JH, Smoth HC, *et al.* (1990) Myocardial infarction and coronary artery occlusion: a prospective 5-year angiographic study. *J Am Coll Cardiol* **15**:218A.

29. Fuster V, Frye RL, Kennedy MA, *et al.* (1979) The role of collateral circulation in the various coronary syndromes. *Circulation* **59**:1137–1144.

30. Glagov S, Weisenberg E, Zarins CK, *et al.* (1987) Compensatory enlargement of human atherosclerotic coronary arteries. *N Engl J Med* **316**:1371–1375.

31. Zarins CK, Weisenberg E, Kolettis G, *et al.* (1988) Differential enlargement of artery segments in response to enlarging atherosclerotic plaques. *J Vasc Surg* **7**:386–394.

32. Goldstein RA, Kirkeeide RL, Demer LL, *et al.* (1987) Relation between geometric dimensions of coronary artery stenoses and myocardial perfusion reserve in man. *J Clin Invest* **79**:1473–1478.

33. Eggen DA & Solberg LA (1968) Variation of atherosclerosis with age. *Lab Invest* **18**:571–579.

34. Berenson GS, Webber LS, Srinivasan SR, *et al.* (1984) Black-white contrasts as determinants of cardiovascular risk in childhood: precursors of coronary artery and primary hypertensive diseases. *Am Heart J* **108**:672–683.

35. Burke AP, Kolodgie FD, Farb A, *et al.* (2001) Healed plaque ruptures and sudden coronary death: evidence that subclinical rupture has a role in plaque progression. *Circulation* **103**:934–940.

36. Kolodgie FD, Gold HK, Burke AP, *et al.* (2003) Intraplaque hemorrhage and progression of coronary atheroma. *N Engl J Med* **349**:2316–2325.

37. Schwartz SM, deBlois D, & O'Brien ER (1995) The intima. Soil for atherosclerosis and restenosis. *Circ Res* **77**:445–465.

38. Moreno PR, Purushothaman KR, Fuster V, *et al.* (2004) Plaque neovascularization is increased in ruptured atherosclerotic lesions of human aorta: implications for plaque vulnerability. *Circulation* **110**:2032–2038.

39. Chatzizisis YS, Coskun AU, Jonas M, *et al.* (2007) Role of endothelial shear stress in the natural history of coronary atherosclerosis and vascular remodeling: molecular, cellular, and vascular behavior. *J Am Coll Cardiol* **49**:2379–2393.

40. Meade TW, North WR, Chakrabarti R, *et al.* (1980) Haemostatic function and cardiovascular death: early results of a prospective study. *Lancet* **1**:1050–1054.

41. Yarnell JW, Baker IA, Sweetnam PM, *et al.* (1991) Fibrinogen, viscosity, and white blood cell count are major risk factors for ischemic heart disease. The Caerphilly and Speedwell collaborative heart disease studies. *Circulation* **83**:836–844.

42. Ernst E (1993) The role of fibrinogen as a cardiovascular risk factor. *Atherosclerosis* **100**:1–12.

43. Aviram M & Brook JG (1987) Platelet activation by plasma lipoproteins. *Prog Cardiovasc Dis* **30**:61–72.

44. Miller GJ (1992) Hemostasis and cardiovascular risk. The British and European experience. *Arch Pathol Lab Med* **116**:1318–1321.

45. Loscalzo J (1990) Lipoprotein(a). A unique risk factor for athero-thrombotic disease. *Arteriosclerosis* **10**:672–679.

46. Scanu AM (1991) Lp(a) as a marker for coronary heart disease risk. *Clin Cardiol* **14**:I35–39.

47. Virmani R, Burke AP, Farb A, *et al.* (2006) Pathology of the vulnerable plaque. *J Am Coll Cardiol* **47**:C13–18.

48. Kolodgie FD, Burke AP, Farb A, *et al.* (2001) The thin-cap fibroatheroma: a type of vulnerable plaque: the major precursor lesion to acute coronary syndromes. *Curr Opin Cardiol* **16**:285–292.

49. Sugiyama S, Okada Y, Sukhova GK, Virmani R, Heinecke JW, & Libby P (2001) Macrophage myeloperoxidase regulation by granulocyte macrophage colony-stimulating factor in human atherosclerosis and implications in acute coronary syndromes. *Am J Pathol* **158**:879–891.

50. Falk E (1989) Morphologic features of unstable atherothrombotic plaques underlying acute coronary syndromes. *Am J Cardiol* **63**:114E–120E.

51. Fuster V, Badimon L, Cohen M, *et al.* (1988) Insights into the pathogenesis of acute ischemic syndromes. *Circulation* **77**:1213–1220.

52. Ambrose JA, Winters SL, Arora RR, *et al.* (1986) Angiographic evolution of coronary artery morphology in unstable angina. *J Am Coll Cardiol* **7**:472–478.

53. Hao H, Ropraz P, Verin V, *et al.* (2002) Heterogeneity of smooth muscle cell populations cultured from pig coronary artery. *Arterioscler Thromb Vasc Biol* **22**:1093–1099.

54. Farb A, Tang AL, Burke AP, *et al.* (1995) Sudden coronary death. Frequency of active coronary lesions, inactive coronary lesions, and myocardial infarction. *Circulation* **92**:1701–1709.

55. Farb A, Burke AP, Tang AL, *et al.* (1996) Coronary plaque erosion without rupture into a lipid core: a frequent cause of coronary thrombosis in sudden coronary death. *Circulation* **93**:1354–1363.

56. Burke AP, Weber DK, Kolodgie FD, *et al.* (2001) Pathophysiology of calcium deposition in coronary arteries. *Herz* **26**:239–244.

57. Swaye PS, Fisher LD, Litwin P, *et al.* (1983) Aneurysmal coronary artery disease. *Circulation* **67**:134–138.

58. Manginas A & Cokkinos DV (2006) Coronary artery ectasias: imaging, functional assessment and clinical implications. *Eur Heart J* **27**:1026–1031.

59. Sorrel VL (1996) Origins of coronary artery ectasia. *Lancet* **20**:136–137.

60. England JF (1981) Herbicides and coronary artery ectasia (letter). *M J Aust* **68**:260.

61. Lamblin N, Bauters C, Hermant X, *et al.* (2002) Polymorphisms in the promoter regions of MMP-2, MMP-3, MMP-9 and MMP-12 genes as determinants of aneurysmal coronary artery disease. *J Am Coll Cardiol* **40**:43–48.

62. Srivatsa SS, Edwards WD, Boos CM, *et al.* (1997) Histologic correlates of angiographic chronic total coronary artery occlusions: influence of occlusion duration on neovascular channel patterns and intimal plaque composition. *J Am Coll Cardiol* **29**:955–963.

63. Katsurgawa M, Fujiwara H, Miyamae M, *et al.* (1993) Histologic studies in percutaneous transluminal coronary angioplasty for chronic total occlusion: comparison of tapering and abrupt types of occlusion and short and long occluded segments. *J Am Coll Cardiol* **21**:604–611.

64. Stone GW, Kandzari DE, Mehran R, *et al.* (2005) Percutaneous recanalization of chronically occluded coronary arteries: a consensus document: part I. *Circulation* **112**:2364–2372.

65. Sueishi K, Yonemitsu Y, Nakagawa K, *et al.* (1997) Atherosclerosis and angiogenesis. Its pathophysiological significance in humans as well as in an animal model induced by the gene transfer of vascular endothelial growth factor. *Ann N Y Acad Sci* **811**:311–322.

66. van der Wal AC (2007) Coronary artery pathology. *Heart* **93**:1484–1489.

67. Elming H & Kober L (1999) Spontaneous coronary artery dissection. Case report and literature review. *Scand Cardiovasc J* **33**:175–179.

68. Kuijpers TW, Biezeveld M, Achterhuis A, *et al.* (2003) Longstanding obliterative panarteritis in Kawasaki's disease: lack of cyclosporin A effect. *Pediatrics* **112**:986–992.

69. Bobryshev YV & Lord RS (2001) Vascular-associated lymphoid tissue (VALT) involvement in aortic aneurysm. *Atherosclerosis* **154**:15–21.

27 Computed Tomography for the Detection of Coronary Artery Disease

Dieter S. Ropers

University of Erlangen, Erlangen, Germany

Introduction

Noninvasive imaging of the coronary arteries would obviously be of tremendous clinical interest. However, the evaluation of the coronary arteries is challenged by their complex anatomy and their small dimensions, in combination with their incessant and constant rapid motion during the cardiac cycle. A high spatial and temporal resolution is therefore a prerequisite for every imaging modality that attempts coronary artery visualization. Thus, invasive coronary angiography has set an extremely high standard with a spatial resolution of 0.2 mm and a temporal resolution of 8 ms. Computed tomography (CT) requires X-ray attenuation data from a multitude of angles to reconstruct one image. The need for mechanical rotation of the gantry limited image acquisition speed, and it was not until recently that image acquisition times below 1 s could be achieved. However, multidetector CT (MDCT) technology has been improved tremendously in the past 8 years. The newest generation of scanners equipped with two X-ray tube/detector units provides a temporal resolution of up to 83 ms with an isotropic spatial resolution of 0.4 mm. As well as accurate detection and quantitation of coronary artery calcifications, modern CT technology allows high-quality contrast-enhanced visualization of the coronary arteries up to their very distal parts. The significant improvement in image quality, reliability, and diagnostic accuracy has resulted in a growing clinical interest.

Computed tomography technology

Multidetector CT scanners first became available in 1998 when four-slice CT systems were introduced. During the following years the technical progress has been impressive. The currently accepted standard for cardiac CT imaging is 64-slice CT [1–3]. These scanners provide rotation times of

Cardiovascular Interventions in Clinical Practice. Edited by Jürgen Haase, Hans-Joachim Schäfers, Horst Sievert and Ron Waksman. © 2010 Blackwell Publishing.

between 300 and 420 ms. With half-scan reconstruction, their temporal resolution is approximately 165–210 ms. So-called multisegment reconstruction algorithms can be used to improve temporal resolution by combining data sampled during several consecutive heart beats [2]. Even though the temporal resolution of CT imaging has improved substantially, it is still somewhat limited with respect to the rapid motion of the heart and especially the coronary arteries. As there is a clear relationship between heart rate and image quality, it is currently recommended to lower the patients' heart rate to less than 60 beats per minute [1,2,4–8]. Oral or intravenous beta blockade is most often used to lower heart rate in preparation for CT coronary angiography (CTCA), but the need to lower heart rate is frequently perceived as a major limitation of CTCA.

Interestingly, although all manufacturers of CT equipment followed the same development from four- to 16-slice CT and now offer 64-slice scanners, they pursue different approaches to improve technology beyond 64-slice CT. One manufacturer has presented a 320-slice system, which allows coverage of the entire heart in one or two single heart beats [9]. This approach makes cardiac CT imaging less susceptible to arrhythmias, requires less contrast, and has the potential to reduce radiation dose. Another manufacturer has made a "dual-source CT" (DSCT) system available. This system combines two X-ray tubes and detectors in a single gantry, arranged at an angular offset of 90° [10]. Only one-quarter rotation is necessary to collect the X-ray data necessary for reconstruction of an axial image, and the system thus provides a temporal resolution of up to 83 ms, a twofold increase in temporal resolution compared with 64-slice CT. Initial publications demonstrate that this noticeably reduces problems caused by motion artifacts [11–14].

Coronary artery calcification

In the coronary arteries, calcifications occur almost exclusively in the context of atherosclerotic changes [15,16]. The only exception are patients in renal failure, in whom medial (nonatherosclerotic) calcification of the coronary artery wall is thought to occur in addition to atherosclerotic calcification. As a surrogate parameter for coronary atherosclerotic plaque

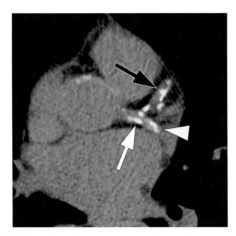

Figure 27.1 Detection of coronary artery calcium using computed tomography (64-slice multidetector CT). Without the injection of contrast agent, calcifications in the left main (white arrow), in the left anterior descending coronary artery (black arrow), and in the circumflex coronary artery (arrowhead) can be visualized.

burden, CT allows the noninvasive assessment of subclinical atherosclerosis (Fig. 27.1) [17]. However, the presence of coronary calcium is not closely associated with the propensity of an individual atherosclerotic plaque to rupture, and calcification is a sign neither of stability nor of instability of a plaque [15]. Some researchers assume calcium to be a sign of previous plaque hemorrhage, although this is disputed by others [18]. Plaques with healed ruptures usually contain calcium, whereas plaques with erosions (a less frequent mechanism of acute coronary syndromes) are often not calcified. Although the relationship between calcium and the mechanisms of acute coronary syndromes is not clearly established, the correlation of calcium with the presence and amount of coronary atherosclerotic plaque makes coronary calcium an interesting target for risk stratification purposes. In the vast majority of patients with acute coronary syndromes, some

coronary calcium can be detected, and the amount of calcium in these patients is substantially greater than in matched control subjects without coronary artery disease [19–21]. Although the relationship between the amount of coronary artery calcium and the likelihood of significant coronary artery disease has been confirmed, there is no close correlation between the amount of coronary calcium assessed by CT and the degree or location of coronary artery stenoses [16]. However, even though high amounts of coronary calcium do not necessarily predict the presence of coronary stenoses, the complete absence of coronary calcium makes the presence of significant luminal obstruction unlikely [17].

Technique

Images are acquired without injection of contrast and at a relatively low radiation dose (about 0.7–3.0 mSv) [22]. The amount of calcium is quantified using the so-called "Agatston score." Several large reference data sets are available that describe the distribution of Agatston scores found in the population, stratified by age and gender [20,23–25]. The volume and mass of calcium are alternative measures of coronary calcification, but they are not widely used even though they display a slightly better reproducibility than the Agatston score. Interscan variability for calcium quantitation can be high, especially for patients with small amounts of calcium. A recent study in 3355 individuals found an average variability of 20% for the Agatston score and 18% for calcified plaque volume [26].

Clinical significance

Several retrospective and prospective studies have demonstrated that the ability of coronary calcium in asymptomatic individuals detected by CT to predict cardiovascular events during the following 3–5 years is more accurate and independent than traditional atherosclerotic risk factors (Table 27.1) [20,27–42]. A meta-analysis demonstrated that a calcium

Table 27.1 Relationship between cardiovascular events and coronary calcium detected by computed tomography in prospective studies.

Reference	Patients	Follow-up (years)	1–100	101–399	>400	400–1000	>1000
Kondos [27]	8855	3.1	1.8	2.6	3.7		
Greenland [29]	1461	7.0	1.5	2.0	3.5		
Arad [30]	4613	4.3	1.9	10.5	26.5		
Vliegenhardt [31]	2013	3.9	1.9	3.5		5.6	10.8
Detrano [34]	6722	3.8	3.6	7.7	9.7		
Budoff [38]	25253	6.8	3.6	3.8		6.5	9.4
LaMonte [39]	10746	3.5	3.5/3.3*	11.1/4.6*	20/9.3*		
Park [40]	1461	6.4	1.7	4.3			
Becker [41]	1726	3.3	1.7/3.3*	4.1/4.5*	6.8/7.9*		

The table includes the relative risk in relation to the amount of coronary calcifications (Agatston Score).
*Male/female.

score of 0 is associated with a very low risk of future myocardial infarction or death due to coronary heart disease (0.4% over 3–5 years) [36]. Agatston scores between 1 and 112 increase the risk of myocardial infarction and coronary artery disease death by 1.9, scores between 100 and 400 by a factor of 4.3, scores between 400 and 999 by a factor of 7.2, and scores of more than 1000 by a factor of 10.8 [37]. In a very recent follow-up study of 25 253 patients observed for a mean period of approximately 7 years, coronary calcium was a substantially better predictor of overall mortality and of the rate of death for any reason, after adjustment for traditional cardiovascular risk factors, than standard risk factors [38]. Interestingly, there is an influence of ethnicity both on the prevalence and on the predictive power of coronary calcification, with African Americans being at highest risk when high calcium scores are present [24,34,39]. Coronary calcification has been found to be progressive over time [43]. The amount of progression correlates to noncoronary atherosclerosis [44], is related to cardiovascular risk factors [45], and shows a genetic association [46]. One study has observed a higher coronary artery disease event rate in individuals who displayed more rapid progression of coronary artery calcium [47]. A number of trials have evaluated the influence of lipid-lowering therapy on the progression of coronary calcium, but they have reported conflicting results [48–53]. Currently, no sufficiently strong data are available to support the use of repeated calcium scans to guide the intensity of risk factor modification. Together with the relatively high measurement variability, especially for small amounts of calcification, this currently prevents clinical applications of repeat coronary calcium scanning [54,55].

Recommendations

Coronary calcium is closely associated to coronary atherosclerosis, and the predictive value of coronary calcium concerning the occurrence of future cardiovascular disease events in asymptomatic individuals is widely accepted [38,55,56]. However, it is less clear which patients or individuals will profit from having a coronary artery calcium scan. It is currently assumed that individuals who are clearly at high risk will not profit from coronary calcium imaging because they need intensive treatment, regardless of the result [57]. Low-risk individuals will not profit from "screening" either. Patients at intermediate risk for future coronary events according to traditional risk categories (risk of hard events at 10 years of 6–20%) will be most likely to profit from coronary calcium imaging as a means of noninvasive testing for subclinical atherosclerosis and to determine whether intensive risk modification is necessary [57]. The potential of coronary calcium detection using MDCT as a useful tool to improve risk prediction for asymptomatic subjects with intermediate pretest probability has been embraced by large professional societies such as the European Society of Cardiology and the American College of Cardiology/American Heart Association. Coronary artery calcium scanning has been incorporated in the European guidelines on Cardiovascular Disease Prevention in Clinical Practice, stating that coronary artery calcium scanning is especially suited for patients at medium risk [56]. Information from the calcium detection could be used to refine the assessment of risk on the basis of traditional algorithms, allowing matching of the intensity of therapy to the risk profile of the individual. However, further research must confirm that calcium detection is cost-effective, especially in comparison with other diagnostic modalities, for the assessment of subclinical atherosclerosis (e.g., carotid intima–media thickness). Unselected "screening" or patient self-referral is uniformly not recommended [37,55,56].

Contrast-enhanced computed tomography coronary angiography

Improvements in scanner technology have led to an improved diagnostic accuracy of CTCA for the detection of coronary artery stenoses and a significantly lower rate of nonevaluable scans. The straightforward data acquisition, robust image quality, and high accuracy for the detection of coronary artery stenoses make CTCA an attractive method for noninvasive evaluation of patients with suspected coronary artery disease. Although it is no substitute for stress testing, because CT is unable to assess the functional relevance of a lesion, and it is not applicable in a variety of patients (e.g., with atrial fibrillation or renal failure), there are potential indications for its clinical use.

Technique

The entire process of data acquisition for CTCA usually requires approximately 10–15 min. Patient preparation usually includes premedication to lower the heart rate to preferably <60 beats/min, which has been shown to substantially reduce the occurrence of motion artifact and is most commonly achieved by administering oral or intravenous beta blockers [58]. Sublingual nitrates are given immediately before scanning to dilate the coronary arteries [58]. Acquisition of the data set for coronary artery visualization requires intravenous injection of 50–100 mL of contrast agent (300–400 mg iodine/mL) at a high flow rate (e.g., 5–7 mL/s). Patients need to perform a breath-hold of 6–20 s (depending on the type of scanner used, heart rate, and dimensions of the heart). Scanner settings vary with the model and manufacturer of the equipment, but they will usually be chosen to maximize spatial and temporal resolution (thinnest possible collimation, fastest possible rotation speed). The radiation exposure (effective dose) is estimated to be between 3 and 15 mSv, depending on the scan protocol. Electrocardiography (ECG)-correlated tube current modulation (reduction of tube current in systole) can very effectively reduce radiation exposure by 30–50% [59–64].

From the obtained X-ray attenuation data, image data sets are reconstructed that typically consist of approximately

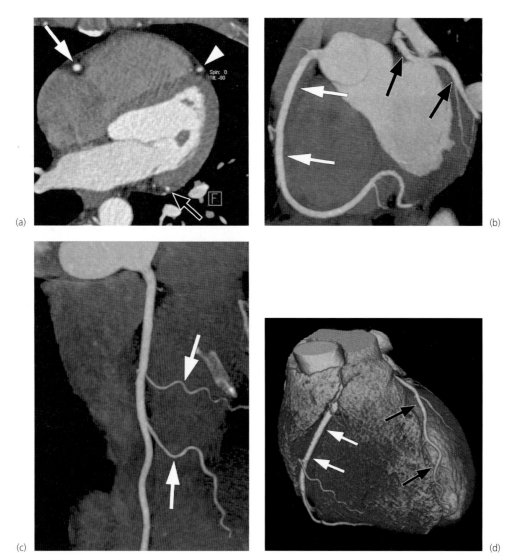

(a)

(b)

(c)

(d)

Figure 27.2 Coronary artery visualization by contrast-enhanced CT (dual-source CT) in a patient without coronary artery disease. (a) Transaxial image (0.75 mm slice thickness) demonstrating cross-sections of the coronary arteries (white arrow, right coronary artery; arrowhead, left anterior descending coronary artery; black arrow, circumflex coronary artery). (b) Double oblique multiplanar reconstruction (8 mm slice thickness) of the right coronary artery (white arrows) demonstrating a normal lumen without coronary artery disease. The black arrows indicate the circumflex coronary artery. (c) Curved multiplanar reconstruction (0.75-mm slice thickness) which shows the course of the right coronary artery. The arrows indicate two small right ventricular branches visualized without motion artifacts. (d) Three-dimensional reconstruction of the heart and the coronary arteries. The right coronary artery (white arrows) and the left anterior descending coronary artery (black arrows) are visualized without motion artifacts.

250–350 transaxial cross-sectional images with a slice thickness between 0.5 and 1.0 mm and a reconstruction increment of less than the slice width so that consecutive images have some overlap. These data sets can be reconstructed at any desired time point in the cardiac cycle. The cardiac phase can have substantial impact on the image quality. In most cases, diastolic reconstructions will yield optimal results, as it is during late diastole, before onset of atrial contraction, that the coronary arteries display the slowest motion. However, in faster heart rates, systolic imaging may provide image quality that is superior to diastolic imaging. Minor alterations in the time point used for image reconstruction can have a

substantial impact on the occurrence of motion artifacts, especially for slower scanner types and, again, patients with high heart rates. Careful identification of the optimal time instant for image reconstruction is therefore of great importance in these situations.

Analysis of the transaxial data set forms the basis of interpretation for CT coronary angiography. Based on the transaxial data set, two-dimensional forms of image reconstruction, such as "multiplanar reconstructions" or "maximum intensity projections," can be applied to facilitate data interpretation (Fig. 27.2). Three-dimensional reconstructions are visually pleasing, but rarely helpful to evaluate the data. Beyond

Table 27.2 Accuracy of 64-slice MDCT and dual-source CT for the detection of significant coronary artery stenoses (defined as a reduction in diameter more than 50%).

Author	Number	Unevaluable (%)	Sensitivity (%)	Specificity (%)	PPV (%)	NPV (%)
Leschka [4]	67	0	100 (47/47)	100 (20/20)	100 (47/47)	100 (20/20)
Leber [67]	59[a]	14	88 (22/25)	85 (17/20)	88 (22/25)	85 (17/20)
Raff [68]	70	0	95 (38/40)	90 (27/30)	93 (38/41)	93 (27/29)
Mollet [69]	52	1	100 (38/38)	92 (12/13)	97 (38/39)	100 (12/12)
Ropers [70]	84	3	96 (25/26)	91 (50/55)	83 (25/30)	98 (50/51)
Schuijf [71]	61	1	94 (29/31)	97 (28/29)	97 (29/30)	93 (27/29)
Nikolaou [72]	72	4	97 (38/39)	79 (23/29)	86 (38/44)	96 (23/24)
Weustink [76]	77	0	99 (76/77)	87 (20/23)	96 (76/79)	95 (20/21)
Leber [77]	90	2	95 (20/21)	90 (60/67)	74 (20/27)	99 (60/61)
Scheffel [75]	30	0	93 (14/15)	100 (15/15)	100 (14/14)	94 (15/16)
Ropers [14]	100	3	98 (39/40)	82 (47/57)	80 (39/49)	98 (47/48)

Patient-based analysis.
[a]Analysis in proximal and mid coronary segments.
NPV, negative predictive value; PPV, positive predictive value.

visualization of the coronary arteries, the ability to reconstruct image data at any desired time instant within the cardiac cycle allows assessment of left ventricular function and wall motion as a "by-product" of CT coronary angiography; it has been shown to allow accurate assessment of global and regional left ventricular function [65,66].

Native coronary arteries

A recent meta-analysis has carefully summarized the accuracy data that are available for CTCA, and the authors demonstrated a clear increase in the accuracy of stenosis detection as scanner technology progressed from four- to 16- and 64-slice equipment (Fig. 27.3) [3]. For 64-slice CT, the pooled data indicated a sensitivity of 93% and specificity of 96% for the detection of coronary artery stenoses on a per-segment level, as well as a sensitivity of 99% and specificity of 93% based on per-patient analysis (Table 27.2). While the available data illustrate the high accuracy of CTCA for the detection of coronary artery stenoses, it needs to be taken into account that most studies were performed in somewhat selected patients with a rather low pretest likelihood of disease, stable sinus rhythm, ability to perform a 10-s breath-hold, and absence of renal failure [67–72]. Also, studies were conducted in experienced centers, usually with tight measures to ensure a low heart rate during the scan. Several trials have convincingly shown that high heart rates and extensive calcification negatively influence accuracy [8,73,74]. For this reason, the high accuracy values may not be extrapolated to unselected patient populations and less experienced centers. Four very recent, small trials have analyzed the diagnostic accuracy of DSCT for the detection of coronary artery stenoses without the use of beta blockade to lower the heart rate. They report sensitivities of 90–96% and specificities of 95–98%

for the detection of coronary stenoses with more than 50% diameter reduction [14,75–77].

Recommendation

As well as the ability to detect significant coronary artery stenoses, it is remarkable that the negative predictive value was uniformly found to be high, ranging from 93% to 100% (Table 27.2). Even though this may partly be influenced by the relatively low prevalence of coronary artery stenoses in most studies, it does indicate the ability when using this method to reliably rule out the presence of coronary artery stenoses. Therefore, the use of MDCT coronary angiography has been suggested in patients with a low to intermediate pretest likelihood of disease (e.g., women of younger age with atypical or even typical symptoms), in whom the ability of CT coronary angiography to rule out stenoses may be clinically beneficial. In these patients, CT coronary angiography will often be able to demonstrate "normal" coronary arteries with absence of coronary stenoses; thus, invasive coronary angiography does not need to be performed. Table 27.3 lists potential circumstances in which CTCA has been considered "appropriate" by a US-based consensus panel of experts from various professional organizations [78]. It can be expected that future, outcome-based studies will better clarify the potential clinical role of CTCA in the setting of suspected coronary artery stenoses.

Coronary artery bypass grafts

Bypass vessels move less rapidly and they are larger in diameter than the native coronary arteries. Thus, they are easier to visualize with CTCA than native coronary arteries (Fig. 27.4). Occlusions of bypass grafts and stenoses in the body of the graft can be detected with very high accuracy,

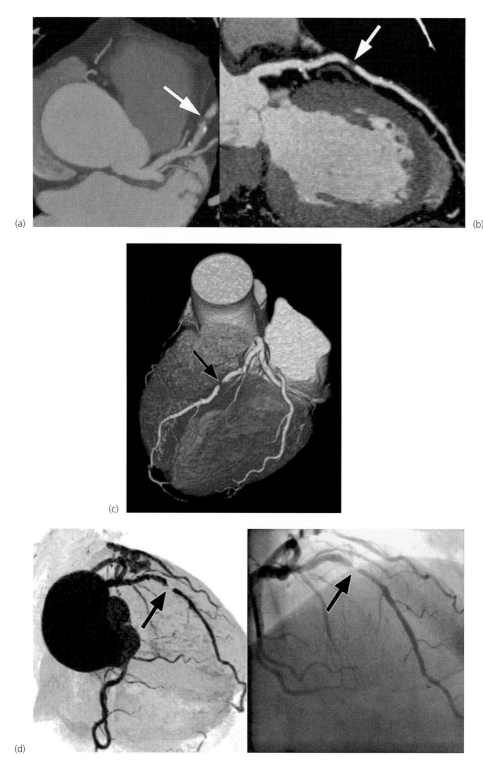

Figure 27.3 Contrast-enhanced 64-slice MDCT in a patient with a high-grade stenosis in the mid part of the left anterior descending coronary artery (LAD). (a) Transaxial image (3 mm slice thickness) demonstrating a severe stenosis (arrow) of the LAD. (b) Curved multiplanar reconstruction (0.75 mm slice thickness) of the LAD. The arrow indicates the significant stenosis. (c) Three-dimensional reconstruction of the heart. The stenosis in the LAD is clearly visualized (arrow). (d) Left: angiographic view of the CT data clearly shows the high-grade lesion in the LAD (arrow). Right: invasive coronary angiography confirms the stenosis (arrow).

Table 27.3 "Appropriate" indications for CT coronary angiography according to an expert consensus document of several cardiovascular societies (ACCF/ACR/SCCT/SCMR/ASNC/NASCI/SCAI/SIR) [78].

Indication	Appropriateness criteria
Detection of CAD with previous test results—evaluation of chest pain syndrome	A (7) Uninterpretable or equivocal stress test result (exercise, perfusion, or stress echocardiography)
Detection of CAD: symptomatic—evaluation of chest pain syndrome	A (8) Intermediate pre-test probability of CAD, ECG uninterpretable or unable to exercise
Detection of CAD: symptomatic—acute chest pain	A (7) Intermediate pre-test probability of CAD, no ECG changes and serial enzymes negative
Evaluation of coronary arteries in patients with new-onset heart failure to assess etiology	A (7)
Evaluation of suspected coronary anomaly	A (9)

A score of 7–9 indicates an appropriate test for specific indication (test is generally acceptable and may be a reasonable approach for indication).
CAD, coronary artery disease; A, Appropriate.

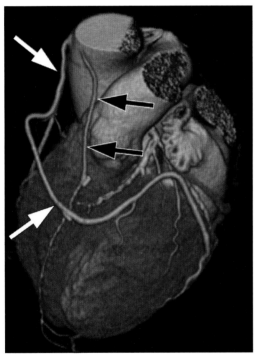

Figure 27.4 Three-dimensional reconstruction of contrast-enhanced MDCT (64-slice MDCT) data in a patient with a patent left internal mammary artery graft (black arrows) to the left anterior descending coronary artery, and a patent venous graft (white arrows) to the first diagonal branch and the second obtuse marginal coronary artery.

close to 100% (Fig. 27.5) [79–85]. Clinically, however, it has to be considered that in most cases it will not be sufficient to merely assess the graft vessels themselves. If a patient who has previously undergone bypass surgery presents with symptoms, it would be necessary to assess the bypass grafts as well as the status of the native coronary arteries distal to the bypass anastomosis and of those branches that did not re-

ceive a bypass graft. Because the coronary arteries in patients after bypass surgery tend to have substantial atherosclerotic changes, often pronounced calcification, and frequently a small caliber, this can be challenging for CTCA (Fig. 27.6) [85]. So far, it has not been conclusively shown that CT imaging permits assessment of the bypass grafts, the anastomotic site, and of the native arteries (Table 27.4). Clinical applications are therefore not backed by sufficient data. The newest scanners have higher temporal and spatial resolution and may thus permit the more reliable assessment of the coronary system in patients with bypass grafts. All the same, a recent study performed by 64-slice CT found a sensitivity and specificity of only 86% and 76%, respectively, for the detection of stenoses in the native coronary arteries after patients with bypass surgery [85]. Assessment of patients with chest pain after bypass surgery is therefore not a current indication for CTCA.

Coronary artery stents

Visualization of stents is possible especially with newer generations of cardiac CT scanner (Fig. 27.7), but image quality will often be impaired in CT. Artifacts can be caused by the high-density stent material. Evaluability of stents is not reliably predictable and depends on many factors, including stent type and material, stent dimensions (especially the diameter), and the vessel the stent has been implanted in [86]. Additional motion artifacts make stents all the more difficult to assess. Using 64-slice and dual-source CT technology, the reported sensitivities and specificities in evaluable stents are high (Table 27.5); however, the positive predictive value is still limited [87–93]. The rate of unevaluable coronary stents as well as the number of false-positive findings clearly limits the use of CT for the evaluation of patients after stent implantation; therefore, a routine clinical use can not be recommended.

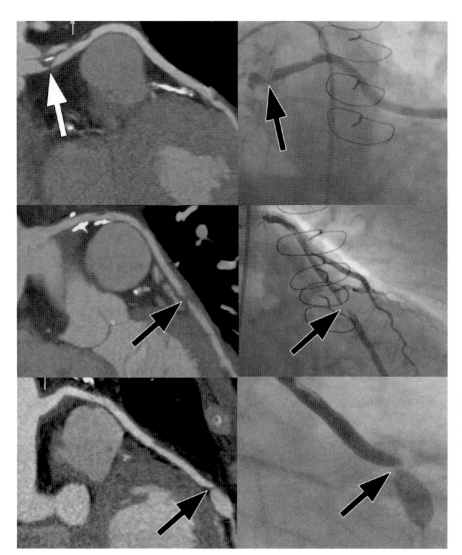

Figure 27.5 Significant stenosis (arrows) in venous bypass-grafts to the left anterior descending coronary artery visualized by curved multiplanar reconstructions of 64-slice MDCT data (left side) confirmed by invasive coronary angiography (right side): First row: stenosis in the proximal part of an 8-year-old venous graft. Second row: stenosis in the distal part of a 5-year-old venous graft. Third row: stenosis at the coronary anastomosis of a 3-year-old venous graft.

Assessment of coronary atherosclerotic plaque

Beyond the detection of coronary artery stenoses, CTCA is able to demonstrate coronary atherosclerotic plaque, both calcified and noncalcified (Fig. 27.8). The ability to visualize noncalcified plaque components has created a great deal of interest because it is assumed that the presence of noncalcified plaque may be more predictive for future cardiovascular events than assessing calcified plaque alone. In addition, CT is thought to potentially contribute to the characterization of noncalcified plaque, in order to identify "vulnerable" plaques at particularly high risk for rupture. However, the accuracy of CTCA to detect noncalcified

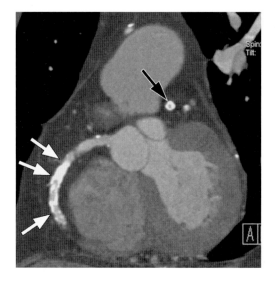

Figure 27.6 (*left*) Severe calcifications in the right coronary artery (white arrows) and the proximal left anterior descending coronary artery (black arrow) in contrast-enhanced 64-sclie MDCT coronary angiograpghy in a patient with a history of bypass surgery 10 years before. The calcifications make a reliable evaluation of the native coronary arteries impossible.

Table 27.4 Accuracy of 16-slice and 64-slice MDCT for evaluation of patients after bypass surgery.

Author	Number of patients/grafts	Evaluation of	Not evaluable (%)	Investigator	Sensitivity (%)	Specificity (%)	PPV (%)	NPV (%)
Nieman [81]	24/60	Graft occlusion	0 (0/60)	Investigator 1	100 (17/17)	100 (42/42)	94 (17/18)	100 (42/42)
			5 (3/60)	Investigator 2	100 (17/17)	98 (39/40)	94 (17/18)	100 (39/39)
		Graft stenosis	10 (4/42)	Investigator 1	60 (3/5)	88 (29/33)	43 (3/7)	94 (29/31)
			5 (2/39)	Investigator 2	83 (5/6)	90 (28/31)	63 (5/8)	97 (28/29)
		Native vessels	34 (65/211)	Investigator 1	90 (71/79)	75 (50/67)	81 (71/88)	86 (50/58)
			31 (61/211)	Investigator 2	79 (54/68)	72 (52/72)	73 (54/74)	79 (52/66)
Stauder [83]	20/ 50	Graft occlusion	0 (0/50)		100 (17/17)	100 (229/229)	100 (17/17)	100 (229/229)
		Graft stenosis	12 (31/240)		99 (92/94)	94 (128/130)	92 (92/94)	99 (128/130)
		Native vessels	31 (81/260)		92 (105/114)	77 (50/65)	88 (105/120)	85 (50/59)
Burgstahler [79]	13/43	Graft occlusion	0 (0/43)		100 (16/16)	100 (27/27)	100 (16/16)	100 (27/27)
		Graft stenosis	5 (2/43)		100 (1/1)	93 (25/27)	33 (1/3)	100 (25/25)
		Native vessels	32 (54/169)		83 (90/108)	59 (36/61)	78 (90/115)	67 (36/54)
Salm [82]	25/67	Graft occlusion	0 (0/67)		100 (25/25)	100 (57/57)	100 (25/25)	100 (57/57)
		Graft stenosis	NI		100 (3/3)	94 (51/54)	50 (3/6)	100 (51/51)
		Native vessels*	8 (17/225)		100 (11/11)	89 (16/18)	85 (11/13)	100 (16/16)
Malagutti [80]	52/109	Graft occlusion**	0 (0/109)		100 (49/49)	98 (59/60)	98 (49/50)	100 (59/59)
		Native vessels	NI		97 (62/64)	86 (50/74)	66 (62/94)	99 (192/194)
Ropers [85]	50/138	Graft occlusion	0 (0/138)		100 (38/38)	100 (100/100)	100 (38/38)	100 (100/100)
		Graft stenosis	0 (0/138)		100 (31/31)	94 (17/19)	92 (31/33)	100 (17/17)
		Native vessels	9 (55/621)		86 (87/101)	76 (354/456)	44 (87/189)	96 (354/368)
Onuma [84]	53/146	Graft occlusion	6 (8/146)		100 (21/21)	100 (117/117)	100 (21/21)	100 (117/117)
		Graft stenosis	6 (8/146)		100 (10/10)	98 (105/107)	83 (10/12)	100 (105/105)
		Native vessels	9 (64/749)		93 (263/282)	88 (353/403)	84 (63/313)	95 (353/372)

Only studies that investigated grafts and native coronary arteries are included. Sensitivities and specificities are calculated for evaluable grafts and native coronary arteries.

NI, information not included; NPV, negative predictive value; PPV, positive predictive value.

*Limited to nongrafted vessels, **defined as a significant graft stenosis or occlusion.

Table 27.5 Accuracy of 64-slice MDCT and dual-source CT for the detection of significant in-stent-restenosis (>50% diameter reduction).

Author	Number of patients/stents	Not evaluable (%)	Sensitivity (%)	Specificity (%)	PPV (%)	NPV (%)
Rixe [88]	64/102	42 (43/192)	86 (6/7)	98 (51/52)	86 (6/7)	98 (51/52)
Rist [91]	25/46	2 (1/46)	75 (6/8)	92 (34/37)	67 (6/9)	94 (34/36)
Oncel [90]	30/39	0 (0/39)	89 (17/19)	95 (19/20)	94 (17/18)	90 (19/21)
Ehara [93]	81/125	12 (15/125)	91 (20/22)	93 (82/88)	77 (20/26)	98 (82/84)
Cademartiri [89]	182/192	7 (14/192)	95 (19/20)	93 (147/158)	63 (19/30)	99 (147/148)
Pugliese [87]	100/178	5 (9/178)	94 (37/39)	92 (128/139)	77 (37/48)	98 (128/130)
Das [92]	53/110	3 (3/110)	97 (31/32)	88 (66/75)	77 (31/40)	98 (66/67)

Per-stent analysis.

NPV, negative predictive value; PPW, positive predictive value.

coronary plaque is not very well known. Sensitivities for the detection of coronary segments with plaque have been reported to be approximately 80–90% [94–97]. The data sets included in these evaluations were preselected, and accuracy for plaque identification in "real life" may be lower. Beyond detection, the characterization of coronary atherosclerotic plaque is possible to a certain extent. One parameter is the CT attenuation of the plaque material. On average, the CT

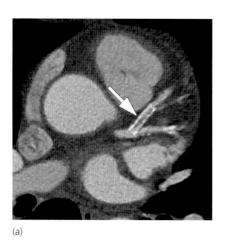
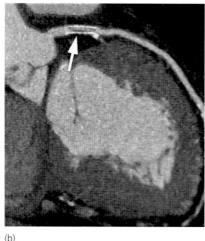
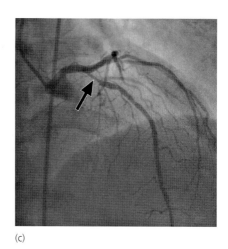

(a) (b) (c)

Figure 27.7 Contrast-enhanced dual-source CT angiography of a patient with a stent in the very proximal part of the left anterior descending coronary artery (LAD) which demonstrates a significant in-stent-stenosis. (a) Transaxial image (1.5 mm slice thickness) demonstrates the stent (arrow) in the proximal LAD. (b) In curved multiplanar reconstruction (0.75-mm slice thickness) the lumen of the stent (arrow) is not completely enhanced by contrast medium indicating a significant in-stent stenosis. (c) Invasive angiography confirms the significant in-stent stenosis (arrow).

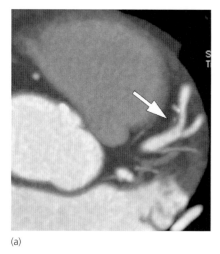
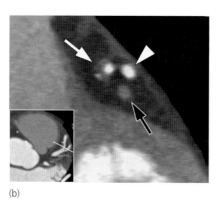
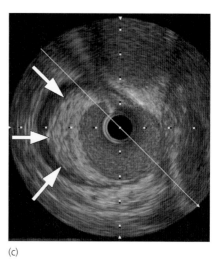

(a) (b) (c)

Figure 27.8 Dual-source CT coronary angiography demonstrating a coronary plaque in the mid left anterior descending coronary artery (LAD) of a 56-year-old female patient. (a) Transaxial image (1.0 mm slice thickness) demonstrates a plaque (arrow) in the mid-LAD shortly after the first diagonal branch is branching off. (b) Trans-section of the LAD (arrow) and the diagonal branch (arrowhead). A significant noncalcified plaque in the LAD which incorporates 270° of the vessels circumference, is clearly visualized. The black arrow indicates the cardiac vein. (c) IVUS of the same vessel area confirms the significant noncalcified plaque (arrows), which envolves two-thirds of the circumference of the artery.

attenuation within plaques classified as "fibrous" by intra-vascular ultrasound (IVUS) (and thus assumed to be relatively stable) is higher than within "lipid-rich" plaques [mean attenuation values of 91–116 Hounsfield units (HU) versus 47–71 HU] [97,98]. However, the variability of density measurements within plaque types is large, which currently prevents accurate classification of noncalcified "plaque types" by CTCA. Other CT-based parameters that might contribute to the detection of "vulnerable" plaques include plaque volume and the degree of remodeling. Both can be assessed by CT [99–103]. However,

especially for plaque volumes measured using CT, interobserver variability has been shown to be quite high (19–37%). Furthermore, clinical data are limited and nearly all studies are performed retrospectively. Therefore, plaque characteristics using CT were compared in patients post acute coronary syndrome with those in patients with stable angina. The authors report a higher percentage of noncalcified plaque and more pronounced positive remodeling in lesions responsible for acute coronary events as opposed to "stable" lesions [104–106]. One single prospective trial concerning the predictive value of plaque seen in CT for future cardiovascular events has recently become available. Pundzuite *et al.* [107] followed 100 patients who underwent CTCA for a mean period of 16 months. They were able to demonstrate that the cardiac event rate was higher in patients with nonobstructive plaque detected by contrast-enhanced CT than individuals without any plaque. Most of these coronary events were "soft" events (revascularizations) and the patient numbers were very small. More data are needed before conclusions about potential clinical applications can be made. Thus, the need for more radiation and contrast agent has to be weighed against a possible substantial advantage over the analysis of traditional risk factors or other markers of atherosclerotic plaque burden (such as coronary calcium) before clinical applications of contrast-enhanced CTCA in asymptomatic individuals for the purpose of risk stratification can be justified. Currently, the use of CTCA in asymptomatic individuals for the purpose of risk stratification is discouraged.

Conclusion

Current MDCT technology with submillimeter slice collimation and high temporal resolution (up to 83 ms) has improved the detection of coronary calcifications as well as the visualization of the coronary artery lumen and wall, including the assessment of luminal obstruction and nonstenotic atherosclerotic noncalcified plaques. The native coronary scan ("calcium score") has been convincingly demonstrated to be associated with the risk of future cardiovascular disease events and death in asymptomatic individuals. It can therefore be used in patients deemed to be at "intermediate risk," based on traditional risk factors, to facilitate a decision on use of intensive risk modification, for example the use of lipid-lowering medication. However, data on clinical utility and cost-effectiveness are not yet available. Contrast-enhanced CTCA allows the detection of coronary artery stenoses with high sensitivity and specificity. Because of a very high negative predictive value, MDCT coronary angiography may be clinically useful in symptomatic patients at low to intermediate risk of significant coronary artery disease for the reliable rule-out of significant coronary artery stenoses. Because of difficulties in reliably visualizing and interpreting the lumen of coronary stents using CT, and because of problems in assessing the anastomotic site of bypass grafts and the distal run-off vessels as well as the nongrafted coronary arteries in patients with a history of bypass surgery, the use of CTCA is not considered "appropriate" in patients after coronary revascularization. It has been shown that CTCA additionally allows the detection and, within certain limits, the characterization of coronary atherosclerotic plaque. However, imaging is not sufficiently robust and accurate enough and the available clinical data are too limited to allow clinical application of CTCA for risk stratification purposes.

References

1. Achenbach S (2007) Cardiac CT: state of the art for the detection of coronary arterial stenosis. *J Cardiovasc Comput Tomogr* **1**:3–20.
2. Schoepf UJ, Zwerner PL, Savino G, Herzog C, Kerl JM, & Costello P (2007) Coronary CT angiography. *Radiology* **244**: 48–63.
3. Vanhoenacker PK, Heijenbrok-Kal MH, Van Heste R, *et al.* (2007) Diagnostic performance of multidetector CT angiography for assessment of coronary artery disease: meta-analysis. *Radiology* **244**:419–428.
4. Leschka S, Wildermuth S, Boehm T, *et al.* (2006) Noninvasive coronary angiography with 64-section CT: effect of average heart rate and heart rate variability on image quality. *Radiology* **241**:378–385.
5. Hoffmann MH, Shi H, Manzke R, *et al.* (2005) Noninvasive coronary angiography with 16-detector row CT: effect of heart rate. *Radiology* **234**:86–97.
6. Herzog C, Arning-Erb M, Zangos S, *et al.* (2006) Multi-detector row CT coronary angiography: influence of reconstruction technique and heart rate on image quality. *Radiology* **238**: 75–86.
7. Ghostine S, Caussin C, Daoud B, *et al.* (2006) Non-invasive detection of coronary artery disease in patients with left bundle branch block using 64-slice computed tomography. *J Am Coll Cardiol* **48**:1929–1934.
8. Wintersperger BJ, Nikolaou K, von Ziegler F, *et al.* (2006) Image quality, motion artifacts, and reconstruction timing of 64-slice coronary computed tomography angiography with 0.33-second rotation speed. *Invest Radiol* **41**:436–342.
9. Rybicki FJ, Otero HJ, Steigner ML, *et al.* (2008) Initial evaluation of coronary images from 320-detector row computed tomography. *Int J Cardiovasc Imaging* **24**:535–546.
10. Flohr TG, McCollough CH, Bruder H, *et al.* (2006) First performance evaluation of a dual-source CT (DSCT) system. *Eur Radiol* **16**:256–268.
11. Achenbach S, Ropers D, Kuettner A, *et al.* (2006) Contrast-enhanced coronary artery visualization by dual-source computed tomography—initial experience. *Eur J Radiol* **57**:331–335.
12. Johnson TR, Nikolaou K, Wintersperger BJ, *et al.* (2006) Dual-source CT cardiac imaging: initial experience. *Eur Radiol* **16**:1409–1415.
13. Reimann AJ, Rinck D, Birinci-Aydogan A, *et al.* (2007) Dual-source computed tomography: advances of improved temporal resolution in coronary plaque imaging. *Invest Radiol* **42**:196–203.
14. Ropers U, Ropers D, Pflederer T, *et al.* (2007) Influence of heart rate on the diagnostic accuracy of dual-source computed tomography coronary angiography. *J Am Coll Cardiol* **50**:2393–2398.
15. Burke AP, Virmani R, Galis Z, *et al.* (2003) Task Force #2—What is the pathologic basis for new atherosclerosis imaging techniques? *J Am Coll Cardiol* **41**:1874–1886.
16. O'Rourke RA, Brundage B, Froelicher VF, *et al.* (2000) ACC/AHA Expert Consensus Document on electron-beam computed tomography for the diagnosis and prognosis of coronary artery disease. *Circulation* **102**:126–140.

17. Redberg RF, Vogel RA, Criqui MH, *et al.* (2003) Task Force #3—What is the spectrum of current and emerging techniques for the noninvasive measurement of atherosclerosis? *J Am Coll Cardiol* **41**:1886–1898.

18. Pham PH, Rao DS, Vasunilashorn F, Fishbein MC, & Goldin JG (2006) Computed tomography calcium quantification as a measure of atherosclerotic plaque morphology and stability. *Invest Radiol* **41**:674–680.

19. Pohle K, Ropers D, Mäffert R, *et al.* (2003) Coronary calcifications in young patients with first, unheralded myocardial infarction: a risk factor matched analysis by electron beam tomography. *Heart* **89**:625–628.

20. Raggi P, Callister TQ, Cooil B, *et al.* (2000) Identification of patients at increased risk of first unheralded acute myocardial infarction by electron-beam computed tomography. *Circulation* **101**:850–855.

21. Schmermund A, Schwartz RS, Adamzik M, *et al.* (2001) Coronary atherosclerosis in unheralded sudden coronary death under age fifty: histopathologic comparison with "healthy" subjects dying out of hospital. *Atherosclerosis* **155**:499–508.

22. Gerber TC, Kuzo RS, & Morin RL (2005) Techniques and parameters for estimating radiation exposure and dose in cardiac computed tomography. *Int J Cardiovasc Imaging* **21**:165–176.

23. Hoff JA, Chomka EV, Krainik AJ, *et al.* (2001) Age and gender distribution of coronary artery calcium detected by electron beam tomography in 35246 adults. *Am J Cardiol* **87**:1335–1339.

24. McClelland RL, Chung H, Detrano R, *et al.* (2006) Distribution of coronary artery calcium by race, gender, and age. Results from the Multi-Ethnic Study of Atherosclerosis (MESA). *Circulation* **113**:30–37.

25. Schmermund A, Mohlenkamp S, Berenbein S, *et al.* (2006) Population-based assessment of subclinical coronary atherosclerosis using electron-beam computed tomography. *Atherosclerosis* **185**:177–182.

26. Detrano RC, Anderson M, Nelson J, *et al.* (2005) Coronary calcium measurements: effect of CT scanner type and calcium measure on rescan reproducibility—MESA study. *Radiology* **236**:477–484.

27. Kondos GT, Hoff JA, Sevrukov A, *et al.* (2003) Electron-beam tomography coronary artery calcium and cardiac events: a 37-month follow-up of (5635) initially asymptomatic low- to intermediate-risk adults. *Circulation* **107**:2571–2576.

28. Shaw LJ, Raggi P, Schisterman E, *et al.* (2003) Prognostic value of cardiac risk factors and coronary artery calcium screening for all-cause mortality. *Radiology* **228**:826–833.

29. Greenland P, LaBree L, Azen SP, *et al.* (2004) Coronary artery calcium score combined with Framingham score for risk prediction in asymptomatic individuals. *JAMA* **291**:210–215.

30. Arad Y, Goodman KJ, Roth M, *et al.* (2005) Coronary calcification, coronary disease risk factors, C-reactive protein, and atherosclerotic cardiovascular disease events: the St. Francis Heart Study. *J Am Coll Cardiol* **46**:158–165.

31. Vliegenthart R, Oudkerk M, Song B, *et al.* (2002) Coronary calcification detected by electron-beam computed tomography and myocardial infarction. The Rotterdam Coronary Calcification Study. *Eur Heart J* **23**:1596.

32. Wong ND, Hsu JC, Detrano RC, *et al.* (2000) Coronary artery calcium evaluation by electron beam computed tomography and its relation to new cardiovascular events. *Am J Cardiol* **86**:495–498.

33. Church TS, Levine BD, McGuire DK, *et al.* (2007) Coronary artery calcium score, risk factors, and incident coronary heart disease events. *Atherosclerosis* **190**:224–312.

34. Detrano R, Guerci AD, Carr JJ, *et al.* (2008) Coronary calcium as a predictor of coronary artery events in four racial or ethnic groups. *N Engl J Med* **358**:1336–1345.

35. Taylor AJ, Bindeman J, Feuerstein I, *et al.* (2005) Coronary calcium independently predicts incident premature coronary heart disease over measured cardiovascular risk factors: mean three-year outcomes in the Prospective Army Coronary Calcium (PACC) project. *J Am Coll Cardiol* **46**:807–814.

36. Pletcher MJ, Tice JA, Pignone M, & Browner WS (2004) Using the coronary artery calcium score to predict coronary heart disease events: a systematic review and meta-analysis. *Arch Intern Med* **164**:1266–1268.

37. Budoff MJ, Achenbach S, Blumenthal RS, *et al.* (2006) Assessment of coronary artery disease by cardiac computed tomography: a scientific statement from the American Heart Association Committee on Cardiovascular Imaging and Intervention, Council on Cardiovascular Radiology and Intervention, and Committee on Cardiac Imaging, Council on Clinical Cardiology. *Circulation* **114**:1761–1791.

38. Budoff MJ, Shaw LJ, Liu ST, *et al.* (2007) Long-term prognosis associated with coronary calcification: observations from a registry of 25 253 patients. *J Am Coll Cardiol* **49**:1860–1870.

39. LaMonte MJ, FitzGerald SJ, Church TS, *et al.* (2005) Coronary artery calcium score and coronary heart disease events in a large cohort of asymptomatic men and women. *Am J Epidemiol* **162**:421–429.

40. Park R, Detrano R, Xiang M, *et al.* (2002) Combined use of computed tomography coronary calcium scores and C-reactive protein levels in predicting cardiovascular events in nondiabetic individuals. *Circulation* **106**:2073–2077.

41. Becker A, Leber A, Becker C, & Knez A (2008) Predictive value of coronary calcifications for future cardiac events in asymptomatic individuals. *Am Heart J* **155**:154–160.

42. Nasir K, Shaw LJ, Liu ST, *et al.* (2007) Ethnic differences in the prognostic value of coronary artery calcification for all-cause mortality. *J Am Coll Cardiol* **50**:953–960.

43. Schmermund A, Baumgart D, Möhlenkamp S, *et al.* (2001) Natural history and topographic pattern of progression of coronary calcification in symptomatic patients. *Arterioscler Thromb Vasc Biol* **21**:421–426.

44. Taylor AJ, Bindeman J, Le TP, *et al.* (2008) Progression of calcified coronary atherosclerosis: relationship to coronary risk factors and carotid intima-media thickness. *Atherosclerosis* **197**:339–345.

45. Kronmal RA, McClelland RL, Detrano R, *et al.* (2007) Risk factors for the progression of coronary artery calcification in asymptomatic subjects: results from the Multi-Ethnic Study of Atherosclerosis (MESA). *Circulation* **115**:2722–2730.

46. Cassidy-Bushrow AE, Bielak LF, Sheedy PF 2nd, *et al.* (2007) Coronary artery calcification progression is heritable. *Circulation* **116**:25–31.

47. Raggi P, Callister TQ, & Shaw LJ (2004) Progression of coronary artery calcium and risk of first myocardial infarction in patients receiving cholesterol-lowering therapy. *Arterioscler Thromb Vasc Biol* **24**:1272–1277.

48. Callister TQ, Raggi P, Cooil B, *et al.* (1998) Effect of HmG-CoA reductase inhibitors on coronary artery disease as assessed by electron-beam computed tomography. *N Engl J Med* **339**:1972–1980.

49. Achenbach S, Ropers D, Pohle K, *et al.* (2002) Influence of lipid-lowering therapy on the progression of coronary artery calcification: a prospective evaluation. *Circulation* **106**:1077–1082.

50. Budoff MJ, Lane KL, Bakhsheshi H, *et al.* (2000) Rates of progression of coronary calcium by electron beam tomography. *Am J Cardiol* **86**:8–11.

51. Raggi P, Davidson M, Callister TQ, *et al.* (2005) Aggressive versus moderate lipid-lowering therapy in hypercholesterolemic postmenopausal women: Beyond Endorsed Lipid Lowering with EBT Scanning (BELLES). *Circulation* **112**:563–571.

52. Schmermund A, Achenbach S, Budde T, *et al.* (2006) Effect of intensive versus standard lipid-lowering treatment with atorvastatin on the progression of calcified coronary atherosclerosis over 12 months: a multicenter, randomized, double-blind trial. *Circulation* **113**:427–437.

53. Arad Y, Spadaro LA, Roth M, *et al.* (2005) Treatment of asymptomatic adults with elevated coronary calcium scores with atorvastatin, vitamin C, and vitamin E: the St. Francis Heart Study randomized clinical trial. *J Am Coll Cardiol* **46**:166–172.

54. Terry JG, Carr JJ, Kouba EO, *et al.* (2007) Effect of simvastatin (80 mg) on coronary and abdominal aortic arterial calcium (from the coronary artery calcification treatment with zocor [CATZ] study). *Am J Cardiol* **99**:1714–1717.

55. Taylor AJ, Bairey Merz CN, & Udelson JE (2003) 34th Bethesda Conference. Executive Summary—Can atherosclerosis imaging techniques improve the detection of patients at risk for ischemic heart disease? *J Am Coll Cardiol* **41**:1860–1862.

56. Greenland P, Bonow RO, Brundage BH, *et al.* (2007) ACCF/AHA 2007 clinical expert consensus document on coronary artery calcium scoring by computed tomography in global cardiovascular risk assessment and in evaluation of patients with chest pain: a report of the American College of Cardiology Foundation Clinical Expert Consensus Task Force (ACCF/AHA Writing Committee to Update the 2000 Expert Consensus Document on Electron Beam Computed Tomography). *Circulation* **115**:402–426.

57. De Backer G, Ambrosioni E, Borch-Johnsen K, *et al.* (2003) European guidelines on cardiovascular disease prevention in clinical practice. Third Joint Task Force of European and Other Societies on Cardiovascular Disease Prevention in Clinical Practice. *Eur Heart J* **24**:1601–1610.

58. Achenbach S (2006) Computed tomography coronary angiography. *J Am Coll Cardiol* **48**:1919–1928.

59. Hunold P, Vogt FM, Schmermund A, *et al.* (2003) Radiation exposure during cardiac CT: effective doses at multi-detector row CT and electron-beam CT. *Radiology* **226**:145–152.

60. Coles DR, Smail MA, Negus IS, *et al.* (2006) Comparison of radiation doses from multislice computed tomography coronary angiography and conventional diagnostic angiography. *J Am Coll Cardiol* **47**:1840–1845.

61. Gerber TC, Stratmann BP, Kuzo RS, Kantor B, & Morin RL (2005) Effect of acquisition technique on radiation dose and image quality in multidetector row computed tomography coronary angiography with submillimeter collimation. *Invest Radiol* **40**:556–563.

62. Hausleiter J, Meyer T, Hadamitzky M, *et al.* (2006) Radiation dose estimates from cardiac multislice computed tomography in daily practice: impact of different scanning protocols on effective dose estimates. *Circulation* **113**:1305–1310.

63. Poll LW, Cohnen M, Brachten S, Ewen K, & Modder U (2002) Dose reduction in multi-slice CT of the heart by use of ECG-controlled tube current modulation ("ECG pulsing"): phantom measurements. *Rofo* **174**:1500–1505.

64. Jakobs TF, Becker CR, Ohnesorge B, *et al.* (2002) Multislice helical CT of the heart with retrospective ECG gating: reduction of radiation exposure by ECG-controlled tube current modulation. *Eur Radiol* **12**:1081–1086.

65. Halliburton SS, Petersilka M, Schvartzman PR, Obuchowski N, & White RD (2003) Evaluation of left ventricular dysfunction using multiphasic reconstructions of coronary multi-slice computed tomography data in patients with chronic ischemic heart disease: validation against cine magnetic resonance imaging. *Int J Cardiovasc Imaging* **19**:73–78.

66. Grude M, Juergens KU, Wichter T, *et al.* (2003) Evaluation of global left ventricular myocardial function with electrocardiogram-gated multidetector computed tomography: comparison with magnetic resonance imaging. *Invest Radiol* **38**:653–661.

67. Leber AW, Knez A, von Ziegler F, *et al.* (2005) Quantification of obstructive and nonobstructive coronary lesions by 64-slice computed tomography: a comparative study with quantitative coronary angiography and intravascular ultrasound. *J Am Coll Cardiol* **46**:147–1454.

68. Raff GL, Gallagher MJ, O'Neill WW, & Goldstein JA (2005) Diagnostic accuracy of noninvasive coronary angiography using 64-slice spiral computed tomography. *J Am Coll Cardiol* **46**:552–557.

69. Mollet NR, Cademartiri F, van Mieghem CA, *et al.* (2005) High-resolution spiral computed tomography coronary angiography in patients referred for diagnostic conventional coronary angiography. *Circulation* **112**:2318–2323.

70. Ropers D, Rixe J, Anders K, *et al.* (2006) Usefulness of multidetector row spiral computed tomography with 64- × 0.6-mm collimation and 330-ms rotation for the noninvasive detection of significant coronary artery stenoses. *Am J Cardiol* **97**:343–348.

71. Schuijf JD, Pundziute G, Jukema JW, *et al.* (2006) Diagnostic accuracy of 64-slice multislice computed tomography in the noninvasive evaluation of significant coronary artery disease. *Am J Cardiol* **98**:145–148.

72. Nikolaou K, Knez A, Rist C, *et al.* (2006) Accuracy of 64-MDCT in the diagnosis of ischemic heart disease. *AJR Am J Roentgenol* **187**:111–117.

73. Grosse C, Globits S, & Hergan K (2007) Forty-slice spiral computed tomography of the coronary arteries: assessment of image quality and diagnostic accuracy in a non-selected patient population. *Acta Radiol* **48**:36–44.

74. Hoffmann U, Moselewski F, Cury RC, *et al.* (2004) Predictive value of 16-slice multidetector spiral computed tomography to

detect significant obstructive coronary artery disease in patients at high risk for coronary artery disease: patient-versus segment-based analysis. *Circulation* **110**:2638–2643.

75. Scheffel H, Alkadhi H, Plass A, Vachenauer R, *et al.* (2006) Accuracy of dual-source CT coronary angiography: first experience in a high pre-test probability population without heart rate control. *Eur Radiol* **16**:2739–2747.

76. Weustink AC, Meijboom WB, Mollet NR, *et al.* (2007) Reliable high-speed coronary computed tomography in symptomatic patients. *J Am Coll Cardiol* **50**:786–794.

77. Leber AW, Johnson T, Becker A, *et al.* (2007) Diagnostic accuracy of dual-source multi-slice CT-coronary angiography in patients with an intermediate pretest likelihood for coronary artery disease. *Eur Heart J* **28**:2354–2360.

78. Hendel RC, Patel MR, Kramer CM, *et al.* (2006) ACCF/ACR/SCCT/SCMR/ASNC/NASCI/SCAI/SIR 2006 appropriateness criteria for cardiac computed tomography and cardiac magnetic resonance imaging: a report of the American College of Cardiology Foundation Quality Strategic Directions Committee Appropriateness Criteria Working Group, American College of Radiology, Society of Cardiovascular Computed Tomography, Society for Cardiovascular Magnetic Resonance, American Society of Nuclear Cardiology, North American Society for Cardiac Imaging, Society for Cardiovascular Angiography and Interventions, and Society of Interventional Radiology. *J Am Coll Cardiol* **48**:1475–1497.

79. Burgstahler C, Beck T, Kuettner A, *et al.* (2006) Non-invasive evaluation of coronary artery bypass grafts using 16-row multi-slice computed tomography with 188 ms temporal resolution. *Int J Cardiol* **106**:244–249.

80. Malagutti P, Nieman K, Meijboom WB, *et al.* (2007) Use of 64-slice CT in symptomatic patients after coronary bypass surgery: evaluation of grafts and coronary arteries. *Eur Heart J* **28**:1879–1885.

81. Nieman K, Pattynama PM, Rensing BJ, Van Geuns RJ, & De Feyter PJ (2003) Evaluation of patients after coronary artery bypass surgery: CT angiographic assessment of grafts and coronary arteries. *Radiology* **229**:749–756.

82. Salm LP, Bax JJ, Jukema JW, *et al.* (2005) Comprehensive assessment of patients after coronary artery bypass grafting by 16-detector-row computed tomography. *Am Heart J* **150**:775–781.

83. Stauder NI, Kuttner A, Schroder S, *et al.* (2006) Coronary artery bypass grafts: assessment of graft patency and native coronary artery lesions using 16-slice MDCT. *Eur Radiol* **16**:2512–2520.

84. Onuma Y, Tanabe K, Chihara R, *et al.* (2007) Evaluation of coronary artery bypass grafts and native coronary arteries using 64-slice multidetector computed tomography. *Am Heart J* **154**:519–526.

85. Ropers D, Pohle FK, Kuettner A, *et al.* (2006) Diagnostic accuracy of noninvasive coronary angiography in patients after bypass surgery using 64-slice spiral computed tomography with 330-ms gantry rotation. *Circulation*:**114**:2334–2341.

86. Maintz D, Seifarth H, Raupach R, *et al.* (2006) 64-slice multi-detector coronary CT angiography: in vitro evaluation of 68 different stents. *Eur Radiol* **16**:818–826.

87. Pugliese F, Weustink AC, Van Mieghem C, *et al.* (2007) Dual-source coronary computed tomography angiography for detecting in-stent restenosis. *Heart* **94**:848–854.

88. Rixe J, Achenbach S, Ropers D, *et al.* (2006) Assessment of coronary artery stent restenosis by 64-slice multi-detector computed tomography. *Eur Heart J* **27**:2567–2572.

89. Cademartiri F, Schuijf JD, Pugliese F, *et al.* (2007) Usefulness of 64-slice multislice computed tomography coronary angiography to assess in-stent restenosis. *J Am Coll Cardiol* **49**:2204–2210.

90. Oncel D, Oncel G, & Karaca M (2007) Coronary stent patency and in-stent restenosis: determination with 64-section multi-detector CT coronary angiography—initial experience. *Radiology* **242**:403–409.

91. Rist C, von Ziegler F, Nikolaou K, *et al.* (2006) Assessment of coronary artery stent patency and restenosis using 64-slice computed tomography. *Acad Radiol* **13**:1465–1473.

92. Das KM, El Menyar AA, Salam AM, *et al.* (2007) Contrast-enhanced 64-section coronary multidetector CT angiography versus conventional coronary angiography for stent assessment. *Radiology* **245**:424–432.

93. Ehara M, Kawai M, Surmely JF, *et al.* (2007) Diagnostic accuracy of coronary in-stent restenosis using 64-slice computed tomography: comparison with invasive coronary angiography. *J Am Coll Cardiol* **49**:951–959.

94. Schroeder S, Kopp AF, Baumbach A, *et al.* (2001) Noninvasive detection and evaluation of atherosclerotic coronary plaques with multislice computed tomography. *J Am Coll Cardiol* **37**:1430–1435.

95. Schroeder S, Kopp AF, & Burgstahler C (2007) Noninvasive plaque imaging using multislice detector spiral computed tomography. *Semin Thromb Hemost* **33**:203–209.

96. Achenbach S, Moselewski F, Ropers D, *et al.* (2004) Detection of calcified and noncalcified coronary atherosclerotic plaque by contrast-enhanced, submillimeter multidetector spiral computed tomography: a segment-based comparison with intravascular ultrasound. *Circulation* **109**:14–17.

97. Leber AW, Knez A, Becker A, *et al.* (2004) Accuracy of multi-detector spiral computed tomography in identifying and differentiating the composition of coronary atherosclerotic plaques: a comparative study with intracoronary ultrasound. *J Am Coll Cardiol* **43**:1241–1247.

98. Pohle K, Achenbach S, Macneill B, *et al.* (2007) Characterization of non-calcified coronary atherosclerotic plaque by multi-detector row CT: comparison to IVUS. *Atherosclerosis* **190**:174–180.

99. Leber AW, Becker A, Knez A, *et al.* (2006) Accuracy of 64-slice computed tomography to classify and quantify plaque volumes in the proximal coronary system: a comparative study using intravascular ultrasound. *J Am Coll Cardiol* **47**:672–677.

100. Schoenhagen P, Tuzcu EM, Stillman AE, *et al.* (2003) Non-invasive assessment of plaque morphology and remodeling in mildly stenotic coronary segments: comparison of 16-slice computed tomography and intravascular ultrasound. *Coron Artery Dis* **14**:459–462.

101. Moselewski F, Ropers D, Pohle K, *et al.* (2004) Comparison of measurement of cross-sectional coronary atherosclerotic plaque and vessel areas by 16-slice multidetector computed tomography versus intravascular ultrasound. *Am J Cardiol* **94**:1294–1297.

102. Schmid M, Pflederer T, Jang IK, *et al.* (2008) Relationship between degree of remodeling and CT attenuation of plaque in

coronary atherosclerotic lesions: an in-vivo analysis by multi-detector computed tomography. *Atherosclerosis* **197**:457–464.

103. Hoffmann U, Moselewski F, Nieman K, *et al.* (2006) Noninvasive assessment of plaque morphology and composition in culprit and stable lesions in acute coronary syndrome and stable lesions in stable angina by multidetector computed tomography. *J Am Coll Cardiol* **47**:1655–1662.

104. Leber AW, Knez A, White CW, *et al.* (2003) Composition of coronary atherosclerotic plaques in patients with acute myocardial infarction and stable angina pectoris determined by contrast-enhanced multislice computed tomography. *Am J Cardiol* **91**:714–718.

105. Motoyama S, Kondo T, Sarai M, *et al.* (2007) Multislice computed tomographic characteristics of coronary lesions in acute coronary syndromes. *J Am Coll Cardiol* **50**:319–326.

106. Schuijf JD, Beck T, Burgstahler C, *et al.* (2007) Differences in plaque composition and distribution in stable coronary artery disease versus acute coronary syndromes; non-invasive evaluation with multi-slice computed tomography. *Acute Card Care* **9**:48–53.

107. Pundziute G, Schuijf JD, Jukema JW, *et al.* (2007) Prognostic value of multislice computed tomography coronary angiography in patients with known or suspected coronary artery disease. *J Am Coll Cardiol* **49**:62–70.

28 Invasive Coronary Arteriography for Assessment of Coronary Artery Disease

Jürgen Haase

Kardiocentrum Frankfurt, Klinik Rotes Kreuz, Frankfurt/Main, Germany

Historical background

The origin of cardiac catheterization started with the pioneering work of Werner Forssman, who performed the first right heart catheterization in 1929 in Erberswalde [1]. The first determination of cardiac output in human beings was carried out by Klein in Prague [2]. Physiologic studies using right heart catheterizations were also performed by Cournand and co-workers in New York [3–5]. James Warren was among the first to use cardiac catheterization for diagnostic purposes in Atlanta [6]. The catheterization of the left side of the heart was developed by Henry Zimmerman in Cleveland [7]. Subsequently, many investigators started to test angiographic techniques to visualize coronary arteries in animals and humans [8–21]. The first selective coronary arteriogram was carried out by Mason Sones in Cleveland in 1958 [19]. In the late 1960s invasive coronary arteriography became the diagnostic standard for the assessment of coronary artery disease and the selection of patients for coronary artery bypass surgery [22,23]. With the introduction of percutaneous transluminal coronary angioplasty (PTCA) by Andreas Grüntzig in Zürich in 1977 [24], invasive coronary angiography took over the role of a peri-interventional technique to estimate lesion characteristics [25], to directly assess the result of percutaneous coronary interventions (PCIs), and to appreciate the long-term outcome by angiographic follow-up. The development of quantitative coronary angiography (QCA) enabled cardiologists to accurately measure the angiographic dimensions of coronary artery lesions and to overcome interobserver variability in the visual assessment of coronary artery stenoses [26].

Indications for diagnostic invasive coronary arteriography

Invasive coronary arteriography should be performed in patients with suspected coronary artery disease based on severe stable angina (Canadian Cardiovascular Society [CCS]) class III or IV) or those who have less severe symptoms but show "high-risk" criteria for an adverse outcome on noninvasive testing. High-risk criteria include a stress electrocardiogram demonstrating significant ST-segment depression (1 mV or more in at least two precordial leads) or hypotension associated with decreased exercise capacity [27] as well as resting or exercise-induced left ventricular dysfunction. High risk for an adverse outcome is also suspected in the case of moderate or large perfusion defects on stress imaging, multiple defects, a large perfusion defect in the presence of left ventricular dilation or increased lung uptake, or extensive stress or dobutamine-induced wall motion abnormalities. Invasive coronary arteriography should also be carried out in patients who were resuscitated from sudden cardiac death. Coronary calcifications on fluoroscopy or a high calcium score during MSCT without symptoms or signs of ischemia do not represent an indication for invasive coronary arteriography.

Patients with unstable angina who demonstrate recurrent symptoms despite medical therapy or those who are at intermediate or high risk for death or myocardial infarction are also candidates for invasive coronary arteriography. High-risk criteria include sustained chest pain (>20 min), pulmonary congestion, worsening mitral insufficiency, arterial hypotension, and dynamic ST-segment depression (1 mV or more). Intermediate-risk criteria include angina at rest (>20 min) relieved with sublingual nitroglycerine, angina associated with dynamic ECG changes, recent-onset angina with a high likelihood of coronary artery disease, pathologic Q-waves, ST-segment depression in multiple leads, and age older than 65 years.

Patients with an ST-segment elevation myocardial infarction (STEMI) or a non-ST-segment elevation myocardial infarction (NSTEMI), or those with unstable angina who show spontaneous ischemia or ischemia at a minimal workload should undergo invasive coronary arteriography [28]. Additional indications in patients with acute myocardial infarctions are the development of congestive heart failure, cardiac arrest, mitral insufficiency, or a ventricular septal defect. Patients with unstable or provokable angina after a myocardial infarction are also candidates for coronary arteriography.

Cardiovascular Interventions in Clinical Practice. Edited by Jürgen Haase, Hans-Joachim Schäfers, Horst Sievert and Ron Waksman. © 2010 Blackwell Publishing.

Patients who suffer from chest pain of unclear etiology, especially in the presence of high-risk criteria on noninvasive testing, may benefit from coronary arteriography to diagnose or exclude significant coronary artery disease. Patients with a history of revascularization should undergo coronary arteriography if they develop recurrent angina that meets high-risk criteria on noninvasive testing.

Patients who are scheduled to undergo noncardiac surgery who show high-risk criteria of coronary artery disease on noninvasive testing, who have angina nonresponsive to medical therapy, who develop unstable angina, or who demonstrate equivocal noninvasive test results and are scheduled for high-risk surgery should undergo coronary arteriography.

Invasive coronary arteriography is also recommended in patients scheduled to undergo cardiac surgery for valvular or congenital heart disease, particularly in the presence of multiple risk factors or infective endocarditis when coronary embolization is suspected.

Coronary arteriography often provides important information about the presence of coronary artery disease in patients who present with intractable dysrhythmias before electrophysiological testing or in patients who present with dilated cardiomyopathy of unknown etiology.

Invasive coronary arteriography is the basic requirement for planning and preparation of PCIs as well as the peri-interventional evaluation of procedural progress and outcome (see Peri-interventional coronary arteriography, below).

Contraindications and risks of invasive coronary arteriography

Relative contraindications for coronary arteriography include untreated infections, unexplained fever, severe anemia (hemoglobin <8 mg/dL), uncontrolled systemic hypertension, digitalis toxicity, previous allergic contrast reaction without corticosteroid pretreatment, ongoing stroke, acute renal failure, decompensated heart failure, severe intrinsic or iatrogenic coagulopathy (international normalized ratio >2.0), and active endocarditis.

Risk factors for complications after coronary arteriography include advanced age as well as several general medical, cardiac, and vascular characteristics listed in Table 28.1. Coronary arteriography should be deferred until important comorbidities have been stabilized, unless there is evidence of significant ongoing myocardial necrosis. If coronary arteriography is performed under emergency conditions, it is associated with a higher risk of procedural complications. Risks and benefits of the procedure and its alternatives should be carefully evaluated before coronary arteriography is undertaken in the presence of relative contraindications. Potential complications of invasive coronary arteriography are listed in Table 28.2.

Table 28.1 Risk factors for complications after invasive coronary arteriography.

Increased general medical risk
age >70 years
Complex congenital heart disease
Morbid obesity
General debility or cachexia
Uncontrolled glucose intolerance
Arterial oxygen desaturation
Severe chronic obstructive airway disease
Renal insufficiency (creatinine >1.5 mg/dL)

Increased cardiac risk
Three-vessel coronary artery disease
Left main coronary artery disease
Heart failure functional class IV
Significant mitral or aortic valve disease or mechanical prosthesis
Left ventricular ejection fraction <35%
Left ventricular end-diastolic pressure >25 mmHg
High risk stress test (severe ischemia or hypotension)
Pulmonary hypertension

Increased vascular risk
Bleeding diathesis or anticoagulation
Uncontrolled arterial hypertension
Severe peripheral artery disease
Recent stroke
Severe aortic insufficiency

Adapted from reference 27.

Table 28.2 Incidence of complications with invasive coronary arteriography.

Complication	SCAI Registry (%)
Mortality	0.11
Myocardial infarction	0.05
Cerebrovascular accident	0.07
Arrhythmias	0.38
Vascular complications	0.43
Allergic contrast reaction	0.37
Hemodynamic complications	0.26
Other complications	0.28

SCAI, Society for Cardiac Angiography and Intervention.
Adapted from reference 27.

Invasive coronary arteriography versus computed tomography coronary arteriography

Although computed tomography coronary arteriography (CTCA) offers a noninvasive tool for the assessment of coronary artery disease (see Chapter 27), this technique is limited by various factors. The spatial and temporal resolution of CTCA are clearly below the resolution of invasive coronary arteriography, the radiation exposure of CTCA exceeds the radiation exposure of invasive coronary arteriography, and angiographic visualization of coronary artery stenoses may be disturbed by beam hardening in the presence of coronary calcium or at the site of previously implanted metallic stents [29–31]. Moreover, owing to the complexity of image processing, CTCA cannot be used for repeated peri-interventional angiographic evaluations as required during PCIs.

The above-mentioned limitations of CTCA explain why invasive coronary arteriography remains the gold standard for the assessment of coronary artery disease, especially in the field of interventional cardiology [32–35]. While CTCA is going to take over part of the diagnostic role, predominantly in patients with a low pretest likelihood of disease, in whom coronary artery stenoses should be ruled out, the main role of invasive coronary arteriography is represented by the exact luminographic assessment of coronary artery disease as well as peri-interventional angiographic evaluations. In conjunction with QCA, invasive coronary arteriography guides the interventional cardiologist in the preparation and performance of PCIs. It allows the correct sizing of interventional devices (balloons, atherectomy devices, embolic protection devices, stents, etc.), provides visualization of the actual position of such devices, and gives an immediate angiographic result at any stage of the procedure including functional information by the visualization of coronary flow.

Patient preparation

Before invasive coronary arteriography, a baseline ECG, electrolyte and renal function tests, complete blood cell count, and coagulation panel should be reviewed. If the patient needs to be prepared for PCI, an oral dose of aspirin (100–500 mg) should be administered at least 2 h before the procedure. Warfarin should be discontinued at least 2 days before elective coronary arteriography, and the INR should be <2 before the arterial puncture. Patients at increased risk for systemic thromboembolism on withdrawal of warfarin, such as those with atrial fibrillation, mitral valve disease, or a history of systemic thromboembolism, may be treated with intravenous unfractionated heparin or subcutaneous low-molecular-weight heparin in the periprocedural period.

Arterial access site

Various arterial access sites are available for invasive coronary arteriography. The selection depends on operator experience, the presence of peripheral artery disease, and the complexity of subsequent PCIs.

Femoral artery approach

Right or left femoral arteries are the most commonly used access sites for invasive coronary arteriography and PCIs.

The anterior wall of the common femoral artery should be punctured several centimeters below the inguinal ligament but proximal to the bifurcation of the superficial and the profunda femoral artery branches. Puncture of the common femoral artery proximal to the inguinal ligament may lead to bleeding into the retroperitoneal space, whereas puncture distal to the bifurcation may be complicated by aneurysm formation after sheath removal.

The most important advantages of the femoral over the radial or brachial approach are based on the relatively large vessel diameters: the freedom of motion for the introduction and manipulation of PCI devices as well as the fact that practically no limitation exists regarding the dimensions of the introducer sheath. These advantages may become relevant in the case of complex PCIs (use of multiple wires, atherectomy, thrombectomy, or embolic protection devices) or high-risk coronary interventions (need of intra-aortic counterpulsation). In addition, the radiation exposure of the operator is less with the femoral approach, because adequate shielding can be used throughout the procedure.

Brachial and radial approaches

The brachial and radial approaches are preferred over the femoral approach in the presence of severe peripheral vascular disease. The brachial artery allows the insertion of relatively large introducer sheaths up to 8F (1F = 0.33 mm in diameter), and the smaller radial artery is limited to 5–7F catheters. If puncture of the brachial artery is performed instead of surgical preparation, it is recommended to use introducer sheaths no larger than 6F to avoid major bleeding complications at the puncture site.

An Allen test should be carried out before radial artery access is attempted in order to demonstrate ulnar artery patency in the event of radial artery occlusion. Systemic anticoagulation is used for both approaches to prevent catheter thrombosis and intra-arterial application of verapamil or nitroglycerine may be used to reduce brachial or radial artery spasm during manipulation of the catheters.

Catheters

Catheters for diagnostic coronary arteriography and PCI (guiding catheters) are constructed from polyurethane or polyethylene with a fine wire braid within the wall to allow advancement and torque control and to prevent kinking. The outer diameter of the catheters ranges from 4F to 8F. In patients with regular vessel anatomy, diagnostic coronary

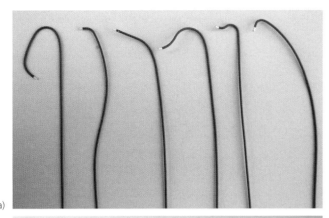

(a)

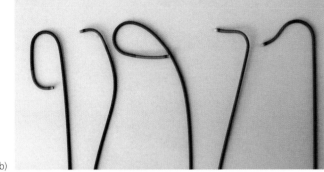

(b)

Figure 28.1 (a) Diagnostic coronary catheters. The most frequently used configurations of 5F diagnostic coronary catheters: Judkins left, Judkins right, multipurpose, Amplatz left, Amplatz right, internal mammary artery catheter (from left to right) (courtesy of Medtronic Europe, Tolochenaz, Switzerland). (b) Coronary guiding catheters. Frequently used configurations of 6F coronary guiding catheters: Judkins left, Judkins right, EBU left, Amplatz right, Amplatz left (from left to right). In comparison with Judkins configurations, Amplatz and EBU configurations provide superior catheter backup during coronary interventions (courtesy of Medtronic Europe, Tolochenaz, Switzerland).

arteriography can be carried out with 4F catheters from the femoral access site, which allows ambulation after 1 h of pressure bandage following the procedure, provided no anticoagulation was used. Superior torque control and stability are provided by 5F, in the presence of a dilated aortic root, aortic aneurysms, or kinkings. For peri-interventional coronary angiography 6F guiding catheters are recommended, in case of complex percutaneous coronary interventions (PCI of bifurcation lesions, chronic total occlusions) 7F may be required. The various shapes of diagnostic and guiding catheters are shown in Figure 28.1.

Contrast agents

For invasive coronary arteriography and PCI, ionic contrast agents are no longer used because of the high incidence of side-effects, predominantly resulting from their high osmolarity (about 1900 mosmol/kgH_2O). The side-effects are much less frequent with nonionic contrast agents (290–600 mosmol/

kgH_2O). They include hot flushing, nausea, vomiting, and arrhythmias. For patients with impaired renal function, the use of an isosmolar contrast medium (Iodixanol, Visipaque) is recommended.

Engagement of coronary artery and bypass ostia for diagnostic versus peri-interventional coronary angiography

The diagnostic or therapeutic goal of these procedures determines the selection not only of catheter dimensions, but also of catheter configuration. Whereas diagnostic angiography focuses on optimal imaging of the coronary artery segments, the equipment used for peri-interventional coronary arteriography has to be selected according to the requirements of the intervention. Variability of the degree of friction within the coronary artery segment, which depends on vessel tortuosity and the presence of wall irregularities (calcifications), means that optimal catheter backup is required to enhance the pushability of guidewires and interventional devices. Potential changes in interventional strategies during the procedure (necessity of rotational atherectomy owing to vessel wall calcifications) should be anticipated by an adequate selection of the guiding catheter (inner lumen of the guiding catheter matched to the diameter of potentially required atherectomy devices). Moreover, a stable position of the guiding catheter tip is crucial for precise positioning of imaging catheters (e.g., motorized pull-back of intravascular ultrasound [IVUS] catheters) or coronary stents.

Left coronary ostium

Cannulation of the left coronary ostium is carried out in an left anterior oblique (LAO) projection. The Judkins left 4.0 coronary catheter is most frequently used for diagnostic angiography of the left coronary artery (LCA), even if left anterior descending (LAD) and left circumflex coronary artery (LCx) have separate ostia. A Judkins left 3.5 coronary catheter may be required when the aortic arch is small or the take-off of the LCA is high. A Judkins left 5.0 coronary catheter may be useful in the presence of an ectatic ascending aorta or for cannulation of a separate take-off of the LCx. Alternatively, an Amplatz left coronary catheter may be helpful in these circumstances. The Amplatz left coronary catheter may require more manipulation to engage the left main trunk than the standard Judkins left catheter. The secondary curve of the Amplatz left 1 or 2 is positioned on the right coronary cusp of the aortic valve with the catheter tip pointing to the left aortic cusp. Alternating advancement and retraction of the catheter with clockwise rotation allows the catheter tip to move slowly along the left sinus of Valsalva to enter the left coronary ostium. At the end of this procedure, the catheter tip can be stabilized by slight retraction of the catheter. For PCI in the LAD or the LCx, a left extra backup (EBU) configuration (EBU left 3.5–5.0) normally provides optimal back-up if the catheter is adequately sized

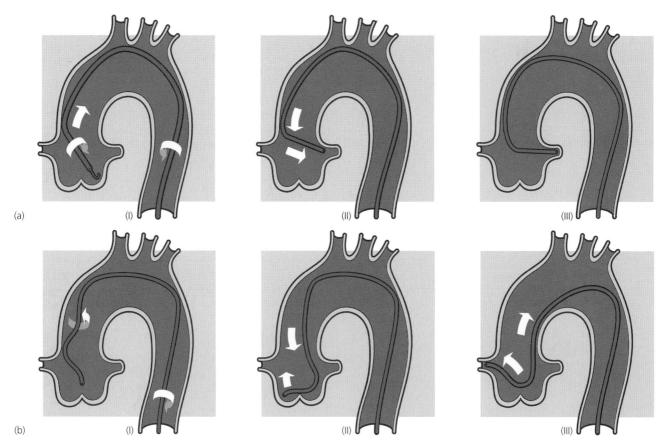

(a)   (I)   (II)   (III)

(b)   (I)   (II)   (III)

Figure 28.2 Peri-interventional coronary arteriography. (a) Cannulation of the left coronary artery with EBU guiding catheter: The left EBU catheter is advanced with the J-wire to the aortic root, where the guidewire is removed. Intubation in the ostium of the left main is accomplished by slight retraction and rotation of the catheter tip (I). When in coaxial position to the left main trunk, the catheter is carefully advanced by a few millimeters (II and III). (b) Cannulation of the RCA with Amplatz left I guiding catheter. The Amplatz catheter is advanced to the aortic root and rotated clockwise to the right coronary ostium (I). For intubation of the coronary ostium the secondary curve of the catheter is pushed on the right coronary cusp of the aortic valve moving the catheter tip into a cephalad direction (II) Following insertion of the tip the catheter is slightly retracted allowing coaxial penetration in the ostium of the RCA (III).

(Fig. 28.2a). Adequate sizing of left EBU guiding catheters is achieved if the catheter tip penetrates at least 3–5 mm into the left main. Amplatz as well as EBU configurations are superior to the Judkins left when strong catheter backup is required. In selected cases, however, the Judkins left backup may be enhanced by a deep intubation into the LAD with the secondary curve forming a loop in the aortic root.

Right coronary ostium

Engagement of the right coronary artery ostium is also performed in an LAO view. While the Judkins left catheter naturally directs to the left coronary ostium when advanced to the aortic root, Judkins right coronary catheters as well as Amplatz catheters need to be rotated clockwise to the right coronary ostium after having reached the aortic root. When the ostium of the right coronary artery (RCA) atypically takes off at a more superior and anterior location, an Aplatz left I or multipurpose catheter may alleviate cannulation of the right coronary origin. Both catheters also have to be rotated clockwise after having reached the proximal portion of the

ascending aorta to cannulate the RCA. When PCI is planned at the RCA, EBU as well as Amplatz configurations may improve catheter backup (Fig. 28.2b). If a dominant RCA has to be treated in the presence of an ectatic aortic root, Amplatz left I or Amplatz left II guiding catheters may be required to provide adequate catheter backup.

Aortocoronary bypass grafts

Saphenous vein grafts to RCA normally originate at the right anterolateral side of the ascending aorta about 5 cm above the sinotubular ridge and steeply descend to the distal anastomosis [36]. They are best cannulated with a multipurpose catheter, which is first advanced to the aortic root and subsequently pulled back during clockwise rotation to the right anterolateral wall (Fig. 28.3a). Saphenous vein grafts to the LAD or the diagonal branches originate at the anterior wall of the ascending aorta, approximately 7 cm above the sinotubular ridge. Saphenous vein grafts to the circumflex coronary system normally originate from the left anterolateral portion of the ascending aorta about 10 cm above the sinotubular ridge and turn to their posterolateral

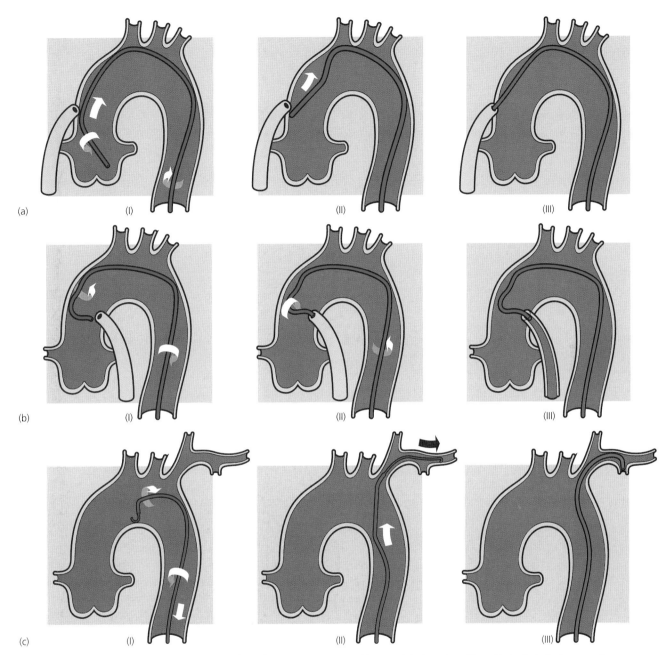

Figure 28.3 Peri-interventional coronary bypass angiography.
(a) Cannulation of an aortocoronary bypass to the right coronary artery. The tip of the multipurpose catheter is advanced to the aortic root and then rotated clockwise to the anterolateral wall of the ascending aorta (I). In this position the catheter is pulled back several centimeters, keeping in touch with the anterolateral wall of the aorta (II). Slight rotation may be required to intubate a bypass-graft to the RCA (III). (b) Cannulation of an aortocoronary bypass to the left coronary artery. An Amplatz left I guiding catheter is advanced to the proximal portion of the aortic root and turned clockwise to the ostium of the aortocoronary graft to the left coronary artery (I). Following insertion of the catheter tip, a counterclockwise rotation helps to achieve coaxial orientation of the catheter tip in the bypass ostium (II and III). (c) Cannulation of the left internal mammary artery. The IMA guiding catheter is first positioned in the aortic arch and then pulled back under counter-clockwise rotation to intubate the left subclavian artery (I). When intubation is accomplished, the J-wire is advanced to the distal portion of the left subclavian artery (II). The tip of the guiding catheter is advanced to a position distal to the take-off of the left internal mammary artery. Following removal of the wire, the catheter-tip is carefully pulled back under counter-clockwise rotation to engage the LIMA ostium (III). Intubation of the LIMA ostium may require a slight LAO and a 30° RAO projection.

direction. They may be cannulated with either a regular Judkins right 4, an Amplatz left I, or a multipurpose catheter (Fig. 28.3b). Multipurpose, hockey stick, or Amplatz guiding catheters normally provide sufficient backup for saphenous vein graft interventions. Aortocoronary bypass grafts should be imaged in at least two projections with special focus on the aortic ostium, the entire course, the distal anastomosis, and the supplied native vessel (see Projections of invasive coronary arteriography, below). For percutaneous interventions within the body of saphenous vein grafts, the extension of a landing zone for distal embolic protection devices (e.g., filters) has to be documented.

Internal mammary artery grafts

Engagement of the left internal mammary artery (LIMA) is achieved via the left subclavian artery. To cannulate the left subclavian artery, the mammary artery catheter is first advanced on the guidewire into the aortic arch. Subsequently, the guidewire is removed and the mammary artery catheter is pulled back under counterclockwise rotation, directing the catheter tip to the outer curve of the aortic arch. Several maneuvers of clockwise and counterclockwise rotation of the catheter tip may be required to engage the ostium of the left subclavian artery. The guidewire is carefully advanced to avoid cannulation of the left carotid artery. Guidewire and mammary artery catheter are positioned in the left subclavian artery with the guidewire and mammary artery catheter tip distal to the suspected origin of the LIMA. After removal of the guidewire, the catheter is slowly pulled back with slight counterclockwise rotation until it enters the LIMA ostium (Fig. 28.3c). Similarly, the right internal mammary artery is cannulated via the right subclavian artery. Mammary artery guiding catheters normally provide sufficient backup for PCI via both internal mammary arteries. To improve insufficient backup for such procedures, a brachial approach may be selected. As with aortocoronary bypass grafts, the angiographic recording should include imaging of the ostium, the entire course, the distal anastomoses, as well as the supplied native vessel (see Projections of invasive coronary arteriography, below).

Gastroepiploic artery

The right gastroepiploic artery was transiently used as an alternative *in situ* arterial graft to the posterior descending coronary artery (PDA) in patients undergoing coronary artery bypass surgery. The right gastroepiploic artery arises from the gastroduodenal artery, which originates from the common hepatic artery in 75% of cases (it may also arise from the celiac trunk or from the left or right hepatic artery). Cannulation of the right gastroepiploic artery is performed using a Cobra catheter engaging the common hepatic artery first. A coronary guidewire with hydrophilic coating is advanced to the gastroduodenal artery and then to the gastroepiploic artery. The Cobra catheter is then exchanged for a multipurpose or Judkins right coronary catheter to selectively cannulate the right gastroepiploic artery [36].

Projections of invasive coronary arteriography

Although the original description of angiographic projections is oriented to the direction of the X-ray beam from the X-ray source located below the patient toward the image intensifier located above the patient, it has become generally accepted among cardiologists to name the individual angiographic projection according to the position of the image intensifier [37]; The picture obtained is that which the viewer would have if he or she were in the same position as the image intensifier. In a right anterior oblique (RAO) view, the viewer looks at the right anterior side of the chest, and in a left anterior oblique cranial (LAO CRAN) view the coronary tree is visualized as if the viewer were looking over the left shoulder of the patient. The cranial RAO view allows one to look at the coronary arteries from a position over the right shoulder, and the caudal RAO (RAO CAUD) and caudal LAO (LAO CAUD) allow views from the liver and spleen, respectively. The degree of rotation in the transverse plain is measured from the midline (i.e., a left lateral projection is a 90° LAO) and angulation in the sagittal plane from the vertical.

Baseline angiographic projections

Invasive coronary arteriography should primarily be based on a series of baseline views aiming at optimal visualization of the various portions of the coronary artery segments in a sequence that is oriented to minimize the potential risk of the investigation while detecting the location of potential coronary artery lesions.

It is recommended that the first injection is made into the left coronary artery in a shallow RAO projection to allow visualization of any major left main disease immediately (RAO 10°). In addition, the projection gives an overview over the left coronary artery system (Fig. 28.4a). If there is no major left main disease, the second injection should be made in the left lateral projection (LAO 90°), which depicts the unforeshortened course of the LAD (Fig. 28.4b). The third injection should use the LAO cranial view (LAO 50°, CRAN 20°), which shows the take-off of the diagonal branches and also the proximal portion of the left circumflex system (Fig. 28.4c). If there is no major disease visible so far, the last injection into the left coronary artery should be made in a RAO caudal view (RAO 20°, CAUD 20°), depicting the LCx largely unforeshortened (Fig. 28.4d).

The angiographic examination of the RCA should start with an LAO projection (LAO 60°) to detect RCA-ostial disease during the first injection (Fig. 28.4e). In case of a right dominant or codominant coronary system, the second injection should be made in an LAO cranial view (LAO 40°, CRAN 30°), to visualize the RCA bifurcation and the course of PDA as well as the right posterolateral branches (RPLB) (Fig. 28.4f). The investigation of the RCA should be completed with an RAO 30° view (Fig. 28.4g). The above-mentioned routine projections are listed in Table 28.3. These projections are modified according

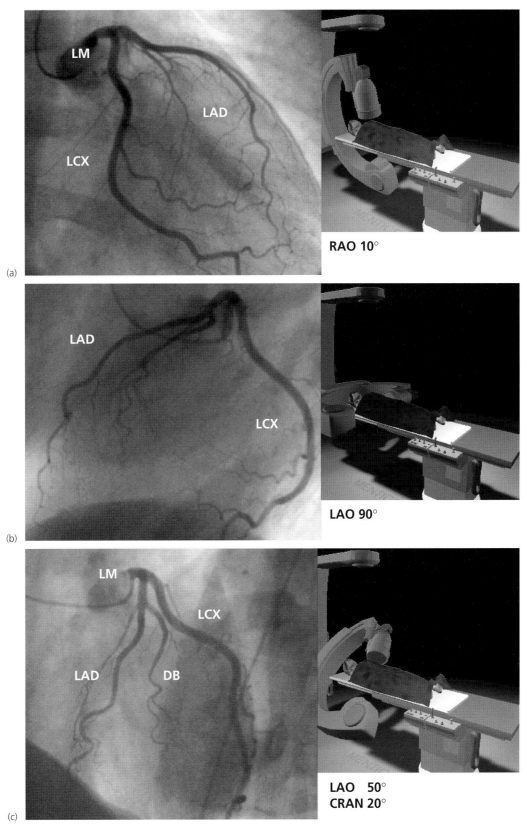

Figure 28.4 Projections of coronary arteriography. (a) Left coronary artery in RAO 10°. This view displays the left main trunk without foreshortening. (b) Left coronary artery in LAO 90°. In this view the entire course of the LAD is visualized without foreshortening. (c) Left coronary artery in LAO 50° with 20° cranial angulation. This view allows to differentiate between diagonal and septal branches; however LAD as well as its side branches are visualized foreshortened.

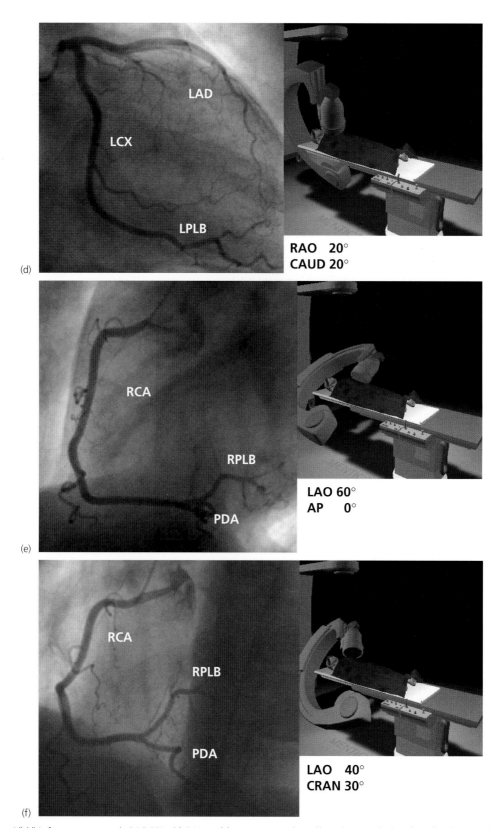

Figure 28.4 (cont'd) (d) Left coronary artery in RAO 20° with 20° caudal angulation. This view displays the entire course of the LCx in a largely unforeshortened way. (e) Right coronary artery in LAO 60°. This view shows the entire course of the proximal segment of the RCA, however PDA and posterolateral branches are displayed in a foreshortened and frequently overlapped fashion. (f) Right coronary artery in LAO 40° with 30° cranial angulation. This view displays the bifurcation of the RCA at the crux cordis and allows a clear differentiation between PDA and RPLB.

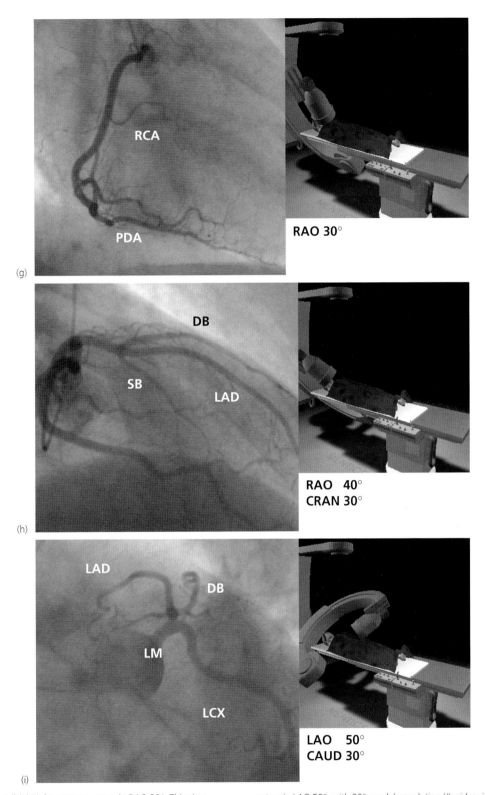

Figure 28.4 *(cont'd)* (g) Right coronary artery in RAO 30°. This view displays the entire course of the PDA without foreshortening. (h) Left coronary artery in RAO 40° with 30° cranial angulation. This view displays the proximal and mid segment of the LAD as well as the take off of diagonal and septal branches. In contrast to the LAO cranial projection, LAD as well as diagonal branches are visualized without foreshortening. (i) Left coronary artery in LAO 50°, with 30° caudal angulation ("spider view"). This view displays the bifurcation of the left main trunk as well as the origin of LAD and LCx. (DB, diagonal branch; LAD, left anterior descending coronary artery; LCx, left circumflex coronary artery; LM, left main trunk; LPLB, left posterolateral branch; PDA, posterior descending coronary artery; RCA, right coronary artery; RPLB, right posterolateral branch; SB, septal branch).

Table 28.3 Baseline angiographic projections.

Left coronary artery
RAO 10°
LAO 90°
LAO 50°, CRAN 20°
RAO 20°, CAUD 20°

Right coronary artery
LAO 60°
LAO 40°, CRAN 30°
RAO 30°

CRAN, cranial angulation; CAUD, caudal angulation; LAO, left anterior oblique projection; RAO, right anterior oblique projection.

to the individual anatomy and the clinical condition of the patient. If the patient cannot tolerate a full coronary angiogram, the selection of views has to be tailored to focus on the individual problem and reduce the load of contrast medium.

Special angiographic projections

If in any of the primary projections a coronary artery lesion has been detected, the angiographic schedule should be further modified in optimally visualize the region of interest. The corresponding coronary artery segment should be imaged in at least two possibly orthogonal projections, with one of them showing the lesion without foreshortening (projection perpendicular to the course of the segment) or overlap and with at least one other projection showing the maximal degree of lumen reduction.

Left main coronary artery

Angiographic visualization of the left main coronary artery is critical and sometimes problematic. If left main disease is visible with the primary shallow RAO view, an additional shallow LAO view projecting the left main on the spine frequently provides important information. If the left main stenosis is located at the site of the bifurcation, a "spider view" (or "spleen shot") is required (LAO 50°, CAUD 30°; Fig. 28.4i). This projection is also indispensable in the case of ostial disease of the LAD, the LCx, or an intermediate branch. Additional views to visualize left main disease are an LAO cranial projection (LAO 45°, CRAN 30°) and an RAO caudal view (RAO 20°, CAUD 20°). In the case of eccentric distal left main stenosis, a frontal view with cranial angulation (e.g., 30°) may be useful. If a high-grade left main stenosis is detected, the total number of injections should be limited to a minimum (two or three) and intracoronary injection of aspirin (500 mg) is recommended.

Left anterior descending coronary artery

Ostial disease of the LAD is visualized in the spider view (LAO 50°, CAUD 30°), an RAO caudal projection (RAO 30°,

CAUD 30°), or an RAO cranial view (RAO 40°, CRAN 30°). The RAO cranial projection is also important for the differentiation between diagonal and septal branches and serves best during PCI of bifurcation lesions (Fig. 28.4h). Additional projections for the estimation of LAD bifurcation lesions are the cranial LAO view (LAO 50°, CRAN 20°) as well as a frontal view with 30° cranial angulation. In rare cases, an additional RAO caudal view is required to fully visualize an LAD bifurcation lesion.

Left circumflex coronary artery

Angiographic visualization of the LCx should be based on at least one RAO caudal view (e.g., RAO 20°, CAUD 20°) and one LAO view (e.g., LAO 60°). For estimation of the ostium of the LCx, an additional "spider view" (LAO 50°, CAUD 30°) is normally helpful. If the left circumflex system is dominant, visualization of peripheral stenoses may require an LAO cranial projection (LAO 40°, CRAN 30°) in conjunction with an RAO caudal view (RAO 30°, CAUD 30°).

Right coronary artery

Visualization of the take-off of the RCA as well as the ostium of the PDA may be difficult. When the take-off from the aorta is quite anterior, a steep LAO or RAO cranial view may be useful. If portions of the proximal or mid segments of the vessel are insufficiently visualized in the above-mentioned standard views, a lateral projection (LAO 90°) may be helpful. The ostium of the PDA may also be visualized in an RAO cranial view (RAO 30°, CRAN 30°).

Quantitative coronary angiography

Although visual assessment of the severity of coronary artery stenoses represents the standard procedure in most institutions, high interobserver and intraobserver variability has been well documented [38]. These observations gave rise to the development and validation of computer-based systems for objective quantitative analysis of geometric parameters at the site of coronary artery lesions [26,39,40]. QCA became the reference technique for evaluation of angiographic multicenter studies on the efficacy of new interventional devices and restenosis [32–35]. Contour detection algorithms of QCA systems are based on weighted first- and second-derivative functions on the brightness profile of scan lines perpendicular to a previously defined center line within the coronary contrast image. The contrast-filled tip of the guiding catheter is used for calibration of the measurement systems providing a calibration factor (mm/pixel). The detected contour points are connected to contour lines delineating the luminal vessel borders within a two-dimensional angiographic image. From these contour lines, reference diameters in the proximal or distal portion of the "normal" vessel as well as the minimal luminal diameter at the site of the lesion are calculated. The two-dimensional QCA approach has recently been transformed to a three-dimensional system to improve the estimation

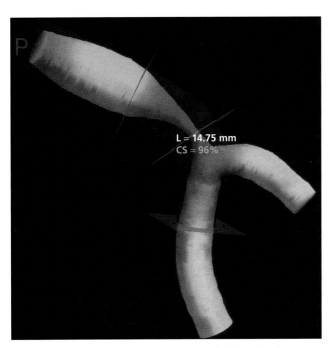

Figure 28.5 Three-dimensional reconstruction of a bifurcational coronary lesion based on QCA (courtesy of Siemens Medical Solutions, Forchheim, Germany).

Table 28.4 Angiographic lesion classification.

Type A lesion criteria (high success, low risk)
Short (<10 cm)
Concentric
Readily accessible
Nonangulated segment (<45°)
Smooth contour
Little or no calcium
Less than totally occlusive
Not ostial in location
No major side branch involvement
No thrombus

Type B lesion criteria (moderate success, moderate risk)
Tubular (10–20 mm length)
Eccentric
Moderate tortuosity of proximal segment
Moderately angulated (45°–90°)
Irregular contour

Type C lesion criteria (low success, high risk)
Diffuse (>20 mm length)
Excessive tortuosity of proximal segment
Extremely angulated (>90°)
Chronic total occlusion (>3 months old)
Involvement of major side branch
Degenerated vein graft (friable lesion)

Adapted from reference 41.

of complex coronary lesions such as bifurcational stenoses (Fig. 28.5).

Angiographic lesion characteristics

Angiographic features of atherosclerotic coronary lesions have been identified to determine the complexity as well as the risk of PCI. The primary definition of lesion characteristics published by an American College of Cardiology and American Heart Association (ACC/AHA) task force suggested that a number of different lesion criteria would predict procedural success and complication rates (Table 28.4) [41]. Despite refinement of interventional procedures, including the introduction of IIb/IIIa inhibitors, distal protection devices and drug-eluting stents, basic criteria of lesion complexity have remained important predictors of the long-term outcome. These criteria include lesion length, ostial location, bifurcation lesions, lesion angulation, lesion calcification, thrombotic lesions, and degenerated saphenous vein graft lesions.

Peri-interventional coronary arteriography

Luminographic assessment of coronary artery lesions in at least two projections is the prerequisite of any PCI. This angiographic procedure is performed with the same guiding catheter that is used for insertion of guidewires as well as interventional devices. The choice of the guiding catheter is crucial for the success of the PCI because its backup in conjunction with the mechanical properties of the corresponding guidewire provides secure access to the site of the intervention.

Before angiographic recording of the arterial segment of interest, intracoronary nitroglycerine should be administered to achieve maximal vasodilation. The still images of two possibly orthogonal angiographic views of the vessel segment of interest serve as road maps for the subsequent intervention. They should display both an angiographic image of the vessel segment without foreshortening or overlap with other structures and an angiographic image of the maximal degree of the lumen narrowing (documentation of lesion eccentricity). The two road map images should be taken with the patient not breath-holding so that they can easily be compared with angiographic injections during the procedure. On-line QCA can be used to exactly determine reference diameter and minimal luminal diameter of the stenosis. Such measurements alleviate the correct sizing of balloons, atherectomy devices, distal embolic protection systems as well as stents. Angiographic landmarks (side branches) may also help to guide the positioning of interventional devices.

Peri-interventional angiographic injections allow the visualization of intracoronary thrombi (filling defects) and dissections, thereby guiding the operator's decision as to whether thrombectomy might become necessary or an additional stent should be implanted. The velocity of contrast run-off indicates whether coronary artery perfusion is normal or whether additional measures are required to overcome peri-interventional flow disturbances. Rare complications of PCI, such as coronary artery perforations, are also visualized by peri-interventional angiographic injections. Adequate angiographic imaging allows the assessment of the location and severity of the perforation guiding the operator's decision regarding a pharmacologic and/or mechanical treatment approach (administration of protamine sulfate, long balloon inflation, or implantation of a polytetrafluoroethylene membrane-covered stent graft for sealing of the perforation).

At the end of the procedure, the result of PCI is angiographically documented using the same two projections that served as a road map during the intervention. The final angiographic images should be recorded after complete removal of the guidewire and following another dose of intracoronary nitroglycerine.

Summary

Invasive coronary arteriography represents the reference technique for the assessment of coronary artery disease. It allows a detailed visualization of coronary artery lumen and contours, and thus providing essential information as required for any revascularization procedure. Invasive coronary arteriography is indispensable for the planning and preparation of percutaneous coronary interventions as well as the peri-interventional evaluation of procedural progress and outcome. In conjunction with quantitative coronary angiography exact and reproducible assessment of luminal dimensions is provided.

Acknowledgment

The technical support for preparation of illustrations from Medtronic Europe (Tolochenaz, Switzerland) is gratefully acknowledged.

References

1. Forsmann W (1929) The catheterization of the right side of the heart. *Klin Wochenschr* **8**:2085.
2. Klein O (1939) Determining human cardiac output (minute volume) using Fick's principle (extraction of mixed venous blood by cardiac catheterization). *Med Wochenschr* **77**:1311.
3. Cournand A (1975) Cardiac catheterization: development of the technique, its contributions to experimental medicine, and its initial applications in man. *Acta Med Scand* (Suppl.) **7**:579.
4. Cournand A & Ranges HA (1941) Catheterization of the right auricle in man. *Proc Soc Exp Biol Med* **46**:462.
5. Cournand A, Lauson HD, Bloomfield RA, Breed ES, & Baldwin E de F (1944) Recording of right heart pressures in man. *Proc Soc Exp Biol Med* **55**:34.
6. Warren JV & Stead EA (1944) Fluid dynamics in chronic congestive heart failure: an interpretation of the mechanisms producing edema, increased plasma volume and elevated venous pressure in certain patients with prolonged congestive failure. *Arch Intern Med* **73**:138.
7. Zimmerman HA, Scott RW, & Becker NO (1950) Catherization of the left side of the heart in man. *Circulation* **1**:357.
8. Moniz E, DeCarvalho L, & Lima A (1931) Angiopneumographie. *Presse Med* **39**:996.
9. Reboul H & Racine M (1933) La ventriculographie cardiaque expérimentale. *Presse Med* **1**:763.
10. Radner S (1945) An attempt at the roentgenologic visualization of the coronary blood vessels in man. *Acta Radiol* **26**:497.
11. DiGuglielmo L & Guttaduro M (1952) Roetgenologic study of coronary arteries in living. *Acta Radiol (Suppl.)(Stockh)* 97.
12. DiGugliemo L & Guttaduro M (1954) Visualization of arteries in living: review of 413 observations. *Radiol Med* **40**:945.
13. Dotter CT & Frische LH (1958) Visualization of the coronary circulation by occlusion aortography: a practical method. *Radiology* **76**:502.
14. Arnulf G & Chacornac R (1958) Communication to La Société de Chirurgie de Lyon, November 14, 1957, in Arnulf G: L'arteriographie méthodique des artères coronairies grâce à l'utilisation de l'acetylcholine: données expérimentales et cliniques. *Bull Acad Natl Med (Paris)* **661**:25–26.
15. Richards LS & Thal AP (1958) Phasic dye injection control system for coronary arteriography in the human. *Surg Gynecol Obstet* **107**:739.
16. Bellman S, Frank HA, Lambert PB, Littman D, & Williams JA (1960) Differential opacification of the aortic stream catheters of special design–experimental development. *N Engl J Med* **262**:325.
17. Nordenstrom B (1960) Contrast examination of the cardiovascular system during increased intrabronchial pressure *Acta Radiol (Stockh)* (Suppl.) **200**:110.
18. Bilgutay AM, Gannon P, Sterns LP, Ferlic R, & Lillehei CW (1964) Coronary arteriography: New method under induced hypotension by pacing–experimental and clinical application. *Arch Surg* **89**:899.
19. Sones FM Jr (1959) *Coronary Arteriography*. Read before the Eighth Annual Convention of the American College of Cardiology, Philadelphia.
20. Sones FM Jr (1959) Cine coronary arteriography. In Abstracts of the 32nd Scientific Session of the American Heart Association. *Circulation* **20**:773.
21. Ricketts HJ & Abrams HL (1962) Percutaneous selective coronary cine arteriography. *JAMA* **181**:620.
22. Favaloro RG (1969) Saphenous vein graft in the surgical treatment of coronary artery disease. *J Thorac Cardiovasc Surg* **58**:178.
23. Johnson WD, Flemma RJ, Lepley T Jr, *et al.* (1969) Extended treatment of severe coronary artery disease: a total surgical approach. *Ann Surg* **170**:460.
24. Grüntzig AR, Senning A, & Siegenthaler WE (1979) Nonoperative dilatation of coronary artery stenosis: percutaneous transluminal coronary angioplasty. *N Engl J Med* **301**:61.
25. Ellis S, Vandormael M, Cowley M, *et al.* (1990) Coronary morphologic and clinical determinants of procedural outcome with angioplasty for multivessel coronary artery disease. Implications for patient selection. *Circulation* **82**:1193.

26. Serruys PW, Booman F, Troost J, *et al.* (1982) Computerized quantitative coronary angiography applied to percutaneous transluminal coronary angioplasty: advantages and limitations. In: Kaltenbach M, Grüntzig A, Rentrop K, & Bussmann WD (eds). Transluminal Coronary Angioplasty and Intracoronary Thrombolysis—Heart Disease IV. Berlin: Springer, p. 110.

27. Scanlon P, Faxon D, Audet A, *et al.* (1999) ACC/AHA guidelines for coronary angiography. *J Am Coll Cardiol* **33**:1756–1824.

28. Braunwald E, Antman E, Beasley J, *et al.* (2002) ACC/AHA guideline update for the management of patients with unstable angina and non-ST segment elevation myocardial infarction—summary article: a report of the American College of Cardiology/American Heart Association task force on practice guidelines (Committee on the Management of Patients with Unstable Angina). *J Am Coll Cardiol* **40**:1366–1374.

29. Ropers D, Baum U, Pohle U, *et al.* (2003) Detection of coronary artery stenoses with thin-slice multi-detector row spiral computed tomography and multiplanar reconstruction. *Circulation* **107**:664–666.

30. Leber AW, Knez A, von Ziegler F, *et al.* (2005) Quantification of obstructive and nonobstructive coronary lesions by 64-slice computed tomography: a comparative study with quantitative coronary angiography and intravascular ultrasound. *J Am Coll Cardiol* **46**:147–154.

31. Hamon M, Biondi-Zoccai GG, Malagutti P, Agostoni P, Morello R, & Valgimigli M (2006) Diagnostic performance of multislice spiral computed tomography of coronary arteries as compared with conventional invasive coronary angiography: a meta-analysis. *J Am Coll Cardiol* **48**:1896–1910.

32. Morice MC, Serruys PW, Sousa JE, *et al.,* for the RAVEL study group (2002) A randomized comparison of a sirolimus-eluting stent with a standard stent for coronary revascularization. *N Engl J Med* **346**:1773–1780.

33. Waksman R, Ajani AE, White RL, *et al.* (2002) Intravascular gamma radiation for in-stent restenosis in saphenous vein bypass grafts. *N Engl J Med* **346**:1194–1199.

34. Moses JW, Leon MB, Popma JJ, *et al.,* for the SIRIUS investigators (2003) Sirolimus eluting stents versus standard stents for treatment of patients with stenosis in a native coronary artery. *N Engl J Med* **349**:1315–1323.

35. Stone GW, Ellis SG, Cox DA, *et al.,* for the TAXUS-IV investigators (2004) A polymer-based paclitaxel-eluting stent in patients with coronary disease. *N Engl J Med* **350**:221–223.

36. Popma JJ (2008) Coronary arteriography and intravascular Imaging. In: Libby P, Bonow RO, Mann DL, Zipes DP, & Braunwald E (eds) *Braunwald's Heart Disease: A Textbook of Cardiovascular Medicine,* 8th edn. Philadelphia: Saunders Elsevier, pp. 465–508.

37. Douglas JS & King SB III (1985) New radiographic views for imaging the coronary anatomy. In: King SB III & Douglas JS (eds). Coronary arteriography and angioplasty. New York: McGraw-Hill, pp. 275–287.

38. DeRouen TA, Murray JA, & Owen W (1977) Variability in the analysis of coronary arteriograms. *Circulation* **55**:324.

39. Reiber JHC, van der Zwet PMJ, Koning G, *et al.* (1991) Quantitative coronary measurements from cine and digital arteriograms; methodology and validation results. 4th International Symposium on Coronary Arteriography, Rotterdam, June 23–25. Rotterdam: Erasmus University Press, p. 36.

40. Haase J, Di Mario C, Slager CJ, *et al.* (1992) In vivo validation of on-line and off-line geometric coronary measurements using insertion of stenosis phantoms in porcine coronary arteries. *Cathet Cardiovasc Diagn* **27**:16.

41. Adapted from Ryan TJ, Bauman WB, Kennedy JW, *et al.* (1993) Guidelines for percutaneous coronary angioplasty. A report of the AHA/ACC Task Force on Assessment of Diagnostic and Therapeutic Cardiovascular Procedures (Subcommittee on Percutaneous Transluminal Coronary Angioplasty). *Circulation* **88**:2987.

29 Stress Echocardiography for Functional Assessment of Coronary Artery Disease

Uwe Nixdorff

European Prevention Center, Duisburg, Germany

Introduction of methodology

In principle, stress echocardiography offers pre- and post-interventional diagnostic information influencing decision-making. Therefore, it is complementary to the invasive diagnostic findings. The diagnostic advantages of stress echocardiography within the decision process of coronary artery disease (CAD) are:

- cost-effectiveness,
- noninvasive approach and lack of radiation exposure,
- availability and applicability of technique,
- low complication rate,
- time-effective examination,
- very high positive and negative predictive accuracy.

Sensitivity and specificity for detecting hemodynamically relevant CAD, defined as a reduction in the lumen of the coronary vessel of >50%, are established to be approximately 88% and 83%, respectively [1]. Sensitivity is highest for stenoses of the left anterior descending artery (LAD), followed by the right coronary artery (RCA), and is least for stenoses of the circumflex artery (Cx) [1]. In comparison with other imaging modalities, the specificity of stress echocardiography is relatively high [2]; in particular, the negative predictive value is extremely high, i.e., a negative test means that a coronary event is extremely unlikely. The expected event rate among patients with a normal dynamic stress echocardiogram is <1%/year [3]. Those patients do not require further diagnostic approaches including invasive coronary arteriography.

For patients who are capable of performing an exercise test, exercise rather than pharmacologic stress is recommended, as exercise capacity is an important predictor of outcome (Fig. 29.1) [1]. In patients who cannot exercise, dobutamine (DSE) and vasodilator stress (dipyridamole, adenosine) are alternatives. Although vasodilators may have advantages for assessment of myocardial perfusion, dobutamine is preferred when the test is based on assessment of regional wall motion (RWM). A graded dobutamine infusion starting at 5 μg/kg/min and increasing at 3-min intervals to 10, 20, 30, and 40 μg/kg/min is the standard for DSE (Fig. 29.2). The inclusion of low-dose stages facilitates recognition of viability and ischemia in segments with abnormal function at rest. Additional atropine, in divided doses of 0.25–0.5 mg to a total of 2.0 mg, should be used as needed to achieve target heart rate.

Imaging interpretation consists of visual assessment of endocardial excursion as well as myocardial thickening on a segment-based model. The 16- [4] or the 17-segment model of the left ventricle may be used (Fig. 29.3) [5]. The 17-segment model includes an "apical cap", a segment beyond the level at which the left ventricular cavity is seen. The 17-segment model is recommended if myocardial perfusion is evaluated or if echocardiography is compared with another imaging modality, such as cardiac magnetic resonance imaging (CMR) or multidetector computed tomography (MDCT). Function in each segment is graded at rest and with stress as normal or hyperdynamic, hypokinetic, akinetic, dyskinetic, or aneurysmal. Images from low or intermediate stages should be compared with peak stress images to maximize the sensitivity for detection of CAD (Fig. 29.2) [1]. The timing of wall motion abnormality (WMA) should also be assessed. Ischemia delays the onset of both contraction and relaxation and slows the velocity of contraction in addition to decreasing the maximum amplitude of contraction. Hypokinesis can refer to delay in the velocity or onset of contraction (tardo-kinesis) and reduction in the maximum amplitude of contraction. In principle, the consideration of timing of contraction (asynchrony, postsystolic thickening) enhances diagnostic accuracy. In addition to the evaluation of segmental function, the global left ventricular response to stress should be assessed (changes in left ventricle shape, cavity size [especially end-systolic volume], and global contractility).

Qualification of examiners

A crucial issue is qualification of examiners because diagnostic accuracy depends on it. Interpretation of stress echocardiograms requires extensive experience in echocardiography and should

Cardiovascular Interventions in Clinical Practice. Edited by Jürgen Haase, Hans-Joachim Schäfers, Horst Sievert and Ron Waksman. © 2010 Blackwell Publishing.

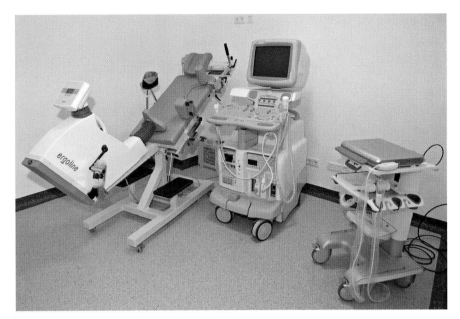

Figure 29.1 Instrumental setting of a stress echocardiographic laboratory. A special ergometer that enables the patient to remain stable in the supine position while tilting the couch in an anteroposterior as well as left-sided direction is typically used for the dynamic or exercise approach (left). Such an ergometer configuration guarantees optimal echogenicity. For the echo platform, a high-end machine is preferred (middle) but a hand-held, portable machine may also be appropriate (right) providing stress echo software (enabling an ECG triggered and synchronized quad screen).

be performed only by physicians with specific training in the technique. To achieve the minimum level of competence for independent interpretation, training should include interpretation of at least 100 stress echocardiograms under the supervision of an expert [1,6]. To maintain competence, it is recommended that examiners interpret a minimum of 100 stress echocardiograms per year [1].

Extent of myocardial ischemia

The Task Force Summary of the European Guidelines for Percutaneous Coronary Interventions (PCI) is introduced as follows: "In patients with stable CAD, PCI can be considered a valuable initial mode of revascularization in all patients *with objective large ischemia* in the presence of almost every lesion subset" (class of recommendation and level of evidence IA) [7]. In particular, a substudy of the Clinical Outcomes Utilizing Revascularization and Aggressive Drug Evaluation (COURAGE) trial [8], the Swiss Interventional Study on Silent Ischemia Type II (SWISS-II) study [9], as well as the Angioplasty Compared to Medicine (ACME) study [10] demonstrated the requirement of measuring the extent of myocardial ischemia. Only if the extent is significant and a clear therapeutic reduction in ischemia is achieved a clinical and prognostic benefit of interventional procedures can be expected. A very thorough study in 10 627 patients with a follow-up of 1.9 ± 0.6 years confirmed this by differentiating several groups with ischemia of various extents [11]. This study concluded that revascularization compared with medical therapy had greater survival benefit (absolute and relative) in patients with moderate to large amounts of inducible ischemia (>10%

myocardial ischemic area) (Fig. 29.4). The following key findings in stress echocardiography indicate a poorer prognosis and provide valuable information in the decision process for pre-interventional diagnosis [1]:

- high wall motion score index at prestress (more than five segments);
- reduced or lack of increase in left ventricular systolic function;
- absence of a reduction or even an increase in end-systolic volume;
- ischemia in several supplying areas;
- low stress at induction of ischemia;
- detection of ischemia at left ventricular hypertrophy;
- ischemic territories within the supplying area of the left main stem or LAD.

As well as enabling interpretation of the extent of ischemic stress, echocardiography allows topographic correlation of myocardial areas and their supplying coronary arteries (for which exercise electrocardiography [ECG] is much less reliable). Thus, in multivessel CAD, this method may provide important information about which lesions require intervention and which do not.

Borderline coronary lesion

Qualitative or quantitative coronary angiography (QCA) provides anatomic data about coronary stenoses, but not necessarily information about the physiologic relevance of the lesions. Increasingly, data suggest that revascularization can safely be deferred if fractional flow reserve (FFR) is not substantially decreased [13]—usually considered to be FFR >0.75—or if

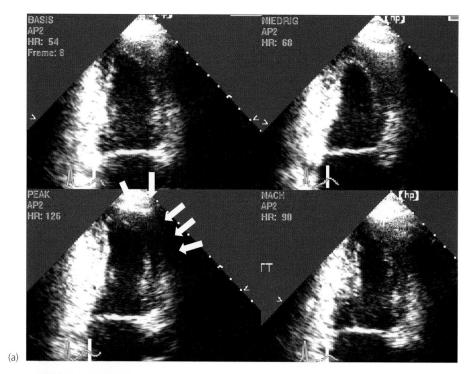

(a)

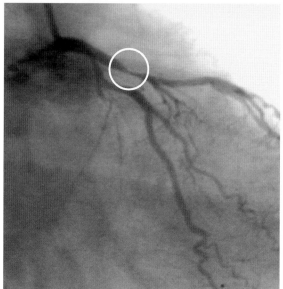

(b)

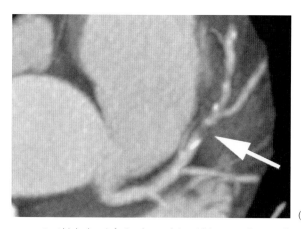

(c)

Figure 29.2 A 67-year-old female patient suffering from angina pectoris, nondiagnostic exercise ECG due to insufficient heart rate increase. (a) DSE documented by two-chamber view (ECG-triggered and ECG-synchronized end-systolic images by quad-screen display; titration steps: preinfusion, left upper corner; low-dose infusion, right upper corner; high-dose infusion, left lower corner; postinfusion, right lower corner). Induced hypo- to akinesia of anterolateral, apical, and inferoapical segments at high-dose infusion (arrows). In addition, note increased end-systolic volume in comparison with a low dose and post infusion. (b) Invasive coronary arteriography showing high-grade stenosis of LAD (circle). (c) Maximum intensity projection by EBCT coronary angiography demonstrating high-grade stenosis in the proximal LAD (arrow). Note also multiple calcified plaques within this vessel segment.

ischemia has been excluded by noninvasive imaging such as stress echocardiography [14] in patients with borderline stenosis. The so-called "oculostenotic reflex" can be avoided if such functional information is considered in the decision-making process.

Hibernating myocardium

Myocardial viability within the infarct zone is an important determinant of left ventricular function recovery after

LEFT VENTRICULAR SEGMENTATION

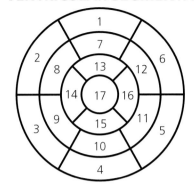

1 Basal anterior
2 Basal anteroseptal
3 Basal inferoseptal
4 Basal inferior
5 Basal inferolateral
6 Basal anterolateral
7 Mid anterior
8 Mid anteroseptal
9 Mid inferoseptal
10 Mid inferior
11 Mid inferolateral
12 Mid anterolateral
13 Apical anterior
14 Apical septal
15 Apical inferior
16 Apical lateral
17 Apex

(a)

CORONARY ARTERY TERRITORIES

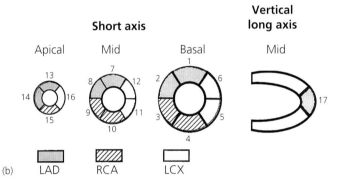

(b)

Figure 29.3 Standardized myocardial segmentation and nomenclature for tomographic imaging of the heart by the Cardiac Imaging Committee of the Council on Clinical Cardiology of the American Heart Association [5].

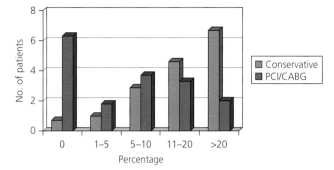

Figure 29.4 Revascularization-relevant myocardial ischemia. Note that at least 10% ischemic myocardium might be mandatory if, in principle, an interventional or surgical approach is expected to be of any prognostic utility. Note also that less than 10% ischemic myocardium might be detrimental as the interventional or surgical approach might increase mortality [11].

Table 29.1 Principal comparison of both pathophysiologic postmyocardial infarction situations of lacking contraction but maintained viability.

Criteria	Stunning	Hibernation
Concept	Experimental	Clinical evaluation
Function	↓	↓
Flow	=	↓
Reversibility	Spontaneous	After revascularization
Electron microscopy	Normal	Reduction of myofibrils
Mechanism	Oxygen radicals	Undefined, downregulation

interventional coronary revascularization. Echocardiographic techniques are extremely valuable in identifying hibernation, especially in conjunction with dobutamine titration. Low doses may detect the inotropic reserve by significant enhancement of segmental WMA, but high doses may surpass the ischemic threshold and wall motion deteriorate (biphasic response). According to the Stress Echocardiographic Appropriateness Criteria issued by the American Heart Association in conjunction with other related societies, stress echocardiography is officially recommended for the purpose of clinical decision-making in respect to revascularization therapies (appropriateness score 8 from a scoring system ranging from 1 to 9) [15]. It is well established that this applies in particular to DSE and to the subacute infarct period as well as specifically in chronic left ventricular dysfunction due to CAD. In contrast to just stunning the interventional challenging noncontracting but viable myocardium is the hibernating myocardium, first described

by Rahmitoola [16]. It is defined as a viable chronically underperfused myocardium with distorted metabolism and function that is potentially reversible on restoration of an adequate blood flow; this may imply the need for interventional or surgical coronary revascularization [17]. For clinical decision-making with respect to interventional therapy, there is high diagnostic demand that should not focus only on viability but more specifically on hibernation. The still ongoing pathophysiologic discussion about the definitions of stunning and hibernation [18] should not affect the clinical respose (Table 29.1). If hibernation can also be interpreted as repetitive stunning [18] this might be of minor clinical importance because the underlying reasons for repetitive stunning should be ischemia-provoking events (exercise, unstable plaque) which also would require revascularization. However, the main focus of the diagnostic approach remains the differentiation between stunning and hibernation as, in principle, only the latter necessitates revascularization therapy (Table 29.1). Initial work has already confirmed the highly valuable diagnostic information provided by DSE by predicting functional success of postinfarct PCI in 72% of cases; non- or monophasic response accounted for 13% and 15% of successful

Table 29.2 Prediction of functional recovery post revascularization by DSE in comparison with nuclear techniques [21].

Technique	Sensitivity (%)	Specificity (%)	No. of patients	Studies
DSE	84 (82–86)	81 (79–84)	448	16
$^{99}Tc^m$	83 (78–87)	69 (63–74)	207	10
Tl-201 stress redistribution	86 (83–89)	47 (43–51)	209	7
PET	88 (84–91)	73 (69–74)	327	12
Tl-201 rest-redistribution	90 (87–93)	54 (49–60)	145	8

PCI cases, respectively [19]. Indeed, recent data [20] have histologically defined the specific echocardiographic response of hibernation by transmural biopsies taken intraoperatively during bypass surgery after preoperative DSE ($r = -0.78$; $P < 0.05$).

None of the other established available techniques for identifying viable myocardial zones, including the nuclear approach, can really be considered unequivocally superior to DSE (Table 29.2) [21]. Sensitivity is similar for all the techniques, but the specificity is highest with DSE and lowest with thallium-201 studies. The superiority of DSE may largely depend on methodology as the detection of inotropic reserve is closer to the clinically most interesting end point of functional recovery. Positron emission tomography (PET) measures metabolism whereas the other nuclear modalities (thallium-201 single-photon emission computed tomography [SPECT], technetium-99 SEPCT) focus on cellular and mitochondrial membrane integrity. A fundamental study [22] compared DES, PET, and SPECT in patients with severe left ventricular dysfunction (ejection fraction [EF] 14.5% ± 5.2%) who underwent heart transplantation. The explanted hearts were studied histologically and viable myocardium was quantitated within the segments examined by the various techniques. The nuclear methods detected relatively more segments with only small and minor extended amounts of viability. This may have no clinical relevance as these segments will not recover, which explains the poorer specificities. Existing evidence supports the concept that functional recovery is dependent on a threshold level of viable contracting myocardium, whereas metabolic integrity and perfusion will be detected at a level below that which is necessary for functional recovery.

Indeed, the threshold of the myocardial area showing inotropic reserve is very important in that it can be used clinically to predict recovery of left ventricular function after successful revascularization. Bax *et al.* [23] demonstrated that improvement in contractility of at least four of the standardized 16 segments (echocardiographic 16-segment model according the American Society of Echocardiography (ASE) [4]) on catecholaminergic challenge is needed to predict recovery of left ventricular function. Notably, these authors have found similar findings for myocardial perfusion SPECT [24].

Viability can also be ruled by assessing wall thickness on the resting echocardiogram. Segments that are thinned

(≤0.5 or 0.6 cm) and bright (likely a result of advanced fibrosis) rarely recover [25].

Postinterventional control

Stress echocardiography can predict restenosis or graft occlusion, detect native unrevascularized CAD, and assess adequacy of revascularization [26], for which indications the sensitivity of exercise stress echocardiography ranges between 67% and 87% and specificity between 83% and 95% [26–28]. Positive stress echocardiography after PCI identifies patients at high risk for recurrence of angina. Ischemia detected by stress echocardiography is incrementally predictive of cardiac events [29]. In patients who have previously undergone coronary artery bypass graft (CABG), the addition of the exercise echocardiographic variables, abnormal left ventricular end-systolic volume response, and exercise EF to clinical information, resting echocardiography, and exercise ECG provides further information aiding the prediction of cardiac events.

For increased diagnostic implications of stress echocardiography within the workflow of PCI, serial assessments have been proposed. Such an approach enables documentation of ischemia just before the intervention, improved exercise tolerance immediately after the intervention, and, in addition, ischemia reactions in the further follow-up due to restenoses. In addition, such a serial assessment could help avoid misinterpretation of positive findings as being due to restenoses when they are, in fact, the result of further untreated lesions in multivessel disease.

New technical approaches

In spite of the well-established diagnostic accuracy of stress echocardiography [1,15] there has always been criticism on the grounds of its subjectivity and interobserver variability [30]. In principle, two aspects of solution for the problem were addressed by introducing quantitation of regional wall motion and the improvement of image quality. Today echocardiography is well able to compete with other imaging modalities [30]. The technical development of echo machines consisted in a significant increase in temporal resolution up to 70–150 Hz in the two-dimensional (2-D) and 20–40 Hz in the three-dimensional (3-D) approach, combined with improved endocardial and epicardial wall delineation by tissue harmonic imaging either with or without echo contrast material [31]. This reduces near-field artifacts, improves resolution, enhances myocardial signals, and is superior to fundamental imaging for endocardial visualization. The significant improvement in endocardial and epicardial visualization achieved with harmonic imaging has decreased interobserver variability and improved sensitivity of the method progressively over the last 10 years.

Tissue Doppler and strain/strain rate echocardiography

It is claimed that ischemia can be quantitated, and thus made an objective finding by the tissue Doppler echocardiographic technique, especially by strain and strain rate imaging or myocardial textural analysis by speckle imaging or 2-D strain resembling myocardial deformation [32]. Thus, adequate 2-D or, in the near future, 3-D image quality is mandatory for a consistent and reproducible measurement. The methods are prone to artifacts and are hampered by limited echogenicity, suggesting, in the case of parametric imaging by tissue Doppler echocardiography and its derived parameters—tissue velocity, strain and strain rate—considerable Doppler angle dependence. Textural analysis is much better at demonstrating involvement of the anterior wall than the inferior wall [32]. General clinical applicability awaits multicenter validations and further simplification of applicability within the echo machines.

Myocardial contrast echocardiography

Improved delineation of the endocardial borders, especially in cases of limited echogenicity, can be provided by left-sided echo contrast, which significantly improves sensitivity (usually not specificity) by reducing the number of uninterpretable segments as well as test-to-test and interobserver variability [30]. Contrast should be used when two or more segments are not well visualized. A further diagnostic by-product is myocardial perfusion analysis, whether by triggered technique or real-time techniques by low mechanical index, enabling simultaneous perfusion and contraction analysis. The flash techniques that use sequential single ultrasound waves with a high mechanical index, sufficient to destroy intramyocardial contrast echo bubbles, enables the qualitative or even quantitative analyses of refilling kinetics [33]. However, the diagnostic robustness of those techniques has been shown only in the setting of publishing competence centers and is not yet established in a broader basis.

Three-dimensional echocardiography

In principle and de facto, multidimensional registration of the left ventricle offers some advantages, especially in distorted left ventricular geometry, as in the postmyocardial infarction situation (remodeling, aneurysm). There is the possibility of generating multiple short axes similar to CMR by reformatting the 3-D data sets [34]. In this way, the accuracy of global and regional left ventricular volume and function analysis can be increased [34]. However, limitations may not be completely overcome because of the lower spatial and temporal resolution of the 3-D transducers in comparison with the 2-D ones as well as occasional rhythm artifacts. Further developments in future transducer generations will provide the basis for more widespread application of this modality.

References

1. Pellikka PA, Nagueh SF, Ehlendy AA, Kühl CA, & Sawada SG (2007) American Society of Echocardiography recommendations for performance, interpretation, and application of stress echocardiography. *J Am Soc Echocardiogr* **20**:1021–1041.
2. Nixdorff U, Küfner C, Achenbach S, *et al.* (2008) Head-to-head comparison of dobutamine stress echocardiography and cardiac computed tomography for the detection of significant coronary artery disease. *Cardiology* **110**:81–86.
3. Bangalore S, Yao MHA, Puthumana J, & Chaudhry FA (2006) Incremental prognostic value of stress echocardiography over clinical and stress electrocardiographic variables in patients with prior myocardial infarction: "Warranty time" of a normal stress echocardiogram. *Echocardiography* **23**:455–464.
4. Lang RM, Bierig M, Devereux RB, *et al.* (2005) Recommendations for chamber quantification: a report from the American Society of Echocardiography´s Guidelines and Standards Writing Group, developed in conjunction with the European Association of Echocardiography, a branch of the European Society of Cardiology. *J Am Soc Echocardiogr* **18**:1440–1463.
5. Cerqueira MD, Weissman NJ, Dilsizian V, *et al.* (2002) Standardized myocardial segmentation and nomenclature for tomographic imaging of the heart: a statement for healthcare professionals from the Cardiac Imaging Committee of the Council on Clinical Cardiology of the American Heart Association. *Circulation* **105**:539–542.
6. Nixdorff U, Buck T, Engberding R, *et al.* (2006) Position paper for qualification and certification of examiners in echocardiography. *Clin Res Cardiol* **1**(Suppl.):96–102.
7. Silber S, Albertsson P, & Avilés FF (2005) Guidelines for percutaneous coronary interventions. The Task Force for Percutaneous Coronary Interventions of the European Society of Cardiology. *Eur Heart J* **26**:804–847.
8. Shaw LJ, Berman DS, Maron DJ, *et al.* (2008) Optimal medical therapy with or without percutaneous coronary intervention to reduce ischemic burden: results from the Clinical Outcomes Utilizing Revascularization and Aggressive Drug Evaluation (COURAGE) trial nuclear substudy. *Circulation* **117**:1283–1291.
9. Erne P, Schönenberger AW, Burckhardt D, *et al.* (2007) Effects of percutaneous coronary interventions in silent ischemia after myocardial infarction: the SWISS II randomized controlled trial. *JAMA* **297**:1985–1991.
10. Folland ED, Hartigan PM, & Parisi AF (1997) Percutaneous transluminal coronary angioplasty versus medical therapy for stable angina pectoris: outcomes for patients with double-vessel versus single-vessel coronary artery disease in a Veterans Affairs

Cooperative randomized trial. Veterans Affairs ACME Investigators. *J Am Coll Cardiol* **29**:1505–1511.

11. Hachamovitch R, Hayes SW, Friedman JD, Cohen I, & Berman DS (2003) Comparison of the short-term survival benefit associated with revascularization compared with medical therapy in patients with no prior coronary artery disease undergoing stress myocardial perfusion single photon emission computed tomography. *Circulation* **107**:2900–2907.

12. Boden WE, O'Rourke RA, Teo KK, *et al.* for the COURAGE Trial Research Group (2007) Optimal medical therapy with or without PCI for stable coronary disease. *N Engl J Med* **356**:1503–1516.

13. Berger A, Botman K-J, MacCarthy PA, *et al.* (2005) Outcome after fractional flow reserve-guided percutaneous coronary intervention in patients with multivessel disease. *J Am Coll Cardiol* **46**:438–442.

14. Giesler T, Lamprecht S, Voigt J-U, *et al.* (2002) Long term follow up after deferral of revascularisation in patients with intermediate coronary stenosis and negative dobutamine stress echocardiography. *Heart* **88**:645–646.

15. Douglas PS, Khandheria B, Stainback RF, *et al.* (2008) ACCF/ASE/ACEP/AHA/ASNC/SCAI/SCCT/SCMR (2008) Appropriateness criteria for stress echocardiography. *Circulation* **117**:1478–1497.

16. Rahmitoola SH (1989) The hibernating myocardium. *Am Heart J* **117**:211–221.

17. Nixdorff U (2004) Stress echocardiography: basis and non-invasive assessment of myocardial viability. *J Intervent Cardiol* **17**:349–355.

18. Völler H, Nixdorff U, & Flachskampf FA (2000) Assessment of myocardial viability by dobutamine echocardiography: an overview. *Z Kardiol* **89**:921–931.

19. Afridi I, Kleiman NS, Raizner AE, *et al.* (1995) Dobutamine echocardiography in myocardial hibernation. Optimal dose and accuracy in predicting recovery of ventricular function after coronary angioplasty. *Circulation* **91**:663–670.

20. Hennessy T, Diamond P, Holligan B, *et al.* (1997) Assessment of inotropic reserve using dobutamine stress echocardiography and it's relation to myocardial histological changes in dysfunctional myocardial segments. *Eur Heart J* **18**(Suppl.):243–250.

21. Bax JJ, Wijns W, Cornel JH, *et al.* (1997) Accuracy of currently available techniques for prediction of functional recovery after revascularization in patients with left ventricular dysfunction due to chronic coronary artery disease: comparison of pooled data. *J Am Coll Cardiol* **30**:1451–1460.

22. Baumgartner H, Porenta G, Lau YK, *et al.* (1998) Assessment of myocardial viability by dobutamine echocardiography, positron emission tomography and thallium-201 SPECT: correlation with histopathology in explanted hearts. *J Am Coll Cardiol* **32**:1701–1708.

23. Bax JJ, Poldermans D, Ehlendy A, *et al.* (1999) Improvement of left ventricular ejection fraction, heart function symptoms and prognosis after revascularization in patients with chronic coronary artery disease and viable myocardium detected by dobutamine stress echocardiography. *J Am Coll Cardiol* **34**:163–169.

24. Bax JJ, Visser FC, Poldermans D, *et al.* (2001) Relationship between preoperative viability and postoperative improvement in LVEF and heart failure symptoms. *J Nucl Med* **42**:79–86.

25. Biagini E, Galema T, Schinkel A, Vletter W, Roelandt J, & Ten Cate F (2004) Myocardial wall thickness predicts recovery of contractile function after primary coronary intervention for acute myocardial function. *J Am Coll Cardiol* **43**:1489–1493.

26. Mertes H, Erbel R, Nixdorff U, Mohr-Kahaly S, Krüger S, & Meyer J (1993) Exercise echocardiography for the evaluation of patients after nonsurgical coronary artery revascularization. *J Am Coll Cardiol* **21**:1087–1093.

27. Aboul-Enein H, Bengtson JR, Adams DB, *et al.* (1991) Effect of the degree of effort on exercise echocardiography for the detection of restenosis after coronary artery angioplasty. *Am Heart J* **122**:430–436.

28. Hecht HS, DeBord L, Shaw R, *et al.* (1993) Supine bicycle stress echocardiography versus tomographic thallium-201 exercise imaging for the detection of coronary artery disease. *J Am Soc Echo* **6**:177–185.

29. Bountioukos M, Ehlendy A, van Domburg R, *et al.* (2004) Prognostic value of dobutamine stress echocardiography in patients with previous coronary revascularization. *Heart* **90**:1031–1035.

30. Hoffmann R, von Bardeleben S, Kasprzak JD, *et al.* (2006) Analysis of regional left ventricular function by cineventriculography, cardiac magnetic resonance imaging, and unenhanced and contrast-enhanced echocardiography: a multicenter comparison of methods. *J Am Coll Cardiol* **47**:121–128.

31. Nixdorff U, Matschke C, Winkelmaier M, *et al.* (2001) Native tissue second harmonic imaging improves endocardial and epicardial border definition in dobutamine stress echocardiography. *Eur J Echocardiogr* **2**:52–61.

32. Hanekom L, Cho GY, Leano R, Jeffriess L, & Marwick TH (2007) Comparison of two-dimensional speckle and tissue Doppler strain measurement during dobutamine stress echocardiography: an angiographic correlation. *Eur Heart J* **28**:1765–1772.

33. Moir S, Haluska B, Jenkins C, Fathi R, & Marwick T (2004) Incremental benefit of myocardial contrast to combine dipyridamole-exercise stress echocardiography for the assessment of coronary artery disease. *Circulation* **110**:1108–1113.

34. Kühl H, Schreckenberger M, Rulands D, *et al.* (2004) High-resolution transthoracic real-time three-dimensional echocardiography: quantitation of cardiac volumes and function using semi-automatic border detection and comparison with cardiac magnetic resonance imaging. *J Am Coll Cardiol* **43**:2083–2090.

30   MRI for Functional Assessment of Coronary Artery Disease

Juerg Schwitter

Center of the University Hospital Lausanne, Lausanne, Switzerland

Introduction

In the field of coronary artery disease (CAD) treatment options have improved considerably during the past years, ranging from systematic management of risk factors to efficient strategies of revascularizations mainly employing drug-eluting stents. Fortunately, there is growing evidence that newer diagnostic approaches could catch up with these therapeutic developments. The confirmation of a substantial amount of ischemic myocardium is considered to be one of the most relevant indications for revascularization procedures, i.e., a class IA indication based on sound evidence [1]. Diagnostic tests should therefore detect myocardial ischemia reliably and independent of observer. In addition, such tests ideally should bring no harm to the patient, should be low in costs, and should be repeatable, as CAD, being a chronic disease, should ideally be monitored over several decades.

Cardiac magnetic resonance (CMR) for detection and monitoring of CAD meets most of these prerequisites, which will be discussed in detail. Two main concepts for ischemia detection by CMR are currently available. One detects ischemia-induced myocardial dysfunction and the other evaluates myocardial perfusion in a pharmacologically induced hyperemic state.

For all the CMR applications discussed below, some safety aspects should be considered. Electronic devices such as pacemakers and implantable cardioverter–defibrillators are a contraindication for CMR [2]. Coronary stents are safe, as are mechanical heart valves (for valves implanted decades ago, exceptions exist). Some gadolinium-chelated magnetic resonance contrast media are associated with the incidence of nephrogenic systemic fibrosis in patients with severe impairment of kidney function. For detailed information, the reader should consult specific literature [3].

Magnetic resonance coronary angiography was found to be successful for stenosis detection in several single-center

Cardiovascular Interventions in Clinical Practice. Edited by Jürgen Haase, Hans-Joachim Schäfers, Horst Sievert and Ron Waksman. © 2010 Blackwell Publishing.

studies, but a larger multicenter trial revealed inadequate robustness of the technique [4]; this application will not be discussed further in this chapter, as a clinical application can only be recommended for detection of coronary anomalies (inter-aortopulmonary course) but not for detection/exclusion of CAD.

Detection of ischemia-induced myocardial dysfunction by cardiac magnetic resonance

This approach is, in fact, similar in most aspects to the examination that utilizes transthoracic echocardiography (stress echocardiography). As for the echocardiographic study, the patient is subject to a positive inotropic (and chronotropic) stimulus, most often achieved by dobutamine infusion. As in stress echocardiography, dobutamine is administered at increasing doses of 10, 20, 30, and 40 µg/kg/min for 3 min each, and myocardial function is monitored at each stage by acquiring typically three long-axis and three short-axis cine loops, each of the imaging planes collected during a short breath-hold. The functional data are evaluated as the study progresses and the examination is stopped if significant wall motion abnormalities are observed or, in a negative test, if the patient reaches submaximal heart rate ($[220 - age] \times 0.85$) without detection of relevant dysfunction. To achieve submaximal heart rate, atropine is administered if needed (as in stress echocardiography). In addition to ischemia, criteria for test termination are a drop in systolic blood pressure of ≥ 20 mmHg or an increase to $\geq 240/120$ mmHg, arrhythmias, or intractable symptoms.

For this type of stress testing, the advantage of utilizing CMR lies in its excellent image quality in most cases, irrespective of, for example, body habitus. With this CMR technique, cine loops are acquired within a breath-hold of 5–10 s duration (depending on heart rate) applying steady-state free-precession (SSFP) sequences showing blood as bright signal contrasted with dark-gray myocardium. Most often, the studies are read visually by grading the wall motion in a 17-segment model [5] as normal (=1), slightly hypokinetic (=2), severely hypokinetic (=3), akinetic (=4), or dyskinetic [5]. A milestone study in

1999, using a fast gradient-echo CMR technique (which is inferior to the currently used SSFP sequences), demonstrated a high sensitivity and specificity to detect ischemic regions of 86% and 86%, respectively. For the comparison of the diagnostic performance of CMR versus stress echocardiography it is of major importance to note that CMR outperformed echocardiography, particularly in patients with suboptimal echo windows. From these results and others it can be concluded that CMR is most valuable as a first-line tool for CAD diagnostics in patients with suboptimal echo quality, as supported by the meta-analysis by Nandular *et al.* [6] (although it should be recognized that meta-analyses cannot eliminate systematic limitations of trials and publication bias if present). Hundley *et al.* [7] demonstrated in this patient population with suboptimal echo quality that a negative stress-CMR study (no ischemia, ejection fraction >60%) predicted an excellent outcome with an annual event rate for cardiac death and nonfatal myocardial infarction of 0.8%/year (and 1%/year with ejection fraction >40%), whereas patients with ischemia demonstrated a substantial event rate of 10.6%/year. These prognostic data were confirmed in a recent CMR study, in which the event rates in patients without ischemia were as low as 0.7%/year [8].

With regard to safety of the stress-CMR examination, several larger studies have documented a very low event rate [7]. However, safety data from multicenter studies or registries are not (yet) available, most likely because no contrast media are required for this technique, and, thus, no approval from official authorities is required to document test performance and safety.

The image quality of CMR, which is in general high, allows for a reliable reading. For such a visual approach for SSFP images, a good interobserver reproducibility was reported with a kappa value of 0.59 (range among four readers: 0.52–0.76). As the SSFP technique is robust and easy to apply, intercenter variability is expected to be low, although data for this comparison are currently lacking. Nevertheless, an observer-independent analysis of the functional data is still missing. The state-of-the-art SSFP sequences delineate the trabeculated endocardial border with high-temporal and spatial resolution, but variable overestimation of systolic thickening can occur due to "compaction" of these trabeculae during systole, which hampers the development of automatic algorithms for analysis.

Another CMR technique to assess myocardial deformation is called "tissue-tagging" [9]. In these ECG-triggered acquisitions, typically a "grid-like" pattern is imprinted onto the myocardium a few milliseconds after detection of the R-wave (Fig. 30.1). This grid-like pattern is then preserved within the myocardial tissue during systole into mid-diastole. Deformation of this grid pattern is then monitored during the cardiac cycle and allows for assessment of myocardial deformation (e.g., separating it from bulk cardiac motion and/or tethering). Ultrafast tagging techniques currently allow us to acquire these data within a short breath-hold, even during pharmacologic [10,11] and

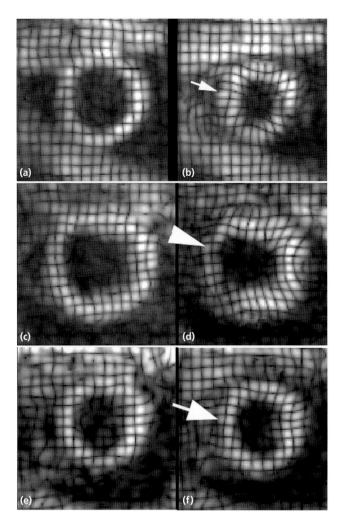

Figure 30.1 Example of tagging images acquired in (a and b) a normal volunteer, (c and d) a patient with left bundle branch block, and (e and f) a patient after anteroseptal myocardial infarction. The images on the left (a, c, e) were acquired a few milliseconds after the onset of the R-wave; the images on the right (b, d, f) represent myocardial deformation at the time of aortic valve closure. These are extracted from a full 3-D data set covering the entire heart every 34 ms, acquired with three breath-holds. In the control subject, uniform deformation is present at end-systole (small arrow pointing to the septum), but, in the patient with left bundle branch block, stretching of the septum occurs (arrowhead) as a result of hypercontraction in the lateral wall. In the patient with an infarct, no deformation in the interventricular septum occurs (large arrow). Images courtesy of Rutz A, MSc, ETH Zurich, Zurich, Switzerland. Localized deformation parameters are extracted from such data sets by HARP strategies within minutes [15].

physical stress [12]. As the tagging technique encodes tissue deformation as phase changes in the frequency domain, such tagging data can be analyzed by novel (semi-)automatic algorithms called "harmonic phase imaging" (HARP) [13,14] or by further modifications of HARP [15]. In a study by Kuijpers *et al.* [11], stress tagging data were used for visual analysis of deformation, and a specificity of 96% for detection of CAD was achieved. Because the CMR results in that study determined the need for invasive coronary angiography, no sensitivity was given. However, the event-free survival for patients without ischemia on CMR and with normal resting function was 0.7%/year [11]. To our knowledge, automatic postprocessing procedures of tagging data for ischemia detection during high-dose dobutamine have not yet been evaluated. The latest developments in tagging techniques even allow for the acquisition of full 3-D-deformation data of the entire heart (acquired within three breath-holds only) [16]. This technique, although unlikely to be applicable during stress, appears promising for the evaluation of dyssynchrony with respect to cardiac resynchronization therapy. By combining 3-D-deformation data with 3-D viability data, an in-depth assessment of CAD patients with suspected dyssynchrony becomes feasible [17].

Perfusion cardiac magnetic resonance

This CMR approach takes advantage of the high-speed performance of current CMR hardware and software to monitor the passage of contrast media through the myocardium during hyperemic conditions [18,19]. Hyperemia is generally induced by a standard dose of 0.14 mg/kg/min adenosine administered over 3 min intravenously. At this time point, maximum hyperemia in the myocardium is expected to occur and the contrast medium is administered into a peripheral vein (at rates of 4–5 mL/s) and image acquisition is started simultaneously as the patient is instructed to hold his/her breath. After a few seconds, the contrast medium then reaches the coronary arteries and the myocardial first pass of contrast medium lasts another 5–10 s. Thus, within 10–15 s the complete perfusion information is acquired over 3–7 short-axis slices covering the left ventricular myocardium every one to two heart beats. These perfusion pulse sequences are run with a spatial resolution of 1.5–3 mm × 1.5–3 mm, thus providing perfusion information within the various layers of the myocardium. Several studies demonstrated superior diagnostic performance for CAD detection when analyzing subendocardial data versus transmural perfusion data [20,21]. To preserve the nominally high spatial resolution of the CMR acquisition, cardiac and respiratory motion must be controlled. As the crucial perfusion information is acquired during the wash-in phase of the contrast media, i.e., within 15 s or so, respiratory motion can be avoided by breath-holding. Careful instruction of the patient and spending some time testing the patient's cooperation are essential to achieve a near-100% success rate for perfusion CMR studies. Control of cardiac motion is more challenging, as two conflicting goals are pursued: (1) limiting the acquisitions to cardiac phases with minimal cardiac motion, for which the periods of mid-diastole and mid to end-systole appear available, and (2) acquiring as many slices of the left ventricular myocardium as possible, which goes along with increasing acquisition duration per cardiac cycle. Several

studies have demonstrated that extended cardiac coverage with five or more slices, which require acquisitions during phases with substantial cardiac motion, severely degrades image quality and renders such protocols inferior to protocols with fewer slices [22–24]. Conversely, three or four short-axis slices of 8–10 mm thickness (separated by 4-mm gaps to account for systolic long-axis shortening) covered up to 5.2 cm of the left ventricular long axis during systole and yielded excellent sensitivities and specificities for CAD detection [22,23]. In a study comparing perfusion CMR with both PET and X-ray coronary angiography, sensitivities/specificities of 91%/94% and 87%/85% were achieved, respectively [20]. A slightly modified technique was then evaluated in a multi-center, single-vendor trial (Fig. 30.2), which fully confirmed the single-center results [22]. Furthermore, this multicenter trial showed that doses of a conventional magnetic resonance contrast medium of 0.1–0.15 mmol/kg body weight yielded best results for CAD detection (CAD defined as > 50% diameter stenoses on X-ray coronary angiography), but lower doses caused inadequate signal responses, and thus low diagnostic performance (Fig. 30.3a).

Applications of CMR are generally characterized by their broad range of versatility, as several dozen parameters need to be optimized to achieve best results for any given clinical question. Accordingly, the variety of pulse sequences and parameters among vendors regarding perfusion CMR techniques is large, and a multicenter, multivendor trial was designed to evaluate the technique's performance in conditions approaching real-world clinical situations. In this trial, called MR-IMPACT (Magnetic Resonance Imaging for Myocardial Perfusion Assessment in Coronary Artery disease Trial), 18 centers participated and perfusion CMR was compared with SPECT utilizing invasive X-ray coronary angiography as the standard of reference [25]. Perfusion CMR yielded a high diagnostic accuracy with an area under the receiver operator characteristics curve of 0.86 ± 0.06, which was significantly superior to SPECT (Fig. 30.3b) [25]. The superiority of perfusion CMR over SPECT was also demonstrated for multivessel disease [25]. Furthermore, the SPECT results of the MR-IMPACT are in good agreement with earlier multicenter nuclear trials yielding sensitivities of 77–87% and specificities of 36–58% [26–29]. Given that the MR-IMPACT is the largest multicenter trial on SPECT published so far, with 18 centers involved, the results provide strong evidence for the recommendation of perfusion CMR as the first-line technique to confirm or exclude CAD, if it is available.

As demonstrated by Figure 30.3a, contrast medium dose is a major determinant of maximum signal response in the myocardium, and thus of test performance. But, in addition, the type of the pulse sequence and the imaging parameters also strongly modify the signal response [24]. Therefore, any (semi-)automatic perfusion data analysis requires exact definition of these parameters and adequate adaptation of the analysis algorithm in case any imaging parameters or the

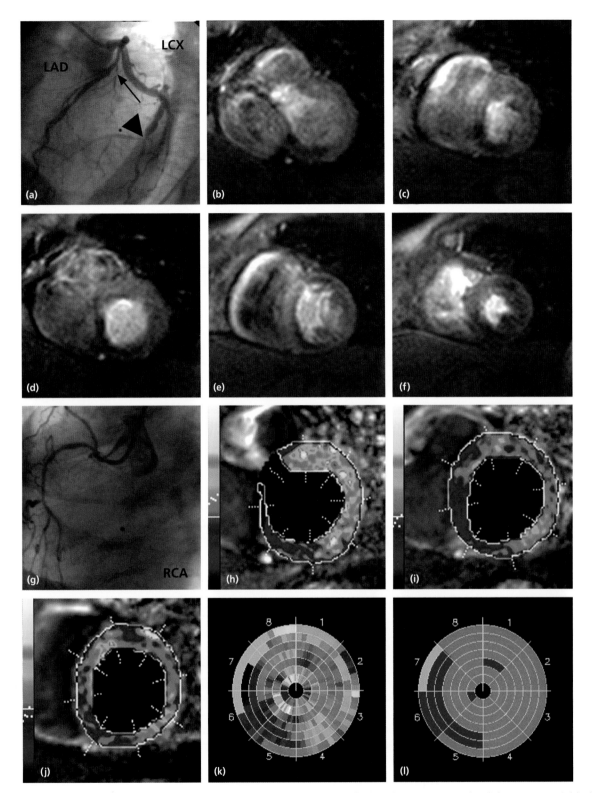

Figure 30.2 In a patient with stenoses in the small first diagonal branch of the LAD (arrow in a) and the large left circumflex coronary artery (LCx, arrowhead in a), a perfusion CMR scan (with 0.15 mmol/kg gadolinium-diethylenetriamine penta-acetic acid bismethyl-amide, Gd-DTPA-BMA) shows a subendocardial perfusion deficit in the inferior wall from the base to the apes (b–f) and a small deficit in the anterior wall (e and f). The right coronary artery (RCA) shows no stenosis (g). These perfusion deficits are also detected by the semiautomatic upslope analysis, with ischemia shown as blue areas (red = normal, h–j). (k) and (l) show, respectively, pixel-wise and segmental polar maps of the subendocardium of the left ventricular myocardium [22]. Reproduced with permission from the European Society of Cardiology and Oxford University Press.

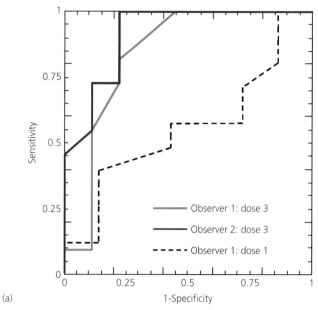

(a)

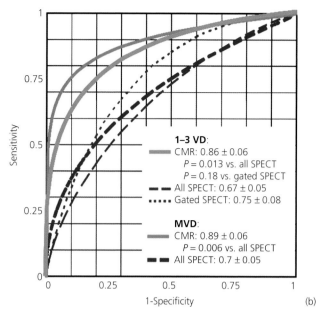

(b)

Figure 30.3 Performance of perfusion CMR. The area under the receiver–operator characteristics curve represents diagnostic performance in the detection of coronary artery disease (defined as ≥50% diameter stenosis in any vessel >2 mm in invasive coronary angiography). The single-vendor multicenter trial shows that the best performance was achieved at the highest contrast medium dose of 0.15 mmol/kg (=dose 3) [22]. Dose 1, 0.05 mmol/kg gadolinium-diethylenetriamine penta-acetic acid (Gd-DTPA); dose 3, 0.15 mmol/kg Gd-DTPA. (b) In the multivendor multicenter trial MR-IMPACT (Magnetic Resonance Imaging for Myocardial Perfusion Assessment in Coronary Artery Disease Trial), the diagnostic performance of perfusion CMR was found to be superior to that of SPECT in all patients (1–3 VD: $P = 0.013$) and in the subset of multivessel disease patients (MVD: $P = 0.006$) [25]. VD, vessel disease. Reproduced with permission from the European Society of Cardiology and Oxford University Press.

dose, rate or site of contrast medium injection are changed. Keeping these precautions in mind, CMR perfusion data appear well suited for (semi-)automatic analysis as respiratory and cardiac motion can effectively be controlled. In addition, residual respiratory motion such as a diaphragmatic drift during breath-holding can easily be corrected using current algorithms provided by various vendors. Furthermore, CMR perfusion data are not compromised by any signal attenuation in patients with various habitus (which still poses a problem in SPECT). Spatially dependent signal reception by the surface coils [20] is taken into account by all current state-of-the-art analysis software packages.

Newest developments in data acquisition exploiting temporospatial correlations of the signals in k-space currently deliver excellent data quality with up to 8 pixels across the left ventricular wall [31–33]. Such high-resolution data may further improve the efficiency and accuracy of automatic algorithms. However, visual readings of these data by experienced observers have demonstrated that detection of ischemia (represented by the area under the receiver operator characteristics curve: area under the curve, AUC) cannot be further improved with these newer techniques over conventional techniques, even when combined with higher field strength of 3 T, most likely demonstrating that the current perfusion CMR has reached optimum performance in comparison with invasive X-ray coronary angiography [34]. Residual "inaccuracy" (i.e., AUC is smaller than 1.0 versus coronary angiography)

most likely reflects the fact that coronary anatomy is not always in agreement with perfusion, i.e., hemodynamic significance does not always correlate with stenosis severity for each lesion. Taking this into consideration, probably the best parameter for assessment of perfusion test performance would be its prognostic power. Therefore, more data on this aspect would be highly valuable. In one study performed by Jahnke and co-workers [8], a normal perfusion scan was associated with an excellent prognosis and an event rate of only 0.7%/year. Also, in the emergency room, Ingkanisorn *et al.* [35] found that perfusion CMR was of remarkable value in predicting CAD (>50% diameter stenosis on invasive study), an abnormal SPECT study, new myocardial infarction, or death during a follow-up period of 1 year (sensitivity and specificity of 100% and 93%, respectively). Thus, perfusion CMR is an excellent test in experienced centers to exclude or detect CAD because of its high data quality, its reliability, and its lack of ionizing radiation, which allows for repetitive studies during the course of CAD over many decades. A current list of indications for CMR can be found in the booklet "CMR-Update" [36].

Assessment of myocardial viability by cardiac magnetic resonance

If the efforts to prevent, to diagnose, and to treat coronary lesions have failed, and myocardial infarction has occurred,

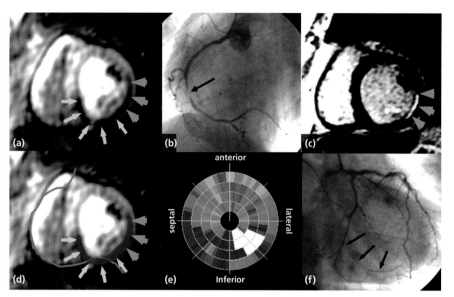

Figure 30.4 Application of perfusion CMR and LGE for viability assessment in a female patient. (a) A representative short-axis slice; perfusion is reduced in the subendocardium of the inferior, inferoseptal, and lateral wall. (b) Invasive coronary angiography confirms a severe stenosis in the right coronary artery (RCA, arrow). Further viability testing (c) demonstrates a subendocardial scar in the lateral wall (green arrows), which explains the finding of hypoperfusion. (d) The course of the RCA is projected on the perfusion image in red, demonstrating the supply territory of the RCA (yellow arrows). The hypoperfused zone in the lateral wall (green arrows) is not supplied by the RCA. (e) This perfusion and viability information is combined into a polar map of the left ventricular subendocardium (colors as in Figure 30.2, white area = scar tissue). Coronary angiography (f) confirms occlusion of the second posterolateral branch of the circumflex with retrograde filling (arrows).

the assessment of myocardial viability and scar is essential for further adequate patient management. Several studies demonstrated convincingly that revascularization of viable, not contracting (i.e. hibernating) myocardium is improving the outcome versus drug treatment alone [37–39]. CMR is an excellent technique to detect and quantify acute myocardial necrosis owing to the fact that conventional extracellular magnetic resonance contrast media are excluded from viable cells with intact cell membranes [40–42]. In acute cell damage, the magnetic resonance contrast media can enter the intracellular compartment, thereby expanding their distribution volume with the result that the high concentration of contrast media delineates acute myocyte necrosis. Several clinical studies demonstrated that this so-called late gadolinium enhancement (LGE) mechanism detects acute myocardial infarction with high accuracy and also predicts recovery of function and remodeling during the healing process [43,44]. In the chronic myocardial infarction situation, fibrous tissue has replaced acute myocyte necrosis. In scar tissue consisting of a large extracellular space and containing a small intracellular compartment made up of fibrocytes, the distribution volume of the magnetic resonance contrast media is even larger than in acute necrosis, and thus chronic infarcts appear bright using the LGE technique. Owing to the high spatial resolution of this LGE application of CMR, the transmurality of the scar tissue can be visualized with excellent contrast versus viable myocardium. In particular, the transmural ratio of scar versus viable rim tissue appears to predict the potential to recover systolic function following

revascularization [45–47]. It was also shown that not only did this ratio predict outcome, but also the absolute thickness of viable rim tissue, as well as the absolute thickness of scar formation at the endocardium [48]. Segments with thick subendocardial scar (approximately >4mm) and/or thin viable rim myocardium (approximately <4mm) are unlikely to recover any function after revascularization [48].

In the setting of known CAD with regional impairment of contractile function, it is recommended to assess both the presence of ischemia and the presence of scar tissue in each segment of the left ventricular myocardium. As shown in the example in Figure 30.4, the perfusion CMR module localizes areas with impaired hyperemic perfusion (e.g., in the inferior and lateral wall in this patient). The LGE module then demonstrates viable tissue in the inferior wall (myocardium that would experience ischemia during inotropic challenge), and scar tissue in the subendocardium of the lateral wall indicates that hypoperfusion is due to the scar tissue, and most likely revascularization would not be required for this lateral wall. This combination of perfusion CMR (with a stress-only protocol) followed by a viability study provides excellent information on the status of all myocardial segments of the left ventricle from which treatment decisions can be derived. To be able to match regions with hypoperfusion with scar distribution, a high spatial resolution is mandatory. With CMR collecting perfusion and viability information in the 2–3mm range, it is possible to detect very small territories of ischemia and/or scar. Wagner *et al.* [49] demonstrated that scar detection was similar for CMR and SPECT for nearly transmural infarcts, whereas in the case of smaller subendocardial scars, which are readily detected by CMR, up to 80% were missed by SPECT in animals and in ~50% in humans. Although the prognostic significance of such small areas of ischemia is not yet known, Kwong *et al.* [50] found an approximately eight times higher risk for major cardiac events (MACEs) in patients with infarcts as small as 1.4% of the total left ventricular mass. However, it is not only the size of an infarction that seems to predict outcome. There is growing evidence that the extent of a dark core in the infarcted tissue, often observed in the acute phase of myocardial necrosis, is even more closely related to outcome than the entire mass of tissue necrosis. This dark core, generally referred to as zone of microvascular obstruction, has been shown to be highly predictive for MACEs, indicating that the composition of the infarcted area provides prognostic information [51]. In particular, the mode of death in the infarct zone may influence infarct healing, remodeling, and, thus, outcome. As small infarcts of a few grams of tissue can now be studied noninvasively and serially in patients, the CMR technique will certainly become an important tool for research as well to assess treatment outcomes in the acute myocardial infarction setting. For example, in a recent multicenter study in patients undergoing percutaneous coronary interventions (PCI) in acute myocardial infarction, the effect of a novel fibrin-derived peptide on a potential reperfusion injury was evaluated by CMR measuring the infarct size as the primary study end point.

In summary, the LGE application of CMR yields excellent results for viability assessment in the clinical setting, and it will certainly become an important research tool for the assessment of novel treatment strategies in acute myocardial infarction. It should be noted that viability assessment is also highly valuable in patients with severely impaired left ventricular function for differentiation between CAD and dilated cardiomyopathy (CMP) [36,52]. Finally, the LGE technique provides high sensitivity to detect thrombi in the cardiac cavities after infarction [36,53], and can identify or exclude myocarditis in patients with chest pain and normal coronary angiograms [36,54–56].

The role of cardiac magnetic resonance in the workup and management of patients with suspected or known coronary artery disease

It is obvious that treatment regimens in cardiology are instituted primarily for two reasons: (1) to reduce symptoms and (2) to improve the patient's prognosis. However, the latter goal requires (1) a diagnostic test that can estimate the patient's prognosis and, (2) even more importantly, that the influence of different treatment regimens on prognosis for any given patient is known to enable the optimum management to be selected. For this purpose, the dichotomous diagnostics of "no disease" (associated with low event rates) and "disease present" (associated with increased risk for complications) is not sufficient because most (or all) therapeutic interventions are also handicapped by their own complication rate. Selecting the optimum treatment strategy (optimum with respect also to costs) requires that the spontaneous course of the disease in an individual patient is known, and the treatment selected should be associated with a lower complication rate than the spontaneous course and/or other treatment options. To assess the spontaneous course of CAD, data from the "preinterventional" era were analyzed [57–59] and an exponential relationship between the degree of stenosis and the frequency of complete occlusion was found, as shown in Figure 30.5 [60]. Although low-degree, and thus hemodynamically nonsignificant, plaques can rupture and suddenly occlude a vessel, the rate of complete occlusion is rather low in the case of such nonobstructive lesions, whereas the occlusion rate increases exponentially with increasing stenosis [60]. Assuming that lesions causing ischemia detectable by SPECT cause diameter reduction in the range 50–99%, we see a strong agreement between these SPECT perfusion data [61] and the anatomical data (Fig. 30.5). One might argue that this stenosis severity versus occlusion curve does not take account of the much higher prevalence of low-degree stenosis in a given patient compared with severe stenosis. This consideration is highly relevant for cost-effectiveness calculations. If the total numbers of both low- and high-degree stenoses are considered (for the invasive studies shown in Fig. 30.5), and if one further assumes that a lesion treated mechanically (e.g., by PCI and stenting) is no longer at risk for occlusion, 187 low-degree stenoses would need to be treated (number needed to treat, NNT) to prevent one occlusion compared with an NNT of 11 to prevent one occlusion in the case of high-degree lesions. These considerations clearly suggest that mechanical treatment of low-degree stenoses is not cost-effective.

But what about the treatment of high-degree stenosis? Here, the complication rates of the interventions also need to be considered. Without any doubt, some aspects of the COURAGE trial [62] are controversial, but the results still merit consideration, particularly in view of the spontaneous course of the disease. As shown in Figure 30.5, the complication rate for PCI in COURAGE was close to that of the spontaneous course, which suggests that a significant advantage over medical treatment cannot be expected. A similar picture is shown by the AVERT trial [63], in which the outcome for balloon dilation was again close to the spontaneous course of the disease. From these examples, it can be derived that patients with stenosis of low and intermediate degree are unlikely to benefit from PCI, but that potential benefit increases (exponentially) with increasing lesion severity. Although stenosis severity is predictive of the likelihood of an occlusion, it does not take account of the extent of myocardium at risk, and thus the extent of potential myocardial

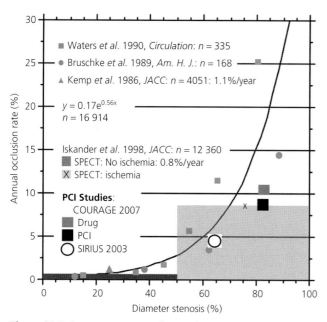

Figure 30.5 Spontaneous course of CAD. The relationship between the degree of diameter stenosis detected by invasive X-ray quantitative coronary angiography and annual occlusion rate (at the site of quantified stenosis) in 4554 prospectively studied patients is shown [57–59]. The relationship between pathologic/normal SPECT scans (light- and dark-gray bars, respectively) and complication rate per year (deaths or nonfatal myocardial infarctions) in 12 360 patients is also shown [61]. On SPECT scans, ischemia was defined as stenosis amounting to =≥50% diameter reduction (mean 75% stenosis) and a normal scan was defined as <50% diameter reduction (mean 25% stenoses). Even though the clinical complications in patients after SPECT testing cannot be related to specific locations of stenoses, the SPECT data provide indirect support that low- and high-grade stenoses are associated, respectively, with a low and high risk of occlusion. Overall, these data from more than 16 000 patients [57–59,61] demonstrate a considerable (i.e., exponential) increase in the risk of complications with increasing stenosis severity (an exponential curve). The results of PCI trials are added to the figure. The complication rates in the COURAGE (Clinical Outcomes Utilizing Revascularization and Aggressive Drug Evaluation) trial [62] and the Sirius trial [67] are close to the spontaneous course of disease (when stenosis degree is considered). This exponential curve is meant as a rough estimation of CAD course, as it averages populations with different risk profiles (e.g., patients with diabetes) and does not consider lesion characteristics, which determine complication rate and would modify (shift) the exponential curve accordingly. Adapted from reference 60, with permission from Future Medicine Ltd.

loss in the case of an occlusion. Assessment of the ischemic myocardium (e.g., by perfusion CMR) is therefore highly advantageous as it both detects high-degree stenoses (and thus, lesions with a high risk for occlusion) and quantifies the potential extent of myocardial loss in the case of occlusion; perfusion tests, for example, also show collateral flow into the area at risk. Perfusion CMR may become an important tool to assess both a patient's risk for a coronary occlusion and its consequences, with regard to the extent of potentially

infarcted myocardium. As both aspects affect he final complication rate, perfusion CMR appears to be ideal for the accurate prediction of outcome, and thus may provide a valuable basis for treatment decisions.

In conclusion, there is growing evidence that the diagnostic performance of perfusion CMR is excellent and superior to that of other techniques such as SPECT. In addition, CMR does not expose patients to any ionizing radiation, and therefore does not subject the patients to an increased risk of cancer development [64–66]. Although these results are encouraging, larger prospective trials are needed to identify the best test or test combination to design the best treatment strategy for any individual patient, e.g., medical treatment only versus medical plus PCI or medical plus bypass surgery.

References

1. Silber S, Albertsson P, Avile's F, *et al.* (2005) Guidelines for percutaneous coronary interventions. The Task Force for Percutaneous Coronary Interventions of the European Society of Cardiology. *Eur Heart J* **26**:804–847.
2. Roguin A, Schwitter J, Vahlhaus V, *et al.* (2008) Magnetic resonance imaging in individuals with cardiovascular implantable electronic devices. *Europace* **10**:336–743.
3. Shellock F (2008) *Reference Manual for Magnetic Resonance Safety, Implants, and Devices: 2008.* Los Angeles: Biomedical Research Publishing Group.
4. Kim WY, Danias PG, Stuber M, *et al.* (2001) Coronary magnetic resonance angiography for the detection of coronary stenoses. *N Engl J Med* **345**:1863–1869.
5. Cerqueira M, Weissman N, Dilsizian V, *et al.* (2002) Standardized myocardial segmentation and nomenclature for tomographic imaging of the heart: a statement for healthcare professionals from the Cardiac Imaging Committee of the Council on Clinical Cardiology of the American Heart Association. *Circulation* **105**:539–542.
6. Nandalur KR, Dwamena BA, Choudhri AF, Nandalur MR, & Carlos RC (2007) Diagnostic performance of stress cardiac magnetic resonance imaging in the detection of coronary artery disease: a meta-analysis. *J Am Coll Cardiol* **50**:1343–1353.
7. Hundley WG, Morgan TM, Neagle CM, Hamilton CA, Rerkpattanapipat P, & Link KM (2002) Magnetic resonance imaging determination of cardiac prognosis. *Circulation* **106**:2328–2333.
8. Jahnke C, Nagel E, Gebker R, *et al.* (2007) Prognostic value of cardiac magnetic resonance stress tests: adenosine stress perfusion and dobutamine stress wall motion imaging. *Circulation* **115**:1769–1776.
9. Zerhouni E, Parish D, Rogers W, Yang A, & Shapiro E (1988) Human heart: tagging with MR imaging: a method for non-invasive assessment of myocardial motion. *Radiology* **169**:59–63.
10. Power T, Kramer C, Shaffer A, *et al.* (1997) Breath-hold dobutamine magnetic resonance myocardial tagging: normal left ventricular response. *Am J Cardiol* **80**:1203–1207.
11. Kuijpers D, Ho K, van Dijkman P, Vliegenthart R, & Oudkerk M (2003) Dobutamine cardiovascular magnetic resonance for the

detection of myocardial ischemia with the use of myocardial tagging. *Circulation* **107**:1592–1597.

12. Ryf S, Schwitter J, Spiegel MA, *et al.* (2005) Accelerated tagging for the assessment of left ventricular myocardial contraction under physical stress. *J Cardiovasc Magn Reson* **7**:693–703.

13. Osman N, Kerwin W, McVeigh E, & Prince J (1999) Cardiac motion tracking using CINE harmonic phase (HARP) magnetic resonance imaging. *Magn Reson Med* **42**:1048–1060.

14. Garot J, Bluemke D, Osman N, *et al.* (2000) Fast determination of regional myocardial strain fields from tagged cardiac images using harmonic phase MRI. *Circulation* **101**:981–988.

15. Ryf S, Tsao J, Schwitter J, Stuessi A, & Boesiger P (2004) Peak-combination HARP: a method to correct for phase errors in HARP. *J Magn Reson Imaging* **20**:874–880.

16. Rutz A, Ryf S, Plein S, Boesiger P, & Kozerke S (2008) Accelerated whole-heart 3D CSPAMM for myocardial motion quantification. *Magn Reson Med* **59**:755–763.

17. Rutz AK, Manka R, Kozerke S, Roas S, Boesiger P, & Schwitter J (2008) Left ventricular dyssynchrony in patients with left bundle branch block and patients after myocardial infarctions: Integration of mechanics and viability by cardiac magnetic resonance. *Eur Heart J* **30**:2117–2127.

18. Schwitter J (2003) CMR of Myocardial Perfusion: In: Lardo AC, Fayad ZA, Chronos NAF, & Fuster V (eds). *Cardiovascular Magnetic Resonance: Established and Emerging Applications.* London: Martin Dunitz, Taylor and Francis, p. 111–126.

19. Schwitter J (2005) Myocardial Perfusion in Ischemic Heart Disease. In: Higgins CB & de Roos A (eds). *MRI and CT of the Cardiovascular System,* 2nd edn. Lippincott Williams and Wilkins.

20. Schwitter J, Nanz D, Kneifel S, *et al.* (2001) Assessment of myocardial perfusion in coronary artery disease by magnetic resonance: a comparison with positron emission tomography and coronary angiography. *Circulation* **103**:2230–2235.

21. Keijer JT, van Rossum AC, Wilke N, *et al.* (2000) Magnetic resonance imaging of myocardial perfusion in single-vessel coronary artery disease: implications for transmural assessment of myocardial perfusion. *J Cardiovasc Magn Reson* **2**:189–200.

22. Giang T, Nanz D, Coulden R, *et al.* (2004) Detection of coronary artery disease by magnetic resonance myocardial perfusion imaging with various contrast medium doses: first European multicenter experience. *Eur Heart J* **25**:1657–1665.

23. Nagel E, Klein C, Paetsch I, *et al.* (2003) Magnetic resonance perfusion measurements for the noninvasive detection of coronary artery disease. *Circulation* **108**:432–437.

24. Bertschinger KM, Nanz D, Buechi M, *et al.* (2001) Magnetic resonance myocardial first-pass perfusion imaging: parameter optimization for signal response and cardiac coverage. *J Magn Reson Imaging* **14**:556–562.

25. Schwitter J, Wacker C, van Rossum A, *et al.* (2008) MR-IMPACT: comparison of perfusion-cardiac magnetic resonance with single-photon emission computed tomography for the detection of coronary artery disease in a multicentre, multivendor, randomized trial. *Eur Heart J* **29**:480–489.

26. Hendel RC, Berman DS, Cullom SJ, *et al.* (1999) Multicenter clinical trial to evaluate the efficacy of correction for photon attenuation and scatter in SPECT myocardial perfusion imaging. *Circulation* **99**:2742–2749.

27. Van Train KF, Garcia EV, Maddahi J, *et al.* (1994) Multicenter trial validation for quantitative analysis of same-day rest-stress technetium-99m-sestamibi myocardial tomograms. *J Nucl Med* **35**:609–618.

28. Zaret BL, Rigo P, Wackers FJ, *et al.* (1995) Myocardial perfusion imaging with ^{99m}Tc tetrofosmin. Comparison to 201Tl imaging and coronary angiography in a phase III multicenter trial. Tetrofosmin International Trial Study Group. *Circulation* **91**:313–319.

29. He ZX, Iskandrian AS, Gupta NC, & Verani MS (1997) Assessing coronary artery disease with dipyridamole technetium-99m-tetrofosmin SPECT: a multicenter trial. *J Nuc Med* **38**:44–48.

30. Schwitter J (2006) Myocardial perfusion imaging by cardiac magnetic resonance. *J Nucl Cardiol* **13**:841–854.

31. Plein S, Ryf S, Schwitter J, Radjenovic A, Boesiger P, & Kozerke S (2007) Dynamic contrast-enhanced myocardial perfusion MR imaging accelerated with k-t SENSE. *Magn Reson Med* **58**:777–785.

32. Plein S, Kozerke S, Suerder D, *et al.* (2008) High spatial resolution myocardial perfusion cardiac magnetic resonance for the detection of coronary artery disease. *Eur Heart J* **29**:2148–2155.

33. Kellman P, Derbyshire J, Agyeman K, McVeigh E, & Arai A (2004) Extended coverage first-pass perfusion imaging using slice-interleaved TSENSE. *Magn Reson Med* **51**:200–204.

34. Plein S, Schwitter J, Suerder D, Greenwood J, Boesiger P, & Kozerke S (2008) k-t SENSE-accelerated myocardial perfusion MR imaging at 3.0 Tesla–comparison with 1.5 Tesla. *Radiology* in press.

35. Ingkanisorn W, Kwong R, Bohme N, *et al.* (2006) Prognosis of negative adenosine stress magnetic resonance in patients presenting to an emergency department with chest pain. *J Am Coll Cardiol* **47**:1427–1432.

36. Schwitter J (ed.). (2009) *CMR-Update,* 1st edition. Zurich: J. Schwitter. http://herz-mri.ch

37. Beanlands RS, Ruddy TD, deKemp RA, *et al.* (2002) Positron emission tomography and recovery following revascularization (PARR-1): the importance of scar and the development of a prediction rule for the degree of recovery of left ventricular function. *J Am Coll Cardiol* **40**:1735–1743.

38. Bonow RO (1996) Identification of viable myocardium. *Circulation* **94**:2674–2680.

39. Pasquet A, Robert A, D'Hondt AM, Dion R, Melin JA, & Vanoverschelde JL (1999) Prognostic value of myocardial ischemia and viability in patients with chronic left ventricular ischemic dysfunction. *Circulation* **100**:141–148.

40. Judd R, Lugo-Olivieri C, Arai M, *et al.* (1995) Physiological basis of myocardial contrast enhancement in fast magnetic resonance images of 2-day-old reperfused canine infarcts. *Circulation* **92**:1902–1910.

41. Schwitter J, Saeed M, Wendland MF, *et al.* (1997) Influence of severity of myocardial injury on distribution of macromolecules: extravascular versus intravascular gadolinium-based magnetic resonance contrast agents. *J Am Coll Cardiol* **30**:1086–1094.

42. Rehwald WG, Fieno DS, Chen EL, Kim RJ, & Judd RM (2002) Myocardial magnetic resonance imaging contrast agent concentrations after reversible and irreversible ischemic injury. *Circulation* **105**:224–229.

43. Kim RJ, Fieno DS, Parrish TB, *et al.* (1999) Relationship of MRI delayed contrast enhancement to irreversible injury, infarct age, and contractile function. *Circulation* **100**:1992–2002.

44. Choi KM, Kim RJ, Gubernikoff G, Vargas JD, Parker M, & Judd RM (2001) Transmural extent of acute myocardial infarction

predicts long-term improvement in contractile function. *Circulation* **104**:1101–1107.

45. Kim RJ, Wu E, Rafael A, *et al.* (2000) The use of contrast-enhanced magnetic resonance imaging to identify reversible myocardial dysfunction. *N Engl J Med* **343**:1445–1453.

46. Klein C, Nekolla SG, Bengel FM, *et al.* (2002) Assessment of myocardial viability with contrast-enhanced magnetic resonance imaging: comparison with positron emission tomography. *Circulation* **105**:162–167.

47. Wu E, Judd RM, Vargas JD, Klocke FJ, Bonow RO, & Kim RJ (2001) Visualisation of presence, location, and transmural extent of healed Q-wave and non-Q-wave myocardial infarction. *Lancet* **357**:21–28.

48. Knuesel PR, Nanz D, Wyss C, *et al.* (2003) Characterization of dysfunctional myocardium by positron emission tomography and magnetic resonance: relation to functional outcome after revascularization. *Circulation* **108**:1095–1100.

49. Wagner A, Mahrholdt H, Holly TA, *et al.* (2003) Contrast-enhanced MRI and routine single photon emission computed tomography (SPECT) perfusion imaging for the detection of subendocardial myocardial infarcts: an imaging study. *Lancet* **361**:374–379.

50. Kwong RY, Chan AK, Brown KA, *et al.* (2006) Impact of un-recognized myocardial scar detected by cardiac magnetic resonance imaging on event-free survival in patients presenting with signs or symptoms of coronary artery disease. *Circulation* **113**:2733–2743.

51. Wu KC, Zerhouni EA, Judd RM, *et al.* (1998) Prognostic significance of microvascular obstruction by magnetic resonance imaging in patients with acute myocardial infarction. *Circulation* **97**:765–772.

52. Assomull R, Prasad S, Lyne J, *et al.* (2005) Cardiovascular magnetic resonance, fibrosis, and prognosis in dilated cardio-myopathy. *J Am Coll Cardiol* **48**:1977–1985.

53. Mollet N, Dymarkowski S, Volders W, *et al.* (2002) Visualization of ventricular thrombi with contrast-enhanced magnetic resonance imaging in patients with ischemic heart disease. *Circulation* **106**:2873–2876.

54. Mahrholdt H, Goedecke C, Wagner A, *et al.* (2004) Cardiovascular magnetic resonance assessment of human myocarditis: a comparison to histology and molecular pathology. *Circulation* **109**:1250–1258.

55. Mahrholdt H, Wagner A, Deluigi CC, *et al.* (2006) Presentation, patterns of myocardial damage, and clinical course of viral myocarditis. *Circulation* **114**:1581–1590.

56. Ingkanisorn WP, Paterson DI, Calvo KR, *et al.* (2006) Cardiac magnetic resonance appearance of myocarditis caused by high dose IL-2: similarities to community-acquired myocarditis. *J Cardiovasc Magn Reson* **8**:353–360.

57. Waters D, Lesperance J, Francetich M, *et al.* (1990) A controlled clinical trial to assess the effect of a calcium channel blocker on the progression of coronary atherosclerosis. *Circulation* **82**:1940–1953.

58. Bruschke AV, Kramer JR Jr, Bal ET, Haque IU, Detrano RC, & Goormastic M (1989) The dynamics of progression of coronary atherosclerosis studied in 168 medically treated patients who underwent coronary arteriography three times. *Am Heart J* **117**:296–305.

59. Kemp H, Kronmal R, Vlietstra R, & Frye R (1986) Seven year survival of patients with normal or near normal coronary arteriograms: a CASS registry study. *J Am Coll Cardiol* **7**:479–483.

60. Schwitter J (2006) Future strategies in the management of coronary artery disease. *Future Cardiol* **2**:555–565.

61. Iskander S & Iskandrian AE (1998) Risk assessment using single-photon emission computed tomographic technetium-99m sestamibi imaging. *J Am Coll Cardiol* **32**:57–62.

62. Boden W, O'Rourke R, Teo K, *et al.* (2007) Optimal medical therapy with or without PCI for stable coronary artery disease. *N Engl J Med* **356**:1503–1516.

63. Pitt B, Waters D, Brown W, *et al.* (1999) Aggressive lipid-lowering therapy compared with angioplasty in stable coronary artery disease. *N Engl J Med* **341**:70–76.

64. Cardis E, Vrijheid M, Blettner M, *et al.* (2005) Risk of cancer after low doses of ionising radiation: retrospective cohort study in 15 countries. *Br Med J* **331**:77–82.

65. Committee to Assess Health Risks from Exposure to Low Levels of Ionizing Radiation NRCNAoS (2006) Health risks from exposure to low levels of ionizing radiation: BEIR VII–Phase 2. Executive Summary. Available at: http://www.nap.edu/catalog/11340.html:1–424.

66. Einstein A, Henzlova M, & Rajagopalan S (2007) Estimating risk of cancer associated with radiation exposure from 64-slice computed tomography coronary angiography. *JAMA* **298**:317–323.

67. Moses J, Leon M, Popma J, *et al.* (2003) Sirolimus-eluting stents versus standard stents in patients with stenosis in a native coronary artery. *N Engl J Med* **349**:1315–1323.

68. Nijveldt R, Beek A, Hirsch A, *et al.* (2008) Functional recovery after acute myocardial infarction: a comparison between angiography, electrocardiography and cardiovascular magnetic resonance measures of microvascular injury. *J Am Coll Cardiol* **52**:181–189.

31   Grayscale Intravascular Ultrasound and Virtual Histology of the Unstable Coronary Lesion

Hector M. Garcia-Garcia, Nieves Gonzalo, Anne L. Gaster & Patrick W. Serruys

Thoraxcenter, Erasmus Medical Center, Rotterdam, The Netherlands

Introduction

The ability to detect vulnerable plaques *in vivo* is essential to study their natural history and to evaluate potential therapeutic interventions that may ultimately favorably impact on acute coronary syndrome and death. Coronary angiography offers valuable information on the long-term behavior of complex coronary lesions but does have several limitations. Goldstein *et al.* [1] reported that the incidence of recurrent acute coronary syndrome during the year after STEMI was higher in patients with ST-segment elevation myocardial infarction (STEMI) and multiple complex lesions than in patients with a single complex lesion (19.0% vs. 2.6%, respectively, $P < 0.001$). Taking this into consideration, however, angiography permits only a two-dimensional (2-D) view of the arteries and is unable to give precise details about the vessel wall. Grayscale intravascular ultrasound (IVUS) is used along with angiography as an assessment tool to better study the vessel wall and ultimately guide treatment of coronary atherosclerotic lesions. Research enterprises in tissue characterization are seeking to develop methods that complement the information provided by grayscale IVUS in assessing the composition of plaques. Virtual Histology™ allows characterization of four different tissue types (i.e., fibrofatty tissue, necrotic core, fibrous tissue, and dense calcium tissue). This chapter will provide a contemporary review of grayscale IVUS and IVUS Virtual Histology (IVUS-VH) with particular reference to their use in the assessment of unstable lesions.

Grayscale intravascular ultrasound

For intracoronary imaging, IVUS is currently the "gold standard." IVUS provides cross-sectional images of the vessel wall,

Cardiovascular Interventions in Clinical Practice. Edited by Jürgen Haase, Hans-Joachim Schäfers, Horst Sievert and Ron Waksman. © 2010 Blackwell Publishing.

allowing the visualization of the luminal border, the atherosclerotic plaque, the media (that appears as an anechoic structure), and the hyperechoic adventitia [2]. Visual assessment of plaque echogenicity provides semiquantitative tissue characterization [3]. Calcification can be identified with a sensitivity and specificity of approximately 90%, as bright echo signals with acoustic shadowing [4]. Lipid deposits, visualized as echolucent zones, can be detected with high sensitivity (78–95%), but low specificity (30%) [5,6]. Plaques can be classified in four categories by grayscale IVUS: (1) soft plaque (lesion echogenicity less than the surrounding adventitia), (2) fibrous plaque (intermediate echogenicity between soft [echolucent] atheromas and highly echogenic calcified plaques), (3) calcified plaque (echogenicity higher than the adventitia with acoustic shadowing), and (4) mixed plaques (when they contain more than one acoustical subtype) (Fig. 31.1) [2].

Large eccentric plaques containing an echolucent zone by grayscale IVUS were associated with the development of acute coronary syndrome in a prospective study [7]. Furthermore, it has been reported also that culprit lesions in acute coronary syndromes are associated with expansive remodeling (outward expansion of the external elastic membrane). In turn, coronary lesions in patients with stable angina pectoris are associated with constrictive remodeling (reduction of external elastic membrane dimensions) [8]. Expansively remodeled plaques contain greater amounts of metalloproteinases, a critical factor in fibrous cap rupture [9]. In the following section, remodeling is explained in more detail.

Remodeling assessment

Vessel remodeling can readily be evaluated with IVUS [10–12]. Grayscale IVUS examination allows the identification of positive or outward vascular remodeling that is defined as a compensatory enlargement of the coronary artery vessel wall in response to an increase in plaque area [13]. Pathologic studies have established a relationship between positive vessel remodeling and plaque vulnerability, showing an increase

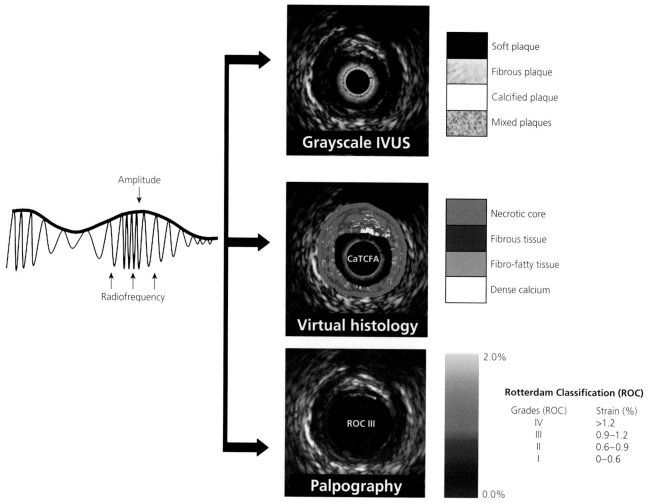

Figure 31.1 Grayscale IVUS image formed by the envelope (amplitude) of the radiofrequency signal. The frequency and power of the signal commonly differ between tissues, regardless of similarities in the amplitude. From the backscatter radiofrequency data, two different types of information can be retrieved: Virtual Histology and palpography. Using grayscale, atherosclerotic plaque can be classified into four categories: soft, fibrotic, calcified, and mixed plaques. Virtual Histology is able to detect four tissue types: necrotic core, fibrous, fibrofatty and dense calcium. Palpography plaque deformability is reported in strain values, which are subsequently categorized into four grades according to the Rotterdam Classification. Grayscale IVUS, Virtual Histology, and palpography are acquired with a single IVUS pullback.

in inflammatory marker concentrations, larger lipid cores, paucity of smooth muscle cells and medial thinning in positively remodeled vessels [14–16]. In several IVUS studies, positive vessel remodeling has been identified as one of the features associated with culprit coronary lesions [12], and is also frequently observed in ruptured plaques [17,18]. It occurs significantly more often in patients with acute coronary syndrome than in those with stable coronary artery disease [19,20]. In patients with unstable angina, outward remodeling has been defined as a significant independent predictor of major adverse cardiac events [21], and a prospective IVUS study in this group of patients observed that plaques exhibiting positive remodeling more often had thrombus or signs of rupture [22]. The remodeling pattern has also been correlated with the plaque composition. Tauth *et al.* [23] showed that soft plaques were associated with positive remodeling but that fibrocalcific

plaques more often showed constrictive remodeling. These results have been confirmed recently using IVUS radiofrequency data (RFD) analysis, a technique developed specifically for tissue characterization. Rodriguez-Granillo *et al.* [24] found a positive correlation between outward remodeling and necrotic core and a negative correlation between outward remodeling and fibrous tissue.

In conclusion, the plaques that have been associated with vulnerability in grayscale IVUS are eccentric, with hypoechoic areas and associated positive remodeling. Nevertheless, the ability of IVUS to identify plaques susceptible to rupture is limited by its axial resolution (150–200 μm), which does not allow the identification of thin fibrous caps (<65 μm) and has limited accuracy for tissue composition characterization. New IVUS-derived techniques have been developed to overcome limitations such as IVUS-VH.

Plaque rupture

Pathologic findings

Autopsy studies have shown that acute coronary syndromes result from spontaneous plaque rupture or erosion and subsequent thrombosis [25–27]. A recent pathologic study using a novel longitudinal tissue section approach reported 0.45 plaque ruptures per heart in patients who died of cardiovascular cause. Among those patients with at least one ruptured plaque, one or more additional ruptured plaques were present in almost 30% [28]. Most of these ruptured plaques were located in the proximal portions of the left anterior descending artery (LAD) and left circumflex artery (LCx), with plaques being less common and more disperse in the right coronary artery (RCA) [28].

Prevalence and distribution

Several IVUS studies have reported the frequency and distribution of plaque ruptures in the three coronary epicardial vessels. Rioufol *et al.* [29] studied 24 patients (72 arteries) with acute coronary syndrome and found a mean prevalence of two ruptured plaques per patient. Interestingly, 12.5% of these patients had ruptured plaques in the three major coronary arteries. Only 37.5% of the ruptured plaques were located on the culprit lesion, and 79% of the patients also had a ruptured plaque somewhere other than on the culprit lesion. In a similar study in 45 patients with acute myocardial infarction (AMI), plaque rupture was observed in 21 patients (47%) at the culprit site, and 17 additional plaque ruptures were found at remote sites in 11 patients (24%) [30]. Hong *et al.* [31] evaluated the incidence of plaque rupture depending on the clinical presentation. They performed three-vessel IVUS examination in 235 patients (122 with AMI and 113 with stable angina pectoris [SAP]). Plaque rupture of infarct-related or target lesions occurred in 66% of patients with AMI and in 27% of patients with SAP. Noninfarct-related or nontarget artery plaque ruptures occurred in 17% of patients with AMI and in 5% of patients with SAP. Multiple plaque ruptures were observed in 20% of patients with AMI and 6% of those with SAP. The same authors evaluated the distribution of plaque rupture in native coronary arteries in 392 patients (231 with acute coronary syndrome and 161 with SAP). Three-vessel IVUS imaging showed that plaque ruptures in the LAD occurred mainly in proximal segments (83% of LAD ruptured plaques), in the RCA occurred in the proximal and distal segments (48% and 32% of RCA ruptured plaques, respectively), and in the LCx occurred throughout the entire vessel [32]. These results are in line with another study that included 104 patients and studied 160 ruptured plaques in the LAD; the majority were located within the proximal 30 mm of the artery [33].

Pathologic studies have found that ruptured plaques are mainly located in the proximal portions of the LAD and LCx, and are more disperse in the RCA [28]. The tendency of advanced plaques to develop preferentially in these locations

has been explained by the low shear stress conditions generated in areas of tortuosity or with many branches. Low shear stress may induce the migration of lipids and monocytes into the vessel wall, leading to the progression of the lesion toward a plaque with a high risk of rupture [34].

A study aimed at characterizing plaque ruptures in the left main coronary artery (LMCA) found 16 plaque ruptures in 17 patients (two AMI, 13 unstable angina, and one SAP). The ruptures were located in the distal portion and/or bifurcation of the LMCA, often did not compromise the lumen, and had an angiographic complex appearance. When ruptured plaques involved the bifurcation of LAD and LCx, they occurred opposite the distal flow divider [35].

Ruptured atherosclerotic plaques in native coronary arteries but not in saphenous vein grafts (SVGs) have been well described with intravascular ultrasound. Preintervention IVUS of 791 SVGs found 95 ruptured plaques in 76 SVGs (73 patients), a prevalence of 9.7%. These ruptured plaques were found to be associated with complex angiographic characteristics and positive remodeling [36,37].

In an analysis of 300 ruptured plaques in 254 patients, Maehara *et al.* [17] reported that the presence of ruptured plaques detected by IVUS was strongly correlated with complex angiographic lesion morphology: ulceration in 81%, intimal flap in 40%, thrombus in 7%, and aneurysm in 7%.

Intravascular ultrasound findings in ruptured plaques

Regarding the morphologic IVUS features, different studies have confirmed that plaque ruptures occur at sites of significant plaque accumulation associated with positive remodeling and with nonsignificant lumen compromise [17,18,38]. In an analysis of 51 ruptured plaques, the empty cavity was, on average, larger in lesions associated with positive remodeling and showed a linear relation with lesion plaque and vessel size but not with the degree of narrowing [39]. It has also been reported that ruptured plaques have a more eccentric distribution [18] and that the presence of thrombus is more common among culprit lesions in patients with unstable angina or AMI and in multiple ruptures [17,40]. Ruptured plaques in culprit lesions in acute coronary syndrome are also associated with a smaller lumen, greater plaque burden and area of stenosis, and positive remodeling [40]. Gender also influences the characteristics and clinical presentation of ruptured plaques; in women, coronary plaque ruptures are more often associated with thrombus and acute presentations [41]. The tear of the rupture in the fibrous cap can be identified in approximately 60% of the cases and occurs more often at the shoulder of the plaque than in the center [17,42,43]. Recently, it has been postulated that the longitudinal location of the rupture in the plaque can be a determinant of coronary artery occlusion. In a study of 72 patients with acute coronary syndrome, patients with plaques ruptured in the proximal shoulder showed more frequently TIMI 0 in the angiogram than patients with plaques ruptured in the center of the

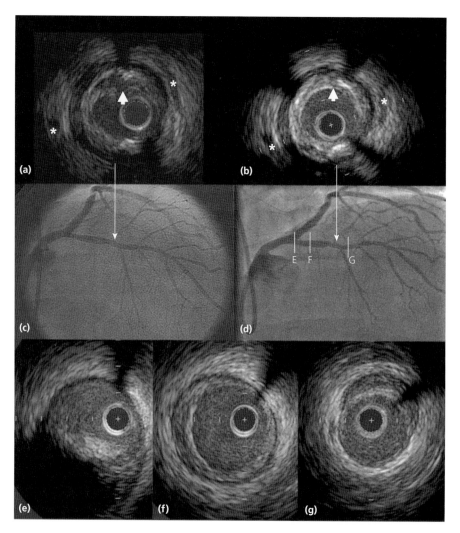

Figure 31.2 The heterogeneous nature of the atherosclerotic disease and the fate of an untreated plaque rupture. The patient presented with stable angina due to a significant lesion in the right coronary artery, which was stented (not shown). (a) A ruptured plaque. The arrowhead indicates the remnants of the fibrous cap and the entry of the cavity. (b) The healed plaque after 18 months; the arrowhead indicates the area where the rupture was. Asterisks in (a) and (b) indicate the same anatomical landmarks. (c) A grayscale IVUS pullback in the left anterior descending (LAD) artery was performed to better characterize the mild lesion present in its mid-segment. (d) The unchanged angiographic appearance of the mid-LAD after 18 months. (e) An eccentric and calcified lesion, located at the ostium of the LAD. (f) A concentric lesion in the proximal LAD. (g) An eccentric, mild lesion in the mid-LAD.

lesion or in the distal shoulder [44]. Regarding the calcification patterns, ruptured plaques had quantitatively less calcium (in particular superficial calcium) but a larger number of small (<90° arc) calcium deposits (in particular deep calcium deposits) [45].

Fate of ruptured plaques

Intravascular ultrasound also allows the study of the evolution of ruptured plaques (Fig. 31.2). Rioufol *et al.* [46] showed that approximately 50% of the ruptured plaques detected in a first acute coronary syndrome healed with medical therapy, without significant plaque modification. Hong *et al.* [47] studied the natural evolution of nonculprit/nontarget ruptured plaques and assessed the impact of statin therapy. Twenty-eight patients with nonstenotic ruptured plaques underwent IVUS examination at baseline and at 12 months' follow-up. Half of the population was treated with statins. The majority (89%) of nonculprit plaque ruptures remained stable without the need for revascularization for up to 1 year, even if the ruptured cavities did not entirely heal. Overall,

72% nonculprit/nontarget lesion plaque ruptures did not change, 17% healed completely or partially, and 11% progressed to stenosis. Lesions that progressed to require revascularization showed an increase in plaque area. This is consistent with previous pathologic studies that showed multiple layers of plaque rupture and healing within the same area, suggesting that healed ruptures may contribute to stenosis progression [48]. Complete plaque rupture healing was observed in 29% of the patients receiving statin treatment and incomplete healing was observed in the patients who did not receive statins [47].

Intravascular ultrasound-derived techniques

Intravascular ultrasound radiofrequency analysis

Palpography

Palpography allows the assessment of local mechanical tissue properties. At any given pressure, soft tissue (e.g., lipid-rich)

components will deform more than hard tissue components (e.g., fibrous, calcified) [49,50]. Radiofrequency data obtained at different pressure levels are compared to determine the local tissue deformation. Each palpogram represents the strain information for a certain cross-section over the full cardiac cycle. Palpograms are acquired using a 20-MHz phased-array IVUS catheter (Eagle Eye™ 20 MHz catheter, Volcano Therapeutics, Rancho Cordova, CA, USA). Digital radiofrequency data are acquired using the same console as for Virtual Histology (see below). The local strain is calculated from the gated radiofrequency traces, using cross-correlation analysis, and displayed in color coded form: blue for 0% strain to red to yellow for 2% strain [51]. Plaque strain values are assigned a Rotterdam Classification (ROC) score ranging from 1 to 4 (ROC I, 0 to <0.6%; ROC II, 0.6% to <0.9%; ROC III, 0.9% to <1.2%; ROC IV, ≥1.2%) (Fig. 31.1) [52].

Our group has demonstrated that palpography has a high sensitivity (88%) and specificity (89%) to detect vulnerable plaques *in vitro* [49]. Postmortem coronary arteries were investigated with intravascular elastography, and were subsequently processed for histology. There was a positive correlation between the level of strain and the degree of macrophage infiltration ($P < 0.006$), and an inverse relation between the number of smooth muscle cells and strain ($P < 0.0001$). Vulnerable plaques identified by palpography had a thinner cap than nonvulnerable plaques ($P < 0.0001$). In a subsequent study, 55 patients with either stable or unstable angina or acute myocardial infarction were analyzed. The prevalence of deformable plaques per vessel was significantly lower (0.6 ± 0.6) among patients with stable angina than in patients presenting with unstable angina (1.6 ± 0.7, $P = 0.0019$) or with acute myocardial infarction (2.0 ± 0.7, $P < 0.0001$). In the Integrated Biomarker and Imaging Study I (IBIS-I) on palpography, both the absolute number of high-strain spots (grade III/IV) in the region of interest (ROI; $P = 0.009$) and the density per centimeter ($P = 0.012$) decreased significantly between baseline and follow-up. This decrease in the overall population was largely driven by changes in the subgroup of patients with STEMI; this group had both the highest number of high-strain spots at baseline and the most marked relative decrease during follow-up compared with patients with other clinical presentations [53].

The potential value of IVUS palpography is currently under evaluation in two international multicenter prospective studies: the Providing Regional Observations to Study Predictors of Events in the Coronary Tree (PROSPECT) and Integrated Biomarker and Imaging Study II (IBIS-II) trials. These two studies have also obtained IVUS-VH during the same IVUS pullback, allowing for the assessment of both morphologic and biomechanical properties of a particular plaque. Assessing several characteristics of a given plaque could potentially enhance invasive risk stratification by identifying very high-risk plaques, thereby reducing the number of vulnerable plaques that need to be serially followed and ultimately treated (Fig. 31.1).

Shear stress mapping

Angiographic three-dimensional (3-D) reconstruction requires assumptions about the shape of the lumen cross-sections and therefore has limited applicability. The ANGUS method offers an attractive alternative for 3-D coronary artery reconstruction; this method combines high-resolution IVUS imaging and biplane angiography. In particular, the ability to reconstruct the arterial wall is of great value because this allows new *in vivo* studies relating spatial wall characteristics with hemodynamic parameters derived from computational fluid dynamics applied to the lumen reconstructions to be conducted [54,55].

In our center, we have studied the role of shear stress in the more advanced stages of atherosclerosis. To this end, we imaged 13 native coronary arteries with biplane angiography and IVUS to obtain the 3-D shape of the lumen and the vessel wall. Wall thickness data were used to identify a total of 31 plaques, and lumen data were combined with computational fluid dynamics to obtain the 3-D shear stress over the plaques. Palpography was applied to measure radial strain, which served as a surrogate marker for plaque composition. Each plaque was subdivided into four regions (upstream, throat, shoulder, and downstream), and the average normalized shear stress and strain were determined in each region. In the downstream regions, both the shear stress and the strain were lower than in the other regions. The values for upstream, shoulder, and throat did not differ significantly. However, if we combine all the low shear stress regions and determine the average strain, and do this for the medium and high shear stress regions as well, we get a strong positive correlation: low strain at low shear stress, and high strain in the regions with high shear stress. In conclusion, we found that shear stress correlates with strain, and that the shear stress a plaque is exposed to can be associated with different plaque compositions. A limitation in the application of the ANGUS method is the fact that the acquisition set-up requires biplane imaging, a sheath-based catheter type, and a motorized stepped pullback device. In addition, the current inability to incorporate side branches in the reconstruction does not allow complete vessel reconstruction.

Vasa vasorum imaging with intravascular ultrasound

The vasa vasorum is the microvascular bed responsible for nourishing a portion of the walls of arteries and veins. It is now well recognized that pathologic neovascularization occurs during plaque development, and that the resulting microvessels have abnormal spatial distributions and branching patterns. Further, this may provide an indication of lesion vulnerability [56]. There is, therefore, considerable interest in targeting the neovascular vasa vasorum as a therapeutic strategy as well as in improving understanding of the potentially deleterious effects that other angiogenically active therapies may have on the plaque vasa vasorum. Although imaging has been successful in detecting carotid artery vasa vasorum [57], at present there are no established methods of *in vivo* imaging of the vasa vasorum in coronary arteries. IVUS is one candidate imaging modality for accomplishing this. The first specifically targeted acoustic contrast agents for ultrasound molecular imaging were liquid perfluorocarbon (PFC) nanoparticle emulsions [58], followed by echogenic liposomes [59]. Later studies with targeted microbubbles also have shown promise for sensitive molecular imaging [60–64], although their relatively large size (typically in the order of microns), their susceptibility to destruction by insonant mechanical waves, and their nonlinear response render quantitation problematic.

To date, IVUS imaging of contrast agents has been limited, with the focus being to enhance lumen boundary detection [65] or to perform molecular imaging [66]. There have been several reports of extraluminal image enhancement after the bolus injection of contrast agent, which has been attributed to the presence of vasa vasorum [67]. Although these results are promising, it has yet to be established if the enhancement is associated with perivascular microvessels. The basis of this approach is to compare postcontrast injection images with a baseline image derived from a single point in the cardiac cycle. The sensitivity and robustness of this approach ultimately relys on the assumption of similarity between images acquired at the same point in the cardiac cycle and, as such, it is susceptible to a cyclical catheter vessel motion or non-uniform rotation velocity of the transducer element. This motivated the development of contrast IVUS detection techniques based on bubble-specific signatures, which are dominant at lower frequencies [68]. To this end, a prototype nonlinear IVUS contrast imaging system has been developed in our center [69]. The feasibility of subharmonic contrast intravascular ultrasound imaging was investigated using a prototype nonlinear IVUS system and the commercial contrast agent Definity™. The system employed a mechanically scanned commercial catheter with a custom transducer element fabricated to have sensitivity at both 15 and 30 MHz. Experiments were conducted at a fundamental frequency of 30 MHz (F30; 25% bandwidth), with on-axis pressures ranging from 0.12 to 0.79 MPa, as measured with a needle hydrophone. *In vitro* characterization experiments demonstrated the detection of 15-MHz subharmonic signals (SH15) when pressure levels reached 360 kPa. The formation of SH15 images was shown, with tissue signals suppressed to near the noise floor, and contrast to tissue ratios were improved by up to 30 dB relative to F30. *In vivo* experiments were performed using the atherosclerotic rabbit aorta model. After the bolus injection of contrast agent upstream of the imaging catheter, agent was detected within the aorta, vena cava, and the perivascular space. These results provide a first *in vivo* demonstration of subharmonic contrast IVUS and suggest its potential as a new technique for imaging of the vasa vasorum [69].

Virtual Histology

Description of the technique

The main technological difference between grayscale IVUS and Virtual Histology is that grayscale IVUS imaging is formed only by the envelope (amplitude) of the radiofrequency signal, discarding a considerable amount of information lying beneath and between the peaks of the signal. The frequency and power of the signal commonly differ between tissues, regardless of similarities in the amplitude (Fig. 31.1). IVUS-VH (Volcano Therapeutics) involves spectral analysis of the data to construct tissue maps that classify plaque into four major components: fibrous (green), fibrofatty (light green), necrotic core (red), and dense calcium (white) [70]. Although this classification was initially evaluated *in vitro*, more recently pre- and postprocedure IVUS-VH findings have also been correlated with pathologic atherectomy specimens, revealing good correlation for all four tissue types [71]. As assessed by IVUS-VH, the sensitivity and specificity, respectively, were 86% and 90.5% for fibrous tissue, 79.3% and 100% for fibrofatty tissue, 67.3% and 92.9% for the necrotic core, and 50% and 98.9% for dense calcium. More recently, these tissue maps have been validated *ex vivo* using, for comparison, 899 histological sections of selected regions ($n = 94$ plaques): 471 fibrous tissue, 130 fibrofatty tissue, 132 necrotic core, and 156 dense calcium tissue regions. The overall predictive accuracies were 93.5% for fibrous tissue, 94.1% for fibrofatty tissue, 95.8% for necrotic core, and 96.7% for dense calcium, with sensitivities and specificities ranging from 72% to 99%. The kappa statistic was calculated to be 0.845, indicating very high agreement with histology [72].

Data from IVUS-VH are currently acquired using a commercially available 64-element phased-array catheter (Eagle Eye™ 20 MHz catheter, Volcano Therapeutics). Using an automated pullback device, the transducer is withdrawn at a continuous speed of 0.5 mm/s up to the ostium. IVUS-VH acquisition is electrocardiogram (ECG)-gated at the R-wave peaks using a dedicated console. IVUS B-mode images are reconstructed using customized software, and contour detection is performed using cross-sectional views with semiautomatic contour detection software to provide quantitative geometrical and compositional measurements. Owing to the limitations of manual calibration [73], the radiofrequency data are normalized using a technique known as "blind deconvolution," an iterative algorithm that deconvolves the catheter transfer function from the backscatter, thus accounting for catheter-to-catheter variability [74,75].

Plaque characterization

Pathologic lesion classification is based on static images obtained from autopsy specimens. The mechanism underlying lesion progression is the subject of continuous debate. Some believe that atherosclerotic lesion progression starts with pathologic intimal thickening in which lipid accumulates in areas rich in

Table 31.1 IVUS-VH proposed lesion types.

Lesion type	Brief description
Adaptive intimal thickening	<600 µm of intima thickness
Pathologic intimal thickening	≥600 µm thickness for >20% of the circumference with fibrofatty tissue >15%, and no confluent necrotic core or dense calcium
Fibrotic plaque	Dominant fibrous tissue and no confluent necrotic core or dense calcium
Fibrocalcific plaque	>10% Confluent dense calcium with no confluent necrotic core
Fibroatheroma	>10% Confluent necrotic core not at the lumen on three consecutive frames
Thin cap fibroatheroma	>10% Confluent necrotic core at the lumen on three consecutive frames

proteoglycans (lipid pools), but no trace of necrotic core. Others believe that the earliest change of atherosclerosis is the fatty streak, also called intimal xanthoma. The earliest lesion with a necrotic core is the fibroatheroma, and this is the precursor lesion that may give rise to symptomatic heart disease. Thin-capped fibroatheroma (TCFA) is a lesion characterized by a large necrotic core containing numerous cholesterol clefts. The overlying cap is thin and rich in inflammatory cells, macrophages and T-lymphocytes, with few smooth muscle cells. Plaques prone to rupture are those with thin cap thickness, large lipid–necrotic core, and severe inflammatory infiltrate. A study by Burke *et al.* [76] identified a cut-off value for cap thickness of <65 µm for vulnerable coronary plaque definition.

Virtual Histology can potentially identify TCFAs. In addition, the progression of the disease can also be followed up. Table 31.1 outlines the Virtual Histology plaque and lesion types that are proposed based on the above pathologic data.

Our group evaluated the incidence of IVUS-derived thin-cap fibroatheroma (IDTCFA) using IVUS-VH [77]. Two independent IVUS analysts defined IDTCFA as a lesion fulfilling the following criteria in at least three consecutive cross-sectional areas: (1) necrotic core ≥10% without evident overlying fibrous tissue, and (2) lumen obstruction ≥40%. In this study, 62% of patients had at least one IDTCFA in the interrogated vessels. The number of IDTCFAs per coronory artery was significantly higher in patients with acute coronary syndrome than in stable patients: 3.0 (interquartile range [IQR] 0.0–5.0) versus 1.0 (IQR 0.0–2.8) (*P* = 0.018). Finally, a clear clustering pattern was seen along the coronary arteries, with 66.7% of all IDTCFAs located in the first 20 mm, whereas further along the vessels the incidence was significantly lower (33.3%, *P* = 0.008). This distribution of IDTCFAs is consistent with previous *ex vivo* and clinical studies, with a clear clustering pattern from the ostium demonstrating a nonuniform distribution of vulnerable plaques along the coronary tree [78]. Patients presenting with acute coronary syndrome had a significantly higher prevalence of IDTCFA even in nonculprit vessels, supporting the concept of a multifocal process [79]. Of note, the proportion of the lesion area affected by stenosis and the mean area of necrotic core of the IDTCFAs detected by IVUS-VH were also similar to previously reported histopatho-logic data (55.9% vs. 59.6% and 19% vs. 23%, respectively) [80].

We have developed software to quantify the amount of necrotic core in contact with the lumen, enabling refinement of our analysis. Our current definition of an IVUS-derived TCFA is a lesion fulfilling the following criteria in at least three consecutive cross-sectional areas (CSAs): (1) plaque burden of ≥40% and (2) confluent necrotic core of ≥10% in direct contact with the lumen (i.e. no visible overlying tissue) in the investigated CSA. All consecutive CSAs having the same morphologic characteristics are considered as part of the same IDTCFA lesion [81]. In a study using this refined definition of TCFA, as assessed by IVUS-VH, in patients with acute coronary syndrome who underwent IVUS of all three epicardial coronaries, there were, on average, two IVUS-derived TCFAs per patient, with half of them showing outward remodeling (Fig. 31.3) [81].

The PROSPECT (Providing Regional Observations to Study Predictors of Events in the Coronary Tree) trial is a first-of-its-kind multicenter, natural history study of acute coronary syndrome (ACS) patients. All patients underwent PCI in their culprit lesion at baseline. Following the PCI procedure, an angiogram and a detailed IVUS (including virtual histology and palpography) image was captured in the three major coronary arteries. Patients were clinically followed up for three years.

The highest risk PROSPECT plaque type being VH Thin Cap Fibroatheromas with a minimum lumen area of ≤4 mm^2 and a large plaque burden (≥70%), had a 17.2% likelihood of causing an event within 3 years [HR 10.8 (95% CI 4.3–27.2), *P* < 0.001].

Lipoprotein-associated phospholipase A$_2$ (Lp-PLA$_2$) is expressed abundantly in the necrotic core of coronary lesions and products of its enzymatic activity may contribute to inflammation and cell death, rendering plaque vulnerable to rupture.

IBIS 2 study compared the effects of 12 months of treatment with darapladib (oral Lp-PLA$_2$ inhibitor, 160 mg daily) or placebo on coronary atheroma deformability (IVUS-palpography) and plasma hsCRP in 330 patients with angiographically documented coronary disease. Secondary end-points included changes in necrotic core size (IVUS-VH), atheroma size

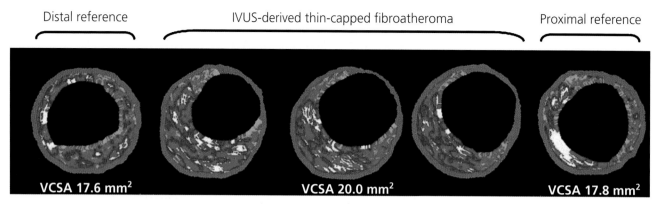

Distal reference | IVUS-derived thin-capped fibroatheroma | Proximal reference

VCSA 17.6 mm²   VCSA 20.0 mm²   VCSA 17.8 mm²

Figure 31.3 An IVUS-derived thin capped fibroatheroma is shown in the three central frames. Of note, a considerable amount of confluent necrotic core (red) is adjacent to the lumen. The vessel cross-sectional area (VCSA) at the frame with the minimum luminal area (MLA) is 20 mm². Within side branches, the two least diseased frames, one proximal and one distal, were found. The remodeling index is calculated as follows: VCSA at the MLA site divided by the mean VCSA of the two reference frames. In this example, the remodeling index is 1.13.

(IVUS-grayscale), and blood biomarkers. Background therapy was comparable between groups, with no difference in LDL-cholesterol at 12 months (placebo: 88 ± 34 and darapladib: 84 ± 31 mg/dL, $P = 0.37$). In contrast, Lp-PLA$_2$ activity was inhibited by 59% with darapladib ($P < 0.001$ versus placebo). After 12 months, there were no significant differences between groups in plaque deformability ($P = 0.22$) or plasma hsCRP ($P = 0.35$). In the placebo-treated group, however, necrotic core volume increased significantly, whereas darapladib halted this increase, resulting in a significant treatment difference of −5.2 mm³ ($P = 0.012$). These intra-plaque compositional changes occurred without a significant treatment difference in total atheroma volume ($P = 0.95$). Despite adherence to a high level of standard of care treatment, the necrotic core continued to expand among patients receiving placebo. In contrast, Lp-PLA$_2$ inhibition with darapladib prevented necrotic core expansion [82].

Virtual Histology and plaque rupture

Our group [83] described the ruptured plaque profile as assessed by IVUS-VH in a prospective study of 40 patients referred for cardiac catheterization (Fig. 31.4). There were 13 patients with stable angina, 12 with unstable angina, and 15 with acute myocardial infarction. The risk factors were fairly typical of patients with coronary artery disease: 10% of patients had diabetes, 73% were male, 38% were smokers, and 50% had elevated cholesterol. Although three-vessel IVUS was the goal in all patients, only two-vessel characterization was possible in 9 of the 40 patients. Ruptured plaque was identified in 26 patients and, as expected, was more frequent in patients with acute myocardial infarction and unstable angina. Patients with ruptured plaques had a larger body mass index than those without plaque rupture and were more likely to be smokers, and patients with ruptures had more widespread calcification and a larger area of necrotic core. Of note, the location of plaque ruptures in this study mirrors the pathologic findings [83]. In our study, the LAD was the most common

site of plaque rupture, in which it was usually proximal, whereas in the RCA, rupture was as frequently found mid-artery as in the proximal segment. In a pathologic series of 79 ruptures, Burke *et al.* [84] found that, out of 34 ruptures in the LAD, 25 (74%) were in the proximal segment. In contrast, out of 28 ruptures in the RCA, only 10 (36%) were in the proximal segment, 12 in the mid-artery, and six in the distal segment. Similarly, in pathologic studies and in our study, in the LCx only one-fourth were located in the proximal part, with the rest located distally or in the obtuse marginal branches.

Virtual Histology and coronary embolization

Identification of subclinical high-risk plaques is potentially important because they may be more likely to rupture and result in thrombosis. In 55 patients, a nonculprit vessel with <50% diameter stenosis was studied with IVUS-VH. Mean necrotic core percentage was significantly higher in patients with acute coronary syndrome than in stable patients (12.26% ± 7.0% vs. 7.40% ± 5.5%, $P = 0.006$). In addition, stable patients showed more fibrotic vessels (70.97% ± 9.3% vs. 63.96% ± 9.1%, $P = 0.007$) [85]. However, not only is the amount of necrotic core content larger in patients with acute coronary syndrome, but it appears that necrotic core is also unevenly distributed. In 51 consecutive patients, a nonculprit vessel was investigated using IVUS-VH. The overall length of the region of interest, subsequently divided into 10-mm segments, was 41.5 ± 13 mm. No significant change was observed in terms of relative plaque composition along the vessel with respect to fibrous, fibrofatty, and calcified tissue, whereas the percentage of necrotic core was higher in the first (median 8.75%; IQR 5.7–18) than in the third (median 6.1%; IQR 3.2–12) ($P = 0.036$) and fourth (median 4.5%; IQR 2.4–7.9) ($P = 0.006$) segments. At multivariable regression analysis, distance from the ostium was an independent predictor of relative necrotic content (beta = −0.28 [95% CI −0.15 to −0.41]), together with older age, unstable presentation, no use of statins, and the presence of diabetes mellitus [86].

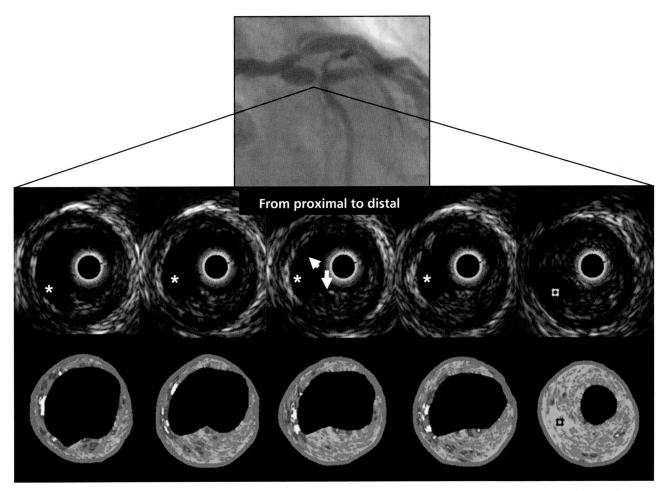

Figure 31.4 This figure shows the grayscale IVUS appearance and IVUS-VH tissue composition of a ruptured plaque in the proximal left anterior descending coronary artery. The grayscale IVUS frames show the cavity (*) of the rupture and the remnants of the fibrous cap and the entry of the cavity (white arrows). The grayscale IVUS and IVUS-VH frames on the right hand side show the presence of thrombus (□) that in IVUS-VH is misclassified as fibrofatty.

Recently, two studies have evaluated the usefulness of IVUS-VH plaque composition to predict the risk of embolization during stenting [87,88]. One included 71 patients with STEMI who underwent primary PCI within 12 h of onset of the symptoms. After crossing the lesion with a guidewire and performing thrombectomy with an aspiration catheter, IVUS-VH of the infarct-related vessel was performed. The stent was then deployed without embolic protection. During stenting, ST segment re-elevation was used as a marker of distal embolization. Eleven patients presented with ST segment re-elevation after stenting. Total plaque volume was similar in both groups, but the necrotic core volume was significantly higher in the group of patients with ST segment re-elevation ($32.9 \pm 14.1 \, \text{mm}^3$ vs. $20.4 \pm 19.1 \, \text{mm}^3$, $P < 0.05$). On receiver operating characteristic curves, necrotic core volume was a better predictor of ST re-elevation after stent deployment than fibrous, fibrofatty, dense calcium, and total plaque volumes. The cut-off point for necrotic core volume that was highly predictive for ST re-elevation was $33.4 \, \text{mm}^3$, with a sensitivity of 81.7% and a specificity of 63.6%. The second study included 44 patients who underwent elective coronary stenting. Plaque composition was assessed with IVUS-VH, and small embolic particles liberated during stenting were detected as high-intensity transient signals (HITS) with a Doppler guidewire. Patients were divided into the tertiles according to the HITS counts. Dense calcium and necrotic core area were significantly larger in the highest tertile. In the multivariate logistic regression analysis, only necrotic core area was an independent predictor of high HITS counts (odds ratio 4.41, $P = 0.045$).

Conclusion

Currently the main purpose of grayscale intravascular ultrasound and Virtual Histology is to improve our understanding of atherosclerotic disease and to define its natural history. Ultimately, the aim is to identify patients at high risk for future cardiovascular events and to evaluate the benefits of either local or systemic therapeutic interventions.

Virtual Histology appears to be very promising and its predictive role is presently under investigation in large international trials.

References

1. Goldstein JA, Demetriou D, Grines CL, Pica M, Shoukfeh M, & O'Neill WW (2000) Multiple complex coronary plaques in patients with acute myocardial infarction. *N Engl J Med* **343**:915–922.

2. Mintz GS, Nissen SE, Anderson WD, *et al.* (2001) American College of Cardiology Clinical Expert Consensus Document on Standards for Acquisition, Measurement and Reporting of Intravascular Ultrasound Studies (IVUS). A report of the American College of Cardiology Task Force on Clinical Expert Consensus Documents. *J Am Coll Cardiol* **37**:1478–1492.

3. Aoki J, Abizaid AC, Serruys PW, *et al.* (2005) Evaluation of four-year coronary artery response after sirolimus-eluting stent implantation using serial quantitative intravascular ultrasound and computer-assisted grayscale value analysis for plaque composition in event-free patients. *J Am Coll Cardiol* **46**:1670–1676.

4. Di Mario C, The SH, Madretsma S, *et al.* (1992) Detection and characterization of vascular lesions by intravascular ultrasound: an in vitro study correlated with histology. *J Am Soc Echocardiogr* **5**:135–146.

5. Potkin BN, Bartorelli AL, Gessert JM, *et al.* (1990) Coronary artery imaging with intravascular high-frequency ultrasound. *Circulation* **81**:1575–1585.

6. Rasheed Q, Dhawale PJ, Anderson J, & Hodgson JM (1995) Intracoronary ultrasound-defined plaque composition: computer-aided plaque characterization and correlation with histologic samples obtained during directional coronary atherectomy. *Am Heart J* **129**:631–637.

7. Yamagishi M, Terashima M, Awano K, *et al.* (2000) Morphology of vulnerable coronary plaque: insights from follow-up of patients examined by intravascular ultrasound before an acute coronary syndrome. *J Am Coll Cardiol* **35**:106–111.

8. Schoenhagen P, Ziada KM, Kapadia SR, Crowe TD, Nissen SE, & Tuzcu EM (2000) Extent and direction of arterial remodeling in stable versus unstable coronary syndromes: an intravascular ultrasound study. *Circulation* **101**:598–603.

9. Schoenhagen P, Vince DG, Ziada KM, *et al.* (2002) Relation of matrix-metalloproteinase 3 found in coronary lesion samples retrieved by directional coronary atherectomy to intravascular ultrasound observations on coronary remodeling. *Am J Cardiol* **89**:1354–1359.

10. Nakamura M, Nishikawa H, Mukai S, *et al.* (2001) Impact of coronary artery remodeling on clinical presentation of coronary artery disease: an intravascular ultrasound study. *J Am Coll Cardiol* **37**:63–69.

11. Maehara A, Mintz GS, Bui AB, *et al.* (2002) Morphologic and angiographic features of coronary plaque rupture detected by intravascular ultrasound. *J Am Coll Cardiol* **40**:904–910.

12. Kotani J, Mintz GS, Castagna MT, *et al.* (2003) Intravascular ultrasound analysis of infarct-related and non-infarct-related arteries in patients who presented with an acute myocardial infarction. *Circulation* **107**:2889–2893.

13. Glagov S, Weisenberg E, Zarins CK, Stankunavicius R, & Kolettis GJ (1987) Compensatory enlargement of human atherosclerotic coronary arteries. *N Engl J Med* **316**:1371–1375.

14. Pasterkamp G, Schoneveld AH, van der Wal AC, *et al.* (1998) Relation of arterial geometry to luminal narrowing and histologic markers for plaque vulnerability: the remodeling paradox. *J Am Coll Cardiol* **32**:655–662.

15. Varnava AM, Mills PG, & Davies MJ (2002) Relationship between coronary artery remodeling and plaque vulnerability. *Circulation* **105**:939–943.

16. Burke AP, Kolodgie FD, Farb A, Weber D, & Virmani R (2002) Morphological predictors of arterial remodeling in coronary atherosclerosis. *Circulation* **105**:297–303.

17. Maehara A, Mintz GS, Bui AB, *et al.* (2002) Morphologic and angiographic features of coronary plaque rupture detected by intravascular ultrasound. *J Am Coll Cardiol* **40**:904–910.

18. von Birgelen C, Klinkhart W, Mintz GS, *et al.* (2001) Plaque distribution and vascular remodeling of ruptured and nonruptured coronary plaques in the same vessel: an intravascular ultrasound study in vivo. *J Am Coll Cardiol* **37**:1864–1870.

19. Jeremias A, Spies C, Herity NA, *et al.* (2000) Coronary artery compliance and adaptive vessel remodelling in patients with stable and unstable coronary artery disease. *Heart* **84**:314–319.

20. Nakamura M, Nishikawa H, Mukai S, *et al.* (2001) Impact of coronary artery remodeling on clinical presentation of coronary artery disease: an intravascular ultrasound study. *J Am Coll Cardiol* **37**:63–69.

21. Gyongyosi M, Yang P, Hassan A, *et al.* (2000) Intravascular ultrasound predictors of major adverse cardiac events in patients with unstable angina. *Clin Cardiol* **23**:507–515.

22. Gyongyosi M, Yang P, Hassan A, *et al.* (1999) Arterial remodelling of native human coronary arteries in patients with unstable angina pectoris: a prospective intravascular ultrasound study. *Heart* **82**:68–74.

23. Tauth J, Pinnow E, Sullebarger JT, *et al.* (1997) Predictors of coronary arterial remodeling patterns in patients with myocardial ischemia. *Am J Cardiol* **80**:1352–1355.

24. Rodriguez-Granillo GA, Serruys PW, Garcia-Garcia HM, *et al.* (2006) Coronary artery remodelling is related to plaque composition. *Heart* **92**:388–391.

25. Virmani R, Kolodgie FD, Burke AP, Farb A, & Schwartz SM (2000) Lessons from sudden coronary death: a comprehensive morphological classification scheme for atherosclerotic lesions. *Arterioscler Thromb Vasc Biol* **20**:1262–1275.

26. Davies MJ & Thomas A (1984) Thrombosis and acute coronary-artery lesions in sudden cardiac ischemic death. *N Engl J Med* **310**:1137–1140.

27. Farb A, Burke AP, Tang AL, *et al.* (1996) Coronary plaque erosion without rupture into a lipid core. A frequent cause of coronary thrombosis in sudden coronary death. *Circulation* **93**:1354–1363.

28. Cheruvu PK, Finn AV, Gardner C, *et al.* (2007) Frequency and distribution of thin-cap fibroatheroma and ruptured plaques in human coronary arteries: a pathologic study. *J Am Coll Cardiol* **50**:940–949.

29. Rioufol G, Finet G, Ginon I, *et al.* (2002) Multiple atherosclerotic plaque rupture in acute coronary syndrome: a three-vessel intravascular ultrasound study. *Circulation* **106**:804–808.

30. Tanaka A, Shimada K, Sano T, *et al.* (2005) Multiple plaque rupture and C-reactive protein in acute myocardial infarction. *J Am Coll Cardiol* **45**:1594–1599.

31. Hong MK, Mintz GS, Lee CW, *et al.* (2004) Comparison of coronary plaque rupture between stable angina and acute myocardial infarction: a three-vessel intravascular ultrasound study in 235 patients. *Circulation* **110**:928–933.

32. Hong MK, Mintz GS, Lee CW, *et al.* (2005) The site of plaque rupture in native coronary arteries: a three-vessel intravascular ultrasound analysis. *J Am Coll Cardiol* **46**:261–265.

33. Pregowski J, Tyczynski P, Mintz GS, *et al.* (2006) Intravascular ultrasound assessment of the spatial distribution of ruptured coronary plaques in the left anterior descending coronary artery. *Am Heart J* **151**:898–901.

34. Cunningham KS & Gotlieb AI (2005) The role of shear stress in the pathogenesis of atherosclerosis. *Lab Invest* **85**:9–23.

35. Tyczynski P, Pregowski J, Mintz GS, *et al.* (2005) Intravascular ultrasound assessment of ruptured atherosclerotic plaques in left main coronary arteries. *Am J Cardiol* **96**:794–798.

36. Pregowski J, Tyczynski P, Mintz GS, *et al.* (2005) Incidence and clinical correlates of ruptured plaques in saphenous vein grafts: an intravascular ultrasound study. *J Am Coll Cardiol* **45**:1974–1979.

37. Pregowski J, Tyczynski P, Mintz GS, *et al.* (2006) Comparison of ruptured plaques in native coronary arteries and in saphenous vein grafts: an intravascular ultrasound study. *Am J Cardiol* **97**:593–597.

38. Fujii K, Mintz GS, Carlier SG, *et al.* (2006) Intravascular ultrasound profile analysis of ruptured coronary plaques. *Am J Cardiol* **98**:429–435.

39. von Birgelen C, Klinkhart W, Mintz GS, *et al.* (2000) Size of emptied plaque cavity following spontaneous rupture is related to coronary dimensions, not to the degree of lumen narrowing. A study with intravascular ultrasound in vivo. *Heart* **84**:483–488.

40. Fujii K, Kobayashi Y, Mintz GS, *et al.* (2003) Intravascular ultrasound assessment of ulcerated ruptured plaques: a comparison of culprit and nonculprit lesions of patients with acute coronary syndromes and lesions in patients without acute coronary syndromes. *Circulation* **108**:2473–2478.

41. Kruk M, Pregowski J, Mintz GS, *et al.* (2007) Intravascular ultrasonic study of gender differences in ruptured coronary plaque morphology and its associated clinical presentation. *Am J Cardiol* **100**:185–189.

42. Jensen LO, Mintz GS, Carlier SG, *et al.* (2006) Intravascular ultrasound assessment of fibrous cap remnants after coronary plaque rupture. *Am Heart J* **152**:327–332.

43. Ge J, Chirillo F, Schwedtmann J, *et al.* (1999) Screening of ruptured plaques in patients with coronary artery disease by intravascular ultrasound. *Heart* **81**:621–627.

44. Tanaka A, Shimada K, Namba M, *et al.* (2008) Relationship between longitudinal morphology of ruptured plaques and TIMI flow grade in acute coronary syndrome: a three-dimensional intravascular ultrasound imaging study. *Eur Heart J* **29**:38–44.

45. Fujii K, Carlier SG, Mintz GS, *et al.* (2005) Intravascular ultrasound study of patterns of calcium in ruptured coronary plaques. *Am J Cardiol* **96**:352–357.

46. Rioufol G, Gilard M, Finet G, Ginon I, Boschat J, & Andre-Fouet X (2004) Evolution of spontaneous atherosclerotic plaque rupture with medical therapy: long-term follow-up with intravascular ultrasound. *Circulation* **110**:2875–2880.

47. Hong MK, Mintz GS, Lee CW, *et al.* (2007) Serial intravascular ultrasound evidence of both plaque stabilization and lesion progression in patients with ruptured coronary plaques: effects of statin therapy on ruptured coronary plaque. *Atherosclerosis* **191**:107–114.

48. Burke AP, Kolodgie FD, Farb A, *et al.* (2001) Healed plaque ruptures and sudden coronary death: evidence that subclinical rupture has a role in plaque progression. *Circulation* **103**:934–940.

49. Schaar JA, de Korte CL, Mastik F, *et al.* (2003) Characterizing vulnerable plaque features with intravascular elastography. *Circulation* **108**:2636–2641.

50. Schaar JA, Regar E, Mastik F, *et al.* (2004) Incidence of high-strain patterns in human coronary arteries: assessment with three-dimensional intravascular palpography and correlation with clinical presentation. *Circulation* **109**:2716–2719.

51. de Korte CL, Carlier SG, Mastik F, *et al.* (2002) Morphological and mechanical information of coronary arteries obtained with intravascular elastography: feasibility study in vivo. *Eur Heart J* **23**:405–413.

52. van Mieghem CAG, Bruining N, Schaar JA, *et al.* (2005) Rationale and methods of the integrated biomarker and imaging study (IBIS): combining invasive and non-invasive imaging with biomarkers to detect subclinical atherosclerosis and assess coronary lesion biology. *Int J Cardiovasc Imaging* (formerly Cardiac Imaging) **21**:425–441.

53. Van Mieghem CA, McFadden EP, de Feyter PJ, *et al.* (2006) Noninvasive detection of subclinical coronary atherosclerosis coupled with assessment of changes in plaque characteristics using novel invasive imaging modalities: the Integrated Biomarker and Imaging Study (IBIS). *J Am Coll Cardiol* **47**:1134–1142.

54. Krams R, Wentzel JJ, Oomen JA, *et al.* (1997) Evaluation of endothelial shear stress and 3D geometry as factors determining the development of atherosclerosis and remodeling in human coronary arteries in vivo. Combining 3D reconstruction from angiography and IVUS (ANGUS) with computational fluid dynamics. *Arterioscler Thromb Vasc Biol* **17**:2061–2065.

55. Slager CJ, Wentzel JJ, Schuurbiers JC, *et al.* (2000) True 3-dimensional reconstruction of coronary arteries in patients by fusion of angiography and IVUS (ANGUS) and its quantitative validation. *Circulation* **102**:511–516.

56. Moreno PR, Purushothaman KR, Fuster V, *et al.* (2004) Plaque neovascularization is increased in ruptured atherosclerotic lesions of human aorta: implications for plaque vulnerability. *Circulation* **110**:2032–2038.

57. Kerwin W, Hooker A, Spilker M, *et al.* (2003) Quantitative magnetic resonance imaging analysis of neovasculature volume in carotid atherosclerotic plaque. *Circulation* **107**:851–856.

58. Lanza GM, Wallace KD, Scott MJ, *et al.* (1996) A novel site-targeted ultrasonic contrast agent with broad biomedical application. *Circulation* **94**:3334–3340.

59. Alkan-Onyuksel H, Demos SM, Lanza GM, *et al.* (1996) Development of inherently echogenic liposomes as an ultrasonic contrast agent. *J Pharm Sci* **85**:486–490.

60. Klibanov AL, Hughes MS, Marsh JN, *et al.* (1997) Targeting of ultrasound contrast material. An in vitro feasibility study. *Acta Radiol Suppl.* **412**:113–120.

61. Villanueva FS, Jankowski RJ, Klibanov S, *et al.* (1998) Microbubbles targeted to intercellular adhesion molecule-1 bind to activated coronary artery endothelial cells. *Circulation* **98**:1–5.

62. Lindner JR, Song J, Xu F, *et al.* (2000) Noninvasive ultrasound imaging of inflammation using microbubbles targeted to activated leukocytes. *Circulation* **102**:2745–2750.

63. Lindner JR, Dayton PA, Coggins MP, *et al.* (2000) Noninvasive imaging of inflammation by ultrasound detection of phagocytosed microbubbles. *Circulation* **102**:531–538.

64. Leong-Poi H, Christiansen J, Klibanov AL, Kaul S, & Lindner JR (2003) Noninvasive assessment of angiogenesis by ultrasound and microbubbles targeted to alpha(v)-integrins. *Circulation* **107**:455–460.

65. Cachard C, Finet G, Bouakaz A, Tabib A, Francon D, & Gimenez G (1997) Ultrasound contrast agent in intravascular echography: an in vitro study. *Ultrasound Med Biol* **23**:705–717.

66. Hamilton AJ, Huang SL, Warnick D, *et al.* (2004) Intravascular ultrasound molecular imaging of atheroma components in vivo. *J Am Coll Cardiol* **43**:453–460.

67. Carlier S, Kakadiaris IA, Dib N, *et al.* (2005) Vasa vasorum imaging: a new window to the clinical detection of vulnerable atherosclerotic plaques. *Curr Atheroscler Rep* **7**:164–169.

68. de Jong N, Bouakaz A, & Ten Cate FJ (2002) Contrast harmonic imaging. *Ultrasonics* **40**(1–8):567–573.

69. Goertz DE, Frijlink ME, Tempel D, *et al.* (2007) Subharmonic contrast intravascular ultrasound for vasa vasorum imaging. *Ultrasound Med Biol* **33**:1859–1872.

70. Nair A, Kuban BD, Tuzcu EM, Schoenhagen P, Nissen SE, & Vince DG (2002) Coronary plaque classification with intravascular ultrasound radiofrequency data analysis. *Circulation* **106**:2200–2206.

71. Nasu K, Tsuchikane E, Katoh O, *et al.* (2006) Accuracy of in vivo coronary plaque morphology assessment: a validation study of in vivo Virtual Histology compared with in vitro histopathology. *J Am Coll Cardiol* **47**:2405–2412.

72. Nair A MP, Kuban BD, & Vince DG (2007) Automated coronary plaque characterization with intravascular ultrasound backscatter: ex vivo validation. *Eurointervention* **3**:113–130.

73. Rodriguez-Granillo GA, Aoki J, Ong AT, *et al.* (2005) Methodological considerations and approach to cross-technique comparisons using in vivo coronary plaque characterization based on intravascular ultrasound radiofrequency data analysis: insights from the Integrated Biomarker and Imaging Study (IBIS). *Int J Cardiovasc Intervent* **7**:52–58.

74. Kaaresen K (1997) Deconvolution of sparse spike trains by iterated window maximization. *IEEE Trans Signal Process* **45**:1173–1183.

75. Kaaresen K & Bolviken E (1999) Blind deconvolution of ultrasonic traces accounting for pulse variance. *IEEE Trans Ultrason Ferroelectr Freq Control* **46**:564–573.

76. Burke AP, Farb A, Malcom GT, Liang YH, Smialek J, & Virmani R (1997) Coronary risk factors and plaque morphology in men with coronary disease who died suddenly. *N Engl J Med* **336**:1276–1282.

77. Rodriguez-Granillo GA, Garcia-Garcia HM, Mc Fadden EP, *et al.* (2005) In vivo intravascular ultrasound-derived thin-cap fibroatheroma detection using ultrasound radiofrequency data analysis. *J Am Coll Cardiol* **46**:2038–2042.

78. Wang JC, Normand SL, Mauri L, & Kuntz RE (2004) Coronary artery spatial distribution of acute myocardial infarction occlusions. *Circulation* **110**:278–284.

79. Rioufol G, Finet G, Ginon I, *et al.* (2002) Multiple atherosclerotic plaque rupture in acute coronary syndrome: a three-vessel intravascular ultrasound study 10.1161/01.CIR.0000025609. 13806.31. *Circulation* **106**:804–808.

80. Virmani R, Burke AP, Kolodgie FD, & Farb A (2002) Vulnerable plaque: the pathology of unstable coronary lesions. *J Interv Cardiol* **15**:439–446.

81. Garcia-Garcia HM, Goedhart D, Schuurbiers JC, *et al.* (2006) Virtual Histology and remodeling index allow in vivo identification of allegedly high risk coronary plaques in patients with acute coronary syndromes: a three vessel intravascular ultrasound radiofrequency data analysis. *Eurointervention* **2**:338–344.

82. Serruys PW, Garcia-Garcia HM, Buszman P, *et al.* (2008) Effects of the direct lipoprotein-associated phospholipase A(2) inhibitor darapladib on human coronary atherosclerotic plaque. *Circulation* **118**:1172–1182.

83. Rodriguez-Granillo GA, Garcia-Garcia HM, Valgimigli M, *et al.* (2006) Global characterization of coronary plaque rupture phenotype using three-vessel intravascular ultrasound radiofrequency data analysis. *Eur Heart J* **27**:1921–1927.

84. Burke AP, Joner M, & Virmani R (2006) IVUS-VH: a predictor of plaque morphology? *Eur Heart J* **27**:1889–1890.

85. Rodriguez-Granillo GA, McFadden EP, Valgimigli M, *et al.* (2006) Coronary plaque composition of nonculprit lesions, assessed by in vivo intracoronary ultrasound radio frequency data analysis, is related to clinical presentation. *Am Heart J* **151**:1020–1024.

86. Valgimigli M, Rodriguez-Granillo GA, Garcia-Garcia HM, *et al.* (2006) Distance from the ostium as an independent determinant of coronary plaque composition in vivo: an intravascular ultrasound study based radiofrequency data analysis in humans. *Eur Heart J* **27**:655–663.

87. Kawaguchi R, Oshima S, Jingu M, *et al.* (2007) Usefulness of virtual histology intravascular ultrasound to predict distal embolization for ST-segment elevation myocardial infarction. *J Am Coll Cardiol* **50**:1641–1646.

88. Kawamoto T, Okura H, Koyama Y, *et al.* (2007) The relationship between coronary plaque characteristics and small embolic particles during coronary stent implantation. *J Am Coll Cardiol* **50**:1635–1640.

32 Optical Coherence Tomography of the Unstable Coronary Lesion

Ron Waksman & Tina L. Pinto Slottow

Washington Hospital Center, Washington, DC, USA

Most cardiac events are triggered by the rupture of vulnerable plaque, frequently at nonobstructive locations in the coronary tree [1–5]. These lesions are characterized by the presence of (1) lipid-rich cores, (2) thin, fibrous caps <65 μm thick, and (3) activated macrophages [1–4,6]. Postmortem studies demonstrate that most fatal acute coronary events occur at the site of a ruptured, macrophage-rich, thin-capped fibroatheroma (TCFA), with a minority due to endothelial erosion [1–4,7,8]. Not all TCFAs will rupture, but, as yet, what instigates plaque rupture in one site as opposed to another is unknown.

Identification and visualization of unstable atherosclerotic plaque is the key to achieving an improved understanding of vulnerable plaque. The ultimate goals are to accurately risk-stratify patients, to target therapy to appropriate areas of vulnerable plaque, and thus to prevent events. Noninvasive imaging modalities, such as multidetector-row computed tomography coronary angiography, and magnetic resonance imaging (MRI), have been limited in resolution when compared with invasive methods, and are poor at imaging distal vessels [9–11]. Likewise, angiography has a resolution of >500 μm and does not allow one to visualize the components of atherosclerotic plaque [12].

A number of invasive imaging modalities are currently in use (intravascular ultrasound [IVUS] and angioscopy) or under investigation (optical coherence tomography [OCT], intracoronary thermography, near-infrared spectroscopy, and intracoronary MRI) for the evaluation of vulnerable plaque. This chapter examines the recently developed, high-resolution technology OCT.

Theory

Optical coherence tomography is an optical analog of IVUS that measures the intensity of reflected light waves and translates these optical echoes into a high-resolution two-dimensional (2D) tomographic image. It was originally designed for use in

transparent tissues, such as those present in the eye, but was found capable of imaging nontransparent tissue through the use of longer wavelength light, which augmented imaging penetration depth [9,11,13]. OCT has the highest resolution of any vascular imaging modality, ranging from 4 to 20 μm, an order of magnitude higher than possible with IVUS [10]. The mathematical principles behind OCT have been well described by Brezinski et al. [11] and Patel et al. [14].

Low-coherence, near-infrared light emanates from a superluminescent diode and is split in half, with part directed toward the tissue sample of interest and part toward a revolving mirror (Fig. 32.1). The wavelength used is approximately 1300 nm, which minimizes absorption of the light waves by water, protein, lipids, and hemoglobin [15]. Light is reflected by the tissue's microstructures and by the mirror toward a detector. As the speed of light is too rapid to measure the echo delay electronically, coherence interferometry is used. When the distance to the tissue and the mirror is identical, light reflected back experiences interference. The detector measures the intensity of the interference as the beams recombine and uses this information to create an image. The motion of the mirror enables reflected intensity to be measured at different depths within the arterial wall [11,13]. Low-coherence interferometry allows echo time delay to be calculated with high accuracy [9]. Low energies of the order of 5–8 mW are applied, so no tissue damage has been demonstrated [15].

As an invasive imaging technique OCT has multiple advantages beyond its excellent resolution. The benefit of a high data acquisition rate (currently 4–8 frames/s) is that it allows real-time imaging. Also, unlike IVUS, OCT can see beyond calcified plaque. It can visualize the intima because of its high resolution, a feature unique to this technology [10]. As the catheter does not require a transducer, but simply an optical fiber, lens, and prism to direct light, the imaging guidewire is small (0.017 inches) and inexpensive [9].

In vitro studies

Optical coherence tomography was first demonstrated to be a feasible tool for vascular imaging by Brezinski and colleagues

Cardiovascular Interventions in Clinical Practice. Edited by Jürgen Haase, Hans-Joachim Schäfers, Horst Sievert and Ron Waksman. © 2010 Blackwell Publishing.

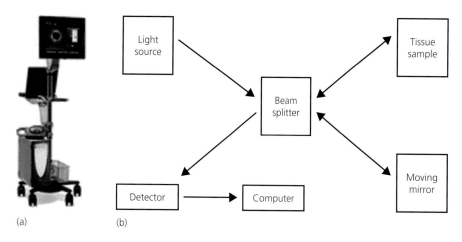

(a)   (b)

Figure 32.1 (a) Photograph of a LightLab optical coherence tomography (OCT) system [37]. (b) OCT schematic [37].

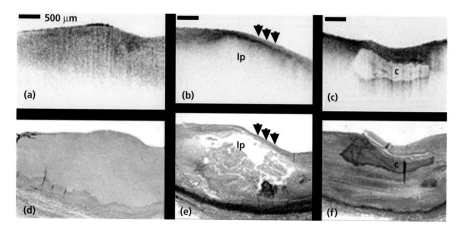

(a)   (b)   (c)

(d)   (e)   (f)

Figure 32.2 Correlation between optical coherence tomography (OCT) images (a–c) and histologic images of postmortem coronary plaques (d–f). Fibrous plaque is shown in (a) and (d), lipid pool (lp) and thin cap (arrows) in (b) and (e), and an area of calcification (C) in (c) and (f) [38].

in the early 1990s when a left anterior descending coronary artery from a cadaver was scanned successfully, and the images obtained corresponded well with the histopathology [16]. Examining postmortem aortas, they discovered that OCT produced a sharp delineation between lipid- and water-based tissues, unlike ultrasound, owing to differences in the amount of reflectivity. As infrared light is less strongly reflected by calcified tissues, it was also possible to image beyond calcified areas of atherosclerotic plaque. Intimal thickness was easily measurable, and fine structural details such as fissuring were readily apparent and consistent with histologic findings (Fig. 32.2) [11].

Comparing OCT images with the IVUS images and histology of postmortem aortas and stenotic coronary arteries revealed multiple advantages [9,17]. OCT had a higher resolution, a sharper delineation between intima and plaque, an ability to see behind calcified tissue, and a superior ability to see lipid pools not captured by IVUS. It provided finer-quality structural details of side branches. Distortion created by multiple echoes ("ring-down artifact") in IVUS images did not materialize with OCT. The trade-off was a shallower depth of penetration, which precluded ascertainment of positive or negative remodeling.

A small study evaluated the ability of OCT to detect the presence of the third important component of the vulnerable

plaque: activated macrophages. Macrophages weaken the structural integrity of vulnerable plaque and have been found near thrombi in patients who died of acute myocardial infarction [3,18]. With the premise that a stronger OCT signal is created by stronger optical scattering as is found in areas with higher heterogeneity, such as areas with large numbers of macrophages, Tearney and colleagues [19] examined 26 aortic and carotid plaques by OCT and histology. A bright speckled appearance on OCT was correlated to the presence of >10% CD68 staining by histology. Owing to the lack of predetermined criteria when calculating sensitivity and specificity, among other concerns [20], further study is necessary to confirm these findings.

Another unique aspect of OCT as an imaging modality is its ability to visualize the intima. Intimal thickening is a harbinger of atherosclerosis, and in examining 54 coronary segments with OCT, IVUS, and histology, Kume and colleagues [21] found that intimal–medial thickening was more accurately measured by OCT than by IVUS, and that intimal thickening could be measured only by OCT. As therapies to stimulate regression of atherosclerosis are developed, this technology may prove to be a method of assessing treatment efficacy.

Yabushita and colleagues [22] examined 357 autopsy segments from 90 cadavers. Fifty OCT images and corresponding

Table 32.1 Optical coherence tomography characteristics of coronary microstructures [22].

Histology	Optical coherence tomography finding
Intima	Signal-rich layer near lumen
Media	Signal-poor layer in middle of artery wall
Adventitia	Signal-rich outer layer of artery wall
Plaque	Loss of normal wall architecture, narrowed lumen
Fibrous	Signal-rich, homogeneous area
Calcified	Well-demarcated, heterogeneous area
Lipid	Signal-poor, poorly demarcated, homogeneous area
Cap	Signal-rich layer overlying signal-poor area

histopathology were used to establish objective criteria to define lipid, fibrous, and fibrocalcific plaques (Table 32.1). Validation by blinded readers of 307 segments revealed good intra- and interobserver reliability ($\kappa = 0.83–0.84$) as well as excellent sensitivity and specificity: 71–79% and 97–98%, respectively, for fibrous plaques; 95–96% and 97%, respectively, for fibrocalcific plaques; and 90–94% and 90–92%, respectively, for lipid-rich plaques. These definitions have formed the basis of plaque composition interpretation in clinical studies of OCT. It was theorized that some predominantly fibrous plaques contained lipid and were incorrectly labeled lipid rich, accounting for the lower sensitivity of OCT for detection of fibrous plaques. The limited depth of penetration may also have caused some thick-capped but predominantly lipid-rich plaques to be classified as fibrous. When compared with IVUS, MRI, and spectroscopy, OCT was the most sensitive and specific imaging modality for vulnerable plaque.

A recent analysis examining 166 coronary sections from 40 cadavers evaluated the sensitivity and specificity of OCT compared with IVUS for differentiating lipid from fibrous and fibrocalcific plaque with histology as the gold standard [23]. Few lipid-rich plaques were misclassified as fibrous or fibrocalcific by OCT, which had a higher sensitivity than IVUS for characterizing lipid-rich plaque (85% vs. 59%, $P = 0.03$), and intra- and interobserver reliability was good ($\kappa = 0.86–0.92$). IVUS was superior in assessing vessel remodeling, imaging deep vascular structures, and in determining the total lipid pool due to OCT's limited depth of penetration. The high resolution of OCT, however, enabled it to detect lipid-rich plaques more accurately.

In vivo studies

Vascular imaging by OCT was first tested *in vivo* in New Zealand in the aortas of white rabbits [24]. It became apparent that flowing blood would obstruct the view of the arterial wall with signal attenuation likely related to light scattering by red blood cells (RBCs). Saline flushes at a rate of 2–3 mL/s

allowed complete visibility of the aortic wall with visualization to a depth slightly over 2 mm. Saline permitted imaging as effectively as air had in *in vitro* studies.

The first study of OCT in human coronaries involved 10 patients undergoing percutaneous coronary intervention (PCI) [10]. Seventeen nonculprit lesion plaques were analyzed by OCT and IVUS, and blinded observers classified plaque as lipid-rich, fibrous, or calcific. OCT identified every finding observed by IVUS and provided better definition of intimal hyperplasia and lipid pools. The depth of penetration was 1.25 mm with OCT and 5 mm with IVUS. No adverse events resulted from performance of OCT. The layered structure of the normal coronary wall (intima, media, adventitia) was absent in areas of atherosclerotic plaques. This study establishes the feasibility of OCT to image vulnerable plaque and potentially to monitor plaque regression during treatment.

Jang and colleagues [25] analyzed OCT images among 57 patients who presented with stable angina pectoris (SAP), acute coronary syndrome, or ST elevation myocardial infarction (STEMI). The STEMI group was more likely than the ACS group, which was more likely than the SAP group, to have a thinner cap, more lipid, and a higher percentage of TCFA by OCT (72% vs. 50% vs. 20%, respectively, $P = 0.012$). The SAP group was more likely than the ACS group, which was more likely than the STEMI group, to have calcification present and evidence of thrombus. These findings support the current understanding of the pathophysiology of coronary artery disease that had previously been based predominantly on postmortem studies: that STEMI and ACS occur at areas of unstable plaque whereas SAP patients tend to have symptoms from more stable plaque. OCT added < 5 min to the procedure and caused no adverse events.

Kubo *et al.* [26] recently evaluated the ability of OCT for assessment of the culprit lesion morphology in acute myocardial infarction (AMI) in comparison with IVUS and coronary angioscopy and found that the high resolution of OCT provides a greater understanding of the intrinsic morphologic features that determine plaque vulnerability. Among 30 patients enrolled with AMI, the incidence of plaque rupture observed by OCT was 73%, and it was significantly higher than that of coronary angioscopy (47%, $P = 0.035$) and IVUS (40%, $P = 0.009$). OCT (23%) was superior to coronary angioscopy (3%, $P = 0.022$) and IVUS (0%, $P = 0.005$) in the detection of fibrous cap erosion. The intracoronary thrombus was observed in all cases by OCT and coronary angioscopy, but it was identified in 33% by IVUS (vs. OCT, $P < 0.001$). The incidence of TCFA was 83% in this population by OCT. Additionally, only OCT could estimate the fibrous cap thickness, which was $49 \pm 21\,\mu m$. The lipid-rich plaque was observed in 93% and the frequency of TCFA was 83% in the OCT findings. When compared with conventional imaging techniques, intracoronary OCT allowed authors to identify plaque ruptures, fibrous cap erosions, TCFA, and intracoronary thrombus *in vivo*, which has been demonstrated more frequently and clearly by histology only.

Limitations

Optical coherence tomography has two main disadvantages compared with other invasive imaging techniques. First, it has poor penetration into nontransparent tissues, with visualization limited to 2–3 mm [9,20]. Depth of penetration is adequate to evaluate the intima and plaque composition and to make thin cap measurements, but not to allow assessment of positive or negative remodeling, and the technique cannot fully image the total lipid pool in deep plaques with large necrotic cores. Nonetheless, the depth is sufficient for the purpose of vulnerable plaque evaluation and for coronary microstructure and pathology imaging for most lesions. Despite the better depth of penetration of IVUS, it has not been shown to reliably detect vulnerable plaque, possibly because of its low resolution. Overall, OCT is more sensitive and specific for the detection of unstable plaque [12,27].

The more challenging problem is signal attenuation by RBCs, which is believed to be a result of the mismatch in refractive index between serum and RBC cytoplasm as opposed to artifact from absorption or scattering caused by cellular components such as membranes and hemoglobin. This is supported by data that show that lysed blood does not interfere with OCT imaging [28].

Saline flushes have allowed scanning *in vivo* for up to 2 s at a time, which, coupled with the current imaging speed of 1 mm/s, has severely limited imaging. Employment of balloon occlusion catheters, with saline flushes as needed, resulted in improved imaging. Visualization is still limited for vessel segments shorter than 3.5 cm, as the maximum recommended inflation time is 35 s [29]. Also, retrograde flow from grafts or collaterals can impact image quality, even while a balloon is inflated proximally. It is reasonable to be concerned about the practical utilization of an imaging technology that necessitates prolonged ischemia, and this could hamper clinical use.

Ongoing investigations hope to overcome this problem. First, index matching by infusion of compounds that correct signal attenuation by RBCs has been shown to improve OCT image quality *in vitro* [28]. Dextran and intravenous contrast increased the refractive index of plasma and raised it closer to the intracellular refractive index of erythrocyte cytoplasm. Neither dextran nor intravenous contrast had a strong enough effect to create image quality comparable to scanning in saline. Future compounds may be found that could allow imaging without the need to clear blood from the field.

A second area of technologic improvement is Fourier-domain OCT (FD-OCT) imaging, which is described in more detail below. Briefly, it would increase the speed of image acquisition so that the amount of time that the vessel would have to be free of blood would be in the order of a few seconds [29].

Guiding percutaneous coronary intervention

Another clinical application of OCT is to assist with PCI. Angiography is limited in the ability to define intracoronary pathology, such as dissection, presence of thrombus, stent malapposition, and tissue prolapse. The high resolution of OCT gives it the potential to be an excellent tool in the interventionalist's armamentarium. OCT can nicely define the areas of eccentric and highly calcified plaque that can lead to asymmetric stent deployment; it is possible that use of OCT could improve procedural and clinical results. Bouma and colleagues [30] imaged 42 stents placed in 39 patients with OCT and IVUS. OCT provided more detailed coronary structural information than did IVUS although the clinical relevance of the information is yet unknown.

Optical coherence tomography has revealed flaps of tissue present owing to the use of cutting balloons that were not observed by angiography or IVUS [31]. In a comparison of OCT, IVUS, and histopathology in a patient with a history of stent placement who died from noncardiovascular causes, neointimal formation and stent apposition detected by histology were more closely approximated by OCT than by IVUS [32]. Diaz-Sandoval and colleagues [33] performed OCT and IVUS in 10 patients before and after PCI to determine how the vessel wall responds to angioplasty. OCT revealed vessel wall disruption after angioplasty and, subsequent to PCI, unveiled dissection, tissue prolapse, and incomplete stent apposition more frequently than did IVUS. Before intervention, ulcerated plaques were also more clearly defined and were assessed to be more complicated than they appeared on angiograms, with intimal disruption and clot often present.

These preliminary findings intimate that OCT would be an excellent modality to use in the study of stent design and to aid with real-time stent apposition (Fig. 32.3). This principle has been explored by Regar and colleagues [34], who placed an OCT imaging wire within the stent scanned with the balloon inflated to different pressures to evaluate stent diameter and acute recoil during stent deployment. Final stent area and recoil were easily assessed in real time.

As stent strut distribution affects drug delivery in drug-eluting stents, Suzuki and colleagues [35] performed OCT after deployment of a sirolimus- and a paclitaxel-eluting stent in silicon tubing and analyzed the interstrut angles. Stent architecture can affect procedural success and risk of restenosis, and OCT can provide clear images of stent struts, so this technology could be helpful in the early stages of stent design.

Ongoing technologic investigations

A collaborative effort between scientists and engineers at Light-Lab Imaging, Inc. (Westford, MA, USA) and the Massachusetts

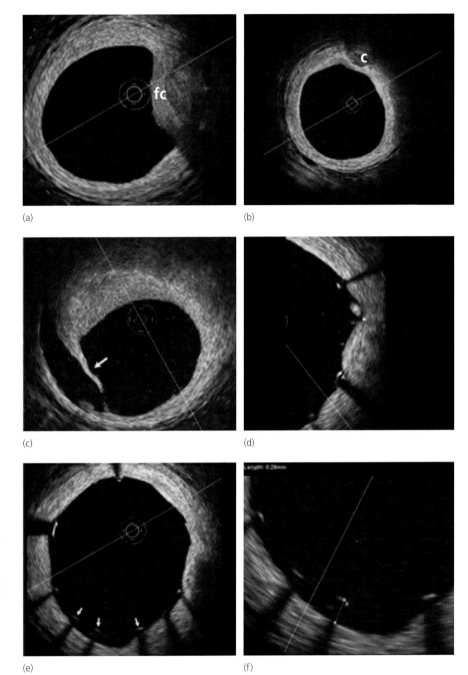

Figure 32.3 (a) Fibrous cap (fc) can be easily measured by optical coherence tomography (OCT). (b) Calcium (C) appears as a sharply defined, signal-poor region. (c) Dissection flap (arrow) is clearly shown. (d) OCT reveals tissue prolapse past stent struts. (e) Stent malapposition (arrows) can be evaluated. (f) High-power view of (e) to measure extent of stent malapposition. Images courtesy of LightLab, Inc. [37].

Institute of Technology is FD-OCT imaging, which is in an early stage of development, but shows promise [29]. As described above, the chief limitation of OCT is the need to interrupt blood flow to the heart, which adds complexity and risk to the imaging procedure. FD-OCT enables images to be acquired at a speed of 15 mm/s, 15 times faster than systems currently in use (Table 32.2). Faster pullback would greatly decrease the amount of time during which an artery needed to be clear of blood, making the procedure comparable to the brief seconds that arteries are contrast-filled during routine angiography.

In standard OCT, reflected light waves are detected sequentially and a mirror is rotated to generate different optical delays. As a mechanical process is involved, the maximum scan rate is limited. In FD-OCT, optical echoes from all time delays are detected simultaneously and Fourier transformations of the interference signals are used to create an image from all sample depths simultaneously. This does not require the mirror to move and thus allows extremely rapid acquisition rates and improved image quality (Fig. 32.4). FD-OCT is anticipated to be available for use in humans in 2–3 years [36]. Given the high grade of device miniaturization, combination

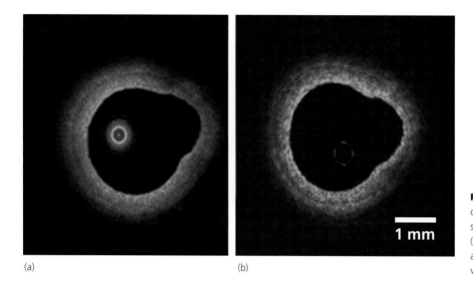

(a)

(b)

1 mm

Figure 32.4 Comparison of optical coherence tomography (OCT) images of the same cross-section of a pig artery acquired with (a) the prototype Fourier domain-OCT system and (b) a conventional OCT scanner. Adapted with permission from ref. 28.

Table 32.2 Performance of FD-OCT prototype compared with the LightLab OCT M2 system.

Characteristic	FD-OCT prototype	OCT M2 system
Line scan rate	45 kHz	3.1 kHz
Maximum frame rate	80 frames/s at 562 lines/frame	15.6 frames/s at 200 lines/frame
Scan diameter	7.2 mm	6.8 mm
Axial resolution	11–17 μm	15 μm

Adapted with permission from ref. 29.

diagnostic or therapeutic devices could eventually be incorporated into the OCT catheter and allow, for example, spectroscopy or atherectomy capabilities [15].

Our institution is involved in a prospective multicenter study of the OCT imaging system that uses occlusion balloon catheters to improve image quality and to allow longer scan times than is possible with saline flushing alone. It compares OCT images with IVUS and evaluates the safety of OCT as an invasive imaging modality. The goal is to image 115 patients undergoing PCI by OCT and IVUS, and examine image quality in detection of minimum lumen area. Secondary end points will include detection of intracoronary pathology such as stent malapposition, edge dissection, and tissue prolapse, as well as quality of visualization of the vessel wall, examining presence of calcium, degree of in-stent restenosis, stent endothelialization, and intimal hyperplasia. As balloon occlusion can cause ischemia, safety end points include angina, ST segment changes, spasm, arrhythmia, myocardial infarction, thrombus formation, and distal embolization.

Conclusion

Optical coherence tomography is an invasive imaging modality that uses optical echoes to create a tomographic image.

Advantages include high resolution; small, inexpensive catheters; real-time imaging; and visualization of the intima and fibrous cap thickness. *In vitro* and *in vivo* studies have demonstrated the feasibility of OCT to visualize vulnerable plaque and to guide PCI. It is more sensitive and specific than IVUS, especially for identification of the lipid-rich areas that are the hallmark of vulnerable plaque. It provides significant details of coronary microstructure and stent architecture, which could be harnessed to improve procedural and clinical outcomes and to facilitate stent design. Technologic advances hope to improve scan time and allow imaging in the presence of blood. In the future, once a move is made from diagnosis to focal or systemic treatment of vulnerable plaque, OCT may also become a prominent tool for quantification of treatment response and plaque regression.

References

1. Burke AP, Farb A, Malcom GT, *et al.* (1997) Coronary risk factors and plaque morphology in men with coronary disease who died suddenly. *N Engl J Med* **336**:1276–1282.
2. Virmani R, Kolodgie FD, Burke AP, *et al.* (2000) Lessons from sudden coronary death: a comprehensive morphological classification scheme for atherosclerotic lesions. *Arterioscler Thromb Vasc Biol* **20**:1262–1275.

3. Davies MJ, Richardson PD, Woolf N, *et al.* (1993) Risk of thrombosis in human atherosclerotic plaques: role of extracellular lipid, macrophage, and smooth muscle cell content. *Br Heart J* **69**:377–381.

4. Kolodgie FD, Virmani R, Burke AP, *et al.* (2004) Pathologic assessment of the vulnerable human coronary plaque. *Heart* **90**:1385–1391.

5. Kotani J, Mintz GS, Castagna MT, *et al.* (2003) Intravascular ultrasound analysis of infarct-related and non-infarct-related arteries in patients who presented with an acute myocardial infarction. *Circulation* **107**:2889–2893.

6. Virmani R, Burke AP, Farb A, *et al.* (2002) Pathology of the unstable plaque. *Prog Cardiovasc Dis* **44**:349–356.

7. Arbustini E, Grasso M, Diegoli M, *et al.* (1991) Coronary atherosclerotic plaques with and without thrombus in ischemic heart syndromes: a morphologic, immunohistochemical, and biochemical study. *Am J Cardiol* **68**:36B–50B.

8. Farb A, Burke AP, Tang AL, *et al.* (1996) Coronary plaque erosion without rupture into a lipid core. A frequent cause of coronary thrombosis in sudden coronary death. *Circulation* **93**:1354–1363.

9. Brezinski ME, Tearney GJ, Weissman NJ, *et al.* (1997) Assessing atherosclerotic plaque morphology: comparison of optical coherence tomography and high frequency intravascular ultrasound. *Heart* **77**:397–403.

10. Jang IK, Bouma BE, Kang DH, *et al.* (2002) Visualization of coronary atherosclerotic plaques in patients using optical coherence tomography: comparison with intravascular ultrasound. *J Am Coll Cardiol* **39**:604–609.

11. Brezinski ME, Tearney GJ, Bouma BE, *et al.* (1996) Optical coherence tomography for optical biopsy. Properties and demonstration of vascular pathology. *Circulation* **93**:1206–1213.

12. Brezinski M (2002) Characterizing arterial plaque with optical coherence tomography. *Curr Opin Cardiol* **17**:648–655.

13. Huang D, Swanson EA, Lin CP, *et al.* (1991) Optical coherence tomography. *Science* **254**:1178–1181.

14. Patel NA, Stamper DL, Brezinski ME (2005) Review of the ability of optical coherence tomography to characterize plaque, including a comparison with intravascular ultrasound. *Cardiovasc Intervent Radiol* **28**:1–9.

15. Regar E, Schaar JA, Mont E, *et al.* (2003) Optical coherence tomography. *Cardiovasc Radiat Med* **4**:198–204.

16. Brezinski ME, Tearney GJ, Bouma BE, *et al.* (1996) Imaging of coronary artery microstructure (in vitro) with optical coherence tomography. *Am J Cardiol* **77**:92–93.

17. Patwari P, Weissman NJ, Boppart SA, *et al.* (2000) Assessment of coronary plaque with optical coherence tomography and high frequency ultrasound. *Am J Cardiol* **85**:641–644.

18. van der Wal AC, Becker AE, van der Loos CM, *et al.* (1994) Site of intimal rupture or erosion of thrombosed coronary atherosclerotic plaques is characterized by an inflammatory process irrespective of the dominant plaque morphology. *Circulation* **89**:36–44.

19. Tearney GJ, Yabushita H, Houser SL, *et al.* (2003) Quantification of macrophage content in atherosclerotic plaques by optical coherence tomography. *Circulation* **107**:113–119.

20. Stamper D, Weissman NJ, Brezinski M (2006) Plaque characterization with optical coherence tomography. *J Am Coll Cardiol* **47**:C69–C79.

21. Kume T, Akasaka T, Kawamoto T, *et al.* (2005) Assessment of coronary intima-media thickness by optical coherence tomography: comparison with intravascular ultrasound. *Circ J* **69**:903–907.

22. Yabushita H, Bouma BE, Houser SL, *et al.* (2002) Characterization of human atherosclerosis by optical coherence tomography. *Circulation* **106**:1640–1645.

23. Kume T, Akasaka T, Kawamoto T, *et al.* (2006) Assessment of coronary arterial plaque by optical coherence tomography. *Am J Cardiol* **97**:1172–1175.

24. Fujimoto JG, Boppart SA, Tearney GJ, *et al.* (1999) High resolution in vivo intra-arterial imaging with optical coherence tomography. *Heart* **82**:128–133.

25. Jang IK, Tearney GJ, MacNeill B, *et al.* (2005) In vivo characterization of coronary atherosclerotic plaque by use of optical coherence tomography. *Circulation* **111**:1551–1555.

26. Kubo T, Imanishi T, Takarada S, *et al.* (2007) Assessment of culprit lesion morphology in acute myocardial infarction. Ability of optical coherence tomography compared with intravascular ultrasound and coronary angioscopy. *J Am Coll Cardiol* **50**:933–939.

27. MacNeill BD, Lowe HC, Takano M, *et al.* (2003) Intravascular modalities for detection of vulnerable plaque: current status. *Arterioscler Thromb Vasc Biol* **23**:1333–1342.

28. Brezinski M, Saunders K, Jesser C, *et al.* (2001) Index matching to improve optical coherence tomography imaging through blood. *Circulation* **103**:1999–2003.

29. Schmitt JM, Huber R, Fujimoto JG (2004) Limiting ischemia by fast Fourier-Domain imaging. In: Waksman R, Serruys PW, (eds). *Handbook of the Vulnerable Plaque*. New York: Informa Health Care.

30. Bouma BE, Tearney GJ, Yabushita H, *et al.* (2003) Evaluation of intracoronary stenting by intravascular optical coherence tomography. *Heart* **89**:317–320.

31. Ito S, Itoh M, Suzuki T (2005) Intracoronary imaging with optical coherence tomography after cutting balloon angioplasty for instent restenosis. *J Invasive Cardiol* **17**:369–370.

32. Kume T, Akasaka T, Kawamoto T, *et al.* (2005) Visualization of neointima formation by optical coherence tomography. *Int Heart J* **46**:1133–1136.

33. Diaz-Sandoval LJ, Bouma BE, Tearney GJ, *et al.* (2005) Optical coherence tomography as a tool for percutaneous coronary interventions. *Catheter Cardiovasc Interv* **65**:492–496.

34. Regar E, Schaar J, Serruys PW (2006) Images in cardiology. Acute recoil in sirolimus eluting stent: real time, in vivo assessment with optical coherence tomography. *Heart* **92**:123.

35. Suzuki Y, Ikeno F, Yeung AC (2006) Drug-eluting stent strut distribution: a comparison between Cypher and Taxus by optical coherence tomography. *J Invasive Cardiol* **18**:111–114.

36. Zhang S. July 11, 2006, personal communication.

33   Thermography of the Unstable Coronary Lesion

Konstantinos Toutouzas, Maria Drakopoulou & Christodoulos Stefanadis

Hippokration Hospital, Athens Medical School, Athens, Greece

Initiated early in life, atherosclerosis is a continuous process, which gradually progresses with potentially devastating consequences: atherosclerotic plaque rupture is the most common underlying pathologic mechanism creating acute ischemic coronary syndromes [1]. This term refers to the process whereby the endothelial surface of the plaque is disrupted to expose the underlying prothrombotic vessel wall to circulating platelets and coagulation factors.

In order to identify the high-risk plaque *in vivo*, we need to recognize the specific morphologic and functional characteristics. The morphologic characteristics have been identified in several human histopathologic and *in vivo* studies, and include (1) a large lipid core ($\geq$40% plaque volume) composed of free cholesterol crystals, cholesterol esters, and oxidized lipids impregnated with tissue factor, (2) a thin fibrous cap depleted of smooth muscle cells and collagen, (3) an outward (positive) remodeling, (4) inflammatory cell infiltration of fibrous cap and adventitia (mostly monocyte macrophages, activated T-cells and mast cells), and (5) increased neovascularity. The terms vulnerable, unstable, and "high risk" are now widely used to describe plaques that exhibit such features, irrespective of whether rupture of the fibrous cap is present [2]. Unfortunately, coronary angiographic techniques routinely used to identify stenotic atherosclerotic lesions are unable to identify high-risk plaques, prone to rupture. This is partly because the majority of culprit lesions that produce acute coronary syndromes are not severely stenotic, possibly as a result of significant positive remodeling [3]. In addition, the risk of plaque rupture is more closely related to plaque content than to plaque size. Currently, there is no ideal method for the identification of all these morphologic features [4]. Thus, several invasive and noninvasive methods have been developed for the recognition of these plaques. However, all methods have important advantages and limitations in their ability to identify the mentioned morphologic characteristics. Thus, there is an urgent need for methods that can identify plaques at risk of rupture and creation of acute coronary events.

The identification of functional characteristics of the unstable plaque appears to be even more complex. The role of local inflammatory activation in the process of plaque destabilization is well defined, and the infiltration of the atherosclerotic plaque by inflammatory cells has been recognized as one of the leading causes of plaque vulnerability resulting in plaque disruption, thrombus formation and the development of an acute coronary syndrome [5]. By the time the inflammatory cells exhaust their supply of oxygen, anaerobic metabolism ensues, leading to local acidosis [6]. In addition, many areas of atherosclerotic plaques are known to be ischemic, and the lack of oxygen can lead to ineffective metabolism of nutrients and greater loss of energy in the form of heat instead of adenosine triphosphate (ATP) production [7]. Moreover, neovessel formation increases blood flow within the atheromatous arterial wall, producing higher local temperatures [8,9]. Based on these observations, intracoronary thermography was introduced as a technique for identification of the vulnerable plaque. Since inflammation has been closely related to increased heat production, temperature elevation in atherosclerotic plaques may reflect the intensity of the local inflammatory process. The increased heat production from unstable plaques has been confirmed in several *ex vivo* human studies (Table 33.1), in experimental models, and in human *in vivo* studies.

Thermal heterogeneity of atherosclerotic plaques

Human ex vivo studies

Ex vivo carotid artery intimal surface temperatures were assessed first by Casscells *et al.* [10], revealing several regions in which the surface temperature differences within each sample varied from 0.2°C to 2.2°C. In particular, surface temperatures were measured during surgical endatherectomy using a sensitive needle thermistor at 20 sites in 50 samples of carotid plaques. In the absence of blood flow, surface temperature of plaques at different points showed marked and

Cardiovascular Interventions in Clinical Practice. Edited by Jürgen Haase, Hans-Joachim Schäfers, Horst Sievert and Ron Waksman. © 2010 Blackwell Publishing.

Table 33.1 Human *ex vivo* thermography studies.

Reference	Year	Main finding
Casscells *et al.* [10]	1996	Living atherosclerotic plaques show thermal heterogeneity. Temperature correlated positively with cell density and inversely with the distance of the cell clusters from the luminal surface
Madjid *et al.* [12]	2002	No significant association between temperature heterogeneity and *Chlamydia pneumoniae* was found. After incubation of the plaques with indomethacin a gradual decrease in plaque heat production was observed over 5 h, suggesting inflammatory origin of heat production in atherosclerotic plaques
Naghavi *et al.* [13]	2002	pH Heterogeneity in atheromatous plaques: low pH in the detection of plaque vulnerability
Toutouzas *et al.* [11]	2003	A significant increase in serum matrix metalloproteinases-1, -3, and -9 were found in samples with high temperature differences

reproducible thermal heterogeneity. Moreover, temperature heterogeneity could also be confirmed using an infrared camera *in vivo*. Most importantly, the measured temperature was directly correlated with cell density and inversely correlated with the depth of the cell clusters. Thus, this was the first study demonstrating that heat is generated from inflamed atheromatous plaques in humans. These observations were also confirmed in preliminary clinical studies combining temperature measurements with directional atherectomy of the same specimens. In addition, a correlation between the serum matrix metalloproteinase (MMP)-1, -3, and -9 concentrations and temperature differences has been reported [11]. In this study, samples were obtained through direct coronary atherectomy in eight patients and a significant increase in serum MMPs was found in samples showing high temperature differences. However, the strength of the relationship between serum levels of serum MMPs and focal activity of such enzymes at the plaque level remains to be determined.

In an attempt to investigate the potential impact of infections on the generation of hot plaques, the genus-specific monoclonal antibody CF-2 against *Chlamydia pneumoniae* (now known as *Chlamydophila pneumoniae*) was used in carotid artery specimens [12]. However, no significant association between temperature heterogeneity and *Chlamydia pneumoniae* was found. In addition, the gross color of the lumen surface of human atherosclerotic carotid plaques could not predict the underlying temperature [12]. After incubation of the plaques with indomethacin, a gradual decrease in plaque heat production was observed over 5 h, suggesting inflammatory origin of heat production in atherosclerotic plaques [12].

In a recent study, lower pH readings in vulnerable plaques of human carotid endarterectomy specimens and atherosclerotic rabbit aortas have been observed [13]. In these samples, a lower pH was associated with a higher temperature ($r = 0.7$; $P < 0.01$). Lipid-rich areas had a lower pH and a higher temperature, whereas calcified areas showed a higher pH and a lower temperature. Temperature and pH were inversely correlated ($r = 0.94$; $P < 0.01$). This finding is in line with the

assumption that lipid-rich vulnerable areas may have a more acidic environment.

Animal studies

In animal models, several investigators have applied devices for intraluminal thermography. Although there are significant differences in the technologic characteristics of each device, we obtained important pathophysiologic insights in the development of unstable plaque. Naghavi *et al.* [14] developed a contact-based "thermobasket" catheter for measuring *in vivo* the temperature at several points on the vessel wall in the presence of blood flow (Fig. 33.1a) [14,15]. This thermocouple-based basket catheter is equipped with four small, flexible wires with built-in thermocouples and a thermal sensor in its central wire for simultaneous monitoring of the blood temperature. The device has a thermal resolution of 0.02°C, thermal accuracy of 0.02°C with a sampling rate of 20 temperature readings per second, and contains seven sensors. The system was applied in a canine and a rabbit model of atherosclerosis. In inbred cholesterol-fed dogs with femoral atherosclerosis, marked thermal heterogeneity was found on the surface of atherosclerotic regions but not on disease-free regions ($P < 0.05$). Marked temperature heterogeneity was also observed in the aortas of atherosclerotic Watanabe rabbits but not in normal rabbits. The catheters showed satisfactory accuracy, reproducibility, and safety [14].

Verheye *et al.* [16] developed an over-the-wire thermography catheter with four thermistors. Twenty New Zealand rabbits were randomized to either a normal diet or a cholesterol-rich diet for 6 months. Marked temperature heterogeneity (up to 1°C) was found in the hypercholesterolemic rabbits at sites of thick plaques (assessed by intravascular ultrasound), in which histology showed a high macrophage density. Temperature heterogeneity was absent at sites of plaques with a low macrophage density. The temperature heterogeneity detected in hypercholesterolemic rabbits was reduced significantly after 3 months of cholesterol-lowering therapy and paralleled changes in plaque histology, which showed a marked loss of macrophages. In a recently published study, *in vivo* temperature heterogeneity was found

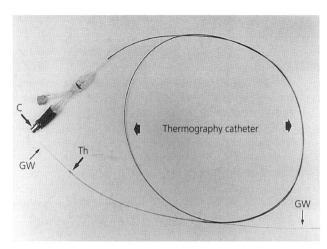

Figure 33.1 Photographs of thermography catheters for intravascular measurement of vessel wall temperature. (a) Thermosensor basket catheter in open condition. (b) Intracoronary thermography catheter. C, connector; GW, guidewire; Th, thermistor.

to be associated with plaque regions of increased inflammatory activity. The plaques were experimentally induced in rabbit aortas, and, at the day of sacrifice, a pullback was performed with a thermography catheter. *In vivo* temperature measurements detected plaques that contained more macrophages, less smooth muscle cell concentration, and a higher MMP-9 activity (Table 33.2) [17].

Human in vivo studies

Intracoronary thermography catheters

The first intracoronary thermography catheter allowing *in vivo* temperature measurements was designed and developed at our institution and is now being manufactured (Epiphany catheter, Medispes Sw AG, Zug, Switzerland) (Fig. 33.1b) [18–26]. The Epiphany coronary thermography catheter contains two lumens. The first lumen runs through the distal 20 cm of the device and is used for insertion of a 0.014-inch guidewire by monorail technique. In the second lumen, the thermistor leads are inserted. At the distal part of the

thermography catheter, a thermistor is positioned that attaches the vessel wall. To date, many different types of catheters have been designed to record *in vivo* the coronary vessel wall temperature. The thermography basket catheter (Volcano Therapeutics Inc., Rancho Cordova, CA, USA) consists of a 3F shaft with an expandable and externally controllable basket with built-in thermocouple [14,27]. Another thermography catheter has been developed by Thermocore (Thermocore Medical Systems NV, Ghent, Belgium). The over-the-wire catheter consists of a functional end that can be engaged by retracting a covering sheath. Four flexible nitinol strips with four dedicated thermistors are placed at the distal end. Once engaged, the nitinol strips expand, ensuring contact of the thermistor with the endoluminal surface of the vascular wall [16,28]. Guidewire-based systems also have been proposed as an alternative method to measure intracoronary temperature [29]. The ThermoCoil system (Imetrx, Mountain View, CA, USA) consists of a 0.014-inch guidewire, pullback handle, and data acquisition system [30]. The temperature sensor is located in the tip of the wire and has a resolution of 0.08°C. The tip of the wire is prebent in an angled curve 10 mm proximal to the tip, which brings the tip into contact with the vessel wall. The signals are converted to temperature readings and displayed in real time as a digital readout and in graphical form.

The first human study with *in vivo* intracoronary thermography was published in 1999 [19]. In this study, 90 patients were included. Temperature was constant within the arteries of the control subjects, whereas most atherosclerotic plaques showed a higher temperature than healthy vessel walls. Temperature differences between atherosclerotic plaque and a healthy vessel wall increased progressively from patients with stable angina to those with acute myocardial infarction. Plaque temperature heterogeneity was present in 20%, 40%, and 67% of the patients with stable angina, unstable angina, and acute myocardial infarction, respectively, and did not correlate with the degree of stenosis. Temperature heterogeneity was absent in the control group. Moreover, increased plaque temperature was observed for an extended period after myocardial infarction, indicating that the inflammatory

Table 33.2 Animal thermography studies.

Referemce	Year	Main finding
Verheye *et al.* [16]	2002	Modifying the cell composition of rabbit atherosclerotic plaques by lowering dietary cholesterol influences temperature heterogeneity
Naghavi *et al.* [14]	2003	Marked temperature heterogeneity was observed in the aortas of atherosclerotic Watanabe rabbits
Verheye *et al.* [28]	2004	Intracoronary thermography using a dedicated catheter is safe and feasible with a similar degree of de-endothelialization as intravascular ultrasound. Temperature heterogeneity remained unchanged under normal physiologic flow conditions allowing clinical use of thermography
Krams *et al.* [17]	2005	*In vivo* temperature measurements enable to detect plaques that contain more macrophages, less smooth muscle cells, and a higher metalloproteinase activity

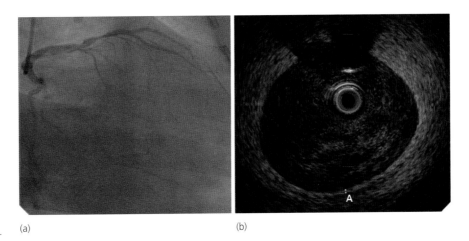

Figure 33.2 The angiography of a patient with acute coronary syndrome (a) and the optical coherence tomography image showing a lesion with thin fibrous cap (b) (A = 0.40 mm).

(a)   (b)

process is sustained after plaque rupture [31]. In this study 55 patients were enrolled. In patients with recent myocardial infarction thermal heterogeneity was 0.19 ± 0.18°C, but in patients with stable angina thermal heterogeneity was 0.10 ± 0.08°C (*P* = 0.03).

Temperature heterogeneity also has been associated with vascular remodeling [26]. Using intravascular ultrasound in 81 consecutive patients (48 with acute coronary syndromes and 33 with stable angina) a strong and positive correlation between the coronary remodeling index (defined as the ratio of the external elastic membrane area at the lesion, to that at the proximal site) and the temperature difference between the atherosclerotic plaque and healthy vascular wall was found in patients with acute coronary syndromes. In particular, patients with acute coronary syndrome had greater remodeling index than patients with stable angina (1.15 ± 0.18°C vs. 0.90 ± 0.12°C; *P* < 0.01), as well as an increased temperature difference (0.08 ± 0.03°C vs. 0.04 ± 0.02°C; *P* < 0.01). Moreover, patients with positive remodeling had higher thermal heterogeneity than patients with negative remodeling (0.07 ± 0.03°C vs. 0.04 ± 0.02°C; *P* < 0.001) [26]. In patients with negative remodeling there was no difference in thermal heterogeneity between acute coronary syndrome and stable angina. Patients with plaque rupture had increased temperature difference compared with patients without (0.09 ± 0.03°C vs. 0.05 ± 0.02°C; *P* < 0.01). Thus, culprit lesions with plaque rupture and positive arterial remodeling have increased thermal heterogeneity, although in certain patients a discrepancy between morphologic and functional characteristics was observed. These results confirm the concept that there is no ideal method for identification of unstable or high-risk lesions. However, this study showed that a combination of morphologic and functional examination may offer additional diagnostic information. In a recent study [32], intracoronary thermography and optical coherence tomography were performed in culprit lesions of patients with acute coronary syndrome. In plaques with increased thermal heterogeneity fibrous caps were thinner than plaques without temperature

increase. Moreover, the incidence of intraluminal thrombus was not related to plaque temperature (Fig. 33.2).

Prognosis

The impact of intracoronary thermography on risk stratification of patients undergoing percutaneous coronary intervention was also investigated [33]. The relationship of temperature difference between the atherosclerotic plaque and the healthy vessel wall and event-free survival was studied in 86 patients undergoing a successful percutaneous intervention. The patients had stable angina (34.5%), unstable angina (34.5%), or acute myocardial infarction (30%). The temperature difference increased progressively from stable angina to acute myocardial infarction. Over a median clinical follow-up of 17.8 ± 7.1 months, temperature difference was a strong predictor of adverse cardiac events (odds ratio 2.14, *P* = 0.043). Increased local temperature in atherosclerotic plaques was found to be a strong predictor of an unfavorable clinical outcome in patients with coronary artery disease undergoing percutaneous interventions.

Impact of diabetes mellitus

Especially in patients with diabetes, inflammation is significantly pronounced, and increased infiltration of inflammatory cells is observed in atheromatous lesions. We therefore investigated whether patients with coronary artery disease and diabetes had increased local heat generation compared with patients without diabetes. In this study we enrolled 45 patients with diabetes and 63 patients without diabetes [34,35]. Patients with diabetes mellitus had increased temperature differences compared with patients without diabetes. Moreover, patients with diabetes mellitus suffering from acute coronary syndromes or stable angina showed increased local inflammatory involvement compared with patients without diabetes mellitus. This study demonstrated that, in culprit lesions of patients with diabetes mellitus, an increased inflammatory activation is present, suggesting that diabetes mellitus may have a strong impact on plaque destabilization via inflammation.

Impact of statins

The only cardiovascular medication with proved anti-inflammatory action in atheromatous plaques is statins. Therefore, increased interest has been recently directed toward preventing rather than healing plaque rupture by administration of statins. Intracoronary thermography has shown to be effective in evaluating the effect of diet and medications on the thermal heterogeneity of atherosclerotic plaques. Statins have well-recognized anti-inflammatory effects and can reduce the number of macrophages while increasing the collagen content in atherosclerotic plaques, hence stabilizing the plaque [36]. We investigated a possible stabilizing effect of statins on hot plaques [23]. The study population included 72 patients: 37 patients receiving statins for >4 weeks and 35 not receiving statins. It was found that thermal heterogeneity was lower in patients treated with statins, independent of the clinical syndrome. This effect on temperature was also independent of the serum cholesterol level at hospital admission. Furthermore, patients with diabetes mellitus receiving statins showed smaller temperature differences than untreated patients, suggesting that statins have a favorable effect on culprit lesions in patients with diabetes [35]. These findings support the hypothesis that aggressive treatment with statins may be essential for stabilization of the vulnerable atherosclerotic plaque in patients with coronary artery disease, including those in whom percutaneous coronary intervention is planned, as increased culprit plaque temperature at the time of intervention is associated with a poor prognosis. Moreover, the effect of statins on nonculprit lesion inflammation has been recently investigated. Temperature differences were smaller in patients treated with statins in both clinical groups.

Recently, Rzeszutko *et al.* [37] performed intracoronary thermography in 40 patients with acute coronary syndrome, using a thermography catheter containing five thermocouples measuring vessel wall temperature and one thermocouple measuring blood temperature (accuracy 0.05°C). Temperature gradients between blood temperature and the maximum wall temperature were assessed. In 40% of the patients, temperature gradients were found to be >0.10°C. Schmermund *et al.* [27] used a nonoccluding thermography catheter (Volcano Therapeutics, Rancho Cordova, CA, USA). Nineteen patients were included in the study, of whom 11 had stable angina and eight had unstable angina. Focal high temperature was determined by comparing the temperature between arterial wall thermocouples against a central thermocouple. The recorded temperature differences ranged from 0.14°C to 0.36°C. Focal temperature heterogeneity was observed in 50% of patients with unstable angina and in 27% of patients with stable angina. This study showed a difference between the two groups; however, there was still a considerable overlap. Wainstein *et al.* [30] used a different thermography catheter (ThermoCoil Guidewire, Imetrx, Mountain View, CA, USA). Thirteen patients presenting with either acute coronary syndromes or chronic stable angina with indication for percutaneous coronary intervention were evaluated by intracoronary thermography, intravascular ultrasound, and angiography. In addition, directional atherectomy was performed in two patients and histopathologic tissue analysis was carried out. Intra-arterial temperature rises between 0.1°C and 0.3°C were noted in four subjects. Intravascular ultrasound findings and atherectomy tissue histology showed correlates of plaque vulnerability in plaques with elevated temperature.

Dudek *et al.* [38] recently reported a study including 40 patients with acute coronary syndrome using a multisensor thermography basket catheter with five wall thermocouples and a central blood thermocouple. The temperature difference was measured, defined as the maximum temperature difference between blood and any thermal couple. Mean temperature difference was 0.09 ± 0.03°C. Average temperature difference at the culprit segment was 0.092 ± 0.03°C, which was significantly higher than temperature differences recorded in nonculprit lesions (0.06 ± 0.01°C, range 0.03°C to 0.28°C; $P < 0.01$). Temperature differences showed an inverse correlation with blood flow during thermal mapping. In this study, the presence of blood flow led to a significant decrease in the recorded temperature difference between culprit and nonculprit segments [38]. Recently, Takumi *et al.* [39] generated the hypothesis that the site of maximal temperature, as measured by the thermal wire, coincides with the location of a culprit plaque as detected by intravascular ultrasound in patients with acute myocardial infarction. In this study, the angiographic occlusive site was significantly more proximal but the maximal temperature site coincided with the culprit plaque detected by intravascular ultrasound (Fig. 33.3).

Cooling effect

Although inflammation leads to increased heat release from the atherosclerotic plaque, higher temperature differences have been observed with *ex vivo* rather than *in vivo* temperature measurements [10,28]. Coronary flow may exert a "cooling effect" on measured coronary temperature. Complete obstruction of blood flow may increase the degree of detected temperature heterogeneity by 60–76% [20]. However, other studies have shown that normal physiologic flow conditions reduce temperature heterogeneity only by 8–13% compared with the surface temperature of the plaque measured in the absence of flow [28]. A mathematical simulation of a model of a coronary artery segment containing a heat source predicted that measured temperature is strongly affected by blood flow and also by cap thickness, source geometry, and maximal flow velocity. In particular, maximal temperature differences at the lumen wall increased when the source volume increased and blood flow was acting as a coolant to the lumen wall. Additionally, when cap thickness increased, maximal temperatures decreased and the influence of flow increased [40,41]. On the basis of these studies, the potential influence of coronary blood flow has been further investigated using temperature measurements during complete interruption of flow [42].

- LAD total occlusion

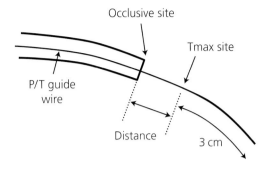

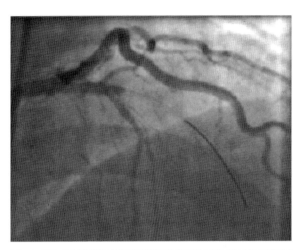

(a)

- LAD reperfusion

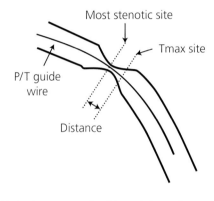

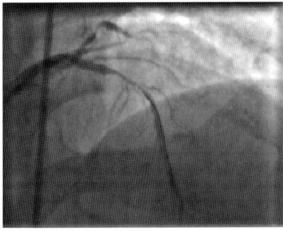

(b)

Figure 33.3 Methods to measure the distance between the maximal temperature (T_{max}) site by the pressure/temperature (P/T) guidewire and the occlusive site by angiography in patients with left anterior descending coronary artery (LAD) total occlusion (a) and that between the T_{max} site and the most stenotic site in patients with LAD reperfusion (b).

During vessel occlusion, the assessed temperature was elevated both in patients with stable angina and in patients with acute coronary syndromes, strongly implying that coronary flow has a "cooling effect" on thermal heterogeneity, which may lead to underestimation of local heat production [20,42]. To eliminate this shortcoming, especially in intermediate lesions in which attachment of the thermistor cannot be ensured, new catheter designs were recently introduced. A balloon thermography catheter, with the thermistor opposite to the inflated balloon, facilitates contact of the thermistor to the plaque surface [42]. Using this catheter, temperature elevations up to 59% were recorded in stable lesions. Moreover, Belardi et al. [43] presented preliminary results with a new basket catheter with multiple thermistors, which can also measure atheromatous plaque temperature during complete interruption of coronary blood flow. All of these devices would need to be investigated in a large number of patients in order to draw conclusions regarding their safety, their reliability, and the prognostic value of the obtained measurements.

Widespread inflammation

The concept that inflammation is not a local phenomenon restricted to the culprit atherosclerotic plaque, but widespread in the coronary arteries, especially in patients with acute coronary events, has recently emerged. In a preliminary study Webster et al. [44] found more than one "hot" spot in the same vessel. Moreover, recent studies support the hypothesis that plaque instability may not represent a mere random "vascular accident," but reflect a "pancoronary" process due to widespread inflammatory activation. We studied serum inflammatory biomarkers in 60 patients with stable angina, unstable angina, and acute myocardial infarction, and compared them with the findings in 20 gender- and age-matched control subjects without coronary artery disease [18]. In this study, there was a strong correlation between C-reactive protein (CRP) and serum amyloid A levels, with detected differences in temperature. In a recent study, we presented an increased thermal heterogeneity in nonculprit intermediate lesions (Fig. 33.4). We also found that local inflammatory

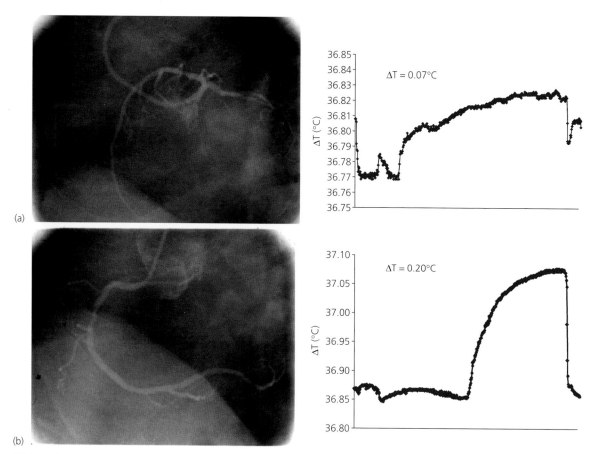

Figure 33.4 Angiographic images and thermography measurements of a patient with multivessel disease. (a) Culprit lesion at the proximal segment of the left anterior descending artery with thermal heterogeneity of 0.07°C. (b) Nonculprit lesion at the middle segment of the right coronary artery with thermal heterogeneity of 0.20°C. Thermal heterogeneity was higher at the nonculprit lesion.

activation in nonculprit intermediate lesions correlates well with the systemic inflammation, as documented by the concomitant assessment of CRP levels ($r = 0.46$, $P < 0.01$) [24]. In the same study, patients with acute coronary syndromes had increased thermal heterogeneity in both culprit and nonculprit lesions, supporting a pancoronary inflammatory activation. Rzeszutko *et al.* [37] performed intracoronary thermography in 40 patients with acute coronary syndrome, and in 23 patients (57.5%) the highest temperature difference was found in the culprit segment. Also, the highest temperature differences between culprit and adjacent nonculprit segments was observed in patients with transient blood flow interruption during thermography (0.11 ± 0.03 vs. 0.08 ± 0.01; $P = 0.04$), in contrast to patients with preserved flow (0.07 ± 0.03 vs. 0.06 ± 0.02; $P = 0.058$). The investigators used a thermography catheter containing five thermocouples measuring vessel wall temperature, and one thermocouple measuring blood temperature. Wainstein *et al.* [30] found an apparently higher mean CRP level in patients with higher temperature heterogeneity than in those without elevated temperature (14.0 vs. 6.2 mg/L). These results provide new

insights supporting the concept of diffuse destabilization of coronary atherosclerotic plaques: although a single lesion is clinically symptomatic, acute coronary syndromes are associated with diffuse thermal heterogeneity.

To evaluate whether this widespread coronary inflammation increases temperature of the blood as it flows into the coronary artery tree and empties into the coronary sinus, blood temperature differences were measured between the coronary sinus and the right atrium in patients with symptomatic coronary artery disease. The thermographic catheter was designed in our institution and briefly consists of a steering arm with a connector for the thermistor lead wires attached to the proximal part of the catheter. The steering arm passes through the lumen of the catheter and is attached to its tip. The distal 7 cm of the catheter shaft consists of a soft nonthrombogenic material. The thermistor lead wires end at the connector and pass through another lumen of the catheter. A thermistor probe is positioned at the center of the catheter tip. The thermistor has a sensitivity of 0.05°C and a time constant of 300 ms. We included 53 patients with acute coronary syndrome, 25 patients with stable angina, and 22 subjects without coronary

Table 33.3 Human *in vivo* thermography studies.

Reference	Year	Main finding
Stefanadis *et al.* [19]	1999	Temperature differences between atherosclerotic plaque and healthy vessel wall increased progressively with the clinical syndrome
Stefanadis *et al.* [18]	2000	Positive correlation between C-reactive protein and serum amyloid A with the temperature difference of the plaque
Stefanadis *et al.* [33]	2001	Increased local temperature in atherosclerotic plaques is a strong predictor of an unfavorable clinical outcome in patients with coronary artery disease undergoing percutaneous interventions
Stefanadis *et al.* [23]	2002	Statins seem to have a favorable effect on heat release from atherosclerotic plaques
Stefanadis *et al.* [20]	2003	Thermal heterogeneity is underestimated in atherosclerotic plaques owing to the "cooling effect" of coronary blood flow
Stefanadis *et al.* [42]	2003	*In vivo* atherosclerotic plaque temperature recording was feasible with the new balloon-thermography catheter. Increased temperature difference after complete interruption of blood flow by inflation of the balloon
Stefanadis *et al.* [46]	2004	Coronary sinus temperature was increased in patients with coronary artery disease and was found to be a prognostic factor for mid-term clinical outcome
Toutouzas *et al.* [31]	2004	Increased plaque temperature is observed for an extended period after myocardial infarction, indicating that the inflammatory process is sustained after plaque rupture. Statins have a beneficial effect on plaque temperature after myocardial infarction
Dudek *et al.* [38]	2005	No ability to differentiate between lesions at risk, despite a selection of lesions that should appear most distinct to differentiate
Toutouzas *et al.* [45]	2006	Systemic inflammation is well correlated with coronary sinus temperature independently of the extent of the disease
Toutouzas *et al.* [35]	2005	Patients with diabetes have increased temperature difference compared with patients without diabetes. Patients with diabetes under statins showed decreased temperature difference compared with untreated patients
Toutouzas *et al.* [25]	2006	Heat is generated in nonculprit lesions progressively increasing from patients with acute coronary syndrome to patients with stable angina
Rzeszutko *et al.* [37]	2006	Intracoronary thermography was safe and feasible. No ability to differentiate between lesions at risk, despite a selection of lesions that should appear most distinct to differentiate
Wainstein *et al.* [30]	2007	Thermography using a guidewire-based system can be performed safely, and detect lesions of which the intravascular and/or atherectomy findings suggest plaques at high risk of rupture
Toutouzas *et al.* [24]	2007	Local inflammatory activation in nonculprit lesions is correlated with systemic inflammation. Statins have a beneficial effect on nonculprit lesion heat production
Toutouzas *et al.* [24]	2007	Culprit lesions with plaque rupture and positive arterial remodeling have increased thermal heterogeneity
Takumi *et al.* [39]	2007	Temperature measurement enables accurate localization of the culprit plaque in patients with acute myocardial infarction and coronary total occlusion

artery disease [45]. Temperature differences were greater in patients with acute coronary syndrome and with stable angina than in the control group. The acute coronary syndrome group had greater thermal heterogeneity than the stable angina group, although the difference did not reach statistical significance ($P = 0.09$). The levels of CRP correlated well with thermal heterogeneity ($r = 0.35$, $P < 0.01$) supporting a potential relationship between systemic inflammation and coronary sinus temperature. Moreover, coronary sinus blood temperature was found to be greater than right atrium blood temperature in patients with angiographically significant lesions, independently of the site of the lesion, but not in subjects without coronary artery disease (Table 33.3).

Clinical implications and limitations of the method

Intracoronary thermography is a method for "functional imaging" of atherosclerotic plaques with a potential for detection of vulnerable plaques and identifying vulnerable patients. However, there are several different aspects that deserve further investigation. The obvious limitations of intravascular thermography by any means in analyzing individual plaque stability include the inability to provide direct imaging of plaque components, such as the lipid pool, the thickness of the fibrous cap, or the degree of positive remodeling. In addition, it is essential in intracoronary thermography for accurate assessment of thermal heterogeneity that the thermistor is in direct contact with the vessel wall, a prerequisite that implies the risk of endothelial disruption.

Discrepancies between *ex vivo* and *in vivo* temperature measurements suggest a cooling effect of coronary blood flow, which raises concern about the accuracy of this technique *in vivo* and the potential underestimation of the true heat production in several plaques. The correct interpretation of intravascular thermographic measurements might require knowledge of data with respect to flow and morphologic characteristics of the atherosclerotic plaque that are not simultaneously available at this stage. Another potential limitation of intravascular thermography, or any invasive means of identifying vulnerable plaque, is that coronary atherosclerosis represents a diffuse rather than a focal phenomenon. The inflammatory process is not restricted to one unstable lesion, particularly in patients with acute coronary syndromes. Moreover, it remains challenging to clarify whether and how this information may be incorporated into clinical decision-making. Obviously, a number of clinical trials with different designs are needed to answer these questions. Vulnerable plaques have multiple characteristics, and a combination of thermography with anatomical imaging methods, such as intravascular ultrasound, elastography, or optical coherence tomography, may be required for their correct assessment.

Conclusion

Plaque rupture is probably the most important mechanism underlying the sudden onset of an acute coronary event. Soft, lipid-rich plaques, heavily infiltrated by macrophages are possibly more prone to rupture. Early detection of the high-risk lesion may lead to the most favorable local or systemic treatment selection that will prevent the sequel of events resulting in acute coronary syndrome. Intracoronary thermography is a promising method for the functional assessment of vulnerable plaque and has been introduced into clinical practice, with a good predictive value for clinical events in patients with increased temperature in the atherosclerotic plaque.

References

1. Rosamond W, Flegal K, Furie K, *et al.* (2008) Heart disease and stroke statistics—2008 update: a report from the American Heart Association Statistics Committee and Stroke Statistics Subcommittee. *Circulation* **117**:e25–146.
2. Naghavi M, Libby P, Falk E, *et al.* (2003) From vulnerable plaque to vulnerable patient: a call for new definitions and risk assessment strategies: Part II. *Circulation* **108**:1772–1778.
3. Ambrose JA, Tannenbaum MA, Alexopoulos D, *et al.* (1998) Angiographic progression of coronary artery disease and the development of myocardial infarction. *J Am Coll Cardiol* **12**:56–62.
4. Tan KT & Lip GY (2008) Imaging of the unstable plaque. *Int J Cardiol* **127**:157–165.
5. Ross R (1999) Atherosclerosis—an inflammatory disease. *N Engl J Med* **340**:115–126.
6. Heinle H (1987) Metabolite concentration gradients in the arterial wall of experimental atherosclerosis. *Exp Mol Pathol* **46**:312–320.
7. Kockx M, Knaapen MWM, Martinet W, *et al.* (2000) Expression of the uncoupling protein UCP-2 in macrophages of unstable human atherosclerotic plaques. *Circulation* **102**:E99.
8. Tenaglia AN, Peters KG, Sketch MH, *et al.* (1998) Neovascularization in atherectomy specimens from patients with unstable angina: implications for pathogenesis of unstable angina. *Am Heart J* **135**:10–14.
9. Madjid M, Willerson JT, & Casscells SW (2006) Intracoronary thermography for detection of high-risk vulnerable plaques. *J Am Coll Cardiol* **47**:C80–85.
10. Casscells W, Hathorn B, David M, *et al.* (1996) Thermal detection of cellular infiltrates in living atherosclerotic plaques: possible implications for plaque rupture and thrombosis. *Lancet* **347**:1447–1451.
11. Toutouzas K, Spanos V, Ribichini F, *et al.* (2003) A correlation of coronary plaque temperature with inflammatory markers obtained from atherectomy specimens in humans. *Am J Cardiol* **92**:476.
12. Madjid M, Naghavi M, Malik BA, *et al.* (2002) Thermal detection of vulnerable plaque. *Am J Cardiol* **90**:36L-39L.
13. Naghavi M, John R, Naguib S, *et al.* (2002) pH Heterogeneity of human and rabbit atherosclerotic plaques; a new insight into detection of vulnerable plaque. *Atherosclerosis* **164**:27–35.
14. Naghavi M, Madjid M, Gul K, *et al.* (2003) Thermography basket catheter: in vivo measurement of the temperature of atherosclerotic plaques for detection of vulnerable plaques. *Catheter Cardiovasc Interv* **59**:52–59.
15. Zarrabi A, Gul K, Willerson JT, *et al.* (2002) Intravascular thermography: a novel approach for detection of vulnerable plaque. *Curr Opin Cardiol* **17**:656–662.
16. Verheye S, De Meyer GR, Van Langenhove G, *et al.* (2002) In vivo temperature heterogeneity of atherosclerotic plaques is determined by plaque composition. *Circulation* **105**:1596–1601.
17. Krams R, Verheye S, van Damme LC, *et al.* (2005) In vivo temperature heterogeneity is associated with plaque regions of increased MMP-9 activity. *Eur Heart J* **26**:2200–2205.
18. Stefanadis C, Diamantopoulos L, Dernellis J, *et al.* (2000) Heat production of atherosclerotic plaques and inflammation assessed by the acute phase proteins in acute coronary syndromes. *J Mol Cell Cardiol* **32**:43–52.
19. Stefanadis C, Diamantopoulos L, Vlachopoulos C, *et al.* (1999) Thermal heterogeneity within human atherosclerotic coronary arteries detected in vivo: a new method of detection by application of a special thermography catheter. *Circulation* **99**:1965–1971.
20. Stefanadis C, Toutouzas K, Tsiamis E, *et al.* (2003) Thermal heterogeneity in stable human coronary atherosclerotic plaques is underestimated in vivo: the "cooling effect" of blood flow. *J Am Coll Cardiol* **41**:403–408.
21. Stefanadis C, Toutouzas K, Tsiamis E, *et al.* (2001) Thermography of human arterial system by means of new thermography catheters. *Catheter Cardiovasc Interv* **54**:51–58.
22. Stefanadis C, Toutouzas K, Tsiamis E, *et al.* (2007) Relation between local temperature and C-reactive protein levels in patients

with coronary artery disease: effects of atorvastatin treatment. *Atherosclerosis* **192**:396–400.

23. Stefanadis C, Toutouzas K, Vavuranakis M, *et al.* (2002) Statin treatment is associated with reduced thermal heterogeneity in human atherosclerotic plaques. *Eur Heart J* **23**:1664–1669.

24. Toutouzas K, Drakopoulou M, Markou V, *et al.* (2007) Correlation of systemic inflammation with local inflammatory activity in non-culprit lesions: beneficial effect of statins. *Int J Cardiol* **119**:368–373.

25. Toutouzas K, Drakopoulou M, Mitropoulos J, *et al.* (2006) Elevated plaque temperature in non-culprit de novo atheromatous lesions of patients with acute coronary syndromes. *J Am Coll Cardiol* **47**:301–306.

26. Toutouzas K, Synetos A, Stefanadi E, *et al.* (2007) Correlation between morphologic characteristics and local temperature differences in culprit lesions of patients with symptomatic coronary artery disease. *J Am Coll Cardiol* **49**:2264–2271.

27. Schmermund A, Rodermann J, & Erbel R (2003) Intracoronary thermography. *Herz* **28**:505–512.

28. Verheye S, De Meyer GR, Krams R, *et al.* (2004) Intravascular thermography: immediate functional and morphological vascular findings. *Eur Heart J* **25**:158–165.

29. Courtney BK, Nakamura M, Tsugita R, *et al.* (2004) Validation of a thermographic guidewire for endoluminal mapping of atherosclerotic disease: an in vitro study. *Catheter Cardiovasc Interv* **62**:221–229.

30. Wainstein M, Costa M, Ribeiro J, *et al.* (2007) Vulnerable plaque detection by temperature heterogeneity measured with a guidewire system: clinical, intravascular ultrasound and histopathologic correlates. *J Invasive Cardiol* **19**:49–54.

31. Toutouzas K, Vaina S, Tsiamis E, *et al.* (2004) Detection of increased temperature of the culprit lesion after recent myocardial infarction: the favorable effect of statins. *Am Heart J* **148**:783–788.

32. Toutouzas K, Riga MI, Vaina S, *et al.* (2007) Abstract 1989: Optical coherence tomography in patients with acute coronary syndromes. Increased local inflammatory activation in ruptured plaques with thin fibrous cap. *Circulation* **116**: II–430.

33. Stefanadis C, Toutouzas K, Tsiamis E, *et al.* (2001) Increased local temperature in human coronary atherosclerotic plaques: an independent predictor of clinical outcome in patients undergoing a percutaneous coronary intervention. *J Am Coll Cardiol* **37**:1277–1283.

34. Toutouzas K, Markou V, Drakopoulou M, *et al.* (2005) Patients with type two diabetes mellitus: increased local inflammatory activation in culprit atheromatous plaques. *Hellenic J Cardiol* **46**:283–288.

35. Toutouzas K, Markou V, Drakopoulou M, *et al.* (2005) Increased heat generation from atherosclerotic plaques in patients with type 2 diabetes: an increased local inflammatory activation. *Diabetes Care* **28**:1656–1661.

36. Libby P (2002) Lipid-lowering therapy stabilizes plaque, reduces events by limiting inflammation. *Am J Manag Care Suppl.* **1**:4.

37. Rzeszutko L, Legutko J, Kaluza GL, *et al.* (2006) Assessment of culprit plaque temperature by intracoronary thermography appears inconclusive in patients with acute coronary syndromes. *Arterioscler Thromb Vasc Biol* **26**:1889–1894.

38. Dudek D, Rzeszutko L, Legutko J, *et al.* (2005) High-risk coronary artery plaques diagnosed by intracoronary thermography. *Kardiol Pol* **62**:383–389.

39. Takumi T, Lee S, Hamasaki S, *et al.* (2007) Limitation of angiography to identify the culprit plaque in acute myocardial infarction with coronary total occlusion utility of coronary plaque temperature measurement to identify the culprit plaque. *J Am Coll Cardiol* **50**:2197–2203.

40. ten Have AG, Draaijers EB, Gijsen FJ, *et al.* (2007) Influence of catheter design on lumen wall temperature distribution in intracoronary thermography. *J Biomech* **40**:281–288.

41. ten Have AG, Gijsen FJ, Wentzel JJ, *et al.* (2004) Temperature distribution in atherosclerotic coronary arteries: influence of plaque geometry and flow (a numerical study). *Phys Med Biol* **49**:4447–4462.

42. Stefanadis C, Toutouzas K, Vavuranakis M, *et al.* (2003) New balloon-thermography catheter for in vivo temperature measurements in human coronary atherosclerotic plaques: a novel approach for thermography? *Catheter Cardiovasc Interv* **58**:344–350.

43. Belardi JA, Albertal M, Cura FA, *et al.* (2005) Intravascular thermographic assessment in human coronary atherosclerotic plaques by a novel flow-occluding sensing catheter: a safety and feasibility study. *J Invasive Cardiol* **17**:663–666.

44. Webster M, Stewart J, & Ruygrok P (2002) Intracoronary thermography in stable and unstable coronary disease. *Circulation* **106**:657.

45. Toutouzas K, Drakopoulou M, Markou V, *et al.* (2006) Increased coronary sinus blood temperature: correlation with systemic inflammation. *Eur J Clin Invest* **36**:218–223.

46. Stefanadis C, Tsiamis E, Vaina S, *et al.* (2004) Temperature of blood in the coronary sinus and right atrium in patients with and without coronary artery disease. *Am J Cardiol* **93**:207–210.

34   Coronary Stent Technology

Neville Kukreja, Yoshinobu Onuma & Patrick W. Serruys

Thoraxcenter, Erasmus Medical Center, Rotterdam, The Netherlands

Introduction

Percutaneous revascularization for coronary artery disease has seen rapid and drastic technologic advances since its introduction 30 years ago. The technique has been adopted worldwide and is now the most common modality of revascularization, with increasing numbers of patients being treated each year. The first stents were initially used as bailout devices to deal with complications of balloon angioplasty. However, the beneficial effects on restenosis coupled with easier to use devices have resulted in stent implantation as a default strategy in the majority of procedures [1]. The initial shortcomings of acute stent thrombosis were rapidly resolved, leaving restenosis due to neointimal hyperplasia as the major potential drawback of stent implantation. The acute complications of contemporary percutaneous intervention are now very low, with mortality rates of 0.3%, emergency coronary artery bypass graft (CABG) rates of 0.2%, and myocardial infarction rates of 0.6% [1]. In 2002, the field of interventional cardiology entered a new era with the advent of the first commercially available drug-eluting stent (DES) [2]. These expensive and novel devices were quickly embraced by cardiologists and have already had a major impact on coronary revascularization. However in 2006, worrisome data on late stent thrombosis in the first generation of DES emerged. Physician-driven registries with long follow-up suggest an unabated rate of late and very late stent thrombosis even up to 4 years [3–6]. New pharmacologic strategies (e.g., nonpolymeric reservoirs, dual drug elution with antithrombotic and anti-inflammatory agents) and new bioabsorbable metallic or nonmetallic platforms are currently being tested. Rather than the complete abolition of neointimal hyperplasia, the primary goal of DES is the restitution of a healthy, functionally active endothelial lining without inducing excessive neointimal hyperplasia. Each DES comprises three components: the stent platform, the active pharmacologic compound, and a drug carrier vehicle (usually a polymer), which controls drug elution. Research for the development of the next generations of DES has focused on each of these components. In this chapter, we aim to describe the currently available bare and drug-eluting stents, while also providing an insight into exciting new developments which may eventually reach everyday clinical practice.

Plain old balloon angioplasty and the arrival of coronary stents

Balloon dilation as a treatment for obstructive coronary artery disease was first performed in 1977 [7]. The initial shortfalls of this therapy included acute recoil and abrupt vessel closure, which frequently necessitated emergency surgical revascularization [8]. The advent of intracoronary stents in 1986, initially as a "bailout" for complications of balloon angioplasty but subsequently used as a default revascularization strategy, addressed these problems by providing a mechanical scaffold, thereby reducing rates of emergency bypass surgery to <0.5% and reducing restenosis rates from 30–40% with balloon angioplasty to 20–25% with bare metal stents (BMSs) [9–11]. However, the iatrogenic problem of acute stent thrombosis rapidly became evident, with reocclusion rates of up to 18% within the first 2 weeks [12]. Coronary stents are foreign bodies and, as such, trigger platelet adhesion and activation of the coagulation cascade. Furthermore, high-pressure implantation may cause vessel injury, exposing the thrombogenic subintima, media, and atherosclerotic plaque components to the circulation. Stent thrombosis occurred despite the use of aggressive anticoagulation regimes involving heparin, aspirin, dipyridamole, dextran, and vitamin K antagonists, which ironically led to a high incidence of bleeding complications. The balance has been resolved with the standard use of dual antiplatelet therapy with aspirin and a thienopyridine (either ticlopidine or clopidogrel) until the thrombogenic stent struts have been endothelialized (within 30 days for conventional stents) [13–15]. With these clear advantages, stent usage gradually increased, and in 2005 they had been implanted in 88% of 912 801 percutaneous revascularization procedures performed in Europe [1]. However, restenosis due to neointimal

Cardiovascular Interventions in Clinical Practice. Edited by Jürgen Haase, Hans-Joachim Schäfers, Horst Sievert and Ron Waksman. © 2010 Blackwell Publishing.

hyperplasia with bare metal stents still remains a concern. This is an exaggerated healing response to vessel trauma resulting from the angioplasty and stent procedure and has been the major limitation of percutaneous coronary intervention (PCI) in the bare metal stent era, occurring in 20–30% of cases [16], and has therefore been the pre-eminent focus of recent developments, including DESs, which utilize the stent itself as a vehicle for local intracoronary drug delivery.

Developments in bare metal stent technology

The first experiences with coronary stents used the self-expanding flexible coil design Wallstent® (Boston Scientific, Natick, MA, USA), which was first implanted in human coronary arteries in 1986 [9]. Despite initial difficulties with acute stent thrombosis, these devices were remarkably effective in reducing in-stent restenosis with a mean late lumen loss (LLL: difference in minimum lumen diameter after implantation and at angiographic follow-up) of 0.72 mm and binary angiographic restenosis (BAR: percentage diameter stenosis greater than 50%) of only 14% [12]. However, a number of balloon-expandable flexible coil design stents, including the Gianturco–Roubin stent (Cook Cardiology, Bloomington, IN, USA) and Wiktor stent (Medtronic, Minneapolis, MN, USA), exhibited higher degrees of acute recoil than the alternative slotted-tube design [17–20].

The initial balloon-mounted slotted tube stent was developed in 1985 by Palmaz [21,22]. The modified 15-mm length Palmaz-Schatz stent (Cordis, Warren, NJ, USA) consisted of two segments of a 7-mm stainless-steel slotted tube connected by a 1-mm bridging strut and was the forerunner of all currently used stents [23]. The majority of currently available stainless-steel stents feature a similar structural design, although they are premounted on a delivery balloon.

Cobalt–chromium alloy bare metal stents

The initial coronary stents were composed of 316L stainless-steel alloy, since this material is radiopaque with adequate radial strength to maintain adequate arterial scaffolding and low degrees of acute recoil. However, cobalt–chromium (CoCr) exhibits superior radial strength and improved radiopacity, allowing for thinner stent struts, which may reduce restenosis and target lesion revascularization (TLR) while reducing device profile and hence improving its deliverability to the target lesion [24–26]. CoCr is the platform for the widely used Driver (Medtronic Inc., Minneapolis, MN, USA) and Multi-link Vision® (Abbot Vascular, Santa Clara, CA, USA) stents, both of which feature thin struts, excellent deliverability, and acceptable clinical efficacy (Multi-link Vision: 0.0032 inches, BAR 15.7%, LLL 0.83 mm, 6-month TLR 6.7%; Driver: 0.0036 inches, in-stent LLL 0.94 mm, BAR rate 15.7% and 9-month TLR rate 7.0%) [26,27].

Covered stents

The concept of a coronary stent covered with autologous vein was initially used as a treatment for coronary aneurysms [28,29]. Subsequently, specialized stents have been produced for the treatment of aneurysms and perforations, and should ideally be available in every interventional cardiology suite.

The balloon-expandable Jostent coronary stent graft (JoMed International, Sweden) is composed of a polytetrafluoro-ethylene (PTFE) layer sandwiched between two stainless-steel stents and is effective in sealing perforations or occluding aneurysms. However, the BAR rate of 31.6% is higher than for conventional stents [30]. Although this stent was investigated to treat saphenous vein graft lesions, it was not superior to a conventional stent, with no differences in postprocedure thrombolysis in myocardial infarction (TIMI) flow rate and a trend toward higher LLL and incidence of late occlusion in one study [31] and a higher incidence of periprocedural myocardial infarction in another [32]. Moreover, the PTFE barrier results in delayed endothelialization with the consequent risk of late stent thrombosis, so most operators advise long-term dual antiplatelet therapy. Implantation of a DES within the covered stent is feasible, and reduces the rate of restenosis: in a series of 14 patients, BAR was only 7.7% and LLL 0.18 mm [33].

The Symbiot self-expanding stent (Boston Scientific, Natick, MA, USA), consisting of a nickel–titanium (nitinol) stent sandwiched between two layers of PTFE, was developed for the treatment of friable saphenous vein graft lesions, with the concept of preventing distal embolization. Although this stent appeared effective, with 6-month target vessel revascularization (TVR) rates of 14.3% [34], it was associated with a trend toward increased restenosis when compared with a conventional bare stent without any beneficial effect on in-hospital adverse events [35].

Passive coated stents

A number of "passive" coatings have been applied to stent surfaces with the aim of decreasing thrombosis and restenosis. The Benestent II trial using heparin-coated Palmaz–Schatz stents combined with dual antiplatelet therapy (as opposed to more aggressive antithrombotic regimes) confirmed the superiority of coronary stenting over balloon angioplasty, with 16% BAR and LLL of 0.8 mm [36].

Gold exhibits attractive properties *in vitro*, including reduced neointimal formation, reduced thrombogenicity, and improved endothelialization, but a gold-coated stainless steel stent *in vivo* resulted in excessive neointimal hyperplasia (LLL 1.61 mm vs. 1.34 mm, BAR 50% vs. 38%) compared with an uncoated stent [37]. A different gold-coated stent gave similar results, with more neointimal hyperplasia than an uncoated stent [38]. Furthermore, gold increases radiopacity, which may aid stent positioning in the catheterization laboratory but makes noninvasive coronary imaging impossible because of the excessive "blooming" effect.

Silicon carbide exhibits antithrombotic properties *in vitro*, but failed to demonstrate any significant differences when compared with conventional stents [39]. A carbon-coated stent showed no differences in angiographic or clinical outcomes when compared with stainless-steel stents [40].

A titanium–nitric oxide alloy-coated stent (using physical vapor deposition), which had been shown to decrease platelet aggregation and encourage endothelial cell growth, has been compared with stainless-steel stents with encouraging results: a 40% reduction in neointimal hyperplasia compared with conventional BMS (LLL 0.55 mm for the coated stent vs. 0.9 mm for the uncoated stent, BAR 33% vs. 15%) [41]. Most recently, the Titan 2 Bio-active stent (Hexacath, Rueil-Malmaison, France) was compared with the Taxus paclitaxel-eluting stent (Boston Scientific) in the setting of primary PCI for acute myocardial infarction: after 6 months, there were no differences in composite major adverse cardiac events (MACEs), but the rate of stent thrombosis

was nonsignificantly lower with the Titan stent (0.5% vs. 3.3%) [42].

First generation drug-eluting stents

In 2002–2003, DESs were approved by regulatory bodies in Europe and the USA after initial studies showed a dramatic reduction in rates of restenosis compared with BMSs [2,43–45]. Subsequent data from patients with more challenging lesions and clinical presentations have confirmed this benefit, with a reduction in restenosis of 60–80% across the board [46–49]. Consequently, the use of DES was swiftly embraced, with market penetration of up to 90% in certain countries. In Europe, >220 000 DESs were implanted in 2005 [1].

The sirolimus-eluting Cypher® stent (Cordis, Warren, NJ, USA) is approved for use in the USA, Europe, and Japan (Table 34.1). The stent consists of a stainless steel platform

Table 34.1 Drug-eluting stents in clinical use or under investigation.

Drug category	Drug	Stent platform	Coating	Stent name	Company	Approval status
mTOR Inhibitors	Sirolimus	SS	DP	Cypher Select	Cordis	FDA/CE
		SS	BP	Supralimus	Sahajanand	CE
		SS	BP	CURA	Orbus Neich	
		SS	BP	Exel	JW Medical	
		SS	None	Yukon	Translumina	CE
		CoCr	BP	Supralimus-Core	Sahajanand	
	Everolimus	SS	BP	Future	Biosensors	Trial
		CoCr	DP	Xience V	Abbott	CE
		PLLA	BP	Absorb	Abbott	Trial
	Zotarolimus	CoCr	DP	Endeavour	Medtronic	FDA/CE
		CoCr	DP	Endeavour resolute	Medtronic	Trial
	Biolimus A9	SS	BP	Biomatrix	Biosensors	CE
		SS	BP	Nobori	Terumo	CE
		CoCr	BP	Xtent	Xtent	Trial
		Nitinol	BP	Axxess Plus	Devax	Trial
Calcineurin Inhibitors	Tacrolimus	SS	None	Janus	Sorin	CE
		CoCr	BP	Maharoba	Kaneka	Trial
	Pimecrolimus	CoCr	BP	Corio	Conor	
		CoCr	BP	Prolimus	Biotronik	Trial
		Magnesium	BP	Dreams	Biotronik	Trial
Microtubule stabilizer	Paclitaxel	SS	DP	Taxus Liberte	Boston Scientific	FDA/CE
		SS	BP	Infinnium	Sahajanand	CE
		CoCr	BP	CoStar	Conor	CE
		Tyrosine polycarbonate	BP	REVA	REVA	Trial
Other	Anti-CD34	SS	DP	Genous	Orbus Neich	CE
	Anti-VEGF	SS	DP		Biosensors	Trial

BP, biodegradable polymer; CE, Conformité Européenne; CoCr, cobalt–chromium; DP, durable polymer; EPC, endothelial progenitor cell; FDA, Food and Drug Administration; mTOR, mammalian target of rapamycin; PLLA, poly-L-lactic acid; SS, stainless steel; VEGF, vascular endothelial growth factor.

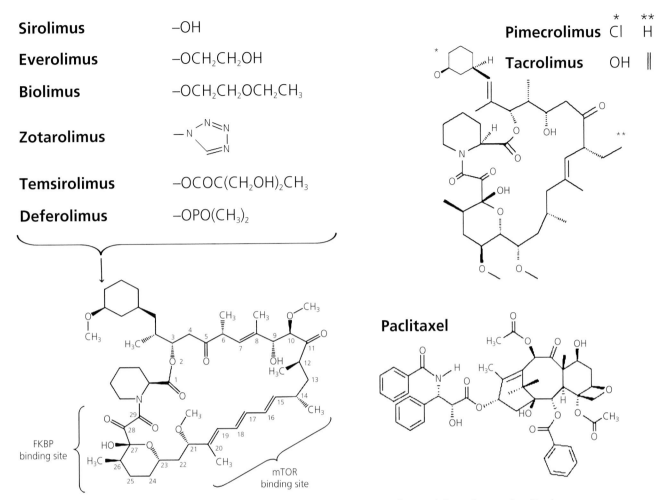

Sirolimus   –OH

Everolimus   –OCH₂CH₂OH

Biolimus   –OCH₂CH₂OCH₂CH₃

Zotarolimus

Temsirolimus   –OCOC(CH₂OH)₂CH₃

Deferolimus   –OPO(CH₃)₂

Pimecrolimus Cl   H

Tacrolimus   OH   ‖

Paclitaxel

Figure 34.1 Chemical structures of the antirestenotic sirolimus family mTOR inhibitors: tacrolimus and pimecrolimus, and paclitaxel.

coated with a permanent polymer (polyethylene-co-vinyl acetate [PEVA] and poly-n-butyl methacrylate [PBMA]) containing sirolimus 140 μg/cm², 80% of which is released in 30 days [2,50]. Sirolimus (also known as rapamycin) is a naturally occurring macrolide, which is also a potent immunosuppressant licensed for use in transplant recipients (Fig. 34.1) [51]. The lipophilic sirolimus binds to FK506-binding protein 12 (FKBP12) and subsequently the mammalian target of rapamycin (mTOR) and thereby blocks the cell cycle, inhibiting the transition from the G1 to S phase, resulting in inhibition of smooth muscle cell (SMC) migration and proliferation [52–54]. The initial reports of the sirolimus-eluting stent (SES) demonstrated almost complete abolition of neointimal growth [55,56], which was confirmed in the landmark RAVEL trial (LLL −0.01 mm vs. 0.8 mm, $P < 0.001$ and BAR 0% vs. 26.6%, $P < 0.001$) [2]. This profound effect on restenosis and repeat revascularization has subsequently been confirmed in larger industry-sponsored randomized trials as well as physician-driven registries including more complex lesions and patients

[43,46,48,57–62]. However, potential adverse biologic actions of sirolimus include accelerated senescence of endothelial progenitor cells (EPCs), the upregulation of tissue factor, and an increase in the expression of plasminogen activator inhibitor 1 (PAI-1) [63–65]. In clinical practice, SES has been found to unfavorably affect endothelial function, which may contribute to adverse clinical events [66–69].

The Taxus (Boston Scientific) paclitaxel-eluting stent (PES) has also been widely studied in a range of patient and lesion subsets (Table 34.1) [44,45,70–74]. This stent also incorporates a stainless-steel platform with a permanent polymer coating (poly[styrene-b-isobutylene-b-styrene]) combined with 1 μg/mm² paclitaxel [50]. The release of paclitaxel is biphasic, with a 48-h early burst followed by low-level release for 2 weeks; however, 90% of the drug remains bound to the polymer [75]. Paclitaxel (Fig. 34.1) is an antimitotic microtubule inhibitor which suppresses cell division in the G0/G1 and G2/M phases, resulting in disruption of SMC migration and proliferation. However, paclitaxel also increases expression of

Table 34.2 Registries comparing drug-eluting and bare metal stents.

Registry	Author	Recruitment period	Follow-up (months)	DES (n)	BMS (n)	Adjusted HR (95% CI), DES vs. BMS mortality
DEScover	Williams	2005	12	6509	397	0.52 (0.33–0.81)
SCAAR	Lagerqvist	2003–04	36	6033	13738	1.18 (1.04–1.35)
Western Denmark	Jensen	2002–05	15	3548	8847	0.90 (0.75–1.09)
Ontario	Tu	2003–05	36	3751	3751	0.68 (0.57–0.82)
NHLBI dynamic registry	Abbott	2004	12	1460	1763	0.97 (0.66–1.43)
REAL	Marzocchi	2002–05	24	3064	7565	0.91 (0.77–1.07)
Wake Forest	Applegate	2002–05	24	1285	1164	0.71 (0.54–0.92)

BMS, bare metal stent; DES, drug-eluting stent.

tissue factor in endothelial cells and increases the expression of PAI-1 [65,76]. In a landmark randomized controlled trial, the PES demonstrated lower rates of in-stent LLL (0.29 mm vs. 0.92 mm, $P < 0.001$), BAR (7.9% vs. 26.6%, $P < 0.001$), and TLR (3.0% vs. 11.3%, $P < 0.001$) compared with the bare metal stent platform [44].

Safety concerns and scope for improvement

Despite the beneficial effects of DES on restenosis and repeat revascularization, there are concerns regarding late (>30 days) and very late (>1 year) stent thrombosis due to delayed endothelialization despite prolonged dual antiplatelet therapy [6,77–79]. Long-term follow-up suggests that this risk continues for at least 3 years with no evidence of diminution [6,80]. Features associated with an increased risk of stent thrombosis include small minimal lumen diameter, stent malapposition (either immediately after implantation or as a result of positive remodeling), increasing stent length, residual dissections, geographical miss of the diseased target, poor left ventricular function, diabetes mellitus, increasing age, acute coronary syndrome at presentation, renal failure, treatment of bifurcations, and treatment of in-stent restenosis (ISR) [5,6,80–84].

Pathologic autopsy studies have shown an association between lack of neointimal strut coverage and stent thrombosis [85,86]. More recently, from a registry totaling 81 human autopsies of drug-eluting stents, Finn et al. [78] demonstrated that the most powerful histologic predictor of stent thrombosis was incomplete endothelial coverage. Recent angioscopic studies also support this association, demonstrating incomplete neointimal coverage as long as 2 years after implantation of SESs [87,88]. Therefore, one of the targets in current research is restitution of a healthy but not hyperproliferative endothelial lining.

To permit controlled drug release, the first generation DESs were coated with a permanent polymer, which persisted after drug release. The presence of such a polymer coating may contribute to stent thrombosis as a result of delayed healing and a hypersensitivity reaction in some cases [86,89–91]. Since these hypersensitivity reactions can occur >4 months after DES implantation (long after the period of drug release), it is possible that these events are due to the polymer coating [86]. A principal target of current research is the evaluation of biocompatible polymer coatings, with the aim of permitting controlled drug release while minimizing any such adverse effects (see later). Another alternative is to avoid the use of polymers altogether.

Nevertheless, the exact risk posed by DESs remains unclear. A collaborative network analysis of 38 trials enrolling >18 000 patients found no difference in mortality between SESs, PESs, and BMSs (SES vs. BMS: hazard ratio [HR] 1.00, 95% CI 0.82–1.25; PES vs. BMS: HR 1.03, 95% CI 0.84–1.22; SES vs. PES: HR 0.96, 95% CI 0.83–1.24) [92]. The risk of myocardial infarction was actually lower with SES than with either BMSs (HR 0.81, 95% CI 0.66–0.97) or PESs (HR 0.83, 95% CI 0.71–1.00). Although there were no differences in overall stent thrombosis rates, late thrombosis rates were higher with PES. There have also been several large-scale registries that have failed to demonstrate an excess in mortality or stent thrombosis after DES implantation when compared with BMSs, as shown in Table 34.2 [93–97]. The exception was the Swedish SCAAR registry, which showed increased mortality with DESs in patients undergoing PCI in 2003–04 [79]. However, in the 2005 patient cohort, with an increase in DES use from 22% in 2003 to 53% in 2005, mortality was reduced with DESs, perhaps indicating that DES use in 2003–04 was reserved for the highest risk patients [98]. "Off-label" DES implantation (e.g., bifurcations, primary PCI for acute myocardial infarction, treatment of saphenous vein graft [SVG] disease) is associated with worse outcomes (including mortality and stent thrombosis) than "on-label" indications [84,99]. However "off-label" indications may account for approximately 50% of all cases of DES implantation, and DESs still perform better than BMSs in these situations, with significant reductions in restenosis without any excess of adverse events [100–103].

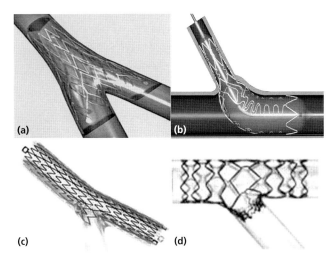

(a)

(b)

(c)

(d)

Figure 34.2 Dedicated bifurcation stents. (a) The AXXESS Plus (Devax, Irvine, CA, USA) self-expanding biolimus-A9 eluting nitinol stent; (b) the balloon-expandable bare metal cobalt–chromium Tryton side-branch stent (Tryton Medica, Newton, MA, USA); (c) the Stentys (Stentys SAS, France) self-expanding nitinol stent; (d) the balloon-expandable stainless-steel AST petal (Boston Scientific, Natick, MA, USA).

Second-generation drug-eluting stents

Two second-generation DESs are commonly used in Europe at the time of writing. Both utilize a CoCr platform to improve deliverability to the target lesion and biocompatible polymer coatings.

The Endeavor® (Medtronic Vascular, Santa Rosa, CA, USA) zotarolimus-eluting stent (ZES) is currently commercially available in both Europe and the USA (Table 34.1). This uses the CoCr Driver stent platform loaded with a permanent "biomimetic" phosphorylcholine polymer and the sirolimus analog zotarolimus (70% released over 30 days) (Figs. 34.1 and 34.3). In the first-in-man (FIM) trial, 12-month angiography demonstrated an LLL of 0.61 mm and 5.4% BAR [104].

Although the LLL is higher than for other DESs, the clinical efficacy was excellent, with a 12-month major adverse cardiac event (MACE) rate of only 2%. Four-year follow-up of the FIM trial has indicated an excellent long-term safety record, with a 4-year TLR rate of 3.1% and stent thrombosis rate of 1% [105]. In a large-scale randomized trial, the benefits compared with BMSs were confirmed, with a reduction in 9-month in-stent LLL (0.61 mm vs. 1.03 mm, $P < 0.001$) and TLR (4.6% vs. 11.8%, $P = 0.0001$) [106]. This benefit was maintained after 24 months with a continued reduction in TLR (6.5% vs. 14.7%, $P < 0.0001$) and overall MACE (10.0% vs. 18.7%, $P < 0.0001$). However, in a further randomized controlled trial, the ZES was unable to match the neointimal suppression of SES after 8 months (in-stent LLL 0.6 mm vs. 0.15 mm, $P < 0.001$; BAR 9.2% vs. 2.1%, $P = 0.02$). Although TLR rates were higher with ZES after 9 months (6.3% vs. 3.5%, $P = 0.04$), there were no differences in target vessel failure (12% vs. 11.5%, $P = 1.0$) or MACE (defined as death, myocardial infarction, or TLR: 7.6% vs. 7.1%, $P = 1.0$) [107].

The Xience™ V (Abbott Vascular, Santa Clara, CA, USA) everolimus-eluting stent (EES) consists of the Multi-Link Vision CoCr platform with a nonerodable polymer and $100\,\mu g/cm^2$ everolimus, a synthetic analog of sirolimus (40-O-[2-hydroxyethyl]-rapamycin) [108] (Table 34.1 and Fig. 34.1). The polymer is composed of acrylic and fluoro polymers and releases approximately 75% of the drug within 30 days. In the FIM study, after 6 months the EES demonstrated an LLL of 0.1 mm and 0% BAR, compared with 0.87 mm and 26% for the bare metal Vision stent [109,110]. After 2 years' follow-up, the TLR rate was 7.7% vs. 21.4% without any cases of stent thrombosis [111]. This degree of neointimal inhibition was confirmed in a larger randomized controlled trial (SPIRIT II), comparing the EES with the PES (LLL 0.11 vs. 0.36, $P < 0.0001$). There were no significant differences between the two stents in terms of major adverse clinical events after 6 months (2.7% vs. 6.5%) [112].

PC Technology   BioLinx

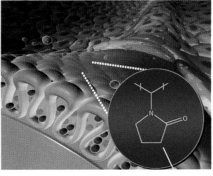

Figure 34.3 The phosphorylcholine and Biolinx polymer coatings for the Endeavor (a) and Endeavor Resolute (b) stents.

(a)   The phosphorylcholine (PC) Headgroup

(b)   Vinyl pyrrolidinone groups

New permanent metallic platforms

The Conor DES (Conor Medsystems, Menlo Park, CA, USA) utilized initially a stainless-steel and subsequently a CoCr platform with multiple intrastrut wells (Table 34.1). The stent struts are linked to flexible sinusoidal bridges by specially contoured features called ductile hinges. Stent deformation during deployment is confined to the 10% of the stent constituting the ductile hinges, rendering the struts as passive elements, allowing them to utilize reservoirs for drug delivery with no detrimental effect on the strength or crush resistance of the struts. The advantage is that these holes can be loaded with polymer/drug that will not deform or separate from the stent during expansion [113,114]. Elution of the drug from the wells is controlled by bioabsorption of a fully absorbable PLGA (polylactic-co-glycolic acid) polymer matrix. The low-dose Conor CoCr paclitaxel-eluting stent (10 μg paclitaxel released over 30 days) demonstrated excellent clinical efficacy with LLL of 0.28 mm and 12-month TLR of 2.8% [115].

In addition to novel "workhorse" DES platforms, new stents are under evaluation for specific lesion types, which historically are associated with worse angiographic and clinical outcomes, namely bifurcations and small vessels.

The Cardiomind self-expanding nitinol stent (Cardiomind, Sunnyvale, CA, USA) has been designed to improve deliverability to distal or tortuous segments of the coronary tree. The stent is mounted on a 0.014-inch guidewire and has a far lower crossing profile than balloon-expandable stents. The clinical feasibility of a bare Cardiomind stent has already been tested with promising results, and the evaluation of a biodegradable polymer-coated stent has recently commenced [116].

Another novel concept is the Xtent custom NX stent (Xtent, Menlo Park, CA, USA). This is a CoCr platform coated with polylactic acid (PLA) and Biolimus A9 (Table 34.1 and Fig. 34.1). The unique feature is that the stent consists of multiple 6-mm interdigitating segments, which can be deployed either in combination or separately. This system allows for *in situ* customization of stent length instead of relying on fixed-length stents. This stent has already been investigated in humans, with further studies in progress [117].

Bifurcation stents

The anatomy of bifurcation lesions produces difficulties in ensuring adequate scaffolding while preserving the side-branch ostium—stent underexpansion at this site is common and is associated with increased restenosis and thrombosis rates [118]. A number of dedicated devices which provide scaffolding for the carina are under investigation.

The bare metal stainless-steel Multi-link Frontier bifurcation stent (Abbott Vascular) has been successfully used to treat bifurcation lesions. This device covers the main branch proximally and distally, while also scaffolding the side branch ostium [119]. The in-segment BAR rates were 29%, with LLL 0.84 mm and 0.34 mm in the main and side branches, respectively. The next-generation CoCr everolimus-eluting version is currently undergoing preclinical evaluation [120].

The Axxess Plus stent (Devax, Irvine, CA, USA) is a self-expanding thin-strut (0.006 inches, 0.015 mm) conical nitinol (nickel–titanium) stent, coated with abluminal PLA and biolimus A9, another sirolimus analog (Table 34.1 and Fig. 34.1). The stent is designed to expand into the bifurcation covering the proximal main branch and the carina (Fig. 34.2a). If required, conventional stents can then be deployed into the distal main and/or side branches either sequentially or simultaneously (in a V-stent fashion) [121]. The initial clinical results have shown a 6-month in-stent LLL of 0.19 mm, a TLR rate of 7.5%, with 7.1% BAR in the main branch and 9.2% of patients needing a side branch stent [122]. Intravascular ultrasound analysis confirmed effective lesion coverage and neointimal suppression after 6 months [123].

The CoCr balloon-expandable bare metal Tryton side-branch stent (Tryton Medica, Newton, MA, USA) is currently undergoing clinical evaluation (Fig. 34.2b). The Tryton stent is deployed into the side branch with a central transition zone straddling the side branch origin. A conventional stent is then deployed in the main branch through the Tryton stent. In the Tryton 1 FIM trial, the angiographic success rate for this stent was 96.7% using 6F guiding catheters [124]. After 6 months' follow-up, the overall MACE rate was 9.9%. In the proximal main branch, LLL was 0.25 mm, in the distal main branch it was 0.00 mm, and in the side branch it was 0.17 mm. The in-segment BAR was 4.3% [125].

The Stentys coronary bifurcation stent (Stentys SAS, France) is a self-expanding nitinol stent which is deployed in the main branch (Fig. 34.2c). The stent structure is that of a Z-shaped mesh linked by small interconnections that can be disconnected by a PTCA balloon inflated into the side branch, thus allowing side branch access and scaffolding of the side branch ostium. In a similar method to provisional T-stenting, a further conventional stent can then be deployed at the side branch ostium if required [126].

Another dedicated bifurcation device is the stainless steel AST petal (Boston Scientific), which is mounted on two balloons and advanced over two guidewires (Fig. 34.2d). The FIM study demonstrated the feasibility of this stent [127]. Although the BAR rates were approximately 50%, the 4-month TVR rate was 18%.

Novel stent coatings

The first generation of DESs incorporated a permanent polymer to allow controlled drug release. The next generations of DESs are utilizing more complex biocompatible materials to achieve these aims. For example, the phosphorylcholine polymer used in the second-generation Endeavor ZES, although nondegradable, is a natural component of the cell membrane and, as such, is considered biocompatible (Fig. 34.3). A multitude of new stents have been investigated incorporating fully biodegradable polymers—the most commonly used polymers are PLA and PLGA—which are fully metabolized to water and carbon dioxide, leaving *in situ* a BMS after all the drug has been released. Preliminary promising data are available on three different stainless-steel stents coated with sirolimus and PLA—Excel (JW Medical Systems, China), Cura (Orbus Neich, Fort Lauderdale, FL, USA)—and Supralimus (Sahajanand Medical Technologies, India), although large-scale trials have yet to be performed [128,129] (Table 34.1). Paclitaxel has also shown encouraging results when incorporated with PLGA (Conor Medsystems, Menlo Park, CA, USA), as already described [115], and PLA (Infinnium; Sahajanand Medical Technologies, India) (Table 34.1) [130].

Everolimus (the drug used in the Xience V second-generation stent) had previously been evaluated in the PLA-coated stainless-steel S stent (Biosensors international, Singapore), which was effective in the FIM trial (LLL 0.10 mm vs. 0.85 mm for the BMS, $P < 0.0001$) [131,132] (Table 34.1 and Fig. 34.1). This stent releases 70% of the 197 $\mu g/cm^2$ everolimus within 30 days, and 85% within 90 days. A pooled analysis of 106 patients randomized in two clinical trials demonstrated the beneficial effect of EES regardless of vessel size [133].

The Endeavor Resolute (Medtronic Vascular, Santa Rosa, CA, USA) is the next version of the currently available Endeavor ZES, currently undergoing clinical evaluation (Table 34.1). This uses the Driver CoCr stent platform, but uses the Biolinx polymer (Fig. 34.3)—a blend of three different polymers (the hydrophobic C_{10} polymer to control drug release, the biocompatible and hydrophilic C_{19} polymer, and polyvinyl pyrrolidone to allow an early burst of drug release) [134]. Within 60 days, 85% of the drug is released: the remainder is released within 180 days. Porcine studies demonstrated no difference in inflammation or healing between the Endeavor Resolute and bare metal Driver stent. The FIM study showed impressive 4-month angiographic results with LLL of 0.12 mm and 0% BAR.

Other concepts include avoiding the use of a polymer completely. A microporous stainless-steel stent (Yukon, Translumina, Germany) offers the potential to customize drug doses and combinations [135] (Table 34.1). The system is therapeutically effective with rapamycin [136]. A nanoporous hydroxyapatite (a biocompatible crystalline derivative of calcium phosphate) coating, which can be impregnated with antirestenotic drugs, is currently under development [137]. A stainless-steel stent coated with nanoporous aluminum oxide and tacrolimus showed disappointing results, however, with evidence of particle debris shed from the coating contributing to increased neointimal hyperplasia [138].

New drugs and combinations

Another sirolimus analogue under investigation is biolimus A9 (Fig. 34.1). This has been evaluated in two biodegradable (PLA) polymer-coated stainless-steel stents (Biomatrix, Biosensors International, Singapore, and Nobori, Terumo, Japan), in which approximately 70% of the drug is eluted over 30 days followed by sustained release with polymer degradation over several months (Table 34.1). In both stents, the drug is applied to the abluminal surface only. The 6-month angiographic results of the Biomatrix FIM study showed an LLL of 0.26 mm vs. 0.74 mm and 3.9% BAR vs. 7.7% compared with the bare metal stent platform [139,140]. The Nobori stent demonstrated superior neointimal inhibition after 9 months when compared with a PES (LLL 0.15 mm vs. 0.32 mm, $P = 0.006$) [141].

Tacrolimus is another macrolide immunosuppressant drug licensed for recipients of organ transplantation (Fig. 34.1). However, the cellular mechanisms of tacrolimus differ from sirolimus: tacrolimus acts by binding FKBP12 and subsequently inhibiting calcineurin (and thereby decreasing the expression of proinflammatory cytokines (e.g., interleukin 2, IL-2) and suppressing T-cell proliferation [51]. The cellular effect is to hold cells in the G0 phase, where they are able to function but unable to replicate. Furthermore, tacrolimus has a preferential effect on SMCs as opposed to endothelial cells but, unlike the mTOR inhibitors and paclitaxel, does not increase expression of tissue factor [63,76,142,143]. However, a stainless-steel stent loaded with tacrolimus in abluminal reservoirs (Janus; Sorin Biomedica Cardio, Italy) performed no better than a BMS [144]. A CoCr stent coated with PLGA and tacrolimus (Mahoroba; Kaneka, Japan) is currently under investigation (Table 34.1) [145].

Pimecrolimus, a tacrolimus analog, has been investigated on its own and also in combination with paclitaxel. It exerts multiple anti-inflammatory effects including inhibition of IL-2 synthesis via calcineurin inhibition (Table 34.1 and Fig. 34.1).

The Synchronnium stent (Sahajanand Medical Technologies, India) consists of a stainless-steel stent coated with a biodegradable polymer incorporating heparin and sirolimus. The addition of heparin aims to decrease the thrombogenicity of the stent. Both drugs are released simultaneously over approximately 50 days. The initial clinical results are promising.

Genistein, a natural isoflavanoid phytoestrogen, is currently under investigation in combination with sirolimus. Flavanoids have a number of potentially beneficial characteristics including antiplatelet aggregation, anti-inflammatory properties, and antioxidant properties.

An alternative approach, concentrating on healing as opposed to SMC inhibition, is used in the Genous endothelial progenitor cell (EPC) capture stent (Orbus Neich, Fort Lauderdale, FL, USA). This is a stainless-steel stent coated with murine monoclonal antihuman CD34 antibodies, which attract circulating EPCs, thereby encouraging rapid endothelialization and reducing the risk of thrombosis (Table 34.1). The EPC capture stent appears to be effective in stable patients [146–148] and also in the setting of acute myocardial infarction [149].

Another novel target is the local delivery of anti-VEGF (vascular endothelial growth factor) antibodies, which might decrease the formation of vasa vasorum and thereby promote atheromatous plaque stability (Table 34.1). The anti-VEGF bevacizumab (Avastin) eluting BiodivYsio 316L stainless-steel stent (Biocompatibles Ltd, London, UK) uses a phosphorylcholine polymer impregnated with bevacizumab, 80% of which is released within 48 h. When used in patients with acute coronary syndromes, the LLL was 0.2 mm after 9 months; all 20 patients in the FIM study remained free of adverse clinical events during this follow-up period [150,151].

Fully biodegradable platforms

An option that is currently attracting a great deal of interest is the development of fully biodegradable stents. The required characteristics are the ability for controlled, sustained drug release, sufficient mechanical strength to prevent negative vessel remodeling and avoid stent deformity or strut fractures, and compatibility with noninvasive coronary angiography (magnetic resonance imaging [MRI] and computed tomography [CT]). Conceptually, once they are fully absorbed, only the healed vessels are left behind, with no residual prosthesis and therefore no potential adverse interactions with the coronary artery. Accordingly, long-term antiplatelet therapy may not be warranted as the risk of late or very late stent thrombosis should be low. Additionally, after absorption, vasomotion is restored, and there is less difficulty with future percutaneous or surgical revascularization.

The safety of an uncoated fully degradable poly-L-lactic acid (PLLA) stent (Igaki-Tamai; Igaki Medical Planning, Japan) has already been established [152]. The deployment procedure is technically more complex than for a typical balloon-expandable metal stent (the Igaki-Tamai stent is partially self-expanding, but deployment requires the use of a balloon containing heated contrast). Although the acute recoil of the stent was measured as 22% by quantitative coronary angiography, the clinical results were encouraging, with a target lesion revascularization rate of 10.5% after 6 months.

An everolimus-eluting PLLA stent (BVS; Abbott Laboratories, IL, USA) has recently undergone clinical evaluation, with promising results (Table 34.1). The stent consists of a PLLA backbone with a poly-DL-lactic acid (PDLLA)-everolimus coating [153,154]. Both polymers are hydrolyzed to lactic acid, which is then metabolized by the Krebs' cycle. In a porcine model, the mass loss was about 30% at 12 months, with further reduction to 60% mass loss by 18 months after implantation. The mechanical properties of the stent appear favorable:

acute recoil (the difference between mean diameter during balloon dilation and mean diameter at the end of the procedure) was similar to a CoCr EES (6.9% vs. 4.9%) [155]. The stent is radiolucent, but contains two platinum markers at each end, to allow identification on both conventional and noninvasive angiography [153,156]. Optical coherence tomography demonstrated that 99% of struts were covered by tissue after 6 months, suggesting a low risk of very late stent thrombosis [154]. After 6 months, the angiographic LLL was 0.44 mm, which was mainly due to an 11.8% decrease in the stent area, suggesting that, as the stent degrades, the scaffolding properties may become insufficient to prevent chronic recoil.

Another polymer-based degradable stent currently undergoing clinical evaluation is the tyrosine-derived polycarbonate REVA stent (REVA medical, San Diego, CA, USA). This has the advantage of being radiopaque, permitting direct visualization under standard fluoroscopy. The stent structure is unique and utilizes a "slide and lock" design rather than the usual material deformation for deployment.

Apart from polymer-based fully degradable stents, magnesium is a promising alternative. The absorbable metal stent (AMS; Biotronik, Bülach, Switzerland) consists of a bioabsorbable magnesium alloy, with similar mechanical properties to stainless steel (recoil <8%) and complete degradation within 56 days [157]. The stent is completely radiolucent: accurate positioning during deployment is possible because of two radiopaque markers at the balloon ends. Although clearly visible on intravascular ultrasound, the stent itself is not visible by conventional or noninvasive imaging [158,159]. However, the clinical results of the bare AMS were disappointing, with a 4-month in-stent LLL of 1.08 mm and 12-month TLR of 45% [157]. A drug-eluting version is eagerly anticipated, although a possible reason for the high TLR rate is that stent degradation is too rapid, resulting in an inadequate duration of scaffolding. Different magnesium alloy compositions and stent designs are currently under investigation to address these issues.

When should drug-eluting stents be used?

Unfortunately, this is a difficult question, and the answer depends on numerous patient and economic factors. There is no doubt that DESs reduce restenosis, but are they really necessary for everybody? In patients requiring noncardiac surgery or with other life-limiting conditions, or those whose compliance with long-term dual antiplatelet therapy is questionable, a BMS may be a safer option. Perhaps the best guidance comes from the National Institute for Clinical Excellence in the UK, which in 2008 recommended DESs for on-label indications in lesions <3.0 mm diameter or >15 mm length provided that the cost difference between DES and BMS is less than £300 (approximately €400 or $600 at the time of writing) [160]; this guidance takes into account the fact that in patients with large vessels and short lesions the risk of restenosis is low, even with BMSs, while acknowledging that DESs are costly devices.

Cost-effective analysis of landmark randomized trials found that for SESs, the cost per quality-adjusted life year (QALY) gained was $27 540 (assuming a BMS cost of $900 and SES cost $2900). The incremental cost-effectiveness ratio (ICER) for SESs was $1650 per repeat revascularization [161]. For PESs, the ICER per TVR was $4678 and $47 798 per QALY gained (assuming costs of BMS and PES of $800 and $2700 respectively) [162]. However, among patients assigned to clinical follow-up alone, the ICER per TVR was $760 and $5105 per QALY gained.

Analysis of data from all-comer patients (rather than carefully selected patients enrolled in randomized clinical trials) in the RESEARCH (Rapamycin-eluting Stent Evaluated and Rotterdam Cardiology Hospital) registry showed that, for SESs, the ICER per TVR avoided was €29 373 at 1 year and €22 267 at 2 years (assuming a stent cost of €1929 per SES and €692 per BMS) [163]. The authors calculated that the price per SES would have to fall to €1023 to become cost neutral. The Basel Stent Kosten Effektivitäts Trial (BASKET) comparing the BMS, SES, and PES found that after 18 months the ICER was €64 732 to prevent one major adverse cardiac event and €40 467 per QALY gained (mean price: SES €2275, PES €1935, BMS €1260) [164]. However, DES were more effective and less expensive in vessels of < 3.0 mm diameter. For vessels of > 3.0 mm diameter, although the overall cost per QALY was €39 641, subgroup analysis revealed that the cost per QALY was €6863 for off-label use, €3471 for lesions ≥ 24 mm in length, and €300 for patients aged ≥ 65 years.

Thus, it seems that with these stent prices, DESs are cost-effective in certain subgroups, although not for *every* patient. Hopefully, market forces and the development and production of DES in the developing world (e.g., China and India) are likely to bring down the costs.

The future

From these historical developments, we can see that the ideal coronary stent should have several properties. The first is to provide a scaffold to prevent acute recoil and to seal any significant dissection flaps. The stent itself should be deliverable and visible, with adequate radiopacity (or the presence of radiopaque markers) to enable precise positioning under X-ray fluoroscopic guidance. The second is to allow sufficient functional endothelialization to prevent stent thrombosis while minimizing the natural vessel healing reaction, which results in neointimal hyperplasia [165]. To achieve this fine balance, the next generations of DESs utilize biocompatible and biodegradable polymer coatings. Fully degradable stents offer potential solutions to these conundrums, while the use of

new or combinations of drugs has the theoretical advantage of producing less toxicity.

Conclusion

The technologic advances in stent technology have been rapid, especially since the commercial introduction of DESs in 2002; the DES has emerged as the default treatment for many patients with coronary artery disease. However, the provision of a permanent mechanical scaffold with complete inhibition of the endothelium no longer seems sufficient. Nonetheless, despite safety concerns about stent thrombosis, and as more evidence accumulates, the first generation of DESs appear to be more effective than BMSs. A large number of devices are currently under investigation, with particular emphasis on new metallic platforms, biocompatible stent coatings, new drug combinations, and fully biodegradable platforms. A review of historical developments should remind us, however, that many stents that appear promising *in vitro* fail to reproduce their beneficial effects in real life. The optimal composition of the next generation of stents has yet to be resolved.

Note

All authors have approved the final manuscript, which has not been published and is not under consideration elsewhere. There are no conflicts of interest.

References

1. Praz L, Cook S, & Meier B (2008) Percutaneous coronary interventions in Europe in 2005. *EuroIntervention* **3**:442–446.
2. Morice MC, Serruys PW, Sousa JE, *et al.* (2002) A randomized comparison of a sirolimus-eluting stent with a standard stent for coronary revascularization. *N Engl J Med* **346**:1773–1780.
3. McFadden EP, Stabile E, Regar E, *et al.* (2004) Late thrombosis in drug-eluting coronary stents after discontinuation of antiplatelet therapy. *Lancet* **364**:1519–1521.
4. Ong AT, McFadden EP, Regar E, de Jaegere PP, van Domburg RT, & Serruys PW (2005) Late angiographic stent thrombosis (LAST) events with drug-eluting stents. *J Am Coll Cardiol* **45**:2088–2092.
5. Iakovou I, Schmidt T, Bonizzoni E, *et al.* (2005) Incidence, predictors, and outcome of thrombosis after successful implantation of drug-eluting stents. *JAMA* **293**:2126–2130.
6. Daemen J, Wenaweser P, Tsuchida K, *et al.* (2007) Early and late coronary stent thrombosis of sirolimus-eluting and paclitaxel-eluting stents in routine clinical practice: data from a large two-institutional cohort study. *Lancet* **369**:667–678.
7. Grüntzig A (1978) Transluminal dilatation of coronary-artery stenosis. *Lancet* **1**:263.
8. Grüntzig A, Senning A, & Siegenthaler W (1979) Nonoperative dilatation of coronary-artery stenosis: percutaneous transluminal coronary angioplasty. *N Engl J Med* **301**:61–68.

9. Sigwart U, Puel J, Mirkovitch V, Joffre F, & Kappenberger L (1987) Intravascular stents to prevent occlusion and restenosis after transluminal angioplasty. *N Engl J Med* **316**:701–706.

10. Serruys PW, de Jaegere P, Kiemeneij F, *et al.* (1994) A comparison of balloon-expandable-stent implantation with balloon angioplasty in patients with coronary artery disease. *N Engl J Med* **331**:489–495.

11. Fischman DL, Leon MB, Baim DS, *et al.* (1994) A randomized comparison of coronary-stent placement and balloon angioplasty in the treatment of coronary artery disease. *N Engl J Med* **331**:496–501.

12. Serruys PW, Strauss BH, Beatt KJ, *et al.* (1991) Angiographic follow-up after placement of a self-expanding coronary-artery stent. *N Engl J Med* **324**:13–17.

13. Schomig A, Neumann F-J, Kastrati A, *et al.* (1996) A randomized comparison of antiplatelet and anticoagulant therapy after the placement of coronary-artery stents. *N Engl J Med* **334**:1084–1089.

14. Colombo A, Hall P, Nakamura S, *et al.* (1995) Intracoronary stenting without anticoagulation accomplished with intravascular ultrasound guidance. *Circulation* **91**:1676–1688.

15. Bertrand ME, Rupprecht H-J, Urban P, Gershlick AH, & Investigators ftC (2000) Double-blind study of the safety of clopidogrel with and without a loading dose in combination with aspirin compared with ticlopidine in combination with aspirin after coronary stenting: the clopidogrel aspirin stent international cooperative study (CLASSICS). *Circulation* **102**:624–629.

16. Rajagopal V & Rockson SG (2003) Coronary restenosis: a review of mechanisms and management. *Am J Med* **115**:547–553.

17. Flueckiger F, Sternthal H, Klein GE, Aschauer M, Szolar D, & Kleinhappl G (1994) Strength, elasticity, and plasticity of expandable metal stents: in vitro studies with three types of stress. *J Vasc Interv Radiol* **5**:745–750.

18. Lossef SV, Lutz RJ, Mundorf J, & Barth KH (1994) Comparison of mechanical deformation properties of metallic stents with use of stress-strain analysis. *J Vasc Interv Radiol* **5**:341–349.

19. Okabe T, Asakura Y, Ishikawa S, Asakura K, Mitamura H, & Ogawa S (1999) Evaluation of scaffolding effects of five different types of stents by intravascular ultrasound analysis. *Am J Cardiol* **84**:981–986.

20. Carrozza JP, Jr., Hosley SE, Md DJC, & Baim DS (1999) *In vivo* assessment of stent expansion and recoil in normal porcine coronary arteries: differential outcome by stent design. *Circulation* **100**:756–760.

21. Palmaz JC, *et al.* (1985) Expandable intraluminal graft: a preliminary study. Work in progress. *Radiology* **156**:73–77.

22. Schatz RA, Palmaz JC, Tio FO, Garcia F, Garcia O, & Reuter S (1987) Balloon-expandable intracoronary stents in the adult dog. *Circulation* **76**:450–457.

23. Schatz RA, Baim DS, Leon M, *et al.* (1991) Clinical experience with the palmaz-schatz coronary stent: initial results of a multicenter study. *Circulation* **83**:148–161.

24. Kastrati A, Mehilli J, Dirschinger J, *et al.* (2001) Intracoronary Stenting and Angiographic Results: Strut Thickness Effect on Restenosis Outcome (ISAR-STEREO) Trial. *Circulation* **103**:2816–2821.

25. Pache Ju, Kastrati A, Mehilli J, *et al.* (2003) Intracoronary Stenting and Angiographic Results: Strut Thickness Effect on Restenosis Outcome (ISAR-STEREO-2) Trial. *J Am Coll Cardiol* **41**:1283–1288.

26. Kereiakes DJ, Cox DA, Hermiller JB, *et al.* (2003) Usefulness of a cobalt chromium coronary stent alloy. *Am J Cardiol* **92**:463–466.

27. Sketch JMH, Ball M, Rutherford B, Popma JJ, Russell C, & Kereiakes DJ (2005) Evaluation of the Medtronic (Driver) cobalt-chromium alloy coronary stent system. *Am J Cardiol* **95**:8–12.

28. Wong SC, Kent KM, Mintz GS, *et al.* (1995) Percutaneous transcatheter repair of a coronary aneurysm using a composite autologous cephalic vein-coated Palmaz-Schatz biliary stent. *Am J Cardiol* **76**:990–991.

29. Stefanadis C & Toutouzas P (1995) Percutaneous implantation of autologous vein graft stent for treatment of coronary artery disease. *Lancet* **345**:1509.

30. Gercken U, Lansky AJ, Buellesfeld L, *et al.* (2002) Results of the Jostent coronary stent graft implantation in various clinical settings: procedural and follow-up results. *Catheter Cardiovasc Interv* **56**:353–360.

31. Schächinger V, Hamm CW, Munzel T, *et al.* (2003) A randomized trial of polytetrafluoroethylene-membrane-covered stents compared with conventional stents in aortocoronary saphenous vein grafts. *J Am Coll Cardiol* **42**:1360–1369.

32. Stankovic G, Colombo A, Presbitero P, *et al.* (2003) Randomized evaluation of polytetrafluoroethylene-covered stent in saphenous vein grafts: the Randomized Evaluation of Polytetrafluoroethylene Covered stent in Saphenous Vein Grafts (RECOVERS) Trial. *Circulation* **108**:37–42.

33. Papafaklis M, Sianos G, Cost B, *et al.* (2006) Clinical and angiographic follow-up after overlapping implantation of polytetrafluoroethylene covered stents with drug eluting stents. *EuroIntervention* **2**:218–223.

34. Laarman GJ, Kiemeneij F, Mueller R, *et al.* (2005) Feasibility, safety, and preliminary efficacy of a novel ePTFE-covered self-expanding stent in saphenous vein graft lesions: the Symbiot II trial. *Catheter Cardiovasc Interv* **64**:361–368.

35. Turco MA, Buchbinder M, Popma JJ, *et al.* (2006) Pivotal, randomized US study of the Symbiot covered stent system in patients with saphenous vein graft disease: eight-month angiographic and clinical results from the Symbiot III trial. *Catheter Cardiovasc Interv* **68**:379–388.

36. Serruys PW, van Hout B, Bonnier H, *et al.* (1998) Randomised comparison of implantation of heparin-coated stents with balloon angioplasty in selected patients with coronary artery disease (Benestent II). *Lancet* **352**(9129):673–681.

37. Kastrati A, Schomig A, Dirschinger J, *et al.* (2000) Increased risk of restenosis after placement of gold-coated stents: results of a randomized trial comparing gold-coated with uncoated steel stents in patients with coronary artery disease. *Circulation* **101**:2478–2483.

38. vom Dahl J, Haager PK, Grube E, *et al.* (2002) Effects of gold coating of coronary stents on neointimal proliferation following stent implantation. *Am J Cardiol* **89**:801–805.

39. Unverdorben M, Sippel B, Degenhardt R, *et al.* (2003) Comparison of a silicon carbide-coated stent versus a noncoated stent in human beings: the Tenax versus Nir Stent Study's long-term outcome. *Am Heart J* **145**:E17.

40. Haase J, Storger H, Hofmann M, Schwarz CE, Reinemer H, & Schwarz F (2003) Comparison of stainless steel stents coated

with turbostratic carbon and uncoated stents for percutaneous coronary interventions. *J Invasive Cardiol* **15**:562–565.

41. Windecker S, Simon R, Lins M, *et al.* (2005) Randomized comparison of a titanium-nitride-oxide-coated stent with a stainless steel stent for coronary revascularization: the *TiNOX Trial. Circulation* **111**:2617–2622.

42. Giraud-Sauveur Y (2007) *TITAN 2* bio-active stent (BAS) with titanium-NO. *EuroIntervention* **3**:526–528.

43. Moses JW, Leon MB, Popma JJ, *et al.* (2003) Sirolimus-eluting stents versus standard stents in patients with stenosis in a native coronary artery. *N Engl J Med* **349**:1315–1323.

44. Stone GW, Ellis SG, Cox DA, *et al.* (2004) A polymer-based, paclitaxel-eluting stent in patients with coronary artery disease. *N Engl J Med* **350**:221–231.

45. Stone GW, Ellis SG, Cannon L, *et al.* (2005) Comparison of a polymer-based paclitaxel-eluting stent with a bare metal stent in patients with complex coronary artery disease: a randomized controlled trial. *JAMA* **294**:1215–1223.

46. Serruys PW, Ong ATL, Morice M-C, *et al.* (2005) Arterial Revascularisation Therapies Study Part II–Sirolimus-eluting stents for the treatment of patients with multivessel de novo coronary artery lesions. *EuroIntervention* **1**:147–156.

47. Ong AT, Serruys PW, Aoki J, *et al.* (2005) The unrestricted use of paclitaxel- versus sirolimus-eluting stents for coronary artery disease in an unselected population: one-year results of the Taxus-Stent Evaluated at Rotterdam Cardiology Hospital (T-SEARCH) registry. *J Am Coll Cardiol* **45**:1135–1141.

48. Daemen J, Ong AT, Stefanini GG, *et al.* (2006) Three-year clinical follow-up of the unrestricted use of sirolimus-eluting stents as part of the Rapamycin-Eluting Stent Evaluated at Rotterdam Cardiology Hospital (RESEARCH) registry. *Am J Cardiol* **98**: 895–901.

49. Daemen J & Serruys PW (2007) Drug-eluting stent update (2007): Part I: a survey of current and future generation drug-eluting stents: meaningful advances or more of the same? *Circulation* **116**:316–328.

50. Finn AV, Nakazawa G, Joner M, *et al.* (2007) Vascular responses to drug eluting stents: importance of delayed healing. *Arterioscler Thromb Vasc Biol* **27**:1500–1510.

51. Halloran PF (2004) Immunosuppressive drugs for kidney transplantation. *N Engl J Med* **351**:2715–2729.

52. Burke SE, Lubbers NL, Chen YW, *et al.* (1999) Neointimal formation after balloon-induced vascular injury in Yucatan minipigs is reduced by oral rapamycin. *J Cardiovasc Pharmacol* **33**:829–835.

53. Gallo R, Padurean A, Jayaraman T, *et al.* (1999) Inhibition of intimal thickening after balloon angioplasty in porcine coronary arteries by targeting regulators of the cell cycle. *Circulation* **99**:2164–2170.

54. Marx SO & Marks AR (2001) Bench to bedside: the development of rapamycin and its application to stent restenosis. *Circulation* **104**:852–855.

55. Sousa JE, Costa MA, Abizaid A, *et al.* (2001) Lack of neointimal proliferation after implantation of sirolimus-coated stents in human coronary arteries: a quantitative coronary angiography and three-dimensional intravascular ultrasound study. *Circulation* **103**:192–195.

56. Rensing BJ, Vos J, Smits PC, *et al.* (2001) Coronary restenosis elimination with a sirolimus eluting stent: first European human experience with 6-month angiographic and intravascular ultrasonic follow-up. *Eur Heart J* **22**:2125–2130.

57. Schofer J, Schluter M, Gershlick AH, *et al.* (2003) Sirolimus-eluting stents for treatment of patients with long atherosclerotic lesions in small coronary arteries: double-blind, randomised controlled trial (E-SIRIUS). *Lancet* **362**(9390):1093–1099.

58. Schampaert E, Cohen EA, Schluter M, *et al.* (2004) The Canadian study of the sirolimus-eluting stent in the treatment of patients with long de novo lesions in small native coronary arteries (C-SIRIUS). *J Am Coll Cardiol* **43**:1110–1115.

59. Lemos PA, Hoye A, Goedhart D, *et al.* (2004) Clinical, angiographic, and procedural predictors of angiographic restenosis after sirolimus-eluting stent implantation in complex patients: an evaluation from the Rapamycin-Eluting Stent Evaluated At Rotterdam Cardiology Hospital (RESEARCH) Study. *Circulation* **109**:1366–1370.

60. Urban P, Gershlick AH, Guagliumi G, *et al.* (2006) Safety of coronary sirolimus-eluting stents in daily clinical practice: one-year follow-up of the e-cypher registry. *Circulation* **113**: 1434–1441.

61. Kastrati A, Mehilli J, Pache J, *et al.* (2007) Analysis of 14 trials comparing sirolimus-eluting stents with bare-metal stents. *N Engl J Med* **356**:1030–1039.

62. Spaulding C, Daemen J, Boersma E, Cutlip DE, & Serruys PW (2007) A pooled analysis of data comparing sirolimus-eluting stents with bare-metal stents. *N Engl J Med* **356**:989–997.

63. Steffel J, Latini RA, Akhmedov A, *et al.* (2005) Rapamycin, but not FK-506, increases endothelial tissue factor expression: implications for drug-eluting stent design. *Circulation* **112**:2002–2011.

64. Imanishi T, Kobayashi K, Kuki S, Takahashi C, & Akasaka T (2006) Sirolimus accelerates senescence of endothelial progenitor cells through telomerase inactivation. *Atherosclerosis* **189**:288–296.

65. Muldowney JA, 3rd, Stringham JR, Levy SE, *et al.* (2007) Antiproliferative agents alter vascular plasminogen activator inhibitor-1 expression: a potential prothrombotic mechanism of drug-eluting stents. *Arterioscler Thromb Vasc Biol* **27**:400–406.

66. Togni M, Windecker S, Cocchia R, *et al.* (2005) Sirolimus-eluting stents associated with paradoxic coronary vasoconstriction. *J Am Coll Cardiol* **46**:231–236.

67. Hofma SH, van der Giessen WJ, van Dalen BM, *et al.* (2006) Indication of long-term endothelial dysfunction after sirolimus-eluting stent implantation. *Eur Heart J* **27**:166–170.

68. Obata JE, Kitta Y, Takano H, *et al.* (2007) Sirolimus-eluting stent implantation aggravates endothelial vasomotor dysfunction in the infarct-related coronary artery in patients with acute myocardial infarction. *J Am Coll Cardiol* **50**:1305–1309.

69. Fuke S, Maekawa K, Kawamoto K, *et al.* (2007) Impaired endothelial vasomotor function after sirolimus-eluting stent implantation. *Circ J* **71**:220–225.

70. Stone GW, Ellis SG, Cox DA, *et al.* (2004) One-year clinical results with the slow-release, polymer-based, paclitaxel-eluting TAXUS Stent: the TAXUS-IV Trial. *Circulation* **109**:1942–1947.

71. Ong ATL, Serruys PW, Aoki J, *et al.* (2005) The unrestricted use of paclitaxel- versus sirolimus-eluting stents for coronary artery disease in an unselected population: one-year results of the Taxus-Stent Evaluated at Rotterdam Cardiology Hospital (T-SEARCH) registry. *J Am Coll Cardiol* **45**:1135–1141.

72. Grube E, Dawkins KD, Guagliumi G, *et al.* (2007) TAXUS VI 2-year follow-up: randomized comparison of polymer-based paclitaxel-eluting with bare metal stents for treatment of long, complex lesions. *Eur Heart J* **28**:2578–2582.

73. Daemen J, Tsuchida K, Stefanini GG, *et al.* (2006) Two-year clinical follow-up of the unrestricted use of the paclitaxel-eluting stent compared to the sirolimus-eluting stent as part of the Taxus-Stent Evaluated at Rotterdam Cardiology Hospital (T-SEARCH) Registry. *EuroIntervention* **2**:330–337.

74. Daemen J, Spaulding C, Jacob S, Boersma E, Varenne O, & Serruys P (2007) A pooled safety analysis of data comparing paclitaxel-eluting stents with bare-metal stents. *EuroIntervention* **3**:392–399.

75. Colombo A, Drzewiecki J, Banning A, *et al.* (2003) Randomized study to assess the effectiveness of slow- and moderate-release polymer-based paclitaxel-eluting stents for coronary artery lesions. *Circulation* **108**:788–794.

76. Stahli BE, Camici GG, Steffel J, *et al.* (2006) Paclitaxel enhances thrombin-induced endothelial tissue factor expression via c-Jun terminal NH2 kinase activation. *Circ Res* **99**:149–155.

77. Mauri L, Hsieh W-h, Massaro JM, Ho KKL, D'Agostino R, & Cutlip DE (2007) Stent thrombosis in randomized clinical trials of drug-eluting stents. *N Engl J Med* **356**:1020–1029.

78. Finn AV, Joner M, Nakazawa G, *et al.* (2007) Pathological correlates of late drug-eluting stent thrombosis: strut coverage as a marker of endothelialization. *Circulation* **115**:2435–2441.

79. Lagerqvist B, James SK, Stenestrand U, *et al.* (2007) Long-term outcomes with drug-eluting stents versus bare-metal stents in Sweden. *N Engl J Med* **356**:1009–1019.

80. de la Torre-Hernandez JM, Alfonso F, Hernandez F, *et al.* (2008) Drug-eluting stent thrombosis: results from the multicenter Spanish registry ESTROFA (Estudio Espanol sobre Trombosis de stents Farmacoactivos). *J Am Coll Cardiol* **51**:986–990.

81. Kuchulakanti PK, Chu WW, Torguson R, *et al.* (2006) Correlates and long-term outcomes of angiographically proven stent thrombosis with sirolimus- and paclitaxel-eluting stents. *Circulation* **113**:1108–1113.

82. Park D-W, Park S-W, Park K-H, *et al.* (2006) Frequency of and risk factors for stent thrombosis after drug-eluting stent implantation during long-term follow-up. *Am J Cardiol* **98**:352–356.

83. Okabe T, Mintz GS, Buch AN, *et al.* (2007) Intravascular ultrasound parameters associated with stent thrombosis after drug-eluting stent deployment. *Am J Cardiol* **100**:615–620.

84. Win HK, Caldera AE, Maresh K, *et al.* (2007) Clinical outcomes and stent thrombosis following off-label use of drug-eluting stents. *JAMA* **297**:2001–2009.

85. Farb A, Burke AP, Kolodgie FD, & Virmani R (2003) Pathological mechanisms of fatal late coronary stent thrombosis in humans. *Circulation* **108**:1701–1706.

86. Joner M, Finn AV, Farb A, *et al.* (2006) Pathology of drug-eluting stents in humans: delayed healing and late thrombotic risk. *J Am Coll Cardiol* **48**:193–202.

87. Awata M, Kotani J-i, Uematsu M, *et al.* (2007) Serial angioscopic evidence of incomplete neointimal coverage after sirolimus-eluting stent implantation: comparison with bare-metal stents. *Circulation* **116**:910–916.

88. Kotani J-i, Awata M, Nanto S, *et al.* (2006) Incomplete neointimal coverage of sirolimus-eluting stents: angioscopic findings. *J Am Coll Cardiol* **47**:2108–2111.

89. van der Giessen WJ, Lincoff AM, Schwartz RS, *et al.* (1996) Marked inflammatory sequelae to implantation of biodegradable and nonbiodegradable polymers in porcine coronary arteries. *Circulation* **94**:1690–1697.

90. Virmani R, Guagliumi G, Farb A, *et al.* (2004) Localized hypersensitivity and late coronary thrombosis secondary to a sirolimus-eluting stent: should we be cautious? *Circulation* **109**:701–705.

91. Nebeker JR, Virmani R, Bennett CL, *et al.* (2006) Hypersensitivity cases associated with drug-eluting coronary stents: a review of available cases from the Research on Adverse Drug Events and Reports (RADAR) project. *J Am Coll Cardiol* **47**:175–181.

92. Stettler C, Wandel S, Allemann S, *et al.* (2007) Outcomes associated with drug-eluting and bare-metal stents: a collaborative network meta-analysis. *Lancet* **370**(9591):937–948.

93. Williams DO, Abbott JD, Kip KE, for the DI (2006) Outcomes of 6906 patients undergoing percutaneous coronary intervention in the era of drug-eluting stents: report of the DEScover Registry. *Circulation* **114**:2154–2162.

94. Jensen LO, Maeng M, Kaltoft A, *et al.* (2007) Stent thrombosis, myocardial infarction, and death after drug-eluting and bare-metal stent coronary interventions. *J Am Coll Cardiol* **50**:463–470.

95. Tu JV, Bowen J, Chiu M, *et al.* (2007) Effectiveness and safety of drug-eluting stents in Ontario. *N Engl J Med* **357**:1393–1402.

96. Marzocchi A, Saia F, Piovaccari G, *et al.* (2007) Long-term safety and efficacy of drug-eluting stents: two-year results of the REAL (registro angioplastiche dell'emilia romagna) multicenter registry. *Circulation* **115**:3181–3188.

97. Abbott JD, Voss MR, Nakamura M, *et al.* (2007) Unrestricted use of drug-eluting stents compared with bare-metal stents in routine clinical practice: findings from the national heart, lung, and blood institute dynamic registry. *J Am Coll Cardiol* **50**:2029–2036.

98. Serruys PW & Daemen J (2007) The SCAAR registry or the Swedish yo-yo. *EuroIntervention* **3**:297–300.

99. Beohar N, Davidson CJ, Kip KE, *et al.* (2007) Outcomes and complications associated with off-label and untested use of drug-eluting stents. *JAMA* **297**:1992–2000.

100. Spaulding C, Henry P, Teiger E, *et al.* (2006) Sirolimus-eluting versus uncoated stents in acute myocardial infarction. *N Engl J Med* **355**:1093–1104.

101. Laarman GJ, Suttorp MJ, Dirksen MT, *et al.* (2006) Paclitaxel-eluting versus uncoated stents in primary percutaneous coronary intervention. *N Engl J Med* **355**:1105–1113.

102. Marroquin OC, Selzer F, Mulukutla SR, *et al.* (2008) A comparison of bare-metal and drug-eluting stents for off-label indications. *N Engl J Med* **358**:342–352.

103. Roy P, Buch AN, Javaid A, *et al.* (2008) Impact of "off-label" utilization of drug-eluting stents on clinical outcomes in patients undergoing percutaneous coronary intervention. The *Am J Cardiol* **101**(3): pp. 293–299.

104. Meredith IT, Ormiston JA, Whitbourn R, *et al.* (2005) First-in-human study of the Endeavor ABT-578-eluting phosphorylcholine-encapsulated stent system in de novo native coronary artery lesions: Endeavor I Trial. *EuroIntervention* **1**:157–164.

105. Meredith IT, Ormiston J, Whitbourn R, *et al.* (2007) Four-year clinical follow-up after implantation of the endeavor zotarolimus-eluting stent: ENDEAVOR I, the first-in-human study. *Am J Cardiol*. Integrating Safety into the Practice of Drug-Eluting Stent Deployment **100**(8, Suppl. 2):S56–S61.

106. Fajadet J, Wijns W, Laarman G-J, *et al.* (2006) Randomized, double-blind, multicenter study of the endeavor zotarolimus-eluting phosphorylcholine-encapsulated stent for treatment of native coronary artery lesions: clinical and angiographic results of the ENDEAVOR II trial. *Circulation* **114**:798–806.

107. Kandzari DE, Leon MB, Popma JJ, *et al.* (2006) Comparison of zotarolimus-eluting and sirolimus-eluting stents in patients with native coronary artery disease: a randomized controlled trial. *J Am Coll Cardiol* **48**:2440–2447.

108. Schuler W, Sedrani R, Cottens S, *et al.* (1997) SDZ RAD, a new rapamycin derivative: pharmacological properties in vitro and *in vivo*. *Transplantation* **64**:36–42.

109. Serruys PW, Ong ATL, Piek JJ, *et al.* (2005) A randomized comparison of a durable polymer Everolimus-eluting stent with bare metal coronary stent: the SPIRIT first trial. *EuroIntervention* **1**:58–65.

110. Tsuchida K, Piek JJ, Neumann F, *et al.* (2005) One-year results of a durable polymer everolimus-eluting stent in de novo coronary narrowings (The SPIRIT FIRST Trial). *EuroIntervention* **1**:266–272.

111. Beijk MA, Neumann F, Wiemer M, *et al.* (2007) Two-year results of a durable polymer everolimus-eluting stent in de novo coronary artery stenosis (the SPIRIT FIRST Trial). *EuroIntervention* **3**:206–212.

112. Serruys PW, Ruygrok P, Neuzner J, *et al.* (2006) A randomised comparison of an everolimus-eluting coronary stent with a paclitaxel-eluting coronary stent: the SPIRIT II trial. *EuroIntervention* **2**:286–294.

113. Aoki J, Ong ATL, Abizaid A, *et al.* (2005) One-year clinical outcome of various doses and pharmacokinetic release formulations of paclitaxel eluted from an erodable polymer–insight in the Paclitaxel In-Stent Controlled Elution Study (PISCES). *EuroIntervention* **1**:165–172.

114. Serruys PW, Sianos G, Abizaid A, *et al.* (2005) The effect of variable dose and release kinetics on neointimal hyperplasia using a novel paclitaxel-eluting stent platform: the Paclitaxel In-Stent Controlled Elution Study (PISCES). *J Am Coll Cardiol* **46**:253–260.

115. Dawkins K, Verheye S, Schühlen H, *et al.* (2007) The European Cobalt Stent with Antiproliferative for Restenosis Trial (Euro-STAR): 12 month results. *EuroIntervention* **3**:82–88.

116. Abizaid AC, De Ribamar Costa J, Whitbourn RJ, & Chang JC (2007) The CardioMind coronary stent delivery system: stent delivery on a.014″ guidewire platform. *EuroIntervention* **3**:154–157.

117. Evans LW, Doran P, & Marco P (2007) XTENT® Custom NX™ drug eluting stent systems. *EuroIntervention* **3**:158–161.

118. Ormiston JA, Webster MWI, Jack SE, *et al.* (2006) Drug-eluting stents for coronary bifurcations: bench testing of provisional side-branch strategies. *Catheter Cardiovasc Interv* **67**:49–55.

119. Lefevre T, Ormiston J, Guagliumi G, *et al.* (2005) The FRONTIER stent registry: safety and feasibility of a novel dedicated stent for the treatment of bifurcation coronary artery lesions. *J Am Coll Cardiol* **46**:592–598.

120. Duchamp J & Boeke-Purkis K (2007) Abbott Vascular's everolimus eluting side branch access stent. *EuroIntervention* **2**:509–511.

121. Verheye S & Trauthen B (2007) AXXESS™ Biolimus A9® eluting bifurcation stent system. *EuroIntervention* **2**:506–508.

122. Grube E, Buellesfeld L, Neumann FJ, *et al.* (2007) Six-month clinical and angiographic results of a dedicated drug-eluting stent for the treatment of coronary bifurcation narrowings. *Am J Cardiol* **99**:1691–1697.

123. Miyazawa A, Ako J, Hassan A, *et al.* (2007) Analysis of bifurcation lesions treated with novel drug-eluting dedicated bifurcation stent system: intravascular ultrasound results of the AXXESS PLUS trial. *Catheter Cardiovasc Interv* **70**:952–957.

124. Kaplan A, Ramcharitar S, Louvard Y, *et al.* (2007) Tryton I, First-In-Man (FIM) study: acute and 30 day outcomes: preliminary report. *EuroIntervention* **3**:54–9.

125. Onuma Y, Müller R, Ramcharitar S, *et al.* (2008) Tryton I, First-In-Man (FIM) study: six month clinical and angiographic outcome, analysis with new quantitative coronary angiography dedicated for bifurcation lesions. *EuroIntervention* **3**:546–552.

126. Laborde J-C, Borenstein N, Behr L, & Ramcharitar S (2007) Stentys coronary bifurcation stent. *EuroIntervention* **3**:162–165.

127. Ormiston J, Webster M, El-Jack S, McNab D, & Plaumann SS (2007) The AST petal dedicated bifurcation stent: first-in-human experience. *Catheter Cardiovasc Interv* **70**:335–340.

128. Ge J, Qian J, Wang X, *et al.* (2007) Effectiveness and safety of the sirolimus-eluting stents coated with bioabsorbable polymer coating in human coronary arteries. *Catheter Cardiovasc Interv* **69**:198–202.

129. Lee CH, Lim J, Low A, *et al.* (2007) Sirolimus-eluting, bioabsorbable polymer-coated constant stent (Cura) in acute ST-elevation myocardial infarction: a clinical and angiographic study (CURAMI Registry). *J Invasive Cardiol* **19**:182–185.

130. Vranckx P, Serruys PW, Gambhir S, *et al.* (2006) Biodegradable-polymer-based, paclitaxel-eluting Infinnium™ stent: 9-month clinical and angiographic follow-up results from the SIMPLE II prospective multi-centre registry study. *EuroIntervention* **2**:310–317.

131. Grube E, Sonoda S, Ikeno F, *et al.* (2004) Six- and twelve-month results from first human experience using everolimus-eluting stents with bioabsorbable polymer. *Circulation* **109**:2168–2171.

132. Costa RA, Lansky AJ, Mintz GS, *et al.* (2005) Angiographic results of the first human experience with everolimus-eluting stents for the treatment of coronary lesions (the FUTURE I trial). *Am J Cardiol* **95**:113–116.

133. Tsuchiya Y, Lansky AJ, Costa RA, *et al.* (2006) Effect of everolimus-eluting stents in different vessel sizes (from the pooled FUTURE I and II trials). *Am J Cardiol* **98**:464–469.

134. Meredith I, Worthley S, Whitbourn R, *et al.* (2007) The next-generation Endeavor™ Resolute™ stent: 4-month clinical and angiographic results from the Resolute™ first-in-man trial. *EuroIntervention* **3**: pp. 50–53.

135. Wessely R, Hausleiter J, Michaelis C, *et al.* (2005) Inhibition of neointima formation by a novel drug-eluting stent system that allows for dose-adjustable, multiple, and on-site stent coating. *Arterioscler Thromb Vasc Biol* **25**:748–753.

136. Mehilli J, Kastrati A, Wessely R, *et al.* (2006) Randomized trial of a nonpolymer-based rapamycin-eluting stent versus a polymer-based paclitaxel-eluting stent for the reduction of late lumen loss. *Circulation* **113**:273–279.

137. Rajtar A, Kaluza G, Yang Q, *et al.* (2006) Hydroxyapatite-coated cardiovascular stents. *EuroIntervention* **2**:113–115.

138. Kollum M, Farb A, Schreiber R, *et al.* (2005) Particle debris from a nanoporous stent coating obscures potential antiproliferative effects of tacrolimus-eluting stents in a porcine model of restenosis. *Catheter Cardiovasc Interv* **64**:85–90.

139. Grube E, Hauptmann K-E, Buellesfeld L, Lim V, & Abizaid A (2005) Six-month results of a randomized study to evaluate safety and efficacy of a biolimus A9 eluting stent with a biodegradable polymer coating. *EuroIntervention* **1**:53–57.

140. Costa RA, Lansky AJ, Abizaid A, *et al.* (2006) Angiographic results of the first human experience with the biolimus A9 drug-eluting stent for de novo coronary lesions. The *Am J Cardiol* **98**:443–446.

141. Chevalier B, Serruys PW, Silber S, *et al.* (2007) Randomised comparison of Nobori™, biolimus A9-eluting coronary stent with a Taxus®, paclitaxel-eluting coronary stent in patients with stenosis in native coronary arteries: the Nobori 1 trial. *EuroIntervention* **2**:426–434.

142. Matter CM, Rozenberg I, Jaschko A, *et al.* (2006) Effects of tacrolimus or sirolimus on proliferation of vascular smooth muscle and endothelial cells. *J Cardiovasc Pharmacol* **48**:286–292.

143. Mohacsi PJ, Tuller D, Hulliger B, & Wijngaard PL (1997) Different inhibitory effects of immunosuppressive drugs on human and rat aortic smooth muscle and endothelial cell proliferation stimulated by platelet-derived growth factor or endothelial cell growth factor. *J Heart Lung Transpl* **16**:484–492.

144. Morice M-C, Bestehorn H-P, Carrie D, *et al.* (2006) Direct stenting of *de novo* coronary stenoses with tacrolimus-eluting versus carbon-coated carbostents. The randomized JUPITER II trial. *EuroIntervention* **2**:45–52.

145. Tanimoto S, van der Giessen W, van Beusekom H, *et al.* (2007) MAHOROBA™: Kaneka's tacrolimus eluting coronary stent. *EuroIntervention* **3**:149–153.

146. Aoki J, Serruys PW, van Beusekom H, *et al.* (2005) Endothelial progenitor cell capture by stents coated with antibody against CD34: the HEALING-FIM (Healthy Endothelial Accelerated Lining Inhibits Neointimal Growth-First In Man) registry. *J Am Coll Cardiol* **45**:1574–1579.

147. Duckers HJ, Silber S, Winter RD, *et al.* (2007) Circulating endothelial progenitor cells predict angiographic and intravascular ultrasound outcome following percutaneous coronary interventions in the HEALING-II trial: evaluation of an endothelial progenitor cell capturing stent. *EuroIntervention* **3**:67–75.

148. Duckers HJ, Soullié T, Heijer PD, *et al.* (2007) Accelerated vascular repair following percutaneous coronary intervention by capture of endothelial progenitor cells promotes regression of neointimal growth at long term follow-up: final results of the Healing II trial using an endothelial progenitor cell capturing stent (Genous R stent)™. *EuroIntervention* **3**:350–358.

149. Co M, Tay E, Lee CH, *et al.* (2008) Use of endothelial progenitor cell capture stent (Genous Bio-Engineered R Stent) during primary percutaneous coronary intervention in acute myocardial infarction: intermediate- to long-term clinical follow-up. *Am Heart J* **155**:128–132.

150. Stefanadis C, Toutouzas K, Stefanadi E, Kolodgie F, Vermani R, & Kipshidze N (2006) First experimental application of bevacizumab-eluting PC coated stent for inhibition of vasa vasorum of atherosclerotic plaque: angiographic results in a rabbit atheromatic model. *Hellenic J Cardiol* **47**:7–10.

151. Stefanadis C, Toutouzas K, Tsiamis E, Vavuranakis M, Stefanadi E, & Kipshidze N (2007) First-in-man study with bevacizumab-eluting stent: a new approach for the inhibition of atheromatic plaque neovascularisation. *EuroIntervention* **3**:460–464.

152. Tamai H, Igaki K, Kyo E, *et al.* (2000) Initial and 6-month results of biodegradable poly-l-lactic acid coronary stents in humans. *Circulation* **102**:399–404.

153. Ormiston JA, Webster MW, & Armstrong G (2007) First-in-human implantation of a fully bioabsorbable drug-eluting stent: the BVS poly-L-lactic acid everolimus-eluting coronary stent. *Catheter Cardiovasc Interv* **69**:128–31.

154. Ormiston JA, Serruys PW, Regar E, *et al.* (2008) A bioabsorbable everolimus-eluting coronary stent system for patients with single de-novo coronary artery lesions (ABSORB): a prospective open-label trial. *Lancet* **371**:899–907.

155. Tanimoto S, Serruys PW, Thuesen L, *et al.* (2007) Comparison of in vivo acute stent recoil between the bioabsorbable everolimus-eluting coronary stent and the everolimus-eluting cobalt chromium coronary stent: insights from the ABSORB and SPIRIT trials. *Catheter Cardiovasc Interv* **70**:515–523.

156. Kukreja N, Otsuka M, van Mieghem C, Ligthart J, Sianos G, & Serruys P (2006) Biodegradable drug eluting stents: invasive and non-invasive imaging. *EuroIntervention* **2**:403.

157. Erbel R, Di Mario C, Bartunek J, *et al.* (2007) Temporary scaffolding of coronary arteries with bioabsorbable magnesium stents: a prospective, non-randomised multicentre trial. *Lancet* **369**:1869–1875.

158. Eggebrecht H, Rodermann J, Hunold P, *et al.* (2005) Novel magnetic resonance-compatible coronary stent: the absorbable magnesium-alloy stent. *Circulation* **112**:e303–304.

159. Bose D, Eggebrecht H, & Erbel R (2006) Absorbable metal stent in human coronary arteries: imaging with intravascular ultrasound. *Heart* **92**:892.

160. National Institute for Health and Clinical Excellence (2008) Final appraisal determination: drug-eluting stents for the treatment of coronary artery disease. Available at: http://www.nice.org.uk/nicemedia/pdf/TA152Guidance.pdf

161. Cohen DJ, Bakhai A, Shi C, *et al.* (2004) Cost-effectiveness of sirolimus-eluting stents for treatment of complex coronary stenoses: results from the sirolimus-eluting balloon expandable stent in the treatment of patients with de novo native coronary artery lesions (SIRIUS) trial. *Circulation* **110**:508–514.

162. Bakhai A, Stone GW, Mahoney E, *et al.* (2006) Cost effectiveness of paclitaxel-eluting stents for patients undergoing percutaneous coronary revascularization: results from the TAXUS-IV Trial. *J Am Coll Cardiol* **48**:253–261.

163. Ong AT, Daemen J, van Hout BA, *et al.* (2006) Cost-effectiveness of the unrestricted use of sirolimus-eluting stents vs. bare metal stents at 1 and 2-year follow-up: results from the RESEARCH registry. *Eur Heart J* **27**:2996–3003.

164. Brunner-La Rocca HP, Kaiser C, Bernheim A, *et al.* (2007) Cost-effectiveness of drug-eluting stents in patients at high or low risk of major cardiac events in the Basel Stent KostenEffektivitats Trial (BASKET): an 18-month analysis. *Lancet* **370**(9598):1552–1559.

165. van Beusekom HM, Saia F, Zindler JD, *et al.* (2007) Drug-eluting stents show delayed healing: paclitaxel more pronounced than sirolimus. *Eur Heart J* **28**:974–979.

35   Adjunctive Techniques for PCI

Suntharo Ly, Seth Assar & Richard Heuser

St. Luke's Medical Hospital and Medical Center, Phoenix, AZ, USA

Introduction

Percutaneous transluminal coronary angioplasty (PTCA) with and without coronary stents is the definitive treatment in many patients presenting with acute coronary syndromes. However, not all coronary lesions are easily treated with PTCA and/or stenting. Some lesions are complex and require adjunctive devices to debulk or modify the plaque before balloon angioplasty and/or stenting. Treatment of native coronary or vein graft vessels associated with thrombus poses the risks of distal embolization, abrupt vessel closure, and the no-reflow phenomenon. These complex coronary lesions can include heavily calcified, diffusely diseased, non-dilatable, ostial and bifurcation lesions, as well as chronic total occlusions. Although adjunctive devices were originally created to battle restenosis, they have evolved to facilitate the maximal benefit of PTCA and stents. This chapter will discuss the specialization of atherotomy devices (score plaque), atherectomy devices (remove plaque), thrombectomy devices (remove thrombus), and embolic protection devices (remove debris).

Atherotomy

Cutting balloon atherotomy

Numerous endeavors have been made to solve the problem of in-stent restenosis and general postprocedural restenosis in percutaneous coronary intervention (PCI). While drug-eluting stents such as the sirolimus-eluting stent have been proven to be the best solution to in-stent restenosis to date, high device cost has stimulated the demand for a cost-effective approach to treatment. Cutting balloon atherotomy (CBA), a technique theorized in 1980 [1], involves a balloon catheter equipped to incise and score the vessel lumen during angioplasty, reducing barotrauma due to high hoop stresses and controlling microfissures—factors associated with neointimal hyperplasia in conventional PTCA (Fig. 35.1) [2].

Despite the fact that CBA is seemingly optimal for intervention in hyperplasia-susceptible ostial lesions, evidence has yet to be produced giving grounds to CBA as an effective method of treatment [3]. However, a small trial ($n = 87$) has shown promise: CBA was associated with a significantly reduced rate of restenosis (40%) compared with conventional PTCA (67%) following its use in the treatment of bifurcation lesions [4].

Typically, cutting balloon catheters feature three or four blades, or atherotomes, longitudinally mounted with pads onto a balloon catheter. The mounting pads allow the atherotomes to remain fixed to the balloon, while permitting greater flexibility. Typically less compliant than conventional catheters, CBA devices are limited in traversing tortuous anatomy. Furthermore, the presence of atherotomes poses a risk for balloon rupture, blade fracture, and retention, as well as laceration of the coronary artery [5]. These risks are minimized through proper catheter guidance and multiple low-pressure (<8 atm), slow inflations, as recommended by the manufacturer.

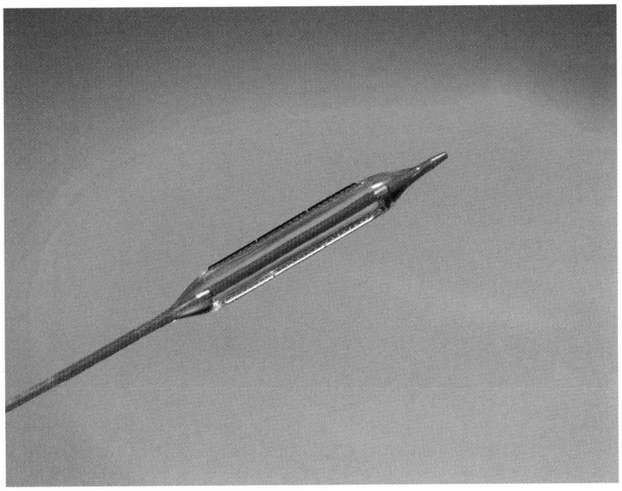

Cardiovascular Interventions in Clinical Practice. Edited by Jürgen Haase, Hans-Joachim Schäfers, Horst Sievert and Ron Waksman. © 2010 Blackwell Publishing.

Figure 35.1 Boston Scientific Flextome cutting balloon catheter. Image courtesy of Boston Scientific, USA.

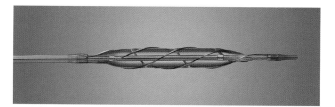

Figure 35.2 AngioSculpt PTCA cutting balloon catheter. Image courtesy of AngioScore Inc.

The first CBA products to be introduced to the market were the Cutting Balloon Ultra-2 and the Flextome Cutting Balloon, both manufactured by Boston Scientific (Natick, MA, USA) [6]. The balloons range in thickness from 2.00 to 3.25 mm in the case of those with three atherotomes and from 3.5 to 4.0 mm for those with four atherotomes, with lengths of 6, 10, and 15 mm, and feature longitudinally mounted atherotomes.

Cumulatively, studies evaluating CBA have shown considerable variation in results. These results have been expressed largely by the angiographic restenosis rate, although 30-day major adverse cardiac event (MACE) rate, 30-day myocardial infarction rate, and 30-day mortality rate end points have also been explored. The Cutting Balloon vs. Conventional Angioplasty (CUBA) study ($n = 194$) reported a 41% of 6-month angiographic restenosis rate [7]. However, large multicenter investigations such as the Cutting Balloon Global Randomized Trial (GRT) ($n = 1238$), conducted in 1997, have found no difference in technique, with angiographic restenosis rates for CBA and PTCA of 31.4% and 30.4%, respectively [8].

Innovative cutting balloon catheters hold promise for improving clinical outcomes. One such device is the AngioSculpt, which uses rectangular nitinol atherotomes spiraled about a semicompliant balloon catheter (Fig. 35.2). Although the device is still relatively new, with recent FDA pre-market approval, initial evaluations are certainly promising, boasting significantly lower balloon slippage rates than conventional PTCA balloons, greater luminal gains than both predilations or direct stenting, and successes in type C lesions [9].

Atherectomy

Atherectomy techniques include directional coronary atherectomy (DCA), rotational atherectomy, and laser atherectomy as represented by Excimer laser coronary angioplasty (ELCA) (Figs. 35.3 and 35.4).

Directional coronary atherectomy

Directional coronary atherectomy is a technique that removes or debulks coronary atheroma in preparation for balloon angioplasty and/or stenting. Luminal diameter gain is achieved from both plaque removal and angioplasty [10,11]. DCA was first used in the coronary arteries in 1986 using the Flex-Cut

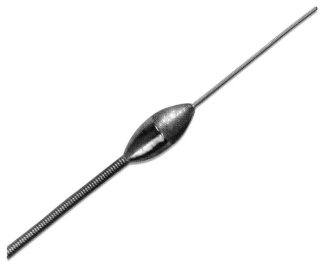

Figure 35.3 Rotablator rotational atherectomy system. Image courtesy of Boston Scientific, USA.

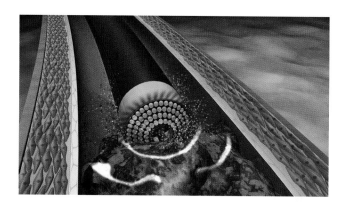

Figure 35.4 Mechanism of action for the Spectranetics ELCA laser catheter system. Images courtesy of Spectranetics Corporation.

device atherectomy device (Guidant Corporation, Santa Clara, CA, USA), approved by the FDA in 1990 [10,12].

Stand-alone DCA versus PTCA trials include the Canadian Coronary Atherectomy Trial (CCAT) [13] and Coronary Angioplasty Versus Excisional Atherectomy Trial I (CAVEAT I) [14] in native coronaries and the Coronary Angioplasty Versus Excisional Atherectomy Trial II (CAVEAT II) in saphenous vein grafts [15].

With a total study population of approximately 1000 patients, the CAVEAT I also compared DCA with PTCA, showing less residual restenosis early on with higher procedural success and larger luminal diameter gains in the DCA group. However, at 1-year follow-up, myocardial infarctions in native coronary arteries were higher in the DCA group than in the PTCA group (8.9% vs. 4.4%, respectively, $P = 0.005$) with no difference in restenosis (50% vs. 57%, respectively) [14].

The CAVEAT II trial moved away from native coronaries to compare DCA with PTCA in saphenous vein grafts (SVGs), initially showing a higher procedural success in the DCA group, with larger luminal gains (1.45 mm vs. 1.12 mm) but more frequent early complications of distal embolization (13.4% vs. 5.1%, $P = 0.012$) and a trend toward more myocardial infarction (16.1 vs. 9.6%) with no difference in repeat procedures or restenosis (46–51%) at 6 months between the two groups. These results were similar to the CAVEAT I trial [14,15].

Subsequent trials combined the technique of aggressive DCA debulking followed by PTCA with and without IVUS-guided DCA, and aggressive DCA with and without stents in hopes of achieving a lower residual restenosis.

The Adjunctive Balloon Angioplasty Following Coronary Atherectomy Study (ABACAS) evaluated whether intravascular ultrasound (IVUS)-guided DCA with or without PTCA reduced restenosis. Both groups had debulking of atheroma to <30% angiographically or to 46% of the cross-sectional area as determined by IVUS. One group went on to have adjunctive PTCA and the other group no further treatment. Although the adjunctive PTCA group had an initial increased minimal luminal diameter (MLD) of 2.73 ± 0.55 mm compared with 2.51 ± 0.52 mm ($P = 0.03$), there was no difference of MLD or restenosis at 6 months (23.6% in DCA with PTCA vs. 19.6% DCA alone) [16].

The Optimal Atherectomy Restenosis Study (OARS) hypothesized that a more aggressive "optimal" atherectomy, defined as a residual stenosis of <15% with adjunctive PTCA, would reduce restenosis rates. A 7% postprocedural residual diameter stenosis was lower than that seen in the CCAT and CAVEAT I trials (32% and 29%, respectively). Six-month angiographic restenosis rates were 28.9% [13,14,17].

DCA trials have shown an immediate postprocedural luminal gain and early lower angiographic restenosis but do not result in any clinical or angiographic long-term benefit compared with PTCA.

Rotational atherectomy

In contrast to DCA, rotational atherectomy (Boston Scientific, Natick MA, USA) is useful for calcified lesions as well as lesions unresponsive to PTCA, and fibrotic or restenotic lesions. Rotational atherectomy has four basic components: a guidewire, an advancer, a burr, and a console. The rotational atherectomy device has an elliptically shaped brass burr with diamond chips attached to the leading end. The drive shaft is rotated by a turbine which is driven by compressed air. The atherectomy device requires a Rotawire, which is a stainless-steel 0.0009-inch-diameter monofilament wire that comes in a floppy or extra support version. There is also a Rota Floppy Gold version that is gold coated to the distal wire segment at 12.5 cm. Burr sizes vary in diameter from 1.25 mm to 2.5 mm. The rotational speed of 160 000–180 000 rpm for 15–45 s is recommended. Guiding catheters of 6F, 7F, or 8F are used depending on the burr size [18,19].

Complications of rotational atherectomy include bradycardia (especially with RCA lesions), perforations, no reflow, and

postprocedural increase of creatinine phosphokinase-MB levels. Temporary pacing wires are recommended, especially for RCA lesions. Wire bias commonly occurs in tortuous coronary vessels due to the increased force of the wire and burr to the inner curvature of the vessel, especially if the lesion is not concentric. To reduce complications, starting with a small burr size of 1.25–1.50 mm and increasing by no >0.5 mm per burr step-up size is advised. In addition, a maximal burr to artery ratio of 0.7 is recommended. More aggressive burr to artery ratios (>0.7) are associated with an increased frequency of complications. Rotational atherectomy is contraindicated in a thrombus-containing vessel, SVG, diffuse disease, coronary lesions with poor distal runoff, and in patients with severely reduced left ventricular function. In addition, lesions with bends of >60° should not be attempted with rotational atherectomy because of the increased risk of perforation and dissection.

The question of aggressive versus moderate rotational atherectomy was answered in the Study to Determine Rotablator and Transluminal Angioplasty Strategy (STRATAS), which compared aggressive rotational atherectomy (burr–artery ratio 0.7–0.9) with no- or low-pressure balloon inflation (1 atm) and conventional rotational atherectomy (burr–artery ratio 0.6–0.8) with adjunctive balloon inflation (balloon–artery ratio 1.1–1.3, 3 atm) in native coronary vessels. At 6 months, there was no significant difference in death, myocardial infarction, target lesion revascularization (TLR,) or restenosis rates, except for a trend toward more non Q-wave myocardial infarction (11% vs. 7%) and restenosis (58% vs. 52%) in the aggressive than in the conventional arm. From this, aggressive burr sizing was not favored [20].

While the STRATAS trial studied lesions <20 mm in length and vessels <3.25 mm in diameter, the Dilation versus Ablation Revascularization Trial (DART) looked at lesions <20 mm long but at a smaller vessel diameter of 2.0–2.9 mm. The DART trial studied rotational atherectomy versus balloon angioplasty for noncomplex native coronary lesions in type A or B1 lesions. The rotational atherectomy group showed less major dissection (8% vs. 16%, $P < 0.05$) and bailout stenting (6% vs. 14%, $P < 0.01$), but more slow flow/no reflow (8% vs. 0.5%) than the PTCA group with no difference in restenosis rates [21].

The Stenting Post Rotational Atherectomy Trial (SPORT) randomized 735 patients to rotational atherectomy or PTCA before stenting. Results showed an initial procedural success in the rotational atherectomy plus stent group (93.6% vs. 88%, $P = 0.01$). However, there was no difference in TLR, TVR or clinical end points at 6 months' follow-up [22].

Available data on the use of rotational atherectomy for in-stent restenosis are conflicting. The multicenter Angioplasty Versus Rotational Atherectomy for Treatment of Diffuse In-stent Restenosis Trial (ARTIST) sought to compare and evaluate PTCA with and without rotational atherectomy in 298 patients with in-stent restenosis. PTCA with rotational atherectomy used low-pressure balloon inflation of 6 atm. A subset of 86 patients (45 PTCA and 41 PTCA with rotational atherectomy) used IVUS during the intervention and on 6 months' follow-up. The results demonstrated superiority of PTCA alone compared with low-inflation PTCA with rotational atherectomy. The 6-month primary end point showed a higher MLD (0.67 mm vs. 0.45 mm, $P < 0.0019$) in the PTCA alone group than in the PTCA with rotational atherectomy group. In addition, the 6-month secondary end points showed a decrease in binary restenosis (51% vs. 65%, $P = 0.039$) and an increase in event-free survival (91.3% vs. 79.6%, $P = 0.0052$) in the PTCA group.

As with directional coronary atherectomy, rotational atherectomy trials appear to show improved acute luminal gain with better procedural success. However, there are no differences in restenosis or late outcomes compared with balloon angioplasty. Aggressive rotational atherectomy tended toward more non Q-wave myocardial infarctions. Rotational atherectomy may be helpful in selected difficult lesions; these include heavily calcified (superficial calcium), nondilatable (not responding to balloon inflations of 10–12 atm), jailed side branch, or chronic total occlusion lesions. Despite limited data from randomized trials, rotational atherectomy has been recommended in bifurcation and aorto-ostial lesions before stenting [23,24].

Excimer laser coronary atherectomy

Laser technology was first applied to coronaries in the early 1980s [25,26]. Laser angioplasty was originally thought to produce less restenosis, but studies have not shown superiority compared with PTCA. Lasers for coronary angioplasty can be characterized as a continuous-wave system or the newer pulsed wave system. The pulsed-wave system should reduce in theory heating of surrounding tissue, but some thermal effects are still produced [27,28]. They can be ultraviolet lasers (xenon chloride [XeCl] excimer) or infrared lasers (holmium: YAG). The ablative effects of laser can cause photothermal (tissue vaporization), photoacoustic (shock wave can cause ejection of debris), or photochemical (direct breakdown of molecules) effects. The medium in which lasers travel can dictates their effects. Water is strongly absorbed by infrared light, whereas blood and contrast agents absorb UV light [29]. XeCl used in coronary angioplasty first became available in 1983.

Excimer laser coronary angioplasty (ELCA) was introduced in 1988. The term "excimer" is derived from excited dimer (in which a high-voltage electrical discharge is placed across a mixture of gases to produce high-energy light of a uniform wavelength). XeCl operates at 308 nm wavelength, which is in the ultraviolet electromagnetic spectrum. Radiation at 308 nm is absorbed by water and nonaqueous components of atherosclerotic plaque [6]. Blood and contrast media are strong absorbers of excimer light at 308 nm wavelength, forming "fast bubbles," an insoluble gas that rapidly expands and implodes, thought to contribute to coronary perforations and dissections. Some energy is converted into the process of photochemical dissociation; most is converted to heat. The laser causes heat and intracellular water is then vaporized, causing cells to explode [30,31].

The Excimer laser, Rotational atherectomy, Balloon Angioplasty Comparison (ERBAC) study was a randomized prospective single-center German study that enrolled 685 patients divided into three groups to compare the procedural success of excimer laser, rotational atherectomy, and balloon angioplasty. The primary end point of immediate procedural success was 89% in the rotational atherectomy group, 80% in the balloon angioplasty group, and 77% in the excimer laser angioplasty group. At 6 months, revascularization of the original target lesion was more frequent in the atherectomy and excimer laser group than in the balloon angioplasty group (42.4% and 46% vs. 31.9%, $P = 0.013$). The results showed that both laser and rotational atherectomy provided no clinical or angiographic benefit in late outcomes [32].

Lasers were originally thought to mainly have a photochemical effect, but it has now been shown that the photoacoustic effects predominate [33]. Because of the ability of laser angioplasty to heat vascular tissue, the concept of thermal welding was thought to seal coronary dissections; however, it resulted in unacceptable rates of coronary perforation and long-term restenosis [34]. Are lasers better in specific lesions? In the ERBAC trial, laser treatment of calcified lesions, such as type B and C lesions, resulted in more complications than rotational atherectomy and PTCA; thus, laser angioplasty is not recommended for calcified lesions [32]. Laser treatment of total occlusions was evaluated in the AMRO trial, which included a subset of patients with total occlusion and found no benefit of lastr treatment, in terms of reduced restenosis, compared with balloon angioplasty [35]. Laser angioplasty was initially thought to decrease restenosis rates, but restenosis rates of approximately 50% have been reported [36].

Thrombectomy

There are several different mechanical approaches to dealing with coronary vessels containing thrombus, such as simple mechanical compression against the coronary vessel wall using balloon angioplasty or mechanical removal using specialized catheters. Distal embolization occurs in 15% of patients presenting with ACS treated with primary percutaneous coronary intervention [37].

In the setting of ST-segment elevation myocardial infarction (STEMI), reduction in ST-segment elevation of >70% is considered a good indicator of myocardial perfusion [38]. Mechanical thrombectomy devices can be categorized into the aspiration devices, cut-and-aspirate devices, Venturi–Bernoulli devices, and ultrasonic devices.

Aspiration thrombectomy

Aspiration catheters, in general, have similar designs that have a distal primary lumen used to suck thrombus, with a secondary lumen through which the guidewire enters. They are easy to use and have a relatively low profile. The primary lumen is attached to a suction device, usually a 60-mL syringe attached to a valve to create a vacuum suction. Examples of suction thrombectomy catheters include the Export catheter (Medtronic Inc., Minneapolis, MN, USA), Diver CE (Invatec, Roncadelle, Italy), the Rescue catheter (Boston Scientific, Natick, MA, USA), the Pronto catheter (Vascular Solutions, Minneapolis, MN, USA), and the Rinspirator catheter (Kerberos Proximal Solutions, Mountainview, CA, USA) [33]. The Rinspirator catheter is unique because it can infuse saline while aspirating, which may facilitate a more efficient removal of thrombus.

The Dethrombosis to Enhance Acute Reperfusion in Myocardial Infarction (DEAR-MI) Study evaluated 148 patients presenting with STEMI randomly assigned to primary PCI (PPCI) or manual thrombus aspiration with the Pronto extraction catheter before PPCI and compared outcomes. The results showed better ST-segment resolution (50% vs. 68%, $P < 0.05$) and angiographic myocardial blush grade 3 (44% vs. 88%, $P < 0.0001$), with lower no reflow (15% vs. 3%, $P < 0.05$) and angiographic embolization (19% vs. 5%, $P < 0.05$), in the "thrombectomy before PPCI" group [39].

Siddiqui and colleagues [40] were able to successfully use the Pronto thrombectomy device in three patients with stent thrombosis. Burzotta and colleagues [41] used the Diver C.E. thrombectomy device to reduce the thrombus burden in 50 patients presenting with STEMI, non-STEMI (NSTEMI), and angiographic evidence of thrombus.

The recently published Thrombus Aspiration during Primary Percutaneous Coronary Intervention Study (TAPAS) compared mechanical aspiration of thrombus during PCI with conventional PCI. It was a prospective single-center randomized study conducted at the University Medical Center Groningen, the Netherlands. Patients presenting with STEMI were randomly assigned either to the thrombus aspiration group followed by PCI or to the conventional PCI group before any angiography was performed. Aspirated thrombus obtained was then evaluated by microscopy. The 6F Export Aspiration Catheter (Medtronic Inc., Minneapolis, MN, USA) was used in the thrombus aspiration group. All stents placed were bare metal. A total of 1071 patients were enrolled and 1007 patients (502 thrombus aspiration group, 503 conventional PCI group) underwent PCI. The primary end point of post-procedural myocardial blush grade of 0 or 1 was achieved in 17.1% of the thrombus aspiration group and in 26.3% of the conventional PCI group ($P < 0.001$). Complete ST-segment resolution occurred in 56.6% in the thrombus aspiration group and 44.2% in the conventional PCI group ($P < 0.001$). Aspiration was defined as effective or not effective depending on whether or not the aspirated material included athero-

thrombotic material; atherothrombotic material was aspirated from 331 patients (72.9%). There was no difference in 30-day mortality or MACE rate between the two groups, but there was a significant difference in 30-day mortality and MACE between groups with different myocardial blush grades. Mortality rates in groups with blush grade 0/1, 2, and 3 were 5.2%, 2.9%, and 1%, respectively ($P = 0.003$) whereas MACE rates were 14.1%, 8.8%, and 4.2%, respectively ($P < 0.001$). This study supports the important notion that microvascular obstruction may be related to embolization of thrombotic material downstream. Mechanical removal of thrombus can therefore reduce embolization [42].

Cut-and-aspirate

The transluminal extraction catheter (TEC) was previously recommended for thrombectomy of native coronaries and vein grafts. The main niche application appeared to be the treatment of diseased degenerated SVGs. However, rates of complications and restenosis were high. The TEC catheter is no longer available.

Another example of the cut-and-aspirate thrombectomy device is the X-Sizer catheter (eV3). The X-sizer mechanical thrombectomy system functions to remove thrombus from vessels using a patented helical cutter housed in the tip of a small catheter combined with a vacuum bottle. It is a fully assembled self-contained battery-powered unit that is disposable after use. The helical cutter diameter comes in two sizes, a 1.5 mm fitting a minimal introducer sheath of 6F and a 2.0 mm fitting a minimal introducer sheath of 7F. The rotational speed of the cutter is 2100 rpm.

The Prospective Randomized Trial of Thromboatherectomy With the X-sizer in Native Coronary Arteries and Saphenous Vein Grafts (X-TRACT) enrolled 797 patients with diseased SVGs or thrombus-containing native coronary vessels and compared the outcomes with and without use of the X-sizer thrombectomy device before stenting. The SVGs made up 72% and native coronary vessels 28%. The results showed no difference in MACE rates at both 30 days and 1 year [43].

In 2002, the X-sizer was approved for use in native coronaries and SVGs in Europe, but not in the USA; instead, the X-sizer catheter was FDA approved in September 2004 for removal of thrombus in synthetic hemodialysis grafts in the USA.

Venturi–Bernoulli

Rheolytic thrombectomy using the Possis Angiojet (Possis Medical, Inc., Minneapolis, MN, USA) catheter is based on the Venturi–Bernoulli vacuum principle (Fig. 35.5). The Angiojet uses pulsed high-pressure saline (10 000 psi) at a rate of 60 mL/min to disrupt and extract thrombus particles. Infused saline connected to a hypotube to the stainless-steel tip producing a high-pressure jet that is ejected back toward the mouth of the catheter to create a low-pressure region (-760 to 860 mmHg) that pulls and removes thrombus fragments from the vessel. Once the Angiojet catheter is placed at the distal

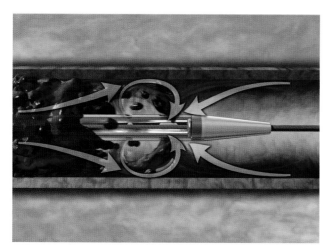

Figure 35.5 Mechanism of action for the Possis AngioJet catheter. Image courtesy of Possis Medical Inc.

end of the thrombus, the catheter is withdrawn at a rate of 0.5–1.0 mm/s, and the procedure then repeated as necessary.

The Vein Graft Angiojet Study I (VEGAS I) trial was a pilot study designed to evaluate the Possis Angiojet rheolytic thrombectomy system in removing coronary thrombus in ischemic coronary disease. The 90 patients enrolled had stable or unstable angina with vessel (native or vein grafts) lesions with a reference diameter of >2.5 mm. Approximately one-third of patients had had an acute myocardial infarction (AMI) and 7% had cardiogenic shock. visual assessment of the vessel to receive intervention revealed >70% stenosis, with 39 native and 52 vein grafts treated. Device success was defined as >20% improvement in MLD with a final diameter stenosis of ≤50%, and TIMI 3 flow. Procedural success encompassed device success after all treatments, including adjunctive stents used in 90% of patients. The results showed that thrombus area was reduced from 81.8 mm^2 to 21.4 mm^2 with the Angiojet device with procedural success of 86.8%. There was no significant difference in mortality between patients with and without myocardial infarction. The overall 1-year mortality was 4.4%. The effectiveness of the Angiojet system in VEGAS I led to the VEGAS II trial [44,45].

The VEGAS II study was a multicenter, randomized trial that compared rheolytic thrombectomy with thrombolytic therapy for angiographic evidence of thrombus. The rheolytic thrombectomy arm received treatment with the Angiojet system followed by definitive therapy. The thrombolytic arm received continuous intracoronary infusion of urokinase for >6 h. The primary end point was 30-day success, defined as >20% improvement in MLD, reaching a final diameter stenosis of ≤50% with TIMI 3 flow and freedom from MACEs. Abciximab was discouraged in both groups, but was received by 12% and 15% in the rheolytic and thrombolytic group, respectively. Both treatment modalities reached the primary end point effectively, but procedural success was significantly higher in the Angiojet group (86.3% vs. 72.7%) and freedom

from MACE at 30 days was also higher (82.2% vs. 65.7%). The originally planned enrollment of 520 patients was terminated early since 30-day freedom from MACE was higher in the Angiojet group after enrollment of only 300 patients, reaching a final enrollment of 349 patients. Both the VEGAS I and II studies established the safety and efficacy of the Angiojet device. The Angiojet device was FDA approved in June 1998 [44,45].

The Angiojet Rheolytic Thrombectomy in Patients Undergoing Primary Angioplasty for Acute Myocardial Infarction (AIMI) Trial compared infarct size in patients presenting with STEMI treated within 12 h with Angiojet thrombectomy followed by definitive treatment versus immediate primary PCI. A total of 480 patients were enrolled in the study, 240 patients in each group. Angiojet thrombectomy followed by PCI was hypothesized to reduce myocardial infarct size compared with PCI alone by reducing the thrombus burden. Infarct size was measured by ^{99m}Tc^m-sestamibi SPECT imaging. The primary end point was infarct size at 14–28 days. Eptifibatide was given in 95% of patients. In contrast to the VEGAS I and II trials, the results of the AIMI trial showed a worse outcome for the Angiojet group with significantly larger infarct size (12.5% ± 12.1% vs. 9.8% ± 10.9%), significantly higher 30-day MACE (6.7% vs. 1.7%), and significantly higher 30-day mortality (4.6% vs. 0.8%) than in the primary PCI group. In addition, postprocedure TIMI 3 rates were lower in the Angiojet group (92% vs. 97%) than in the PCI group [46]. A limitaton of the trial was its open-label nature: as randomization occurred after identification of angiographic thrombus, the larger thrombi may have been treated by rheolytic thrombectomy. Moreover, procedural time was, on average, 16 min longer because of the time required to set up the device.

Trial results suggest that thrombectomy devices appear more promising than atherectomy devices, as evidenced by the recent TAPAS trial. As with all devices, routine use is not recommended. Patients presenting with an AMI with a large filling defect consistent with thrombus should probably be treated with a thrombectomy device. Selectivity seems appropriate.

Embolic protection devices

Coronary embolism due to atherosclerotic debris is a rather common cause of postprocedural complications. In a more general sense, emboli are frequently the cause of end-organ failure [33]. Thrombosis aside, cholesterol clefts, foam cells, and the acellular debris beneath the fibrous cap of atherosclerotic lesions encompass the majority of emboli histology. These debris typically ranged from 25 μm to 2 mm [47].

Within SVG interventions, elevated cardiac enzymes (CK-MB, troponin) and the no-reflow phenomenon account for the greatest incidents of complication, 17% and 8%, respectively [48,49]; both are associated with impaired myocardial perfusion. These benchmarks are thought to be compounded by microvascular spasms. MACEs encompass these complications, as well as others, including sudden death.

Although evidence has shown that both arterial vasodilators and platelet glycoprotein inhibitors are ineffective against post- and periprocedural embolism [50], mechanical interventional devices have been shown to reduce 30-day MACE rates. Distal devices, such as distal filtration and distal and proximal occlusion balloons, in particular, have shown promising evidence of improving left ventricular function during acute periprocedural myocardial infarctions (PMIs) [51].

Distal occlusion devices

The distal occlusion balloon was the first approach to embolic protection. The intervention involves placement of a low-pressure (<2 atm) balloon distal to the lesion of interest. Antegrade flow is temporarily interrupted while the lesion is treated. Shaknovich and colleagues [52] developed the distal occlude washout (DOW) method for subsequent saline infusion coupled with debris aspiration. Distal flow is then restored. Total occlusion time (TOT) depends on the complexity of the lesion and skill of the operator.

Distal occlusion presents a unique set of benefits and limitations. The benefits of the distal occlusion method include, theoretically, a more complete capture of embolic debris, and currently the lowest lesion crossing profile, with device calibers ranging about approximately 0.026 inches. Limitations include distal ischemia due to prolonged interruption in antegrade flow and vessel injury due to the occlusion balloon. Furthermore, emboli shunting into side branches can occur, as well as incomplete aspiration of the stagnant debris field. In practice, distal occlusion balloon embolic protection requires greater procedural complexity than its distal filter counterparts. Finally, balloon placement assumes that there is an adequate landing site distal to the lesion. Operator skill can ameliorate several of these limitations while advancement in device design attempts continue.

Preliminary reports by Oesterle and associates [53] reported no complications in porcine models undergoing PTCA under distal occlusion. In addition to this, a lower than expected (4%) cardiac enzyme elevation was reported. The first distal occlusion device to be described was the PercuSurge GuardWire (Medtronic Vascular, Minneapolis, MN, USA) in 2003 (Fig. 35.6). The device consisted of a 0.014-inch radiopaque-tipped nitinol balloon wire coupled with a monorail aspiration catheter called the Export. The first large-scale (*n* = 801) randomized

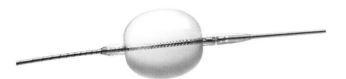

Figure 35.6 Medtronic PercuSurge GuardWire temporary occlusion and aspiration system. Image courtesy of Medtronic Vascular, Inc.

trial of the GuardWire system was termed Saphenous Vein Graft Angioplasty Free of Emboli, Randomized (SAFER) trial, which challenged conventional guidewire lesion crossing to the balloon occlusion wire. The study showed a statistically significant reduction in MACE rate from 16.9% to 9.6% (*P* = 0.004). In addition, the no-reflow phenomenon was reduced by over 50%: from 8.3% to 3.3% (*P* = 0.02). These results were attributed to a combination of a reduction in non-Q-wave myocardial infarction, reduction in creatine kinase elevations, as well as reduction in other humoral mediators [54].

Succeeding generation devices (innovative new occlusion devices) are undergoing evaluation. The GuardDOG (Possis Medical, Coon Rapids, MN, USA), which pairs a balloon catheter with their AngioJet thrombectomy ingestion/inspiration catheter, is currently being evaluated.

In addition to the powerful application of distal occlusion systems in PCI, there is strong preliminary evidence to support the use of the device in carotid interventions despite fears of ischemic damage [55].

Distal filters

Mounted on conventional 0.014-inch guidewire shafts, distal filtration systems utilise a similar intervention method to distal occlusion. In this procedure, a delivery/recovery sheath catheter deploys an expandable filter device approximating the lumen, which is later removed after PTCA or stent placement in retroversion.

The variety of existing rather novel filter designs typically feature a wire mounted umbrella-type filter consisting of laser-drilled micropores design varied, averaging approximately 100 μm.

The primary benefit of distal filtration is the uninterruption of antegrade flow. In addition, operators report a greater ease of use and lower procedural complexity; contrast injections proceed in normal fashion. Complications of the design theory include the possibility of exceeding filter capacity, large thrombosis clogging, incomplete apposition (or transient loss thereof) of the filter to the vessel wall, allowing filtrate to bypass the device, and, most notably, a significantly larger caliber ranging from 0.035 to 0.040 inches. Overcoming device limitations is largely a design factor.

Intuitively, distal filtration should provide less embolic protection than devices that cause antegrade flow to cease, such as the distal occlusion balloon. However, Functional Improvement through the Revascularization of the Extremities (FIRE), the first large-scale (*n* = 656) clinical trial of the industry's first filtration device, the FilterWire EX (Boston Scientific–EPI, Santa Clara, CA, USA), proved equivalent to the GuardWire technique, evaluated in terms of 30-day MACE (Fig. 35.7). This strengthens the hypothesis that soluble factors, such as the no-reflow phenomenon, do not significantly contribute to MACE events [56]. The greater ease of use and maintenance of FilterWire have allowed the device to emerge as the premier embolic protection device, largely replacing GuardWire.

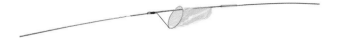

© 2008 Boston Scientific Corporation

Figure 35.7 Boston Scientific FilterWire EZ catheter shown deployed. Image courtesy of Boston Scientific, USA.

Advancement of filter design, in particular the subsequent generation of the 2003 FilterWire EX, has brought about the FilterWire EZ. This device incorporates an innovative filtrate centering design, in addition to a freely rotating suspension arm, allowing for greater lumen approximation and a reduction in wall shear stress endothelial injury. Preliminary results are promising, with a further reduction of MACE to 5.7% in the BLAZE registry [56]. In addition, derivatives of FilterWire are being developed for smaller-caliber (<3 mm) vessels. Other filters include Angioguard (Cordis, Miami Lakes, FL, USA) as well as CardioShield (MedNova Ltd., Galway, Ireland), the subject of the CardioShield Application Protects During Transluminal Intervention of Vein Grafts by Reducing Emboli (CAPTIVE) trial, which went as far as to nearly show noninferiority (P = 0.054) to GuardWire [57]. Subsequent generations of filters will likely incorporate opening and closing devices proximal on the wire, removing the need for a delivery/retrieval sheath, lowering crossing profile, and enhancing ease of use.

Proximal occlusion devices

It is postulated that some, if not a significant portion of, postprocedural complications involving distal embolic protection devices arise in the crossing of the lesion. Thus, a solution of proximal protection has been proposed. Proximal occlusion follows a nearly identical implementation as distal occlusion. A low-pressure (<2 atm) balloon is placed proximal to the lesion, impeding antegrade flow of the vessel, including the vicinity of the lesion itself. Contrast can be injected after flow occlusion, but usually before a wire or stent crosses the lesion. Further contrast injection should be avoided until a full iteration of debris aspiration is complete. The liberated potential emboli from the subsequent intervention remain suspended in the blood, rather than flowing into distal microcirculation. After the primary procedure, a saline rinsing catheter can be used to encourage debris mobilization proximally toward a suction aspiration catheter. Interestingly, collateral vessels encourage a slight backflow within the dispersion.

Unlike distal occlusion, proximal devices allow for vessel protection before lesion crossing, a great advantage in cases involving thrombus or vulnerable plaque. Furthermore, proximal occlusion allows for bifurcation lesion protection, or more generally, side branch protection. Similar to distal occlusion, the cessation of antegrade flow and, consequently, the risk of ischemic injury persist. In practice, proximal occlusion is the most difficult method for embolic protection and thus intervention, often requiring the use of two operators.

The first proximal protection to enter practice was Arteria (Parodi, San Francisco, CA, USA), designed for carotid interventions. For PCI, the Proxis occlusion device (Velocimed–ev3, Minneapolis, MN, USA) has emerged and has shown promising results at reducing MACE in the Proximal Protection During Saphenous Vein Graft Intervention Using the Proxis Embolic Protection System (PROXIS, St. Jude Medical, St. Paul, MN, USA) and Feasibility And Safety Trial, European Registry (FASTER) (n = 35) trials. Under FASTER, Proxis delivered a reduction in MACE to 4% [58]. Larger trials designed to show equivalence or noninferiority to other methods of embolic protection are currently under way.

Although substantial research is still needed, interventionalists are advised to always use embolic protection devices in SVG interventions. In addition to its adjunctive role in PCI, embolic protection is currently being investigated in carotid and renal artery settings, in which ischemic stroke and renal failure are common postprocedural complications. In fact, Cordis's Angioguard combined with carotid stenting has proved noninferior to carotid endarterectomy for high embolic-risk patients [59]. Furthermore, Accunet (Guidant, Santa Clara, CA, USA) has been FDA approved for carotid interventions based on the results of the Acculink for Revascularization of Carotids in High Risk Patients (ARCHER) trial [60].

In contrast to typical embolic protection device results, the Enhanced Myocardial Efficacy and Removal by Aspiration of Liberated Debris (EMERALD) trial failed to show a reduction in myocardial blush, ST-segment resolution, and radionuclide infarct size, despite emboli recovery using the distal occlusion GuardWire device and various distal filters [61]. This suggests that embolic protection may not be effective in native coronary artery myocardial infarctions.

Conclusion

Difficult complex plaques sometimes have to be modified or debulked and thrombus removed in both native coronaries and SVGs. Although PTCA and stenting is effective, adjunctive devices are sometimes required for optimal PTCA, stent deployment, and prevention of distal embolization. The goal of adjunctive devices is not massive debulking but compliance changes to facilitate optimal PTCA and proper stent deployment. Attempts to place stents without proper vessel preparation (predilation, plaque modification, or debulking) run the risk of stent entrapment or stent underexpansion, leading to higher rates of restenosis. The main concern of these adjunctive devices lies in safety and efficacy.

Bittl and colleagues [62] looked at 16 trials in a meta-analysis of atherectomy, laser, or cutting balloon versus balloon angioplasty and concluded that mechanical approaches of plaque ablation or sectioning were not associated with improved clinical outcomes or reduced restenosis.

Burzotta and colleagues [63] conducted a meta-analysis of 18 prospective randomized trials involving 3180 patients with STEMI treated with different adjunctive devices in primary or rescue PCI. Although heterogeneity was documented in the majority of analyses, they concluded that the use of adjunctive devices may be associated with lower rates of angiographic distal embolization, improved myocardial blush score and ST-segment reduction, and an overall trend toward better results.

Kunadian and colleagues [64] conducted a meta-analysis of 14 randomized trials of thrombectomy and distal protection devices compared with standard PCI in native vessel acute myocardial infarction and concluded that the use of these anti-embolic devices did not reduce early mortality or reinfarction.

Many studies have produced conflicting results. Overall, adjunctive devices do not appear superior to PTCA or stents. However, efficacy varies with the device. Nevertheless, adjunctive devices play an important role in coronary intervention of complex lesions. More trials and refinements of adjunctive devices are still needed.

References

1. Lary BG (1980) Coronary artery incision and dilation. *Arch Surg* **115**:1478–1480.

2. Giugliano GR, Cox N, & Popma J (2005) Cutting balloon entrapment during treatment of in-stent restenosis: an unusual complication and its management. *J Invasive Cardiol* **17**:168–170.

3. Smith SC Jr, Feldman TE, Hirschfeld JW Jr, *et al.* (2006) ACC/AHA/SCAI 2005 guideline update for percutaneous coronary intervention: a report of the American College of Cardiology/American Heart Association Task Force on Practice Guidelines (ACC/AHA/SCAI Writing Committee to Update 2001 Guidelines for Percutaneous Coronary Intervention). *Circulation* **113**:e166–286.

4. Takebayashi H, Haruta S, Kohno H, *et al.* (2004) Immediate and 3-month follow-up outcome after cutting balloon angioplasty for bifurcation lesions. *J Interv Cardiol* **17**:1–7.

5. Bejarano J (2004) The cutting balloon for in-stent restenosis: a review. *J Interv Cardiol* **17**:203–209.

6. Topol EJ (2008) *Textbook of Interventional Cardiology*, 5th edn. Philadelphia: Saunders/Elsevier.

7. Ellis SG & Holmes DR (2006) *Strategic Approaches in Coronary Intervention*, 3rd edn. Philadelphia: Lippincott Williams & Wilkins.

8. Mauri L, Bonan R, Weiner BH, *et al.* (2002) Cutting balloon angioplasty for the prevention of restenosis: results of the Cutting Balloon Global Randomized Trial. *Am J Cardiol* **90**:1079–1083.

9. Costa RA, Mooney MR, Teirstein PS, *et al.* (2006) Final results from the multi-center trial of the angiosculpt scoring balloon catheter for the treatment of complex coronary artery lesions. *Cardiovas Revasc Med* **7**:112.

10. Baim DS, Hinohara T, Holmes D, *et al.* (1993) Results of directional coronary atherectomy during multicenter preapproval testing. The US Directional Coronary Atherectomy Investigator Group. *Am J Cardiol* **72**:6E–11E.

11. Penny WF, Schmidt DA, Safian RD, Erny RE, & Baim DS (1991) Insights into the mechanism of luminal improvement after directional coronary atherectomy. *Am J Cardiol* **67**:435–437.

12. Hinohara T, Selmon MR, Robertson GC, Braden L, & Simpson JS (1990) Directional atherectomy. New approaches for treatment of obstructive coronary and peripheral vascular disease. *Circulation* **81**(3 Suppl.):IV79–91.

13. Adelman AG, Cohen EA, Kimball BP, *et al.* (1993) A comparison of directional atherectomy with balloon angioplasty for lesions of the left anterior descending coronary artery. *N Engl J Med* **329**:228–233.

14. Topol EJ, Leya F, Pinkerton CA, *et al.* (1993) A comparison of directional atherectomy with coronary angioplasty in patients with coronary artery disease. The CAVEAT Study Group. *N Engl J Med* **329**:221–227.

15. Holmes DR Jr, Topol EJ, Califf RM, *et al.* (1995) A multicenter, randomized trial of coronary angioplasty versus directional atherectomy for patients with saphenous vein bypass graft lesions. CAVEAT-II Investigators. *Circulation* **91**:1966–1974.

16. Suzuki T, Hosokawa H, Katoh O, *et al.* (1999) Effects of adjunctive balloon angioplasty after intravascular ultrasound-guided optimal directional coronary atherectomy: the result of Adjunctive Balloon Angioplasty After Coronary Atherectomy Study (ABACAS). *J Am Coll Cardiol* **34**:1028–1035.

17. Simonton CA, Leon MB, Baim DS, *et al.* (1998) 'Optimal' directional coronary atherectomy: final results of the Optimal Atherectomy Restenosis Study (OARS). *Circulation* **97**:332–339.

18. Ahn SS, Auth D, Marcus DR, & Moore WS (1988) Removal of focal atheromatous lesions by angioscopically guided high-speed rotary atherectomy. Preliminary experimental observations. *J Vasc Surg* **7**:292–300.

19. Fourrier JL, Bertrand ME, Auth DC, Lablanche JM, Gommeaux A, & Brunetaud JM (1989) Percutaneous coronary rotational angioplasty in humans: preliminary report. *J Am Coll Cardiol* **14**:1278–1282.

20. Whitlow PL, Bass TA, Kipperman RM, *et al.* (2001) Results of the study to determine rotablator and transluminal angioplasty strategy (STRATAS). *Am J Cardiol* **87**:699–705.

21. Mauri L, Reisman M, Buchbinder M, *et al.* (2003) Comparison of rotational atherectomy with conventional balloon angioplasty in the prevention of restenosis of small coronary arteries: results of the Dilatation vs Ablation Revascularization Trial Targeting Restenosis (DART). *Am Heart J* **145**:847–854.

22. Buchbinder M, FR, Sharma S, *et al.* (2000) Debulking prior to stenting improves acute outcomes: early results from the SPORT trial. *Circulation* **35**(Suppl. A):8a.

23. Moses JW, Carlier S, & Moussa I (2004) Lesion preparation prior to stenting. *Rev Cardiovasc Med* **5**(Suppl. 2):S16–21.

24. Rihal CS, Garratt KN, & Holmes DR Jr (1998) Rotational atherectomy for bifurcation lesions of the coronary circulation: technique and initial experience. *Int J Cardiol* **65**:1–9.

25. Kern MJ, Donohue TJ, Aguirre FV, *et al.* (1995) Clinical outcome of deferring angioplasty in patients with normal translesional pressure-flow velocity measurements. *J Am Coll Cardiol* **25**:178–187.

26. de Bruyne B, Bastunek J, Sys SU, *et al.* (1996) Simultaneous coronary pressure and flow velocity measurements in humans.

Feasibility, reproducibility, and hemodynamic dependence of coronary flow velocity reserve, hyperemic flow versus pressure slope index, and fractional flow reserve. *Circulation* **94**:1842–1849.

27. Isner JM, Rosenfeld K, White CJ, *et al.* (1992) In vivo assessment of vascular pathology resulting from laser irradiation. Analysis of 23 patients studied by directional atherectomy immediately after laser angioplasty. *Circulation* **85**:2185–2196.

28. Clarke RH, Isner JM, Donaldson RF, & Jones G, 2nd (1987) Gas chromatographic-light microscopic correlative analysis of excimer laser photoablation of cardiovascular tissues: evidence for a thermal mechanism. *Circ Res* **60**:429–437.

29. Bonner R, Smith PD, & Prevosti LD (1989) New sources for laser angioplasty: Er:YAG, excimer lasers, and nonlaser hot-tip catheters, in interventional cardiology: future directions. In: Vogel JH & King SB (eds). St Louis: Mosby, pp. 101–118.

30. Grundfest WS, Litvack F, Forrester JS, *et al.* (1985) Laser ablation of human atherosclerotic plaque without adjacent tissue injury. *J Am Coll Cardiol* **5**:929–933.

31. Isner JM, Donaldson RF, Deckelbaum LI, *et al.* (1985) The excimer laser: gross, light microscopic and ultrastructural analysis of potential advantages for use in laser therapy of cardiovascular disease. *J Am Coll Cardiol* **6**:1102–1109.

32. Reifart N, Vandormael M, Krajcar M, *et al.* (1997) Randomized comparison of angioplasty of complex coronary lesions at a single center. Excimer Laser, Rotational Atherectomy, and Balloon Angioplasty Comparison (ERBAC) Study. *Circulation* **96**:91–98.

33. Baim DS & Grossman W (2006) *Grossman's Cardiac Catheterization, Angiography, and Intervention*, 7th edn. Philadelphia: Lippincott Williams & Wilkins, xvii:807, [4] of plates.

34. King SB & Yeung AC (2007) *Interventional Cardiology*. New York: McGraw-Hill Medical, xvii:846.

35. Appelman YE, Pick JJ, David GK, *et al.* (1996) Randomised trial of excimer laser angioplasty versus balloon angioplasty for treatment of obstructive coronary artery disease. *Lancet* **347**(8994):79–84.

36. Bittl JA, Kuntz RE, Estella P, Sanborn TA, & Baim DS (1994) Analysis of late lumen narrowing after excimer laser-facilitated coronary angioplasty. *J Am Coll Cardiol* **23**:1314–1320.

37. Henriques JP, Zijlstra F, Ottervanger JP, *et al.* (2002) Incidence and clinical significance of distal embolization during primary angioplasty for acute myocardial infarction. *Eur Heart J* **23**:1112–1117.

38. Sharma SK & Chen V (2006) Coronary interventional devices: balloon, atherectomy, thrombectomy and distal protection devices. *Cardiol Clin* **24**:201–215, vi.

39. Silva-Orrego P, Colombo P, Bigi R, *et al.* (2006) Thrombus aspiration before primary angioplasty improves myocardial reperfusion in acute myocardial infarction: the DEAR-MI (Dethrombosis to Enhance Acute Reperfusion in Myocardial Infarction) study. *J Am Coll Cardiol* **48**:1552–1559.

40. Siddiqui DS, Choi CJ, Tsimikas S, & Mahmud E (2006) Successful utilization of a novel aspiration thrombectomy catheter (Pronto) for the treatment of patients with stent thrombosis. *Catheter Cardiovasc Interv* **67**:894–899.

41. Burzotta F, Trani C, Romagnoli E, *et al.* (2006) A pilot study with a new, rapid-exchange, thrombus-aspirating device in patients with thrombus-containing lesions: the Diver C.E. study. *Catheter Cardiovasc Interv* **67**:887–893.

42. Svilaas T, Vlaar PJ, van der Horst IC, *et al.* (2008) Thrombus aspiration during primary percutaneous coronary intervention. *N Engl J Med* **358**:557–567.

43. Stone GW, Cox DA, Babb J, *et al.* (2003) Prospective, randomized evaluation of thrombectomy prior to percutaneous intervention in diseased saphenous vein grafts and thrombus-containing coronary arteries. *J Am Coll Cardiol* **42**:2007–2013.

44. Kuntz RE, Baim DS, Cohen DJ, *et al.* (2002) A trial comparing rheolytic thrombectomy with intracoronary urokinase for coronary and vein graft thrombus (the Vein Graft AngioJet Study [VeGAS 2]). *Am J Cardiol* **89**:326–330.

45. Popma J, Carrozza J, Ho K, *et al.* (1997) One-year outcomes for the vein graft angiojet study I (VEGAS I) pilot trial. *Ciculation* **96**:216-I–217-I.

46. Ali A, Cox D, Dib N, *et al.* (2006) Rheolytic thrombectomy with percutaneous coronary intervention for infarct size reduction in acute myocardial infarction: 30-day results from a multicenter randomized study. *J Am Coll Cardiol* **48**:244–252.

47. Webb JG, Carere RG, Virmani R, *et al.* (1999) Retrieval and analysis of particulate debris after saphenous vein graft intervention. *J Am Coll Cardiol* **34**:468–475.

48. Hong MK, Mehran R, Dangas G, *et al.* (1999) Creatine kinase-MB enzyme elevation following successful saphenous vein graft intervention is associated with late mortality. *Circulation* **100**:2400–2405.

49. Piana RN, Paik GY, Moscucci M, *et al.* (1994) Incidence and treatment of 'no-reflow' after percutaneous coronary intervention. *Circulation* **89**:2514–2518.

50. Ellis SG, Lincoff AM, Miller D, *et al.* (1998) Reduction in complications of angioplasty with abciximab occurs largely independently of baseline lesion morphology. EPIC and EPILOG Investigators. Evaluation of 7E3 for the Prevention of Ischemic Complications. Evaluation of PTCA To Improve Long-term Outcome with abciximab GPIIb/IIIa Receptor Blockade. *J Am Coll Cardiol* **32**:1619–1623.

51. Haery C, Exaire JE, Bhatt DL, *et al.* (2004) Use of PercuSurge GuardWire in native coronary arteries during acute myocardial infarction. *J Invasive Cardiol* **16**:152–154.

52. Shaknovich A, Forman AT, Parikh MA, *et al.* (1999) Novel distal occluder washout method for prevention of no-reflow during stenting of saphenous vein grafts. *Catheter Cardiovasc Interv* **47**:397–403.

53. Oesterle SN, Hayase M, Baim DS, *et al.* (1999) An embolization containment device. *Catheter Cardiovasc Interv* **47**:243–250.

54. Baim DS, Wahr D, George B, *et al.* (2002) Randomized trial of a distal embolic protection device during percutaneous intervention of saphenous vein aorto-coronary bypass grafts. *Circulation* **105**:1285–1290.

55. Gruberg l (2004) *PRIDE: A Prospective Randomized Controlled Trial of Distal Protection With the Kensey-Nash TriActiv System*. Available at: www.medscape.com/viewarticle/491695.

56. Stone GW, Rogers C, Hermiller J, *et al.* (2003) Randomized comparison of distal protection with a filter-based catheter and a balloon occlusion and aspiration system during percutaneous intervention of diseased saphenous vein aorto-coronary bypass grafts. *Circulation* **108**:548–553.

57. Holmes D (2004) CardioShield Application Protects During Transluminal Interventions in Vein Grafts by Reducing Emboli (CAPTIVE) trial. Presented at Transcatheter Cardiovascular Therapeutics; Washington, DC.

58. Sievert H, Wahr DW, Schuler G, *et al.* (2004) Effectiveness and safety of the Proxis system in demonstrating retrograde coronary blood flow during proximal occlusion and in capturing embolic material. *Am J Cardiol* **94**:1134–1139.

59. Hobson RW 2nd (1998) Status of carotid angioplasty and stenting trials. *J Vasc Surg* **27**:791.

60. Wholey M (2003) The ARCHeR trial: prospective clinical trial for carotid stenting in high surgical risk patients—preliminary 30-day results. Presented at the American College of Cardiology annual meeting, Chicago, IL.

61. Stone G (2004) The Emerald Trial—Lessons Learned. Presentation at the American College of Cardiology annual meeting. March; New Orleans.

62. Bittl JA, Chew DP, Topol EJ, *et al.* (2004) Meta-analysis of randomized trials of percutaneous transluminal coronary angioplasty versus atherectomy, cutting balloon atherotomy, or laser angioplasty. *J Am Coll Cardiol* **43**:936–942.

63. Burzotta F, Testa L, Giannico F, *et al.* (2008) Adjunctive devices in primary or rescue PCI: a meta-analysis of randomized trials. *Int J Cardiol* **123**:313–321.

64. Kunadian B, Dunning J, Vijayalakshmi K, *et al.* (2007) Meta-analysis of randomized trials comparing anti-embolic devices with standard PCI for improving myocardial reperfusion in patients with acute myocardial infarction. *Catheter Cardiovasc Interv* **69**:488–496.

36 Percutaneous Coronary Intervention for Acute Myocardial Infarction

Jürgen Haase

Kardiocentrum Frankfurt, Klinik Rotes Kreuz, Frankfurt/Main, Germany

Historical background

Continuous progress in the treatment of patients with acute ST-segment elevation myocardial infarction (STEMI) has reduced overall in-hospital mortality from >20% at the time of exclusively conservative management strategy to about 5% in the era of percutaneous coronary interventions [1–5].

The first major step in this development was the introduction of thrombolysis with the publication of the Italian Group for the Study of the Survival of Myocardial Infarction (Gruppo Italiano per lo Studio della Sopravvivenza nell'Infarto Miocardico; GISSI) trial in 1987 [6]. Systemic thrombolysis with streptokinase, when performed within the first 6h after onset of symptoms, was shown to recanalize thrombotic occlusions in the infarct-related coronary artery, to restore blood flow, to reduce infarct size, and to improve myocardial function and survival [7]. However, despite the introduction of fibrin-specific thrombolytics, the individual outcome of thrombolytic therapy remained unpredictable, with about 25% of patients failing to respond with continuous infarct artery patency [8–10]. In addition, severe and partially fatal bleeding complications may occur [11].

The introduction of primary percutaneous coronary intervention (PCI) for the treatment of acute STEMI has fundamentally changed the preferred management strategy from a purely pharmacologic to an interventional approach, with predictable infarct artery patency in >95% of patients [12]. Today, primary PCI represents the most effective treatment approach for patients with acute STEMI.

Pathophysiology

Acute coronary artery occlusion due to thrombosis may be caused by various mechanisms, such as plaque rupture or plaque erosion [13]. The rupture of an unstable coronary

plaque (thin-cap fibroatheroma) represents the most important cause of sudden thrombotic coronary occlusion and is encountered in >60% of these cases [14]. Plaque disruption leads to the exposure of substances that promote platelet activation and aggregation, thrombin generation, and thrombus formation [15,16]. The resultant thrombus interrupts coronary blood flow and leads to an imbalance between myocardial oxygen supply and demand and, if this imbalance is severe and persistent, to necrosis of myocardial tissue. In the absence of collateral blood flow, the extension of myocardial necrosis due to total coronary occlusion represents a time-dependent process which starts in the endocardial layers of the ventricular wall and is completed by 6–12h [17]. The duration of this time interval as well as the biochemical markers of infarct size correlate with late mortality [18–20]. Thus, the potential success of primary PCI in terms of infarct size limitation as well as reduction of late mortality appears to be inversely related to the time interval between symptom onset and recanalization of the infarct-related coronary artery (Fig. 36.1).

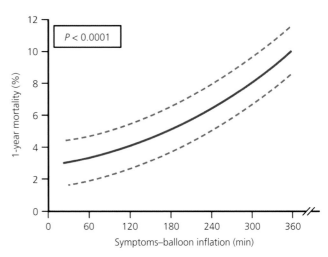

Figure 36.1 After adjusting for baseline risk, there is a curvilinear relationship between the time elapsed from the onset of symptoms to balloon inflation and the rate of mortality at 1 year. For every 30-min delay from onset of symptoms to primary PCI, there is an 8% increase in the relative risk of 1-year mortality. Flanking curves indicate 95% confidence intervals. Reproduced from De Luca G *et al.* [18], with permission from American Heart Association.

Cardiovascular Interventions in Clinical Practice. Edited by Jürgen Haase, Hans-Joachim Schäfers, Horst Sievert and Ron Waksman. © 2010 Blackwell Publishing.

Indications

Acute ST-segment elevation myocardial infarction

Primary PCI is the therapy of choice in patients presenting with a history of chest pain or chest discomfort of duration less than 12 h who show STEMI or a presumed new bundle branch block on electrocardiography (ECG). Primary PCI represents a class I A recommendation when available within 90 min after the first medical contact and also in patients in whom fibrinolytic therapy is contraindicated [21,22]. Transportation of patients with acute STEMI from a hospital without PCI capability to a specialized PCI center improves the clinical outcome compared with on-site thrombolysis [23,24]. Even after 12 h, primary PCI may reduce infarct size, as residual flow in the presence of collaterals and/or an incomplete occlusion of the infarct-related artery may widen the time window available for myocardial salvage [25]. In patients in whom thrombolysis after STEMI has failed, rescue PCI should be undertaken [26] and even after successful thrombolysis, early PCI may reduce ischemic complications [27].

Primary PCI may also be indicated in patients presenting with cardiogenic shock, where it has demonstrated to improve survival rates [28]. In addition, it may be of special advantage in elderly patients, in whom systemic fibrinolyisis is associated with an increased risk of intracerebral bleeding [11].

Acute non-ST segment elevation myocardial infarction

In patients with an acute non-ST-segment myocardial infarction (NSTEMI), the indication for PCI depends on a variety of parameters by which the risk–benefit ratio of the procedure is determined [29,30].

Urgent invasive strategy

An urgent invasive strategy is required in patients who are early in the process of developing major myocardial necrosis escaping the ECG (e.g., occlusion of the circumflex artery) or who are judged to be at high risk of rapid progression to vessel occlusion. These patients present with refractory angina (e.g., evolving myocardial infarction without ST-segment abnormalities), recurrent angina despite intense antianginal treatment associated with ST-segment depression (>0.2 mV) or deep negative T-waves, clinical symptoms of heart failure, hemodynamic instability, or life-threatening arrhythmias (ventricular fibrillation or ventricular tachycardia).

Early invasive strategy

An early invasive strategy (routine coronary arteriography within 72 h) is recommended in patients who initially respond to antianginal therapy but are at increased risk. They are characterized by elevated troponin or creatine kinase, creatine kinase myocardial band isoenzyme (CK-MB) levels, dynamic ST-segment or T-wave changes, diabetes mellitus, impaired renal function (glomerular filtration rate [GFR] < 60 mL/1.73 m²), depressed left ventricular ejection fraction (EF < 40%), early postmyocardial infarction angina, PCI within the last 6 months, previous coronary artery bypass graft operation, or an intermediate to high Global Registry of Acute Coronary Events (GRACE) risk score [31–33].

Technical aspects

Reducing the time interval between symptom onset and percutaneous coronary intervention

Optimal timing of primary PCI requires a strategy that aims at reducing the time interval between symptom onset and intervention to a minimum [18]. Such treatment strategy depends on multiple factors such as patient response to the symptoms, transportation to the hospital, in-hospital decision-making, transfer to a PCI center if required, and the door to balloon time [34–36]. Accordingly, the strategy to reduce the time interval between symptom onset and PCI should include patient education, improvement of prehospital diagnosis (if possible using wireless ECG transmission from emergency medical services to the emergency department to accelerate treatment planning on a prehospital basis) [37,38], a well established coordination of patient transmission to PCI centers [39], and a reduction of the door-to balloon time to a minimum. If diagnosis of STEMI is made before admission using a 12-lead ECG by emergency medical services or achieved by wireless ECG transmission, door-to-balloon times can be effectively minimized as the patient, if in a stable clinical condition, may circumvent the emergency room and be admitted directly to the catheterization laboratory [40]. Important prerequisite of such a strategy is a 24-h service of an experienced PCI team 7 days per week [41].

Emergency coronary arteriography

When emergency coronary arteriography is required in acute STEMI, the patient may present with severe chest pain, respiratory failure, and hemodynamic instability. If needed, anesthesia, mechanical ventilation, intravenous catecholamines, and intra-aortic balloon counterpulsation should be initiated before the angiographic procedure is started. The performance of emergency angiography does not differ from the routine procedure (see Chapter 28). However, the patient should be on aspirin and heparin, and the number of angiographic views should be limited to minimize the consumption of contrast medium. Left ventricular angiography should be performed after completion of PCI to correctly assess baseline left ventricular ejection fraction or omitted if the patient remains hemodynamically unstable.

Adjunctive pharmacotherapy

Patients with acute STEMI who undergo primary PCI are pretreated with aspirin (500 mg i.v.) and unfractured heparin

(5000–7500 units). Before mechanical recanalization of the infarct artery, intracoronary injection of a weight-adjusted bolus of abciximab is recommended. If distal run-off remains impaired despite successful recanalization of the occlusion site, owing to distal vasospasm or microvascular flow disturbances, intracoronary nitrates or verapamil may be administered. The use of these vasodilators may be limited by the side-effect of arterial hypotension, which may require volume administration if left ventricular function is only slightly reduced or catecholamines if ventricular function is severely impaired. Immediately after successful primary PCI, the patient receives an oral loading dose of clopidogrel (600 mg) [22].

Adjunctive pharmacotherapy for patients with NSTEMI who undergo percutaneous coronary intervention implies similar components in a different order of application. Patients are pretreated with aspirin, heparin, and an intravenous bolus injection and infusion of small-molecule glycoprotein IIb/IIIa receptor blockers (e.g., eptifibatide, tirofiban). In addition, the loading dose of clopidogrel is administered before the interventional procedure. A continuous intravenous infusion of the same IIb/IIIa inhibitor is continued over 18 h. In selected patients at high risk for stent thrombosis and in particular in patients who are assumed to be clopidogrel non-responders, prasugrel may be used as an alternative to clopidogrel [42]. Prasugrel may be associated with an increased risk of bleeding complications especially in underweight and older patients (<60 kg; >75 years) and should not be applied in this subset of patients. The use of prasugrel is not indicated in patients with prior stroke. Adjunctive pharmacotherapy during PCI is described in more detail in Chapter 41.

Recanalization of the infarct-related coronary artery (primary percutaneous coronary intervention)

The primary PCI procedure for recanalization of the infarct-related coronary artery starts with the intubation of the coronary ostium using a 6F guiding catheter, which is selected to provide access for guidewire, thrombus aspiration catheters, balloons, and stents and to allow sufficient catheter backup that is needed to advance such devices into the relevant coronary artery segment. Optimal guiding catheter backup is mostly provided by an extra backup (EBU) left catheter for the left anterior descending artery (LAD) and the left circumflex (LCx) artery and an Amplatz right or left catheter for the right coronary artery (RCA) (see Chapter 28).

Crossing of the occlusion should be attempted first with a floppy-tip guidewire (e.g., 0.014-inch Hi-Torque Balance Middleweight™ guidewire; Boston Scientific, Natick, MA, USA). If required, the floppy wire may be exchanged for a soft-tip guidewire with hydrophilic coating (e.g., 0.014-inch Hi-Torque Pilot™ 50 guidewire; Boston Scientific). Once the guidewire has crossed the lesion and has been advanced to the distal portion of the vessel, the subsequent injection of contrast medium mostly demonstrates TIMI flow I to II (according to the classification of the Thrombolysis In Myocardial Infarction trial) across the previous occlusion owing to partial removal of the clot. At this point of the procedure we recommend intracoronary injection of a weight-adjusted bolus of abciximab, which normally helps to further dissolve the occluding thrombus and improve coronary flow [43]. Conventional primary PCI includes the subsequent use of balloon dilation before stenting. Instead of balloon dilation, an attempt can be made to remove the thrombotic material using a manual aspiration catheter, as shown in Figure 36.2 [44]. It consists of a tapered tip with an eccentric guidewire canal and a large lumen for the suction of thrombotic material form the occlusive coronary lesion. The catheter is inserted using the monorail technique and connected with a 20-cm^3 syringe for the collection of aspirated material. It is recommended that continuous negative pressure is applied to the aspiration catheter until it has been completely removed from the guiding catheter to prevent embolization of aspirated material. After thrombus aspiration, most of the previously occluded lesions can be directly stented [45]. If thrombectomy was successful, a drug-eluting stent may be implanted, especially when lesion morphology (e.g., long lesion, small vessel diameter) predicts a high risk of restenosis [46–48]. If residual thrombotic material is suspected or the vessel diameter is relatively large (> 3.0 mm), a bare metal stent may be used. Direct stenting using high expansion pressures (> 15 atm) is preferred over pre- or postdilation using additional balloon inflations to avoid dislodgement of residual wall adherent thrombi or cellular debris. The interventional recanalization of an occluded right coronary artery with an inferior myocardial infarction is illustrated in Figure 36.3.

Plain balloon angioplasty instead of stenting may be of advantage for patients in whom clopidogrel is contraindicated because of thrombocytopenia or the presence of severe left main or extensive multivessel disease, and who may require bypass surgery within days after successful primary PCI. Balloon angioplasty may also be preferred when the lesion at the infarct-related artery is not suitable for stent implantation due to mechanical reasons or an extremely small vessel diameter (e.g., <2 mm).

Primary percutaneous coronary intervention in multivessel coronary artery disease

It is recommended that interventional treatment of acute myocardial infarctions be confined to primary PCI of the infarct-related artery, even in the presence of multivessel disease. Because more than one lesion may be involved in an acute coronary syndrome, primary PCI of more than one unstable coronary lesion may be required in selected cases. Invasive evaluation of coronary lesions of questionable instability using intravascular ultrasound [49], optical coherence tomography [50], or thermography [51] may be useful;

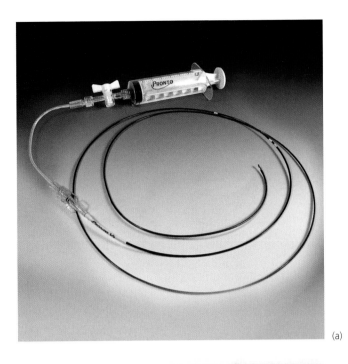

(a)

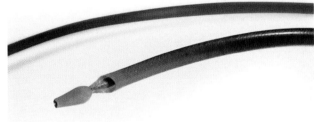

(b)

Figure 36.2 The thrombus aspiration catheter Pronto V3 (Vascular Solutions, Minneapolis, MN, USA) is designed for manual thrombus aspiration during primary PCI. After flushing with saline, its proximal end is connected to a 20-cm³ syringe (a). The distal catheter tip is asymmetrically tapered (b) while the distal portion of the catheter contains both an eccentric monorail canal for the guidewire and a large lumen for thrombus aspiration as shown in the cross-section (c).

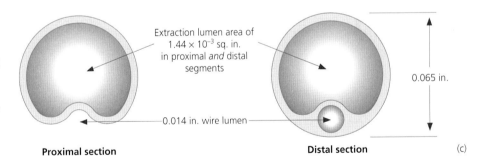

Extraction lumen area of 1.44×10^{-3} sq. in. in proximal *and* distal segments

0.065 in.

0.014 in. wire lumen

Proximal section

Distal section

(c)

however, the prognostic value of multivessel PCI in the setting of acute coronary syndromes still needs to be evaluated. When patients with coronary multivessel disease present with an acute coronary syndrome, the severity of stenosis in noninfarct-related coronary arteries may be overestimated owing to vasospasm or reduced flow due to enhanced microvascular coronary resistance [52]. This phenomenon may be a consequence of increased levels of circulating catecholamines or other coronary vasoconstrictors, such as serotonin, endothelin, angiotensin, and thromboxane [53,54]. In turn, oxidant stress reduces the vasodilatory effects of nitric oxide, adenosine, and prostacyclin.

Primary percutaneous coronary intervention in cardiogenic shock

Cardiogenic shock in acute myocardial infarction represents a life-threatening condition, which requires adjunctive measures to stabilize the patient immediately before primary PCI [55,56]. Because the infarct-related coronary artery cannot be safely recanalized in the presence of coronary hypoperfusion, arterial pressures have to be normalized before and during the interventional procedure. This can be achieved using continuous catecholamine infusions, but repetitive additional bolus injections may be required. The insertion of an intra-aortic balloon pump (IABP), using a contralateral

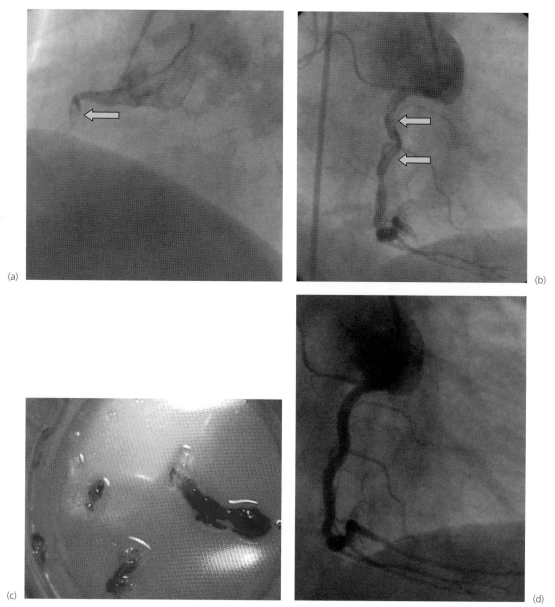

(a)

(b)

(c)

(d)

Figure 36.3 Acute inferior wall myocardial infarction (STEMI) treated with primary PCI. The proximal occlusion of the dominant right coronary artery shows intraluminal contrast lucency (arrow) typical of thrombotic material (a). After insertion of a soft-tip extra-support guidewire and intracoronary injection of abciximab, coronary flow is established and large thrombus masses (arrows) become visible (b). Manual aspiration using a Pronto V3 catheter (shown in Figure 36.2) removes the thrombotic material (c). Final angiography after implantation of two cobalt–chromium stents (d).

femoral access, may help to achieve hemodynamic stabilization before PCI. In our experience, it is frequently possible to achieve sufficient hemodynamic stability during emergency coronary angiography and primary PCI using repetitive bolus injections of catecholamines (e.g., epinephrine). The IABP may then be inserted after an exchange of the introducer sheath using the primary femoral access site after completion of the PCI procedure. This approach may help to accelerate the revascularization procedure and reduce postoperative bleeding complications. The balloon for intra-aortic counterpulsation is placed in the descending aorta with its tip below the distal portion of the aortic arch and its proximal end above the take off of the renal arteries (Fig. 36.4). Intra-aortic balloon counterpulsation should be continued after successful primary PCI for a period of 48–72 h. Contraindications for intra-aortic balloon pumping include severe aortic insufficiency, aortic aneurysms, severe kinkings of the aorta and/or the common iliac arteries, or significant peripheral artery disease.

Postoperative care

After primary PCI the patient is transferred to the coronary care unit and monitored until full hemodynamic stability is

Figure 36.4 Contemporary intra-aortic balloon pump (IABP) console (a), designed for ECG-triggered balloon counterpulsation (Arrow, Reading, PA, USA) with gas injection into the balloon during diastole and deflation during systole. The IABP catheter (b) is inserted via femoral approach into the descending aorta with the distal tip of the balloon positioned distal to the aortic arch, and the proximal tip proximal to the take-off of the renal arteries.

achieved and creatinine kinase levels have normalized. The introducer sheath is manually removed as soon as partial thromboplastin time (PTT) values approach the normal range. When 6F introducer sheaths were used, a pressure bandage and bed rest in supine position is required over 6 h after sheath removal. When pressure bandages cannot be tolerated by the patient, percutaneous closure devices may be used. A continuous intravenous infusion of glycoprotein IIb/IIIa receptor blockers is recommended after the interventional procedure (over 12 h with abciximab, and over 18 h with eptifibatide or tirofiban). In addition to aspirin and clopidogrel, a medical regimen with beta-blockers, angiotensin-converting enzyme (ACE) inhibitors and statins should be initiated [57–59]. The initiation of beta-blockers and ACE inhibitors depends on hemodynamic stability, and the dosage must be adapted to individual heart rate and blood pressure. Dual antiplatelet therapy (clopidogrel 75 mg and aspirin 100 mg/day) is of crucial importance to prevent stent thrombosis and should be maintained over a period of 12 months [60].

Results

Primary PCI versus thrombolysis

Initial randomized trials comparing primary PCI with intravenous thrombolysis in patients with acute STEMI indicated the potential advantage of the interventional treatment approach [61–65]. A significant reduction in scintigraphic infarct size using primary PCI in conjunction with glycoprotein IIb/IIIa receptor blockers compared with thrombolysis was first reported by the randomized Stent or Percutaneous Transluminal Coronary Angioplasty for Occluded Coronary Arteries in Patients with Acute Myocardial Infarction Ineligible for Thrombolysis (STOP-AMI) trial [66]. The clinical superiority of primary PCI over thrombolytic therapy was clearly documented by a meta-analysis of 23 randomized trials on 7739 patients comparing both management strategies [5]. The study revealed an overall reduction in short-term death from 9% to 7% ($P = 0.0002$) and after exclusion of shock patients from 7% to 5% ($P = 0.0003$). Nonfatal reinfarctions were reduced from 7% to 3% ($P < 0.0001$), strokes from 2% to 1% ($P = 0.0004$), and the combined end point of death, nonfatal reinfarctions, and stroke was reduced from 14% to 8% ($P < 0.0001$). The superiority of primary PCI in the short term (4–6 weeks) was maintained after a mean follow-up period of 6–18 months.

Treatment with primary PCI also appears to reduce infarct rupture. In a meta-analysis of the Global Utilization of Streptokinase and Tissue Plasminogen Activator (alteplase) for Occluded Coronary Arteries (GUSTO-I) and Primary Angioplasty in Myocardial Infarction (PAMI) I/II trials, primary PCI resulted in an 86% reduction in the risk of mechanical complications compared with intravenous thrombolysis [67]. There was a significant reduction in acute mitral insufficiency (0.31% vs. 1.73%; $P < 0.0001$) and ventricular septal defects (0.0% vs. 0.47%; $P < 0.001$). In a multivariate analysis of 1375 patients, treatment with primary PCI was independently associated with a lower risk of free ventricular wall rupture [68].

In the Danish Trial in Acute Myocardial Infarction (DANAMI), the potential benefit of an immediate transfer of patients to specialized PCI centers was investigated in comparison with on-site thrombolysis [23]. The study included 1572 patients with acute STEMI who where randomized to receive either angioplasty or an accelerated treatment with alteplase; 1129 patients were enrolled at 24 referral hospitals and 443 patients at five specialized PCI centers. The primary end point was a composite of death, reinfarction, or disabling stroke at 30 days. Among patients who underwent randomization at referral hospitals, the primary end point was reached in 8.5% in the PCI group, compared with 14.2% of those in the fibrinolysis group ($P = 0.002$). The results were similar in patients who were enrolled in specialized PCI centers: the primary end point was reached in 6.7% of patients in the angioplasty group versus 12.3% of patients in the fibrinolysis group ($P = 0.05$). Among all patients the better outcome after primary PCI was driven primarily by a reduction of the rate of reinfarction (1.6% in the angioplasty group vs. 6.3% in the fibrinolysis group; $P < 0.001$); no significant differences were observed in the rate of death (6.6% vs. 7.8%, $P = 0.35$) and stroke (1.1% vs. 2.0%, $P = 0.15$). Ninety-six percent of patients were transferred from referral hospitals to an invasive treatment center within 2h. The benefit of transfer for primary PCI was sustained after 3 years [69], with a combined end point met by 19.6% of patients in the invasive treatment group versus 25.2% in the fibrinolysis group ($P = 0.006$). Among patients transferred to a PCI center compared with those receiving on-site thrombolysis, the combined end point occurred in 20.1% versus 26.7% ($P = 0.007$).

A similar comparison was made in a multicenter trial from Poland [24,70], where 401 patients with STEMI admitted to 13 community hospitals (radius 20–150 km from catheterization laboratory) were randomized to receive either on-site thrombolysis or transport to a PCI center and tirofiban pretreatment (10 μg/kg bolus i.v. plus i.v. infusion 0.1 μg/kg/min). Primary end points were total mortality, recurrent myocardial infarction, and stroke during 1 year follow-up. Delay to reperfusion, defined as the time interval between admission and start of fibrinolysis or primary PCI, was 35 and 145 min ($P < 0.0001$). The mean duration of tirofiban infusion until PCI in the transfer group was 122.3 ± 35.7 min. Mortality was not different during hospitalization and at 30 days, with a trend toward lower mortality at 1 year in the PCI group (12.5% vs. 7.0%, $P = 0.061$). There were no differences in the rate of recurrent myocardial infarctions and stroke, with a trend toward lower incidence of recurrent myocardial infarctions in the PCI group at 1 year (7.5% vs. 3.5%, $P = 0.073$). The composite of death, recurrent myocardial infarction, and stroke was higher in the on-site thrombolysis group at 30 days (15.5% vs. 8%; $P = 0.019$), at 1 year (21.5% vs. 11.4%, $P = 0.006$), and also after 5 years of follow-up (53% vs. 40%, $P < 0.001$).

The role of PCI in patients in whom reperfusion fails to occur has been outlined in a randomized trial on 427 patients who were assigned to either repeat thrombolysis, conservative treatment, or rescue PCI [26]. The composite end point was death, reinfarction, or severe heart failure within 6 months. The rate of event-free survival among patients treated with rescue PCI was 84.6%, as compared with 70.1% among those receiving conservative therapy and 68.7% among those undergoing repeated thrombolysis ($P = 0.004$). The adjusted hazard ratio for the occurrence of the primary end point for repeated thrombolysis versus conservative therapy was 1.09 (95% CI 0.71–1.67; $P = 0.69$), as compared with adjusted hazard ratios of 0.43 (95% CI 0.26–0.72; $P = 0.001$) for rescue PCI versus repeated thrombolysis and 0.47 (95% CI 0.28–0.79; $P = 0.004$) for rescue PCI versus conservative therapy.

In the Trial of Routine Angioplasty and Stenting after Fibrinolysis to Enhance Reperfusion in Acute Myocardial Infarction (TRANSFER-AMI), 1059 STEMI patients who underwent fibrinolysis in hospitals that did not have the capability to perform primary PCI were randomized to either standard treatment (including rescue PCI if required) or immediate transfer to a specialized center for PCI within 6 hours after thrombolysis [27]. The primary end point was the composite of death, reinfarction, recurrent ischemia, new or worsening congestive heart failure or cardiogenic shock within 30 days. The primary end point occurred in 11.0% of the patients who were assigned to routine early PCI and in 17.2% of the patients with standard treatment (95% CI 0.47–0.87; $P = 0.004$).

These trials indicate that immediate transfer of patients with STEMI to a specialized PCI center appears to be the superior treatment strategy compared with on-site thrombolysis; however, early PCI following thrombolysis still offers clinical benefit irrespective whether or not the thrombolytic approach was successful.

Stenting versus percutaneous transluminal coronary angioplasty

After primary balloon angioplasty for acute STEMI, the presence of dissection or residual stenosis of >30% has been shown to be a major predictor of recurrent ischemia and infarct artery reocclusion [71,72]. The implantation of stents provides sealing of dissections and restoration of vessel geometry and blood flow. Accordingly, stenting of the infarct artery lowers the rates of restenosis and the frequencies of recurrent angina and repeated revascularization procedures. After early promising results of pilot studies and small randomized trials [73–75], this was shown by the randomized PAMI trial, in which 900 patients with acute myocardial infarctions were treated either with conventional balloon angioplasty or with balloon angioplasty combined with implantation of heparin-coated stents [76]. After 6 months, fewer patients in the stent group than in the angioplasty group had angina (11.3% vs. 16.9%, $P < 0.02$) or needed target vessel revascularization because of ischemia (7.7% vs. 17.0%, $P < 0.001$). In addition, the combined primary end point of death, reinfarction, disabling stroke, or target vessel revascularization because of ischemia occurred in fewer patients in the stent group than in the angioplasty group (12.6% vs. 20.1%, $P < 0.01$). The decrease in the combined end point was due entirely to the decreased need for target vessel revascularization. Angiographic follow-up at 6.5 months demonstrated a lower incidence of restenosis in the stent group than in the angioplasty group (20.3% vs. 33.5%, $P < 0.001$).

The superior outcome of stenting compared with plain balloon angioplasty in primary PCI was also demonstrated by the large randomized multicenter Controlled Abciximab and Device Investigation to Lower Late Angioplasty Complications (CADILLAC) trial comparing plain balloon angioplasty with stenting with or without abciximab in 2082 patients with acute myocardial infarction [45]. In this trial, the combined end point of death, reinfarction, disabling stroke, and ischemia driven by revascularization of the target vessel had occurred in 20.0% of patients after plain balloon angioplasty (percutaneous transluminal coronary angioplasty, PTCA), in 16.5% after PTCA plus abciximab, in 11.5% after stenting, and in 10.2% after stenting plus abciximab ($P < 0.001$). The rates of death, stroke, and reinfarction were not different among the groups. The variation in the incidence of the primary end point was entirely related to different rates of target vessel revascularization, ranging from 15.7% after PTCA to 5.2% after stenting plus abciximab ($P < 0.001$). The 7-month angiographic restenosis rate was 40.8% after PTCA and 22.2% after stenting ($P < 0.001$).

In a meta-analysis on 4120 patients treated with stenting compared with plain balloon angioplasty, the clinical advantage of stent implantation was confirmed [77]. The composite incidence of major adverse cardiac events at 6–12 months was significantly reduced (13.3% vs. 22.5%; $P < 0.001$), driven by a reduction in target vessel revascularization (9.2% vs. 18.7%; $P < 0.001$). As a consequence of these results, stenting of the infarct-related artery has evolved as the preferred treatment strategy in primary PCI.

When compared with bare metal stents, drug-eluting stents appear to reduce further the rates of restenosis within 12 months after primary PCI [78,79]. In the Paclitaxel-Eluting Stent versus Conventional Stent in Myocardial Infarction with ST-Segment Elevation (PASSION) trial, 619 patients with acute STEMI were randomly assigned to receive a paclitaxel-eluting stent or an uncoated stent [46]. The primary end point was a composite of death from cardiac causes, recurrent myocardial infarction, or target lesion revascularization at 1 year. There was a trend toward a lower rate of serious adverse events in the paclitaxel stent group than in the uncoated stent group (8.8% vs. 12.8%; $P = 0.09$). A nonsignificant trend was also detected in favor of the paclitaxel stent group, compared with the uncoated stent group, in the rate of death from cardiac causes or recurrent myocardial infarction (5.5% vs. 7.2%; $P = 40$) and in the rate of target lesion revascularization (5.3% vs. 7.8%; $P = 0.23$). The incidence of stent thrombosis was the same in both groups (1.0%).

In the Trial to Assess the use of the Cypher Stent in Acute Myocardial Infarction Treated with Balloon Angioplasty (TYPHOON), 712 patients with acute STEMI were randomly assigned to receive a sirolimus-eluting stent or an uncoated stent [47]. The primary end point was target vessel failure at 1 year, defined as target vessel-related death, recurrent myocardial infarction, or target vessel revascularization. A follow-up angiographic substudy at 8 months was performed among 174 patients from selected centers. The rate of the primary end point was significantly lower in the sirolimus stent group (7.3% vs. 14.3%; $P = 0.004$). This reduction was driven by a decrease in the rate of target vessel revascularization (5.6% vs. 13.4%; $P < 0.001$). There was no significant differ-

ence between the two groups in the rate of death (2.3% vs. 2.2%; $P = 1.00$), reinfarction (1.1% vs. 1.4%; $P = 1.00$), or stent thrombosis (3.4% vs. 3.6%; $P = 1.00$). The degree of neointimal proliferation, as assessed by the mean in-stent late luminal loss, was significantly lower in the sirolimus stent group (0.14 ± 0.49 mm vs. 0.83 ± 0.52 mm) than in the uncoated stent group ($P < 0.001$).

In a large-scale propensity-score matching study on 7217 patients with acute myocardial infarction [80] the 2-year risk-adjusted mortality rates were lower for drug-eluting stents than for bare-metal stents among all patients with myocardial infarction (10.7% vs. 12.8%; $P = 0.02$), among patients with STEMI (8.5% vs. 11.6%; $P = 0.008$), and among patients with NSTEMI (12.8% vs. 15.6%; $P = 0.04$).

These data indicate that drug-eluting stents can be used safely in the setting of primary PCI and are likely to reduce the need for repeated revascularization. However, the results do not demonstrate that criteria for selecting a drug-eluting stent should differ from those for elective procedures (e.g., diabetes, long lesions, small vessels).

Glycoprotein IIb/IIIa receptor blockers

Various studies have shown that abciximab may prevent abrupt vessel closure after percutaneous coronary revascularization procedures [81]. In a small randomized trial of patients with acute myocardial infarctions, the potential of abciximab to improve the recovery of microvascular perfusion and to enhance the contractile function in the myocardial area at risk was demonstrated [43].

The randomized Abciximab Before Direct Angioplasty and Stenting in Myocardial Infarction Regarding Acute and Long-Term Follow-up (ADMIRAL) study demonstrated that abciximab in combination with stent implantation may reduce both the incidence of acute ischemic events as well as the incidence of end points related to clinical restenosis [82]. In this study, 300 patients with acute myocardial infarction were randomized to receive either abciximab plus stenting or placebo before they underwent coronary angiography. At 30 days, the primary end point, a composite of death, reinfarction, or urgent revascularization of the target vessel, had occurred in 6.0% of the patients in the abciximab group, compared with 14.6% of those in the placebo group ($P = 0.01$); at 6 months the corresponding figures were 7.4% and 15.9% ($P = 0.02$). The better clinical outcomes in the abciximab group were related to the greater frequency of grade III coronary flow in this group than in the placebo group.

The beneficial effect of glycoprotein IIb/IIIa receptor blockers was confirmed by a meta-analysis on 1101 patients presenting for primary PCI and stenting in acute STEMI who were randomized to abciximab or placebo [83]. The primary end point of death or reinfarction was reduced from an estimated cumulative hazard rate of 19.0% with placebo to 12.9% with abciximab ($P = 0.008$). The mortality rate was reduced from an estimated cumulative hazard rate of 14.3% in the placebo arm to 10.9% in the abciximab arm ($P = 0.052$) and reinfarctions were reduced from an estimated cumulative hazard rate of 5.5% with placebo to 2.3% with abciximab ($P = 0.013$). In addition, abciximab provided a significant benefit on the primary end point for diabetics ($P = 0.022$).

Thrombus aspiration in primary percutaneous coronary intervention

Distal embolization of atherothrombotic material during primary PCI may lead to microvascular obstruction and impairment of myocardial perfusion contributing to late mortality after acute STEMI [84]. In particular, myocardial blush grade after primary PCI was identified as a predictor of late mortality [85]. Embolic protection during PCI in acute myocardial infarctions has been tested with various devices in small and medium-sized trials with conflicting results [86–94]. This variation in results may in part be explained by the individual device mechanism, as trials involving manual aspiration have all shown favorable effects on myocardial perfusion variables [90–92].

In a large randomized prospective trial on patients with acute STEMIs, a total of 1071 patients were randomly assigned to be treated with manual thrombus aspiration or conventional PCI [44]. Aspiration was considered to be successful if there was histopathologic evidence of atherothrombotic material. Angiographic and electrocardiographic signs of myocardial reperfusion, as well as clinical outcome, were assessed. The primary end point of the study was myocardial blush grade of 0 or 1, defined as absent or minimal myocardial reperfusion, respectively. A myocardial blush grade of 0 or 1 occurred in 17.1% of the patients in the thrombus aspiration group and in 26.3% of those in the conventional PCI group ($P < 0.001$). Complete resolution of ST-segment elevation occurred in 56.6% versus 44.2% ($P < 0.001$). At 30 days, the rate of death in patients with a myocardial blush grade of 0 or 1, 2, and 3 was 5.2%, 2.9%, and 1.0%, respectively ($P = 0.003$), and the rate of adverse events was 14.1%, 8.8%, and 4.2%, respectively ($P < 0.001$). Histopathologic examination confirmed successful aspiration in 72.9% of patients.

The study demonstrated that manual thrombus aspiration can be performed in a large majority of patients presenting with acute STEMI irrespective of their clinical and angiographic features (e.g., visible thrombus on angiography) and that this adjunctive procedure may result in improved myocardial reperfusion and clinical outcome compared with conventional PCI.

In a meta-analysis of nine trials involving 2417 patients comparing manual thrombectomy with conventional primary PCI in acute STEMI, adjunctive manual thrombectomy was associated with a significant increase in postprocedural TIMI III flow (87.1% vs. 81.2%, $P < 0.0001$) and postprocedural myocardial blush grade 3 (52.1% vs. 31.7%; $P < 0.0001$), less distal embolization (7.9% vs. 19.5%; $P < 0.0001$), and a reduction in 30-day mortality (1.7% vs. 3.1%; $P = 0.04$) [95].

Primary percutaneous coronary intervention versus coronary artery bypass graft in patients with cardiogenic shock

Cardiogenic shock complicates 7–10% of myocardial infarctions and is associated with a 70–80% mortality rate [96,97]. It represents the leading cause of death in patients hospitalized with acute myocardial infarctions [98,99]. Nonrandomized studies have reported markedly lower mortality rates among patients receiving revascularization therapy [100–105].

In the Should we Emergently Revascularize Occluded Coronaries for Cardiogenic Shock? (SHOCK) trial, 302 patients with acute myocardial infarction complicated by cardiogenic shock were randomized to receive either emergency revascularization or initial medical stabilization [106]. Revascularization was accomplished by PCI or coronary artery bypass grafting. Intra-aortic balloon pumping was performed in 86% of the patients in both treatment groups. The primary end point of the study was all-cause mortality; a secondary end point was 6-month survival. Overall mortality did not differ significantly between the revascularization and the medical treatment group (46.7% vs. 56.0%; $P = 0.11$). However, after 6 months, mortality was lower in the revascularization than in the medical therapy group (50.3% vs. 63.1%; $P = 0.027$).

In the SHOCK trial, patients randomized to revascularization were individually selected for PCI or bypass surgery. Eighty-one patients (63.3%) underwent PCI and 47 (36.7%) underwent CABG. There were relatively more patients with diabetes (48.9% vs. 26.9%; $P = 0.02$), three-vessel disease (80.4% vs. 60.3%; $P = 0.03$), and left main coronary disease (41.3% vs. 13.0%; $P = 0.001$) in the CABG group than in the PCI group. The survival rates were 55.6% in the PCI group compared with 57.4% in the CABG group ($P = 0.86$) and 51.9% compared with 46.8%, respectively, at 1 year, ($P = 0.71$). More than 80% of the patients enrolled in the SHOCK trial were younger than 75 years. Among these patients, all subgroups based on clinical, hemodynamic, and echocardiographic characteristics derived benefit from early revascularization.

The SHOCK trial registry on 884 patients admitted with left ventricular pump failure demonstrated a lower in-hospital mortality among patients treated with interventional or surgical revascularization [107]. In this registry, 276 patients (31.2%) underwent PCI and 109 (12.3%) underwent CABG. The in-hospital mortality rate was 78.0% in patients treated medically, 46.4% in those treated with PCI, and 23.9% in those treated with CABG ($P < 0.001$). Among patients with single-vessel disease, the in-hospital mortality rate was similar regardless of whether they were treated with PCI or GABG (32.9% vs. 33.3%); in-hospital mortality was higher in those treated with PCI than in those who underwent CABG among both patients with two-vessel disease (42.2% vs. 17.7%, $P = 0.025$) and patients with three-vessel disease (59.35% vs. 29.6%; $P < 0.0001$). In-hospital mortality was strikingly lower among those patients who underwent IABP placement and subsequent revascularization with PCI or CABG than in patients in whom IABP therapy was not applied (39% vs. 78%, $P < 0.001$).

Although the relative clinical benefit of PCI may have been blunted in these cohorts of patients by a limited use of stents and glycoprotein IIb/IIIa receptor blockers (33% and 69.4% in the SHOCK trial), the important conclusion is that both interventional as well as surgical revascularization appear to provide a mortality benefit in patients with cardiogenic shock. The two approaches seem to represent complementary treatment strategies when selected individually with regard to the presence of diabetes and variability in patient anatomy.

Percutaneous coronary intervention in non-ST-segment myocardial infarctions

A meta-analysis of seven randomized trials (including studies before the widespread use of stents and multidrug adjunctive therapy) comparing routine angiography ($n = 4608$) followed by revascularization with a more conservative strategy (invasive therapy only in patients with recurrent or inducible ischemia, $n = 4604$) found reduced rates of death and myocardial infarction at the end of follow-up (12.2% vs. 14.4%; $P < 0.001$) for routine invasive versus selective invasive treatment [108]. Although no reduction in mortality was observed, there were fewer myocardial infarctions (7.3% vs. 9.4%, $P < 0.001$) in the invasive treatment group. These results were obtained despite an early hazard observed during initial hospitalization in the routine invasive group, when a significantly higher risk of death and death and myocardial infarction was noted (1.8% vs. 1.1%, $P = 0.007$ for death; 5.2% vs. 3.8%, $P = 0.002$ for death and MI). The beneficial effect was actually achieved from hospital discharge to the end of follow-up, with a significant reduction in the risk of death and myocardial infarction being observed for routine invasive versus selective invasive treatment (3.8% vs. 4.9%, $P = 0.01$ for death; 7.4% vs. 11.0%, $P < 0.001$ for death and MI). Over a mean follow-up of 17 months, recurrent angina was reduced by 33% and rehospitalization by 34% in the routine invasive group.

In another meta-analysis including six contemporary trials, the odds ratio was 0.84 (95% confidence interval [CI] 0.73–0.97) for early invasive versus conservative strategy. The benefit of the routine invasive strategy was apparent in patients with elevated troponins at baseline, but not in troponin-negative patients [109–111].

A more recent meta-analysis including seven trials involving 8375 patients available for analysis showed, after a mean follow-up of 2 years, a significant reduction in all-cause mortality (4.9% vs. 6.5%, $P = 0.001$) for early invasive versus conservative treatment without excess death at 1 month [112]. At 2 years' follow-up, the incidence of nonfatal myocardial infarction was 7.6% versus 9.1% ($P = 0.012$). Long-term mortality reduction was confirmed in the follow-up of Randomized Intervention Trial of Unstable Angina (RITA)

3 trial at 5 years [113] and in the Fragmin during Instability in Coronary artery disease (FRISC) 2 trial at 2 and 5 years [109,111]. More recently, another meta-analysis has confirmed the existence of a trend toward an early excess of mortality with an invasive strategy (relative risk [RR] 1.59, 95% CI 0.96–2.54), but with a significant long-term benefit in terms of death (RR 0.75, 95% CI 0.62–0.92) or myocardial infarction (RR 0.75, 95% CI 0.62–0.91) with invasive versus conservative treatment at 2–5 years' follow-up [114].

In all randomized trials, a large proportion of patients in the conservative arm eventually underwent revascularization ("crossover"), such that the true benefit of revascularization appears to be underestimated [115].

Percutaneous coronary intervention in elderly patients

Elderly patients undergoing primary PCI for acute myocardial infarction present with numerous comorbid conditions known to portend an adverse prognosis. Despite these risk factors, success rates of primary PCI are similar in elderly and young patients.

A small randomized trial on 87 patients older than 75 years comparing primary PCI with streptokinase demonstrated an impressive reduction in the primary combined end point of death, reinfarction, and stroke from 29% to 9% ($P < 0.01$) in favor of PCI [116]. In addition, 30-day (7% vs. 22%, $P = 0.04$) and 1-year mortality (11% vs. 29%, $P = 0.03$) were considerably reduced.

Despite this advantage of primary PCI over thrombolysis, the Controlled Abciximab and Device Investigation to Lower Late Angioplasty Complications (CADILLAC) trial revealed an exponential increase in 1-year mortality among patients older than 65 years (1.6% for patients <55 years, 2.1% for 55–65 years, 7.1% for 65–75 years, 11.1% for patients >75 years; $P < 0.0001$). One-year rates of ischemic target revascularization (7.0% vs. 17.6%, $P < 0.0001$) and subacute or late thrombosis (0% vs. 2.2%, $P < 0.005$) were reduced with stenting compared with balloon angioplasty [45].

In the Senior PAMI trial, 481 patients older than 70 years were randomized to primary PCI with abciximab versus thrombolysis [117]. In-hospital recurrent ischemia (4.8% vs. 31%, $P = 0.0001$), reinfarction (1.2% vs. 4.4%, $P = 0.032$), and the 30-day end point of death, reinfarction, and stroke (11.6% vs. 18%, $P = 0.05$) were significantly reduced with primary PCI. This benefit, however, was confined to the age group 70–80 years; no benefit was seen in patients older than 80 years. A similar lack of benefit from primary PCI was also seen in a small randomized study of 120 patients aged 80 years and older compared with conservative treatment over a 3-year follow-up period [118].

Obviously, in the subgroup of very old patients, the decision about interventional versus conservative treatment options should include a thorough consideration of functional status and comorbidities.

Conclusion

Primary PCI of the infarct-related coronary artery with stent implantation and administration of glycoprotein IIb/IIIa receptor blockers within the first 12 h after onset of symptoms has evolved as the most effective therapy for patients presenting with acute STEMI. The treatment is directed to reverse acute thrombotic occlusion of the infarct artery, to safely restore vessel patency and coronary blood flow, and to minimize myocardial infarct size and mortality. Primary PCI represents a class IA recommendation when available within 90 min after the first medical contact. However, even after 12 h of symptom duration, primary PCI may provide clinical benefit for patients with STEMI. Adjunctive manual thrombus aspiration before stent implantation appears to improve the clinical outcome. The use of drug-eluting stents should be oriented to the expected risk of restenosis and the feasibility of a 12-month dual antiplatelet therapy protocol. In patients with NSTEMI, PCI represents the preferred treatment strategy when a high risk of adverse clinical outcome is anticipated.

References

1. Brown KWG, McMillian RL, Forbath N, Mel'Grano F, & Scott JW (1963) Coronary unit: an intensive care center for acute myocardial infarction. *Lancet* **2**:349.

2. Nachlass MM & Miller DI (1965) Closed-chest cardiac resuscitation in patients with acute myocardial infarction. *Am Heart J* **69**:448.

3. Rogers WJ, Canto JG, Lambrew CT, *et al.* (2000) Temporal trends in the treatment of over 1.5 million patients with myocardial infarction in the U.S. from 1990 through 1999: the National Registry of Myocardial Infarction 1, 2 and 3. *J Am Coll Cardiol* **36**:2056–2063.

4. Furman MI, Dauerman HL, Goldberg RJ, Yarzebski J, Lessard D, & Gore JM (2001) Twenty-two year 1975–1997 trends in the incidence, in-hospital and long-term case fatality rates from initial Q-wave and non-Q-wave myocardial infarction: a multi-hospital, community-wide perspective. *J Am Coll Cardiol* **37**:1571–1580.

5. Keeley E, Boura JA, & Grines CL (2003) Primary angioplasty versus intravenous thrombolytic therapy for acute myocardial infarction: a quantitative review of 23 randomised trials. *Lancet* **361**:13–20.

6. Rovelli F, De Vita C, Feruglio GA, Lotto A, Selvini A, & Tognoni G (1987) GISSI trial: early results and late follow up. Gruppo Italiano per la Sperimentazione della Streptochinasi nell'Infarto Myocardico. *J Am Coll Cardiol* **10**(5 Suppl. B):33B–39B.

7. Boersma E, Mercado N, Polderman D, Gardien M, Vos J, & Simoons ML (2003) Acute myocardial infarction. *Lancet* **361**:847–858.

8. The GUSTO Angiographic Investigators (1994) The effects of tissue plasminogen activator, streptokinase, or both on coronary artery patency, ventricular function, and survival after acute myocardial infarction. *N Engl J Med* **331**:277–278.

9. Anderson JL, Karagounis LA, Becker LC, Sorensen SG, &

Menlove RL (1993) TIMI perfusion grade 3 but not grade 2 results in improved outcome after thrombolysis for myocardial infarction: ventriculographic, enzymatic, and electrocardiographic evidence from the TEAM-3 Study. *Circulation* **87**:1829–1839.

10. Gibson CM, Karha J, Murphy SA, *et al.* (2003) Early and long-term clinical outcomes associated with reinfarction following fibrinolytic administration in the Thrombolysis in Myocardial Infarction trials. *J Am Coll Cardiol* **42**:7–16.

11. Ahmed S, Antmann EM, Murphy SA, *et al.* (2006) Poor outcomes after fibrinolytic therapy for ST-segment elevation myocardial infarction: impact of age (a meta-analysis of a decade of trials). *J Thromb Thrombolysis* **21**:119–129.

12. Keeley EC & Hillis LD (2007) Primary PCI for myocardial infarction with ST-segment elevation. *N Engl J Med* **356**:47–54.

13. Virmani R, Burke AP, Kolodgie FD, & Farb A (2002) Vulnerable plaque: the pathology of unstable coronary lesions. *J Interven Cardiol* **15**:439–446.

14. Ohtani T, Ueda Y, Mizote I, *et al.* (2006) Number of yellow plaques detected in a coronary artery is associated with future risk of acute coronary syndrome: detection of vulnerable patients by angioscopy. *J Am Coll Cardiol* **47**:2194.

15. Malek AM, Alper SL, & Izumo S (1999) Hemodynamic shear stress and its role in atherosclerosis. *JAMA* **282**:2035.

16. Rosenberg RD & Aird WC (1999) Vascular-bed-specific hemostasis and hypercoagulable states. *N Engl J Med* **340**:1555.

17. Reimer KA, Lowe JE, Rasmussen MM, & Jennings RB (1977) The wavefront phenomenon of ischemic cell death: myocardial infarct size versus duration of coronary occlusion in dogs. *Circulation* **56**:786–794.

18. De Luca G, Suryapranata H, Ottervanger JP, & Antman EM (2004) Time delay to treatment and mortality in primary angioplasty for acute myocardial infarction: every minute of delay counts. *Circulation* **109**:1223–1225.

19. Lindahl B, Toss H, Siegbahn A, *et al.* (2000) Markers of myocardial damage and inflammation in relation to long-term mortality in unstable coronary artery disease. FRISC study group. Fragmin during instability in coronary artery disease. *N Engl J Med* **343**:1139–1147.

20. Halkin A, Stone GW, Grines CL, *et al.* (2006) Prognostic implications of creatine kinase elevation after primary percutaneous coronary intervention for acute myocardial infarction. *J Am Coll Cardiol* **47**:951–961.

21. Van de Werf F, Ardissino D, Betriu A, *et al.* (2003) Management of acute myocardial infarction in patients presenting with ST-segment elevation. *Eur Heart J* **24**:28–66.

22. Antman EM, Hand M, Armstrong PW, *et al.* (2008) 2007 focused update of the ACC/AHA 2004 guidelines for the management of patients with ST-elevation myocardial infarction: a report of the American College of Cardiology/American Heart Association Task Force on Practice Guidelines: developed in collaboration With the Canadian Cardiovascular Society endorsed by the American Academy of Family Physicians: 2007 Writing Group to Review New Evidence and Update the ACC/AHA 2004 Guidelines for the Management of Patients With ST-Elevation Myocardial Infarction, Writing on Behalf of the 2004 Writing Committee. *Circulation* **117**:296–329.

23. Andersen HR, Nielsen TT, Rasmussen K, *et al.* (2003) A comparison of coronary angioplasty with fibrinolytic therapy in acute myocardial infarction. *N Engl J Med* **349**:733–742.

24. Widimsky P, Budesinski T, Vorac D, *et al.* (2003) Long distance transport for primary angioplasty vs. immediate thrombolysis in acute myocardial infarction. Final results of the randomized national multicenter trial—PRAGUE-2. *Eur Heart J* **24**:94–104.

25. Schömig A, Mehilli J, Antonucci D, *et al.* (2005) Mechanical reperfusion in patients with acute myocardial infarction presenting more than 12 hours from symptom onset. *JAMA* **293**: 2865–2872.

26. Gershlick AH, Stephens-Lloyd A, Hughes S, *et al.* (2005) Rescue angioplasty after failed thrombolytic therapy for acute myocardial infarction. *N Engl J Med* **353**:2758–2768.

27. Cantor WJ, Fitchett D, Borgundvaag B, *et al.*, for the TRANSFER-AMI trial investigators. (2009) Routine early angioplasty after fibrinolysis for acute myocardial infarction. *N Engl J Med* **360**: 2705–2718.

28. Hochmann JS, Sleeper LA, Webb JG, *et al.* (1999) Early revascularization in acute myocardial infarction complicated by cardiogenic shock. *N Engl J Med* **341**:625–634.

29. Bassand JP, Hamm CW, Ardissino D, *et al.* (2007) Guidelines for the diagnosis and treatment of non-ST-segment elevation acute coronary syndromes. *Eur Heart H* **28**:1598–1660.

30. Anderson JL, Adams CD, Antman EM, *et al.* (2007) ACC/AHA guidelines for the management of patients with unstable angina/non-ST-elevation myocardial infarction—executive summary. *J Am Coll Cardiol* **50**:652–726.

31. Eagle KA, Lim MJ, Dabbous OH, *et al.* (2004) A validated prediction model for all forms of acute coronary syndromes: estimating the risk of 6-month postdischarge death in an international registry. *JAMA* **291**:2727–2733.

32. Fox KA, Dabbous OH, Goldberg RJ, *et al.* (2006) Prediction of risk of death and myocardial infarction in the six months after presentation with acute coronary syndrome: prospective multinational observational study (GRACE). *BMJ* **333**:1091.

33. Granger CB, Goldberg RJ, Dabbous O, *et al.* (2003) Predictors of hospital mortality in the global registry of acute coronary events. *Arch Intern Med* **163**:2345–2353.

34. Cannon CP, Gibson CM, Lambrew CT, *et al.* (2000) Relationship of symptom-onset-to-balloon time and door-to-balloon time with mortality in patients undergoing angioplasty for acute myocardial infarction. *JAMA* **283**:2941–2947.

35. De Luca G, Suryapranata H, Zijlstra F, *et al.* (2003) Symptom-onset-to-balloon time and mortality in patients with acute myocardial infarction treated by primary angioplasty. *J Am Coll Cardiol* **42**: 991–997.

36. McNamara RL, Wang Y, Herrin J, *et al.* (2006) Effect of door-to-balloon time on mortality in patients with ST-segment elevation myocardial infarction. *J Am Coll Cardiol* **47**:2180–2186.

37. Dhruva VN, Abdelhadi SI, Anis A, *et al.* (2007) ST-segment analysis using wireless technology in acute myocardial infarction (STAT-MI) trial. *J Am Coll Cardiol* **50**:509–513.

38. Le May MR, So DY, Dionne R, *et al.* (2008) A citywide protocol for primary PCI in ST-segment elevation myocardial infarction. *N Engl J Med* **358**:231–240.

39. Henry TD, Sharkey SW, Burke N, *et al.* (2007) A regional system to provide timely access to percutaneous coronary intervention for ST-elevation myocardial infarction. *Circulation* **116**:721–728.

40. Khot UN, Johnson ML, Ramsey C, *et al.* (2007) Emergency department physician activation of the catheterization laboratory and immediate transfer to a immediately available catheteriza-

tion laboratory reduce door-to-balloon time in ST-elevation myocardial infarction. *Circulation* **116**:67–76.

41. Canto JG, Every NR, Magid DJ, *et al.* (2003) The volume of primary angioplasty procedures and survival after acute myocardial infarction. *N Engl J Med* **342**:1573–1580.

42. Wiviott SD, Braunwald E, McCabe CH, *et al.*, for the TRITON-TIMI 38 investigators. (2007) Prasugrel versus clopidogrel in patients with acute coronary syndromes. *N Engl J Med* **357**:2001–2015.

43. Neumann FJ, Blasini R, Schmitt C, *et al.* (1998) Effect of glycoprotein IIb/IIIa receptor blockade on recovery of coronary flow and left ventricular function after the placement of coronary artery stents in acute myocardial infarction. *Circulation* **98**:2695–2701.

44. Svilaas T, Vlaar PJ, van der Horst IC, *et al.* (2008) Thrombus aspiration during primary percutaneous coronary intervention. *N Engl J Med* **358**:557–567.

45. Stone GW, Grines CL, Cox DA, *et al.* (2002) Comparison of angioplasty with stenting, with or without abciximab, in acute myocardial infarction. *N Engl J Med* **346**:957–966.

46. Laarman GJ, Suttorp MJ, Dirksen MT, *et al.* (2006) Paclitaxel-eluting versus uncoated stents in primary percutaneous coronary intervention. *N Engl J Med* **355**:1105–1113.

47. Spaulding C, Henry P, Teiger E, *et al.* (2006) Sirolimus-eluting versus uncoated stents in acute myocardial infarction. *N Engl J Med* **355**:1093–1104.

48. Sianos G, Papafaklis MI, Daemen J, *et al.* (2007) Angiographic stent thrombosis after routine use of drug-eluting stents in ST-segment elevation myocardial infarction. *J Am Coll Cardiol* **50**:573–583.

49. Hong MK, Mintz GS, Lee CW, *et al.* (2004) Comparison of coronary plaque rupture between stable angina and acute myocardial infarction: a three-vessel intravascular ultrasound study in 235 patients. *Circulation* **110**:928–933.

50. Kubo T, Imanishi T, Takarada S, *et al.* (2007) Assessment of culprit lesion morphology in acute myocardial infarction. *J Am Coll Cardiol* **50**:933–939.

51. Stefanadis C, Toutouzas K, Tsiamis E, *et al.* (2001) Increased local temperature in human coronary atherosclerotic plaques: an independent predictor of clinical outcome in patients undergoing a percutaneous coronary intervention. *J Am Coll Cardiol* **37**:1277–1283.

52. Hanratty CG, Koyama Y, Rasmussen HH, Nelson GIC, Hansen PS, & Ward MR (2002) Exaggeration of nonculprit stenosis severity during acute myocardial infarction: implications for immediate multivessel revascularization. *J Am Coll Cardiol* **40**:911–916.

53. Gibson CM, Ryan KA, Murphy SA, *et al.* (1999) Impaired coronary blood flow in non-culprit arteries in the setting of acute myocardial infarction. The TIMI study group. Thrombplysis In Myocardial Infarction. *J Am Coll Cardiol* **34**:974–982.

54. Gregorini L, Marco J, Kozakova M, *et al.* (1999) Alpha-adrenergic blockade improves recovery of myocardial perfusion and function after coronare stenting in patients with acute myocardial infarction. *Circulation* **99**:482–490.

55. Goldberg RJ, Samad NA, Yarzebski J, Gurwitz J, Bigelow C, & Gore JM (1999) Temporal trends in cardiogenic shock complicating myocardial infarction. *N Engl J Med* **340**:1162–1168.

56. Hochman JS (2003) Cardiogenic shock complicating acute myocardial infarction. *Circulation* **107**:2998–3002.

57. Chen ZM, Pan HC, Chen YP, *et al.* (2005) Early intravenous then oral metoprolol in 45 852 patients with acute myocardial

infarction: randomized placebo-controlled trial. *Lancet* **366**: 1622–1632.

58. ACE Inhibitor Myocardial Infarction Collaboration Group. (1998) Indications for ACE-inhibitors in the early treatment of acute myocardial infarction: systematic overview of individual data from 100 000 patients in randomized trials. ACE Inhibitor Myocardial Infarction Collaborative Group. *Circulation* **97**:2202–2212.

59. Mega JL, Morrow DA, Cannon CP, *et al.* (2006) Cholesterol, C-reactive protein, and cerebrovascular events following intensive and moderate statin therapy. *J Thromb Thrombolysis* **22**:71–76.

60. Zeymer U, Gitt AK, Jünger C, *et al.* (2006) Effect of clopidogrel on 1-year mortality in hospital survivors of acute ST-segment elevation myocardial infarction in clinical practice. *Eur Heart J* **27**:2661–2666.

61. Grines CL, Browne MJ, Marco J, *et al.* (1993) A comparison of immediate angioplasty with thrombolytic therapy for acute myocardial infarction. *N Engl J Med* **328**:673–679.

62. Zijlstra F, de Boer MJ, Hoorntje JCA, Reiffers S, Reiber JHC, & Suryapranata H (1993) A comparison of immediate coronary angioplasty with intravenous streptokinase in acute myocardial infarction. *N Engl J Med* **328**:680–684.

63. The Global Use of Strategies to Open Occluded Coronary Arteries in Acute Coronary Syndromes (GUSTO IIb) Angioplasty Substudy Investigators (1997) A clinical trial comparing primary coronary angioplasty with tissue plasminogen activator for acute myocardial infarction. *N Engl J Med* **336**:1621–1628.

64. Zijlstra F, Hoorntje JCA, de Boer MJ, *et al.* (1999) Long-term benefit of primary angioplasty as compared with thrombolytic therapy for acute myocardial infarction. *N Engl J Med* **341**:1413–1419.

65. Nunn CM, O'Neil WW, Rothbaum D, *et al.* (1999) Long-term outcome after primary angioplasty: report from the Primary Angioplasty in Myocardial Infarction (PAMI-I) trial. *J Am Coll Cardiol* **33**:640–646.

66. Schömig A, Kastrati A, Dirschinger J, *et al.* (2000). Coronary stenting plus platelet glycoprotein IIb/IIIa blockade compared with tissue plasminogen activator in acute myocardial infarction. *N Engl J Med* **343**:385–391.

67. Kinn JW, O'Neil WW, Benzuly KH, *et al.* (1997) Primary angioplasty reduces the risk of myocardial rupture compared to thrombolysis for acute myocardial infarction. *Cathet Cardiovasc Diagn* **42**:151.

68. Moreno R, Lopez-Sendon J, Garcia E, *et al.* (2002) Primary angioplasty reduces the risk of left ventricular free wall rupture compared with thrombolysis in patients with acute myocardial infarction. *J Am Coll Cardiol* **39**:598.

69. Busk M, Maeng M, Rasmussen K, *et al.* (2008) The Danish multicenter randomized study of fibrinolytic therapy vs. primary angioplasty in acute myocardial infarction (the DANAMI-2 trial): outcome after 3 years follow-up. *Eur Heart J* **29**:1259–1266.

70. Widimsky P, Bilkova D, Penicka M, *et al.* (2007) Long-term outcomes of patients with acute myocardial infarction presenting to hospitals without catheterization laboratory and randomized to immediate thrombolysis or interhospital transport for primary percutaneous coronary intervention. Five year's follow-up of the PRAGUE-2 trial. *Eur Heart J* **28**:679–684.

71. O'Keefe JH, Rutherford BD, McConahay DR, *et al.* (1989) Early and late results of coronary angioplasty without antecedent thrombolytic therapy for acute myocardial infarction. *Am J Cardiol* **64**:1221–1230.

72. Benzuly KH, O'Neill WW, Brodie B, *et al.* (1996) Predictors of maintained infarct artery patency after primary angioplasty in high risk patients in PAMI-2. *J Am Coll Cardiol* **27**(Suppl. A):279 A.

73. Schömig A, Neumann FJ, Walter H, *et al.* (1997) Coronary stent placement in patients with acute myocardial infarction: comparison of clinical and angiographic outcome after randomization to antiplatelet or anticoagulant therapy. *J Am Coll Cardiol* **29**:28–34.

74. Saito S, Hosokawa FG, Kim K, Tanaka S, & Miyake S (1996) Primary stent implantation without coumadin in acute myocardial infarction. *J Am Coll Cardiol* **28**:74–81.

75. Suryanapranata H, van't Hof AWJ, Hoorntje JCA, de Boer MJ, & Zijlstra F (1998) Randomized comparison of coronary stenting with balloon angioplasty in selected patients with acute myocardial infarction. *Circulation* **97**:2502–2505.

76. Grines LG, Cox DA, Stone GW, *et al.* (1999) Coronary angioplasty with or without stent implantation for acute myocardial infarction. *N Engl J Med* **341**:1949–1956.

77. Zhu MM, Feit A, Chadow H, Alam M, Kwan T, & Clark LT (2001) Primary stent implantation compared with primary balloon angioplasty for acute myocardial infarction: a meta-analysis of randomized clinical trials. *Am J Cardiol* **88**:297–301.

78. Saia F, Lemos PA, Lee CH, *et al.* (2003) Sirolimus-eluting stent implantation in ST-elevation acute myocardial infarction: a clinical and angiopgraphic study. *Circulation* **108**:1927–1929.

79. Lemos PA, Saia F, Hofma SG, *et al.* (2004) Short- and long-term clinical benefit of sirolimus-eluting stents compared to conventional bare stents for patients with acute myocardial infarction. *J Am Coll Cardiol* **43**:704–708.

80. Mauri L, Silbaugh TS, Garg P, *et al.* (2008) Drug-eluting or bare-metal stents for acute myocardial infarction. *N Engl J Med* **359**:1330–1342.

81. Adgey AA (1998) An overview of the results of clinical trials with glycoprotein IIb/IIIa inhibitors. *Eur Heart J* **19**(Suppl. D): D10–D21.

82. Montalescot G, Barragan P, Wittenberg O, *et al.* (2001) Platelet glycoprotein IIb/IIIa inhibition with coronary stenting for acute myocardial infarction. *N Engl J Med* **344**:1895–1903.

83. Montalescot G, Antonucci D, Kastrati A, *et al.* (2007) Abciximab in primary coronary stenting of ST-elevation myocardial infarction: a European meta-analysis on individual patients' data with long-term follow-up. *Eur Heart J* **28**:443–449.

84. Henriques JPS, Zijlstra F, Ottervanger JP, *et al.* (2002) Incidence and clinical significance of distal embolization during primary angiolasty for acute myocardial infarction. *Eur Heart J* **23**:1112–1117.

85. Stone GW, Peterson MA, Lansky AJ, Dangas G, Mehran R, & Leon MB (2002) Impact of normalized myocardial perfusion after successful angioplasty in acute myocardial infarction. *J Am Coll Cardiol* **39**:591–597.

86. Napodano M, Pasquetto G, Saccà S, *et al.* (2003) Intracoronary thrombectomy improves myocardial reperfusion in patients undergoing direct angioplasty for acute myocardial infarction. *J Am Coll Cardiol* **42**:1395–1402.

87. Antonucci D, Valenti R, Migliorini A, *et al.* (2004) Comparison of rheolytic thrombectomy before direct infarct artery stenting versus direct stenting alone in patients undergoing percutaneous coronary intervention for acute myocardial infarction. *Am J Cardiol* **93**:1033–1035.

88. Lefèvre T, Garcia E, Reimers B, *et al.* (2005) X-sizer for thrombectomy in acute myocardial infarction improves ST-segment resolution. *J Am Coll Cardion* **46**:246–252.

89. Stone GW, Webb J, Cox DA, *et al.* (2005) Distal microcirculatory protection during percutaneous coronary intervention in acute ST-segment elevation myocardial infarction: a randomized controlled trial. *JAMA* **293**:1063–1072.

90. Burzotta F, Trani C, Romagnoli E, *et al.* (2005) Manual thrombus-aspiration improves myocardial reperfusion: the randomized evaluation of the effect of mechanical reduction of distal embolization by thrombus-aspiration in primary and rescue angioplasty (REMEDIA) trial. *J Am Coll Cardiol* **46**:371–376.

91. De Luca G, Suryapranata H, Chiariello M, *et al.* (2006) Aspiration thrombectomy and primary percutaneous coronary intervention. *Heart* **92**:867–869.

92. Silva-Orrego P, Colombo P, Bigi R, *et al.* (2006) Thrombus aspiration before primary angioplasty improves myocardial reperfusion in acute myocardial infarction: the DEAR-MI (Dethrombosis to Enhance Acute Reperfusion in Myocardial Infarction) study. *J Am Coll Cardiol* **48**:1552–1559.

93. Ali A, Cox D, Dib N, *et al.* (2006) Rheolytic thrombectomy with percutaneous coronary intervention for infarct size reduction in acute myocardial infarction: 30-day results from a multicenter randomized study. *J Am Coll Cardiol* **48**:244–252.

94. Kaltoft A, Bottcher M, Nielsen SS, *et al.* (2006) Routine thrombectomy in percutaneous coronary intervention for acute ST-segment elevation myocardial infarction: a randomized controlled trial. *Circulation* **114**:40–47.

95. De Luca G, Dudek D, Sardella G, *et al.* (2008) Adjunctive manual thrombectomy improves myocardial perfusion and mortality in patients undergoing primary percutaneous coronary intervention for ST-elevation myocardial infarction: a meta-analysis of randomized trials. *Eur Heart J* **29**:3002–3010.

96. Goldberg RJ, Gore JM, Alpert JS, *et al.* (1991) Cardiogenic shock after acute myocardial infarction: incidence and mortality from a community-wide perspective:1975–1988. *N Engl J Med* **325**:1117–1122.

97. Killip T III & Kimbal JT (1967) Treatment of myocardial infarction in a coronary care unit: a two year experience with 250 patients. *Am J Cardiol* **20**:457–467.

98. Holmes DR, Bares ER, Kleiman NS, *et al.* (1995) Contemporary reperfusion therapy for cardiogenic shock: the GUSTO-I trial experience. *J Am Coll Cardiol* **26**:668–674.

99. Becker RC, Gore JM, Lambrew C, *et al.* (1996) A composite view of cardiac rupture in the United States National Registry of Myocardial Infarction. *J Am Coll Cardiol* **27**:1321–1326.

100. Lee L, Bates ER, Pitt B, Walton JA, Laufer N, & O'Neill WW (1988) Percutaneous transluminal coronary angioplasty improves survival in acute myocardial infarction complicated by cardiogenic shock. *Circulation* **78**:1345–1351.

101. Verna E, Repetto S, Boscarini M, Ghezzi I, & Binaghi G (1989) Emergency coronary angioplasty in patients with severe left ventricular dysfunction or cardiogenic shock after acute myocardial infarction. *Eur Heart J* **10**:958–966.

102. Moosvi AR, Khaja F, Villanueva L, Gheorghiade M, Douthat L, & Goldstein S (1992) Early revascularization improves survival in cardiogenic shock complication acute myocardial infarction. *J Am Coll Cardiol* **19**:907–914.

103. Hibbard MD, Holmes DR, Baily KR, Reeder GS, Bresnahan JF, & Gersh BJ (1992) Percutaneous transluminal coronary angioplasty in patients with cardiogenic shock. *J Am Coll Cardiol* **19**:639–646.

104. Antonucci D, Valenti R, Santoro GM, *et al.* (1998) Systematic direct angioplasty and stent-supported direct angioplasty for cardiogenic shock complicating acute myocardial infarction. *Am J Cardiol* **31**:294–300.

105. Himbert D, Juliard JM, Steg PG, Karrillon GJ, Aumont MC, & Gourgon R (1994) Limits of reperfusion therapy for immediate cardiogenic shock complicating acute myocardial infarction. *Am J Cardiol* **74**:492–494.

106. Hochmann JS, Sleeper LA, Webb JG, *et al.* (1999) Early revascularization in acute myocardial infarction complicated by cardiogenic shock. *N Engl J Med* **341**:625–634.

107. Hochmann JS, Buller CE, Sleeper LA, *et al.* (2000) Cardiogenic shock complicating acute myocardial infarction–etiologies, management and outcome: a report from the SHOCK trial registry. *J Am Coll Cardiol* **36**:1063–1070.

108. Metha SR, Cannon CP, Fox KA, *et al.* (2005) Routine vs selective invasive strategies in patients with acute coronary syndromes: a collaborative meta-analysis of randomized trials. *JAMA* **293**:2908–2917.

109. Lagerqvist B, Husted S, Kontny F, Stahle E, Swahn E, & Wallentin L (2006) 5-year outcomes in the FRISC-II randomized trial on an invasive versus a non-invasive strategy in non-ST-segment elevation acute coronary syndrome: a follow-up study. *Lancet* **368**:998–1004.

110. Diderholm E, Andren B, Frostfeld G, *et al.* (2002) The prognostic and therapeutic implications of increased troponin T levels and ST depression in unstable coronary artery disease: the FRISC-II invasive troponin T electrocardiogram substudy. *Am Heart J* **143**:760–767.

111. Lagerqvist B, Husted S, Kontny F, *et al.* (2002) A long-term perspective on the protective effects of an early invasive strategy in unstable coronary artery disease: two year follow-up of the FRISC-II invasive study. *J Am Coll Cardiol* **40**:1902–1914.

112. Bavry AA, Kumbhani DJ, Rassi AN, Bhatt DL, & Askari AT (2006) Benefit of early invasive therapy in acute coronary syndromes: a meta-analysis of contemporary randomized clinical trials. *J Am Coll Cardiol* **48**:1319–1325.

113. Fox KA, Poole-Wilson P, Clayton TC, *et al.* (2005) 5-year outcome of an interventional strategy in non-ST-elevation acute coronary syndrome: the British Heart Foundation RITA 3 randomized trial. *Lancet* **366**:914–920.

114. Hoenig MR, Doust JA, Aroney CN, & Scott IA (2006) Early invasive versus conservative strategies for unstable angina & non-ST-elevation myocardial infarction in the stent era. *Cochrane Database Syst Rev* **3**: CD004815.

115. Cannon CP (2004) Revascularization for everyone? *Eur Heart J* **25**:1471–1472.

116. De Boer MJ, Ottvanger JP, van't Hof AW, *et al.* (2002) Reperfusion therapy in elderly patients with acute myocardial infarction: a randomized comparison of primary angioplasty and thrombolytic therapy. *J Am Coll Cardiol* **39**:1732.

117. Grines C (2005) Senior PAMI: a prospective randomized trial of primary angioplasty and thrombolytic therapy in elderly patients with acute myocardial infarction (presented at TCT Washington, DC, October 19:2005).

118. Minari K, Horie H, Takahashi M, *et al.* (2002) Long-term outcome of primary percutaneous transluminal coronary angioplasty for low-risk acute myocardial infarction in patients older than 80 years old: a single-center open randomized trial. *Am Heart J* **143**:497.

37 Complex Percutaneous Coronary Interventions—Left Main, Bifurcation, and Ostial Disease

Savio D'Souza, Peter Barlis, Giuseppe Ferrante & Carlo Di Mario
Royal Brompton Hospital, London, UK

Introduction

The late German–Swiss radiologist Andreas Grüntzig performed the first balloon percutaneous transluminal coronary angioplasty (PTCA) in 1977 [1]. Thirty years on, interventional cardiology has progressed in leaps and bounds. Over the years, various technical devices have been added to the interventionist's armory, ranging from plain balloon angioplasty to bare metal stents (BMSs) and to the now widely used drug-eluting stents (DESs) [2]. The zest for extending percutaneous coronary intervention (PCI) to various lesions in the coronary tree continues unperturbed. Technologic advances have permitted complex interventions on multivessel coronary disease, chronic total occlusions, bifurcation lesions, ostial disease, and the unprotected left main coronary artery (ULM) stenosis. However, the intended result has not always been sustained, and the indication for PCI as an alternative to surgery remains controversial for the most complex lesions and patient subsets. In this chapter, we review the percutaneous strategies in the treatment of ULM, bifurcation, and ostial lesions, along with the technique and results from the literature, including some of our own case series.

Coronary left main stem stenosis

Significant left main coronary artery disease is a high-risk lesion that can compromise between 70% and 100% of the myocardial left ventricular blood supply based on the type of coronary dominance. Its prevalence in patients undergoing coronary angiography ranges from 2.5% to 10%, and it quite typically coexists with atherosclerotic disease of other segments of the coronary tree, with mortality varying between 43.6% after 24 months and 73.6% after 42 months of follow-up

Cardiovascular Interventions in Clinical Practice. Edited by Jürgen Haase, Hans-Joachim Schäfers, Horst Sievert and Ron Waksman. © 2010 Blackwell Publishing.

[3–5]. Generally, >50% narrowing of the left main is considered clinically significant and associated with a poor prognosis when treated medically, with improved prognosis after coronary artery bypass grafting (CABG). The disease process can typically affect the left main coronary artery anywhere from its ostium or body to its distal segment, with or without bifurcation involvement. Two of Grüntzig's first five patients reportedly had significant left main coronary disease, and one of these died from procedural complications, rapidly leading the pioneers in the field to conclude that left main stenosis was a contraindication to PTCA [6]. Bare metal coronary artery stenting improved acute results and restenosis rates compared with balloon angioplasty, but repeat revascularization rates remained as high as 25–30% [7–9]. The advent of drug-eluting coronary artery stenting in 2002, and the associated dramatic reduction in restenosis, has led to a resurgence of interest in ULM stenting worldwide.

The guidelines

The European Society of Cardiology (ESC) as well as the American Heart Association/American College of Cardiology (AHA/ACC) consider the presence of stenosis in the ULM as a class IIb or IIa indication for PCI only if CABG is contraindicated, deemed a high risk, or declined by the patient [8,10]. The American guidelines unequivocally state that patients eligible for CABG have a class III indication for a PCI (i.e., in these patients angioplasty should not be considered). Surgery is not without risk, particularly in elderly patients undergoing repeat CABG and in those with comorbidities including left ventricular dysfunction and renal impairment. The ESC guidelines specify that stenting should be considered when the EuroScore is greater than 10. However, most cardiac surgeons argue that, even in this cohort of patients, modern surgical and anesthetic techniques have improved outcome in comparison with the historical EuroScore index.

In practice, there is a wide variability in application of guidelines to individual cases. An issue then arises as to who decides a patient to be at a high surgical risk: the cardiologist who initially manages the patient, builds a personal rapport with the patient, but may also have a direct involvement in the PCI procedure, or the surgeon who has limited background information of the clinical situation and has a vested interest in increasing his or her patient base.

Quite appropriately, the patient should have a final say, although his or her judgment can be confounded depending on the information imparted. In most centers this is limited to informing the patient that he or she needs surgery, preceded by a scary discussion on their higher risk on medical therapy. Very few patients tend to be told about PCI alternatives. Conversely, in active interventional centers, PCI and surgery can be offered as equally valid alternatives so that most patients would instinctly avoid surgical revascularization based on the fear of pain, prolonged disability, and an immediate risk but without full understanding of the limited long-term data available for DESs in ULM disease.

Discussing individual patients in a multidisciplinary team forum appears to be an ideal and impartial solution. These tend to involve surgeons and anesthetists, as well as cardiologists. After discussing the merits of an intervention, a consensus is achieved and a full written report is then generated and presented to the patient, who should have the right to discuss with the various consultants involved and have the final say. This open discussion should refrain from partisan interpretation of trial results and adamant claims that left main coronary artery stenosis is always a surgical disease, accusing the cardiologists applying PCI in this condition (<20% in the USA, >30% in Europe) of being irresponsible. The patients should be made aware that the consensus decision of treatment is not binding and his or her final decision will always be respected and best medical care will always be administered.

Diagnosis

Pivotal to the optimum management of left main disease is making the correct diagnosis. Although coronary angiography is accepted as the gold standard for evaluation of coronary artery disease, visual angiographic assessment of the severity of disease of the left main coronary artery is prone to error [11]. This is especially true for eccentric lesions of intermediate severity involving the ostium or the bifurcation of the left main. It is not uncommon to see patients who have received multiple grafts, often all occluded, with 20–30% left main stenosis because of errors from inexperienced angiographers who panic because of pressure damping on the first left coronary injection, leading to grossly inadequate and misleading angiograms.

Two diagnostic techniques complementary to angiography and too seldom used are intracoronary measurement of myocardial fractional flow reserve (FFR) and intravascular ultrasound (IVUS). An FFR value below 0.75 reliably identifies a stenosis associated with inducible ischemia [12]. A gray zone exists with FFR values between 0.75 and 0.80, but there is unequivocal evidence that left main lesions with FFR > 0.80 should be not treated but carefully monitored. A minimal lumen area (MLA) on IVUS of < 6.0 mm² is commonly used as the criterion to determine the significance of the lesion and is well correlated with a functional measurement of lesion severity (FFR < 0.75) [13]. The role of IVUS and its indications is possibly less established for want of expertise in image interpretation and accurate, reproducible measurements. IVUS allows accurate assessment of the reference vessel size, extent of atheroma burden, and composition of the lesion along with its length up to the distal bifurcation, and provides valuable information to guide and optimize the ULM angioplasty. Although believed to overdiagnose a severe lesion, less than half of intermediate left main lesions are found to be significant with IVUS [14].

Percutaneous intervention

Technique

Techniques differ according to the severity, characteristics, and especially position of the left main lesion. Lesions at the

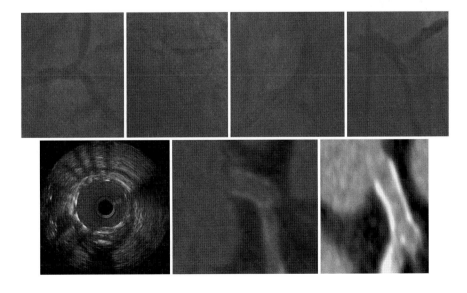

Figure 37.1 This 73-year-old patient had a 3.5 × 26-mm Taxus stent deployed from the left main artery to the LAD, followed by post dilation to 4 mm and kissing balloons (3.5 mm to LAD and 3.5 mm to LCx) with a good result confirmed on intravascular ultrasound from the LAD to the left main. The stent was confirmed patent at 6 months on a 64-multislice computerized tomography scan with specks of calcium seen in the proximal LCx.

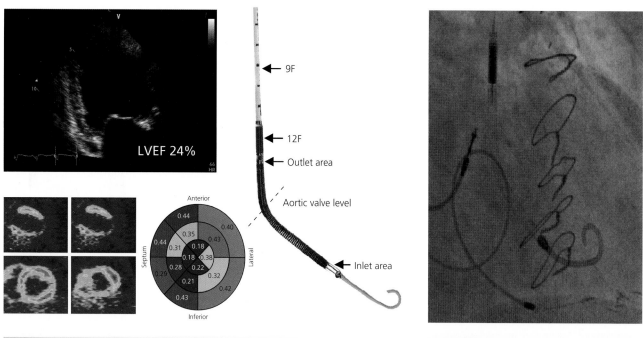

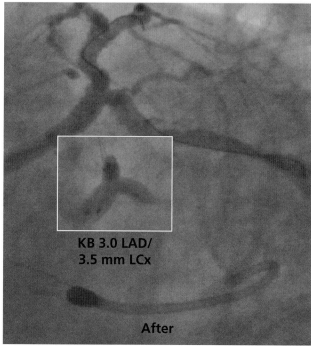

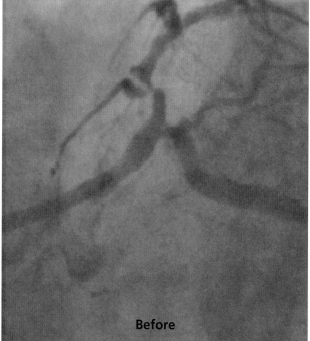

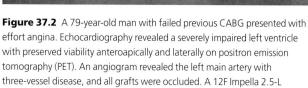

Figure 37.2 A 79-year-old man with failed previous CABG presented with effort angina. Echocardiography revealed a severely impaired left ventricle with preserved viability anteroapically and laterally on positron emission tomography (PET). An angiogram revealed the left main artery with three-vessel disease, and all grafts were occluded. A 12F Impella 2.5-L catheter was inserted as a left ventricular unloading device via the femoral artery. Angiographic appearance before and after the Endeavor Resolute 4.0 × 24-mm stent, from the left main artery into the LCx post expansion to 4.5 mm, finished with kissing balloons (KB) to LAD and LCx. An additional Endeavour Resolute stent was deployed to the LAD.

ostium or body without involvement of the bifurcation are treated with a single stent. Distal left main bifurcation disease is treated based on the lesion characteristics and the operator's preference and experience using either crossover stenting or various techniques of T-stenting, V-stenting, or crush stenting, and is usually completed with kissing balloon inflations (Figs. 37.1 and 37.2). Standard antiplatelet therapy including bivalirudin or unfractionated heparin monitored by activated clotting time is essential. There is no evidence suggesting greater risk of stent thrombosis for ULM treatment

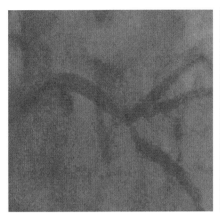
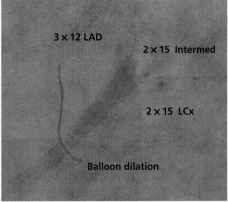
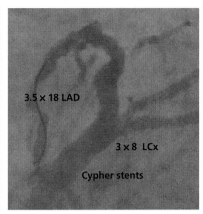

Figure 37.3 A 68-year-old man presenting with stable angina had a distal left main disease extending into the proximal LAD and proximal LCx but sparing the intermediate artery (Intermed). After a trissing balloon (Maverick) predilation, Cypher stents were deployed in the left main artery to the LAD and the left main artery to the LCx. This was then completed with trissing balloons (Maverick) post dilation with 2.5 × 15 mm to the LCx, 2.5 × 15 mm to intermediate artery and 3.5 × 20 mm to LAD. An excellent angiographic result was confirmed on IVUS.

or reporting advantages after prolonged and dual antiplatelet therapy for left main disease. Still, most interventionists will recommend "lifelong" therapy to prevent late thrombosis. Again, evidence for this strategy is flimsy and superstitious, but in part justified by the low incidence of adverse bleeding events observed in patients tolerating 1 year of dual antiplatelet therapy [15].

During stenting, IVUS provides important information regarding the extent, composition, and distribution of plaque, arterial remodeling, vascular responses at the edges, and stent apposition. Minimum stent area (MSA), another IVUS-derived lumen dimension after stent deployment, is a consistent predictor of in-stent restenosis [16] and has been used to predict long-term stent patency [17].

Atherectomy catheters were developed to clear atherosclerotic plaque by grinding, aspirating, or cutting. Atherectomy may be performed instead of or in addition to other procedures and has been suggested to improve both the immediate and long-term success of balloon angioplasty and stenting. There have been a series of studies in which patients with ULM lesions were subjected to either rotational atherectomy or directional coronary atherectomy (DCA). However, lack of conclusive evidence from controlled studies has led to the withdrawal of the DCA catheter (Flextome®, Boston Scientific, Natick, MA, USA) used more commonly in the coronaries. The rotablator certainly has a role for calcific, undilatable lesions, especially those positioned at the left main ostium. A recent Japanese study on debulking of chronic coronary total occlusions with rotational or directional atherectomy before stenting (DOCTORS study) showed that although present plaque debulking (138 patients) versus nondebulking (128 patients) tends to have a higher 30-day major adverse cardiac event (MACE) rate (15.9% vs. 8.5%, P = 0.07) owing to higher periprocedural infarcts, it is associated with a favorable mid-term outcome with lower target vessel revascularization (TVR) and 1-year MACE rate (27.5% vs. 39.8%; P = 0.033) [18]. These

outcomes, however, belong to the pre-DES era, and few centers still use DCA before DESs. Anecdotal reports of persistent pseudoaneurysms after DCA and DESs have not helped the cause in favor of DCA. Other operators, avoid the complexity of rotational atherectomy and use cutting balloons or simple high-pressure balloons (Quantum™, Maverick®, Boston Scientific, Natick, MA, USA; Schweiger, Winterthur, Switzerland) that can reach pressures of ≥ 30 atm.

Intra-aortic balloon pump (IABP) support is recommended in patients with impaired left ventricular systolic function or anticipated complexity of ULM lesion treatment. Recently, active percutaneous left ventricle assist devices have been introduced (TandemHeart, Cardiac Assist Inc., Pittsburgh, PA, USA; Impella, ABIOMED Inc., Danvers, MA, USA) that are more effective than an IABP. The potential for life-saving grace in few procedures leading to transient occlusion of the left main must be balanced against their definitive higher risk of bleeding complications. The TandemHeart, requires a trans-septal insertion of a large cannula in addition to a very large arterial cannula. The Impella is able to deliver blood flow at 2.5 L/min or 4.5 L/min. The 14F, 2.5-L Impella has received significant interest as a life-saving device in cardiogenic shock, and use during high-risk angioplasty is increasing (Fig. 37.3).

Bare metal stents

Over the years, many registries have assessed the feasibility and safety of BMSs in revascularizing the ULM [9,19], particularly in good surgical candidates with a low EuroScore. However, in-stent restenosis remained a major problem, limiting long-term outcomes and freedom from MACE and mortality [20,21]. In the Unprotected Left Main Trunk Investigation Multicenter Assessment (ULTIMA) registry study, low-risk patients (age < 65 years, left ventricular ejection fraction > 30%, and absence of cardiogenic shock from AMI) had 1-year mortality of 3.4% [9]. Similarly, Takagi *et al.* [20] reported a 3-year cardiac mortality of 4.2%, and Park *et al.*

Table 37.1 Clinical and procedural characteristics and outcome of DES implantation for left main stenosis in eight registries/randomized studies.

Author/country	Park et al. [68]/ Korea	Chieffo et al. [24]/ Italy	Valgimigli et al. [67]/ Netherlands	Lee et al. [25]/ USA	Price et al. [26]/ USA	Erglis et al. [22]/ Australia	Buszman et al. [28]/ Poland	Meliga et al. [29]/ EU and USA
No. of patients	102	85	95	50	50	53	18	358
Inclusion criteria	Suitable for stent placement	Suitable anatomy, high risk for CABG	Discussed with surgeons (consecutive)	High risk for CABG	High risk for CABG	Suitable for CABG or stent	Suitable for CABG or stent	Suitable for stent placement (consecutive)
Exclusion criteria	LVEF ≤40, AMI	AMI		—	—	—	AMI, EuroScore >8	
Age (years)	60.3	63.2	64	72	69	61	60	66
Diabetes mellitus (%)	28	21	30	36	26	6	19	30
Ejection fraction (%)	60.4	51.1	41	51	<40 in 24%	56	53	49
Stable/unstable angina/primary PCI (%)	40/50/10	69/31/0	48/33/20 (Shock;12)	34/46/20	66/33/1	43/10/0	36/52/0	44/42/–
Unprotected (%)	100	100	84	100	100	98	100	100
Distal location (%)	71	81	65	60	94	43	56	74
EuroScore >6 and/or Parsonnet >15	No data	45%	Parsonnet 19 on average	64%	58%	No data	No data	20%
SES/Cypher stent (%)	100	48	55	84	100	0	No data	55
PES/Taxus stent (%)	0	52	45	16	0	100	No data	45
Single stent (%)	60	40	73	20	16	98	—	57
Kissing stent/ V stenting (%)	24	14	2.1	10	68	19	—	8
T-stenting (%)	1.4	4.7	11	4	0	2	—	4
Crush stenting (%)	15	35	3.1	24	16	—	0	27
Culotte stenting (%)	0	5.9	9.4	2	0	—	4	4
Angiographic success (%)	100	100	99	98	100		98	100
Overall angiographic restenosis (%)	7	19	No data	No data	44*	6	5.5	No data
Long-term follow-up (months)	12	6	16	6	9	6	24	36
Cardiac death (%)	0	3.5	10.5	4	10	2	5.7	9
Myocardial infarction (Q and non-Q) (%)	0	1	4	No data	2	9	—	9
TLR (%)	2	14.1	6 (all in bifurcation)	10	38 (ischemia driven 18%)	2	9.6	6
MACE-free survival (%)	98	75.3	76	89	56	87	71	74

*23% in the left main artery to LAD and 35% in the LCx location.

AMI, acute myocardial infarction; CABG, coronary artery bypass graft; LAD, left anterior descending artery; LCx, left circumflex artery; LM, left main; LVEF, left ventricular ejection fraction; MACE, major adverse cardiac event; PCI, percutaneous coronary intervention; PES, paclitaxel-eluting stent; SES, sirolimus-eluting stent; TLR, target lesion revascularization.

[21] reported a 20-month total mortality of 3.1% in low-risk patients. By contrast, the cumulative 1-year mortality for the high-risk group was >20% in first two studies.

For a select proportion of elective patients, PCI may be an alternative to a CABG and may also be appropriate for highly symptomatic inoperable patients. In a single-center randomized study of 103 patients with ULM stenosis, implantation of paclitaxel eluting stents (*n* = 53) was found to be superior to BMSs (*n* = 50) in the large-diameter left main vessel at 6 months [22]. Breakdown analysis showed binary restenosis in 11 (22%) patients with BMSs and in three (6%) patients with PESs (*P* = 0.021). With IVUS, neointimal volume obstruction at 6 months was reduced from 25.2% ± 22.0% with BMSs to 16.6% ± 17.2% with PESs (*P* = 0.02). At 6 months, MACE-free survival rate was 70% in patients with BMSs and 87% in patients with PESs (*P* = 0.036).

Drug-eluting stents

A number of registries and nonrandomized studies (summarized in Table 37.1) have confirmed safety and effectiveness of DESs for ULM. Some of the early registries of DESs for ULM dealt with a rather select group of patients considered at low operative risk (e.g., left ventricular ejection fraction >40%) who would also be expected to have good short- and long-term outcomes from CABG. Results showed left main ostial and body lesions to have excellent prognosis with DESs, whereas results were more questionable for PCI to left main distal lesions if two stents were required.

Valgimigli *et al.* [23] compared the sirolimus-eluting stent (SES) with the paclitaxel-eluting stent (PES) in an analysis from the Rapamycin-Eluting and Taxus Stent Evaluated At Rotterdam Cardiology Hospital (RESEARCH and T-SEARCH) registry studies of 110 patients treated for ULM. The cumulative incidence of MACE was similar in both groups: 25% in the SES group versus 29% in the PES group (hazard ratio 0.88; 95% CI 0.43–1.82; *P* = 0.74). Angiographic in-stent late loss (mm), evaluated in 73% of the SES group and in 77% of the PES group, was 0.32 ± 74 in the main and 0.36 ± 0.59 in the side branch in the SES group versus 0.46 ± 0.57 (*P* = 0.36) and 0.52 ± 0.42 (*P* = 0.41) in the PES group, respectively, with the authors concluding that the PES may perform closely to the SES both in terms of angiographic and long-term clinical outcome.

Chieffo *et al.* [24] studied 85 patients with ULM stenosis, including patients in whom CABG was contraindicated, and electively implanted a SES or a PES. The DES group was also compared with a historical group of consecutive patients treated with BMSs. High mortality risk scores (EuroScore >6) were present in 45% of the patient population. The 6-month cardiac mortality rate and MACE-free survival were 3.5% and 75%, respectively. Further, despite the higher-risk patients and lesion profiles in the DES group, the incidence of MACE at a 6-month clinical follow-up was lower in the DES than in the BMS group (20.0% vs. 35.9%, respectively; *P* = 0.039).

Moreover, cardiac deaths occurred in 3 (3.5%) patients in the DES group, compared with 6 (9.3%) in the BMS group (*P* = 0.17).

Lee *et al.* [25] studied 50 patients with DES-treated ULM disease and 123 with CABG-treated left main artery disease. High-risk patients (Parsonnet score >15) constituted 46% of the CABG group and 64% of the DES group (*P* = 0.04). The 30-day major adverse cardiac and cerebrovascular events (MACCE) rate for CABG and the DES was 17% and 2% (*P* < 0.01), respectively. The mean follow-up was 6.7 ± 6.2 months in the CABG group and 5.6 ± 3.9 months in the DES group (*P* = 0.26). The estimated MACCE-free survival at 6 months and 1 year, respectively, was 83% and 75% in the CABG group versus 89% and 83% in the DES group (*P* = 0.20). The Parsonnet score, diabetes, and CABG were independent predictors of MACCE, and despite a higher percentage of high-risk patients, PCI with a DES for ULM disease was not associated with an increase in immediate or medium-term complications compared with CABG.

Price *et al.* [26] studied clinical and angiographic outcomes of 50 patients undergoing SES implantation for ULM disease. The lesions were predominantly distal bifurcation (94%) treated with a double-stent technique. Over a mean follow-up of 276 ± 57 days, TLR occurred in 19 (38%) patients. Angiographic follow-up at 3 and 6 months revealed restenosis of 23% in the left main artery to the left anterior descending artery (LAD) and 35% in the left circumflex artery (LCx), with an overall restenosis rate of 42% in any vessel. The authors concluded that restenosis is a frequent finding when serial angiographic follow-up is performed after SES implantation for distal ULM lesions and is usually focal, often involving the ostial LCx and often asymptomatic. Although alarming, this study confirms the need for meticulous surveillance of patients receiving a DES for ULM, even if they remain asymptomatic.

The impact of preprocedural cardiogenic shock was evaluated in one of our own series, in 20 consecutive symptomatic patients with >50% angiographic stenosis of the ULM who underwent PCI with a DES [27]. Five of these patients had presence of cardiogenic shock and sixteen had absence of preprocedural cardiogenic shock. Sixteen (80%) of 20 patients were at high risk for CABG because of comorbidity, advanced age, or cardiogenic shock. Three of five patients in cardiogenic shock (60%) died in hospital and the two surviving patients experienced no MACE at follow-up (median 14 months). In the absence of cardiogenic shock, there was no in-hospital MACE, but one patient died suddenly 8 weeks post procedure (cumulative MACE of 7% [1/15]). The study demonstrated the feasibility of ULM treatment with a DES with acceptable medium-term outcomes and could be considered in those who are at high risk.

In another study comparing the DES or CABG by Buszman *et al.* [28], 105 patients with ULM disease were randomized to PCI (*n* = 52) or CABG (*n* = 53). PCI was associated with a lower 30-day risk of major adverse events (*P* < 0.006) and

MACCE ($P = 0.03$), with shorter hospitalizations ($P = 0.0007$). At 1 year, left ventricular ejection fraction had improved significantly only in the PCI group (3.3% ± 6.7% after PCI vs. 0.5% ± 0.8% after CABG; $P = 0.047$). After >2 years, MACE-free survival was similar in both groups, with a trend toward improved survival after PCI [28]. Further, more recent data by Meliga et al. [29] on long-term outcomes (3 years) after DES implantation in over 350 consecutive patients analyzed retrospectively across Europe and the USA in the DELFT (DES for Left Main Artery) registry appeared favorable. Stent thrombosis occurred in two patients, MACE-free survival was 74%, cardiac death 9%, and TLR 6%.

Seung et al. reported a 3 year follow-up of 1536 patients in the Korean MAIN-COMPARE registry (Unprotected Left Main Coronary Artery Stenosis: Comparison of Percutaneous Coronary Angioplasty versus Surgical Revascularization) in the wave II study with either DES ($n = 784$) or CABG ($n = 690$) [30]. In 396 propensity matched pairs, there was no significant difference of death (hazard ratio, 1.36; 95% CI 0.80–2.30) or of the composite outcome of death, Q-wave MI and stroke (hazard ratio 1.40; 95% CI 0.88–2.22). The rates of target-vessel revascularization were significantly higher in the DES group (hazard ratio 5.96; 95% CI 2.80–8.11).

Serruys et al., in the Synergy between PTI with Taxus and Cardiac Surgery (SYNTAX) study, randomized 1500 consecutive patients with de novo triple vessel disease or LM disease, equally to either PCI or CABG in assessing the optimal revascularization strategy [31]. At 12 months, the rates of death and myocardial infarction were similar between the two groups and stroke was significantly more likely to occur with CABG (2.2%, vs. 0.6% with PCI; $P = 0.003$). However, MACCE including all causes of death, documented fatal MI, cerebral stroke, and revascularization rates at 12 months were significantly higher in the PCI group (17.8% vs. 12.4% for CABG; $P = 0.002$), largely due to an increased rate of repeat revascularization (13.5% vs. 5.9%, $P < 0.001$); as a result, the criterion for non-inferiority was not met and led the authors to conclude that CABG remains the standard of care for patients with three-vessel or left main coronary artery disease.

Patient follow-up

The role of multislice computed tomography (MSCT) as a noninvasive modality to assess stents is particularly appealing if the in-stent luminal diameter is greater than 3 mm, but this technique is still an experimental alternative in this phase (Fig. 37.1). Most operators still prefer conventional angiography, but the serial assessments at 4 and/or 9–12 months used at the time of BMSs are now rarely used with DESs; a single control angiogram at 6–9 months is the most frequently applied method. Thereafter, follow-up should be either office or telephone based, as per the clinical situation, and at the operator's discretion.

Future trends

Although the increasing use of DESs in ULM has produced encouraging short- and mid-term results, long-term outcomes are still lacking. Randomized multicenter trials are required to settle the argument of whether PCI with a DES is equivalent or superior to CABG in the longer term for patients with de novo ULM. Until their results are available, cardiologists must make individual decisions based on clinical presentation, lesion morphology, anatomy, and the overall operative risk, with frank discussions with the surgeon and patient. PCI with a DES can offer a less invasive procedure and completed with a lower risk in select patients, particularly those not ideal for CABG owing to comorbidities, advanced age, acute myocardial infarction, or cardiogenic shock. These indications may soon be extended in good surgical candidates if there is favorable anatomy for PCI.

Coronary bifurcation lesions

Coronary bifurcation disease accounts for up to 15% of all current PCIs [32]. The greater frequency of stenotic disease at these sites occurs predominantly secondary to a combination of blood flow turbulence and shear stress. Until the mid-1990s, bifurcation lesions were considered relatively contraindicated for PCI and the recommended treatment was surgery. With technologic advances in the mid-1990s, coronary stenting of the main vessel with provisional stenting of the side branch has been the technique of choice for treating most bifurcation lesions. Attempts with various techniques of bifurcation stenting have historically been less successful. The increasing use of the DES has seen improved angiographic and clinical outcomes of both provisional and double-stenting techniques compared with previous outcomes using BMSs, although the high prevalence of restenosis at the side branch ostium and late thrombosis remain an issue.

Classification

Two important determinants in the classification of a bifurcation lesion are lesion location and the angulation between the main vessel and the side branch.

Angulation of vessels

The angle of the side branch to the main vessel has implications for intervention [33]. A Y-angulation (<70°) allows easy wire access to the side branch, but plaque shifting is potentially more pronounced, and precise stent placement with complete ostial coverage is often difficult or geometrically impossible. The converse is generally true in T-shaped lesions for which, less often, the angle between the main vessel and side branch is >70°; wire access to the side branch is usually more difficult but there is less chance of ostial occlusion after main vessel stenting. The use of crush stenting, as described below, is contraindicated in such lesions because of risk of

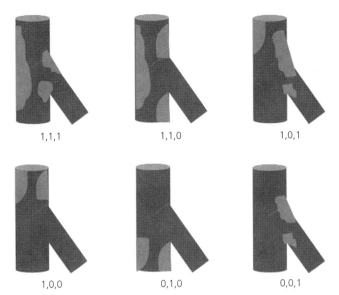

1,1,1   1,1,0   1,0,1

1,0,0   0,1,0   0,0,1

Figure 37.4 Medina classification of coronary bifurcation lesions according to the presence of plaque in the proximal main vessel, distal main vessel, and side branch. A 1 or 0 indicates the presence or absence, respectively, of a lesion at the segment.

stent distortion, irreversibly causing poor apposition [34] and poor long-term clinical outcomes [35].

Lesion location

After multiple and complex classifications (Duke, Lefevre, Syntax) failed to become established, the Medina classification (Fig. 37.4) quickly gained recognition and endorsement from the European Bifurcation Club. This classification is based on the angiographic presence of > 50% stenosis in the three segments constituting the bifurcation. A score of 1 indicates the presence and of 0 indicates the absence of stenosis ≥ 50% for each segment after the other in sequence, i.e., the proximal main vessel, distal main vessel, and side branch. Any combination of main vessel and side branch with ≥ 50% disease identifies a "true" bifurcation lesion. Furthermore, plaque at the side branch ostium with stenosis ≥ 50% is more likely to result in side branch deterioration after main vessel intervention and should be considered for a double-stenting technique if the side branch is large enough or the ostial stenosis is long and severe. Angiographically, when a lesion with > 50% stenosis is present in any segment of a bifurcation, techniques such as IVUS invariably show the presence of plaque in the remaining segments.

Plaque shift

Anatomical studies show that the carina is most often disease free in bifurcation lesions. After predilation and/or stent deployment in the main vessel, compromise of the side branch ostium is most often due to displacement of the carina to the side branch ostium rather than to true plaque shift (Fig. 37.5). Hence, single stenting and kissing balloon dilation is often effective and sufficient. Side branch occlusion, which is said to occur in 4.5–26% of cases, is more frequent in those with a smaller side branch vessel diameter (< 1.4 mm) and in patients presenting with acute coronary syndromes [36]. Occlusion of the side branch can lead to chest pain of varying severity together with a rise in cardiac enzymes, which in itself can have a negative impact on long-term outcome. Despite the immediate side branch occlusion, more than three-quarters of these will have restoration of patency at angiographic follow-up [36].

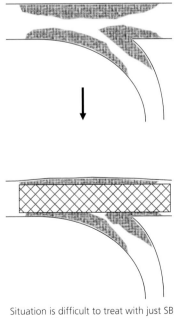

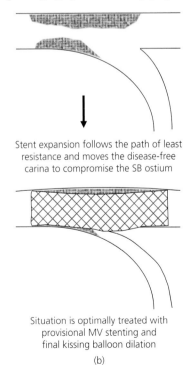

Stent expansion follows the path of least resistance and moves the disease-free carina to compromise the SB ostium

Situation is difficult to treat with just SB balloon dilation; conceptually a stent is required to prevent recoil

(a)

Situation is optimally treated with provisional MV stenting and final kissing balloon dilation

(b)

Figure 37.5 Representation of plaque "shift." MV, main vessel; SB, side branch.

Percutaneous intervention

Bare metal stents

The prognosis after PCI is worse in the case of bifurcation lesions than with nonbifurcation lesions. This has been consistently reported in numerous studies, including the 1000 patients of the National Heart, Lung, and Blood Institute (NHLBI) Registry [37], in which the event-free survival at 12 months among patients treated with BMSs for bifurcation lesions was 67.9% versus 74.3% in those with nonbifurcation lesions ($P < 0.05$). Clinical and angiographic outcomes using BMSs are additionally hampered when a second stent is required in the side branch, with significantly higher rates of restenosis compared with single-stent strategies [37]. The safety of a simple stenting strategy, described next, was confirmed in the French provisional T-stenting for coronary bifurcation lesion prospective evaluation (TULIPE) multicenter study of tubular stents and was associated with a low TLR rate of 16% at 7 months, despite use of a BMS [38].

Drug-eluting stents—strategies and techniques

The DES has had a significant impact on angiographic and clinical outcomes. The use of the DES has led to reduced rates of restenoses, especially in the main vessel, with less need for repeat interventions. Ostial side branch stenoses continue to be problematic, and restenosis rate is higher than with the DES used for different indications. Two strategies are followed in bifurcation PCI depending on the size of the side branch and length and severity of ostial side branch disease—simple and complex stenting.

Simple stenting strategy—one stent

Simple stenting is also referred to as provisional stenting, one-stent technique, or cross-over technique; it is used in situations in which the side branch is small (<2 mm) and/or has limited or no disease at the ostium. Stenting of the side branch is not elected to be the initial strategy of choice and is undertaken only if there is persistent side branch deterioration after balloon predilation or stent implantation resulting in severe residual lesion or dissection with less than TIMI grade 3 flow, electrocardiographic changes, or persistent intraprocedural angina. If deterioration of the ostium or side branch stenosis occurs and the operator chooses to treat the side branch, then this may be accomplished by some techniques of complex stenting described next (T-stenting, Culotte, etc.). All such procedures, however, depend on being able to successfully recross the side branch through the stent struts in the main vessel. Maintaining a wire in the side branch during implantation of the main vessel stent provides more than a visual indication of the target to rewire; it straightens the angle between the main vessel and side branch, holds dissections/flaps (maintaining flow), and facilitates progression of the second wire. However, if after predilation of the main vessel or side branch a severe stenosis or dissection develops, the order of stent insertion can be reversed with the side branch stent implanted first.

Complex stenting strategy—two or more stents

To ensure complete lesion coverage, especially at the side branch ostium, the stenting strategy has evolved. Most operators cross through the stent struts and deploy a second balloon if ≥50–60% side branch stenosis is present. Others limit treatment to side branch as a salvage if TIMI 1 or TIMI 0 flow occurs. The usefulness of universal kissing balloon dilation is under evaluation in a prospective randomized trial NORDIC Bifurcation Study. However, it is generally accepted that kissing balloons should be used when a severe stenosis or slow flow develops after main vessel stenting. A larger sized side branch (>2 mm) with a sufficient territory of distribution justifies stenting the side branch when a poor result is expected, with a single stent on the main vessel and presence of long lesions in the side branch. Stenting the side branch because of its superior acute angiographic result and the intuitive belief that it will yield a better long-term symptomatic and/or prognostic outcome is not acceptable; there is no advantage for restenosis and clinical end points with the universal use of two stents for bifurcation lesions [39,40]. In a multivessel stenting trial without angiographic follow-up, the presence of bifurcations did not affect 1-year outcome after SES implantation, and the outcomes in true versus partial bifurcations and using one versus two stents were similar when the treatment strategies were left to the operator's discretion [41]. Furthermore, the NORDIC bifurcation study, using a SES in 413 patients, compared a simple stenting strategy (stenting main vessel and optional side branch) with a complex strategy (both main vessel and side branch stenting). The single-stent strategy appeared effective in most cases (crossover <20%) [42], with a low incidence of TLR of main vessel and side branch in both groups. The two-stent strategy prolonged procedure and fluoroscopy times and increased the rate of procedure-related biomarker elevation. In a multicenter prospective, randomised study in 500 patients presented at TCT 2008, the British Bifurcation Coronary study: Old, New and Evolving strategies (BBC ONE) comparison of simple, provisional T-stenting using Taxus DES versus complex DES for bifurcation lesions using crush or culotte techniques, is associated with a lower rate of death, MI, and target-vessel failure one year, driven largely by increased procedural MI in the latter group (unpublished data).

A jailed wire in the side branch is strongly recommended in complex lesions, and kissing balloons are used routinely in complex bifurcations, especially in a double-stenting technique [43].

A number of two-stent and even three-stent techniques are currently in use. These include T-stenting and its variations—TAP stenting (T-stenting and small protrusion), crush stenting, modified, classical or reverse T-stenting, the Culotte, simultaneous kissing stenting (V-stent), and Y-stents. The main,

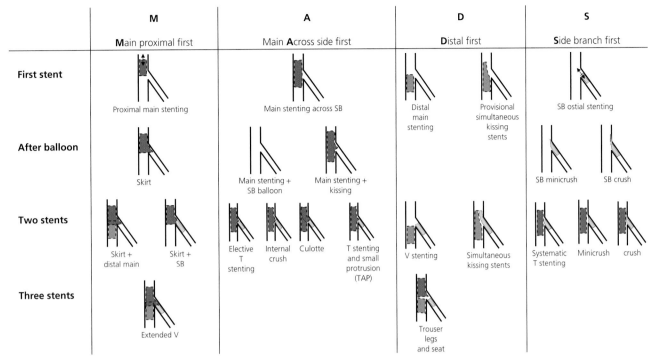

Figure 37.6 MADS classification of bifurcation treatment. Adapted from the European Bifurcation Club [44]. SB, side branch.

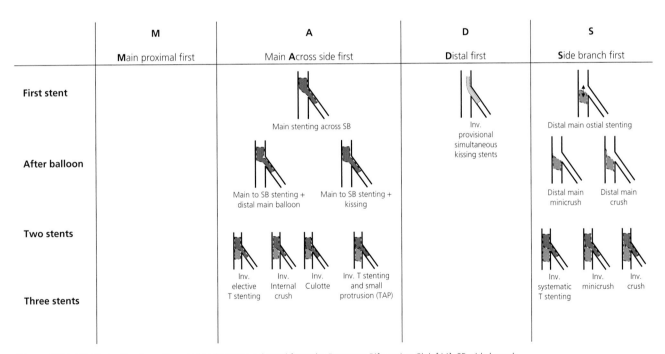

Figure 37.7 MADS classification of inverted techniques. Adapted from the European Bifurcation Club [44]. SB, side branch.

across, distal, side (MADS) classification of bifurcation treatment (Figs. 37.6 and 37.7) reports all the possible variants according to the order that the first stent is placed—in the main vessel proximal to the side branch (M), in main vessel across the side branch (A), in the main vessel distal to the side branch (D) or in the side branch (S).

T-stenting

The *systematic T-stenting* technique begins with positioning a stent at the ostium of the side branch first, being careful to avoid excessive stent protrusion into the main vessel and to cover the ostium of the side branch. Some operators leave a balloon in the main vessel to further help delineate the main vessel and avoid protrusion of the side branch stent into the main vessel. After deployment of the stent and removal of the balloon and wire from the side branch, a second stent is deployed in the main vessel. A wire is then readvanced into the side branch and final kissing balloon inflation is performed.

Modified T-stenting is a variation performed by simultaneously positioning stents in the side branch and the main vessel [45,46]. The side branch stent is deployed first and, after wire and balloon removal from the side branch, the main vessel stent is deployed.

A *provisional* or reverse *T-stenting* technique is used when there is no initial commitment to implant a second stent in the side branch, and this is done because the side branch deteriorates after stent deployment in the main vessel. This requires recrossing the side branch through the main vessel stent struts, followed by ballooning and stenting of the side branch. Final kissing balloon inflations are recommended. This technique popularized by the group at Massy (Lefevre, Louvard), is probably the most widely applied method to treat bifurcational lesion and is generally considered a gold standard against which new methods should be compared.

A novel modification of the provisional T-stenting technique is *TAP stenting*, in which, after stenting of the main vessel, the side branch stent is intentionally made to protrude minimally into the main vessel [47]. Final kissing balloon inflation is performed, using the balloon kept deflated in the main vessel before the side branch is stented to ensure ostial coverage and facilitate final kissing balloon inflation.

T-stenting is simple, technically less demanding, and can be accomplished via a 6F sheath. However, most bifurcations have a vessel angulation of <70° (far from the ideal 90°), so this technique will lead to incomplete stent coverage and geographic miss at the ostium of the side branch, and hence forfeiture of the expected DES advantages of lower restenosis and TLR.

Crush stenting

The *crush technique*, popularized by Colombo *et al.* [46], ensures complete lesion coverage at the side branch ostium. Using a 7F or 8F guiding catheter, two stents are placed in the main vessel and the side branch, with the former placed more proximally than the latter. As in the modified T-stenting technique, the side branch stent is positioned and deployed first; however, rather than placing the side branch stent at the ostium, the proximal stent marker is placed a few millimeters (3–5 mm) proximal to the bifurcation within the main vessel or, in the modified "minicrush" technique, 1–2 mm proximal to the bifurcation [48].

The stent of the side branch is deployed, and its balloon and wire are removed. The stent subsequently deployed in the main vessel flattens the protruding cells of the side branch stent. Wire recrossing and dilation of the side branch, followed by final kissing balloon inflation, is recommended to obtain better strut contact against the ostium of the side branch, optimizing drug delivery. Final kissing balloon dilation after crush stenting with the DES is associated with more favorable long-term outcomes, reducing side branch restenosis and the need for TLR [49].

The main advantage of the crush is that the immediate patency of both branches is assured. In addition, this technique should provide excellent coverage of the ostium of the side branch. However, the mandatory final kissing balloon inflations make the procedure more laborious because of the need to recross multiple stent struts with a wire and a balloon. Furthermore, the crush technique may be associated with an increased rate of stent thrombosis [50] and a high bifurcation angle (>50°), with no final kissing balloon inflation and severe renal dysfunction being an independent predictor of MACE [35]. However, the recent CACTUS (Coronary bifurcations: Application of the Crushing Technique Using SES) study prospectively evaluated the provisional side branch T-stenting technique versus the crush technique at 6 months and obtained similar results on clinical and angiographic end points with the two techniques, thus the patient is not disadvantaged if two stents are intended to be used from the outset [51].

Culotte stenting

The culotte or trouser technique, introduced by Chevalier *et al.* [52], is a two-stent strategy to ensure complete lesion coverage for bifurcation lesions. Using a 6F guiding catheter, both branches are wired and predilated. First, a stent is deployed across the smaller, more angulated branch, usually the side branch. Next, the nonstented branch is rewired through the struts of the stent and dilated. A second stent is then advanced and expanded in the nonstented branch, usually the main vessel. Finally, kissing balloon inflation is performed. This technique is suitable for all angles of bifurcations and provides near-perfect coverage of the side branch ostium. Although it leads to a high concentration of metal with a double-stent layer at the carina and in the proximal part of the bifurcation, which can be thrombogenic, our own experience using a DES has shown a better angiographic result at the level of the side branch compared with the T-stenting and is associated with a lower TLR rate (9% in the culotte group vs. 27% in the T-stenting group) at 9 months' follow-up [53].

Simultaneous kissing stents and V-stenting

The technique is used when the proximal segment of the main vessel has a reference diameter large enough to accommodate two stents side by side proximal to the bifurcation. It works best if there are two side branch lesions which are just ostial. The branches below the bifurcation are typically of similar diameter. A minimum 7F guiding catheter is required to position both stents side by side creating a "double barrel" configuration and deployed simultaneously minimizing

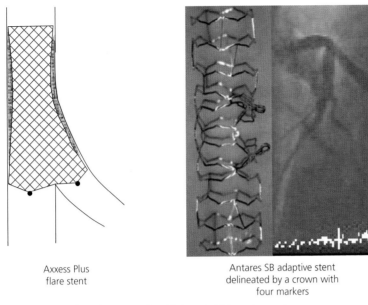

Axxess Plus
flare stent

Antares SB adaptive stent
delineated by a crown with
four markers

Tryton stent. Two markers
delineate a 4-mm zone
between the SB and MV

Figure 37.8 Dedicated bifurcation stents. SB = side branch, MV = main vessel.

plaque shift. Sharma *et al.* [54] reported on 200 consecutive patients (202 lesions) who underwent the simultaneous kissing stent (SKS) technique for true bifurcation lesions in large-caliber vessels using SES. In-hospital and 30-day MACE were 3% and 5%, respectively. At mean follow-up of 9 ± 2 months, the incidence of TLR was 4% in the entire group. Again, in 30 patients who underwent SKS with SES, overall angiographic restenosis at 24 months occurred in 13% at the main vessel and 10% at the side branch. At follow-up angiography, a membranous diaphragm at the carina was identified in 14 patients (47%), but only one of whom was associated with angiographic restenosis [55].

In the V-stenting technique the proximal parts of the stents are positioned to be just abutting each other, thereby creating the classical "V" configuration. The main vessel proximal to the bifurcation must be free of disease to utilize this technique. Both techniques have limited applicability because of the need for relatively narrow bifurcation angles and the use of large size guiding catheters.

Y-stenting

This technique was developed to allow complete lesion coverage but is limited by its procedural complexity and the need to use three stents. Stents are deployed in each of the branch vessels, with a third stent paced in the main vessel proximal to the bifurcation. A registry of 77 patients undergoing Y-stenting demonstrated a 6-month follow-up restenosis rate of 36% and TLR rate of 30%.

Dedicated bifurcation stents

These are dedicated devices aimed at reducing restenosis and thrombosis associated with stents used in bifurcation PCI and

designed to either fit the carina or have a side port or a side branch (Fig. 37.8). They are used primarily to scaffold the ostium of the side branch, thus stabilizing plaque and maintaining access to the side branch.

The AXXESS Plus is a novel self-expanding, flare-shaped, drug-eluting biolimus stent that fits the carina. In a nonrandomized, single-arm, 6-month IVUS analysis in 49 patients, effective lesion coverage with significant neointimal suppression was demonstrated [56]. Furthermore, disease distal to the stent in the main vessel or side branch often requires stenting with a final "Y" technique used for true bifurcation lesions.

Our center is currently enrolling patients into the prospective, single-arm TriReme Antares Sidebranch Adaptive System (Antares SAS) study. This is a BMS, with its crown tailored to match ostial geometry for side-branch access and provisional stenting (Fig. 37.8). The system tracks nicely over a single wire and has a side branch access stabilizing wire with a single balloon and a four radiopaque marker mapping system with alignment points for axial rotation. On deploying the main vessel stent, the ostial crown is automatically deployed to protrude its scaffolding elements 2 mm into the side branch ostium. The primary end point is procedural success, defined as <50% residual stenosis in the main vessel and no in-hospital MACE. Patients have an office follow-up at 1-month and angiographic assessment with IVUS at 6 months.

The Tryton Side-Branch Stent™ is a slotted-tube balloon-deployable stent with a modular design, tracked over a guidewire, and placed in the side branch. Kaplan *et al.* [56] recently presented 6 months' clinical and angiographic results of the device used in conjunction with a standard

Table 37.2 Clinical and procedural characteristics and outcome of DES implantation for bifurcation lesions in four registries/randomized studies.

	SES in NORDIC study (42)		PES in TRUE registry (40)		SES/PES in crush strategy (68)		RES stenting (69)	
	One stent	Two stents	One stent	Two stents	T-stent	Crush stents	One stent	Two stents
No. of patients	207	206	38	109	61	121	47	44
Follow-up (months)	6	6	12	12	8	8	6	6
Angiographic follow-up	176	182	40	118	46	96	41	39
Baseline characteristics								
Age (years)	64	64	62	63	61	62	61	58
Diabetes mellitus (%)	13	12	18	24	26	24	42	39
Hypertension (%)	53	58	68	60	62	64	59	57
LVEF (%)	—	—	56	56	51	53	60	55
Previous PCI (%)	25	26	32	40	—	—	—	—
Previous CABG (%)	4	3	11	11	15	20	—	—
Previous myocardial infarction (%)	—	—	34	49	47	37	19	39
Unstable angina (%)	—	—	39	20	16	21	89	86
Angiographic variables								
Main vessel lesion length (mm)	18.1	17.4	19.2	17.7	16.3	16	—	—
Main vessel stent length (mm)	23.4	23.6	26.2	28.6	27.6	29	25	26
Side branch lesion length (mm)	6.0	6.4	4.4	8.1	11	10.5	—	—
Main vessel reference diameter (mm)	3.3	3.3	2.8	2.9	2.8	2.7	3	2.9
Side branch reference diameter (mm)	2.6	2.6	2.0	2.2	2.6	2.3	2.5	2.5
T-stent/crush/V-stent/culotte	No data		14/43/10/3		33/66/–/–		No data	
Procedure success (%)	97	95	100	100	—	—	94	97
Outcomes								
Main vessel restenosis (%)	4.6	5.1	5	18	13	16	2	10
Side branch restenosis (%)	19.2	11.5	3	27	26.5	8.6*†	5	15
Cardiac death *n* (%)	2(1)	2(1)	0	3(2.7)	0	1(0.8)	0	1(2)
Myocardial infarction (Q and non-Q) *n* (%)	0	1(0.5)	0	1(0.9)	4(6.6)	24(19.9)	2(4)	0
TVR (%)	4(1.9)	4(1.9)	8(21)	20(18.3)	20(33)	20(16.5)	—	—
Stent thrombosis (%)	1(0.5)	0	0	4(3.6)	0	4(3.3)	0	1(2)
TLR (%)	4(1.9)	2(1)	5(13.1)	18(16.5)	19(31)	17(14)*	1(2%)	2(5%)
MACE (%)	2.9	3.4	21	25.5	36	26	6	7

*P significant at <0.05.

†After final kissing balloon.

MACE, major adverse cardiac event; PES, paclitaxel-eluting stent; RES, rapamycin-eluting stents; SES, sirolimus-eluting stent; TLR, target lesion revascularization; TVR, target vessel revascularization.

DES to treat 30 patients with lesions involving large side branches. None of the patients suffered from side branch restenosis. Quantitative analysis reported a late loss of 0.27 ± 0.42 mm in the side branch and 0.12 ± 0.42 mm in the main vessel.

Another promising dedicated bifurcation stent is the Boston Scientific Taxus Petal™ stent, which has a side branch stent that pops up as it is inflated. The stent system has a big balloon and a small balloon, which push the Petal stent into the side branch.

Conclusion

In PCI of the bifurcation lesion, dilation can displace plaque and jeopardize blood flow through plaque shift or dissection, which can affect both the vessels. Hence, in deciding the treatment technique a composite of vessel angulation, plaque distribution and vessel size should be actively considered.

In general, a single stent or provisional stenting strategy is strongly recommended, but if the side branch is also diseased at or near its ostium and is >2 mm in diameter, a two-stent strategy may be a better option. Outcome of DES implantation in bifurcational disease from registries and randomized studies is shown in Table 37.2. Wire both main vessel and side branch branches and dilate both if needed. Stent the vessels followed by high pressure side branch dilation and finish using kissing balloons. Angiographic follow-up is warranted only if clinically indicated. Newer drug eluting dedicated bifurcation stents have recently been introduced and outcomes from registries and randomized control trials are still awaited.

Coronary ostial lesions

A generally accepted definition considers ostial lesions as those arising within 3 mm of the origin of a blood vessel. Ostial lesions that involve the junction of the aorta and the origin of the RCA, left main stem, or a saphenous vein graft are called aorto-ostial lesions (AOLs). The other main type of ostial lesion occurs at the origin of the LAD or the LCx, arising from the bifurcation of the distal left main stem. These lesions tend to be a technically challenging group of coronary disease as they tend to be fibrocalcific and have greater elastic recoil than nonostial lesions. Their anatomical position and propensity for tissue proliferation, especially from the aortic wall in AOLs, along with chronic recoil after stenting, have limited their evaluation to observational studies [58]. In an attempt to overcome these difficulties, rotational atherectomy, directional atherectomy, and cutting balloon PCI have been used to "prepare" the lesions for coronary stenting.

In recent years, a potential method for improving the long-term outcome of stenting in ostial lesions has arrived on the scene—the implantation of a DES. The advantage of a DES in such lesions lies in its potent ability to inhibit this tissue proliferation compared with a BMS. The management of AOLs, being the more complex of ostial lesions, will now be discussed.

Percutaneous intervention

Drug-eluting stents and technique
Before stent implantation, patients are treated with aspirin (300 mg) and clopidogrel (300–600 mg) loading doses, unless on chronic treatment. Aspirin (75 mg) is then continued lifelong and clopidogrel (75 mg) for at least 1 month for BMSs and 12 months for DESs. Intraprocedural intravenous unfractionated heparin (70 IU/kg) should ideally maintain an activated clotting time above 250 s, and use of glycoprotein IIb/IIIa inhibitors is left to the operator's discretion. After wiring the ostial lesion via suitable guiding catheters, a stent is deployed to allow approximately a 1-mm protrusion into the aorta at high pressure (at least 14 atm). Thereafter, further high-pressure dilation with a semicompliant or noncompliant balloon is recommended to ensure optimal stent expansion with flaring performed at the ostium. IVUS guidance for stent

implantation and apposition can be used at the operator's discretion.

Two studies have shown promising results using DESs for AOL, focusing primarily on the SES. Iakovou *et al.* [59] demonstrated favorable angiographic and clinical outcomes in 32 patients treated with SES and, in a more recent study, Park *et al.* [60] confirmed this superiority over BMSs in 184 patients treated primarily with SESs. In our own series of AOLs [61], we showed the benefits of a DES compared with a BMS, by reducing the need for repeat revascularization at 12 months' follow-up, with no difference in mortality or myocardial infarction rate. We retrospectively identified 175 consecutive patients with 175 AOLs involving the left main artery, RCA, or bypass graft. SESs, PESs, and BMSs were implanted in 50, 69 and 56 patients, respectively. Angiographic and procedural success were, respectively, 100% and 97.1% for PESs, 100% and 94% for SESs, 100% and 94.6% for BMSs (not significant). At 12 months, the rates of TLR (8.7% for the PES, 4.0% for the SES) and TVR (3.0% for the PES, 8.0% for the SES) were significantly lower in the DES group than in the BMS group (32.1% and 35.7%, respectively). There was no difference in the rate of death/myocardial infarction in the BMS and DES groups (5.4% vs. 2.4%, $P = 0.32$).

Although routine angiographic follow-up was not performed, the low TLR rates suggest that DESs are effective for the treatment of ostial lesions. However, the gradual increase in MACE rates in the last 2 years suggests that aorto-ostial disease remains problematic, even in the era of DESs using paclitaxel [62]. Unfortunately, it remains unclear if any difference exists between AOLs and ostial lesions of the LAD and the LCx, or whether pretreatment of ostial lesions before stenting has any additional benefit. It is also unclear as to whether vessel size, stent size, and lesion length affect outcomes after DESs compared with BMSs; only a specifically designed, large, randomized trial will address these issues.

Conclusion

Percutaneous interventions to complex coronary lesions are a challenging minefield. The advent of the DES has added to the armory of today's interventionist, making such interventional procedures safer than ever before, extending application of PCI to patients and lesions that would previously have been treated medically or with CABG. In a meta-analyses review of 16 randomized trials ($n = 8695$), comparing SES with PES in coronary artery disease, SES use was associated with a significantly reduced risk of reintervention (hazard ratio 0.74) and of stent thrombosis (hazard ratio 0.66) [63]. These results are at odds with the results of large registries of complex and everyday lesions, with no reported difference in clinical outcomes (MACE rates) up to 14 months [61,64,65].

Although ULM PCI with a DES is considered a strategy still in its infancy, recent reports and studies have generated optimism among interventional cardiologists. Results of randomized trials comparing PCI with traditional CABG are eagerly awaited with the possibility of further propelling this treatment further into mainstream cardiology. Furthermore, the benefits of DESs for bifurcation and ostial lesions have been explicitly laid out with improved angiographic and clinical outcomes. Even so, the issue of late stent thrombosis and restenosis has yet to be fully elucidated and remains a cloud over the current success.

References

1. Gruntzig A (1978) Transluminal dilatation of coronary-artery stenosis. *Lancet* **1**:263.
2. Faltori R, Piva T (2003) Drug-eluting stents in vascular intervention. *Lancet* **361**:247–249.
3. Cohen MV & Gorlin R (1975) Main left coronary artery disease. Clinical experience from 1964–1974. *Circulation* **52**:275–285.
4. Proudfit WL, Shirey EK, & Sones FM Jr (1967) Distribution of arterial lesions demonstrated by selective cinecoronary arteriography. *Circulation* **36**:54–62.
5. Taylor HA, Deumite NJ, Chaitman BR, Davis KB, Killip T, & Rogers WJ (1989) Asymptomatic left main coronary artery disease in the Coronary Artery Surgery Study (CASS) registry. *Circulation* **79**:1171–1179.
6. Gruntzig AR, Senning A, & Siegenthaler WE (1979) Nonoperative dilatation of coronary-artery stenosis: percutaneous transluminal coronary angioplasty. *N Engl J Med* **301**:61–68.
7. Lopez JJ, Ho KK, Stoler RC, et al. (1997) Percutaneous treatment of protected and unprotected left main coronary stenoses with new devices: immediate angiographic results and intermediate-term follow-up. *J Am Coll Cardiol* **29**:345–352.
8. Silber S, Albertsson P, Aviles FF, et al. (2005) Guidelines for percutaneous coronary interventions. The Task Force for Percutaneous Coronary Interventions of the European Society of Cardiology. *Eur Heart J* **26**:804–847.
9. Tan WA, Tamai H, Park SJ, et al. (2001) Long-term clinical outcomes after unprotected left main trunk percutaneous revascularization in 279 patients. *Circulation* **104**:1609–1614.
10. Smith SC Jr, Feldman TE, Hirshfeld JW Jr, et al. (2006) ACC/AHA/SCAI 2005 Guideline Update for Percutaneous Coronary Intervention—summary article: a report of the American College of Cardiology/American Heart Association Task Force on Practice Guidelines (ACC/AHA/SCAI Writing Committee to Update the 2001 Guidelines for Percutaneous Coronary Intervention). *Circulation* **113**:156–175.
11. White CW, Wright CB, Doty DB, et al. (1984) Does visual interpretation of the coronary arteriogram predict the physiologic importance of a coronary stenosis? *N Engl J Med* **310**:819–824.
12. Pijls NH, Van Gelder B, Van der Voort P, et al. (1995) Fractional flow reserve. A useful index to evaluate the influence of an epicardial coronary stenosis on myocardial blood flow. *Circulation* **92**:3183–3193.
13. Jasti V, Ivan E, Yalamanchili V, Wongpraparut N, & Leesar MA (2004) Correlations between fractional flow reserve and intravascular ultrasound in patients with an ambiguous left main coronary artery stenosis. *Circulation* **110**:2831–2836.
14. Sano K, Mintz GS, Carlier SG, et al. (2007) Assessing intermediate left main coronary lesions using intravascular ultrasound. *Am Heart J* **154**:983–988.
15. Bhatt DL, Fox KA, Hacke W, et al. (2006) Clopidogrel and aspirin versus aspirin alone for the prevention of atherothrombotic events. *N Engl J Med* **354**:1706–1717.
16. de Feyter PJ, Kay P, Disco C, & Serruys PW (1999) Reference chart derived from post-stent-implantation intravascular ultrasound predictors of 6-month expected restenosis on quantitative coronary angiography. *Circulation* **100**:1777–1783.
17. Sonoda S, Morino Y, Ako J, et al. (2004) Impact of final stent dimensions on long-term results following sirolimus-eluting stent implantation: serial intravascular ultrasound analysis from the sirius trial. *J Am Coll Cardiol* **43**:1959–1963.
18. Tsuchikane E, Suzuki T, Asakura Y, et al. (2008) Debulking of chronic coronary total occlusions with rotational or directional atherectomy before stenting: final results of DOCTORS study. *Int J Cardiol* **125**:397–403.
19. Silvestri M, Barragan P, Sainsous J, et al. (2000) Unprotected left main coronary artery stenting: immediate and medium-term outcomes of 140 elective procedures. *J Am Coll Cardiol* **35**:1543–1550.
20. Takagi T, Stankovic G, Finci L, et al. (2002) Results and long-term predictors of adverse clinical events after elective percutaneous interventions on unprotected left main coronary artery. *Circulation* **106**:698–702.
21. Park SJ, Lee CW, Kim YH, et al. (2002) Technical feasibility, safety, and clinical outcome of stenting of unprotected left main coronary artery bifurcation narrowing. *Am J Cardiol* **90**:374–378.
22. Erglis A, Narbute I, Kumsars I, et al. (2007) A randomized comparison of paclitaxel-eluting stents versus bare metal stents for treatment of unprotected left main coronary artery stenosis. *J Am Coll Cardiol* **50**:491–497.
23. Valgimigli M, Malagutti P, Aoki J, et al. (2006) Sirolimus-eluting versus paclitaxel-eluting stent implantation for the percutaneous treatment of left main coronary artery disease: a combined RESEARCH and T-SEARCH long-term analysis. *J Am Coll Cardiol* **47**:507–514.
24. Chieffo A, Stankovic G, Bonizzoni E, et al. (2005) Early and mid-term results of drug-eluting stent implantation in unprotected left main. *Circulation* **111**:791–795.
25. Lee MS, Kapoor N, Jamal F, et al. (2006) Comparison of coronary artery bypass surgery with percutaneous coronary intervention with drug-eluting stents for unprotected left main coronary artery disease. *J Am Coll Cardiol* **47**:864–870.
26. Price MJ, Cristea E, Sawhney N, et al. (2006) Serial angiographic follow-up of sirolimus-eluting stents for unprotected left main coronary artery revascularization. *J Am Coll Cardiol* **47**:871–877.
27. Barlis P, Horrigan M, Elis S, et al. (2007) Treatment of unprotected left main disease with drug-eluting stents in patients at high risk for coronary artery bypass grafting. *Cardiovasc Revasc Med* **8**:84–89.
28. Buszman PE, Kiesz SR, Bochenek A, et al. (2008) Acute and late outcomes of unprotected left main stenting in comparison with surgical revascularization. *J Am Coll Cardiol* **51**:538–545.

29. Meliga E, Garcia-Garcia HM, Valgimigli M, *et al.* (2008) Longest available clinical outcomes after drug-eluting stent implantation for unprotected left main coronary artery disease: the DELFT (Drug-eluting stent for LeFT main) Registry. *J Am Coll Cardiol* **51**:2212–2219.

30. Seung KB, Park DW, Kim YH, *et al.* (2008) Stents versus coronary-artery bypass grafting for left main coronary artery disease. *N Engl J Med* **358**:1781–1792.

31. Serruys PW, Morice MC, Kappetein AP, *et al.* for SYNTAX Investigators (2009) Percutaneous coronary intervention versus coronary-artery bypass grafting for severe coronary artery disease. *N Engl J Med* **360**:961–972.

32. Melikian N, Airoldi F, & Di Mario C (2004) Coronary bifurcation stenting. Current techniques, outcome and possible future developments. *Minerva Cardioangiol* **52**:365–378.

33. Lefevre T, Louvard Y, Morice MC, *et al.* (2000) Stenting of bifurcation lesions: classification, treatments, and results. *Catheter Cardiovasc Interv* **49**:274–283.

34. Ormiston JA, Currie E, Webster MW, *et al.* (2004) Drug-eluting stents for coronary bifurcations: insights into the crush technique. *Catheter Cardiovasc Interv* **63**:332–336.

35. Dzavik V, Kharbanda R, Ivanov J, *et al.* (2006) Predictors of long-term outcome after crush stenting of coronary bifurcation lesions: importance of the bifurcation angle. *Am Heart J* **152**:762–769.

36. Poerner TC, Kralev S, Voelker W, *et al.* (2002) Natural history of small and medium-sized side branches after coronary stent implantation. *Am Heart J* **143**:627–635.

37. Al Suwaidi J, Yeh W, Cohen HA, Detre KM, Williams DO, & Holmes DR Jr (2001) Immediate and one-year outcome in patients with coronary bifurcation lesions in the modern era (NHLBI dynamic registry). *Am J Cardiol* **87**:1139–1144.

38. Brunel P, Lefevre T, Darremont O, & Louvard Y (2006) Provisional T-stenting and kissing balloon in the treatment of coronary bifurcation lesions: results of the French multicenter "TULIPE" study. *Catheter Cardiovasc Interv* **68**:67–73.

39. Colombo A, Moses JW, Morice MC, *et al.* (2004) Randomized study to evaluate sirolimus-eluting stents implanted at coronary bifurcation lesions. *Circulation* **109**:1244–1249.

40. Di Mario C, Morici N, Godino C, *et al.* (2007) Predictors of restenosis after treatment of bifurcational lesions with paclitaxel eluting stents: a multicenter prospective registry of 150 consecutive patients. *Catheter Cardiovasc Interv* **69**:416–424.

41. Tsuchida K, Colombo A, Lefevre T, *et al.* (2007) The clinical outcome of percutaneous treatment of bifurcation lesions in multivessel coronary artery disease with the sirolimus-eluting stent: insights from the Arterial Revascularization Therapies Study part II (ARTS II). *Eur Heart J* **28**:433–442.

42. Steigen TK, Maeng M, Wiseth R, *et al.* (2006) Randomized study on simple versus complex stenting of coronary artery bifurcation lesions: the Nordic bifurcation study. *Circulation* **114**:1955–1961.

43. Legrand V, Thomas M, Zelisco M, *et al.* (2007) Percutaneous coronary intervention of bifurcation lesions: state-of-the-art. Insights from the second meeting of the European Bifurcation Club. *EuroIntervention* **3**:44–49.

44. Legrand V, Thomas M, Zelisco M, *et al.* (2007) Percutaneous coronary intervention of bifurcation lesions: state-of-the-art. Insights from the second meeting of the European Bifurcation Club. *EuroIntervention* **3**:44–49.

45. Kobayashi Y, Colombo A, Akiyama T, Reimers B, Martini G, & Di Mario C (1998) Modified "T" stenting: a technique for kissing stents in bifurcational coronary lesion. *Cathet Cardiovasc Diagn* **43**:323–326.

46. Colombo A, Stankovic G, Orlic D, *et al.* (2003) Modified T-stenting technique with crushing for bifurcation lesions: immediate results and 30-day outcome. *Catheter Cardiovasc Interv* **60**:145–151.

47. Burzotta F, Gwon HC, Hahn JY, *et al.* (2007) Modified T-stenting with intentional protrusion of the side-branch stent within the main vessel stent to ensure ostial coverage and facilitate final kissing balloon: the T-stenting and small protrusion technique (TAP-stenting). Report of bench testing and first clinical Italian-Korean two-centre experience. *Catheter Cardiovasc Interv* **70**:75–82.

48. Galassi AR, Colombo A, Buchbinder M, *et al.* (2007) Long-term outcomes of bifurcation lesions after implantation of drug-eluting stents with the "mini-crush technique." *Catheter Cardiovasc Interv* **69**:976–983.

49. Ge L, Airoldi F, Iakovou I, *et al.* (2005) Clinical and angiographic outcome after implantation of drug-eluting stents in bifurcation lesions with the crush stent technique: importance of final kissing balloon post-dilation. *J Am Coll Cardiol* **46**:613–620.

50. Hoye A, Iakovou I, Ge L, *et al.* (2006) Long-term outcomes after stenting of bifurcation lesions with the "crush" technique: predictors of an adverse outcome. *J Am Coll Cardiol* **47**:1949–1958.

51. Colombo A (2008) CACTUS Trial (Coronary Bifurcation: Application of the Crushing Technique Using Sirolimus Eluting Stents). Presented at EuroPCR 2008, Barcelona, Spain.

52. Chevalier B, Glatt B, Royer T, & Guyon P (1998) Placement of coronary stents in bifurcation lesions by the "culotte" technique. *Am J Cardiol* **82**:943–949.

53. Kaplan S, Barlis P, Dimopoulos K, *et al.* (2007) Culotte versus T-stenting in bifurcation lesions: immediate clinical and angiographic results and midterm clinical follow-up. *Am Heart J* **154**:336–343.

54. Sharma SK (2005) Simultaneous kissing drug-eluting stent technique for percutaneous treatment of bifurcation lesions in large-size vessels. *Catheter Cardiovasc Interv* **65**:10–16.

55. Kim YH, Park DW, Suh IW, *et al.* (2007) Long-term outcome of simultaneous kissing stenting technique with sirolimus-eluting stent for large bifurcation coronary lesions. *Catheter Cardiovasc Interv* **70**:840–846.

56. Miyazawa A, Ako J, Hassan A, *et al.* (2007) Analysis of bifurcation lesions treated with novel drug-eluting dedicated bifurcation stent system: intravascular ultrasound results of the AXXESS PLUS trial. *Catheter Cardiovasc Interv* **70**:952–957.

57. Kaplan AV, Ramcharitar S, Louvard Y, *et al.* (2007) Tryton I, First-In-Man (FIM) Study: acute and 30 day outcome. A preliminary report. *EuroIntervention* **3**:54–59.

58. Tsunoda T, Nakamura M, Wada M, *et al.* (2004) Chronic stent recoil plays an important role in restenosis of the right coronary ostium. *Coron Artery Dis* **15**:39–44.

59. Iakovou I, Ge L, Michev I, *et al.* (2004) Clinical and angiographic outcome after sirolimus-eluting stent implantation in aorto-ostial lesions. *J Am Coll Cardiol* **44**:967–971.

60. Park DW, Hong MK, Suh IW, *et al.* (2007) Results and predictors of angiographic restenosis and long-term adverse cardiac events after drug-eluting stent implantation for aorto-ostial coronary artery disease. *Am J Cardiol* **99**:760–765.

61. Barlis P, Kaplan S, Ferrante G, & Di Mario C (2008) Comparison of bare metal and sirolimus- or paclitaxel-eluting stents for aorto-ostial coronary disease. *Cardiology* **111**:270–276.

62. Tsuchida K, Daemen J, Tanimoto S, *et al.* (2007) Two-year outcome of the use of paclitaxel-eluting stents in aorto-ostial lesions. *Int J Cardiol* [Epub ahead of print].

63. Schömig A, Dibra A, Windecker S, *et al.* (2007) A meta-analysis of 16 randomized trials of sirolimus-eluting stents versus paclitaxel-eluting stents in patients with coronary artery disease. *J Am Coll Cardiol* **50**:1373–1380.

64. Simonton CA, Brodie B, Cheek B, *et al.* (2007) Comparative clinical outcomes of paclitaxel- and sirolimus-eluting stents: results from a large prospective multicenter registry—STENT Group. *J Am Coll Cardiol* **50**:1214–1222.

65. Cosgrave J, Melzi G, Corbett S, *et al.* (2007) Comparable clinical outcomes with paclitaxel- and sirolimus-eluting stents in unrestricted contemporary practice. *J Am Coll Cardiol* **49**:2320–2328.

66. Park SJ, Kim YH, Lee BK, *et al.* (2005) Sirolimus-eluting stent implantation for unprotected left main coronary artery stenosis: comparison with bare metal stent implantation. *J Am Coll Cardiol* **45**:351–356.

67. Valgimigli M, van Mieghem CA, Ong AT, *et al.* (2005) Short- and long-term clinical outcome after drug-eluting stent implantation for the percutaneous treatment of left main coronary artery disease: insights from the Rapamycin-Eluting and Taxus Stent Evaluated At Rotterdam Cardiology Hospital registries (RESEARCH and T-SEARCH). *Circulation* **111**:1383–1389.

68. Ge L, Iakovou I, Cosgrave J, *et al.* (2006) Treatment of bifurcation lesions with two stents: one year angiographic and clinical follow up of crush versus T stenting. *Heart* **92**:371–376.

69. Pan M, de Lezo JS, Medina A, *et al.* (2004) Rapamycin-eluting stents for the treatment of bifurcated coronary lesions: a randomized comparison of a simple versus complex strategy. *Am Heart J* **148**:857–864.

38 Percutaneous Coronary Intervention in Multivessel Disease

Yoshinobu Onuma, Neville Kukreja & Patrick W. Serruys

Thoraxcenter, Erasmus Medical Center, Rotterdam, The Netherlands

Historical background

Balloon angioplasty or bare metal stent era

Since percutaneous coronary intervention (PCI) commenced in the late 1970s with the first percutaneous transluminal balloon angioplasty as a nonsurgical alternative [1], PCI has been challenging coronary artery bypass graft surgery (CABG) as the standard treatment for patients with multivessel disease [2–5]. The application of PCI to these patients has been limited mainly by restenosis, which develops in 30–40% of patients who receive treatment with balloon angioplasty and 20–25% of patients who receive treatment with bare metal stents (BMSs) [6].

Between the late 1980s and the early 1990s, six randomized trials compared CABG with balloon angioplasty to investigate the most appropriate revascularization modality [7–12]: Randomized Intervention Treatment of Angina (RITA), German Angioplasty Bypass Surgery Investigation (GABI), Emory Angioplasty versus Surgery Trial (EAST), Coronary Angioplasty versus Bypass Revascularization Investigation (CABRI), Argentine Randomized Trial of Percutaneous Transluminal Coronary Angioplasty Versus Coronary Artery Bypass Surgery in Multivessel Disease (ERACI), and Bypass Angioplasty Revascularization Investigation (BARI). A summary of these trials is presented in Table 38.1. All these trials included patients who were eligible for either a CABG or PCI. A meta-analysis comparing the 1-year and 3-year outcomes of these randomized trials found no significant differences in the rates of death or myocardial infarction [13,14]. As for long-term outcome, Hoffman *et al.* [4] calculated a trend favoring CABG over percutaneous transluminal coronary angioplasty (PTCA) for survival at 5 years (risk difference [RD] 2.3%, confidence interval [CI] 0.29–4.3%, *P* = 0.025) and 8 years (RD 3.4%, CI 0.32–6.4%, *P* = 0.03) in patients with multivessel disease (Fig. 38.1). Ten-year follow-up results from the BARI trial demonstrated that there was no significant difference in

mortality and myocardial infarction event rates between the randomized treatment groups [15].

Subsequent to the initial trials demonstrating better outcome in PCI with coronary stents than in balloon angioplasty [16,17], five randomized controlled trials were performed to compare surgery with PCI with stenting in the mid to late 1990s (Table 38.1): the Arterial Revascularization Therapy Study (ARTS; 2001) [3], the Argentine Randomized Study: Coronary Angioplasty with Stenting versus Coronary Bypass Surgery in Multivessel Disease (ERACI-II; 2001) [18], Stent or Surgery (SoS; 2002) [19], the Angina With Extremely Serious Operative Mortality Evaluation (AWESOME) [20], and the Medicine, Angioplasty or Surgery Study for multivessel coronary artery disease (MASS II) (see Table 38.1) [21].

In the largest trial (ARTS) [3], a total of 1205 patients with the potential for equivalent revascularization were randomly assigned to CABG (*n* = 605) or stent implantation (*n* = 600). The primary end points were measured in terms of major adverse cardiac and cerebrovascular events (MACCE) at 1-year, comprising all-cause death, any cerebrovascular event, nonfatal myocardial infarction, or any repeat revascularization. At 1 year, there was no significant difference between the CABG and stent groups in terms of the rates of death, stroke, or myocardial infarction. For patients who survived without a stroke or a myocardial infarction, 16.8% of those in the stenting group underwent a second revascularization compared with 3.5% of those in the surgery group. At 5 years, there were 48 and 46 deaths in the stent and surgical groups, respectively, (8.0% vs. 7.6%; *P* = 0.83; relative risk [RR] = 1.05 [0.71–1.55]). Importantly, the 5-year outcome from this trial was the first to demonstrate a similar mortality rate for PCI with stenting versus CABG (Fig. 38.2). The incidence of repeat revascularization was significantly higher in the stent group (30.3%) than in the CABG group (8.8%; *P* < 0.001, RR = 3.46 [2.61–4.60]) [5].

In most randomized trials, patients treated with stenting were shown to have similar outcomes to those treated with CABG, in terms of death and myocardial infarction. In a meta-analysis of 1-year patient-based data from ARTS, ERACI II, MASS II, and SoS, Mercado *et al.* [22] reported that the cumulative incidence of death, myocardial infarction, and

Cardiovascular Interventions in Clinical Practice. Edited by Jürgen Haase, Hans-Joachim Schäfers, Horst Sievert and Ron Waksman. © 2010 Blackwell Publishing.

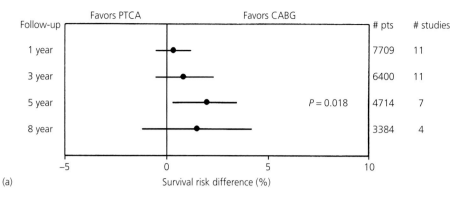

(a)

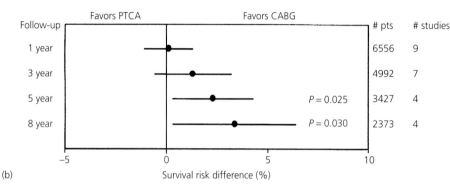

(b)

Figure 38.1 Risk difference for all-cause mortality for years 1, 3, 5, and 8 post initial revascularization. All trials (a) and multivessel coronary artery disease (b). The lines represent 95% confidence intervals. Reproduced from Hoffman *et al.* [4], with permission from Elsevier.

Table 38.1 Summary of randomized trials in the Balloon angioplasty or bare metal stent era.

Trial	Bare metal stent use	Clinical parameters			Angiographic end points	Cost assessment (years)
		Mortality (years)	Angina relief (years)	Repeat revascularization (years)		
GABI	No	No difference (13)	PCI (1)	n/a	No difference	NA
EAST	No	No difference (8)	CABG (3)	CABG (8)	CABG	No difference (8)
RITA	No	No difference (5)	CABG (2.5)	CABG (5)	NA	NA
ERACI	No	No difference (3)	CABG (1)	CABG (3)	NA	PCI (3)
CABRI	No	No difference (1)	CABG (1)	CABG (1)	NA	NA
BARI	No	No difference (10)	n/a	CABG (10)	n NA	No difference (10)
MASS II	Yes	No difference (5)	n/a	CABG (5)	NA	No difference (5)
AWESOME	Yes	No difference (3)	No difference (3)	No difference (3)	NA	NA
ERACI I	Yes	No difference (5)	n/a	CABG (5)	CABG	CABG (5)
SoS	Yes	CABG (3)	CABG (3)	CABG (3)	NA	NA
ARTS	Yes	No difference (5)	n/a	CABG (5)	NA	PCI (3)

ARTS, Arterial Revascularization Therapy Study; AWESOME, Angina With Extremely Serious Operative Mortality Evaluation; BARI, Bypass Angioplasty Revascularization Investigation (1996); CABG, in favor of coronary artery bypass grafting; CABRI, Coronary Angioplasty versus Bypass Revascularization Investigation (1995); EAST, Emory Angioplasty versus Surgery Trial (1994); ERACI, Argentine Randomized Trial of Percutaneous Transluminal Coronary Angioplasty Versus Coronary Artery Bypass Surgery in Multivessel Disease (1996); GABI, German Angioplasty Bypass Surgery Investigation; MASS, Medicine, Angioplasty or Surgery Study for multivessel coronary artery disease; MI, myocardial infarction; NA, not available; PCI, in favor of percutaneous intervention; RITA, Randomized Intervention Treatment of Angina (1993); SoS, Stent or Surgery.

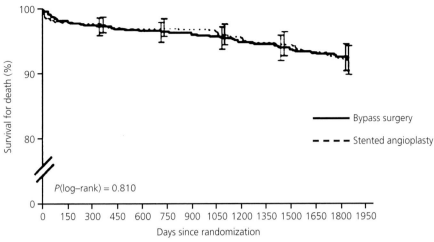

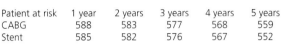

Figure 38.2 Kaplan–Meier curves showing 5-year mortality in the Arterial Revascularization Therapies Study (ARTS). Reproduced from Serruys *et al.* [5], with permission from Elsevier.

Patient at risk	1 year	2 years	3 years	4 years	5 years
CABG	588	583	577	568	559
Stent	585	582	576	567	552

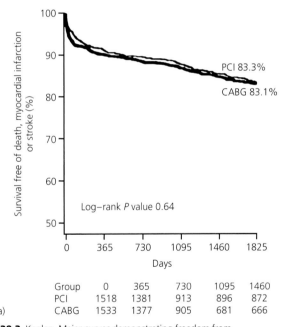

Group	0	365	730	1095	1460
PCI	1518	1381	913	896	872
CABG	1533	1377	905	681	666

(a)

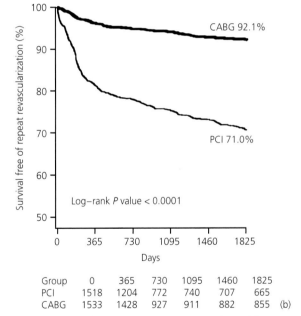

Group	0	365	730	1095	1460	1825
PCI	1518	1204	772	740	707	665
CABG	1533	1428	927	911	882	855

(b)

Figure 38.3 Kaplan–Meier curves demonstrating freedom from death, myocardial infarction or stroke (a), and freedom from repeat revascularization (b). Reproduced from a meta-analysis with 5-year patient level data of the ARTS, ERACI-II, MASS-II and SoS trials, Daemen *et al.* [23], with permission.

stroke at 1-year follow-up was similar in both groups (PCI 8.7% vs. CABG 9.1%, $P = 0.63$). The need for repeat revascularization was considerably higher with PCI (18.0% vs. 4.4%, $P < 0.001$), although the observed gap with CABG surgery had narrowed from approximately 30% reported in the balloon angioplasty era to approximately 18% with BMS. Most recently, a meta-analysis of 5-year data employed from the same trials was available, in which Daemen *et al.* [23] reported that PCI and CABG were associated with a similar

safety profile in terms of death, myocardial infarction, and stroke (PCI 16.7% vs. CABG 16.9%, hazard ratio [HR] 1.05, 95% CI 0.87–1.26) (Fig. 38.3a). However, the need for repeat revascularization procedures still remained significantly greater in the PCI than in the CABG group (PCI 29.0% vs. CABG 7.9%; HR 0.22, 95% CI 0.18–0.28) (Fig. 38.3b).

More recently, Hlatky *et al.* reported a meta-analysis of 7812 individual patient data from 10 randomized trials to evaluate the comparative effectiveness of PCI (either with balloon angioplasty or with bare metal stenting) and CABG, according to baseline clinical characteristics [24]. Overall, the long-term survival of patients with multivessel coronary disease randomized to treatment with CABG or PCI was similar (CABG/PCI: HR = 0.91, 95% CI 0.82–1.02, $P = 0.12$). Patients with diabetes gain a significant survival benefit with CABG (HR 0.71, P for interaction = 0.01). However, although long-term survival is better after CABG than PCI in older patients (HR 0.82 in those older than 65 years, P for interaction = 0.002), long-term survival is better after PCI rather than CABG in younger patients (HR 1.26 in those younger then 55 years).

Another study worth mentioning is a nonrandomized study reported by Hannan *et al.* [25]. They used New York's cardiac registries ($n = 59314$) to determine the rates of death and subsequent revascularization within 3 years after the procedure in various groups. The unadjusted hazard ratio for the long-term risk of death after CABG relative to stent implantation was 0.67 (95% CI 0.59–0.77) for patients with three-vessel disease and a proximal left anterior descending artery (LAD) lesion and 1.05 (95% CI 0.84–1.31) for patients with two-vessel disease without involvement of the proximal LAD. However, inconsistent with other studies, the risk-adjusted survival rates were significantly higher in patients treated with CABG than in those patients treated with coronary stenting in both groups (HR 0.64 [95% CI 0.56–0.74] and 0.76 [95% CI 0.60–0.96], respectively). We have to interpret these data with prudence because baseline characteristics were different between the PCI and CABG groups, in addition to the unadjustable characteristic that the choice of treatment was left to the physician.

Complete revascularization

The concept of complete revascularization arose from the early studies on CABG surgery [26–30]. In a seminal publication from the Coronary Artery Surgery Study (CASS) registry, 3372 patients with three-vessel disease (including left main trunk disease) who underwent isolated a first-time CABG between July 1974 and June 1979 were analyzed with a mean follow-up of 4.9 years, with improved survival and complete revascularization (RR 0.75, 95% CI 0.59–0.94) [30]. Since then, numerous publications have focused on outcomes of complete revascularization and incomplete revascularization with either CABG or PCI [31–35]. However, only one randomized trial compared the prespecified end point of complete revascularization between CABG and PCI: the ARTS trial, in which the possibility for equivalent revascularization was mandatory, has published the 1-year outcomes of patients who were completely or incompletely revascularized. Despite the potential for equivalent revascularization, complete revascularization was more frequently achieved in CABG-treated patients (84.1%) than in stented patients (70.5%, $P < 0.001$). Freedom from MACCE rates were significantly lower in the completely revascularized patients in stented group, driven by an increased need for CABG within the first year of

follow-up (69.4% vs. 76.6%; $P < 0.05$) [36]. This trend was still present after 3 years' follow-up, though it did not reach statistical significance [37].

Although little evidence is available on this aspect of the comparison of CABG and PCI and various definitions are present, the overall trends support complete revascularization. The goal should always be complete revascularization, whether the treatment choice is surgery or PCI, although the presence of chronic total occlusions (CTOs) remains the highest hurdle to overcome to achieve complete revascularization with the percutaneous approach.

Cost-effectiveness

Another crucial aspect to be mentioned is cost-effectiveness. In the Bypass Angioplasty Revascularization Investigation (BARI) randomized trial, the cost of the initial revascularization procedure was 35% lower among PCI patients, but this difference had narrowed to 5% after 5 years of follow-up, mostly as a result of the greater need for additional revascularization procedures among PCI patients. After 10–12 years, these early differences between PTCA and CABG in economic and quality-of-life outcomes were no longer significant [38]. In the EAST, Weintraub *et al.* [39] reported that the cost advantage of PCI in the initial procedure was largely or even completely lost for randomized patients after 8 years' follow-up because of additional procedures after a first revascularization by PCI. In the ERACI trial, the cumulative cost at 3-year follow-up was greater for the bypass surgery group than for the coronary angioplasty group.

Several trials in the stent era have assessed cost-effectiveness. In the MASS II trial, the comparison of CABG and PCI showed no difference in the incidence of death, although the greater occurrence of repeat revascularization procedures in the PCI group elevated its costs to that of CABG after 1 year [40]. In the ARTS trial, the 1-year result demonstrated that PCI was less expensive than CABG and offered the same degree of protection against death, stroke, and myocardial infarction. However, at 3 years the additional costs generated by the higher rate of revascularization in the stented patients reduced the cost saving of €2779 (in favor of stenting observed at 1 year) to €1798 [41]. In the 5-year follow-up of ERACI II, comparison of average cost per patient showed a higher cost with PCI than CABG (PCI $13584 vs. CABG $11362; $P = 0.04$) [42].

Thus, in most trials throughout the balloon angioplasty and BMS era, PCI had an advantage in initial procedure costs, although the advantage in favor of PCI became less significant or lost at long-term follow-up owing to repeat revascularizations.

Diabetic patients

Diabetic patients are known to develop an aggressive form of atherosclerosis and long-term survival following both PCI and CABG is worse than in nondiabetic patients [43–46].

Owing to the smaller vessel size, longer lesion length, and greater plaque burden, diabetic subjects are more likely to suffer from multivessel disease. Furthermore, the restenotic cascade alternative is different from that in nondiabetics and restenosis rates in diabetic patients are higher.

Diabetic patients with multivessel disease who are treated with CABG derive a survival benefit over those treated with balloon angioplasty. The BARI study demonstrated that the 5-year all-cause mortality rate was 34.5% in randomized diabetic patients assigned to PTCA compared with 19.4% in CABG patients ($P = 0.0024$; RR = 1.87); the corresponding cardiac mortality rates were 23.4% and 8.2%, respectively ($P = 0.0002$; RR = 3.10). The CABG benefit was more apparent among patients requiring insulin [47]. The EAST included a small cohort of treated diabetic patients who underwent PCI ($n = 29$) or CABG ($n = 30$) with a nonsignificant trend toward improved 8-year survival in the surgical group (60.1% vs. 75.5%, respectively, $P = 0.23$) [48].

In the BMS era, the survival advantage of CABG was less significant, although PCI was still associated with higher rates of repeat revascularization. In a meta-analysis using pooled patient-level 1-year follow-up data from ARTS, ERACI II, MASS II, and SoS trials, the 1-year mortality rate in the diabetic population was 5.6% in patients allocated to PCI with multiple stenting and 3.5% in those allocated to CABG surgery (HR 1.6, 95% CI 0.72–3.6, $P = 0.3$) [22].

These results are inconclusive because they extracted results from diabetic subgroups without specifically targeting these populations. Furthermore, there seems reason to believe that, owing to the rapid disease progression and greater atherosclerotic burden of the diabetic patient with multivessel disease, CABG should be the preferred treatment, mainly because of its ability to bypass this large amount of plaque burden, which could make future repeat revascularizations less of a necessity.

Current evidence in the drug-eluting stent era

The introduction of drug-eluting stents (DESs) in 2002 has enabled PCI to reduce both angiographic and clinical restenosis to below double figures in simple cases, resulting in a significant reduction in the need for repeat revascularizations [49–51]. Although initial evidence stemming from randomized trials has accumulated on the use of DES in low-risk patients presenting with relatively simple lesions, in real life their use has been extended to higher risk populations and lesions (including diabetic patients, those with diffuse coronary stenoses, and those with chronic total occlusions), who constitute a large proportion of patients with multivessel disease [52,53]. In fact, according to one of the real-world registries, almost 40% of the patients who underwent PCI with DES had multivessel disease [54].

In addition to DESs, new devices have been developed to overcome chronic total occlusions, which has been a major limitation to complete revascularization. In the meantime, CABG has progressed with more effective perioperative management, a higher use of arterial grafting, and contemporary techniques with minimally invasive and off-pump surgery as options [55,56]. Thus, owing to developments in technologies, the findings of the previous trials with balloon angioplasty or bare metal stents cannot be extrapolated to current clinical practice.

Immediately after the revelation of low restenotic rates in PCI using DESs, the first PCI–CABG trials added a DES arm to the historical CABG arms in the previously published trials. The ARTS II trial was one of the first trials to do so, adding a prospectively collected arm of 607 consecutive patients to the ARTS I study [57]. The ARTS I trial randomized 1205 patients with multivessel disease to CABG or PCI with BMSs. The ARTS II 1-year results showed that PCI with a DES was not inferior to CABG with respect to the combined end point of MACCE. The need for repeat revascularizations was still significantly higher than in the historical CABG arm of ARTS I, although overall MACCE rates in ARTS II approached the surgical results and were significantly better than bare metal stenting in ARTS I. The 3-year results of ARTS II [58] demonstrated the same tendency, with similar MACCE rates in ARTS II PCI and ARTS I CABG (80.6 vs. 83.8%, $P = 0.21$). Freedom from revascularization in ARTS II was 85.5%, lower than in ARTS I CABG (93.4%; $P < 0.001$). The ERACI III study was performed using a similar approach as ARTS II by adding a group of 225 DES patients to the ERACI II trial [59]. At 1-year follow-up, freedom from MACCE was significantly greater among patients treated with DES (88%) than in the ERACI II CABG arm (80.5%, $P = 0.038$) and ERACI II PCI patients (78%, $P = 0.006$). However, freedom from repeat revascularization was similar in patients with DES and CABG (91.2% vs. 95.1%, not significant).

Recently, several observational studies have reported the outcome for multivessel disease in patients treated with CABG or PCI using DES [60–62]. In a single-center observational study, including 1680 patients with a high rate of diabetics (over 35%), Javaid *et al.* [61] reported that adjusted outcomes for the nondiabetic subpopulation showed equivalent MACCE (two-vessel disease: HR 1.77, $P = 0.34$; three vessel disease: HR 1.70, $P = 0.19$) and that the diabetic population demonstrated increased MACCE with PCI compared with CABG (two-vessel disease: HR 2.29, $P = 0.01$; three-vessel disease: HR 2.9; $P < 0.001$). In a large observational study by Hannan *et al.* [60] including 17 400 patients using data from the New York state Cardiac Surgery and PCI reporting systems, the authors demonstrated that at 18 months CABG was still associated with lower mortality rates than treatment with DES in the patients with two-vessel disease (adjusted survival rate 96.0% vs. 94.6%, $P = 0.003$) and three-vessel disease (adjusted survival rate

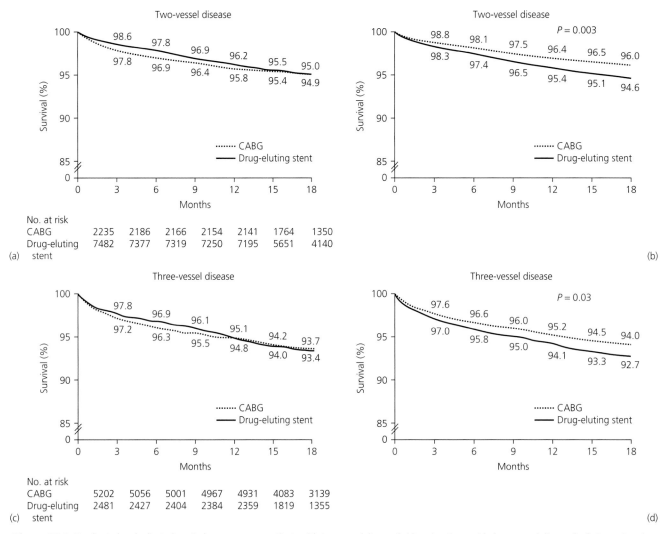

Figure 38.4 Unadjusted and adjusted survival curves among patients with two-vessel disease (a,b) and patients with three-vessel disease (c,d). Reproduced from Hannan *et al.* [60], with permission from Massachusetts Medical Society.

94.0% vs. 92.7%, *P* = 0.03) (Fig. 38.4). However, these observational studies without proper randomization could not eliminate bias result from the inclusion of patients differing with respect to unmeasured confounders such as physician's judgment; therefore, we should await the results of ongoing randomized trials that will help to elucidate the optimal management for patients with multivessel disease in the DES era.

SYNTAX study

The relevance of the previous randomized trials comparing PCI with CABG might be disputable for the following reasons. First, they might not mirror the "real world" because only 2–12% of the patients screened were actually randomized as a result of numerous exclusion criteria and disagreement between the surgeons and the interventional cardiologists [4]; In the "real world," both interventional cardiologists and surgeons are often confronted with complex

anatomy. Second, patients are heterogeneous in terms of severity of coronary artery disease and lesion complexity. For example, a patient with a distal left main trifurcation lesion and an occluded right coronary artery is routinely classified as having "three-vessel disease," as is a patient with three focal lesions in the midportions of the three major coronary arteries. However, the former clearly poses a greater therapeutic challenge for the interventional cardiologist and has a different prognosis from the latter regardless of the revascularization strategy.

Taking these arguments into consideration, the Synergy between Percutaneous Coronary Intervention with Taxus and Cardiac Surgery (SYNTAX) study was planned. SYNTAX is a prospective, multicenter, multinational, randomized clinical trial with an all-comers design [63]. The overall study goal of SYNTAX is to assess the best revascularization treatment for patients with *de novo* three-vessel or left main artery disease by randomizing patients (1:1) to either CABG or PCI using paclitaxel-eluting TAXUS (Express2) stents (Boston Scientific, Natick, MA, USA). Patients were included only if the multidisciplinary medical/surgical conference (the so-called "heart team" conference) determined that equivalent anatomic revascularization could be achieved with either treatment; patients amenable to only one (but not both) treatment option(s) were entered into parallel nested registries (CABG registry for PCI-ineligible patients, $n = 1077$; PCI registry for CABG-ineligible patients, $n = 198$). A noninferiority comparison was performed on the primary end point of binary 12-month MACCE (all-cause death, stroke, myocardial infarction, or revascularization). At 1 year, there were no significant differences between the two treatment groups in all-cause death or myocardial infarction. Strokes were significantly increased in CABG patients ($P = 0.003$), whereas repeat revascularization increased in the PCI arm ($P < 0.001$), causing a significantly higher combined MACCE rate at 12 months overall and in the three-vessel disease cohort. At 1 year, the difference in MACCE rates between PCI and CABG for left main disease or three-vessel disease was 5.5% (upper one-sided CI 8.3%). The prespecified delta was 6.6%, indicating that PCI could not achieve noninferiority to CABG in this patient population.

Of note, SYNTAX employs a unique scoring system named the "SYNTAX score" to quantify the complexity of coronary artery disease [64–67]. It focuses not only on the number of significant lesions and their location, but also on the complexity of each lesion independently. The SYNTAX score is calculated using dedicated software that integrates (1) the number of lesions with their specific weighting factors based on the amount of myocardium distal to the lesion, according to the score of Leaman et al. [68], and (2) the morphologic features of each single lesion, as previously reported [64].

The development of the SYNTAX score should provide guidance to physicians as a predictive tool on the optimal revascularization strategy for patients with multivessel disease as well as left main disease. Although it is an exploratory and hypothesis-generating analysis, the 1-year outcome of the randomized cohort in the SYNTAX trial was stratified according to the SYNTAX score tertiles (Fig. 38.5) [69]. These data would suggest that patients with a low SYNTAX score, regardless of the presence of left main stem disease or three-vessel disease, have similar outcomes after revascularization with PCI or CABG. Thus, the selected revascularization strategy in this group of patients will depend on individual patient characteristics, patient preference, and the physician choice. Patients with three-vessel disease and intermediate SYNTAX scores had a higher MACCE rate after PCI than bypass surgery [70,63]. Ultimately, the final treatment selection in this group will depend on patient characteristics and comorbidity; however, PCI remains as a valid treatment option for those patients with left main disease (Fig. 38.5b). The MACCE rate in patients with high SYNTAX scores (> 33) was significantly higher in PCI than in CABG patients, and therefore it is inferred that PCI is typically limited by a higher

repeat revascularization rate and might be considered as surgical candidates (Fig. 38.5c).

CARDIA

The Coronary Artery Revascularisation in Diabetes (CARDIA) study is a prospective, randomized, multicenter UK investigation of 510 patients with diabetes and is designed to address the hypothesis that PCI with an SES is not inferior to CABG as a revascularization strategy [71]. Preliminary results of the CARDIA trial at 1 year demonstrated no significant difference between CABG and PCI in the composite end points of death, nonfatal myocardial infarction, and nonfatal stroke (10.2% vs. 11.6%, $P = 0.63$) [72]. The individual end point of death (CABG 3.3% vs. PCI 3.2%, $P = 0.83$), nonfatal myocardial infarction (5.7% vs. 8.4%, $P = 0.25$), and nonfatal stroke (2.5% vs. 0.4%, $P = 0.09$) was similar to CABG and PCI but repeat revascularization was higher in the PCI group (9.9%) than in the CABG group (2.0%). When CABG was compared with a subgroup of 179 PCI patients treated with an SES, the composite end point of death, nonfatal myocardial infarction, and nonfatal stroke was 10.2% versus 10.1% ($P = 0.98$). These results would suggest that PCI could be an alternative to CABG in selected patients with diabetes and multivessel coronary artery disease.

Ongoing trials

The Future Revascularization Evaluation in Patients with Diabetes Mellitus: Optimal Management of Multivessel Disease (FREEDOM) trial, a randomized, unblinded, two-sided superiority trial, is enrolling at least 2000 patients with diabetes who have multivessel disease. They are randomized on a 1:1 basis to either CABG or multivessel stenting, using a sirolimus-eluting stent (SES) or a paclitaxel-eluting stent (PES), and observed at 30 days, 1 year, and annually for up to 5 years [73].

Technical aspects

Which lesion should be treated?

Revascularization of a coronary stenosis is indicated if objective evidence of reversible ischemia is present [74,75]. The recommended diagnostic approach includes a number of noninvasive cardiac stress imaging techniques. However, in patients with multivessel coronary artery disease, these noninvasive imaging studies are limited in their ability to localize culprit vessels or lesions [76]. For example, only a minority of patients with severe three-vessel disease exhibit a "multivessel pattern" at gated single-photon emission computed tomography (SPECT) myocardial perfusion imaging [77]. An intracoronary hemodynamic technique, such as fractional flow reserve (FFR), can selectively determine the physiologic significance of a coronary stenosis. It is derived from the ratio of coronary to aortic pressure measurement during maximal

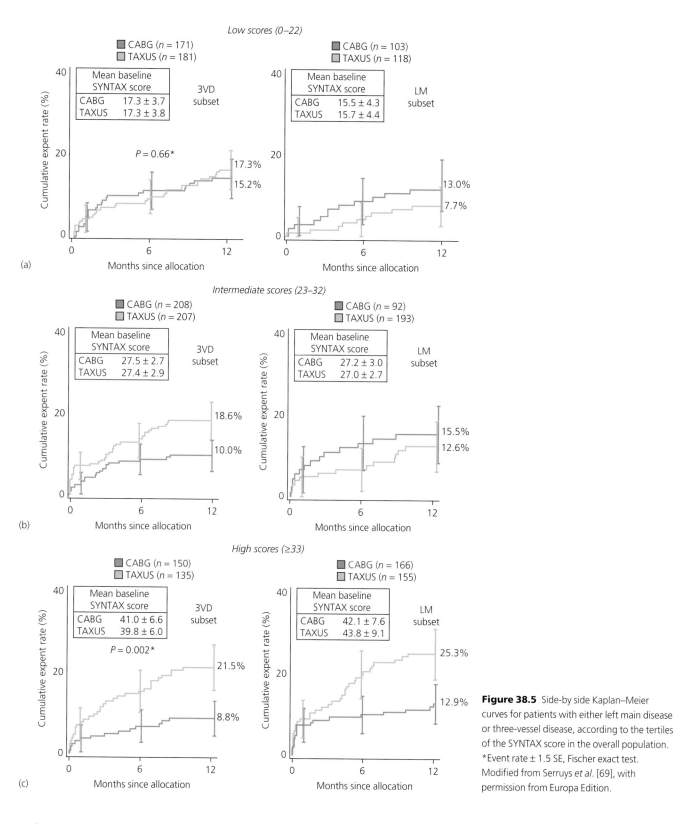

Figure 38.5 Side-by side Kaplan–Meier curves for patients with either left main disease or three-vessel disease, according to the tertiles of the SYNTAX score in the overall population. *Event rate ± 1.5 SE, Fischer exact test. Modified from Serruys *et al.* [69], with permission from Europa Edition.

hyperemia [78]. This technique may be especially useful in a vessel with multiple sequential lesions to help identify which of the potential target lesions require treatment and which can be left alone.

In patients with multivessel disease at angiography, FFR may be superior to SPECT perfusion in detecting a high risk of stenosis for revascularization. Chamuleau *et al.* [79,80] analyzed the clinical follow-up of patients with multivessel disease in whom the myocardial SPECT perfusion imaging showed no perfusion defect in a region supplied by an angiographically intermediate stenosis and in which FFR had been measured. The decision to perform PCI was based on the results of the perfusion scintigram, even if the FFR result was <0.75. The investigators showed that the event rate was significantly higher (relative risk of 3.1) when revascularization was not performed in lesions with an FFR <0.75 but with a normal perfusion scintigram.

Deferral of PCI, based on an FFR cut-off point of 0.75, has been associated with a favorable outcome in patients with multivessel disease [81]. Furthermore, FFR measurements during cardiac catheterization can assist decision-making regarding performing PCI within the same procedure. In the study by Berger et al. [81] of 102 patients with multivessel disease, in whom at least one vessel was treated by PCI and at least one other vessel with an FFR ≥0.75 was deferred, untreated lesions with an FFR ≥0.75 required PCI in 5.9% and 6.3% after 1 and 3 years, respectively. Another retrospective study by Wongpraprut et al. [82] of patients with multivessel disease undergoing PCI compared a group ($n=80$) of patients who underwent PCI based on angiographic guidance with another group ($n=57$) of patients who underwent PCI based on FFR guidance. The average number of vessels treated with PCI and the cost of the procedure were significantly greater in the angiographic-guided group than in the FFR-guided cohort. The 30-month event-free survival was significantly better in the FFR-guided group.

To further compare the clinical outcomes and cost-effectiveness of an FFR-guided PCI strategy to an angiography-guided one in patients with multivessel disease, the FFR Angiography for Multivessel Evaluation (FAME) study was initiated. This was a large, multicenter, randomized trial enrolling 1005 patients to receive PCI with the implantation of DESs guided by either angiography alone or by angiography and FFR measurements [83,84]. In patients assigned to angiography-guided PCI, all indicated lesions were stented, whereas in those assigned to FFR-guided PCI indicated lesions were stented only if the FFR was ≤0.80. The 1-year event rate (death, nonfatal myocardial infarction, and repeat revascularization) was significantly lower in the FFR group (13.2%) than in the angiography group (18.3%, $P=0.02$). Seventy-eight percent of patients in the angiography group were free from angina at 1 year, compared with 81% of patients in the FFR group ($P = 0.20$). Routine measurement of FFR in patients with multivessel disease receiving PCI with DESs, therefore, might reduce the rate of adverse cardiac events at 1 year.

Technical challenge of percutaneous coronary intervention to overcome chronic total occlusions

The presence of a CTO has remained the highest hurdle and the most important technical challenge to overcome to achieve complete revascularization with PCI. CTOs occur relatively frequently, appearing in up to 20% of patients undergoing diagnostic coronary angiography, and constituting 10% of PCIs in the contemporary practice of a tertiary referral catheterization laboratory. Historically, the success rate of crossing CTOs approximates to 60% with conventional techniques [85]. This success rate is dependent on operator experience, the number of attempts performed, anatomic considerations, and the choice of devices available.

Parallel with the emergence of the DES, numerous devices have been developed for the percutaneous treatment of CTOs. Multislice computed tomography coronary angiography has provided additional information such as occlusion length and degree of calcification, and features that predict procedural success and that are often underestimated by conventional coronary angiography [86]. In the randomized TOTAL trial (total Occlusion Trial with Angioplasty by using Laser Guidewire), laser-tipped guidewires were no better than conventional wires [87]. Local delivery of thrombolytic therapy to the site of occlusion via a specialized catheter to facilitate wire crossing was recently reported with promising results [88]. New devices in development include a blunt dissection catheter, a helical screw-like-tipped microcatheter, and a specific system that uses optical coherence reflectometry together with radiofrequency ablation. The retrograde approach using collaterals is also regarded as promising [89–92]. However, high rates of technical success do not result in high rates of procedural success, including the avoidance of complications.

After successful recanalization, the implantation of DES has been shown to improve the midterm outcome of patients with CTOs. Three registries, all with angiographic follow-up, convincingly demonstrate a sustained reduction in restenosis rates, need for reintervention, and occurrence of MACCE with DESs compared with BMSs [85,93,94]. In the recent randomized PRISON II trial (Primary Stenting of Totally Occluded Native Coronary Arteries II), Suttorp et al. [95] showed that the use of SESs was superior to using BMSs, with a significant reduction in angiographic binary in-segment restenosis (SES 11% vs. BMS 41%, $P < 0.0001$), resulting in significantly less necessity for target lesion revascularization.

Conclusion

As outlined above, there is little evidence to believe that PCI would imply a better survival in the general population with multivessel disease. With DESs as well as the multitude of new devices and techniques to overcome CTOs, the ongoing trials will provide new contemporary data on the completeness of revascularization and outcomes in patients randomized to CABG or PCI in multivessel coronary disease. Until the results of these trials are published, the indication for PCI in patients with multivessel disease should be based on the patients' individual risk and anatomy.

References

1. Gruntzig AR, Senning A, & Siegenthaler WE (1979) Nonoperative dilatation of coronary-artery stenosis: percutaneous transluminal coronary angioplasty. *N Engl J Med* **301**:61–68.

2. Favaloro RG (1968) Saphenous vein autograft replacement of severe segmental coronary artery occlusion: operative technique. *Ann Thorac Surg* **5**:334–339.

3. Serruys PW, Unger F, Sousa JE, *et al.* (2001) Comparison of coronary-artery bypass surgery and stenting for the treatment of multivessel disease. *N Engl J Med* **344**:1117–1124.

4. Hoffman SN, TenBrook JA, Wolf MP, Pauker SG, Salem DN, & Wong JB (2003) A meta-analysis of randomized controlled trials comparing coronary artery bypass graft with percutaneous transluminal coronary angioplasty: one- to eight-year outcomes. *J Am Coll Cardiol* **41**:1293–1304.

5. Serruys PW, Ong AT, van Herwerden LA, *et al.* (2005) Five-year outcomes after coronary stenting versus bypass surgery for the treatment of multivessel disease: the final analysis of the Arterial Revascularization Therapies Study (ARTS) randomized trial. *J Am Coll Cardiol* **46**:575–581.

6. Smith SC Jr, Feldman TE, Hirshfeld JW Jr, *et al.* (2006) ACC/AHA/SCAI (2005) Guideline Update for Percutaneous Coronary Intervention—summary article: a report of the American College of Cardiology/American Heart Association Task Force on Practice Guidelines (ACC/AHA/SCAI Writing Committee to Update the (2001) Guidelines for Percutaneous Coronary Intervention). *Circulation* **113**:156–175.

7. Coronary angioplasty versus coronary artery bypass surgery: the Randomized Intervention Treatment of Angina (RITA) trial. *Lancet* (1993) **341**:573–580.

8. King SB 3rd, Lembo NJ, Weintraub WS, *et al.* (1994) A randomized trial comparing coronary angioplasty with coronary bypass surgery. Emory Angioplasty versus Surgery Trial (EAST). *N Engl J Med* **331**:1044–1050.

9. Hamm CW, Reimers J, Ischinger T, Rupprecht HJ, Berger J, & Bleifeld W (1994) A randomized study of coronary angioplasty compared with bypass surgery in patients with symptomatic multivessel coronary disease. German Angioplasty Bypass Surgery Investigation (GABI). *N Engl J Med* **331**:1037–1043.

10. First-year results of CABRI (Coronary Angioplasty versus Bypass Revascularisation Investigation). CABRI Trial Participants. *Lancet* (1995) **346**:1179–1184.

11. Bypass Angioplasty Revascularization Investigation (BARI) Investigators. (1996) Comparison of coronary bypass surgery with angioplasty in patients with multivessel disease. *N Engl J Med* **335**:217–225.

12. Rodriguez A, Mele E, Peyregne E, *et al.* (1996) Three-year follow-up of the Argentine Randomized Trial of Percutaneous Transluminal Coronary Angioplasty Versus Coronary Artery Bypass Surgery in Multivessel Disease (ERACI). *J Am Coll Cardiol* **27**:1178–1184.

13. Sim I, Gupta M, McDonald K, Bourassa MG, & Hlatky MA (1995) A meta-analysis of randomized trials comparing coronary artery bypass grafting with percutaneous transluminal coronary angioplasty in multivessel coronary artery disease. *Am J Cardiol* **76**:1025–1029.

14. Pocock SJ, Henderson RA, Rickards AF, *et al.* (1995) Meta-analysis of randomised trials comparing coronary angioplasty with bypass surgery. *Lancet* **346**:1184–1189.

15. Bypass Angioplasty Revascularization Investigation (BARI) Investigators. (2007) The final 10-year follow-up results from the BARI randomized trial. *J Am Coll Cardiol* **49**:1600–1606.

16. Fischman DL, Leon MB, Baim DS, *et al.* (1994) A randomized comparison of coronary-stent placement and balloon angioplasty in the treatment of coronary artery disease. Stent Restenosis Study Investigators. *N Engl J Med* **331**:496–501.

17. Serruys PW, de Jaegere P, Kiemeneij F, *et al.* (1994) A comparison of balloon-expandable-stent implantation with balloon angioplasty in patients with coronary artery disease. Benestent Study Group. *N Engl J Med* **331**:489–495.

18. Rodriguez A, Bernardi V, Navia J, *et al.* (2001) Argentine Randomized Study: Coronary Angioplasty with Stenting versus Coronary Bypass Surgery in patients with Multiple-Vessel Disease (ERACI II): 30-day and one-year follow-up results. ERACI II Investigators. *J Am Coll Cardiol* **37**:51–58.

19. SoS Investigators (2002) Coronary artery bypass surgery versus percutaneous coronary intervention with stent implantation in patients with multivessel coronary artery disease (the Stent or Surgery trial): a randomised controlled trial. *Lancet* **360**:965–970.

20. Morrison DA, Sethi G, Sacks J, *et al.* (2002) Percutaneous coronary intervention versus repeat bypass surgery for patients with medically refractory myocardial ischemia: AWESOME randomized trial and registry experience with post-CABG patients. *J Am Coll Cardiol* **40**:1951–1954.

21. Hueb W, Lopes NH, Gersh BJ, *et al.* (2007) Five-year follow-up of the Medicine, Angioplasty, or Surgery Study (MASS II): a randomized controlled clinical trial of 3 therapeutic strategies for multivessel coronary artery disease. *Circulation* **115**:1082–1089.

22. Mercado N, Wijns W, Serruys PW, *et al.* (2005) One-year outcomes of coronary artery bypass graft surgery versus percutaneous coronary intervention with multiple stenting for multisystem disease: a meta-analysis of individual patient data from randomized clinical trials. *J Thorac Cardiovasc Surg* **130**:512–519.

23. Daemen J, Boersma E, Flather M, *et al.* (2008) Long-term safety and efficacy of percutaneous coronary intervention with stenting and coronary artery bypass surgery for multivessel coronary artery disease: a meta-analysis with 5-year Patient Level Data from the ARTS, ERACI-II, MASS-II and SoS trials. *Circulation* **118**:1146–1154.

24. Hlatky MA, Boothroyd DB, Bravata DM, *et al.* (2009) Coronary artery bypass surgery compared with percutaneous coronary interventions for multivessel disease: a collaborative analysis of individual patient data from ten randomised trials. *Lancet* **373**:1190–1197.

25. Hannan EL, Racz MJ, Walford G, *et al.* (2005) Long-term outcomes of coronary-artery bypass grafting versus stent implantation. *N Engl J Med* **352**:2174–2183.

26. Tyras DH, Kaiser GC, Barner HB, Pennington DG, Codd JE, & Willman VL (1984) Global left ventricular impairment and myocardial revascularization: determinants of survival. *Ann Thorac Surg* **37**:47–51.

27. Schaff HV, Gersh BJ, Pluth JR, *et al.* (1983) Survival and functional status after coronary artery bypass grafting: results 10 to 12 years after surgery in 500 patients. *Circulation* **68**:II200–204.

28. Cosgrove DM, Loop FD, Lytle BW, *et al.* (1985) Determinants of 10-year survival after primary myocardial revascularization. *Ann Surg* **202**:480–490.

29. Buda AJ, Macdonald IL, Anderson MJ, Strauss HD, David TE, & Berman ND (1981) Long-term results following coronary bypass operation. Importance of preoperative actors and complete revascularization. *J Thorac Cardiovasc Surg* **82**:383–390.

30. Bell MR, Gersh BJ, Schaff HV, *et al.* (1992) Effect of completeness of revascularization on long-term outcome of patients with three-vessel disease undergoing coronary artery bypass surgery. A report from the Coronary Artery Surgery Study (CASS) Registry. *Circulation* **86**:446–457.

31. McLellan CS, Ghali WA, Labinaz M, *et al.* (2005) Association between completeness of percutaneous coronary revascularization and postprocedure outcomes. *Am Heart J* **150**:800–806.

32. Kip KE, Bourassa MG, Jacobs AK, *et al.* (1999) Influence of pre-PTCA strategy and initial PTCA result in patients with multivessel disease: the Bypass Angioplasty Revascularization Investigation (BARI). *Circulation* **100**:910–917.

33. Ijsselmuiden AJ, Ezechiels J, Westendorp IC, *et al.* (2004) Complete versus culprit vessel percutaneous coronary intervention in multivessel disease: a randomized comparison. *Am Heart J* **148**:467–474.

34. Bourassa MG, Yeh W, Holubkov R, Sopko G, & Detre KM (1998) Long-term outcome of patients with incomplete vs. complete revascularization after multivessel PTCA. A report from the NHLBI PTCA Registry. *Eur Heart J* **19**:103–111.

35. Bourassa MG, Holubkov R, Yeh W, & Detre KM (1992) Strategy of complete revascularization in patients with multivessel coronary artery disease (a report from the 1985–1986 NHLBI PTCA Registry). *Am J Cardiol* **70**:174–178.

36. van den Brand MJ, Rensing BJ, Morel MA, *et al.* (2002) The effect of completeness of revascularization on event-free survival at one year in the ARTS trial. *J Am Coll Cardiol* **39**:559–564.

37. Serruys PW, Rensing BJ, Brand MVD, Wittebols K, & Morice M-C (2008) Completeness of revascularisation and event free survival in the ARTS II trial. Paper presented at the SCAI Annual Scientific Sessions in Partnership with ACC i2 Summit. Chicago, IL.

38. Hlatky MA, Boothroyd DB, Melsop KA, *et al.* (2004) Medical costs and quality of life 10 to 12 years after randomization to angioplasty or bypass surgery for multivessel coronary artery disease. *Circulation* **110**:1960–1966.

39. Weintraub WS, Becker ER, Mauldin PD, Culler S, Kosinski AS, & King SB 3rd (2000) Costs of revascularization over eight years in the randomized and eligible patients in the Emory Angioplasty versus Surgery Trial (EAST). *Am J Cardiol* **86**:747–752.

40. Favarato D, Hueb W, Gersh BJ, *et al.* (2003) Relative cost comparison of treatments for coronary artery disease: the first year follow-up of MASS II Study. *Circulation* **108**(Suppl. 1): II21–23.

41. Legrand VM, Serruys PW, Unger F, *et al.* (2004) Three-year outcome after coronary stenting versus bypass surgery for the treatment of multivessel disease. *Circulation* **109**:1114–1120.

42. Rodriguez AE, Baldi J, Fernandez Pereira C, *et al.* (2005) Five-year follow-up of the Argentine randomized trial of coronary angioplasty with stenting versus coronary bypass surgery in patients with multiple vessel disease (ERACI II). *J Am Coll Cardiol* **46**:582–588.

43. West NE, Ruygrok PN, Disco CM, *et al.* (2004) Clinical and angiographic predictors of restenosis after stent deployment in diabetic patients. *Circulation* **109**:867–873.

44. Thourani VH, Weintraub WS, Stein B, *et al.* (1999) Influence of diabetes mellitus on early and late outcome after coronary artery bypass grafting. *Ann Thorac Surg* **67**:1045–1052.

45. Niles NW, McGrath PD, Malenka D, *et al.* (2001) Survival of patients with diabetes and multivessel coronary artery disease after surgical or percutaneous coronary revascularization: results of a large regional prospective study. Northern New England Cardiovascular Disease Study Group. *J Am Coll Cardiol* **37**: 1008–1015.

46. Kip KE, Faxon DP, Detre KM, Yeh W, Kelsey SF, & Currier JW (1996) Coronary angioplasty in diabetic patients. The National Heart, Lung, and Blood Institute Percutaneous Transluminal Coronary Angioplasty Registry. *Circulation* **94**:1818–1825.

47. Detre KM, Guo P, Holubkov R, *et al.* (1999) Coronary revascularization in diabetic patients: a comparison of the randomized and observational components of the Bypass Angioplasty Revascularization Investigation (BARI). *Circulation* **99**:633–640.

48. King SB:3rd, Kosinski AS, Guyton RA, Lembo NJ, & Weintraub WS (2000) Eight-year mortality in the Emory Angioplasty versus Surgery Trial (EAST). *J Am Coll Cardiol* **35**:1116–1121.

49. Babapulle MN, Joseph L, Belisle P, Brophy JM, & Eisenberg MJ (2004) A hierarchical Bayesian meta-analysis of randomised clinical trials of drug-eluting stents. *Lancet* 364:583–91.

50. Dauerman HL (2006) Overview: drug-eluting stents. *Coron Artery Dis* **17**:657–659.

51. Roiron C, Sanchez P, Bouzamondo A, Lechat P, & Montalescot G (2006) Drug-eluting stents: an updated meta-analysis of randomised controlled trials. *Heart* **92**:641–649.

52. Stone GW, Ellis SG, Cannon L, *et al.* (2005) Comparison of a polymer-based paclitaxel-eluting stent with a bare metal stent in patients with complex coronary artery disease: a randomized controlled trial. *JAMA* **294**:1215–1223.

53. Daemen J, Ong AT, Stefanini GG, *et al.* (2006) Three-year clinical follow-up of the unrestricted use of sirolimus-eluting stents as part of the Rapamycin-Eluting Stent Evaluated at Rotterdam Cardiology Hospital (RESEARCH) registry. *Am J Cardiol* **98**:895–901.

54. Beohar N, Davidson CJ, Kip KE, *et al.* (2007) Outcomes and complications associated with off-label and untested use of drug-eluting stents. *JAMA* **297**:1992–2000.

55. Ferguson TB Jr, Hammill BG, Peterson ED, DeLong ER, & Grover FL (2002) A decade of change—risk profiles and outcomes for isolated coronary artery bypass grafting procedures, 1990–1999: a report from the STS National Database Committee and the Duke Clinical Research Institute. Society of Thoracic Surgeons. *Ann Thorac Surg* **73**:480–489; discussion 489–490.

56. Nishida H, Tomizawa Y, Endo M, & Kurosawa H (2005) Survival benefit of exclusive use of in situ arterial conduits over combined use of arterial and vein grafts for multiple coronary artery bypass grafting. *Circulation* **112**:I299–303.

57. Serruys PW, Ong ATL, Morice M-C, *et al.* (2005) Arterial Revascularisation Therapies Study Part II—Sirolimus-eluting stents for the treatment of patients with multivessel de novo coronary artery lesions. *EuroIntervention* **1**:147–156.

58. Serruys PW, Daemen J, Morice M-C, *et al.* (2007) Three-year follow-up of the ARTS-II–sirolimus-eluting stents for the treatment of patients with multivessel coronary artery disease. *EuroIntervention* **3**:450–459.

59. Rodriguez AE, Maree AO, Grinfeld L, *et al.* (2006) Revascularization strategies of coronary multiple vessel disease in the Drug-eluting stent Era: one year follow-up results of the ERACI III Trial. *EuroIntervention* **2**:53–60.

60. Hannan EL, Wu C, Walford G, *et al.* (2008) Drug-eluting stents vs. coronary-artery bypass grafting in multivessel coronary disease. *N Engl J Med* **358**:331–341.

61. Javaid A, Steinberg DH, Buch AN, *et al.* (2007) Outcomes of coronary artery bypass grafting versus percutaneous coronary intervention with drug-eluting stents for patients with multivessel coronary artery disease. *Circulation* **116**:I200–206.

62. Varani E, Balducelli M, Vecchi G, Aquilina M, & Maresta A (2007) Comparison of multiple drug-eluting stent percutaneous coronary intervention and surgical revascularization in patients with multivessel coronary artery disease: one-year clinical results and total treatment costs. *J Invasive Cardiol* **19**:469–475.

63. Serruys PW, Morice MC, Kappetein AP, *et al.* (2009) Percutaneous coronary intervention versus coronary-artery bypass grafting for severe coronary artery disease. *N Engl J Med* **360**:961–972.

64. Sianos G, Morel M-A, Kappetein AP, *et al.* (2005) The SYNTAX Score: an angiographic tool grading the complexity of coronary artery disease. *EuroIntervention* **1**:219–227.

65. Valgimigli M, Serruys PW, Tsuchida K, *et al.* (2007) Cyphering the complexity of coronary artery disease using the syntax score to predict clinical outcome in patients with three-vessel lumen obstruction undergoing percutaneous coronary intervention. *Am J Cardiol* **99**:1072–1081.

66. Ong AT, Serruys PW, Mohr FW, *et al.* (2006) The SYNergy between percutaneous coronary intervention with TAXus and cardiac surgery (SYNTAX) study: design, rationale, and run-in phase. *Am Heart J* **151**:1194–1204.

67. Kappetein AP, Dawkins KD, Mohr FW, *et al.* (2006) Current percutaneous coronary intervention and coronary artery bypass grafting practices for three-vessel and left main coronary artery disease. Insights from the SYNTAX run-in phase. *Eur J Cardiothorac Surg* **29**:486–491.

68. Leaman DM, Brower RW, Meester GT, Serruys P, & van den Brand M (1981) Coronary artery atherosclerosis: severity of the disease, severity of angina pectoris and compromised left ventricular function. *Circulation* **63**:285–299.

69. Serruys PW, Onuma Y, Garg S, *et al.* (2009) Assessment of the SYNTAX score in the Syntax study. *EuroIntervention* **5**:50–56.

70. Banning AP, Westaby S, Morice MC, *et al.* (2009) Diabetic and nondiabetic patients with left main and/or 3-vessel coronary artery disease: comparison of outcomes with cardiac surgery and paclitaxel-eluting stents. *J Am Coll Cardiol*. In-press.

71. Kapur A, Malik IS, Bagger JP, *et al.* (2005) The Coronary Artery Revascularisation in Diabetes (CARDia) trial: background, aims, and design. *Am Heart J* **149**:13–19.

72. Kapur A (2008) Coronary Artery Revascularisation in Diabetes. The CARDia trial. Munich: European Society of Cardiology Congress 2008.

73. Farkouh ME, Dangas G, Leon MB, *et al.* (2008) Design of the Future REvascularization Evaluation in patients with Diabetes mellitus: Optimal management of Multivessel disease (FREEDOM) Trial. *Am Heart J* **155**:215–223.

74. (2008) 2007 Focused update of the ACC/AHA/SCAI 2005 guideline update for percutaneous coronary intervention. A report of the American College of Cardiology/American Heart Association Task Force on Practice Guidelines. *Catheter Cardiovasc Interv* **71**:E1–40.

75. Silber S, Albertsson P, Aviles FF, *et al.* (2005) Guidelines for percutaneous coronary interventions. The Task Force for Percutaneous Coronary Interventions of the European Society of Cardiology. *Eur Heart J* **26**:804–847.

76. Lima RS, Watson DD, Goode AR, *et al.* (2003) Incremental value of combined perfusion and function over perfusion alone by gated SPECT myocardial perfusion imaging for detection of severe three-vessel coronary artery disease. *J Am Coll Cardiol* **42**:64–70.

77. Pijls NH, De Bruyne B, Peels K, *et al.* (1996) Measurement of fractional flow reserve to assess the functional severity of coronary-artery stenoses. *N Engl J Med* **334**:1703–1708.

78. Pijls NH, van Son JA, Kirkeeide RL, De Bruyne B, & Gould KL (1993) Experimental basis of determining maximum coronary, myocardial, and collateral blood flow by pressure measurements for assessing functional stenosis severity before and after percutaneous transluminal coronary angioplasty. *Circulation* **87**:1354–1367.

79. Chamuleau SA, Meuwissen M, Koch KT, *et al.* (2002) Usefulness of fractional flow reserve for risk stratification of patients with multivessel coronary artery disease and an intermediate stenosis. *Am J Cardiol* **89**:377–380.

80. Chamuleau SA, Meuwissen M, van Eck-Smit BL, *et al.* (2001) Fractional flow reserve, absolute and relative coronary blood flow velocity reserve in relation to the results of technetium-99m sestamibi single-photon emission computed tomography in patients with two-vessel coronary artery disease. *J Am Coll Cardiol* **37**:1316–1322.

81. Berger A, Botman KJ, MacCarthy PA, *et al.* (2005) Long-term clinical outcome after fractional flow reserve-guided percutaneous coronary intervention in patients with multivessel disease. *J Am Coll Cardiol* **46**:438–442.

82. Wongpraparut N, Yalamanchili V, Pasnoori V, *et al.* (2005) Thirty-month outcome after fractional flow reserve-guided versus conventional multivessel percutaneous coronary intervention. *Am J Cardiol* **96**:877–884.

83. Fearon WF, Tonino PA, De Bruyne B, Siebert U, & Pijls NH (2007) Rationale and design of the Fractional Flow Reserve versus Angiography for Multivessel Evaluation (FAME) study. *Am Heart J* **154**:632–636.

84. Tonino PA, De Bruyne B, Pijls NH, *et al.* (2009) Fractional flow reserve versus angiography for guiding percutaneous coronary intervention. *N Engl J Med* **360**:213–224.

85. Hoye A, Tanabe K, Lemos PA, *et al.* (2004) Significant reduction in restenosis after the use of sirolimus-eluting stents in the treatment of chronic total occlusions. *J Am Coll Cardiol* **43**:1954–1958.

86. Mollet NR, Hoye A, Lemos PA, *et al.* (2005) Value of preprocedure multislice computed tomographic coronary angiography to predict the outcome of percutaneous recanalization of chronic total occlusions. *Am J Cardiol* **95**:240–243.

87. Serruys PW, Hamburger JN, Koolen JJ, *et al.* (2000) Total occlusion trial with angioplasty by using laser guidewire. The TOTAL trial. *Eur Heart J* **21**:1797–1805.

88. Yang YM, Mehran R, Dangas G, *et al.* (2004) Successful use of the frontrunner catheter in the treatment of in-stent coronary chronic total occlusions. *Catheter Cardiovasc Interv* **63**:462–468.

89. Mario CD, Barlis P, Tanigawa J, *et al.* (2007) Retrograde approach to coronary chronic total occlusions: preliminary single European centre experience. *EuroIntervention* **3**:181–187.

90. Kukreja N, Serruys PW, & Sianos G (2007) Retrograde recanalization of chronically occluded coronary arteries: illustration and description of the technique. *Catheter Cardiovasc Interv* **69**:833–841.

91. Carlino M, Latib A, Godino C, Cosgrave J, & Colombo A (2008) CTO recanalization by intraocclusion injection of contrast: the microchannel technique. *Catheter Cardiovasc Interv* **71**:20–26.

92. Matsumi J & Saito S (2008) Progress in the retrograde approach for chronic total coronary artery occlusion: a case with successful angioplasty using CART and reverse-anchoring techniques

3 years after failed PCI via a retrograde approach. *Catheter Cardiovasc Interv.*

93. Werner GS, Krack A, Schwarz G, Prochnau D, Betge S, & Figulla HR (2004) Prevention of lesion recurrence in chronic total coronary occlusions by paclitaxel-eluting stents. *J Am Coll Cardiol* **44**:2301–2306.

94. Ge L, Iakovou I, Cosgrave J, *et al.* (2005) Immediate and mid-term outcomes of sirolimus-eluting stent implantation for chronic total occlusions. *Eur Heart J* **26**:1056–1062.

95. Suttorp MJ, Laarman GJ, Rahel BM, *et al.* (2006) Primary Stenting of Totally Occluded Native Coronary Arteries II (PRISON II): a randomized comparison of bare metal stent implantation with sirolimus-eluting stent implantation for the treatment of total coronary occlusions. *Circulation* **114**:921–928.

39 Percutaneous Coronary Intervention for Chronic Total Occlusions

Osamu Katoh

Toyohashi Heart Center, Toyohashi, Aichi, Japan

Introduction

Percutaneous coronary intervention (PCI) in chronic total occlusions (CTOs) has not traditionally been attempted by cardiologists, although PCI has developed as an alternative therapy to coronary artery bypass graft (CABG), and many studies have indicated that the presence of a CTO is a major reason for chososing to treat patients with multivessel disease with CABG [1–5]. In fact, some studies have shown that successful PCI of CTOs can reduce the need for CABGs after PCI [5–9]. Is the major reason for this reluctance the question whether a CTO needs to be recanalized for relief of ischemia or whether PCI of CTOs can improve long-term prognosis? These are unlikely to be reasons for concern because nontotal occlusions are currently treated with PCI, despite the fact that its effectiveness in improving long-term prognosis is not yet proven. It is more likely that real reason is that PCI of CTOs is technically more difficult, sometimes leads to unsatisfactory results, and imposes additional stress and cost on both the patient and the operator. For these reasons most interventional cardiologists still have a negative attitude to the procedure [4,10], even after many studies have shown that drug-eluting stent (DES) implantation in CTOs results in favorable long-term outcomes similar to those achieved in conventional lesions [11–16]. However, in the EU and USA [17–21,39,40] experienced operators are now aggressively attempting to treat CTOs following the improvement in long-term results of CTO recanalization with PCI and DES implantation. Although they may be frustrated by current technical limitations, their efforts will undoubtedly bring about a breakthrough in the near future.

In this chapter, the basics of PCI for CTOs and the techniques involved, especially wire techniques currently used for recanalizing a CTO, are reported. In addition, retrograde approaches to CTOs are described; although this approach is largely still under development, it will play a role in the future of CTO PCI.

Cardiovascular Interventions in Clinical Practice. Edited by Jürgen Haase, Hans-Joachim Schäfers, Horst Sievert and Ron Waksman. © 2010 Blackwell Publishing.

Clinical indication and technical consideration

Clinical indication

Because the aim of CTO recanalization is relief of ischemia and improvement of prognosis, objective assessment of ischemia and viable myocardium in the territory of the CTO vessel is imperative for the clinical indication for CTO PCI. However, it should be taken into account that clinical detection of hibernating myocardium, which is usually caused by a CTO, is often difficult on routine examination, especially in patients with multivessel disease (MVD) complicated by congestive heart failure (CHF) [21,22]. The results of the recently published Open Artery Trial (OAT) [23–26] and other studies had a negative impact on the clinical indications for CTO PCI, although interpretation of the data is still subject to debate.

For indications of CTO PCI, not only clinical but also technical considerations, including the possibility of maintaining long-term patency after recanalization, and anatomical factors affecting recanalization, should be considered.

Technical consideration

Although relief of ischemia clearly results in symptom improvement, particularly in patients with single-vessel disease, the effect of revascularization on long-term prognosis is unclear [6,7,24,27–29]. Consequently, a difficult case to decide on CTO recanalization is the patient with MVD in whom CTOs are found incidentally but cannot be proven to be the cause of the ischemia. In the past these patients have received bypass surgery because of the technical difficulties associated with PCI of CTOs [1,4]. Thus, the development of CTO PCI techniques and operator skill remain the major influence on the decision-making process, despite the the drastic reduction in restenosis and reocclusion rates that have been achieved with DESs. Although determining the indication for CTO recanalization in patients with MVD complicated by CHF is difficult, the indication criteria for those patients could be changed by improvements in methods of assessing residual myocardium, such as MRI, and by technical improvements in CTO PCI.

Increasingly, a potential candidate for CTO PCI is the patient with CTO of the native coronary artery after CABG. Instead of performing PCI of the degenerated saphenous vein graft (SVG), the development of technique would enable CTO PCI in the native artery, previously considered to be technically difficult, to be achieved.

It should be emphasized that the indication for CTO PCI continues to change with development of CTO PCI because it is dependent on the balance between clinical indication and technical consideration.

Definition and classification of chronic total occlusion

Definition of chronic total occlusion

When we discuss the technical aspects of CTO PCI, such as initial results, techniques, devices, and so on, the definition of CTO is fundamental; however, there is no formal definition of CTO. Many studies have included subtotal occlusions and recent occlusions within 2 weeks of an acute myocardial infarction (AMI) as CTOs, whereas others have included only completely occluded thrombolysis in myocardial infarction 0 (TIMI 0) CTOs of >3 months' or unknown occlusion duration. Because the clinical results of these subsets are obviously different with the current CTO PCI techniques, the difference in the CTO definition causes confusion, and comparison of CTO PCI results between studies is difficult. Recently the EuroCTO Club proposed a CTO definition which includes only the presence of TIMI 0 flow within the occluded segment with an estimated occlusion duration of >3 months. They discussed the detailed definition of CTO and described their consensus on the definition in their consensus document [20]. Japanese CTO experts accept this CTO definition and believe that it should be respected as a globally authorized definition of CTOs when studying and discussing clinical aspects of CTO PCI.

Classification of chronic total occlusion

Chronic total occlusions involve every kind of coronary lesion (diffuse, small vessel, bifurcation, take-off, calcified, thrombotic lesions, etc.), because CTOs are caused by plaque disruption, which can occur in any kind of lesion, followed by thrombosis with the growth of the thrombi toward the proximal and the distal lumens and eventually leading to organized thrombus. The structure of the CTO plaque also varies because of the different processes involved in its formation. Thus, proper classification of CTOs is necessary to clarify the kind of CTO targeted by devices or techniques when developing CTO devices and discussing technical aspects of CTO PCI. The influential anatomical factors on CTO crossing already reported are applicable to the classification CTOs according to the difficulty level in crossing [6,28]. In the EuroCTO Club consensus document, a reasonable classification is reported. However, 64-multislice computed tomography (MSCT) has recently

been used for the evaluation of CTO plaque and provides valuable information that, in the past, could not be obtained before the procedure [30,31]. The information about CTO structure provided by MSCT (calcium distribution inside the thrombus, vessel size and true extent of occlusion, three-dimensional [3-D] reconstruction of the affected vessel, identifying CTO entry point, and plaque distribution in the segment distal to the CTO) should be applied to CTO classification so that a more detailed classification system reflecting real difficulties of CTO procedures can be established.

Pathology

Neovascular channels have been emphasized as a pathologic finding in CTOs related to wire crossing [32,33]. The neovascular channels connecting to the distal lumen, often seen in tapered CTOs, is considered the basis for wire crossing in CTOs. However, intimal neovasculature in an old CTO with no stump connects to adventitial neovascular channels and not to the distal lumen. A more important finding is that intimal neovascular channels are surrounded by loose fibrous tissue, and dense fibrous tissue exists as a bundle in cross-section, acting as a cross-wall separating loose fibrous tissues [34]. Because a stiff wire cannot follow such a tiny tortuous intimal neovascular channel (100–300 μm), it is reasonable to consider that the stiff wire goes through the loose fibrous tissue. Consequently, the dense fibrous tissue sometimes needs to be punctured by a stiff wire to negotiate a CTO through the intima. This is why the development of stiff and tapered wires has contributed to improvement in wire crossing rates. However, it is difficult to obtain this kind of information on CTO plaque structure before or during the procedure, even when using intravascular ultrasound (IVUS) or MSCT. Furthermore, a physical limitation of stiff and tapered wires is the difficulty in puncturing the cross-wall obliquely facing the tapered wire tip, even when using a stiffer tapered wire. This is a current limitation in CTO PCI elicited by the pathologic findings.

Basics for chronic total occlusion crossing

Although CTO PCI instructions usually focus on wire crossing, it is also important to prepare the conditions to enable wire or other device crossing, such as stability of the guiding catheter, wire maneuverability, and contralateral injections.

Guiding catheter/anchor technique

When selecting a guiding catheter, key points to remember are sufficient backup, stability, coaxial alignment, and low risk of ostial injury. In the LAD, an extra backup guiding catheter is useful for achieving coaxial alignment and sufficient backup, but there is the risk of ostial injury when engaging it. For the left circumflex artery (LCx), an Amplatz left 1.0 or 2.0 catheter (AL-1 or -2) is sometimes better. For the high posterior take-off left coronary artery (LCA), an AL-2 is usually better than a Judkins left catheter or extra backup. In the case of an ostial CTO in the left anterior descending artery (LAD), deep insertion of a Judkins left catheter with a short tip is effective for directing the guidewire to the CTO and providing sufficient backup [35]. In the right coronary artery (RCA), it is more important to obtain coaxial orientation to maintain wire maneuverability. A Judkins right catheter is best for this, but it is often difficult to gain sufficient backup, especially in proximal CTOs. Deep insertion of a Judkins right catheter, exchange for AL-1 or -2, with side hole or the anchor technique using a proximal side branch can be employed to improve the backup, depending on the operator's experience and the anatomy of the origin or the RCA's proximal segment.

To ensure the applicability of various techniques, such as IVUS guidewire-handling technique or the anchor balloon technique, an 8F guiding catheter is usually recommended. For easy cases, a 6F guiding catheter is acceptable. Aortic regurgitation and deterioration in wire maneuverability with the guiding catheter should be noted during the procedure. To improve wire maneuverability with coaxial orientation, the anchor balloon technique is especially useful for a proximal CTO in the RCA.

Guidewire selection/shaping

In Japan, a step-up strategy was often utilized in selecting wires for CTO crossing. However, with the development of dedicated CTO wires and various kinds of wire techniques, the steerability of the CTO wires inside the hard CTO plaque is now emphasized. Therefore, a moderately stiff wire (such as Miracle 3g, Asahi Intecc Co., Ltd., Aichi, Japan) is often chosen as a first wire. However, there are many options for CTO wire selection, as demonstrated by operators in other countries. The most important thing in CTO wire selection is that the wire should be chosen according to the lesion morphology and how you want the chosen wire to perform. Moreover, you should understand the mechanical properties of each CTO wire, the behavior of a stiff CTO wire, such as straightforward advancement, and the mechanisms of wire deflection inside the CTO plaque. In the antegrade approach, one of the keys to easy wire crossing is to avoid entering the subintima when negotiating a CTO. This is true when using either the drilling technique or the penetration technique. Therefore, a tapered stiff wire or a polymer-coated stiff wire should not be selected as a first-choice wire except for straight and short occlusions; the procedure may be quickly done using those wires but there is an increased risk of wire perforation or subintimal tracking.

A tapered soft polymer-coated wire (X-treme™/Fielder™ XT; Asahi Intecc Co., Ltd., Aichi, Japan) is increasingly used as a first choice wire, even in hard CTOs, because it is possible to make a tiny curve (0.3–0.5 mm) on the tip of this wire, which allows it to negotiate a tiny tortuous channel without subintimal tracking.

The tip curve is a crucial factor in negotiating a CTO and avoiding subintimal tracking. The channels in occluded segments are usually associated with tiny curves, even in straight vessels. The bigger tip curve of a stiff wire compared with the tiny curve in the channel results in subintimal tracking; therefore, the size of tip curve should be made as small as possible. However, limitations on the soldering length of a CTO wire often determines how small the curve can be made. It is almost impossible to make a curve < 1.5–2.0 mm at the tip of a CTO wire, although a shrunken CTO vessel with a 2.0–2.5 mm vessel diameter is often observed with IVUS. This is one of the mechanical limitations of CTO wires. A second curve is usually made to access an occluded segment. However, the second curve sometimes deteriorates the control of the wire tip. After accessing or entering a CTO, the second curve should be straightened for precise wire control if wire exchange using a microcatheter, balloon catheter, or Tornus catheter (Asahi Intech, Abbot Vascular, Redwood City, CA, USA) is possible.

Wire handling/wire technique (basics for wire handling)

Two traditional ways to handle a CTO wire are drilling and puncturing. The *drilling technique* involves alternately rotating a wire with a small tip curve clockwise and counterclockwise, always within 180°. This technique is applied for tracking a channel or loose tissue inside the CTO. The wire can be directed by regulating the rotational direction (clockwise/counterclockwise) and combining with the puncturing technique. During drilling, the wire direction should be controlled according to the vessel course extrapolated by simultaneous contralateral injections and confirmed from multiple view angles. To avoid subintimal tracking, it is crucial to repeatedly feel the resistance in the wire tip while pulling back the wire. When the wire tip is in the subintima, it will have a "sticky" sensation. The *puncturing technique* involves pushing a CTO wire, usually toward hard tissue, while avoiding deflection of the wire. This technique is employed when creating a different channel when the correct direction in which to advance the wire is recognized. Although use of a tapered stiff wire is emphasized when employing this technique, any kind of CTO wire should be used with the support of a microcatheter or balloon catheter. This technique of using a tapered stiff wire should be applied in combination with the parallel wire technique.

As mentioned above, it is sometimes difficult and unpredictable to avoid subintimal tracking with the drilling technique owing to the limitation in making a tip curve. Also, with the puncturing technique, wire deflection at the puncture site cannot always be avoided, even when using extra-stiff tapered wires, because the deflection is caused by factors other than stiffness of the tip: the difference in compliance between the hard tissue and the surrounding tissue, the puncture angle to the hard tissue, and so on. Accordingly, wire perforation and subintimal hematoma cannot always be avoided when employing these techniques. Even though no sequela usually accompanies a wire perforation, as long as it occurs in the occluded segment, a subintimal hematoma caused by wire perforation does make the procedure more difficult. These are major limitations in mechanical wire techniques.

To overcome these limitations, several wire techniques for the antegrade approach have been developed, as described below.

Special techniques in the antegrade approach

Side branch technique

If the angle between the wire direction and the distal true lumen is too large, it is quite easy to create a false lumen around the true lumen. In these cases, if there is a side branch forking at the proximal end of distal true lumen, an atttempt should be made from the beginning to advance the wire into the side branch through its ostium. This is the ideal scenario for the side branch technique. After passing the wire into the side branch, a 2.6F Tornus catheter is used to restore blood flow in the parent artery by breaking the plaque. This fracturing may cause recanalization in the parent vessel. Even if recanalization is not obtained, the relative position between the channel created and the distal true lumen can be detected by delivering an IVUS catheter into the side branch. The key point in this technique is to avoid creating a dissection with a balloon at the bifurcation and also in the occluded segment. The IVUS information is useful for returning from the side branch to the parent artery. If a connection is created by the fracturing, the CTO wire should be exchanged for a floppy coil or polymer-coated wire. If the wire goes into the side branch too far from the distal true lumen in the parent vessel, the parallel wire technique or IVUS-guided wire handling technique should be used (described below) to puncture the distal true lumen or to find a correct channel leading to the distal true lumen.

Parallel wire technique

The parallel wire technique [35] is now the standard antegrade approach after the single-wire technique has failed. It can be applied to all CTOs, irrespective of individual lesion characteristics. It is a technique that anyone can perfect as long as they follow the guidelines on wire handling. The parallel wire technique requires the insertion of a second wire into the CTO while the first one is still in place. The principle of this technique is to recognize the target (the proximal end of the distal true lumen) during wire handling using the first wire as a landmark.

Preconditions for the technique

One absolute condition for success is that the distal true lumen must be clearly visible on the angiogram so that the relative positions of the distal true lumen and first wire can be known.

The importance of a support catheter

When inserting the second wire, a 1.5-mm over-the-wire (OTW) balloon catheter, a penetration catheter, or a double-lumen catheter should be used; a bare wire should not be used. This is to avoid twisting the wires and, even more importantly, to maintain maneuverability of the second wire.

Wire handling in theory

Advance the second wire inside the CTO so as to closely follow the course of the first wire, "hugging" it as it goes. It is important to know the exact relative positions of the two wire tips. Care must be taken to ensure that the wires do not get too tangled up with each other inside the CTO, as this will cause wire twisting.

Wire handling in practice

Preferably, the second wire should be stiffer than the first, and will have superior torque transfer. The most commonly used second wires are the Miracle 12g or 6g, or Confianza Pro (Asahi Intecc Co., Ltd.; Asahi Intech, Abbot Vascular). This is, once again, to prevent twisting, to lead the second wire to the correct position for penetrating into the distal true lumen, and to reduce the risk of making a new false lumen or perforating the vessel by using the first wire to secure the position inside the CTO.

Timing and the parallel wire technique

If the single-wire attempt is unsuccessful, rather than to repeatedly and blindly attempt to get through, the parallel wire technique should be immediately employed before creating a large false lumen. This is the most important step for success.

Intravascular ultrasound guidance

The applications of IVUS [35] for wire crossing are (1) locating the true entry to the CTO in case of uncertainty after coronary angiography (CAG) (usually in CTOs at bifurcation) and landmarking this angiographically using the IVUS transducer image and indicating the correct point, and (2) real-time wire-handling guidance using the IVUS catheter, which is positioned parallel to the CTO wire. When using IVUS to locate a CTO ostium, the IVUS catheter is pulled back from the side branch and remains at the position of the ostium. An angiogram is then taken of the best view of the bifurcation and the the ostium is marked on the angiogram. IVUS can be used for leading a CTO wire and checking the entry point with an 8F guiding catheter. For real-time wire-handling guidance, an 8F guiding catheter is essential.

The following is a bailout technique after making a false lumen with a CTO wire around the distal true lumen (not applicable to bifurcation CTOs); however, too large a false lumen makes this bailout technique very difficult. In this technique, after the false lumen created by a CTO wire is dilated with a 2.0- to 2.5-mm balloon, an IVUS catheter is placed into the false lumen, usually beyond the distal end of the CTO because of the IVUS catheter nose. Thus, a phased-array IVUS catheter is usually better than a rotational IVUS catheter to minimize the extent of the distal dissection created by predilation. Using the cross-sectional view and locating the wire in the CTO plaque, the wire is longitudinally advanced using fluoroscopy. Consequently, IVUS cannot lead the wire, but the wire location in cross-section is confirmed and wire movement is tracked by IVUS. This information is essential for escaping from the subintimal space. The major role of IVUS in this technique is to locate plaque extending to the distal true lumen so that a CTO wire (usually a tapered stiff wire) can penetrate that plaque.

Use of multislice computed tomography

As described above, MSCT provides valuable information on CTO vessel structure before the procedure [30,31]. However, it is controversial whether MSCT improves the success rate of CTO crossing. Although there are limitations of MSCT, such as resolution and volume effect in calcification, information on the 3-D distribution of calcification and soft tissue, and on the 3-D structure of the occluded segment and also of the distal vessel, is useful for wire handling. These affect, especially, wire selection (first choice and wire exchange during procedure) and wire course inside a CTO imaged by an operator. MSCT will generally be used not only for preprocedural evaluation, but also as a tool to facilitate CTO crossing in the near future.

Retrograde approaches

The retrograde approach to treating coronary lesions was propounded by the Kansas City group in 1990 [36]. This approach has been traditionally used for recanalizing peripheral CTOs, especially in the iliac vessels. Therefore, it has been well known since the early 1990s that the retrograde approach sometimes facilitates wire crossing in CTOs. However, the access route for the retrograde approach to coronary CTOs was limited, and CTO crossing techniques were primitive in the 1990s. Consequently, this approach was rarely used in the coronary arteries and often failed because there were no reliable techniques for CTO crossing. In 2005, a breakthrough was made using the septal dilation technique and controlled antegrade and retrograde subintimal tracking (CART) technique, in terms of expanding the indication and establishing a reliable method for CTO crossing [37,38].

Retrograde access

For retrograde access to coronary CTOs, the saphenous vein graft (SVG) or a large collateral channel without excessive tortuosity in the atrium, epicardium, or septum has been used. Unfortunately, those access routes are rarely found. Consequently, the indication for retrograde approach has been limited. The first breakthrough was the septal dilation technique [38] and the second was a channel dilation catheter that allowed aggressive use of the epicardial collateral channels. The indication for the retrograde approach could thus be dramatically expanded because tiny collateral channels (350–500 μm in diameter) could now be used as a retrograde access route.

Septal dilation technique

This technique can be applied in 50–60% of CTOs in the RCA or LAD, although the retrograde approach is not needed in all of these cases. Figure 39.1 shows the sequence of the septal dilation technique and optical coherence tomography (OCT) findings after septal collateral channel dilation. The keys to this technique are (1) use of a small balloon (less than 1.3 mm) with sufficient hydrophilic coating for channel dilation, (2) gentle advancement of the balloon when crossing the channel, and (3) dilating the entire length of the collateral channel.

As shown in Figure 39.1, the diameter of the collateral channel after dilation with a 1.3-mm balloon is, at its maximum, 0.8–0.9 mm, so even a 1.5-mm balloon is likely too big. To avoid channel rupture using the septal dilation technique, the use of a very small balloon (0.9, 1.1, 1.25, or 1.3 mm) as well as low-pressure inflation (≤3 atm) is required. More importantly, balloon shaft kinking caused by excessive pushing should be avoided because channel rupture is often caused by the shaft kinking, especially at a bend point. Possible ways to reduce the need for strong push is to use of a good balloon with a nicely tapered tip and with an excellent and durable hydrophilic coating, and to dilate the proximal part of the channel to reduce friction when the balloon cannot be advanced. It should be noted that there is an obvious limitation in channel crossing using either a balloon catheter or a penetration catheter because the excess friction cannot be overcome by simply pushing the catheter, and channel rupture has been reported in about 5–7% of cases in the European multicenter registry [39] and a Japanese registry. To reduce the risk of rupture, a channel dilation catheter (described below) is necessary because it can cross tortuous collateral channels by rotating without the need for undue pushing. It is crucial for modern retrograde CTO crossing techniques such as CART to dilate the entire length of the septal channel to reduce friction when delivering an OTW balloon to the CTO site.

A penetrating catheter or an OTW balloon can be used for retrograde access without the septal dilation technique; however, it is not an ideal technique for ensuring CTO crossing

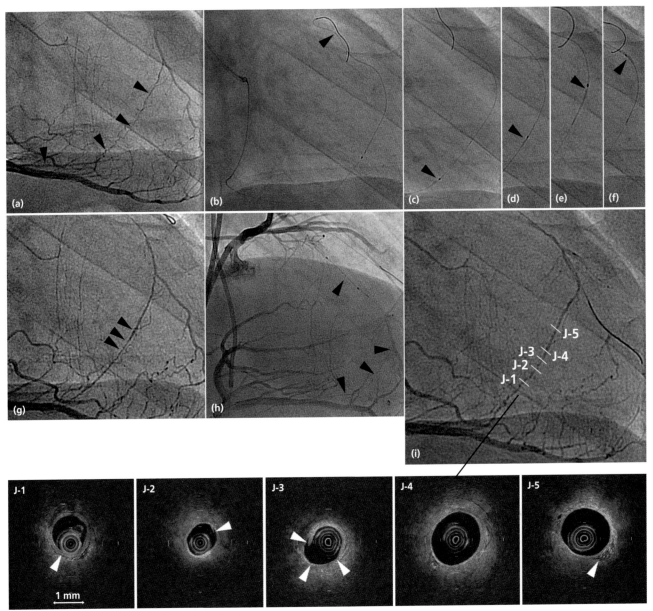

Figure 39.1 Procedure sequence in septal dilation technique and OCT findings of septal channel dilation. (a) Continuous connection 2 (CC2) (Table 39.1) between septal branches. (b) Septal channel was successfully crossed with Fielder FC wires. The wire tip is positioned in the diagonal branch. (c–f) The entire length of septal channel was dilated with low pressure (2–3 atm) using a 1.3-mm balloon. (g) Postdilation. (h) A 2.5-mm OTW balloon was delivered through the dilated channel. (i) After CTO in the left anterior descending artery was crossed with an antegrade wire, the dilated channel was observed with OCT. Inset: (J-1) Dilated septal branch diverging from posterior descending branch. Three layers are seen. (J-2) OCT findings at the connecting site. The small flap (white arrow) created by ballooning and thinned adventitial sheath are seen, but three layer structure is not observed. The diameter of the dilated channel measured by OCT was 0.9 mm. (J-3) Although the disrupted and expanded vessel wall (white arrow) is seen, the adventitial sheath is preserved and no hematoma around the channel is detected. (J-4) The channel is excessively dilated. (J-5) Septal branch diverging from left anterior descending artery. Tree layers and myocardium (white arrow) are shown. Although CC2 channel was used as a retrograde access route in this case, CTO findings showed that the maximum diameter of collateral channel dilated using a 1.3-mm balloon was 0.9 mm. These findings indicate that a ≥1.5-mm balloon could cause channel rupture.

and for providing stability of the retrograde wire, which improves the wire maneuverability. In fact, the use of this technique or a simple retrograde-wire approach without a catheter is a major reason why we have been struggling with the retrograde approach and why the retrograde approach has stayed undeveloped for such a long time.

Appropriate channels for retrograde crossing are found in 50–60% of RCA or LAD CTOs. The diameter of a collateral

Table 39.1 Classification of continuous connection in collateral channels (modified from Werner's definition [41]).

CC0: no continuous connection between donor and recipient artery
CC1: continuous connection, but threadlike connection (≤0.4 mm)
CC2: continuous connection, small side branch-like size of the collateral throughout its course (>0.4 mm)

channel that is classified as a continuous connection (CC) grade 0–2 according to modified Werner's classification (Table 39.1) [41] is not an applicable condition for the septal dilation technique. A septal channel with faint continuous connection classified as CC1 is often appropriate for crossing rather than a CC2 channel. Thus, the septal dilation technique has expanded the indication for the retrograde approach. Tip injection (supeselective) is required for evaluation of applicability because continuity of channel, 3-D anatomy of septal channel, acute bend, corkscrew-like morphology, and bifurcation of a small side branch, which are determinants of successful wire crossing, can be assessed only by superselective tip injection. Mildly corkscrew-like channels with few side branches are ideal, and these are often CC1 channels. Acute bend is a risk factor for channel rupture; consequently, a channel with acute bend, especially at a junction should not be selected, unless a channel dilation catheter is available.

The recognition of channel anatomy checked by tip injection is crucial for wire crossing, and superselective *rotational* tip injection is sometimes needed to assess the anatomy. Another key to wire crossing is the use of a floppy polymer-coated wire in which a tiny tip curve, ideally <0.5 mm, can be made. Fielder™ FC (Asahi Intecc, Co., Ltd) and X-treme/Fielder XT are dedicated wires for collateral channel crossing, as described below. Lack of visualization of the channel during wire

handling or lack of a landmark are additional limitations in channel crossing; however, wedged-tip injections or multiple wire techniques are sometimes helpful.

Guiding catheter, balloons

If an OTW balloon catheter with a long shaft (≥150 cm) is not available, a short guiding catheter (≤90 cm) is needed for the retrograde approach because of the long access route. A long OTW balloon catheter (usually a 2.5-mm balloon) is required for retrograde CTO crossing techniques, rather than a penetrating catheter, to improve retrograde wire maneuverability. This OTW balloon should have excellent hydrophilic coating for ease of delivery to the CTO site; the coating is easily wiped off as a result of strong friction with the dilated channel wall.

Dedicated devices

Floppy coil wires with hydrophilic coating were often used for channel crossing in the early stages; however, the coil wire has been abandoned because the uncovered metal tip is too harmful in a tiny tortuous channel and the relatively large tip curve due to limitations in the soldering length is inappropriate for negotiating a tiny tortuous channel. Although polymer-coated wires with relatively large tip curves have been used for channel crossing instead of the coil wire, new polymer-coated wires dedicated for collateral channel crossing (Fielder FC and Fielder XT/X-treme) have recently been developed. The advantages of these wires are softer tips and smaller tip curves compared with the conventional polymer-coated wires. The short soldering length (<0.3 mm) in both wires enables us to make tip curves of <0.5 mm (Fig. 39.2), and the tapered small tip curve in Fielder XT/X-treme is effective for negotiating a CC1 channel.

The channel dilation catheter has a stainless braiding shaft covered with a polymer and a flexible polymer tip with an

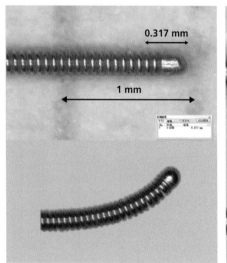
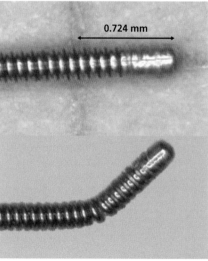

(a)   (b)

Figure 39.2 Comparison of soldering length and tip curve size between Fielder XT and a conventional 0.014-inch wire. (a) Fielder XT, (b) a conventional coil wire (0.014 inches). Because Fielder XT is tapered to 0.009 inches at the tip, it has a smaller metal tip and a tight coil using a thinner string compared with a conventional 0.014-inch wire. The soldering length of Fielder XT is 0.317 mm, which is much shorter than that of the conventional wire (0.724 mm). In the conventional wire it is impossible to make a tip curve smaller than 1.0 mm owing to the long soldering length; however, the short soldering enables the production of a <0.5 mm tip curve in Fielder XT.

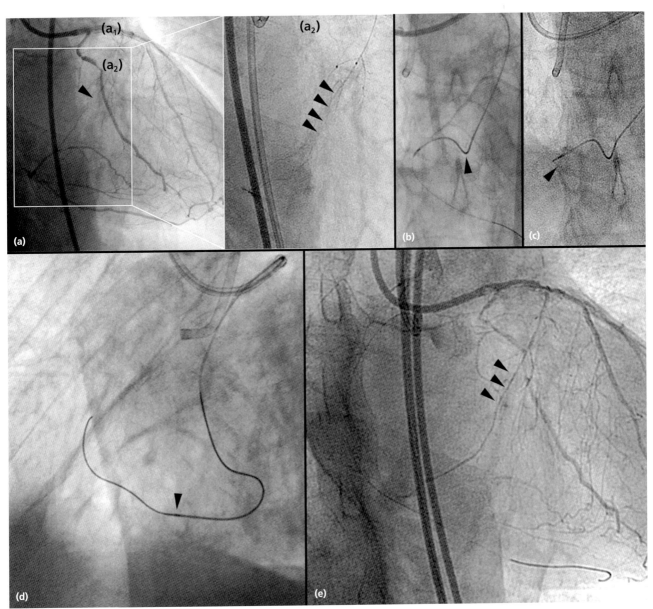

Figure 39.3 A case in which a channel dilation catheter was used for septal channel dilation technique. (a) The first septal branch has continuous connection (black arrow) to the PD branch. inset: The tip injection reveals a CC1 connection (black arrows). (b) The channel dilation catheter passed through the channel along the acute bend (black arrow) and the tip is positioned at the distal bifurcation in the RCA. (c) Tip injection using the channel dilation catheter (black arrow). (d) After the Miracle 3G wire is retrogradely inserted into the CTO, the channel dilation catheter was able to access the CTO. (e) Post recanalization: the smoothly dilated channel with the channel dilation catheter is shown (black arrows). The channel dilation catheter can be advanced along the bend without stretching the bend so that the risk of channel injury is minimized. After crossing the channel, the channel dilation catheter fixed in the CTO can improve the retrograde wire maneuverability.

excellent hydrophilic coating. This catheter can be advanced by counterclockwise rotation, utilizing a screwing effect when crossing tiny channels without the need to push aggressively, and the channels can be dilated using the dottering effect so as to safely open such a tiny tortuous collateral channel (Fig. 39.3). This catheter also provides sufficient backup support for a retrograde wire and improves the wire maneuverability, especially by screwing it into a CTO lesion. The properties of this catheter have drastically simplified and improved the retrograde approach; there is no longer a need for channel dilation with a balloon and for exchange of catheters while improving retrograde wire maneuverability.

Use of epicardial channels (posterolateral channels)
Although the septal dilation technique has expanded the indication for the retrograde approach, other options for

retrograde access are necessary because the septal channel is applicable in only 50–60% of all CTOs. Atrial channels have been used in about 5% of retrograde cases and well-developed epicardial channels have been used even less often. However, CC1 channels located on the posterolateral wall of the left ventricle (posterolateral channels) are often seen, and many of these are mildly corkscrew-like, although they cannotbe dilated by a balloon because of the high risk of cardiac tamponade after channel rupture due to ballooning. After the

channel dilator catheter emerged, posterolateral channels were aggressively attempted because the channel dilation catheter was believed to safely cross and dilate CC1 channels without the need for ballooning, based on the experience in septal channels. Currently, the posterolateral channel is considered to be applicable in about 20% of all CTOs, including LCx CTOs (Fig. 39.4), and the indication for the retrograde approach will likely be expanded by utilizing the posterolateral channels as an alternative access route.

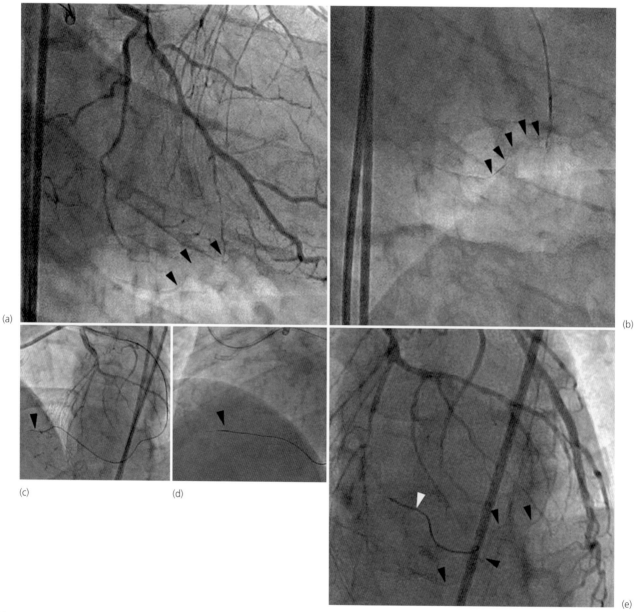

(a)

(b)

(c)

(d)

(e)

Figure 39.4 A case in which CC1 epicardial collateral channel (PL channel) was used as a retrograde access route with a channel dilation catheter. (a) The faint connection (black arrows) is seen between the posterolateral branch in the LCx and the posterolateral branch in the RCA. (b) The tip injection using the channel dilation catheter shows a CC1 continuous connection (black arrows). (c) A Fielder XT could easily get through the channel. (d) The channel dilation catheter advanced into the CTO. (e) Post recanalization: the white arrow indicates the antegrade wire crossing the CTO and the black arrows indicate the dilated epicardial channel with the channel dilator.

Chronic total occlusion crossing techniques in the retrograde approach

Deterioration of wire maneuverability in retrograde fashion due to acute bend and beating is one of the major barriers to the retrograde approach, and used to be a major reason for failure. One way to overcome this limitation is to stabilize the retrograde wire in a CTO vessel. This can be accomplished with the anchor balloon technique, in which an OTW balloon is retrogradely delivered and inflated in the CTO vessel to fix the balloon catheter. The septal dilation technique used to be crucial for safely delivering the OTW balloon, although the process of this procedure was sometimes troublesome because of the difficulty in delivering the balloon due to excess friction, and for exchanging for a bigger balloon according to the CTO vessel size. The channel dilation catheter addresses this problem as described above.

The first step in CTO crossing using the retrograde approach is to retrogradely navigate through the CTO. It is well known from experience in angioplasty of peripheral CTOs that negotiating a CTO is technically easier in retrograde fashion than in antegrade fashion provided maneuverability of the retrograde wire can be preserved. One advantage of the retrograde approach is that there is no need for a stiff wire when negotiating most CTOs. Use of a floppy polymer-coated wire (see the new approach in antegrade approach) is very often useful to avoid wire perforation and to save time.

Retrograde wire crossing technique

This technique is to simply cross a CTO retrogradely with a wire and has been traditionally employed in the retrograde approach. Because the wire maneuverability has improved in the modern retrograde approach, as described above, CTO crossing rates with this technique have increased. However, there are obvious limitations, similarly seen in the antegrade approach. Therefore, the following techniques were developed, although this is still used in the current state because it is the simplest technique.

Kissing wire technique

In the early stages of the retrograde approach, the kissing wire technique was often used [35]. A retrograde wire is placed in a CTO lesion or a distal true lumen as a landmark and an antegrade wire is advanced targeting the retrograde wire to cross the CTO in an antegrade fashion. Since this technique does not always facilitate antegrade wire crossing, it is not usually employed in the current state.

Knuckle wire technique

Originally the knuckle wire technique was developed to create a retrograde subintimal dissection when an OTW balloon was unable to be retrogradely delivered to a CTO vessel before developing the septal dilation technique. In this technique, the retrograde wire, which is usually a polymer-coated wire, is intentionally prolapsed ("knuckle") and simply pushed toward the proximal end while being rotated. The advantages of this technique are easy tracking of a CTO vessel and ensuring formation of a subintimal space similar to the STAR technique [42]. However, this wire technique is very rough and the knuckle wire cannot be controlled, therefore there is a risk of wire perforation or wire trapping that may cause serious complications. Moreover, this technique does not always ensure antegrade wire crossing because the subintimal space created by the knuckle wire is limited.

Controlled antegrade and retrograde subintimal tracking/kissing balloon technique

In order to overcome the limitations of conventional retrograde techniques described above, the CART technique was developed [37]. CART ensures antegrade wire crossing by creating a connection between the antegrade subintimal dissection, created by an antegrade wire, and the retrograde subintimal dissection, created by the retrograde balloon, as shown in Figure 39.5. The challenge of CART is to ensure that both subintimal dissections can be easily connected. However, there is no way to check if the retrograde balloon creates the retrograde subintimal dissection, although the subintimal dissection is crucial for the success of CART. A large balloon, greater than 3.5 mm, is sometimes needed to ensure creation of the subintimal dissection, especially in large-vessel CTOs. This is a disadvantage of CART.

Intravascular ultrasound-guided reverse controlled antegrade and retrograde subintimal tracking

Reverse CART had been tried before CART was developed, i.e. retrograde wire crossing was attempted after making a subintimal dissection with an antegrade balloon. However, this technique was abandoned in the early stages owing to the risk of spiral dissection after subintimal dissection, created by the antegrade balloon, and difficulty in ensuring maneuverability of the retrograde wire, even if using the anchor balloon technique. However, reverse CART was revisited after the channel dilation catheter emerged because this catheter ensures wire exchange during the procedure and improves the retrograde wire maneuverability in most cases. The advantage of reverse CART over other retrograde techniques is that IVUS guidance can be applied when making the subintimal dissection and checking retrograde wire crossing. Locating an appropriate position in which the subintimal dissection is created and optimizing the balloon size with IVUS, the formation of subintimal dissection is ensured and the risk of spiral dissections can be minimized. Also, the results of ballooning can be checked by IVUS, and IVUS guidance facilitates retrograde wire crossing, as shown in Figure 39.6.

Future direction

The retrograde approach has certainly improved the initial success rate of PCI for CTOs (90–95%), as the results of the

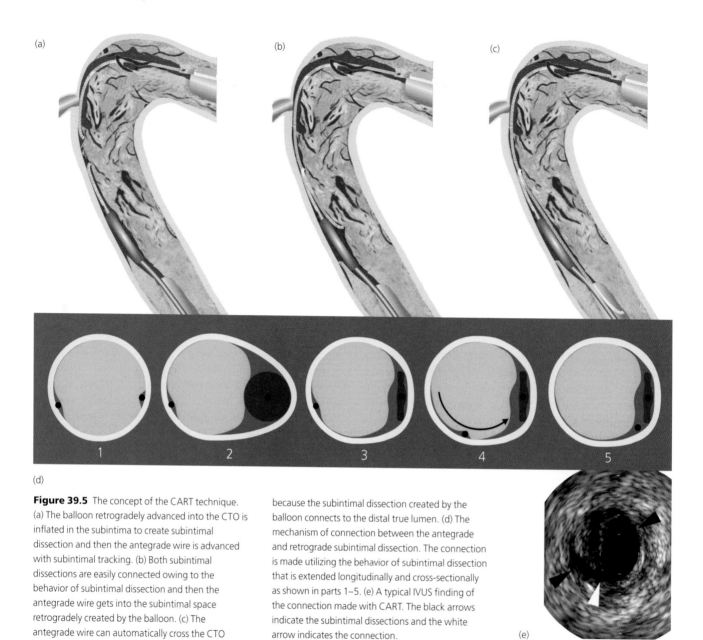

(a)

(b)

(c)

(d)

Figure 39.5 The concept of the CART technique.
(a) The balloon retrogradely advanced into the CTO is
inflated in the subintima to create subintimal
dissection and then the antegrade wire is advanced
with subintimal tracking. (b) Both subintimal
dissections are easily connected owing to the
behavior of subintimal dissection and then the
antegrade wire gets into the subintimal space
retrogradely created by the balloon. (c) The
antegrade wire can automatically cross the CTO

because the subintimal dissection created by the
balloon connects to the distal true lumen. (d) The
mechanism of connection between the antegrade
and retrograde subintimal dissection. The connection
is made utilizing the behavior of subintimal dissection
that is extended longitudinally and cross-sectionally
as shown in parts 1–5. (e) A typical IVUS finding of
the connection made with CART. The black arrows
indicate the subintimal dissections and the white
arrow indicates the connection.

(e)

Figure 39.6 (*opposite*) A case of reverse CART with IVUS guidance.
(a) Preprocedure. The CTO is located in the proximal RCA (between two
black arrows) with an abnormal origin from the left sinus of Valsalva.
(b) The continuous connection 2 (CC2) is seen between the PL branch of
the LCx and the PL branch of the RCA (black arrow). (c) The channel dilation
catheter easily crossed the channel and was advanced to the distal end of
the CTO (black arrow). The anchor technique (white arrow) was applied to
perform predilation with 2.5 mm and to deliver the IVUS catheter. The IVUS
catheter is positioned at the point D. (d) IVUS findings at the point D.
The vessel size in the occluded segment was 5.0 mm and small calcification
was seen at the point D. (e) As an antegrade balloon for creating subintimal
dissection, a 4.5-mm balloon (black arrow) was selected according to
the IVUS findings. (f) After creating the antegrade subintimal dissection with
the 4.5-mm balloon, the retrograde wire (Fielder XT) easily crossed the CTO
(white arrow) with IVUS guidance. Inset: IVUS findings in each point (point
G1–G4). (G1) The subintimal dissection created with the 4.5-mm balloon is

seen (white arrow no. 1). The retrograde wire is located in the subintima
(white arrow no. 2). (G2) The retrograde wire (white arrow no. 2) moved to
the antegrade subintimal space created with the antegrade balloon through
the connection between the antegrade and retrograde subintimal dissection
(white arrow no. 1). (G3 and G4) The retrograde wire passes through
the channel created with the antegrade balloon (white arrow) and reaches
to the proximal true lumen (G4). (g) After the retrograde wire was led to
the guiding catheter, the channel dilation catheter was advanced into
the guiding catheter and the retrograde wire was exchanged for a 300-cm
Rotablator wire (white arrow), which is secured at the right groin for
antegradely delivering the IVUS catheter and the stents. (h) Stenting with
a 3.5-mm Cypher using the 300-cm Rotablator wire. (i) Post stenting.
(j) The channel used for the retrograde access was checked after stenting
(black arrow). No channel injury was detected. Please note that no contrast
media was unnecessary in (c) to (i) because of IVUS guidance, so this
procedure was completed with only 7 mL of contrast medium.

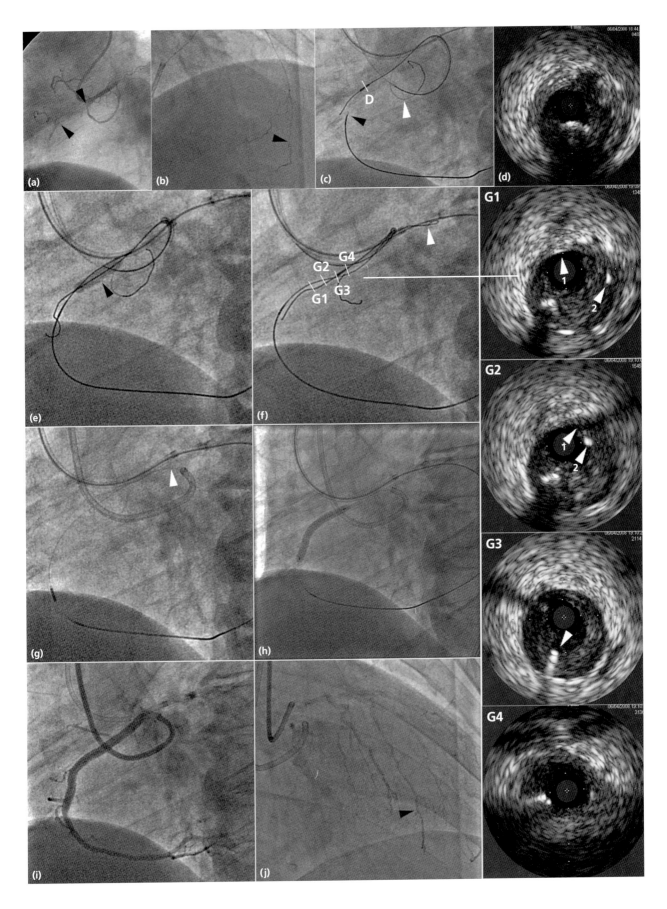

European Multicenter Registry [39], the Japanese registry, and other studies [40] have shown; however, there are many difficulties in performing the retrograde techniques because dedicated devices are limited and there remains much confusion in applying these techniques because of limited operator experience. Nevertheless, IVUS-guided reverse CART is now a means to ensure CTO crossing and saves contrast media and procedure time as long as there is a promising channel for retrograde access. However, there remains the risk of spiral dissection and wire perforation caused by subintimal tracking when the average operator uses this technique. Therefore, a novel method of facilitating CTO crossing without subintimal tracking should be the next stage in development of the retrograde approach.

Other techniques

A few anchor techniques, including the retrograde anchor balloon technique described above, are sometimes useful for the retrograde approach. Another anchor technique often used is to anchor a retrograde wire with an antegrade balloon (2.5- or 3.0-mm balloon is used) inside a guiding catheter engaged in the orifice of the CTO vessel after the retrograde wire passes through the CTO. This technique is the most powerful method for getting backup support for a retrograde balloon or a channel dilation catheter to cross a CTO.

Another technique is the use of a 300-cm Rotablator wire, which is advanced through the antegrade guiding catheter and secured outside the body to deliver an antegrade balloon into the CTO along it. Instead of a 300-cm wire, a coronary snare wire (0.014 inches) can be used to grab the retrograde wire, either in the lumen proximal to the CTO or in the antegrade guiding catheter, and an antegrade balloon then is delivered to the distal lumen along the snare wire.

Specific complications for retrograde approach

Specific complications, such as collateral channel rupture, are described above. If the procedure is performed carefully, septal channel rupture is usually followed by no sequela because a fistula to the ventricle is easily formed and it rarely causes a large intramyocardial hematoma in the septum or inferoposterior wall. The most serious complication is an acute occlusion in the donor artery due to thrombosis or dissection. During the retrograde approach, accelerated coagulation time (ACT) should be monitored and kept at > 300 s. To prevent the dissection, a high-risk lesion in the donor artery should be stented and deep engagement of the retrograde guiding catheter should always be monitored during the procedure.

Chronic total occlusion devices

Many CTO devices have been developed during the past 20 years. Unfortunately, none of them has succeeded in terms of providing an advantage over conventional mechanical wires; however, this does not mean that the concept behind those devices is not viable. Rather, inventors and companies lacked deeper knowledge about CTOs. CTOs involve every kind of coronary lesion and, therefore, no single concept solves all problems associated with CTO PCI; thus the devices never outperform the wires. It is clear that CTO devices should target a specific CTO lesion subset which is formally classified.

The CTO devices currently in use are the Safe Cross-RF™ guidewire (Kensey Nash, Exton, PA, USA), the Frontrunner™ Catheter [43] (Lumend, Redwood City, CA, USA), and the CROSSER™ system (FlowCardia, Sunnyvale, CA, USA), although their use in coronary CTOs is still problematic. The multicenter Guided Radio Frequency Energy Ablation of Total Occlusions (GREAT) registry reported a success rate with the Safe Cross-RF device of 54.3% [44]. The current X-39 Frontrunner (0.03- to 0.04-inch outer diameter, with a 2.8F distal tip) was used in 593 patients and success was achieved in 61% of cases, a rate similar to that achieved with other CTO devices. The clinical results of the CROSSER CTO recanalization system using high-frequency mechanical vibration (21 000 cycles/s) in the prospective European registry have been reported [45]. Technical success was achieved in 56% of 53 patients; however, the success rate improved to 76% using the new version of the device. Even though these devices were tried after a failed procedure using mechanical wires, this is not sufficient to claim the advantages of the CTO devices over the conventional wires.

Drug-eluting stent implantation

Many randomized or nonrandomized studies have demonstrated a drastic reduction in restenosis and reocclusion rates after DES implantation in CTOs [11–16]. However, an unsolved practical problems remains: although full lesion coverage is deemed to be essential for reducing restenosis and reocclusion rates with DES, it is often difficult to fully cover a CTO lesion with a DES because of considerable diffuse plaque. It is also difficult to identify the stent zone for stent deployment in diffuse CTOs. As a result, a "full metal jacket" is often seen, especially when treating a diffuse RCA CTO. The multiple long-stent implantations sometimes result in stent fracture, which causes stent malapposition and might cause late thrombosis. The malapposition after DES implantation in a CTO is also induced by underestimation of CTO vessel size when IVUS is not used. The ideal duration of antiplatelet therapy in CTOs is not identified, but should be longer because stent malapposition is more common than with non-CTO lesions. Whereas the 6-month reocclusion rate after the Cypher stent implantation was reported as 4% in the Primary Stenting of Totally Occluded

Native Coronary Arteries (PRISON) II study [14], probably including the late thrombosis rate, a late stent thrombosis rate of 1% per year was observed in a series of TAXUS® stent implantation in CTOs. DES deployment strategy for CTOs may be changed in the future with the use of IVUS and increased option of DES to prevent the malapposition.

Complications

Although the specific complication for CTO PCI is cardiac tamponade, other major complications, such as acute occlusion, AMI, emergency bypass surgery, and death, could occur [5]. Rates reported by the EuroCTO Club [20] in the 3403 patients treated in 2006 were mortality 0.12%, Q-wave myocardial infarction 0.14%, any myocardial infarction 1.96%, emergency CABG 0.27%, and cardiac tamponade 0.64%, which are similar to the results of the EuroHeart Survey on PCI in 2005 (death 0.3% and myocardial infarction 1.1%), with the exception of a higher incidence of cardiac tamponade (0.64% vs. 0.1% in the EuroHeart Survey). The risk of CTO PCI appears to be similar to that of conventional PCI in terms of major complications. Nevertheless, when trying high-risk CTO in patients with multivessel disease or attempting the retrograde approach, the risk of CTO PCI should be considered higher than with conventional PCI.

The wire exit through an occluded segment during CTO PCI is usually concerning; however, major extravasation resulting in cardiac tamponade is relatively rare, as long as the operator recognizes the event and deals with it appropriately (balloon occlusion, reversal of heparin if needed, and no use of bivalirudin, abciximab, or other glycoprotein IIb/IIIa inhibitors before the procedure). Instead, the common reason for cardiac tamponade is wire perforation in a distal side branch after recanalizing a CTO. This sometimes escapes the attention of an operator when using a polymer-coated wire because no resistance is felt during perforation and no extravasation of contrast is seen on angiography. Even a little extravasation in this type of wire perforation can cause cardiac tamponade because the bleeding does not stop unless it is actively treated, unlike an exit through an occluded segment. Thus, the patient should be monitored for at least 6h, ideally using cardiac echocardiography. The easiest way to achieve hemostasis in this situation is to wedge a penetration catheter with a relatively big profile to the perforated side branch and then appliy negative pressure with reversal of heparin so that the hole created by the wire shrinks completely. Embolization using thrombi, autologous fat tissue from the groin, or coils is useful.

Furthermore, contrast-induced nephropathy and excessive radiation should be noted when a complex strategy is employed. Although the acceptable maximum dose of contrast for each procedure is 400 mL, the use of contrast should be minimized as much as possible in patients with renal dysfunction or diabetes mellitus, or in the case of a second attempt. The amount of contrast can be reduced by using IVUS in combination with superselective tip injections (IVUS-guided wire handling or IVUS-guided reverse CART, shown in Fig. 39.6). However, reduction in radiation during wire handling is still difficult even in the current state [46,47]. Methods of reducing skin radiation include frequently changing the exposure angle during the procedure with low pulsed digital fluoroscopy, using extra beam filtering and low-dose settings, and monitoring irradiation dosage and informing the operator when to stop the procedure by.

Conclusion

The initial results of CTO PCI have been improved with the use of a number of modern techniques, and DES has drastically reduced restenosis and reocclusion rates after successful recanalization of CTOs. A sophisticated approach comprising proper application of various techniques according to the lesion characteristics and a well-thought-out procedural sequence is required for better results because there is no universal technique or device that can be used to recanalize every kind of CTO. Currently, each strategy employed by an operator depends on his/her level of skill and experience. Although this is an obstacle to expansion of CTO PCIs, the lessons from past failures indicate that a hasty simplification of the CTO PCI procedure will never bring about progress.

References

1. Bourassa MG, Roubin GS, Detre KM, *et al.* (1995) Bypass angioplasty revascularization investigation: patient screening, selection, and recruitment. *Am J Cardiol* **75**:3C–8C.
2. Delacretaz E & Meier B (1997) Therapeutic strategy with total coronary artery occlusions. *Am J Cardiol* **79**:185–187.
3. Srinivas VS, Brooks MM, Detre KM, *et al.* (2002) Contemporary percutaneous coronary intervention versus balloon angioplasty for multivessel coronary artery disease: a comparison of the National Heart, Lung and Blood Institute Dynamic Registry and the Bypass Angioplasty Revascularization Investigation (BARI) study. *Circulation* **106**:1627–1633.
4. Christofferson RD, Lehmann KG, Martin GV, Every N, Caldwell JH, & Kapadia SR (2005) Effect of chronic total coronary occlusion on treatment strategy. *Am J Cardiol* **95**:1088–1091.
5. Suero JA, Marso SP, Jones PG, *et al.* (2001) Procedural outcomes and long-term survival among patients undergoing percutaneous coronary intervention of a chronic total occlusion in native coronary arteries: a 20-year experience. *J Am Coll Cardiol* **38**:409–414.
6. Bell MR, Berger PB, Bresnahan JF, Reeder GS, Bailey KR, & Holmes DR Jr (1992) Initial and long-term outcome of 354 patients after coronary balloon angioplasty of total coronary artery occlusions. *Circulation* **85**:1003–1011.

7. Ivanhoe RJ, Weintraub WS, Douglas JS Jr, *et al.* (1992) Percutaneous transluminal coronary angioplasty of chronic total occlusions. Primary success, restenosis, and long-term clinical follow-up. *Circulation* **85**:106–115.

8. Warren RJ, Black AJ, Valentine PA, Manolas EG, & Hunt D (1990) Coronary angioplasty for chronic total occlusion reduces the need for subsequent coronary bypass surgery. *Am Heart J* **120**:270–274.

9. Finci L, Meier B, Favre J, Righetti A, & Rutishauser W (1990) Long-term results of successful and failed angioplasty for chronic total coronary arterial occlusion. *Am J Cardiol* **66**:660–662.

10. Abbott JD, Kip KE, Vlachos HA, *et al.* (2006) Recent trends in the percutaneous treatment of chronic total coronary occlusions. *Am J Cardiol* **97**:1691–1696.

11. Nakamura S, Muthusamy TS, Bae JH, Cahyadi YH, Udayachalerm W, & Tresukosol D (2005) Impact of sirolimus-eluting stent on the outcome of patients with chronic total occlusions. *Am J Cardiol* **95**:161–166.

12. Goy JJ, Stauffer JC, Siegenthaler M, Benoit A, & Seydoux C (2005) A prospective randomized comparison between paclitaxel and sirolimus stents in the real world of interventional cardiology: the TAXi trial. *J Am Coll Cardiol* **45**:308–311.

13. Werner GS, Krack A, Schwarz G, Prochnau D, Betge S, & Figulla HR (2004) Prevention of lesion recurrence in chronic total coronary occlusions by paclitaxel-eluting stents. *J Am Coll Cardiol* **44**:2301–2306.

14. Suttorp MJ, Laarman GJ, Rahel BM, *et al.* (2006) Primary Stenting of Totally Occluded Native Coronary Arteries II (PRISON II): a randomized comparison of bare metal stent implantation with sirolimus-eluting stent implantation for the treatment of total coronary occlusions. *Circulation* **114**:921–928.

15. Lotan C, Almagor Y, Kuiper K, Suttorp MJ, & Wijns W (2006) Sirolimus-eluting stent in chronic total occlusion: the SICTO study. *J Interv Cardiol* **19**:307–312.

16. Migliorini A, Moschi G, Vergara R, Parodi G, Carrabba N, & Antoniucci D (2006) Drug-eluting stent-supported percutaneous coronary intervention for chronic total coronary occlusion. *Catheter Cardiovasc Interv* **67**:344–348.

17. Stone GW, Colombo A, Teirstein PS, *et al.* (2005) Percutaneous recanalization of chronically occluded coronary arteries: procedural techniques, devices, and results. *Catheter Cardiovasc Interv* **66**:217–236.

18. Stone GW, Reifart NJ, Moussa I, *et al.* (2005) Percutaneous recanalization of chronically occluded coronary arteries: a consensus document: part I. *Circulation* **112**:2364–2372.

19. Stone GW, Kandzari DE, Mehran R, *et al.* (2005) Percutaneous recanalization of chronically occluded coronary arteries: a consensus document: part II. *Circulation* **112**:2530–2537.

20. Di Mario C, Werner GS, Sianos G, *et al.* (2007) European perspective in the recanalisation of Chronic Total Occlusion (CTO): consensus document from the EuroCTO Club. *EuroIntervention* **3**:30–43.

21. Moreno R, Conde C, Perez-Vizcayno MJ, *et al.* (2006) Prognostic impact of a chronic occlusion in a noninfarct vessel in patients with acute myocardial infarction and multivessel disease undergoing primary percutaneous coronary intervention. *J Invasive Cardiol* **18**:16–19.

22. van der Schaaf RJ, Vis MM, Sjauw KD, *et al.* (2006) Impact of multivessel coronary disease on long-term mortality in patients with ST-elevation myocardial infarction is due to the presence of a chronic total occlusion. *Am J Cardiol* **98**:1165–1169.

23. Steg PG, Thuaire C, Himbert D, *et al.* (2004) DECOPI (DEsobstruction COronaire en Post-Infarctus): a randomized multicentre trial of occluded artery angioplasty after acute myocardial infarction. *Eur Heart J* **25**:2187–2194.

24. Yousef ZR, Redwood SR, Bucknall CA, Sulke AN, & Marber MS (2002) Late intervention after anterior myocardial infarction: effects on left ventricular size, function, quality of life, and exercise tolerance: results of the Open Artery Trial (TOAT Study). *J Am Coll Cardiol* **40**:869–876.

25. Dzavik V, Buller CE, Lamas GA, *et al.* (2006) Randomized trial of percutaneous coronary intervention for subacute infarct-related coronary artery occlusion to achieve long-term patency and improve ventricular function: the Total Occlusion Study of Canada (TOSCA)-2 trial. *Circulation* **114**:2449–2457.

26. Hochman JS, Lamas GA, Buller CE, *et al.* (2006) Coronary intervention for persistent occlusion after myocardial infarction. *N Engl J Med* **355**:2395–2407.

27. Sirnes PA, Myreng Y, Molstad P, Bonarjee V, & Golf S (1998) Improvement in left ventricular ejection fraction and wall motion after successful recanalization of chronic coronary occlusions. *Eur Heart J* **19**:273–281.

28. Noguchi T, Miyazaki MS, Morii I, Daikoku S, Goto Y, & Nonogi H (2000) Percutaneous transluminal coronary angioplasty of chronic total occlusions. Determinants of primary success and long-term clinical outcome. *Catheter Cardiovasc Interv* **49**:258–264.

29. Hannan EL, Racz M, Holmes DR, *et al.* (2006) Impact of completeness of percutaneous coronary intervention revascularization on long-term outcomes in the stent era. *Circulation* **113**:2406–2412.

30. Mollet NR, Hoye A, Lemos PA, *et al.* (2005) Value of preprocedure multislice computed tomographic coronary angiography to predict the outcome of percutaneous recanalization of chronic total occlusions. *Am J Cardiol* **95**:240–243.

31. Soon KH, Selvanayagam JB, Cox N, Kelly AM, Bell KW, & Lim YL (2006) Percutaneous revascularization of chronic total occlusions: review of the role of invasive and non-invasive imaging modalities. *Int J Cardiol* **116**:1–6.

32. Srivatsa S & Holmes D Jr (1997) The histopathology of angiographic chronic total coronary artery occlusions—changes in neovascular pattern and intimal plaque composition associated with progressive occlusion duration. *J Invasive Cardiol* **9**:294–301.

33. Srivatsa SS, Edwards WD, Boos CM, *et al.* (1997) Histologic correlates of angiographic chronic total coronary artery occlusions: influence of occlusion duration on neovascular channel patterns and intimal plaque composition. *J Am Coll Cardiol* **29**:955–963.

34. Katsuragawa M, Fujiwara H, Miyamae M, & Sasayama S (1993) Histologic studies in percutaneous transluminal coronary angioplasty for chronic total occlusion: comparison of tapering and abrupt types of occlusion and short and long occluded segments. *J Am Coll Cardiol* **21**:604–611.

35. Katoh O (2007) Basic wire-handling strategies for chronic total occlusions. In: King SB 3rd, Yeung AC (eds). *Interventional Cardiology* Columbus, OH: The McGraw-Hill Companies, Inc.

36. Kahn JK & Hartzler GO (1990) Retrograde coronary angioplasty of isolated arterial segments through saphenous vein bypass grafts. *Cathet Cardiovasc Diagn* **20**:88–93.

37. Surmely JF, Tsuchikane E, Katoh O, *et al.* (2006) New concept for CTO recanalization using controlled antegrade and retrograde subintimal tracking: the CART technique. *J Invasive Cardiol* **18**:334–338.

38. Surmely JF, Katoh O, Tsuchikane E, Nasu K, & Suzuki T (2007) Coronary septal collaterals as an access for the retrograde approach in the percutaneous treatment of coronary chronic total occlusions. *Cathet Cardiovasc Interv* **69**:826–832.

39. Sianos G, Barlis P, Di Mario C, *et al.* (2008) European experience with the retrograde approach for the recanalisation of coronary artery chronic total occlusions. A report on behalf of the EuroCTO club. *EuroIntervention* **4**:84–92.

40. Di Mario C, Barlisi P, Tanigawa J, *et al.* (2007) Retrograde approach to coronary chronic total occlusions: preliminary single European center experience. *EuroIntervention* **3**:181–187.

41. Werner GS, Ferrari M, Heinke S, *et al.* (2003) Angiographic assessment of collateral connections in comparison with invasively determined collateral function in chronic coronary occlusions. *Circulation* **107**:1972–1977.

42. Colombo A, Mikhail GW, Michev I, *et al.* (2005) Treating chronic total occlusions using subintimal tracking and reentry: the STAR technique. *Catheter Cardiovasc Interv* **64**:407–411.

43. Whitbourn RJ, Cincotta M, Mossop P, & Selmon M (2003) Intraluminal blunt microdissection for angioplasty of coronary chronic total occlusions. *Catheter Cardiovasc Interv* **58**:194–198.

44. Baim DS, Braden G, Heuser R, *et al.* (2004) Utility of the Safe-Cross-guided radiofrequency total occlusion crossing system in chronic coronary total occlusions (results from the Guided Radio Frequency Energy Ablation of Total Occlusions Registry Study). *Am J Cardiol* **94**:853–858.

45. Grube E, Sütsch G, Lim VY, *et al.* (2006) High-frequency mechanical vibration to recanalize chronic total occlusions after failure to cross with conventional guidewires. *J Invasive Cardiol* **18**:85–91.

46. Suzuki S, Furui S, Kohtake H, *et al.* (2006) Radiation exposure to patient's skin during percutaneous coronary intervention for various lesions, including chronic total occlusion. *Circ J* **70**:44–48.

47. Bell MR, Berger PB, Menke KK, & Holmes DR Jr (1992) Balloon angioplasty of chronic total coronary artery occlusions: what does it cost in radiation exposure, time, and materials? *Cathet Cardiovasc Diagn* **25**:10–15.

40 Percutaneous Coronary Intervention for the Treatment of Saphenous Vein Grafts

Paul Vermeersch[1] & Pierfrancesco Agostoni[2]

[1]Antwerp Cardiovascular Institute Middelheim, Ziekenhuis Netwerk Antwerpen, Antwerp, Belgium
[2]University Medical Center Utrecht, Utrecht, The Netherlands

Historical background

Coronary artery bypass graft (CABG) surgery has had a major impact on the treatment of obstructive coronary artery disease over the past four decades. Although arterial grafts have proven to be superior to saphenous vein grafts (SVGs), the latter remain the conduits most often used in coronary artery bypass surgery.

The treatment of patients with obstructive atherosclerotic disease with coronary saphenous vein bypass grafts remains a challenge in cardiology and cardiac surgery. Within 10 years after surgery, half of all SVGs will have developed significant atherosclerotic disease [1,2], and this often results in patients experiencing severe anginal symptoms, despite optimal pharmacologic therapy [3]. Thus, options to improve the clinical status of these patients are urgently required.

Only two pharmacologic therapies have proven efficacy in the prevention of SVG atherosclerotic progression— antiplatelet agents started at the time of surgery and lipid-lowering therapy with statins—both of which are also effective for long-term secondary prevention [4].

Although most patients with recurrent angina following CABG should be managed medically, coronary catheterization should be performed at the earliest signs of recurrent ischemia to detect critical graft lesions that can be treated before irreversible loss of the graft.

Currently, the two available revascularization alternatives in the case of SVG disease are percutaneous coronary intervention (PCI) and repeat CABG. Percutaneous coronary intervention is the preferred method of treating patients with SVG lesions because there is a significantly higher risk inherent in the redo intervention with repeated CABG surgery [5,6]. Currently, the percutaneous treatment of SVGs accounts for a notable proportion of the caseload in high-volume catheterization laboratories (around 10%) [7].

Cardiovascular Interventions in Clinical Practice. Edited by Jürgen Haase, Hans-Joachim Schäfers, Horst Sievert and Ron Waksman. © 2010 Blackwell Publishing.

Pathophysiology of saphenous vein graft disease

Early and late graft failures, and to a lesser degree progression of native coronary artery disease, are major causes of recurrent angina after surgical revascularization. Reflecting this graft and native vessel attrition, anginal symptoms recur in up to 20% of the patients during the first year after CABG and in around 4% of patients annually during the ensuing 5 years [8]. Further revascularization, either by redo surgery or by PCI, is required in around 4% of patients by 5 years, in 19% of patients by 10 years, and in 31% of patients by 12 years after initial surgery [9].

"Saphenous vein graft disease" comprises three discrete processes: thrombosis, intimal hyperplasia, and atherosclerosis. These processes, although occurring at very different times, are interlinked pathophysiologically in the evolution of vein graft disease.

Early graft failure (from the postoperative period up to around 1 year) is considered to be caused by graft thrombosis and occurs in up to 15% of cases [10]. Immediately during and after the operation a prothrombotic situation occurs, which can be amplified by technical factors that reduce graft flow (intact venous valves, anastomotic stricture, or graft implantation proximal to an atheromatous segment). Harvesting of the venous conduit is associated with focal endothelial disruption, leading to activation of the extrinsic coagulation cascade by tissue factor. Moreover, the inherent antithrombotic properties of veins are comparatively weak compared with coronary arteries. Furthermore, bypass surgery not only impairs the local production of factors influencing hemostasis, but also alters the circulating levels of factors influencing hemostasis, favoring a prothrombotic response. In addition, vein grafts are highly sensitive to circulating vasoconstrictors, further attenuating flow and promoting stasis [11].

Intimal hyperplasia, defined as the accumulation of smooth muscle cells and extracellular matrix in the intimal compartment, is the major disease process in venous grafts between 1 month and 1 year after implantation. Intimal hyperplasia can be seen as a reparative process, a reaction to the trauma and stress that result from transplantation of the vein into the arterial circuit. Nearly all veins implanted will develop intimal thickening within 4–6 weeks, reducing the lumen by up to 25%. After endothelial regeneration, medial smooth muscle cells proliferate in response to a number of growth factors and cytokines released from platelets and from activated endothelial cells and macrophages. This process is followed by migration of smooth muscle cells into the intima, with subsequent further proliferation. Later, synthesis and deposition of extracellular matrix by activated smooth muscle cells leads to a progressive increase in intimal fibrosis and a reduction in cellularity. This process in itself rarely produces significant stenosis; nonetheless, intimal hyperplasia represents the foundation for later development of graft atheroma. The extensive intimal hyperplasia throughout the length of the vein graft may effectively create a diffuse atherosclerosis-prone region [12,13].

Late graft failure (occurring beyond the first year after bypass surgery) is usually associated with degenerative changes of the graft body. Though arterial grafts have a similar risk of acute graft failure, the improved clinical outcome seen with the use of arterial grafts may be explained by the high patency rate at 1-year follow-up (approximately 95%) and the relative protection from late failure [10- to 15-year patency of 80–88%] owing to the far less aggressive degenerative processes [1]. Atherosclerosis is the dominant process underlying the attrition of SVGs. Although necropsy studies have found evidence of atheromatous plaques as early as 1 year after surgery, hemodynamically significant stenoses rarely occur before 3 years [14]. Despite the fundamental process of atheroma development and the fact that the predisposing factors are similar in vein grafts and native coronary arteries, there are several temporal, histologic, and topographic differences compared with native artery disease. Central among these differences is the rapidly progressive nature of the atherosclerotic process in SVGs. A pivotal role in the rapidity of progression of vein graft atheroma is chronic endothelial injury and dysfunction [15]. Histologically, vein graft atheroma contains more foam cells and inflammatory cells than native coronary atheroma. Morphologically, vein graft atherosclerosis tends to be diffuse, concentric, and friable, with a poorly developed or absent fibrous cap and little evidence of calcification [16,17]. *In vivo* intravascular ultrasound evidence suggests that the focal compensatory enlargement observed in atherosclerotic native coronary arteries ("Glagov's law") does not occur in stenotic SVGs. Another common phenomenon is late thrombotic occlusion; late graft thrombosis is a frequent occurrence in old vein grafts with advanced atherosclerotic plaque formation [18]. In a series of 1388 patients, venous graft occlusion was 19% at 1 year and 25% at 5 years. At 15 years, 50% of patients had total venous graft occlusion and, of the remaining 50% of grafts, more than half had significant atherosclerotic disease [1]. Data from the PREVENT IV (Project of *Ex vivo* Vein Graft Engineering via Transfection) trial, involving 1829 patients undergoing CABG surgery with 12- to 18-month angiographic follow-up, recently confirmed a very high (29%) graft failure [2].

Indications for treatment

When dealing with the percutaneous treatment of diseased SVGs, both coronary anatomy and clinical presentation should be considered to optimize the outcome of the patients.

If an acutely occluded vein graft is the culprit lesion in an ongoing acute coronary syndrome, every effort should be made to recanalize the graft. If this strategy is technically or procedurally not possible, the native vessel may also be the target of a PCI. Salvage of the jeopardized myocardial region may depend on a successful restoration of adequate blood flow.

If an occluded vein graft is not responsible for an acute coronary syndrome but is a finding in a patient with stable symptoms, the native vessel should be the primary target for an interventional approach. Percutaneous treatment of chronically occluded grafts has never shown satisfactory results [19]. More aggressive antianginal medical therapy should also be considered as an alternative option if the treatment of the native vasculature is technically infeasible. Indeed, after bypass surgery the major determinant of long-term patient survival is the patency of the left internal mammary artery on the left anterior descending coronary artery [20], whereas patency of the other grafts mainly influences the symptomatic status of the patients without affecting long-term prognosis.

In the case of significantly diseased proximal or distal anastomoses, percutaneous treatment is usually feasible with good acute results.

All stenotic nonoccluded vein grafts are a possible target of percutaneous treatment. However, if the bypasses are degenerated (i.e. diffusely diseased with multiple stenoses along their pathway), an alternative option could be to consider the treatment of the native circulation or, if this is not technically possible, to consider redo CABG, in particular if diffuse disease involves the vein graft to the left anterior descending artery [21].

Several disadvantages after percutaneous treatment of SVGs are evident when compared with the treatment of native vessels: a higher rate of periprocedural myocardial infarctions, an increased incidence of restenosis and of repeated revascularizations, and a faster progression of moderate "nonsignificant" lesions in the same or in other grafts, left untreated during the first intervention [22–23]. Indeed, besides the aforementioned pathologic differences between vein grafts and native coronary arteries, the histopathology of restenosis in SVGs differs from that in native vessels: SVG restenosis is a mixture of cellular hyperplasia, progression of atherosclerosis, local inflammatory reaction, and thrombosis [24–26], whereas in native arteries intimal hyperplasia constitutes the primary determinant of the restenotic process [27].

Results

Percutaneous transluminal coronary angioplasty and bare metal stent

In the early 1990s, several registries assessing percutaneous transluminal balloon angioplasty in SVGs demonstrated the feasibility of this approach and the acceptable early outcome, but in general the results were less favorable than those in native vessels, with a higher percentage of periprocedural and long-term complications and rates of restenosis of around 50% [28]. After the introduction of bare metal stents in clinical practice for selected *de novo* lesions in native vessels in the mid-1990s [29,30], new registries tested these devices in diseased SVGs also [31]. The results were promising, and were substantially confirmed by the two randomized trials comparing percutaneous transluminal balloon angioplasty versus the bare metal stent procedure available to date [the Saphenous Vein De novo trial (SAVED) and the VENESTENT trials] [32,33]. Both trials enrolled a relatively small number of patients (215 and 150, respectively), and both missed the primary angiographic end point, i.e., a significant reduction in the angiographic binary restenosis rate. Notwithstanding this, both studies showed a significant reduction in the rate of major adverse clinical events, mainly because of a trend toward a reduction in the need for a repeated revascularization procedure (Fig. 40.1). Indeed, pooling the two studies using meta-analytic techniques [34,35], a benefit, either angiographic or clinical, of bare metal stent over percutaneous transluminal balloon angioplasty was shown, with a significant reduction in binary restenosis (29.7% vs. 40.4%, $P = 0.05$), repeated revascularization (15.7% vs. 28.3%, $P = 0.004$), and major adverse clinical events (24.9% vs. 39.4%, $P = 0.003$). In light of these results, current percutaneous interventions in SVGs are primarily carried out with elective implantation of bare metal stents, as also recommended by the updated European guidelines for percutaneous coronary interventions, in which bare metal stents in saphenous vein grafts are considered "beneficial, useful and effective" (class IA) [36]. Despite these advantages of bare metal stents compared with balloon angioplasty in patients with SVG lesions, the outcomes in these patients were still inferior to those obtained with bare metal stent implantation in native coronary arteries. The 30-day major adverse clinical event (MACE) rate remained higher than 10% (mainly driven by periprocedural myocardial infarctions due to distal embolization of atherothrombotic material) and the 6-month restenosis rate reached 30%. In light of these observations, new technologic developments have been requested

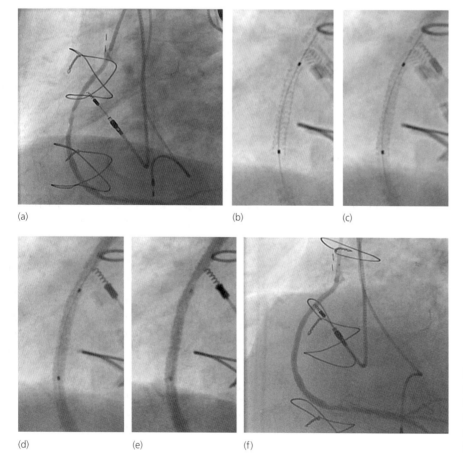

(a)　　　　(b)　　　　(c)

(d)　　　　(e)　　　　(f)

Figure 40.1 Stenting in a saphenous vein graft. (a) Severe stenosis in the mid-portion of a saphenous vein graft to the right coronary artery. (b–e) Stenting of the lesion (enhanced with the StentBoost subtract technology). (f) The final result.

to improve the outcome of the percutaneous treatment of saphenous vein grafts.

Covered stent grafts and embolic protection devices

Covered stent grafts have been developed and proposed as an option to reduce, at the same time, periprocedural embolization of atheromatous material, by entrapping it against the graft wall, and the restenotic process, by limiting neointimal proliferation. The preliminary results from different registries were very promising [37]; however, results from four randomized trials [the Stents in Grafts (STING), the Randomised Evaluation of Polytetrafluoroethylene Covered Stent in Saphenous Vein Grafts (RECOVERS), the SYMBIOT III and the BARRICADE trials], involving >1000 patients, were all negative [38–41]. Once again, using meta-analytic techniques, the pooled results of these four trials clearly show

that no differences between bare metal stents and covered stent grafts are evident in terms of major adverse clinical event and repeated revascularization rates (respectively, 25.1% vs. 28.6%, $P = 0.18$; and 16.3% vs. 18%, $P = 0.81$). There is even a borderline significant ($P = 0.03$) decrease in the rate of angiographic restenosis after a bare metal stent operation, 25.9% versus 32.3% after polytetrafluoroethylene (PTFE)-covered stent procedure. Recently, other strategies to reduce distal embolization were also developed. In particular, the "mechanical" protection of the vasculature distal to the lesion to be treated appeared as a good approach to reduce the downstream spreading of material during the intervention on the graft lesion. So far, three typologies of devices have been developed with this scope.

The first to be tested in SVGs has been a distal occlusion device (Fig. 40.2). Its mechanism is as follows. A compliant

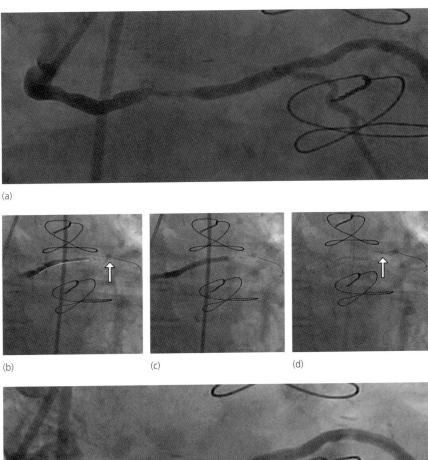

(a)

(b) (c) (d)

Figure 40.2 Distal "occlusion and aspiration" protection device. (a) Severe stenosis in the mid-portion of a saphenous vein graft to the left circumflex coronary artery. (b) Distal occlusion noncompliant and balloon inflated (arrow) with a stent positioned at the level of the lesion (white dotted line). (c) Stent deployed still with inflated distal occlusion balloon in place. (d) Manual debris aspiration (the arrow indicates the tip of the aspiration catheter) still with inflated distal occlusion balloon in place. (e) The final result.

(e)

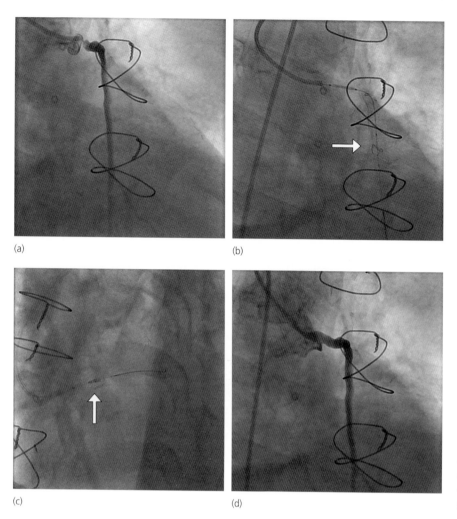

(a)

(b)

(c)

(d)

Figure 40.3 Distal filter. (a) Severe ostial stenosis of a saphenous vein graft to the left circumflex coronary artery. (b) Distal filter (arrow) and stent in place. (c) Filter retrieval from the saphenous vein graft (arrow). (d) Final result.

balloon is positioned distal to the lesion before the PCI and inflated at low pressure during the procedure. Suction of the stagnant blood/debris is performed just after the PCI using an aspiration catheter inserted through the guiding catheter, and the balloon is then deflated. In the randomized SAFER (Saphenous Vein Graft Angioplasty Free of Emboli, Randomized) trial, including 801 patients, this device was shown to significantly reduce the MACE rate at 30 days (9.6% vs. 16.5%, $P = 0.004$) compared with the simple implantation of bare metal stents without distal protection. This benefit was largely driven by a reduction in the rate of periprocedural myocardial infarctions [42]. Some concerns were raised related to the safety of low-pressure inflation of a noncompliant balloon on the SVG vessel wall distal to the lesion to be treated [43]. However, it has been proven in an angiographic study that this inflation, carefully performed in a nonangiographically diseased tract of the SVG is safe and does not produce any major vascular effect directly after the procedure and at 6 months' follow-up [44].

The distal filters utilize the same rationale but have a different mechanism of action with respect to the distal occlusion device (Fig. 40.3). They have of a porous filter, which is placed distal

to the lesion before the PCI, to collect embolic material and retrieve it after the procedure. Their value has been proven in the Filterwire ex Randomized Evaluation (FIRE) trial, another large randomized study, enrolling 651 patients, in which the filter was shown to be noninferior to the previously described "occlusion and aspiration" system. MACE rate at 30 days was 9.9%, compared with 11.6% for the distal filter distal occlusion device (P for noninferiority = 0.0008) [45].

The last type of protection device introduced is the proximal protection device (Fig. 40.4). It is a catheter with a protection balloon on its distal tip that is guided inside a standard guiding catheter up to the ostium of the vein graft, proximal to the lesion site. At this level the balloon is inflated temporarily, occluding blood flow and creating a column of stagnant blood, so that the debris dislodged during the PCI (which is performed through the device itself) can be then aspirated through the same catheter from the vessel. The proximal protection during saphenous vein graft intervention (PROXIMAL) trial, enrolling 600 patients, compared this proximal protection device with the currently available distal protection devices (either occlusion based or filters). The MACE rate at 30 days was 9.2% and 10%, respectively (P for noninferiority

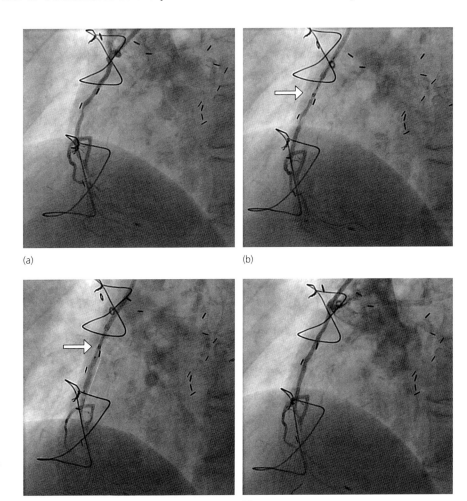

Figure 40.4 Proximal protection device. (a) Severe stenosis in the mid portion of a saphenous vein graft to the right coronary artery. (b) Proximal protection device in place and inflated (the arrow indicates the distal tip of the device, where the noncompliant balloon is): note the stagnant column of contrast downstream. (c) stent inflated (white dotted line) under proximal protection device, still with temporary occlusion of the vessel. (d) final result.

<0.001) [46]. In light of these results, embolic protection devices are currently accepted as the standard therapy for the prevention of distal embolization during percutaneous treatment of SVG disease. Despite this large body of evidence, protection devices remain underutilized in daily practice (<25% of SVGs are treated with PCI) [47]. The high cost of these devices and the steep learning curve required to use them properly seem to be the major explanations for their low utilization.

Of interest, a pooled analysis of five randomized trials, involving 627 patients treated for SVG lesions, found that "pharmacologic" treatment of distal embolization utilizing routinely glycoprotein IIB/IIIA inhibitors did not provide any benefit in terms of reduction in periprocedural complications [48].

Drug-eluting stents

Drug-eluting stents (DESs) have been associated with a significant impact on the restenosis process in selected *de novo* and restenotic native coronary artery lesions when compared with bare metal stents (BMSs). Currently several types of DES are available on the market: eluting sirolimus, paclitaxel, zotarolimus, everolimus, biolimus, or tacrolimus. Large randomized trials have shown a considerable reduction in angio-

graphic restenosis and target lesion revascularization with respect to standard interventional devices [49–51]. However, regarding the treatment of SVG lesions, data are very limited and concern only the use of the sirolimus-eluting stent and paclitaxel-eluting stent. Indeed, almost all of the randomized trials have excluded SVG lesions. The only randomized study allowing SVGs among the inclusion criteria has been the Basel Stent Kosten Effektivitäts Trial (BASKET). In a sub-analysis of this study, the use of DES provided the greatest benefit in patients in whom PCIs were performed in small vessels or venous bypass grafts, use, rather than in large native vessels [52]. However, the absolute number of SVGs included in the trial was low (47 lesions overall), and the specific outcomes in this lesion subset were presented pooled together with the data for small vessels [53]. As previously pointed out, the mechanisms of in-stent restenotic processes in SVGs are different from those in native arteries. In addition, more prothrombotic conditions in the region of the vein graft and the expected delay in endothelial healing after DES placement are cited as possible drawbacks of DES implantation in SVGs, as they can potentially lead to a higher risk of late thrombosis. Thus, clear data concerning the safety and the efficacy of these devices in SVGs are needed before the routine application of DESs in this lesion subset can be approved.

The only randomized study specifically performed in SVGs published to date is the Reduction of Restenosis in Saphenous Vein Grafts with Cypher Sirolimus-eluting Stent (RRISC) trial, which compared a sirolimus-eluting stent and the equivalent uncoated BMS [54]. Overall, 75 patients with 96 *de novo* lesions in 80 grafts were enrolled between 2003 and 2004: 38 patients received 60 sirolimus-eluting stents for 47 lesions, whereas 37 patients received 54 BMSs for 49 lesions. There was an extensive use of distal protection devices (around 80% of the procedures). The primary end point of the study, 6-month in-stent late loss, was significantly lower in the sirolimus-eluting stent group than in the BMS group (0.38 ± 0.51 mm versus 0.79 ± 0.66, $P = 0.001$). In addition, both in-stent and in-segment binary restenosis were lower in the sirolimus-eluting stent group than in the BMS group: in-stent restenosis 11.3% versus 30.6%, respectively (relative risk 0.37, 95% confidence interval [CI] 0.15–0.97, $P = 0.024$); in-segment restenosis 13.6% versus 32.6% (relative risk 0.42, 95% CI 0.18–0.97, $P = 0.031$). This led to a significant reduction in the rate of 6-month repeat revascularization procedures related to the lesion and to the vessel treated: target lesion revascularization was 5.3% compared 21.6% (relative risk 0.24, 95% CI 0.05–1.0, $P = 0.047$) and target vessel revascularization was 5.3% versus 27% (relative risk 0.19, 95% CI 0.05–0.83, $P = 0.012$). During the randomization period, around 20% of the vein graft lesions were excluded because of a vessel diameter larger than 4.0 mm. This issue raises an important problem with currently available DESs: it is not uncommon to treat very large venous bypass grafts, and the placement of a DES in these grafts can be problematic owing to the current lack of adequately sized DESs. The beneficial angiographic and clinical data shown in the RRISC trial were confirmed at a "vascular" level in an intravascular ultrasound (IVUS) substudy [55]. Intravascular ultrasound was performed at 6-month angiographic follow-up in 59 patients with a total of 61 SVGs (29 patients with 40 sirolimus-eluting stents for 34 lesions; 30 patients with 42 BMSs for 39 lesions). Median neo intimal volume was 1.3 mm³ (interquartile range 0–13.1 mm³) in sirolimus-eluting stents compared with 24.5 mm³ (7.8–39.5 mm³) in BMSs ($P < 0.001$). Minimal incomplete stent apposition was detected at only three stent edges (two BMSs, one sirolimus-eluting stent) next to ectatic regions of the SVG. The absence of malapposition in the body of the stents was extremely remarkable, particularly as SVGs are richer in lipids and thrombus, softer, and more friable than native coronary arteries [18]. A potential explanation for this finding can be related to the stent deployment strategy. Some authorities have suggested that stent deployment in SVGs should follow two rules: slight undersizing of the stent and low-pressure inflations to avoid plaque dislodgement and distal embolization, and to "entrap" the plaque between the vessel wall and the stent without squeezing it out [56]. Contrary to this

advice, in the RRISC trial, stents were always deployed with a stent–artery ratio >1 and high-pressure inflations (the mean pressure was >18 atm), and with noncompliant balloon post dilation in around 20% of the cases. The low rate of periprocedural adverse events in the trial (only 4% myocardial infarctions) has confirmed the feasibility of this approach [54].

The results of the RRISC trial suggest that sirolimus-eluting stents for *de novo* SVG lesions are associated with a low rate of restenosis and clinically driven repeated revascularization at mid-term follow-up. However, the long-term safety and effectiveness of DESs in SVGs needs further evaluation, especially in light of reports describing the increased occurrence of DES-associated thrombosis in native coronary arteries after the standard double antiplatelet therapy period [57–59].

To obtain insights into the long-term performance of sirolimus-eluting stents in SVGs, the cohort of patients enrolled in the RRISC study was followed for up to 3 years [60]. At a median follow-up of 32 months, there were 11 deaths among the group that received sirolimus-eluting stents (seven cardiac, of which one was due to very late stent thrombosis and three were sudden) (29%) compared with none in the BMSs = group (0%), an absolute difference of 29% [14–45%] ($P < 0.001$). The long-term rates of myocardial infarction and target vessel revascularization were not different: 18% and 34%, respectively, in the sirolimus-eluting stents group compared with 5% and 38%, respectively, in the BMS group ($P = 0.15$, and $P = 0.74$, respectively). The overall rate of definite angiographically documented stent thrombosis was 5% in the sirolimus-eluting stent group (2 out of 38, both very late, one fatal and one nonfatal) compared with 0% in the BMS group ($P = 0.49$), whereas the rate of any stent thrombosis (including possible stent thrombosis, i.e. sudden death >30 days after stent deployment [61]) was 13% (5 out of 38, two of which were late and three of which were very late) in the sirolimus-eluting stent group compared with 0% in the BMS group (log-rank test = 0.022).

Thus, in this secondary analysis, BMSs were associated with reduced long-term mortality and stent thrombosis compared with sirolimus-eluting stents in patients with SVG disease; in addition, the benefit of sirolimus-eluting stents in terms of a reduction in repeat revascularization at 6 months was lost at longer-term follow-up. However, this was a post hoc analysis and thus should be mainly considered hypothesis generating, requiring further confirmation or refutation from additional studies.

Providing a lower level of evidence than randomized trials, several registries have assessed the mid-term and long-term safety and effectiveness of DESs in SVGs [62–77]. All these studies were retrospective. Some of them were uncontrolled series (Table 40.1). Other registries have compared outcomes in patients treated with BMSs or DESs (Table 40.2), in some cases considering only sirolimus-eluting stents, in others only paclitaxel-eluting stents, and in others considering DESs as a single group regardless of the drug eluted. One registry

Table 40.1 Published uncontrolled series on drug-eluting stents in saphenous vein grafts.

Study	Drug-eluting stent	Enrollment	Follow-up	Death	TLR	TVR	MACE
Hoffmann (multicenter)	344 (100% sirolimus)	2002–2004	6 months	3.5%	NA	18.1%	23.8%
Price (single center)	35 (100% sirolimus)	2003	7.5 months	5.7%	5.7%	5.7%	20%
Hoye (single center)	19 (100% sirolimus)	2002	12 months	5%	5%	5%	16%
Pucelikova (single center)	101 (67% sirolimus)	2004–2005	12 months	6.8%	9.1%	19.3%	31%
Ruchin (single center)	55 (100% paclitaxel)	2003–2005	13 months	8%	2%	6%	18%
Tsuchida (single center)	40 (100% paclitaxel)	2003	15 months	0%	2.5%	5%	10%

MACE, major adverse cardiac event (death, myocardial infarction, and TVR); NA, not available; TLR, target lesion revascularization; TVR, target vessel revascularization.

compared the outcomes of sirolimus-eluting versus paclitaxel-eluting stents (Table 40.3). The design differed between each comparative registry, ranging from contemporary consecutive enrollment to historical matching cohorts. The average timing of the assessment of the outcomes varied widely among all registries, ranging between 6 months and 33 months. Overall, in the studies with a follow-up of less than 1 year, the benefits of DESs seem evident; in the longer term, the effectiveness of these devices is far less evident. Indeed, the majority of the studies have not shown significantly different outcomes between DESs and BMSs, and a few studies have demonstrated only moderate advantages, clearly not comparable to the benefits shown in native coronary arteries. On the other hand, safety issues, such as those shown by the long-term follow-up of the RRISC trial [60], have never been confirmed.

All these data underline the fact that the level of evidence in favor of DESs is not yet sufficient to warrant their routine use in the treatment of SVGs. Future well-designed and well-powered prospective randomized trials are clearly needed to definitively answer the question whether DESs can be safely and effectively implanted in SVGs in place of the currently recommended BMSs.

Technical aspects

When dealing with a lesion in a SVG, pharmacologic pretreatment of the patient is extremely important. Dual antiplatelet therapy (with a thienopyridine given upfront) and statins is mandatory, unless clearly contraindicated. Glycoprotein IIB/IIIA inhibitors, as previously mentioned, seem not to be effective in SVG interventions. However, in the case of acute myocardial infarction due to acute graft closure, we still suggest using these drugs. The choice of the guiding catheter is the first important decision. In our experience, in the case of a vein graft to the right coronary artery, originating from the right anterior surface of the aorta, the multipurpose catheter is giving the best alignment and support. Engagement of the catheter can be performed in the left anterior oblique view. For vein grafts originating from the left anterior surface (usually to the left anterior descending or diagonal arteries, and sometimes to the left circumflex), we prefer Judkins right shape or left coronary bypass catheters (the best-fitting catheter can be determined during diagnostic angiography). In case more support is needed, Amplatz left shape catheters can be used. Engagement is feasible in the right anterior oblique view. Sometimes vein grafts to the circumflex artery originate from the posterior surface of the aorta; in this case Amplatz left, left coronary bypass, or multipurpose guiding catheters are preferred. Also in this case, engagement is performed in the right anterior oblique view. Embolic protection devices should be advocated in any procedure on SVGs; however, for economic reasons, they can be avoided in the case of very focal lesions in small (<3.5 mm) grafts. Instead, a soft-tip coronary guidewire and direct stenting without pre- and post dilation should be the recommended strategy. The choice of the type of protection device depends mainly on the location of the lesion and on the personal experience of the operator with the device itself. For lesions in the mid-body of the graft, any type of protection device can be used. Proximal devices give the hypothetical advantage of a protection before any type of intervention, even the simple crossing with the coronary guidewire. However, in the case of proximal or ostial lesions, distal protection devices should be recommended. A proximal protection device fits better for distal lesions. The theoretical background for these choices relies on the fact that every protection device needs a vein graft disease-free landing zone of around 3–5 cm. For proximal or distal occlusion protection devices, the control of complete occlusion of the vessel is needed. This means that a column of stagnant blood (checked with contrast) should be evident once the device is in place. If a filter is used, we recommend controlling the good deployment of the filter itself and apposition to the vessel wall in two orthogonal views. As previously mentioned, once a protection device is used, undersizing of the stent is not advocated. On the other hand, we always recommend direct stenting, and in case the stent remains underdeployed, poststent high-pressure

Table 40.2 Published comparisons on drug-eluting stents versus bare metal stents in saphenous vein grafts.

Study	BMS	DES	Enrollment	Follow-up	Death		TLR		TVR		MACE		Unadjusted P-values	Adjusted P-values
					BMS	DES	BMS	DES	BMS	DES	BMS	DES		
Ge (single center)	89	61 (57% sirolimus)	2000–2004, historical	6 months	2.2%	1.6%	19.8%	3.3%	23.1%	4.9%	28.1%	11.5%	MACE ($P=0.01$), TLR/TVR ($P=0.003$)	MACE ($P=0.03$)
Hoffman (multicenter)	60	60 (100% paclitaxel)	NA, historical matching	6 months	NA	NA	22%	6%	NA	NA	37%	15%	MACE ($P=0.01$), TLR ($P=0.02$)	Not performed
Lee (single center)	84	139 (73% sirolimus)	2003–2004, contemporary	9 months	4%	1%	NA	NA	37%	10%	37%	10%	Death ($P=0.03$), TVR ($P=0.03$), MACE ($P=0.03$)	Not performed
Chu (single center)	57	48 (100% sirolimus)	2001–2004, historical matching	12 months	7%	6%	7%	6%	11%	13%	18%	21%	Not significant	Not performed
Whorle (single center)	26	13 (100% paclitaxel)	2005, historical matching	12 months	3.8%	0%	26.9%	0%	34.6%	7.7%	38.5%	7.7%	MACE ($P=0.04$)	Not performed
Ellis (multicenter)	175	175 (100% sirolimus)	NA, historical matching	12 months	3.6%	4.7%	9.9%	6.8%	11.8%	6.8%	NA	NA	Not significant	Not performed
Vignali (multicenter)	288	72 (69% sirolimus)	2003–2006, contemporary	14 months	7.8%	3.7%	8.1%	4.3%	11.3%	8.1%	20.3%	17.8%	Not significant	Not significant
Minutello (single center)	50	59 (100% sirolimus)	2000–2005, historical	20 months	12%	6.8%	22%	13.6%	36%	15.3%	50%	25.4%	MACE ($P=0.01$), TVR ($P=0.01$)	MACE ($P=0.03$)
Bansal (single center)	72	37 (95% sirolimus)	2003–2005, contemporary	33 months	22%	19%	38%	30%	42%	35%	50%	46%	Not significant	Not significant

MACE, major adverse cardiac events (death, myocardial infarction, and TVR); NA, not available; TLR, target lesion revascularization; TVR, target vessel revascularization.

Table 40.3 Published comparisons on different types of drug-eluting stents in saphenous vein grafts.

Study	Enrollment	Follow-up	Drug-eluting Stent	Death	TLR	TVR	MACE	Unadjusted P-values	Adjusted P-values
Chu (single center)	NA	6 months	47 sirolimus	4.3%	2.1%	4.3%	8.5%	Not significant	Not performed
	Matching	6 months	42 paclitaxel	5.3%	2.6%	5.3%	10.5%	Not significant	Not performed

MACE, major adverse cardiac event (death, myocardial infarction, and TVR); NA, not available; TLR, target lesion revascularization; TVR, target vessel revascularization.

dilation must be done with a protection device in place. Once the stenting procedure is finished, care should be given to the collection of debris from the protection device. If a proximal device is used, direct aspiration of at least 20 cc of blood from the device should be performed. If a distal occlusion device is used, the specific manual aspiration device should be used and two syringes of 20 cc of blood should be aspirated. If a filter is used, careful complete closure of the filter is necessary before retrieval. We recommend performing the complete procedure under fluoroscopy. If the filter is overloaded with debris and complete closure is not possible, aspiration by means of a manual aspiration device can be a good option. Final angiographic control of the stenting procedure without any device in place is mandatory, in at least two orthogonal views.

Conclusion

In conclusion, the treatment of choice for the percutaneous management of diseased aortocoronary vein grafts is the BMS. However, its use in this lesion subset is still burdened by a high rate of periprocedural complications and by non-satisfactory long-term results. PTFE-covered stent grafts did not fulfill their initial promise and were revealed to be ineffective. The use of embolic protection devices is currently strongly recommended, as they significantly decrease the rate of periprocedural complications. The first data comparing the use of drug-eluting stents versus bare metal stents in saphenous vein grafts are encouraging in the mid term. However, the safety and the benefits of DESs in the longer term are still debated, and the level of evidence in favor of DESs has not yet reached the level at which they can be routinely recommended in the treatment of SVGs.

References

1. Fitzgibbon G, Kafka H, Leach A, *et al.* (1996) Coronary bypass graft fate and patient outcome: angiographic follow-up of 5065 grafts related to survival and reoperation in 1388 patients during 25 years. *J Am Coll Cardiol* **28**:616–626.
2. Alexander JH, Hafley G, Harrington RA, *et al.* (2005) PREVENT IV Investigators. Efficacy and safety of edifoligide, an E2F tran-scription factor decoy, for prevention of vein graft failure following coronary artery bypass graft surgery: PREVENT IV: a randomized controlled trial. *JAMA* **294**:2446–2454.
3. Abbate A, Biondi-Zoccai GG, Agostoni P, *et al.* (2007) Recurrent angina after coronary revascularization: a clinical challenge. *Eur Heart J* 28:1057–1065.
4. Okrainec K, Platt R, Pilote L, *et al.* (2005) Cardiac medical therapy in patients after undergoing coronary artery bypass graft surgery. A review of randomized controlled trials. *J Am Coll Cardiol* **45**: 177–184.
5. Weintraub WS, Jones EL, Morris DC, *et al.* (1997) Outcome of reoperative coronary bypass surgery versus coronary angioplasty after previous bypass surgery. *Circulation* 95:868–877.
6. Morrison DA, Sethi G, Sacks J, *et al.* (2002) Percutaneous coronary intervention versus repeat bypass surgery for patients with medically refractory myocardial ischemia: AWESOME randomised trial and registry experience with post-CABG patients. *J Am Coll Cardiol* 40:1951–1954.
7. Baim D (2003) Percutaneous treatment of saphenous vein graft disease the ongoing challenge. *J Am Coll Cardiol* **42**:1370–1372.
8. Cameron AA, Davis KB, & Rogers WJ (1995) Recurrence of angina after coronary artery bypass surgery: predictors and prognosis (CASS registry). *J Am Coll Cardiol* **26**:895–899.
9. Weintraub WS, Jones EL, Craver JM, *et al.* (1994) Frequency of repeat coronary bypass or coronary angioplasty after coronary artery bypass surgery using saphenous vein grafts. *Am J Cardiol* **73**:103–112.
10. Bourassa MG (1991) Fate of venous grafts: the past, the present and the future. *J Am Coll Cardiol* 17:1081–1083.
11. Cox JL, Chiasson DA, & Gotlieb AL (1991) Stranger in a strange land: the pathogenesis of saphenous vein graft stenosis with emphasis on structural and functional differences between veins and arteries. *Prog Cardiovasc Dis* 34:45–68.
12. Holt CM, Francis SE, Newby AC, *et al.* (1993) Comparison of response to injury in organ culture of human saphenous vein and internal mammary artery. *Ann Thorac Surg* **55**:1522–1528.
13. Allaire E & Clowes AW (1997) Endothelial cell injury in cardio-vascular surgery: the intimal hyperplastic response. *Ann Thorac Surg* 63:582–591.
14. Lie JT, Lawrie GM, & Morris GC (1977) Aortocoronary bypass saphenous vein graft atherosclerosis: anatomic study of 99 vein grafts from normal and hyperlipoproteinemic patients up to 75 months postoperatively. *Am J Cardiol* **40**:906–914.
15. Boyle EM Jr, Lille ST, Allaire E, *et al.* (1997) Endothelial cell injury in cardiovascular surgery: atherosclerosis. *Ann Thorac Surg* **63**:885–894.

16. Webb J, Carere R, Virmani R, *et al.* (1999) Retrieval and analysis of particulate debris following saphenous vein graft intervention. *J Am Coll Cardiol* **34**:461–467.

17. Bryan AJ & Angelini GD (1994) The biology of saphenous vein graft occlusion: etiology and strategies for prevention. *Curr Opin Cardiol* **9**:641–649.

18. Motwani JG & Topol EJ (1998) Aortocoronary saphenous vein graft disease. Pathogenesis, predisposition, and prevention. *Circulation* **97**:916–931.

19. De Feyter PJ, Serruys P, van den Brand M, *et al.* (1989) Percutaneous transluminal angioplasty of a totally occluded venous bypass graft: a challenge that should be resisted. *Am J Cardiol* **64**:88–90.

20. Loop FD, Lytlle BW, Cosgrove DM, *et al.* (1986) Influence of the internal-mammary-artery graft on 10-year survival and other cardiac events. *N Engl J Med* **314**:1–6.

21. Choussat R, Black AJ, Bossi I, *et al.* (2000) Long-term clinical outcome after endoluminal reconstruction of diffusely degenerated saphenous vein grafts with less-shortening wallstents. *J Am Coll Cardiol* **36**:387–394.

22. Ellis SG, Brener SJ, DeLuca S, *et al.* (1997) Late myocardial ischemic events after saphenous vein graft intervention—importance of initially "nonsignificant" vein graft lesions. *Am J Cardiol* **79**:1460–1464.

23. Keeley EC, Velez CA, O'Neill WW, & Safian RD (2001) Long-term clinical outcome and predictors of major adverse cardiac events after percutaneous interventions on saphenous vein grafts. *J Am Coll Cardiol* **38**:659–665.

24. Depre C, Havaux X, & Wijns W (1998) Pathology of restenosis in saphenous bypass grafts after long term implantation. *Am J Clin Pathol* **110**:378–384.

25. Van Beusekom H, Van Der Giessen W, Van Suylen R, *et al.* (1993) Histology after stenting of human saphenous vein bypass grafts: observations from surgically excised grafts 3 to 320 days after stent implantation. *J Am Coll Cardiol* **21**:45–54.

26. Ribichini F, Pugno F, Ferrero V, *et al.* (2008) Long-term histological and immunohistochemical findings in human venous aorto-coronary bypass grafts. *Clin Sci (Lond)* **114**:211–220.

27. Farb A, Sangiorgi G, Carter A, *et al.* (1999) Pathology of acute and chronic coronary stenting in humans. *Circulation* **99**:44–52.

28. De Feyter P, Van Suylen R, De Jaegere P, *et al.* (1993) Balloon angioplasty for the treatment of lesions in saphenous vein bypass grafts. *J Am Coll Cardiol* **21**:1539–1549.

29. Serruys PW, de Jaegere P, Kiemeneij F, *et al.* (1994) A comparison of balloon-expandable-stent implantation with balloon angioplasty in patients with coronary artery disease. Benestent Study Group. *N Engl J Med* **331**:489–495.

30. Fischman DL, Leon MB, Baim DS, *et al.* (1994) A randomized comparison of coronary-stent placement and balloon angioplasty in the treatment of coronary artery disease. Stent Restenosis Study Investigators. *N Engl J Med* **331**:496–501.

31. Wong SC, Baim DS, Schatz RA, *et al.* (1995) Immediate results and late outcomes after stent implantation in saphenous vein graft lesions: the multicenter U.S. Palmaz-Schatz stent experience. The Palmaz-Schatz Stent Study Group. *J Am Coll Cardiol* **26**:704–712.

32. Savage M, Douglas J, Fischman D, *et al.* (1997) Stent placement compared with balloon angioplasty for obstructed coronary bypass grafts. *N Engl J Med* **337**:740–747.

33. Hanekamp C, Koolen J, Den Heijer P, *et al.* (2003) Randomized study to compare balloon angioplasty and elective stent implantation in venous bypass grafts: the VENESTENT study. *Cathet Cardiovasc Interv* **60**:452–457.

34. Vermeersch P & Agostoni P (2005) Should degenerated saphenous vein grafts routinely be sealed with drug-eluting stents? *J Interv Cardiol* **18**:467–473.

35. Biondi-Zoccai GG, Agostoni P, & Abbate A (2003) Parallel hierarchy of scientific studies in cardiovascular medicine. *Ital Heart J* **4**:819–820.

36. Silber S, Albertsson P, Aviles FF, *et al.* (2005) Guidelines for percutaneous coronary interventions: the task force for percutaneous coronary interventions of the European society of cardiology. *Eur Heart J* **26**:804–847.

37. Baldus S, Koster R, Elsner M, *et al.* (2000) Treatment of aortocoronary vein graft lesions with membrane-covered stents: a multicenter surveillance trial. *Circulation* **102**:2024–2027.

38. Schächinger V, Hamm CW, Münzel T, *et al.* (2003) A randomized trial of polytetrafluoroethylene-membrane-covered stents compared with conventional stents in aortocoronary saphenous vein grafts. *J Am Coll Cardiol* **42**:1360–1369.

39. Stankovic G, Colombo A, Presbitero P, *et al.* (2003) Randomized evaluation of polytetrafluoroethylene-covered stent in saphenous vein grafts: the Randomized Evaluation of polytetrafluoroethylene COVERed stent in Saphenous vein grafts (RECOVERS) Trial. *Circulation* **108**:37–42.

40. Turco MA, Buchbinder M, Popma JJ, *et al.* (2006) Pivotal, randomized U.S. study of the Symbiot covered stent system in patients with saphenous vein graft disease: eight-month angiographic and clinical results from the Symbiot III trial. *Catheter Cardiovasc Interv* **68**:379–388.

41. Stone G, Goldberg S, Mehran R, *et al.* (2005) A prospective, randomized U.S. trial of the PTFE-covered JOSTENT for the treatment of diseased saphenous vein grafts: the BARRICADE trial (abstr.). *J Am Coll Cardiol* **45**(Suppl. A):27A.

42. Baim DS, Wahr D, George B, *et al.* (2002) Randomized trial of a distal embolic protection device during percutaneous intervention of saphenous vein aorto-coronary bypass grafts. *Circulation* **105**:1285–1290.

43. Wu CJ, Yang CH, Fang CY, *et al.* (2005) Six-month angiographic results of primary angioplasty with adjunctive PercuSurge GuardWire device support: evaluation of the restenotic rate of the target lesion and the fate of the distal balloon occlusion site. *Catheter Cardiovasc Interv* **64**:35–42.

44. Agostoni P, Vermeersch P, Vydt T, *et al.* (2007) Acute and mid-term local vascular effects of compliant balloon inflation (GuardWire system) on saphenous vein bypass grafts: an angiographic analysis. *Int J Cardiol* **120**:227–231.

45. Stone GW, Rogers C, Hermiller J, *et al.* (2003) Randomized comparison of distal protection with a filter-based catheter and a balloon occlusion and aspiration system during percutaneous intervention of diseased saphenous vein aorto-coronary bypass grafts. *Circulation* **108**:548–553.

46. Mauri L, Cox D, Hermiller J, *et al.* (2007) The PROXIMAL trial: proximal protection during saphenous vein graft intervention using the Proxis Embolic Protection System: a randomized, prospective, multicenter clinical trial. *J Am Coll Cardiol* **50**:1442–1449.

47. Mehta SK, Frutkin AD, Milford-Beland S, *et al.* (2007) American College of Cardiology-National Cardiovascular Data Registry.

Utilization of distal embolic protection in saphenous vein graft interventions (an analysis of 19546 patients in the American College of Cardiology-National Cardiovascular Data Registry). *Am J Cardiol* **100**:1114–1118.

48. Roffi M, Mukherjee D, Chew DP, *et al.* (2002) Lack of benefit from intravenous platelet glycoprotein IIb/IIIa receptor inhibition as adjunctive treatment for percutaneous interventions of aortocoronary bypass grafts: a pooled analysis of five randomized clinical trials. *Circulation* **106**:3063–3067.

49. Moses J, Leon M, Popma J, *et al.* (2003) SIRIUS Investigators. Sirolimus-eluting stents versus standard stents in patients with stenosis in a native coronary artery. *N Eng J Med* **349**:1315–1323.

50. Stone GW, Ellis SG, Cox DA, *et al.* (2004) TAXUS-IV Investigators. A polymer-based, paclitaxel-eluting stent in patients with coronary artery disease. *N Engl J Med* **350**:221–231.

51. Fajadet J, Wijns W, Laarman GJ, *et al.* (2006) ENDEAVOR II Investigators. Randomized, double-blind, multicenter study of the Endeavor zotarolimus-eluting phosphorylcholine-encapsulated stent for treatment of native coronary artery lesions: clinical and angiographic results of the ENDEAVOR II trial. *Circulation* **114**: 798–806.

52. Brunner-La Rocca HP, Kaiser C, & Pfisterer M (2007) BASKET Investigators. Targeted stent use in clinical practice based on evidence from the Basel Stent Cost Effectiveness Trial (BASKET). *Eur Heart J* **28**:719–725.

53. Agostoni P, Vermeersch P, Verheye S, *et al.* (2007) Targeted stent use in clinical practice based on evidence from the Basel Stent Cost Effectiveness Trial (BASKET). *Eur Heart J* **28**:1912–1913.

54. Vermeersch P, Agostoni P, Verheye S, *et al.* (2006) Randomized double-blind comparison of sirolimus-eluting stent versus bare metal stent implantation in diseased saphenous vein grafts: 6-month angiographic, intravascular ultrasound and clinical follow up of the RRISC trial. *J Am Coll Cardiol* **48**:2423–2431.

55. Agostoni P, Vermeersch P, Semeraro O, *et al.* (2007) Intravascular ultrasound assessment of sirolimus-eluting stent versus bare metal stent implantation in diseased saphenous vein grafts (from the RRISC [Reduction of Restenosis In Saphenous vein grafts with Cypher sirolimus-eluting stent] trial). *Am J Cardiol* **100**:52–58.

56. Iakovou I, Dangas G, Mintz GS, *et al.* (2004) Relation of final lumen dimensions in saphenous vein grafts after stent implantation to outcome. *Am J Cardiol* **93**:963–968.

57. Stone GW, Moses JW, Ellis SG, *et al.* (2007) Safety and efficacy of sirolimus- and paclitaxel-eluting coronary stents. *N Engl J Med* **356**:998–1008.

58. Daemen J, Wenaweser P, Tsuchida K, *et al.* (2007) Early and late coronary stent thrombosis of sirolimus-eluting and paclitaxel-eluting stents in routine clinical practice: data from a large two-institutional cohort study. *Lancet* **369**:667–678.

59. Bavry AA, Kumbhani DJ, Helton TJ, *et al.* (2006) Late thrombosis of drug-eluting stents: a meta-analysis of randomized clinical trials. *Am J Med* **119**:1056–1061.

60. Vermeersch P, Agostoni P, Verheye S, *et al.* (2007) Increased late mortality after sirolimus-eluting stents versus bare metal stents in diseased saphenous vein grafts: results from the randomized DELAYED RRISC trial. *J Am Coll Cardiol* **50**:261–267.

61. Mauri L, Hsieh WH, Massaro JM, *et al.* (2007) Stent thrombosis in randomized clinical trials of drug-eluting stents. *N Engl J Med* **356**:1020–1029.

62. Hoffmann R, Hamm C, Nienaber CA, *et al.* (2007) Implantation of sirolimus-eluting stents in saphenous vein grafts is associated with high clinical follow-up event rates compared with treatment of native vessels. *Coron Artery Dis* **18**:559–564.

63. Price M, Sawhney N, Madrid A, *et al.* (2005) Clinical outcomes after sirolimus-eluting stent implantation for de novo saphenous vein graft lesions. *Catheter Cardiovasc Interv* **65**:208–211.

64. Hoye A, Lemos PA, Arampatzis CA, *et al.* (2004) Effectiveness of the sirolimus-eluting stent in the treatment of saphenous vein graft disease. *J Invasive Cardiol* **16**:230–233.

65. Pucelikova T, Mehran R, Kirtane AJ, *et al.* (2008) Short- and long-term outcomes after stent-assisted percutaneous treatment of saphenous vein grafts in the drug-eluting stent era. *Am J Cardiol* **101**:63–68.

66. Tsuchida K, Ong AT, Aoki J, *et al.* (2005) Immediate and one-year outcome of percutaneous intervention of saphenous vein graft disease with paclitaxel-eluting stents. *Am J Cardiol* **96**: 395–398.

67. Ruchin PE, Faddy SC, Muller DW, *et al.* (2007) Clinical follow-up of paclitaxel-eluting (TAXUS) stents for the treatment of saphenous vein graft disease. *J Interv Cardiol* **20**:258–264.

68. Ge L, Iakovou I, Sangiorgi G, *et al.* (2005) Treatment of saphenous vein graft lesions with drug-eluting stents. *J Am Coll Cardiol* **45**:989–994.

69. Hoffmann R, Pohl T, Koster R, *et al.* (2007) Implantation of paclitaxel eluting stents in saphenous vein grafts: clinical and angiographic follow-up results from a multicentre study. *Heart* **93**:331–334.

70. Lee MS, Shah AP, Aragon J, *et al.* (2005) Drug-eluting stenting is superior to bare metal stenting in saphenous vein grafts. *Catheter Cardiovasc Interv* **66**:507–511.

71. Chu WW, Rha SW, Kuchulakanti PK, *et al.* (2006) Efficacy of sirolimus-eluting stents compared with bare metal stents for saphenous vein graft intervention. *Am J Cardiol* **97**:34–37.

72. Wohrle J, Nusser T, Kestler HA, *et al.* (2007) Comparison of the slow release polymer-based paclitaxel-eluting Taxus-Express stent with the bare metal Express stent for saphenous vein graft interventions. *Clin Res Cardiol* **96**:70–76.

73. Ellis SG, Kandzari D, Kereiakes DJ, *et al.* (2007) Utility of sirolimus-eluting Cypher stents to reduce 12-month target vessel revascularization in saphenous vein graft stenoses: results of a multicenter 350-patient case–control study. *J Invasive Cardiol* **19**:404–409.

74. Vignali L, Saia F, Manari A, *et al.* (2008) Long-term outcomes with drug-eluting stents versus bare metal stents in the treatment of saphenous vein graft disease: results from the REAL (REgistro Regionale AngiopLastiche Emilia-Romagna) Registry. *Am J Cardiol* **101**:947–952.

75. Minutello RM, Bhagan S, Sharma A, *et al.* (2007) Long-term clinical benefit of sirolimus-eluting stents compared to bare metal stents in the treatment of saphenous vein graft disease. *J Interv Cardiol* **20**:458–465.

76. Bansal D, Muppidi R, Singla S, *et al.* (2008) Percutaneous intervention on the saphenous vein bypass grafts—long-term outcomes. *Catheter Cardiovasc Interv* **71**:58–61.

77. Chu WW, Kuchulakanti PK, Wang B, *et al.* (2006) Efficacy of sirolimus-eluting stents as compared to paclitaxel-eluting stents for saphenous vein graft intervention. *J Interv Cardiol* **19**:121–125.

41 Pharmacology in the Cardiac Catheterization Laboratory

Sara D. Collins, Asmir I. Syed & Ron Waksman

Washington Hospital Center, Washington, DC, USA

Introduction

Over the last 30 years we have witnessed the development of a new field of pharmacotherapy for the catheterization laboratory. Initially, on-the-shelf drugs were used for percutaneous coronary intervention (PCI) procedures, mainly to prevent thrombosis. Change and progress in the field of cardiovascular pharmacology have led to the introduction and approval of new agents to aid in these procedures. We have seen the development of molecules for the prevention of atherothrombosis, restenosis, and for hemodynamic support, the development of safer contrast agents, and the introduction of agents to prevent nephrotoxicity. Although we do not intend to cover all medications used in the catheterization laboratory in this chapter, we will provide a variety of approaches to different catheterization laboratory situations and suggest pharmacologic therapy solutions. Specific challenges such as the prevention of contrast nephropathy, thrombectomy events, facilitated sedation, hemodynamic support, alleviation of intracardiac spasm, and clinical angina are addressed. Also, this chapter will cover therapies for addressing those with special considerations, such as management of hypertensive emergency and heart failure in the catheterization laboratory.

Nephroprotective agents

There are many factors that predispose patients to contrast-induced nephropathy (CIN). This is defined as an increase of $\geq 25\%$ in serum creatinine within 48 h of receiving contrast. Variables that predispose patients to CIN include patient risk factors, type and volume of contrast agent, ionic content, and contrast viscosity. Patient risk factors include chronic kidney disease, heart failure, diabetes mellitus, age, and anemia. In addition, impaired left ventricular dysfunction can result in hypoperfusion of kidneys, thereby decreasing their ability to

clear the contrast agents. Higher osmotic agents with more iodide content can also be nephrotoxic, although this has been reduced with newer agents. Contrast material may also have a direct effect on the renal arterioles resulting in dye-induced vasoconstriction. Large volumes of contrast used in prolonged interventional procedures also contribute to this process. Practice guidelines recommend obtaining preprocedural serum creatinine levels among patients with renal disease, diabetes, proteinuria, hypertension, gout, or congestive heart failure. In practice, however, most patients who are referred for heart catheterization get a creatinine level check, as these variables can be undiagnosed or progressive.

Certain medications can predispose patients to CIN. It is recommended that metformin be held at least 24 h before the procedure and 48 h post procedure until the creatinine stabilizes. In addition, withholding nephrotoxic agents, such as aminoglycosides and nonsteroidal antiinflammatory agents, is recommended. Hydration with normal saline can prevent renal insufficiency in patients with normal renal function [1,2]. Normal saline is given to inpatients at 1 mL/kg/h for 12 h before the procedure and usually for another 12 h post procedure. Outpatients can get a bolus of 3 mL/kg 1 h before the procedure and then 1 mL/kg/h for the duration of their stay. Hydration alone is often inadequate in patients who have risk factors such as those previously mentioned, and therefore additional protective agents are required.

Currently, there are two agents used in the catheterization laboratory to prevent CIN: N-acetylcysteine (NAC) and sodium bicarbonate ($NaHCO_3$). NAC is an antioxidant that scavenges oxygen-derived free radicals, thus preventing oxidative injury and providing improvement of endothelium-dependent vasodilation. It has Food and Drug Administration (FDA) approval for its mucolytic properties and as an antidote for acetaminophen toxicity. It also has a nephroprotective effect and is used before procedures to prevent renal insufficiency in certain moderate- to high-risk patient populations [3–6]. Its use in the catheterization laboratory is not an official FDA-approved indication; however, numerous trials have shown the benefit of its nephroprotective effect in certain patient subgroups. $NaHCO_3$ infusion can cause urinary alkalinization and can possibly decrease free radical

Cardiovascular Interventions in Clinical Practice. Edited by Jürgen Haase, Hans-Joachim Schäfers, Horst Sievert and Ron Waksman. © 2010 Blackwell Publishing.

renal injury resulting from contrast exposure [7–9]. In a single-center, prospective, randomized trial, Merten *et al.* [7] compared NaHCO₃ with sodium chloride and found a decreased incidence of CIN in patients infused with NaHCO₃. In another study, NaHCO₃ proved even more efficacious than NAC [10]. A combination of these two agents in emergent percutaneous coronary intervention (PCI) seems to be beneficial as well [8,11]. In the Renal Insufficiency Following Contrast Media Administration Trial (REMEDIAL), Briguori *et al.* [11] showed that the combination of these two agents is superior to NAC alone or with the addition of vitamin C.

Pharmacokinetics

NAC is available in oral or intravenous (i.v.) form, although in the USA it is used only in oral form for prevention of CIN. It has a volume of distribution of 0.47 L/kg and is 83% protein bound when given in i.v. form. It has a decreased volume of distribution and protein binding when given orally. It has a half-life of 5.6–6.25 h. The kidney clearance is ~30% of the total clearance of the body. NaHCO₃ comes in a white crystalline, water soluble powder. EVery 84 mg of NaHCO₃ is equal to one milliequivalent each of Na⁺ and HCO₃⁻. NaHCO₃ dissociates into sodium and bicarbonate ions in the blood. Bicarbonate levels are regulated by the kidney and can alkalinize the urine. It raises the blood pH and can reverse acidosis by binding to excess hydrogen ions. If there are adequate levels of hydrogen cations, then bicarbonate is converted to carbonic acid and excreted in the lung as CO_2. Bicarbonate is reabsorbed by the kidneys and <1% is excreted.

Dosing

Various dosing methods have been proposed for NAC. The current standard in most laboratoriess is to give 600 mg twice a day before the procedure and then for 2 days after the procedure. Sodium bicarbonate is usually given as three ampules (154 mEq/L) in 5% dextrose and water. It is given as a bolus of 3 mL/kg for 1 h, and then as an infusion of 1 mL/kg/h during the procedure and for 6 h after the procedure. In patients with heart failure, the duration is shorter.

Route of administration

Currently NAC is given orally. It can also be given intravenously, but this route is not widely used [6]. NaHCO₃ is given intravenously, as described above.

Adverse reactions

Rash, urticaria, pruritus and flushing, and worsening of asthma can be caused by NAC. Anaphylactoid reactions have been described. It has a pregnancy risk factor category of B. There are no well-documented drug interactions. In patients with severe renal insufficiency, NaHCO₃ can cause hydrogen ion retention and thus precipitate or worsen heart failure. It is incompatible with certain medications, and thus caution should be exercised when administering it. Epinephrine, norepinephrine, and calcium can precipitate it and therefore should not be co-administered in the same i.v. line. NaHCO₃ has a pregnancy risk factor category of C. Adverse effects include hypernatremia, metabolic alkalosis, and mechanical complications due to extravasation of solution, resulting in chemical cellulitis.

Agents used in contrast allergy

Allergy can occur with the use of contrast agents in the catheterization laboratory. The severity of contrast allergy can range from mild to severe. Mild reactions can include nausea, vomiting, headache, hives, itching, and flushing. Moderate reactions include shortness of breath, hypotension, and profound cutaneous reactions. Severe reactions can include bronchospasms, arrhythmias, shock, seizures, and cardiac arrest. An anaphylactic reaction is the most serious and is potentially life-threatening. Acute, severe life-threatening symptoms can occur within minutes of administration of contrast. Delayed reactions occur 30 min after contrast administration (30% incidence with ionic agents) and are usually mild. This is less likely to occur with the use of nonionic agents (10% incidence). Nonionic agents, in general, are associated with a lower incidence of allergy [12]. Asthmatics have an increased risk of allergic reactions to contrast agents. Contrast agents have been known to affect fetal thyroid tissue, and should therefore be avoided in pregnant patients if possible. Low-osmolarity, nonionic agents should be used whenever possible; however, because of cost (10 times that of high-osmolarity agents), their use is limited to patients with risk factors as delineated above. Extravasations of contrast can also cause a chemical cellulitis (worse than with ionic agents). Contrary to popular belief, an allergy to shellfish is not considered a risk factor for contrast allergy. Overall, contrast media can cause severe adverse reactions at a rate of 0.2% for ionic agents and 0.04% for lower-osmolality and nonionic agents.

The treatment of allergic reactions is focused on initial assessment and Advanced Cardiac Life Support protocol. Epinephrine (1:1000 dilution given as 0.1–0.3 mg subcutaneously) should be given every 15 min as necessary until an adequate response is observed. If this is inadequate, then intravenous infusion of epinephrine should be instituted (1:10 000 dilution = 100 μg/mL at a rate of 1 μg/min). Corticosteroids should also be administered if bronchospasm is suspected (50 mg i.v. hydrocortisone or methylprednisolone). Combined H₁ (i.v. diphenhydramine 50 mg) and H₂ (i.v. ranitidine 1 mg/kg) receptor blockade provides dramatic relief from symptoms. Glucagon, 1 mg intravenously as a bolus, may be useful in patients who have taken beta-blockers and have ongoing bronchospasm. Continuous infusion of glucagon, 1–5 mg/h, may be given if required. Delayed reactions usually resolve spontaneously and require no treatment.

Prevention of allergic reaction is the main goal for patients in the catheterization laboratory. Patients who have had previous anaphylaxis are at high risk, and identification through history and previous catheterization reports is essential. Prophylactic administration of corticosteroids and H_1 and H_2 blockers prevents minor and moderate reactions from occurring [13,14]. Steroids (prednisone 60 mg) should be given 1 h, 6 h, and 13 h before the procedure. Alternatively, hydrocortisone (100 mg i.v.) can be given 1 h before the procedure. In addition to corticosteroids, diphenhydramine (25–50 mg) orally and ranitidine (150 mg) orally are given before the procedure. Allergy to latex in gloves, catheters, and other devices can further compound the confusion of possible allergy to contrast agents.

Conscious sedation

Conscious sedation is the standard method of analgesia employed in the cardiac catheterization laboratory. The goal of conscious sedation is to achieve a level of consciousness that is mildly depressed, allowing the patient to appropriately respond to verbal commands but without compromise of the airway [15]. Patients are often given oral diazepam (2.5–10 mg) and/or diphenhydramine (25–50 mg) approximately 1 h before the procedure [15]. Intravenous midazolam and fentanyl are the most common agents used for sedation during the catheterization procedure. Standard conscious sedation can be administered by a trained and licensed healthcare professional in the presence of the interventionalist. Patients requiring further anesthesia should undergo induction by a licensed anesthesiologist. If the patient demonstrates signs of respiratory depression, such as hypoxemia not responding to supplemental oxygen or decreased ventilation not responding to gentle stimulation, use of agents to reverse conscious sedation should be considered [15]. Naloxone and flumazenil are the most common agents used in this setting.

Fentanyl
Fentanyl is used as an opioid analgesic in the cardiac catheterization laboratory in combination with midazolam for conscious sedation. Adverse effects include hypotension, bradycardia, nausea, vomiting, and respiratory depression.

Dosing
Twenty-five to fifty micrograms can be given intravenously and may be repeated every 3–5 min until the desired level of consciousness or pain control is achieved. The maximum dose is 500 μg/4 h [16].

Pregnancy risk factor
Fentanyl has a pregnancy risk factor category of C/D.

Midazolam
Midazolam is a benzodiazepine used in the cardiac catheterization laboratory in combination with fentanyl for conscious sedation. Adverse effects include respiratory depression, nausea, and vomiting.

Dosing
An initial dose of ≤2.5 mg can be given in healthy adults <60 years of age; some patients may respond to as little as 1 mg. A total dose of ≤5 mg generally is adequate [17].

Pregnancy risk factor
Midazolam has a pregnancy risk factor category of D.

Naloxone
Naloxone is a pure opiate antagonist used for reversal of opiate intoxication and narcotic overdose. It should be avoided in chronic opioid users because it may precipitate acute withdrawal symptoms and possible cardiovascular instability, such as pulmonary edema and ventricular fibrillation [18].

Dosing
An initial dose of 0.1–0.2 mg, given at 2- to 3-min intervals, can be given until the desired response (i.e., adequate ventilation and alertness without substantial pain or discomfort) is obtained [18].

Pregnancy risk factor
Naloxone has a pregnancy risk factor category of C.

Flumazenil
Flumazenil is a benzodiazepine antagonist used for reversal of conscious sedation. Adverse effects include nausea and vomiting.

Dosing
An initial dose of 0.2 mg is given intravenously over 15 s. Additional 0.2-mg doses may be administered at 1-min intervals until an adequate response is achieved or a cumulative dose of 1 mg during an initial 5-min dosing period is given [19].

Pregnancy risk factor
Flumazenil has a pregnancy risk factor category of C.

Antithrombotic therapy

Antithrombotic therapy remains the cornerstone of adjunctive pharmacology in the cardiac catheterization laboratory. Antiplatelet agents, antithrombin agents, and newer direct factor Xa inhibitors are administered during PCI in an effort to improve early clinical outcomes and prevent procedural complications at the site of intervention [20].

Antiplatelet agents

Aspirin

Mechanism of action/indications

Aspirin produces a functional platelet defect by irreversibly inactivating platelet prostaglandin G/H synthase, therefore suppressing synthesis of the platelet-aggregating protein thromboxane A_2 [21]. Initial studies of aspirin in the setting of PCI focused on preventing restenosis. Although this effect has not been proven, these studies did establish a relationship between aspirin and reduction in short-term ischemic complications after PCI [20,22–26]. There is also overwhelming evidence to support the use of aspirin in the setting of unstable angina, non-ST-elevation myocardial infarction (NSTEMI) [27–30] and ST-elevation myocardial infarction (STEMI) [31]. As a result, aspirin has laid the foundation for antiplatelet therapy in the catheterization laboratory.

Dosing

As no minimum effective dose of aspirin in the setting of PCI has been defined, current recommendations are based on effective dosing that minimizes bleeding risk. Aspirin exerts its inhibitory effect within 60 min of oral administration. This platelet suppression lasts up to 7 days [20]. Current guidelines recommend pretreatment with 75–325 mg of aspirin in patients on long-term aspirin therapy, and 300–325 mg in those who are aspirin naïve at least 2 h, but preferably 24 h, before PCI [32,33]. After implantation of a bare metal stent (BMS), the American College of Cardiology/American Heart Association/Society for Cardiovascular Angiography and Interventions guidelines recommend treatment with 325 mg aspirin for 1 month, then 75–162 mg indefinitely [32,33]. Given the higher risk of late stent thrombosis associated with drug-eluting stent (DES) implantation, prolonged dual therapy with aspirin and clopidogrel is recommended post PCI in patients without high bleeding risk post implantation of a DES [24,25,34–37]. Previous recommendations of dual therapy immediately after stent implantation were based on clinically stable patients with few comorbidities and with short target lesions [24–26,35,38–42]. Patients with high-risk coronary lesions and co-existing conditions, such as renal dysfunction and diabetes mellitus, represent a sicker patient population not previously studied when the initial guidelines for DES implantation were established. This increased incidence of late stent thrombosis often occurs with discontinuation of dual antiplatelet therapy after the initial recommended duration [34–36,38–46]. Experts currently recommend continuing dual antiplatelet therapy for ≥12 months after implantation of a DES in patients who are not at increased bleeding risk [34–39]. Some suggest that dual therapy may be continued indefinitely in these patients [35,37–39], although the ideal duration of dual therapy and the potential increased risk of bleeding with its extended use have not been established [38,39,41,47,48]. Although cleared

with hemodialysis, aspirin use should be avoided in patients with severe renal impairment (creatinine clearance <10).

Pregnancy risk factor
Aspirin has a pregnancy risk factor category of C/D.

Aspirin desensitization
Aspirin hypersensitivity can provide a critical challenge in managing pharmacotherapy in the catheterization laboratory. Aspirin allergies can present as a myriad of symptoms including asthma, rhinitis, urticaria, angioedema, and anaphylactoid reactions [49]. Dual platelet therapy is critical in the management of elective PCI as well as acute coronary syndrome, as discontinuation or avoidance of therapy carries the risk of potentially fatal stent thrombosis. In addition to replacing aspirin with another antiplatelet agent, such as clopidogrel, aspirin desensitization provides another option for managing aspirin hypersensitivity in patients who need long-term therapy. Several different algorithms for aspirin desensitization have been tested, most in small series of patients, with good results [50,51]. Protocols that employ a rapid desensitization (Table 41.1) are appropriate for initiation before catheterization but are not suitable in the management of STEMI, in which reperfusion and antiplatelet agents must be administered immediately [50]. Although there is no universally accepted method, the approach seen in Figure 41.1 to managing cardiovascular patients with aspirin hypersensitivity can be employed in nonemergent cases.

Clopidogrel

Mechanism of action
Thienopyridine derivatives impair platelet aggregation by irreversibly inhibiting the platelet adenosine diphosphate receptor in response to adenosine diphosphate released from activated platelets [52,53]. Aspirin and thienopyridine derivatives work synergistically, and the combination of aspirin and clopidogrel result in greater platelet aggregation than either agent alone [54].

Table 41.1 Arterial septal aneurysm (ASA) challenge/desensitization protocols for patients with ASA-induced cutaneous disease [51].

Time (min)	ASA dose (mg)
0	0.1
15	0.3
30	10.0
45	30.0
60	40.0
85	81.0
110	162.0
135	325.0

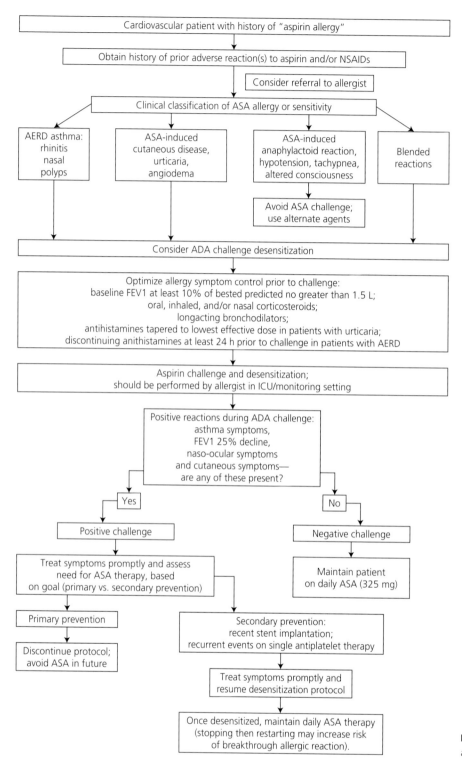

Figure 41.1 Management of patients with aspirin allergy [49].

Ticlopidine versus clopidogrel

Thienopyridine derivatives in combination with aspirin therapy have been proven to reduce the rate of adverse events after PCI versus systemic anticoagulation [55–57]. The most widely used thienopyridine derivatives are ticlopidine and clopidogrel. Initial studies demonstrating lower adverse events after PCI were performed with ticlopidine and aspirin versus anticoagulation [44,55,57]. Clopidogrel has been proven to have similar efficacy to ticlopidine with an improved safety profile [58,59]. Despite the fact that both have been proven to reduce cardiac events with similar efficacy, the increased adverse effects, such as neutropenia and thrombocytopenia, and the ease of use of clopidogrel (daily vs. twice a day dosing) have made clopidogrel the thienopyridine of choice.

Indications and dosing

Clopidogrel is used in the catheterization laboratory for both pretreatment before elective PCI, as well as in the acute settings of unstable angina (UA)/NSTEMI and STEMI [20,27,30,31,60]. Current guidelines recommend a loading dose and then maintenance dose of clopidogrel or glycoprotein IIb/IIIa inhibitor before diagnostic angiography for UA/NSTEMI patients in whom an invasive strategy is selected [27]. Dual therapy with aspirin and clopidogrel 75 mg daily should be initiated in all patients with STEMI, regardless of the method of reperfusion, or whether the patient underwent reperfusion at all. In patients <75 years of age, including those who have received fibrinolytic therapy, a loading dose of 300 mg is recommended [31]. The optimal loading dose of clopidogrel has not yet been established, although most randomized trials demonstrating its efficacy and bleeding risks were performed with a loading dose of 300 mg, followed by a maintenance dose of 75 mg daily [61,62]. Clopidogrel loading doses of 600 and 900 mg have been shown to achieve more rapid and increased levels of platelet inhibition, yet the safety and clinical efficacy of these doses need to be investigated further [63–65]. In a small study of patients with ACS, treatment with a 600-mg loading dose of clopidogrel compared with a 300-mg dose in patients undergoing coronary stenting was associated with a significant reduction in periprocedural myocardial infarctions [66]. Current guidelines recommend a loading dose of 600 mg before or when PCI is performed. This dose may be decreased to 300 mg in patients who have received fibrinolytic therapy within 12–24 h [32].

Late stent thrombosis has been proven to occur more commonly with DESs than with BMSs, even in patients on antiplatelet monotherapy with aspirin [42,45]. Guidelines outlining duration of dual antiplatelet therapy have been modified in an attempt to reduce the incidence of this potentially catastrophic event. For all post-PCI patients receiving a DES, clopidogrel 75 mg should be administered daily for ≥12 months for patients without increased risk of bleeding. Patients receiving a BMS require clopidogrel for ≥1 month and ideally up to 12 months post PCI [22].

Pregnancy risk factor

Clopidogrel has a pregnancy risk factor category of B.

Prasugrel

More novel thienopyridines are currently under study, including prasugrel, which is not yet available in US markets. In a large, randomized controlled trial of prasugrel (60 mg loading and 10 mg maintenance dose) versus clopidogrel (300 mg loading and 75 mg maintenance dose) in patients with ACS, patients who received prasugrel had a reduction in the composite end point of cardiovascular death, myocardial infarction or stroke

at a median follow-up of 14.5 months compared with clopidogrel. A lower rate of stent thrombosis was observed in the prasugrel group; however, a higher rate of significant bleeding occurred [67]. A smaller study was conducted of prasugrel (60 mg loading and 10 mg maintenance dose) versus clopidogrel (at a higher loading dose of 60 mg and 150 mg maintenance dose), which demonstrated more rapid, higher and more consistent antiplatelet effects compared with clopidogrel. More frequent bleeding was also noted in the prasugrel group, although no significant differences were noted [68]. Prasugrel may be beneficial for patients at a higher risk of stent thrombosis, but should be used with caution, if at all, in patients with higher bleeding risk. More studies need to be conducted to further elucidate these concerns before prasugrel is widely accepted for use in the in the USA.

Glycoprotein IIb/IIIa antagonists

Mechanism of action

Glycoprotein (GP) IIb/IIIa antagonists prevent the binding of fibrinogen to the GP IIb/IIIa receptors, thereby inhibiting platelet aggregation [69]. The three approved GP IIb/IIIa antagonists—abciximab, eptifibatide and tirofiban—each have different pharmacokinetic properties. Abciximab is a fragment antigen binding (Fab fragment) fragment of a humanized murine antibody that has a short plasma half-life with a strong affinity for the GP IIb/IIIa receptor. Platelet aggregation usually returns to normal ~24–48 h after discontinuation of the drug [27]. Eptifibatide is a cyclic heptapeptide containing the Lys-Gly-Asp sequence of fibrinogen. Tirofiban is a nonpeptide mimetic of the Arg-Gly-Asp sequence of fibrinogen. Both drugs bind the GP IIb/IIIa receptor with high specificity, but have shorter half-lives of 2–3 h, therefore platelet aggregation returns to normal 4–8 h after their discontinuation [27].

Indications

Overall, the three GP IIb/IIIa receptors licensed in North America reduce clinical events in patients with acute coronary syndrome by 35–50% [20].

Abciximab

In patients with acute coronary syndrome undergoing immediate PCI, abciximab has been shown to decrease rates of myocardial infarction and need for urgent revascularization [70–73]. These benefits do not translate to acute coronary syndrome patients in whom PCI is not planned within 48 h [74]. Therefore, abciximab is an appropriate choice for upstream GP IIb/IIIa therapy if an initial invasive strategy is selected and no delay to PCI is anticipated [27].

Tirofiban

Tirofiban is another GP IIb/IIIa inhibitor approved for the treatment of patients with acute coronary syndrome, in particular patients undergoing PCI [75,76]. This indication is in large part based on a large trial of tirofiban and heparin versus heparin therapy alone in high-risk patients with acute coronary syndrome and undergoing PCI. A decrease in death, myocardial infarction, or refractory ischemia was demonstrated at 7 and 30 days, as well as 6 months, with no difference in major bleeding [76].

Eptifibatide

Eptifibatide is approved for the treatment of patients with UA/NSTEMI who are treated medically or with PCI. The double-bolus regimen of 180 μg/kg 10 min apart followed by an infusion of 2.0 μg/kg/min for 18–24 h was tested in a large study, after trials using smaller bolus regimens were less successful, and is now the standard of care [77]. Another large trial demonstrated a decrease in death or nonfatal myocardial infarction at 6 months in patients treated with eptifibatide [78].

Several large studies have demonstrated a significant reduction in the rate of death or myocardial infarction for patients with UA/NSTEMI managed medically, and also an increased benefit after PCI [27,70,76,78] A meta-analysis was conducted of six large trials comparing GP IIb/IIIa antagonists with placebo in patients with UA/NSTEMI not undergoing urgent revascularization. The study demonstrated the most substantial reduction of death or myocardial infarction in patients at highest risk of thrombotic complications [79]. This evidence provides support for treatment strategies targeted toward GP IIb/IIIa therapy in patients with an elevated troponin level early in their hospital course. This meta-analysis also demonstrated a greater risk reduction in a subgroup of patients undergoing PCI than patients who were medically managed [79]. This provides more support for the fact that GP IIb/IIIa antagonists are of significant benefit in patients with UA/NSTEMI in whom an initial invasive strategy is selected. This benefit becomes less substantial in patients who do not undergo urgent revascularization [27] If an initial invasive strategy is chosen, antiplatelet therapy should be initiated before diagnostic angiography with clopidogrel or a GP IIb/IIIa inhibitor. Eptifibatide or tirofiban are the preferred strategies if any delay to intervention is likely to occur. Abciximab is the GP IIb/IIIa antagonist of choice if there is no anticipated delay to angiography/PCI [27].

Dosing

A 0.25 mg/kg bolus dose of abciximab followed by a 10 μg/min infusion for 12 h [71,80] is given. For eptifibatide, 180 μg/kg double bolus 10 min apart followed by 2.0 μg/kg/min infusion can be given [77,81]. Patients with severe renal impairment (estimated creatinine clearance <50 mL/min) should receive a 180 μg/kg double bolus 10 min apart followed by a 1 μg/kg/min infusion [81]. Tirofiban can be used for acute coronary syndromes intravenously. An initial rate of 0.4 μg/kg/min for 30 min is followed by a rate of 0.1 μg/kg/min. Dosing should be continued through angiography and for 12–24 h after angioplasty or atherectomy. For severe renal

impairment, the dose should be reduced to 50% of the normal rate [82].

Pregnancy risk factors

Abciximab has a pregnancy risk factor category of C, tirofiban has a pregnancy risk factor category of B, and eptifibatide has a pregnancy risk factor category of B.

Antiplatelet drug resistance

Antiplatelet drug resistance, or nonresponsiveness, has been studied for decades but has received increased attention over recent years. Aspirin resistance has been evaluated most extensively [83], although variability in response to other antiplatelet agents, such as clopidogrel and GP IIb/IIIa antagonists has proven to have clinical relevance as well.

Based on the lack of a consensus definition, the incidence of both aspirin and clopidogrel nonresponsiveness is uncertain. Antiplatelet resistance has, however, been associated with poor clinical outcomes. Aspirin resistance in stable cardiovascular patients has been associated with an increased risk of major adverse events [84]. One of the largest prospective studies evaluating aspirin resistance was performed on patients enrolled in the Heart Outcomes Prevention Evaluation (HOPE) study. Aspirin resistance, based on elevated urinary 11-dehydrothromboxane B_2 concentrations was associated with elevated risk of myocardial infarction or cardiovascular death [85]. In addition, dual drug-resistant patients have been shown to have an increased potential risk of thrombotic complications after PCI [86].

Clinical antiplatelet drug resistance can be defined as a recurrence of vascular atherothrombotic events, despite drug compliance [87]. It may be difficult to determine, however, exactly which pathway has been affected and, as a result, which drug has failed. In the laboratory, resistance is defined as post-treatment activity in the target pathway of an antiplatelet agent [87]. Absolute cut-off values for defining resistance are not standardized, however, and vary depending on which platelet drug response assay is used.

A number of tests have been developed to assess platelet function. Biochemical assays use either an enzyme-linked immunosorbent assay (thromboxane) or flow cytometry. Non-biochemical tests measure platelet function directly using light transmittance or electrical impedance [87]. The "gold" standard of platelet function assays is light transmission aggregometry (LTA). These laboratory tests can be costly and labor-intensive, making apparent a need for point-of-care platelet function testing that can provide more convenient and more rapid results [87].

Three point-of-care platelet function tests are used most commonly. The PFA-100 (Dade Behring Inc., Deerfield, IL, USA), used primarily for assessing aspirin resistance, uses arachidonic acid and ADP agonists [88]. VerifyNow (Accumetrics, San

Diego, CA, USA) tests aspirin, clopidogrel, and GP IIb/IIIa responsiveness and has been validated against LTA. The VerifyNow aspirin resistance assay uses arachidonic acid as the agonist, whereas the PDY12 assay uses ADP as the agonist to ascertain the level of platelet function [89]. The Thromboelastogram analyzer (Haemoscope, Niles, IL, USA) measures the shear elasticity of clotting blood and is primarily used in cardiac surgical procedures [90].

Point-of-care platelet function assays have been prospectively studied in both stable and unstable cardiovascular patients undergoing PCI. Patients with aspirin resistance adequately treated with clopidogrel have demonstrated increased risk of myonecrosis after elective PCI [91]. Aspirin resistance has been shown to be an independent predictor of major cardiovascular adverse events in acute myocardial infarction patients undergoing primary PCI [92]. The STRATEGY (High-Dose Bolus Tirofiban and Sirolimus Eluting Stent Versus Abciximab and Bare Metal Stent in Acute Myocardial Infarction) trial assessed platelet responsiveness using both the PFA-100 and LTA assays in STEMI patients undergoing primary PCI treated with GP IIb/IIIa inhibitors. Abnormal platelet function was associated with a 5- to 11-fold increased risk of death, reinfarction, or target vessel revascularization at 1 year [93]. Clopidogrel resistance has been assessed in trials studying variable doses of clopidogrel in stable and unstable patients. Higher loading doses of clopidogrel in both stable and unstable patients after PCI have been shown to improve platelet reactivity [94].

Although platelet nonresponsiveness testing has become less costly and easier to perform at the bedside, differences between testing methods and variable thresholds for nonresponsiveness create challenges in correlating resistance with clinical outcomes. Management of antiplatelet drug resistance is still approached empirically, as little evidence exists to dictate treatment. Trials currently under way are attempting to address the issue of algorithm development to guide antiplatelet therapy based on aspirin and clopidogrel responsiveness.

Anticoagulants

Anticoagulants used in the cardiac catheterization laboratory include heparin and its derivatives, direct thrombin inhibitors, as well as factor Xa inhibitors.

Unfractionated heparin

Mechanism of action

Unfractionated heparin (UFH) is made up of polysaccharide chains of varying molecular weights, resulting in variable anticoagulant activity [20]. It acts by potentiating the action of circulating antithrombin, which inactivates thrombin, in addition to activated coagulation factors IX, X, XI, and XII,

and plasmin. The conversion of fibrinogen to fibrin is also prevented by UFH. These actions prevent the propagation of, but do not lyse, existing thrombi [27].

Indications

Unfractionated heparin is indicated for use in the catheterization laboratory in the setting of elective PCI [20–23,95], UA/NSTEMI [27], and as ancillary therapy for STEMI [31,32]. UFH has been shown to reduce early ischemic events in UA/NSTEMI [80–82,96]. In a meta-analysis of six randomized trials, the combination of aspirin and UFH in the setting of UA/NSTEMI demonstrated a 33% reduction in the risk of myocardial infarction or death compared with aspirin alone [97].

Dosing

As a result of poor bioavailability and highly variable anticoagulant effects, UFH requires monitoring with activated partial thromboplastin time (aPTT) [27]. Initial dosing in the catheterization laboratory, however, is guided by activated clotting time (ACT) because the level of anticoagulation is initially beyond a range measurable with aPTT [20]. Weight-adjusted dosing improves the predictability of anticoagulation compared with a fixed-dose regimen [98,99].

In patients undergoing PCI who have not received initial medical treatment with UFH but who have received a GP IIb/IIIa inhibitor, a UFH bolus of 50–70 IU/kg to achieve a targeted ACT >200 s has been suggested [20]. In UA/NSTEMI, this dose is adjusted to 60–70 U/kg [27]. In patients who do not receive a GP IIb/IIIa inhibitor, UFH should be administered in boluses of 60–100 IU/kg, with a target ACT of 250–350 s [20]. This is adjusted to 100–140 U/kg in the setting of UA/NSTEMI [27]. Postprocedural infusion of UFH is not routinely recommended [20].

Pregnancy risk factor

Unfractionated heparin has a pregnancy risk factor category of C.

Low-molecular-weight heparin: enoxaparin

Mechanism of action

Low-molecular-weight heparins (LMWHs) are derived by chemically or enzymatically depolymerizing the polysaccharide chains of heparin. Low-molecular-weight heparins exert their anticoagulant activity using the same mechanism as UFH, by activating antithrombin [100]. An advantage of LMWHs is that they bind less to plasma proteins and endothelial cells and have a dose-independent clearance. Low-molecular-weight heparins also have a longer half-life than UFH and a more predictable anticoagulation, and therefore require daily or twice-daily dosing. These agents are administered subcutaneously, without requiring laboratory monitoring [100].

Indications

Several LMWHs have been evaluated for use in PCI, the most studied of which is enoxaparin. Enoxaparin has been evaluated for use in both elective PCI [101–103] and as part of an early invasive strategy for treatment of UA/NSTEMI compared with UFH [102,104–106]. Most trials demonstrate noninferiority of enoxaparin, with some revealing increased bleeding risk with enoxaparin use. Enoxaparin has also been studied as ancillary therapy in STEMI patients post reperfusion. One large randomized trial of enoxaparin versus UFH was conducted in patients with STEMI receiving fibrinolytic therapy and subsequent PCI. Patients treated with enoxaparin had a lower rate of death and nonfatal myocardial infarction than patients treated with UFH [107]. Enoxaparin is therefore indicated for use in STEMI [31,32,95] and as part of an early invasive strategy for treatment of UA/NSTEMI [20,95].

Dosing

Enoxaparin is dosed in the cardiac catheterization laboratory, primarily based on the timing of previous treatment. If the last subcutaneous dose of enoxaparin occurred 8–12 h earlier, the patient should receive 0.3 mg/kg enoxaparin intravenously. If the last subcutaneous dose was administered <8 h earlier, no additional dosing is necessary [31,32]. If the last dose of enoxaparin was administered >12 h previously, some authors suggest treatment with conventional heparin therapy [20]. In the setting of UA/NSTEMI, if the patient did not receive previous anticoagulant therapy, he or she should receive 0.5–0.75 mg/kg enoxaparin intravenously [27]. In patients with severe renal impairment (creatinine clearance <30 mL/min), enoxaparin dosing should be adjusted. In the setting of STEMI, the initial bolus should be 30 mg in patients <75 years of age, and should be avoided all together in patients >75 years old [31].

Pregnancy risk factor

Enoxaparin has a pregnancy risk factor category of B.

Direct thrombin inhibitors

Direct thrombin inhibitors (DTIs) are anticoagulants that act more distally in the coagulation cascade than more traditional agents. Three DTIs have been studied as alternatives to heparin during PCI: hirudin, bivalirudin, and argatroban [108–112]. Although hirudin is the prototypical DTI, it has not been evaluated sufficiently in the setting of PCI. Bivalirudin is the only agent approved for routine use with PCI [20,27,31,32,95].

Bivalirudin

Mechanism of action/indications

Bivalirudin is a synthetic 20-amino-acid analog of hirudin that binds reversibly to thrombin and inhibits clot-bound thrombin [20,27]. Bivalirudin has been studied extensively as an alternative to heparin in patients undergoing PCI [108,109]. Bivalirudin has been proven as a safe and effective alternative to UFH and has been associated with less bleeding complications [108–114]. It is therefore indicated as an alternative to UFH and GP IIb/IIIa antagonists in low-risk patients undergoing elective PCI [95]. Bivalirudin is primarily used as the sole anticoagulant in PCI patients not previously treated with GP IIb/IIIa antagonists or UFH [20]. Bivalirudin administered at the time of PCI has also been associated with improved outcomes in patients with acute coronary syndrome pretreated with UFH or LMWH. In the SWITCH (Switching from Enoxaparin to Bivalirudin in Patients with Acute Coronary Syndromes without ST-segment Elevation who Undergo Percutaneous Coronary Intervention) trial, patients pretreated with enoxaparin before to PCI for various durations were switched to bivalirudin infusion at PCI. No difference in major bleeding or need for transfusion was observed [110]. In a substudy of the ACUITY (Acute Catheterization and Urgent Intervention Triage Strategy) trial, patients pretreated with UFH or enoxaparin either remained on heparin or switched to bivalirudin at the time of PCI. Switching from heparin to bivalirudin monotherapy resulted in a roughly 50% reduction in major bleeding, and similar ischemic outcomes to consistent heparin therapy [115]. In patients at high risk, bivalirudin may be used over heparin as an adjunct to GP IIb/IIIa antagonists and is indicated as part of the early invasive strategy for treatment of UA/NSTEMI as an addition to antiplatelet therapy [20,27]. Bivalirudin is also indicated during PCI in the setting of STEMI, when patients have received pretreatment with UFH [31,32].

Dosing

Bolus 0.75 mg/kg bivalirudin is given, followed by bivalirudin infused at 1.75 mg/kg for up to 4 h after the procedure if needed. If the patient has already received pretreatment with an anticoagulant, he or she should receive bolus bivalirudin 0.5 mg/kg, followed by an infusion of 1.75 mg/kg/h for the remainder of the procedure [27]. For patients with severe renal impairment (creatinine clearance 10–29 mL/min), the infusion rate should be adjusted to 1 mg/kg/h. For dialysis-dependent patients, the infusion rate should be reduced to 0.25 mg/kg/h [116].

Pregnancy risk factor

Bivalirudin has a pregnancy risk factor category of B.

Argatroban

Mechanism of action

Argatroban is a small molecule derivative of arginine and acts by targeting the active site of thrombosis [20].

Indication

Argatroban has been compared with heparin in the setting of UA/NSTEMI; however, it has not been extensively evaluated as an alternative to heparin in PCI [20]. This agent has proven effective for use in PCI patients with heparin-induced thrombocytopenia [112] and is indicated to replace heparin in this setting [95].

Dosing

A bolus 350 μg/kg (over 3–5 min), then infuse at 25 μg/kg/min. Check the ACT 5–10 min after bolus infusion; proceed with procedure if the ACT is >300 s. If the ACT is <300 s, give an additional bolus 150 μg/kg, and increase infusion rate to 30 μg/kg/min. Recheck ACT in 5–10 min. If the ACT is >450 s, decrease infusion rate to 15 μg/kg/min. Recheck ACT in 5–10 min. Once therapeutic ACT is achieved, continue infusion at this dose for the remainder of the procedure [117].

Pregnancy risk factor

Argatroban has a pregnancy risk factor category of B.

Factor Xa inhibitors

Fondaparinux

Mechanism of action

This agent suppresses thrombin production by acting proximally in the coagulation cascade and inhibiting the multiplier effects of reaction downstream [27]. Fondaparinux binds less to plasma proteins and endothelial cells, and has dose-independent clearance with a longer half-life. Similar to enoxaparin, this pharmacodynamic profile results in more predictable and sustained anticoagulation and therefore provides advantages over UFH, including fixed-dose, once-daily subcutaneous administration. Fondaparinux also does not require laboratory monitoring [27].

Indications

Fondaparinux has been evaluated for use in patients with both UA/NSTEMI [118] and STEMI [119]. Fondaparinux was proven noninferior to enoxaparin in patients with UA/NSTEMI and was associated with less bleeding [118]. Unfractionated heparin was not used initially in patients undergoing PCI: however, owing to an increased incidence of catheter-associated thrombus, the study protocol was modified to include UFH use at the discretion of the investigator [27,118]. When studied in a large cohort of patients with STEMI, fondaparinux was also associated with increased coronary complications, notably catheter thrombosis [119]. Although the trial design was complicated, the benefit of fondaparinux was confined to patients who did not undergo primary PCI [119]. As a result, although mentioned as part of an early invasive strategy in patients with UA/NSTEMI [27], and in patients with STEMI undergoing PCI [31,32], fondaparinux does not have an official FDA indication for treatment of acute coronary syndrome and should not be used as the sole anticoagulant during PCI. Additional agents with factor IIa activity should be used to relieve the risk of catheter

complications [27,31,32]. Unfractionated heparin is the preferred agent for this purpose, although this recommendation is based on limited data [120].

Dosing

For patients with UA/NSTEMI (Canadian labeling only), 2.5 mg fondaparinux can be given subcutaneously once daily. This should be initiated as soon as possible after diagnosis, and the patient should be treated for up to 8 days or until hospital discharge [121]. For patients with STEMI (Canadian labeling only), a single intravenous dose of 2.5 mg fondaparinux can be given; subsequent doses can be given subcutaneously (2.5 mg once daily). The patient should be treated for up to 8 days or until hospital discharge [121]. A bolus of 50–60 U/kg UFH can be given intravenously during PCI [27].

Pregnancy risk factor

Fondaparinux has a pregnancy risk factor category of B.

Ionotropic agents

Use of ionotropic agents in the catheterization laboratory has been studied extensively. In the setting of acute myocardial infarction, however, use of positive ionotropic agents may actually increase the size of myocardial infarction; thus, ionotropic agents are rarely used in this setting. In many circumstances (such as when the patient is on dobutamine for severe heart failure), the ionotropic agent may be continued throughout the procedure until definitive therapy, PCI, can be carried out. Dobutamine is a selective B1 agonist with a wide range of hemodynamic effects. It increases cardiac output and stroke volume with minimal effect on the heart rate; and increases coronary artery perfusion pressure [122]. It decreases mean capillary wedge pressure and left ventricular end-diastolic pressure [123]. It also decreases systemic vascular resistance and left atrial pressure. It has an onset of 1–2 min when given intravenously and a peak onset of 10 min with a half-life of 2 min. It may be used when there is mild hypotension and can also be used in conjunction with vasopressors if more profound hypotension occurs. Phosphodiesterase inhibitors (milrinone) also have ionotropic effects on the heart by decreasing the breakdown of cyclic adenosine monophosphate and thereby increasing contractility, which can be useful in critically ill patients [124]. It is not as commonly used for heart failure patients because of hypotension and arrhythmias [125], yet may be used in conjunction with a vasopressor in instances in which previous beta blockade makes dobutamine less effective, especially in nonischemic cardiomyopathy [126].

Pharmacokinetics

Dobutamine hydrochloride is a synthetic catecholamine. It is excreted by the kidney after methylation of the catechol and conjugation to inactive particles. Milrinone is a selective peak

III cyclic adenosine monophosphate (cAMP) inhibitor in cardiac and vascular muscle. By inhibiting cAMP isoenzyme, it increases intracellular calcium and thus increases cardiac contractility. It can cause systemic hypotension by the same action on vascular smooth muscle cells and can also improve diastolic function by improving left ventricular diastolic relaxation. It has a half-life of 2.3 h.

Dosing

The rate of infusion of dobutamine ranges from 2.5 to 15 µg/kg/min with a maximum of 40 µg/kg/min. Milrinone infusion can be initiated at 12.5 µg/kg/h in patients with heart failure.

Route of administration

Dobutamine is given intravenously and must be pre-mixed with saline solution. Milrinone can be given intravenously or orally.

Adverse reactions

Ten percent of patients have a 30 beats/min increase in heart rate during dobutamine use; however, most have a mild increase in heart rate. Most patients have a 20 mmHg increase in blood pressure, and 7.5% have an increase in blood pressure of ≥50 mmHg. Dobutamine should not be used in patients who have hypertrophic obstructive cardiomyopathy or have anaphylaxis to the drug. Dobutamine overdose can cause a wide range of effects owing to its ionotropic and chronotropic actions. Nausea, vomiting, and palpitations occur due to supraventricular and ventricular arrhythmias. Hypotension and angina can occur secondary to myocardial ischemia and ventricular fibrillation. Dobutamine can also increase the conduction of atrial fibrillation, thus resulting in recurrent atrial arrhythmias. Propranolol and lidocaine may be used in ventricular arrhythmias due to dobutamine. Milrinone also causes serious ventricular arrhythmias and sudden death, particularly in New York Heart Association class IV patients. Oral milrinone may increase morbidity and mortality, thus it is rarely used [127].

Pregnancy risk factor

Milrinone has a pregnancy risk factor category of C.

Vasopressive agents

Vasopressors are sometimes essential in the catheterization laboratory to stabilize hypotensive patients until more definitive therapy can be instituted. A number of vasopressors are available, including dopamine, norepinephrine, phenylephrine, epinephrine, and vasopressin. Dopamine has a dose-dependent effect on different receptors. A low dose may exert a nephroprotective effect by acting on dopaminergic receptors in the kidneys, although more recent data suggest no clinical benefit

[128]. At higher doses, a B1 agonist exerts most of the beneficial effects seen in clinical practice, and, at a very high dose, vasoconstrictor effects are seen through modulation of α receptors. Norepinephrine is another potent nonselective vasopressor with variable alpha receptor agonist properties and, to a lesser extent, beta receptor agonist properties. Phenylephrine is an α-receptor agonist that causes a marked increase in systolic and diastolic pressures, and sometimes reflex bradycardia. Epinephrine stimulates α and β sympathetic receptors in vascular as well as bronchial and other areas of the body. It has a wide array of hemodynamic and systemic effects. In addition to increasing the sympathetic drive (chronotropic and ionotropic effects), it also causes bronchodilation and can be used in anaphylaxis due to contrast allergy. In the catheterization laboratory, epinephrine can be used for cardiac arrest, as a vasopressor for hypotension, as a chronotropic agent for bradycardia, and for allergic reactions. Vasopressin has recently been shown to be superior when used in combination with epinephrine alone in cardiac arrest [129]. It should not be substituted for epinephrine alone, however [130]. Vasopressin acts on V_1 receptors of the smooth muscles of the arteries, causing vasoconstriction. As with ionotropic agents, a major concern with vasopressor use in the catheterization laboratory is that, in patients with acute myocardial infarction, infarction size may increase. Vasopressors, by increasing the workload on the heart, increase myocardial oxygen consumption, and therefore increase the mismatch of oxygen supply and demand that the heart is already experiencing in acute myocardial infarction. However, circulatory support must be maintained and therefore in certain situations, these agents are essential.

Pharmacokinetics

Dopamine is metabolized in the kidney by monoamine oxidases and catechol-O-methyltransferase to inactive compounds. It can also be converted to norepinephrine and is excreted by the kidney. It has a half-life of 2 min with an onset of action <5 min and duration of action <10 min. Norepinephrine also has a short onset of action and has a duration of action of 1–2 min. Phenylephrine is metabolized in the liver and gastrointestinal tract and has a duration of action of 20 min. Epinephrine is inactivated by enzymes to metanephrines and inactive metabolites which are then conjugated and excreted in the urine. Vasopressin is metabolized by the liver and kidney and excreted in the kidney. It has a half-life of 10–20 min.

Dosing

Dopamine can be started at 2–5 µg/kg/min with β-stimulation occurring at 5–10 µg/kg/min and vasopressor effect (α-agonist) at >10 µg/kg/min, with maximal does of 20 µg/kg/min. Norepinephrine can be started at 1–2 µg/min and titrated up to 160 µg/mL, but usually the maintenance dose is 2–4 µg/min. Phenylephrine can be given as a bolus of 0.04–0.1 mg intravenously or can be started as an infusion of 100–180 µg/min of 1:25 000 or 1:50 000 solution or 10 mg per 250 or 500 mL of D5W or NaCl solution. The maintenance dose is 40–60 μg/min and can be increased at increments of 10 μg/min until adequate blood pressure is achieved. Epinephrine has many uses and, therefore, dosing is dependent on its use. For cardiac arrest, it can be given as 1 mg intravenously (10 mL of 1:10 000 solution) every 5 min as specified by the ACLS protocol. For use in allergic reactions, see the section on contrast allergy. An infusion can be started by using 1 mg intravenously in 250 mL of D5W (4 μg/mL) for infusion at 1–4 μg/min (15–60 mL/h). For hypotension, an infusion at 2–10 μg/min is used to titrate to blood pressure response. Vasopressin can be used in cardiac arrest as a 40-mg intravenous push, then initiating the epinephrine protocol. For profound hypotension, it can be used as an infusion of 20 units in 250 mL of D5W at a rate of 0.01–0.10 units/min.

Route of administration

Vasopressor use in cardiac arrest or hypotension is given intravenously either as a push or as infusion.

Adverse effects

Higher than recommended doses of pressors can cause end-organ hypoperfusion. Vasopressors, even in the normal dosing range, can cause peripheral vasoconstriction in volume depleted patients, resulting in end-organ hypoperfusion. Palpitations due to tachycardia are very frequent, and ventricular arrhythmias can occur. They can also worsen myocardial ischemia.

Pregnancy risk factor

Vasopressors have a pregnancy risk factor category of C.

Vasodilatory agents

Nitroglycerine, nitroprusside, beta-blockers, calcium channel blockers, α-channel blockers, and angiotensin-converting enzyme (ACE) inhibitors are all used in the catheterization lab when blood pressure becomes elevated. Nitroglycerin can be used for controlling blood pressure, decreasing preload in congestive heart failure, and controlling angina in patients with myocardial ischemia periprocedurally [131]. It can be used either sublingually or intravenously. Sodium nitroprusside is also used for uncontrolled hypertension and congestive heart failure.

Dosing

Nitroglycerin can be given as 0.4 mg sublingually or transdermally for angina, but as an antihypertensive it is given as intravenous bolus 12.5–25 μg or as an infusion starting at 5 μg/min intravenously and increasing in increments of 5–20 μg/min every 3–5 min as necessary. Maximal dose is 200 μg/min. It must be used in a glass bottle, which is usually provided by the manufacturer. Nitroprusside infusion (50 mg in 250 mL of D5W) is usually given as 0.1–0.3 μg/kg/min intravenously, with a maximum of 10 mg/kg/min (maximum dose should not be used for > 10 min). Renal dosing is required and should not exceed 3 μg/kg/min if creatinine clearance is < 60 mL/min.

Pharmacokinetics

Nitroglycerine works by direct vasodilator effect by nitric oxide-mediated relaxation of vascular smooth muscles. It has a more pronounced effect on the peripheral veins than arteries, thus reducing preload and myocardial oxygen demand. It also dilates coronary arteries and improves collateral flow to ischemic areas. It has an immediate effect when given intravenously and has a duration of action of 3–5 min. Nitroglycerine is 60% protein bound, has a half-life of 1–4 min, and is excreted in the urine. Nitroprusside has a rapid onset (<2 min) with a short duration of action (1–10 min). It is converted to cyanide ions, which decompose to prussic acid, and in the presence of a sulfur group it becomes thiocyanate. Nitroprusside has a half-life of <10 min and thiocyanate has a half-life of 3–7 days, and is excreted in the urine.

Adverse effects

Prolonged use of nitroglycerin can cause tolerance. It can cause hypotension, paradoxical bradycardia, and worsening of angina. It should not be used with concurrent use of phosphodiesterase-5 inhibitors (sildenafil, tadalafil, or vardenafil). Nitroprusside should not be used in treatment of a compensatory hypertension, such as coarctation of the aorta or arteriovenous shunting, or in high output failure states. Prolonged use or high doses of nitroprusside can lead to cyanide toxicity. If prolonged use (>4 days) is anticipated, monitoring of thiocyanate or cyanide levels is required. Thiocyanate levels are considered therapeutic if they are between 6 and 29 μg/mL, toxic if between 35 and 100 μg/mL, and fatal if > 200 μg/mL. Alternatively, cyanide levels are considered normal if < 0.2 μg/mL (< 0.4 μg/mL in smokers) and toxic if > 2 μg/mL. It should not be administered with alkaline solutions.

Pregnancy risk factor

Nitroprusside has a pregnancy risk factor category of C.

Intracoronary vasodilatory agents

Intracoronary vasodilators used in the catheterization laboratory include nitroglycerin, nitroprusside, calcium channel blockers, and adenosine. Their optimal dose remains uncertain, in part because of the lack of adequately powered clinical trials. Intracoronary nitroglycerin is used for vasospasm that can be catheter-induced or spontaneous, and that does not respond to systemic nitroglycerin [132]. It is diluted to 100–200 μg/mL and given as a 100-μg bolus through the catheter to the coronary artery desired. Intracoronary nitroprusside can also be used for coronary vasospasm and also for slow/no-reflow phenomenon [133]. Administration of intracoronary nitroprusside can induce a sustained coronary hyperemic response without detrimental systemic hemodynamic consequences. In a randomized clinical trial, it failed to show benefit in myocardial perfusion or coronary flow in patients with no-reflow in acute myocardial infarction treated by primary PCI [134]. However, this trial was underpowered and thus the effect of intracoronary nitroprusside on outcomes is still debatable. Calcium channel blockers are occasionally used for coronary no-reflow phenomenon. Nicardipine, diltiazem, and verapamil are currently used. Intracoronary adenosine is also used for no-reflow phenomenon in acute myocardial infarction; however, it failed to show a reduction in the composite primary end point of death, new congestive heart failure, or the first rehospitalization for congestive heart failure [135]. There was a trend toward a reduction in the secondary end point of infarct size, but this did not reach statistical significance.

Dosing

An intracoronary dose of nitroglycerin is usually 100 μg. The intracoronary dose of nitroprusside is controversial. A 60-μg bolus has been reported in clinical trials, but generally 100 μg is given by guiding catheter or selective coronary delivery. The, nicardipine dose is 200 μg (100–200 μg/mL), the diltiazem dose is 1–2.5 mg, and the verapamil dose is 100–200 μg (diluted to 100 μg/mL), although some people believe that 500 μg is more effective. The adenosine dose is 100 μg or an infusion (systemic) of 70 μg/kg/min.

Adverse effects

Nitroglycerin and nitroprusside can cause hypotension. Intracoronary verapamil can cause hypotension or bradycardia (heart block) in 18% of patients in one particular study [136].

Special considerations

Hypertensive emergency

Hypertensive emergencies are usually managed in the catheterization laboratory in the setting of acute coronary syndrome, aortic dissection, or acute pulmonary edema. The choice of parenteral agent for the management of hypertensive emergency in the catheterization laboratory should be tailored to the patient's clinical status [137]. Aggressive blood pressure control is beneficial in most cases; however, caution must be used to avoid excessive reductions in blood pressure, as this can lead to further ischemic complications, such as acute myocardial infarction or stroke [137].

Acute coronary syndromes

In the setting of UA/NSTEMI, severe elevation of blood pressure is a common finding. By contrast, acute elevations in blood pressure can cause myocardial ischemia in patients with otherwise nonobstructive coronary artery disease. This so-called "demand ischemia" occurs as a result of increased left ventricular wall stress and myocardial oxygen consumption. The initial agents of choice for treatment of this hypertensive emergency should be intravenous vasodilators, such as nitroprusside or nitroglycerin [137]. In addition to their moderate hypotensive action, nitrates work to improve coronary perfusion and decrease left ventricular preload [138]. Both of these actions are critical in the management of acute coronary syndrome, especially when left ventricular systolic dysfunction has ensued. Vasodilators can be used in conjunction with intravenous beta-blockers, such as metoprolol and labetalol, which, by decreasing heart rate and blood pressure, reduce myocardial oxygen consumption [137].

Left ventricular failure

When left ventricular failure is associated with volume overload, rapid blood pressure control is critical. Vasodilators should be used in conjunction with loop diuretics for control of volume overload [138].

Aortic dissection

Aortic dissection can be the most fatal hypertensive emergency associated with the most rapid decline. The goal of treatment is to minimize aortic wall stress, by reducing heart rate and blood pressure, and to reduce dP/dT (change in pressure/change in time) [139]. Ideally, intravenous beta-blocker therapy should be initiated before vasodilators to avoid potential reflex tachycardia.

Vasodilators

Sodium nitroprusside

Nitroprusside is a short-acting arteriolar and venous dilator. Its rapid onset of action and intravenous infusion formulation make it an extremely effective agent for treatment of acute hypertension. The risk of hypotension can complicate treatment, but reverses rapidly with discontinuation of the infusion [139]. The major adverse effects of nitroprusside use are cyanate toxicity, hypotension, nausea, and vomiting.

Dosing

The initial recommended starting dose is 0.25–0.5 μg/kg/min and the maximum dose is 8–10 μg/kg/min [140]. Prolonged infusions should not exceed 3 μg/kg/min; thiocyanate concentrations should be monitored if this rate is exceeded for prolonged periods [140]. Use of nitroprusside should be limited in patients with renal impairment to avoid accumulation of thiocyanate. For anuric patients, prolonged infusions should not exceed 1 μg/kg/min (to maintain thiocyanate concentrations <60 μg/mL) [140].

Pregnancy risk factor

Sodium nitroprusside has a pregnancy risk factor category of C.

Nitroglycerin

Nitroglycerin is also administered via intravenous infusion and has a similar action to nitroprusside. This agent produces relatively more venodilation, however, and is therefore more useful for treatment of hypertension in acute coronary syndrome and pulmonary edema. Adverse effects include headache, tachycardia, vomiting, and methemoglobinemia [141].

Dosing

The initial recommended starting dose is 5 μg/min and the maximum dose is 100 μg/min [141].

Pregnancy risk factor

Nitroglycerin has a pregnancy risk factor category of C.

Nicardipine

Nicardipine is a dihydropyridine calcium channel blocker administered by i.v. infusion. This agent is effective in controlled acute hypertension, but has a longer half-life than nitroprusside, which makes it difficult to titrate rapidly. Adverse effects include headache, nausea, flushing, tachycardia and local phlebitis [142].

Dosing

Initial recommended dosing is 5 mg/h, maximum dose 15 mg/h.

Pregnancy risk factor

Nicardipine has a pregnancy risk factor category of C.

Hydralazine

Hydralazine is a direct arteriolar vasodilator that has minimal to no effect on the venous circulation. It is administered as an i.v. bolus and has less predictable hypotensive effects. Reflex tachycardia is a major concern is the setting of aortic dissection and acute coronary syndrome, therefore simultaneous bet blockade is often necessary to minimize reflex sympathetic stimulation. Adverse effects include tachycardia, flushing, headache, vomiting, and progressive angina [143].

Dosing

The recommended dose is 10- to 20-mg i.v. bolus [143].

Pregnancy risk factor

Hydralazine has a pregnancy risk factor category of C.

Urapidil

Urapidil, an α_1 blocker which also has central adrenoreceptor blocking ability (as well as being a serotonin agonist), can also be safely used in hypertensive emergencies [144–146]. Urapidil is an arterial and venous vasodilator but, because of its central action, lacks the reflex tachycardia of other vasodilators. Urapidil is metabolized hepatically [147].

Dosing

Urapidil is dosed 12.5–50 mg as a single i.v. injection. Treatment effect largely depends on the basal α-adrenergic activity.

Pregnancy risk factor

Although it has proven to be safe and effective in pregnancy, it does cross the placenta, and reports of neonatal respiratory depression warrant careful monitoring during treatment of a pregnant patient [148].

Beta-blockers

Labetalol

Labetalol is an α- and β-adrenergic blocker that has particular usefulness for treatment of acute coronary syndrome and aortic dissection secondary to its ability to decrease heart rate and blood pressure and the resultant reduction in myocardial oxygen consumption [149]. Adverse effects include vomiting, dizziness, nausea, heart block, orthostatic hypotension, and bronchospasm [149].

Dosing

Intravenous bolus or infusion is recommended: a dose of 20–80 mg intravenous bolus every 10 min or intravenous infusion of 2 mg/min [149].

Pregnancy risk factor

Labetalol has a pregnancy risk factor of C.

Esmolol

Esmolol hydrochloride is a β-selective adrenergic receptor blocking agent with a short half-life of roughly 9 min. The duration of action is also brief (30 min) and is particularly useful in situations in which rapid titration is necessary. Adverse effects include hypotension, diaphoresis, dizziness, and pain on injection [150].

Dosing

For immediate control of hypertension, 80 mg (1 mg/kg) bolus over 30 s should be given, followed by a 150 μg/kg/min infusion if necessary. The maximum dose is 300 μg/kg/min. For gradual control of hypertension, a loading dose infusion of 500 μg/kg/min for 1 min should be given, followed by a 4-min infusion of 50 μg/kg/min. The loading dose can be repeated with the maintenance infusion increased to 100 μg/kg/min if necessary [150].

Pregnancy risk factor

Esmolol has a pregnancy risk factor category of C.

Metoprolol

Metoprolol is a β_1-selective adrenergic blocking agent that can be used to reduce heart rate acutely in patients with tachycardia, in addition to lowering blood pressure. Adverse effects include hypotension, AV nodal block, bradycardia, and bronchospasm [151].

Dosing

For immediate control of tachycardia, metoprolol tartrate is administered as a rapid intravenous injection of 2.5–10 mg.

Pregnancy risk factor

Metoprolol has a pregnancy risk factor category of C.

Diuretics

Furosemide

Furosemide is a loop diuretic that is particularly useful in treatment of hypertension associated with volume overload and left ventricular failure. This agent should not be administered if volume depletion is initially present [152]. Adverse effects include volume depletion and hypokalemia [153].

Dosing

Furosemide can be given as 20–40 mg intravenous bolus in 1–2 min, with repeated and higher doses with renal insufficiency [153].

Pregnancy risk factor

Furosemide has a pregnancy risk factor category of C.

Special considerations

Heart failure

Diuretics are also commonly used in the catheterization laboratory for pulmonary edema, usually resulting from heart failure. Loop diuretics are the most commonly used because their onset of action is rapid. Thiazide diuretics, aldosterone antagonists, and carbonic anhydrase inhibitors have important uses in cardiovascular medicine; however, they are generally not used in the catheterization laboratory. They may be continued once the procedure is finished. Diuretics are usually withheld the day of the procedure owing to the concern of renal insufficiency. In some instances, however, when the left ventricular end-diastolic pressure or wedge pressure is elevated and the patient becomes symptomatic, loop diuretics can help alleviate the symptoms and avoid respiratory failure. This is especially true in patients with heart failure who have had intravenous fluids the previous night. Loop diuretics include furosemide, bumetanide, ethacrynic acid, and torsemide. Furosemide is the most frequently used agent.

Pharmacokinetics

Loop diuretics inhibit reabsorption of sodium and chloride in proximal and distal tubules and the loop of Henle. About 50% of a dose of furosemide is excreted in unchanged form into the urine, and 50% is bound to glucuronic acid in the kidney [154,155]. This prolongs the half-life of furosemide. It has a bioavailability of 64% in oral form and is 91–99% bound to protein (albumin). It is metabolized to furosemide glucuronide, the half-life of which is 2 h. This is excreted in the urine. The onset of action is 5–10 min (i.v.) and 1 h when given orally. The peak onset is 1–2 h (oral) and 30 min (i.v.). The duration of action is 6–8 h (oral) and 2 h (i.v.).

Adverse effects

Loop diuretics produce large shifts in electrolyte and water balance in the body, therefore monitoring of electrolytes is essential. There are numerous adverse effects associated with the use of furosemide; hypokalemia, hyponatremia, hyperglycemia, electrolyte depletion, and hypovolemia are all common. Reversible and irreversible hearing impairment and/or loss may occur with any of the loop diuretics and occurs with rapid infusion or use of extremely high doses. Cardiovascular effects include chronic aortitis, orthostatic hypotension, and thrombophlebitis. Central nervous system effects include dizziness, fever, headache, paresthesia, and vertigo.

Dosing

It is given as 40 mg intravenously in acute pulmonary edema over 1–2 min. The dose can be increased to 80 mg i.v. if adequate response is not seen. The oral dose is 20–80 mg/day as a single dose and may be repeated every 6–8 h, and depending on the patient's response, this dose can be maintained, reduced, or titrated up to 600 mg/day. The rate of absorption of loop diuretics is slowed in patients with severe heart failure. The maximal response occurs ≥4 h after the oral dose has been administered [156]. In acute pulmonary edema, it is usually used intravenously. Two loop diuretics, bumetanide and torsemide, are largely metabolized by the liver, thus their half-life is not prolonged in patients with renal insufficiency [156].

Pregnancy risk factor

Loop diuretics have a pregnancy risk factor category of C.

References

1. Eisenberg RL, Bank WO, & Hedgock MW (1981) Renal failure after major angiography can be avoided with hydration. *AJR Am J Roentgenol* **136**:859–861.
2. Brown R, Ransil B, & Clark B (1990) Prehydration protects against contrast nephropathy in high-risk patients undergoing cardiac catheterization. *J Am Soc Nephrol* **1**:330A.
3. Tepel M, van der Giet M, Schwarzfeld C, Laufer U, Liermann D, & Zidek W (2000) Prevention of radiographic-contrast-agent-

induced reductions in renal function by acetylcysteine. *N Engl J Med* **343**:180–184.

4. Fishbane S, Durham JH, Marzo K, & Rudnick M (2004) N-acetylcysteine in the prevention of radiocontrast-induced nephropathy. *J Am Soc Nephrol* **15**:251–260.

5. Kay J, Chow WH, Mao CT, *et al.* (2003) Acetylcysteine for prevention of acute deterioration of renal function following elective coronary angiography and intervention: a randomized controlled trial. *JAMA* **289**:553–558.

6. Marenzi G, Assanelli E, Marana I, *et al.* (2006) N-acetylcysteine and contrast-induced nephropathy in primary angioplasty. *N Engl J Med* **354**:2773–2782.

7. Merten GJ, Burgess WP, Gray LV, *et al.* (2004) Prevention of contrast-induced nephropathy with sodium bicarbonate: a randomized controlled trial. *JAMA* **291**:2328–2334.

8. Recio-Mayoral A, Chaparro M, Prado B, *et al.* (2007) The Reno-Protective Effect of Hydration With Sodium Bicarbonate Plus N-Acetylcysteine in Patients Undergoing Emergency Percutaneous Coronary Intervention: The RENO Study. *J Am Coll Cardiol* **49**:1283–1287.

9. Masuda M, Yamada T, Mine T, *et al.* (2008) Comparison of usefulness of sodium bicarbonate versus sodium chloride to prevent contrast-induced nephropathy in patients undergoing an emergent coronary procedure. *Am J Cardiol* **101**:910.

10. Ozcan EE, Guneri S, Akdeniz B, *et al.* (2008) Sodium bicarbonate, N-acetylcysteine, and saline for prevention of radiocontrast-induced nephropathy. A comparison of 3 regimens for protecting contrast-induced nephropathy in patients undergoing coronary procedures. A single-center prospective controlled trial. *Am Heart J* **155**:e31.

11. Briguori C, Airoldi F, D'Andrea D, *et al.* (2007) Renal Insufficiency Following Contrast Media Administration Trial (REMEDIAL): a randomized comparison of 3 preventive strategies. *Circulation* **115**:1211–1217.

12. Katayama H, Yamaguchi K, Kozuka T, Takashima T, Seez P, & Matsuura K (1990) Adverse reactions to ionic and nonionic contrast media. A report from the Japanese Committee on Safety of Contrast Media. *Radiology* **175**:621–628.

13. Greenberger PA & Patterson R (1991) The prevention of immediate generalized reactions to radiocontrast media in high-risk patients. *J Allergy Clin Immunol* **87**:867–872.

14. Lasser EC, Berry CC, Talner LB, *et al.* (1987) Pretreatment with corticosteroids to alleviate reactions to intravenous contrast material. *N Engl J Med* **317**:845–849.

15. Libby P, Bonow RO, Zipes DP, *et al.* (2007) Coronary arteriography and intravascular imaging/technique of coronary arteriography/drugs used during coronary arteriography/analgesics. In: Libby P, Bonow RO, Mann DL, Zipes DP (eds) *Braunwald's Heart Disease: A Textbook of Cardiovascular Medicine*, 8th edn. Philadelphia: Saunders Elsevier.

16. Fentanyl and fentanyl citrate. In: McEvoy GK (ed). AHFS drug information 2004. Bethesda, MD: American Society of Health-System Pharmacists, pp. 2036–2041.

17. Roche Laboratories (2000) Versed® (midazolam hydrochloride) prescribing information. Nutley, NJ.

18. Endo Pharmaceuticals (2003) Narcan® (naloxone hydrochloride injection, USP) prescribing information. Chadds Ford, PA.

19. Roche Laboratories, Inc. (2000) Romazicon® (flumazenil) prescribing information. Nutley, NJ.

20. Popma J, Berger P, Ohman EM, *et al.* (2004) Antithrombotic therapy during percutaneous coronary intervention: The Seventh ACCP Conference on Antithrombotic and Thrombolytic Therapy. *Chest* **126**:576–599.

21. COMMIT collaborative group (2005) Addition of clopidogrel to aspirin in 45 852 patients with acute myocardial infarction: randomised placebo-controlled trial. *Lancet* **366**:1607–1621.

22. Food and Drug Administration (1998) Internal analgesic, antipyretic, and antirheumatic drug products for over-the-counter human use; final rule for professional labeling of aspirin, buffered aspirin, and aspirin in combination with antacid drug products. 21 CFR Part 343. Final rule. [Docket No. 77N-094A] *Fed Regist.* **63**:56802–56819.

23. Lansky A, Hochman J, Ward P, *et al.* (2005) Percutaneous coronary intervention and adjunctive pharmacotherapy in women: a statement for healthcare professionals from the American Heart Association. *Circulation* **111**:940–953.

24. Stone G, Aronow H, *et al.* (2006) Long-term care after percutaneous coronary intervention: focus on the role of antiplatelet therapy. *Mayo Clin Proc* **81**:641–652.

25. Update to FDA Statement on Coronary Drug-Eluting Stents [WWW Document]. URL http://www.fda.gov/cdrh/news/010407.html [Accessed on 10 January 2008].

26. Serruys P, Kutryk M, Ong A, *et al.* (2006) Coronary artery stents. *N Engl J Med* **354**:483–495.

27. Anderson J, Adams C, Antman E, *et al.* (2007) ACC/AHA 2007 Guidelines for the Management of Patients With Unstable Angina/NonST-Elevation Myocardial InfarctionExecutive Summary: A Report of the American College of Cardiology/American Heart Association Task Force on Practice Guidelines (Writing Committee to Revise the 2002 Guidelines for the Management of Patients With Unstable Angina/NonST-Elevation Myocardial Infarction). *J Am Coll Cardiol* **50**:652–726.

28. Lewis H Jr, Davis J, Archibald D, *et al.* (1983) Protective effects of aspirin against acute myocardial infarction and death in men with unstable angina. Results of a Veterans Administration Cooperative Study. *N Engl J Med* **309**:396–403.

29. Théroux P, Ouimet H, McCans J, *et al.* (1988) Aspirin, heparin, or both to treat acute unstable angina. *N Engl J Med* **319**:1105–1111.

30. RISC Group (1990) Risk of myocardial infarction and death during treatment with low dose aspirin and intravenous heparin in men with unstable coronary artery disease. *Lancet* **336**:827–830.

31. Antman E, Hand M, Armstrong P, *et al.* (2008) 2007 Focused Update of the ACC/AHA 2004 Guidelines for the Management of Patients With ST-Elevation Myocardial Infarction: a report of the American College of Cardiology/American Heart Association Task Force on Practice Guidelines, Developed in Collaboration With the Canadian Cardiovascular Society, Endorsed by the American Academy of Family Physicians: 2007 Writing Group to Review New Evidence and Update the ACC/AHA 2004 Guidelines for Management of Patients With ST-Elevation Myocardial Infarction. *J Am Coll Cardiol* **51**:210–247.

32. King S, III, Smith S, Hirshfeld J, *et al.* (2008) 2007 Focused Update of the ACC/AHA/SCAI 2005 Guideline Update for Percutaneous Coronary Intervention: a report of the American College of Cardiology/American Heart Association Task Force on Practice Guidelines: 2007 Writing Group to Review New

Evidence and Update the ACC/AHA/SCAI 2005 Guideline Update for Percutaneous Coronary Intervention. *J Am Coll Cardiol* **51**:172–209.

33. Smith S, Jr, Allen J, & Blair S (2006) AHA/ACC Guidelines for Secondary Prevention for Patients With Coronary and Other Atherosclerotic Vascular Disease: 2006 Update: Endorsed by the National Heart, Lung, and Blood Institute. *Circulation* **113**: 2363–72.

34. Grines C, Bonow R, Casey Jr D, *et al.* (2007) Prevention of premature discontinuation of dual antiplatelet therapy in patients with coronary artery stents. *Circulation* **115**:813–818.

35. Pfisterer M, Brunner-La Rocca H, Buser P, *et al.* For the BASKET-LATE Investigators. (2006) Late clinical events after clopidogrel discontinuation may limit the benefit of drug-eluting stents: an observational study of drug-eluting versus bare metal stents. *J Am Coll Cardiol* **48**:2584–2591.

36. Lüscher T, Steffel J, Eberli F, *et al.* (2007) Drug-eluting stent and coronary thrombosis: biological mechanisms and clinical implications. *Circulation* **115**:1051–1058.

37. Shuchman M (2007) Debating the risks of drug-eluting stents. *N Engl J Med* **356**:325–328. Commentary.

38. Eisenstein E, Anstrom K, Kong D, *et al.* (2007) Clopidogrel use and long-term clinical outcomes after drug-eluting stent implantation. *JAMA* **297**:159–168.

39. Kereiakes D (2007) Does clopidogrel each day keep stent thrombosis away? *JAMA* **297**:209–211, editorial.

40. Kastrati A, Mehilli J, Pache J, *et al.* (2007) Analysis of 14 trials comparing sirolimus-eluting stents with bare metal stents. *N Engl J Med* **356**:1030–1039.

41. Farb A & Boam A (2007) Stent thrombosis redux—the FDA perspective. *N Engl J Med* **356**:984–987, commentary.

42. Stone G, Moses J, Ellis S, *et al.* (2007) Safety and efficacy of sirolimus- and paclitaxel-eluting coronary stents. *N Engl J Med* **356**:998–1008.

43. Spertus JA, Kettelkamp R, Vance C, *et al.* (2006) Prevalence, predictors, and outcomes of premature discontinuation of thienopyridine therapy after drug-eluting stent placement. Results from the PREMIER registry. *Circulation* **113**:2803–2809.

44. Jeremias A, Sylvia B, Bridges J, *et al.* (2004) Stent thrombosis after successful sirolimus-eluting stent implantation. *Circulation* **109**:1930–1932.

45. Ong A, McFadden E, Regar E, *et al.* (2005) Late angiographic stent thrombosis (LAST) events with drug-eluting stents. *J Am Coll Cardiol* **45**:2088–2092.

46. Spaulding C, Daemen J, Boersma E, *et al.* (2007) A pooled analysis of data comparing sirolimus-eluting stents with bare metal stents. *N Engl J Med* **356**:989–997.

47. Maisel W (2007) Unanswered questions—drug-eluting stents and the risk of late thrombosis. *N Engl J Med* **356**:981–984, editorial.

48. Curfman G, Morrissey S, Jarcho J, *et al.* Drug-eluting coronary stents—promise and uncertainty. *N Engl J Med* **356**:1059–1060, editorial.

49. Ramanuja S, Breall J, Kalaria V, *et al.* (2004) Approach to "aspirin allergy" in cardiovascular patients. *Circulation* **110**:e1–e4.

50. Silberman S, Neukirch-Stoop C, Gabriel P, *et al.* (2005) Rapid desensitization procedure for patients with aspirin hypersensitivity undergoing coronary stenting. *Am J Cardiol* **95**:509–510.

51. Wong J, Nagy C, Krinzman S, *et al.* (2000) Rapid oral challenge-desensitization for patients with aspirin-related urticaria-angioedema. *J Allergy Clin Immunol* **105**:997–1001.

52. Hollopeter G, Jantzen H, Vincent D, *et al.* (2001) Identification of the platelet ADP receptor targeted by antithrombotic drugs. *Nature* **409**:202–207.

53. Sharis P, Cannon C, & Loscalzo J (1998) The Antiplatelet Effects of Ticlopidine and Clopidogrel. *Ann Intern Med* **129**:394–405.

54. Herbert J, Dol F, Bernal A, *et al.* (1998) The antiaggregating and antithrombotic activity of clopidogrel is potentiated by aspirin in several experimental models in the rabbit. *Thromb Haemost* **80**:512–518.

55. Schömig A, Neumann F, Kastrati A, *et al.* (1996) A randomized comparison of antiplatelet and anticoagulant therapy after the placement of coronary-artery stents. *N Engl J Med* **334**:1084–1089.

56. Ferguson JJ & Fox R (1997) Meeting highlights—STARS. *Circulation* **95**:761–764.

57. Urban P, Macaya C, Rupprecht H, *et al.* (1998) Randomized evaluation of anticoagulation versus antiplatelet therapy after coronary stent implantation in high-risk patients: the Multicenter Aspirin and Ticlopidine Trial after Intracoronary Stenting (MATTIS). *Circulation* **98**:2126–2132.

58. Bertrand M, Rupprecht H, Urban P, *et al.* For the CLASSICS Investigators (2000) double-blind study of the safety of clopidogrel with and without a loading dose in combination with aspirin compared with ticlopidine in combination with aspirin after coronary stenting: the Clopidogrel Aspirin Stent International Cooperative Study (CLASSICS). *Circulation* **102**:624–629.

59. Müller C, Büttner H, Petersen J, *et al.* (2000) A randomized comparison of clopidogrel and aspirin versus ticlopidine and aspirin after the placement of coronary-artery stents. *Circulation* **101**:590–593.

60. Sabatine M, Cannon C, Gibson C, *et al.* (2005) Effect of clopidogrel pretreatment before percutaneous coronary intervention in patients with ST-elevation myocardial infarction treated with fibrinolytics: the PCI-CLARITY study. *JAMA* **294**:1224–1232.

61. Steinhubl S, Berger P, Tift Mann J, III, *et al.* For the CREDO Investigators (2002) Early and sustained dual oral antiplatelet therapy following percutaneous coronary intervention: a randomized controlled trial. *JAMA* **288**:2411–2420.

62. Mehta S, Yusuf S, Peters R, *et al.* (2001) Effects of pretreatment with clopidogrel and aspirin followed by long-term therapy in patients undergoing percutaneous coronary intervention: the PCI-CURE study. *Lancet* **358**:527–533.

63. Montalescot G, Sideris G, Meuleman C, *et al.* (2006) A randomized comparison of high clopidogrel loading doses in patients with non-ST-segment elevation acute coronary syndromes. *J Am Coll Cardiol* **48**:931–938.

64. von Beckerath N, Taubert D, Pogatsa-Murray G, *et al.* (2005) Absorption, metabolization, and antiplatelet effects of 300-, 600-, and 900-mg loading doses of clopidogrel: results of the ISAR-CHOICE Trial. *Circulation* **112**:2946–2950.

65. Gurbel P, Bliden K, Zaman K, *et al.* (2005) Clopidogrel loading with eptifibatide to arrest the reactivity of platelets: results of the Clopidogrel Loading With Eptifibatide to Arrest the Reactivity of Platelets (CLEAR PLATELETS) Study. *Circulation* **111**:1153–1159.

66. Patti G, Colonna G, Pasceri V, *et al.* (2005) Randomized trial of high loading dose of clopidogrel for reduction of periprocedural

myocardial infarction in patients undergoing coronary intervention: results from the ARMYDA-2 (Antiplatelet therapy for Reduction of MYocardial Damage during Angioplasty) Study. *Circulation* **111**:2099–2106.

67. Wiviott S, Braunwald E, McCabe C, *et al.* (2007) Prasugrel versus clopidogrel in patients with acute coronary syndromes. *N Engl J Med* **357**:2001–2015.

68. Wiviott S, Trenk D, Frelinger A, *et al.*, on behalf of the PRINCIPLE-TIMI 44 Investigators (2007) Prasugrel compared with high loading- and maintenance-dose clopidogrel in patients with planned percutaneous coronary intervention: the Prasugrel in Comparison to Clopidogrel for Inhibition of Platelet Activation and Aggregation-Thrombolysis in Myocardial Infarction 44 trial. *Circulation* **116**:2923–2932.

69. Lefkovits J, Plow E, & Topol E (1995) Platelet glycoprotein IIb/IIIa receptors in cardiovascular medicine. *N Engl J Med* **332**:1553–1559.

70. The CAPTURE investigators (1997) Randomised placebo-controlled trial of abciximab before and during coronary intervention in refractory unstable angina: the CAPTURE study. *Lancet* **349**:1429–1435.

71. The EPIC Investigators (1994) Use of a monoclonal antibody directed against the platelet glycoprotein IIb/IIIa receptor in high-risk coronary angioplasty. *N Engl J Med* **330**:956–961.

72. The EPILOG Investigators (1997) Platelet glycoprotein IIb/IIIa receptor blockade and low-dose heparin during percutaneous coronary revascularization. *N Engl J Med* **336**:1689–1696.

73. Topol E, Moliterno D, Herrmann H, *et al.* (2001) Comparison of two platelet glycoprotein IIb/IIIa inhibitors, tirofiban and abciximab, for the prevention of ischemic events with percutaneous coronary revascularization. *N Engl J Med* **344**:1888–1894.

74. The GUSTO IV-ACS Investigators (2001) Effect of glycoprotein IIb/IIIa receptor blocker abciximab on outcome in patients with acute coronary syndromes without early coronary revascularisation: the GUSTO IV-ACS randomised trial. *Lancet* **357**:1915–1924.

75. The Platelet Receptor Inhibition in Ischemic Syndrome Management (PRISM) Study Investigators (1998) A comparison of aspirin plus tirofiban with aspirin plus heparin for unstable angina. *N Engl J Med* **338**:1498–1450.

76. The Platelet Receptor Inhibition in Ischemic Syndrome Management in Patients Limited by Unstable Signs and Symptoms (PRISM-PLUS) Study Investigators (1998) Inhibition of the platelet glycoprotein IIb/IIIa receptor with tirofiban in unstable angina and non–Q-wave myocardial infarction. *N Engl J Med* **338**:1488–1497.

77. The ESPIRIT Investigators (2000) Novel dosing regimen of eptifibatide in planned coronary stent implantation (ESPRIT): a randomised, placebo-controlled trial. *Lancet* **356**:2037–2044.

78. The Pursuit Trial Investigators (1998) Inhibition of platelet glycoprotein IIb/IIIa with eptifibatide in patients with acute coronary syndromes. *N Engl J Med* **339**:436–443.

79. Boersma E, Harrington R, Moliterno D, *et al.* (2002) Platelet glycoprotein IIb/IIIa inhibitors in acute coronary syndromes: a meta-analysis of all major randomised clinical trials. *Lancet* **359**:189–198.

80. Eli Lilly and Co. (2005) ReoPro® (abciximab) injection for intravenous administration prescribing information. Indianapolis, IN.

81. Millennium (2005) Integrilin® (eptifibatide) injection prescribing information. South San Francisco, CA.

82. Merck & Co. (2004) Aggrastat (trademark) (tirofiban hydrochloride) injection premixed and injection prescribing information. West Point, PA.

83. Helgason C, Tortorice K, Winkler S, *et al.* (1993) Aspirin response and failure in cerebral infarction. *Stroke* **24**:345–350.

84. Gum P, Kandice Kottke-Marchant, Welsh P, *et al.* (2003) A prospective, blinded determination of the natural history of aspirin resistance among stable patients with cardiovascular disease. *J Am Coll Cardiol* **41**:961–965.

85. Eikelboom J, Hirsh J, Weitz J, *et al.* (2002) Aspirin-resistant thromboxane biosynthesis and the risk of myocardial infarction, stroke, or cardiovascular death in patients at high risk for cardiovascular events. *Circulation* **105**:1650–1655.

86. Lev E, Patel R, Maresh K, *et al.* (2006) Aspirin and clopidogrel drug response in patients undergoing percutaneous coronary intervention. *J Am Coll Cardiol* **479**:27–33.

87. Gladding P, Webster M, Ormiston J, *et al.* (2008) Antiplatelet drug responsiveness. *Am Heart J* **155**:591–599.

88. Harrison P, Robinson M, Mackie I, *et al.* (1999) Performance of the platelet function analyzer PFA-100 in testing abnormalities of primary hemostasis. *Blood Coagul Fibrinolysis* **10**:25–31.

89. Dyszkiewicz-Korpanty A, Kim A, Burner J, *et al.* (2007) Comparison of a rapid platelet function assay—Verify Now Aspirin— with whole blood impedance aggregometry for the detection of aspirin resistance. *Thromb Res* **120**:485.

90. Greilich P, Alving B, O'Neill K, *et al.* (1997) A modified thromboelastographic method for monitoring c7E3 Fab in heparinized patients. *Anesth Analg* **84**:31.

91. Chen W, Lee P, Ng W, *et al.* (2004) Aspirin resistance is associated with a high incidence of myonecrosis after non-urgent percutaneous coronary intervention despite clopidogrel treatment. *J Am Coll Cardiol* **43**:1122–1126.

92. Marcucci R, Paniccia R, Antonucci E, *et al.* (2006) Usefulness of aspirin resistance after percutaneous coronary intervention for acute myocardial infarction in predicting one-year major adverse coronary events. *Am J Cardiol* **98**:1156–1159.

93. Campo G, Valgimigli M, Gemmati D, *et al.* (2006) Value of platelet reactivity in predicting response to treatment and clinical outcome in patients undergoing primary coronary intervention. *J Am Coll Cardiol* **48**:2178–2185.

94. Cuisset T, Frere C, Quilici J, *et al.* (2006) Benefit of a 600-mg loading dose of Clopidogrel on platelet reactivity and clinical outcomes in patients with non-ST-segment elevation acute coronary syndrome undergoing coronary stenting. *J Am Coll Cardiol* **48**:1339–1345.

95. Smith S, Jr, Feldman T, Hirshfeld J, *et al.* (2006) ACC/AHA/SCAI 2005 Guideline Update for Percutaneous Coronary Intervention— Summary Article: a report of the American College of Cardiology/American Heart Association Task Force on Practice Guidelines (ACC/AHA/SCAI Writing Committee to Update the 2001 Guidelines for Percutaneous Coronary Intervention). *J Am Coll Cardiol* **47**:216–235.

96. Cohen M, Adams P, Parry G, *et al.* (1994) Combination antithrombotic therapy in unstable rest angina and non-Q- wave infarction in nonprior aspirin users. Primary end points analysis from the ATACS trial. Antithrombotic therapy in Acute Coronary Syndromes Research Group. *Circulation* **89**:81–88.

97. Oler A, Whooley M, & Oler J (1996) Adding heparin to aspirin reduces the incidence of myocardial infarction and death in patients with unstable angina. A meta-analysis. *JAMA* **276**:811–815.

98. Hassan W, Flaker G, Feutz C, *et al.* (1996) Improved anticoagulation with a weight-adjusted heparin nomogram in patients with acute coronary syndromes: a randomized trial. *J Thromb Thrombolysis* **2**:245–249.

99. Becker R, Ball S, Eisenberg P, *et al.* (1999) A randomized, multicenter trial of weight-adjusted intravenous heparin dose titration and point-of-care coagulation monitoring in hospitalized patients with active thromboembolic disease: Antithrombotic Therapy Consortium Investigators. *Am Heart J* **137**:59–71.

100. Weitz J (1997) Low-molecular-weight heparins. *N Engl J Med* **337**:688–698.

101. Rabah M, Premmereur J, Graham M, *et al.* (1999) Usefulness of intravenous enoxaparin for percutaneous coronary intervention in stable angina pectoris. *Am J Cardiol* **84**:1391–1395.

102. Bhatt D, Lee B, Casterella P, *et al.* (2003) Safety of concomitant therapy with eptifibatide and enoxaparin in patients undergoing percutaneous coronary intervention: results of the coronary revascularization using integrilin and single bolus enoxaparin study. *J Am Coll Cardiol* **41**:20–25.

103. Choussat R, Montalescot G, Collet J, *et al.* (2002) A unique, low dose of intravenous enoxaparin in elective percutaneous coronary intervention. *J Am Coll Cardiol* **40**:1943–1950.

104. Ferguson J, Antman E, Bates E, *et al.* (2003) Combining enoxaparin and glycoprotein IIb/IIIa antagonists for the treatment of acute coronary syndromes: final results of the National Investigators Collaborating on Enoxaparin-3 (NICE-3) study. *Am Heart J* **146**:628–634.

105. Miller L, Gupta A, & Bertolet B (2002) Use of clopidogrel loading, enoxaparin, and double-bolus eptifibatide in the setting of early percutaneous coronary intervention for acute coronary syndromes. *J Invasive Cardiol* **14**:247–250.

106. Collet J, Montalescot G, Lison L, *et al.* (2001) Percutaneous coronary intervention after subcutaneous enoxaparin pretreatment in patients with unstable angina pectoris. *Circulation* **103**:658–663.

107. Gibson C, Murphy S, Montalescot G, *et al.* (2007) Percutaneous coronary intervention in patients receiving enoxaparin or unfractionated heparin after fibrinolytic therapy for ST-segment elevation myocardial infarction in the ExTRACT-TIMI 25 trial. *J Am Coll Cardiol* **49**:2238–2246.

108. Lincoff A, Bittl J, Harrington R, *et al.* For the REPLACE-2 Investigators (2003) Bivalirudin and Provisional Glycoprotein IIb/IIIa Blockade Compared With Heparin and Planned Glycoprotein IIb/IIIa Blockade During Percutaneous Coronary Intervention: REPLACE-2 Randomized Trial. *JAMA* **289**:853–863.

109. Lincoff M, Kleiman N, Kottke-Marchant K, *et al.* (2002) Bivalirudin with planned or provisional abciximab versus low-dose heparin and abciximab during percutaneous coronary revascularization: results of the Comparison of Abciximab Complications with Hirulog for Ischemic Events Trial (CACHET). *Am Heart J* **143**:847–853.

110. Waksman R, Wolfram R, Torguson R, *et al.* (2006) Switching from enoxaparin to bivalirudin in patients with acute coronary syndromes without st-segment elevation who undergo percutaneous coronary intervention. Results from SWITCH—a multicenter clinical trial. *J Invasive Cardiol* **18**:370–375.

111. Serruys P, Herrman J, Simon R, *et al.* (1995) A comparison of hirudin with heparin in the prevention of restenosis after coronary angioplasty. *N Engl J Med* **333**:757–764.

112. Lewis B, Matthai W, Jr, Cohen M, *et al.* (2002) Argatroban anticoagulation during percutaneous coronary intervention in patients with heparin-induced thrombocytopenia. *Catheter Cardiovasc Interv* **57**:177–184.

113. Bittl J, Chaitman B, Feit F, *et al.* (2001) On behalf of the Bivalirudin Angioplasty Study Investigators. Bivalirudin versus heparin during coronary angioplasty for unstable or postinfarction angina: final report reanalysis of the Bivalirudin Angioplasty Study. *Am Heart J* **142**:952–959.

114. Burchenal J, Marks D, Tift J, *et al.* (1998) Effect of direct thrombin inhibition with bivalirudin (Hirulog) on restenosis after coronary angioplasty. *Am J Cardiol* **82**:511–515.

115. White H, Chew D, Hoekstra J, *et al.* (2008) Safety and efficacy of switching from either unfractionated heparin or enoxaparin to bivalirudin in patients with non-ST-segment elevation acute coronary syndromes managed with an invasive strategy: results from the ACUITY trial. *J Am Coll Cardiol* **51**:1734–1741.

116. The Medicines Company (2005) Angiomax® (bivalirudin) for injection prescribing information. Cambridge, MA.

117. Encysive (2005) Argatroban injection prescribing information. Bellaire, TX.

118. The Fifth Organization to Assess Strategies in Acute Ischemic Syndromes Investigators (2006) Comparison of fondaparinux and enoxaparin in acute coronary syndromes. *N Engl J Med* **354**:1464–1476.

119. Yusuf S, Mehta S, Chrolavicius S, *et al.* (2006) Effects of fondaparinux on mortality and reinfarction in patients with acute ST-segment elevation myocardial infarction: the OASIS-6 randomized trial. *JAMA* **295**:1519–1530.

120. The CREATE Investigators (2005) Effects of reviparin, a low-molecular-weight heparin, on mortality, reinfarction, and strokes in patients with acute myocardial infarction presenting with ST-segment elevation. *JAMA* **293**:427–435.

121. GlaxoSmithKline (2008) Arixtra® (fondaparinux sodium) injection prescribing information. Ontario, Canada.

122. Meyer S, Curry G, Donsky M, *et al.* (1976) Influence of dobutamine on hemodynamics and coronary blood flow in patients with and without coronary artery disease. *Am J Cardiol* **38**:103–108.

123. Sakai H, Kunichika H, Murata K, *et al.* (2001) Improvement of afterload mismatch of left atrial booster pump function with positive inotropic agent. *J Am Coll Cardiol* **37**:270–277.

124. Prielipp R, MacGregor D, Butterworth J, 4th, *et al.* (1996) Pharmacodynamics and pharmacokinetics of milrinone administration to increase oxygen delivery in critically ill patients. *Chest* **109**:1291–1301.

125. Cuffe M, Califf R, Adams K, Jr, *et al.* (2002) Outcomes of a Prospective Trial of Intravenous Milrinone for Exacerbations of Chronic Heart Failure (OPTIME-CHF) Investigators. Short-term intravenous milrinone for acute exacerbation of chronic heart failure: a randomized controlled trial. *JAMA* **287**:1578–1580.

126. Felker G, Benza R, Chandler A, Leimberger J, *et al.* (2003) For the OPTIME-CHF Investigators. Heart failure etiology and response to milrinone in decompensated heart failure: results from the OPTIME-CHF study. *J Am Coll Cardiol* **41**:997–1003.

127. Packer M, Carver J, Rodeheffer R, *et al.* (1991) Effect of oral milrinone on mortality in severe chronic heart failure: the PROMISE Study Research Group. *N Engl J Med* **325**:1468–1475.

128. Bellomo R, Chapman M, Finfer S, *et al.* (2000) Low-dose dopamine in patients with early renal dysfunction: a placebo-controlled randomised trial. Australian and New Zealand Intensive Care Society (ANZICS) Clinical Trials Group. *Lancet* **356**:2139–2143.

129. Wenzel V, Krismer AC, Arntz HR, Sitter H, Stadlbauer KH, & Lindner KH (2004) A comparison of vasopressin and epinephrine for out-of-hospital cardiopulmonary resuscitation. *N Engl J Med* **350**:105–113.

130. Stiell I, Hebert P, Wells G, *et al.* (2001) Vasopressin versus epinephrine for in-hospital cardiac arrest: a randomised controlled trial. *Lancet* **358**:105–109.

131. Pepine C, Feldman R, & Conti C (1982) Action of intracoronary nitroglycerin in refractory coronary artery spasm. *Circulation* **65**:411–414.

132. Wang H, Lo P, Lin J, *et al.* (2004) Treatment of slow/no-reflow phenomenon with intracoronary nitroprusside injection in primary coronary intervention for acute myocardial infarction. *Catheter Cardiovasc Interv* **63**:171–176.

133. Amit G, Cafri C, Yaroslavtsev S (2006) Intracoronary nitroprusside for the prevention of the no-reflow phenomenon after primary percutaneous coronary intervention in acute myocardial infarction. A randomized, double-blind, placebo-controlled clinical trial. *Am Heart J* **152**:9–14.

134. Ross A, Gibbons R, Stone G, *et al.* (2005) A randomized, double-blinded, placebo-controlled multicenter trial of adenosine as an adjunct to reperfusion in the treatment of acute myocardial infarction (AMISTAD-II). *J Am Coll Cardiol* **45**:1775–1780.

135. Vijayalakshmi K, Whittaker V, Kunadian B, *et al.* (2006) Prospective, randomised, controlled trial to study the effect of intracoronary injection of verapamil and adenosine on coronary blood flow during percutaneous coronary intervention in patients with acute coronary syndromes. *Heart* **92**:1278–1284.

136. Roseia EA, Salvettia M, & Farsang C (2006) European Society of Hypertension Scientific Newsletter: treatment of hypertensive urgencies and emergencies. *J Hypertens* **24**:2482–2485.

137. Vaughan C & Delanty N (2000) Hypertensive emergencies. *Lancet* **356**:411–417.

138. Libby P, Bonow RO, Zipes DP, & Mann DL (2007) *Braunwald's Heart Disease: A Textbook of Cardiovascular Medicine*, 8th edition. Table 41–9: parenteral drugs for treatment of hypertensive emergency. Philadelphia: Saunders.

139. Abbott Laboratories (2000) Nitropress (sodium nitroprusside) injection prescribing information. North Chicago, Il.

140. Neutel J, Smith D, Wallin D, *et al.* (1994) A comparison of intravenous nicardipine and sodium nitroprusside in the immediate treatment of severe hypertension. *Am J Hypertens* **7**:623–628.

141. AHFS drug information 2004. In: McEvoy GK (ed). *Nitroglycerin*. Bethesda, MD: American Society of Health-System Pharmacists, pp. 1689–1692.

142. Wallin J, Fletcher E, Ram C, *et al.* (1989) Intravenous nicardipine for the treatment of severe hypertension. A double-blind, placebo-controlled multicenter trial. *Arch Intern Med* **149**:2662–2669.

143. Par Pharmaceutical, Inc. (2003) Hydralazine hydrochloride tablets prescribing information. Spring Valley, NY.

144. Lehot JJ, Bonnefoy E, Dalmas JP, Filley S, Bastien O, & George M (1995) [Role of urapidil in the treatment of acute hypertension]. *Cah Anesthesiol* **43**:67–76.

145. Ramage AG (1991) The mechanism of the sympathoinhibitory action of urapidil: role of 5-HT1A receptors. *Br J Pharmacol* **102**:998–1002. PMID 1855130.

146. Doods HN, Boddeke HW, Kalkman HO, Hoyer D, Mathy MJ, & van Zwieten PA (1988) Central 5-HT1A receptors and the mechanism of the central hypotensive effect of (+)8-OH-DPAT, DP-5-CT, R28935, and urapidil. J Cardiovasc Pharmacol **11**:432–437.

147. Gillis RA, Kellar KJ, Quest JA, *et al.* (1988) Experimental studies on the neurocardiovascular effects of urapidil. Drugs **35**(Suppl. 6):20–33.

148. Vanhaesebrouck S, Hanssens M, & Allegaert K (2009) Neonatal transient respiratory depression after maternal urapidil infusion for hypertension. *Eur J Pediatr* **168**:221–223.

149. Schering Corporation (1998) Normodyne® (labetalol hydrochloride) injection prescribing information (dated 1997 Feb). In: *Physicians' desk reference*, 52nd edn. Montvale, NJ: Medical Economical Company Inc; (Suppl. A):A280–282.

150. Bedford Laboratories (2008) Esmolol hydrochloride injection prescribing information. Bedford, OH.

151. Novartis (1999) Lopressor® (metoprolol tartrate) tablets and injection prescribing information. East Hannover, NJ.

152. Brater DC (1992) Diuretic pharmacokinetics and pharmacodynamics. In: van Boxtel CJ, Holford NHG, Danhof M (eds). The in vivo study of drug action: principles and applications of kinetic-dynamic modelling. Amsterdam: Elsevier Science, pp. 253–275.

153. Beermann B (1984) Aspects of pharmacokinetics of some diuretics. *Acta Pharmacol Toxicol* (Copenh) **54**(Suppl. 1):17–29.

154. Vasko M, Cartwright D, Knochel J, *et al.* (1985) Furosemide absorption altered in decompensated congestive heart failure. *Ann Intern Med* **102**:314–318.

155. Davies D, Lant A, Millard N, *et al.* (1974) Renal action, therapeutic use, and pharmacokinetics of the diuretic bumetanide. *Clin Pharmacol Ther* **15**:141–155.

156. Brater D, Leinfelder J, & Anderson S (1987) Clinical pharmacology of torasemide, a new loop diuretic. *Clin Pharmacol Ther* **42**:187–192.

42 Magnetic Navigation in Percutaneous Coronary Intervention

Steve Ramcharitar & Patrick W. Serruys

Thoraxcenter, Erasmus Medical Center, Rotterdam, The Netherlands

Introduction

The fundamental technique that bridges all percutaneous intervention is the ability to precisely track a guidewire or a catheter at or through a lesion. In some cases this remains the Achilles heel of the entire procedure as it determines success or failure. To increase success there is a repertoire of wires with varying weights, trackablity, and torque that each cardiologist has in his or her "toolbox." However, there is often a trade-off; wires that excel in one feature, for example the support achieved with a stiffer wire, may lose in another feature, for example its ability to maneuver through the subtle changes in a tortuous vascular anatomy. This provides the rationale for developing systems offering precise distal tip control so as to redirect a wire *in vivo* within the coronary tree without the need to remove it from the patient and reshape the tip [1]. The magnetic navigation system (MNS) uses a magnetically enabled wire tip to have full 360° omni-rotation [2]. This is achieved by using large external permanent magnets to precisely control magnetic vectors created through a dedicated software called Navigant® (Stereotaxis, St. Louis, MO, USA). This novel technology is now firmly established in cardiac electrophysiology and, in addition, has been favorably accepted in neurosurgery following early animal and human studies [3,4]. However, its extension into the competitive world of interventional cardiology has had a cautionary start, despite over 100 systems having been installed worldwide. This may be because the technology still has to define areas in which there are potential benefits over conventional percutaneous coronary interventions (PCIs) to convince the skeptical interventional community [1]. At present, the MNS is an expensive technology that requires a learning phase for both the software and the hardware. Moreover, unlike neurosurgery, targeting a moving structure—for example, the beating heart—presents a challenge for the navigational roadmaps created from static images. Nevertheless, it is postulated that

the system may provide new options to manage challenging and tortuous anatomy such as chronic total occlusions (CTOs): crossing/fluoroscopy time, contrast and materials, targeted stem cell therapies, and ultimately in the realization of remote control PCI [5].

Historical background

The use of magnets to control an intravascular catheter was first reported in 1951 [6]. Exactly 40 years later Ram and Meyer [7] described the first human magnetically guided heart catheterization in a neonate. Several key technologic developments were needed to meet the level of sophistication achieved with the current magnetic MNS [8]. Initially the early magnet designs used large and cumbersome electromagnets to redirect relatively large magnetized wires, which meant that navigation was only permitted in relatively large vessels. It was only with the current smaller permanent magnets that the system allowed tiny magnets (≤0.014 inches) to be deflected at the tip of the wires used for percutaneous coronary interventions. After preclinical evaluation, the Niobe® I system (Stereotaxis, St Louis, MO, USA) received regulatory approval for human clinical use in cardiac electrophysiology and interventional neuroradiology in 2000, and for interventional cardiology in 2003.

The magnetic navigation system

The current magnetic navigation system (MNS) Niobe II consists of two focused-field permanent magnets, one on each side of the body, that create a 0.08-T navigation field (Fig. 42.1). This is integrated with a modified C-arm single planar digital angiography system (AXIOM Artis dFC; Siemens, Forchheim, Germany) or with the Philips Rotational Angiography system (Philips Healthcare, Best, The Netherlands). Both angiography systems have to be specifically adapted to operate within the magnetic field. The flat panel detector (size 20 × 20 cm), flat screen, and the touch screen monitor to "drive" the system are all magnetically shielded. The two rare-earth

Cardiovascular Interventions in Clinical Practice. Edited by Jürgen Haase, Hans-Joachim Schäfers, Horst Sievert and Ron Waksman. © 2010 Blackwell Publishing.

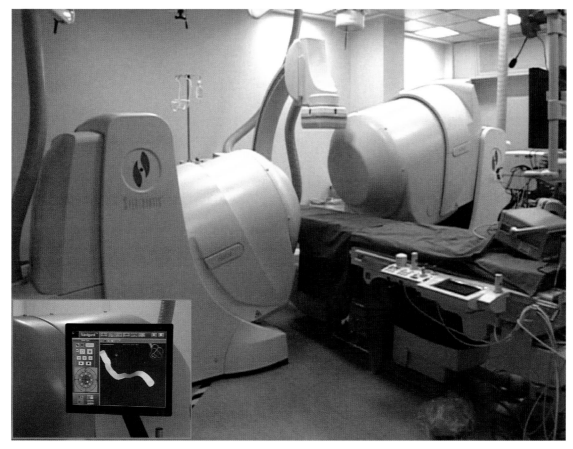

Figure 42.1 Magnetic navigation system with the magnets in the tilt position on either side of the patient. Inserted at the bottom left-hand panel is the touch-screen monitor used to direct the navigation along the chosen vessel.

permanent magnets are mounted on mechanical positioners. These positioners rotate and translate the magnets to generate the specified field direction at the tip of the magnetic device. Each magnet and its respective positioners are contained in a fiberglass cover, which allows the magnets to move within the stationary cover during navigation. When not in use, each magnet can be retracted via semicircular tracks that are permanently installed in the floor. Movement of each magnet can occur along the three different coordinates (x-, y- and z-axes). In addition they can rotate around the z-axis and move toward or away from the navigation volume and tilt. Tilting allows wider angiographic views as the earlier version the Niobe I system was limited to a maximum X-ray imaging angles of 30° left anterior oblique and right anterior oblique. The combination of rotation, translation, and tilting provides a navigation volume resembling a sphere with a diameter of 15 cm between the magnets. Within this magnetic volume, the magnetic vectors are applied to redirect the wire in any direction—360° orientated in all planes. The three-dimensional (3-D) location of the X-ray image is known from the positions of the image intensifier, angiography system, and table. When the magnets are in the stowed position they are retracted 90° from the patient, and the magnetic field in

the operating area is less than 0.0005 T. However, when in the navigational mode they are positioned closest (23.5 inches [59.7 cm]) to the magnets and covers, pointed toward the patient producing a magnetic field of 0.08 T. This field is relatively small, with an order of magnitude 15 times less than that of a standard MRI scanner. Despite this, it is recommended that the MNS should not be used in patients with pacemakers or defibrillators because the eddy currents and heat generated are yet to be fully evaluate in these systems [9].

The magnetic guidewires

The magnetic guidewire used together with the MNS has a nominal diameter of 0.014 inches (0.36 mm) and a nominal length of 185 cm or 300 cm. The wire is configured with a 2- or 3-mm embedded gold encapsulated neodynium–iron–boron magnet at the distal tip (Fig. 42.2). The Cronus™ (Stereotaxis, St. Louis, MO, USA) was a first-generation hydrophilically coated magnetic guidewire that was available in both magnet tip dimensions. When subjected to a magnetic vector, the tiny magnetic tip realigns in the direction of the applied field, and steering of the tip is performed. Once achieved, the wire can be advanced manually until another change of direction is required. This basic principle of wire orientation/guidance

Table 42.1 Characteristics of the Stereotaxis guidewire family.

Guidewire	Distal core	Proximal core	Magnet tip length	Hydrophilic distal coating
Cronus™	Nitinol	Nitinol	2 & 3 mm	25 cm
Titan™	Stainless steel	Stainless steel	2 & 3 mm	10–34 cm
Pegasus™	Nitinol	Stainless steel	2 & 3 mm	40 cm

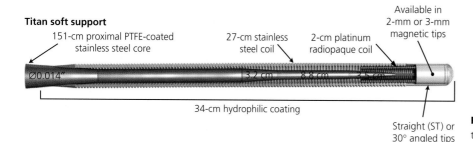

Figure 42.2 The magnetic guidewire with the 2- to 3-mm embedded gold encapsulate neodynium iron boron magnet at the distal tip.

is conserved with the newer generation wires (Table 42.1) that include the Titan™ and the Pegasus™ range (Stereotaxis, St. Louis, MO, USA). Although the basic principle of steering is similar to the Cronus, the newer wires are superior in their ability to deliver a device because of the different materials used in their shafts. Three-point deflection testing performed by supporting the wires at two points and measuring the force required to deflect the midpoint to 4 mm showed that they stiffen quicker to improve device delivery. The Titan soft support wire has a stiffness profile similar to a Balance Medium Weight (BMW; Abbott Vascular Devices, Redwood, CA, USA) moderate support wire, with the even stiffer Titan Assert wire able to deliver a tip load of similar characteristics to a Miracle 3 g wire (Asahi Intecc, Nagoya, Japan). The tip load measures the force needed to buckle the guidewire when applied 1 cm from the tip. In the newest wires, the Pegasus range, the distal shaft is made of nitinol to allow greater shape retention and the proximal shaft is made of stainless steel to maintain pushability. As with other magnetic wires, they are hydrophilically coated to facilitate a smooth wire transit. The three-point deflection test pattern shows that the Pegasus Moderate and Assert have similar support profiles. However, the very distal 2 cm of the Assert is stiffer to transmit more force in the case of crossing tightly or total occlusions.

The mechanical forces exerted on the magnetic wire

Unlike standard nonmagnetized guidewires used in conventional PCI procedures, magnetic wires have different mechanical forces exerted at the tip of the wire [10]. In standard guidewires there is only a push force that the operator uses to direct the wire transit across a lesion. In the magnetic guide-

wire, however, in addition to this push force there is also a deflection force. The deflection force is that applied through the permanent magnet to cause deflection of the magnetic guidewire in the direction of the magnetic field vector. The magnitude of this force can be calculated by combining the torque exerted at the tip of the wire to that acting in the opposite direction of the deflection. The torque (τ) exerted on the tip of the wire is equal to the product of the magnetization vector (M, measured in amperes per meter) of the magnet in the tip of the wire, cross-sectional area (A, measured in square meters) of the magnet in the tip of the wire, magnet length (L, measured in meters), external magnetic field vector (B, measured in teslas), and the sine of the angle between the field and magnetization vectors (θ):

$$\tau = MALB\sin(\theta) \tag{42.1}$$

The torque is also described by two identical forces (F, measured in grams) acting in opposite directions on two poles of the permanent magnet through the moment arm:

$$\tau = 2(L/2)F \tag{42.2}$$

Combining equations (42.1) and (42.2) provides a description of the force exerted by the magnetic field on the distal end of the guidewire:

$$F = MAB\sin(\theta) \tag{42.3}$$

This force is maximal when the wire is perpendicular to the magnetic field (i.e., $\sin(\theta) = 1$) and zero when the wire is parallel to the magnetic field [11].

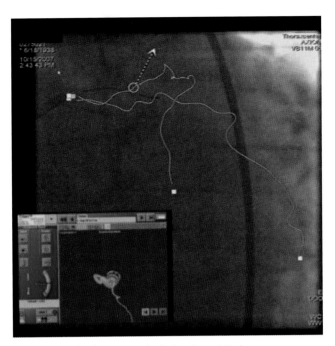

Figure 42.3 The chosen vector is displayed as a dotted arrow on navigational path-line on the live fluoroscopy image. The bottom left panel shows what the operator sees on the touch-screen monitor.

Navigation software

The Navigant software allows several possible modes to navigate through the coronary artery. Broadly speaking, these can be divided into two main groups: the so-called "free mode," in which navigational vectors are manually derived from the two-dimensional (2-D) X-ray angiographic images, and "true vessel" navigation, in which vectors are derived automatically from a 3-D image of the vessel (e.g., a multislice computer tomography [MSCT] data set) or through a dedicated 3-D reconstruction (3-DRC) software package. Regardless of the chosen mode to create the vector, in all cases the operator can manually change a vector using a sterile interactive touch screen monitor located at arms' length at the operation table. With this monitor the operator can also chose for the vector to be automatically updated at a desired incremental distance (1–9 mm). The chosen vector is displayed as a dotted arrow on navigational pathline (centerline) on the live fluoroscopy image (Fig. 42.3). As the vector is updated the dotted arrow moves along the navigational pathline and the permanent magnets rotate about their axes to create a new magnetic field in line with the trajectory of the new coordinate seen as a solid arrow on the live fluoroscopy image (Fig. 42.3). The operator manually pushes the wire forward to follow the preset incremental distance imposed by the desired vector.

Free mode navigation

The "free mode" 2-D navigational modes include the use of "preset navigational vectors" that are adapted to particular coronary anatomies, e.g., left anterior descending and circum-

flex arteries. Other anatomical vasculature can be added if required, such as coronary artery bypass grafts and peripheral arteries. The presets allow relative fast navigation but it lacks accuracy as it is based on the assumption of standardized vasculature. Similarly, the "clock face" navigational mode in which the vectors can move in a chosen direction by touching the periphery of a circle mimicking the dial of a clock is equally simple to use but also lacks accuracy [12]. Its effectiveness depends on the skill of the operator and his or her spatial understanding of coronary anatomy. In combination with a "bull's-eye view," in which the tip of the wire can be made to move along the contours of a dartboard, offers some degree of accuracy and this is particularly useful in locating microchannels within chronic total occlusions (CTOs). Some spatial understanding of the coronary anatomy is required in the more complex "spherical navigational approach," in which the vessel or object is contained within the boundaries of a sphere with regularly spaced polar lines (e.g., latitude and longitude lines). In all the above navigational modes the vectors are generic, as they are not directly created from the anatomy of the vessel being treated. However, "true" anatomical navigation is possible on the vessel being treated by directly introducing two orthogonal fluoroscopic images of the vessel in Navigant®, but such a 2-D image representation of a 3-D structure has obvious limitations [13]. Much more accurate is the creation of a virtual 3-DRC vessel or using MSCT to accurately derive the vector coordinates.

"True" vessel navigation

"True" vessel navigation is an accurate representation of a 3-D navigational roadmap of the coronary artery [14]. Navigant can create such a virtual map from two X-ray images provided that they are 30° apart. To do this, identical points on both images in the same cardiac phase are simultaneously linked to generate the 3-D navigational path or "centerline" through the vessel lumen. This creates a static roadmap that is coregistered with the live fluoroscopy image. It should be noted that if the images are not gated it means that only in the phase in which the images were taken will the navigational road map be perfectly aligned. But, for the purposes of navigation, the trajectory of the vector will be sufficiently good enough to permit the adequate wire transit. The 3-DRC centerline can also be created from two fluoroscopic images using dedicated software (CardiOpB®, Paieon Medical Inc., Rosh Ha'ayin, Israel) that has the added advantage of being able to fine tune the direction of the vector by visualizing subtle changes in the vessel through a virtual lumen—the so-called endoluminal view. A far more accurate 3-D road map can be obtained by employing multislice computer tomography (MSCT) data sets (Fig. 42.4). This imaging modality can also identify vascular anomalies and provide information on coronary plaque composition [15,16]. The vessels can be extracted directly from the MSCT data set through postprocessing software and be directly incorporated,

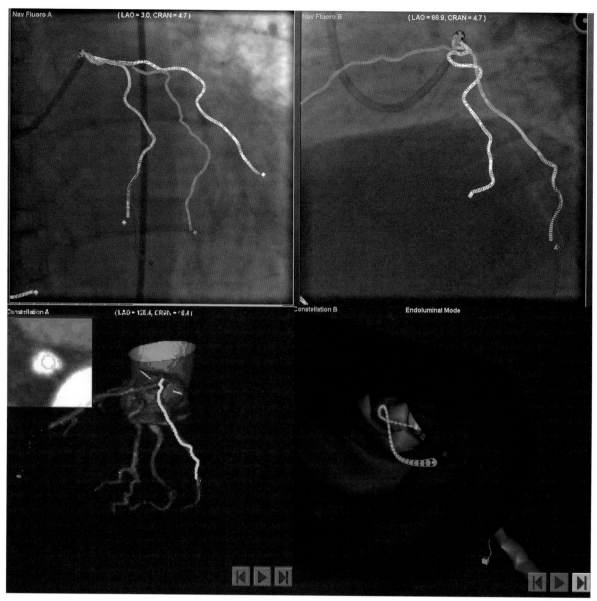

Figure 42.4 Top panels showing the tip of the catheters in fluoroscopy image coregistered with the extracted coronaries derived from the MSCT data set. These give the specific 3-D coordinates that allow integration of the two modalities. Bottom panels showing the extracted coronaries with the centerline together with multiplaner reconstructed cross-section displayed in the Navigant and the endoluminal views for MSCT-based navigation.

coregistered, and aligned to the fluoroscopic image in the Navigant [17].

Current status

It is the intention of the MNS not to revolutionize current practices in PCI, but rather to facilitate in areas in which conventional techniques may be met with difficulty. Potential areas are in the challenging anatomies associated with tortuosity, chronic total occlusions for which the path of the vessel is not visible so the required tip direction is unclear, and in improving the efficacy of myocardial stem cell implantation.

Challenging anatomy

Challenging anatomy often is associated with lower crossing success and higher rates for surgical referral. In a study comparing magnetic and conventional wires in phantom models mimicking tortuous coronary arteries, magnetic wire crossings were found to be superior in the more tortuous phantoms [18]. More than five-fold reduction in crossing times were recorded (201.7 ± 111s to 36.4 ± 13s, $P < 0.001$) compared with standard guidewire techniques. Moreover, the magnetic wires achieved a 98.8% crossing success compared with 68% with the standard guidewires, with considerably fewer wires used (1.3 vs. 5.5) as a result of wire tip damage. But much more interesting was the finding that, in certain cases, operators without prior MNS experience had equally good crossing successes with the magnetic wires compared with senior operators. In the more difficult phantoms however, a learning curve was clearly demonstrable in those operators with limited MNS experience.

In addition to this phantom study, the ability to negotiate challenging anatomy has also been shown in several clinical scenarios in which the procedural success was inherently dependent on the MNS. In a case of hypertrophic obstructive cardiomyopathy (HOCM), the origin of the major septal artery had an unusually extreme angulation (approximately 130°) on coronary angiography that was impossible to access with a conventional guidewire approach [19]. However, by employing MNS guidewire the balloon catheter cannulation of the septal artery made it possible to facilitate a successful transcatheter alcohol septal ablation procedure. MNS guided septal ablation has now been evaluated in a randomized study consisting of 44 consecutive patients [20]. In all cases the procedures were successful, and the only complication was a vessel dissection occurring in the conventional group. Interestingly, as observed in the phantom studies, the time required for guidewire cannulation of the septal branch decreased progressively with increasing experience (third tertile vs. first tertile; 3 min [range 1.25–4.75 min] vs. 10.5 min [range 6–17 min], $P = 0.004$) compared with the conventional group (6 min [range 2–10.25], $P = 0.075$ vs. third tertile), suggesting a learning curve.

Early experience of the magnetic navigation in crossing coronary lesions showed relatively low success (88%) with the first-generation Cronus wires. Although the majority of lesions were relatively straightforward, 4 of the 68 target lesions were complex and had previously failed with conventional wire techniques [21]. When directly compared for the crossing of 21 consecutive simple and straightforward lesions, the magnetic wires had significantly longer crossing times than the standard guidewires (median 120 vs. 40 s, $P = 0.001$; 105 vs. 38 s, $P = 0.001$, respectively) [22]. In addition, the contrast media usage and amount of radiation exposure were also higher with magnetic wires (median, 13 vs. 9 mL, $P = 0.018$; 215 vs. 73 Gy m^2, $P = 0.002$, respectively). Without a demonstrable advantage in simple lesions, many groups have focused on vessels having various degrees of complexity or in cases that were previously met with failure using a conventional wire approach. One of the first studies evaluated 59 patients grouped to attempt MNS guided PCI as a first option ("primary attempt"; $n = 46$) or following failure to pass a conventional guidewire ("secondary attempt"; $n = 13$) [23]. It demonstrated that the target lesion was successfully crossed in 49 of 55 lesions (89%), and in 9 of 13 conventional failed lesions (69%) the MNS was successful, giving procedural successes of 84% and 62%, respectively. As expected, the median crossing, fluoroscopy, and contrast media usage were

longer or higher among the secondary attempt group. Other reports in which MNS was successful in cases that failed conventionally were in recrossing of a crush stent to facilitate kissing balloon post dilation and in crossing a jump saphenous vein graft (SVG), having an acute angulation to a stenosis just before it anastomosed to an obtuse marginal branch and a right posterior descending coronary artery [24,25]. To try to identify other cases that are more likely to be crossed with the magnetic system, a novel complexity scoring system is being evaluated. It uses 3-D information of both the vessel and lesion characteristics in an attempt to address some of the notable limitations encountered with existing classification [26]. Preliminary results have shown that there is a trend to support MNS in more complex vascular anatomies. In one of the largest prospective studies MNS was performed on 439 lesions in 350 consecutive PCI patients predominantly using the radial approach [27]. Successful crossing was accomplished in 93% of the lesions, with 25 of the 35 failures having occurred in the attempted chronic total occlusions. Lesion crossing time was 81 ± 168 s (mean ± SD), and fluoroscopy time was 64 ± 123 s. A clear learning curve was evident after the first 80 patients. In addition, contrast agent usage was reduced when compared with a historical control group. Low success in crossing (sub)chronic total occlusions with magnetic wires was also reported in a study comparing guidewire steering by either 2-D guidance or virtual 3-DRC [28]. In 30 patients with 36 coronary artery lesions, an overall crossing success of 86% (31/36 lesions) was recorded with the five failures occurring in patients having (sub)chronic total occlusions. The study did reveal that significantly less contrast medium was needed to position the magnetic guidewire by using the 3-DRC (60 ± 101 mL vs. 14 ± 15 mL, $P < 0.05$).

Chronic total occlusions

Chronic total occlusions often present a challenge, and their variable success rate (65–80%) is dependent on the skill of the operator, the materials, and the technique used [29]. As a result, a number of strategies have been suggested to facilitate the treatment of CTOs, e.g., intracoronary thrombolytic infusion [30], tapered-tip laser [31], and radiofrequency guidewires [32]. A novel approach to manage a CTO is to integrate the MNS ability to steer a guidewire through the occlusion with a forward-looking technology such as MSCT cross-sections to ensure ideal positioning of the wire in the true lumen (Fig. 42.4). Once the ideal position is accepted, ablative radiofrequency power can be delivered to the tip of the wire to recanalize the CTO [33]. Early evaluation of the MNS-MSCT approach to CTO used magnetic wires without ablative power, and navigation was aided by the bull's eye view to "look forward" at the occlusion—to make the search pattern for microchannels through the occlusion more uniform [34]. Even though the success was limited by the bulkiness of the 2- to 3-mm magnetic tips, the feasibility of using a

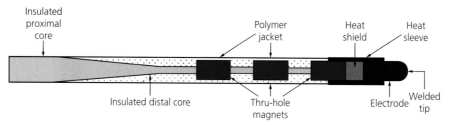

Figure 42.5 The radiofrequency ablating magnetically enabled 0.018-inch wire aimed at addressing chronically occluded vessels.

3-D map generated from an MSCT data set to navigate was demonstrated. This is important because the lack of a fluoroscopic lumenogram in a CTO does not allow navigation using 3-DRC software. With MSCT, both the distal vessel (filled via collaterals) and the tissue attenuation line (the scarred tissue of the original vessel lumen) can be identified. However, the navigational centerline is fixed, and, as a result, the mismatch with the moving artery in the live fluoroscopy image persists, except in the phase in which the navigational path was constructed from the MSCT image. Ordinarily, when navigating through a patent vessel this is not a problem, as the wire is contained within the vessel's lumen so that when the heart moves with each beat the wire can still follow the trajectory of the predetermined vectors. In a CTO, however, the lack of a patent lumen means that, as the heart moves along its axis, the tip of the wire can be perpendicular to the vascular wall and, when pushed, can protrude. Therefore, with magnetically enabled, radiofrequency powered wires, it is crucial to have a dynamic road map (centerline) to superimpose on the live fluoroscopy image, or to ECG phase gate a centerline derived from the MSCT to the fluoroscopic image, following alignment to recognizable landmarks such as the spinal processes and the catheter's tip. This would mean that at all points in the cardiac cycle the centerline would be superimposed on the live fluoroscopic image of the vessel and the advancement of the ablating wire could be achieved safely. The stereotaxis research field is now in its final stages of developing a radiofrequency ablating magnetic enabled wire (Fig. 42.5). This is a 0.018-inch wire with a small radiofrequency electrode at its tip, three small magnets protected by a heat sleeve, and the radiofrequency energy supplied by an external radiofrequency generator.

The nitinol shaft is electrically insulated with asymmetrically coated polytetrafluoroethylene, thinned distally, to provide adequate dielectric strength without affecting the wire's flexibility. The composite metal alloys used in the radiofrequency electrode are encased in a polyurethane polymer jacket for smooth transitions between the different components. *In vivo* studies demonstrated good results in artificially created occlusions (5–8 cm in length and aged 6–8 weeks) in porcine femoral arteries. The first-in-man study assessing the safety and feasibility will first be done in caged CTOs "within stents" and in peripheral vessels.

Stem cell injection

An area in which magnetic navigation is postulated to have an advantage over conventional techniques is intramyocardial injection of stem cells [35]. Current methods for delivery remain inexact despite using electromechanically guided injection. This uses NOGA electromechanical mapping (EMM) of the myocardium to identify the infarction areas for treatment. Appropriate electrical signal strength recorded as the mapping electrode makes a good contact with the myocardium is used as a marker for intramyocardial injection [36]. Although this approach is advantageous, the mapping of remote areas in the heart can be difficult to access, even with very experienced operators. However, by using a magnetically enabled MNS-guided NOGA EMM catheter these remote areas can be effectively mapped. Moreover, the magnetic momentum at the catheter tip is supportive enough to allow the use of softer catheters that are less likely to perforate the myocardium. Preclinical studies on a Stereotaxis-compatible NogaStar® mapping and MyoStar™ injection catheters (Biologics Delivery Systems, Cordis Corporation, Diamond Bar, CA, USA) equipped with a small permanent magnet positioned at the tip have been encouraging, with a 95.8% success rate for intramyocardial injection of mesenchymal precursor cells (MPCs) [37]. The NOGA mapping of the myocardium was performed remotely with a computer-controlled catheter advancement system (Cardiodrive® unit, Stereotaxis St Louis, MO, USA) [38]. This 3-D map was used with Navigant to create the desired navigational vectors needed for the magnetically enabled MyoStar catheter to follow.

Limitations and future developments

The ability of the MNS to precisely direct an *in vivo* device externally makes it a powerful tool that has the potential to benefit several areas of interventional cardiology. At present, it is expensive, technically demanding, and has several drawbacks related to both the software and hardware. Both the operator and technician must overcome the learning curve before maximal gains can be achieved. In addition, current methods used to create the 3-DRC are time-consuming, taking up to 30 min for the navigational pathway to be displayed on the fluoroscopy image. Moreover, this static image has inherent limitations with coregistration and with the accuracy in directing the vectors on static roadmaps. It therefore means that, for the full potential of the MNS to be realized, there must be continuous improvements in both software and hardware design. Some of the major limitations are already being addressed with the next generation of wires/devices. Current magnetic wires suffer from the lack of sophistication that has become widely accepted through the many generations of standard conventional wire designs. The crudeness of the 2- to 3-mm magnet stuck on to the tip of the wire influences the wire's ability to transit smoothly across a lesion. Planned future generation wires will have multi-magnet designs akin to the radiofrequency wire to address this particular limitation. Moreover, different alloy composites are being tested to retain the shape of the wire without compromising its ability to deliver a device. However, a major limitation is the responsiveness of the hardware in executing the vector change demanded by the Navigant. In the earlier versions of the software, the vectors had to be manually updated by pressing an advancing icon on the touch screen monitor. This meant that the operator had a time delay before advancing the magnetic guidewire as the system updated. In the latest version, Navigant 2.11, the vectors are automatically updated at a preset rate—moving at an incremental distance of 1–9 mm over a chosen time in seconds. Although this is a desirable feature, as it frees the operator from performing an additional task, he or she still has to wait for the magnets to move to realign their field in the direction of the vector. This time delay makes the magnetic navigation system slower than conventional wire techniques and this may not be easily solved because of the mechanical limitations in moving large external magnets rapidly and accurately. It is also sometimes not fully appreciated that the operator is still required to manually advance the wire with his/her left hand, and that the MNS is only steering the tip through the external field. By using a Cardiodrive unit attached to the distal part of the wire, automatic advancement is possible. This system has been extensively used in magnetic guided cardiac electrophysiologic procedures and may provide a window for remote control intervention when amalgamated with technologies that can enable accurate device positioning [39]. Such technologies exist but require significant investment to make them magnetically field compatible. In the future, the potential benefits of steering the tip of a guidewire in a desired direction, driving it externally, and accurately knowing the position of a device on the wire will certainly have an impact on the current way of performing PCI [40].

Conclusion

The MNS is a promising technology that, when integrated with 3-D information, can offer new possibilities in performing percutaneous intervention. Key developments are still, however, required in both hardware and software to provide a real challenge to conventional approaches. The versatility of the system, however, in its ability to redirect a device *in vivo*, means that there may be additional benefits in many important aspects of invasive cardiology and patient care.

References

1. Raizner AE (2007) Magnetic navigation: a pivotal technology. *Catheter Cardiovasc Interv* **69**:856.
2. Ramcharitar S, Patterson MS, van Geuns RJ, van Mieghem C, & Serruys PW (2008) Technology insight: magnetic navigation in coronary interventions. *Nat Clin Pract Cardiovasc Med* **5**:148–156.
3. Ernst S, Ouyang F, Linder C, *et al.* (2004) Initial experience with remote catheter ablation using a novel magnetic navigation system: magnetic remote catheter ablation. *Circulation* **109**:1472–1475.
4. Chu JC, Hsi WC, Hubbard L, *et al.* (2005) Performance of magnetic field-guided navigation system for interventional neurosurgical and cardiac procedures. *J Appl Clin Med Phys* **6**:143–149.
5. Patterson MS, Schotten J, van Mieghem C, Kiemeneij F, & Serruys PW (2006) Magnetic navigation in percutaneous coronary intervention. *J Interv Cardiol* **19**:558–565.
6. Llander H (1951) Magnetic guidance of a catheter with articulated steel tip. *Acta Radiol* **35**:62–64.
7. Ram W & Meyer H (1991) Heart catheterization in a neonate by interacting magnetic fields: a new and simple method of catheter guidance. *Cathet Cardiovasc Diagn* **22**:317–319.
8. Gillies GT, Ritter RC, Broaddus WC, Grady MS, & Howard MA (1994) Magnetic manipulation instrumentation for medical physics research. *Rev Sci Instrum* **65**:533–562.
9. Kolb C, Luik A, Hessling G, & Zrenner B (2007) Magnetic catheter navigation system interference with a dual-chamber pacemaker. *J Cardiovasc Electrophysiol* **18**:892–893.
10. Wood BJ, Zhang H, Durrani A, *et al.* (2005) Navigation with electromagnetic tracking for interventional radiology procedures: a feasibility study. *J Vasc Interv Radiol* **16**:493–505.
11. Schiemann M, Killmann R, Kleen M, Abolmaali N, Finney J, & Vogl TJ (2004) Vascular guide wire navigation with a magnetic guidance system: experimental results in a phantom. *Radiology* **232**:475–481.
12. Hertting K, Ernst S, Stahl F, *et al.* (2005) Use of the novel magnetic navigation system Niobe™ in percutaneous coronary interventions: the Hamburg experience. *EuroIntervention* **1**:336–339.
13. Ramcharitar S, Daeman J, Patterson M, *et al.* (2008) First direct in vivo comparison of two commercially available three-dimensional quantitative coronary angiography systems. *Catheter Cardiovasc Interv* **71**:44–50.
14. Tsuchida K, van der Giessen W, Patterson M, *et al.* (2007) In vivo validation of a novel three-dimensional quantitative coronary angiography system (CardiOp-B): comparison with a conventional two-dimensional system (CAAS II) and with special reference to optical coherence tomography. *EuroIntervention* **3**:100–108.
15. Hoffmann MH & Lessick J (2006) Multidetector-row computed tomography for noninvasive coronary imaging. *Expert Rev Cardiovasc Ther* **4**:583–594.
16. Fishman EK & Horton KM (2007) The increasing impact of multidetector row computed tomography in clinical practice. *Eur J Radiol* **62**(Suppl.):1–13.

17. Ramcharitar S, Pugliese F, Patterson M, *et al.* (2008) Advanced magnetic navigation: multi-slice computer tomography-guided percutaneous coronary intervention in a patient with triple-vessel disease. *EuroIntervention* in press.

18. Ramcharitar S, Patterson MS, van Geuns RJ, *et al.* (2007) A randomised controlled study comparing conventional and magnetic guidewires in a two-dimensional branching tortuous phantom simulating angulated coronary vessels. *Catheter Cardiovasc Interv* **70**:662–668.

19. Bach RG, Leach C, Milov SA, & Lindsay BD (2006) Use of magnetic navigation to facilitate transcatheter alcohol septal ablation for hypertrophic obstructive cardiomyopathy. *J Invasive Cardiol* **18**:E176–178.

20. Buergler JM, Alam S, Spencer W, *et al.* (2007) Initial experience with alcohol septal ablation using a novel magnetic navigation system. *J Interv Cardiol* **20**:559–563.

21. Tsuchida K, García-García H, Tanimoto S, *et al.* (2005) Feasibility and safety of guidewire navigation using a magnetic navigation system in coronary artery stenoses. *EuroIntervention* **1**:329–335.

22. Tsuchida K, Garcia-Garcia HM, van der Giessen WJ, *et al.* (2006) Guidewire navigation in coronary artery stenoses using a novel magnetic navigation system: first clinical experience. *Catheter Cardiovasc Interv* **67**:356–363.

23. Atmakuri SR, Lev EI, Alviar C, *et al.* (2006) Initial experience with a magnetic navigation system for percutaneous coronary intervention in complex coronary artery lesions. *J Am Coll Cardiol* **47**:515–521.

24. Patterson MS, Ramcharitar S, & Serruys PW (2007) Magnetically supported PCI: success after failed surgery and conventional PCI. *Cath Lab Digest* **15**:1–14.

25. Ramcharitar S, Patterson MS, van Geuns RJ, & Serruys PW (2007) Magnetic navigation system used successfully to cross a crushed stent in a bifurcation that failed with conventional wires. *Catheter Cardiovasc Interv* **69**:852–855.

26. Patterson S, Hoeks S, Tanimoto S, Van Mieghem C, Ramcharitar S, Van Domburg R, Serruys PW. A simple score for predicting prolonged crossing times to select patients who would benefit from a magnetic percutaneous coronary intervention. European Heart Journal:2007; 28 (Abstract Supplement P(4762):847–848.

27. Kiemeneij F, Patterson MS, Amoroso G, Laarman G, & Slagboom T (2008) Use of the stereotaxis Niobe magnetic navigation system for percutaneous coronary intervention: results from 350 consecutive patients. *Catheter Cardiovasc Interv* **71**(4):510–516.

28. Schneider MA, Hoch FV, Neuser H, *et al.* (2008) Magnetic-guided percutaneous coronary intervention enabled by two-dimensional guidewire steering and three-dimensional virtual angioscopy: initial experiences in daily clinical practice. *J Interv Cardiol* **21**:158–166.

29. Di Mario C, Werner GS, Sianos G, *et al.* (2007) for the EuroCTO Club JS. European perspective in the recanalisation of chronic total occlusions (CTO): consensus document from the EuroCTO Club. *EuroIntervention* **3**:30–43.

30. Abbas AE, Brewington SD, Dixon SR, Boura JA, Grines CL, & O'Neill WW (2005) Intracoronary fibrin-specific thrombolytic infusion facilitates percutaneous recanalization of chronic total occlusion. *J Am Coll Cardiol* **46**:793–798.

31. Serruys PW, Hamburger JN, Koolen JJ, *et al.* (2000) Total occlusion trial with angioplasty by using laser guidewire. The TOTAL trial. *Eur Heart J* **21**:1797–1805.

32. Werner GS, Fritzenwanger M, Prochnau D, *et al.* (2007) Improvement of the primary success rate of recanalization of chronic total coronary occlusions with the Safe-Cross system after failed conventional wire attempts. *Clin Res Cardiol* **96**:489–496.

33. Baim DS, Braden G, Heuser R, *et al.* (2004) Utility of the Safe-Cross-guided radiofrequency total occlusion crossing system in chronic coronary total occlusions (results from the Guided Radio Frequency Energy Ablation of Total Occlusions Registry Study). *Am J Cardiol* **94**:853–858.

34. Garcia-Garcia HM, Tsuchida K, van Mieghem C, *et al.* (2007) Multi-slice computed tomography and magnetic navigation-initial experience of cutting edge new technology in the treatment of chronic total occlusions. *EuroIntervention* **3**:188–196.

35. Perin EC (2006) Stem cell therapy for cardiovascular disease. *Tex Heart Inst J* **33**:204–208.

36. Perin EC, Dohmann HF, Borojevic R, *et al.* (2003) Transendocardial, autologous bone marrow cell transplantation for severe, chronic ischemic heart failure. *Circulation* **107**:2294–2302.

37. Perin E, Silva G, Fernandes M, *et al.* (2007) First experience with remote left ventricular mapping and transendocardial cell injection with a novel integrated magnetic navigation-guided electro-mechanical mapping system. *EuroIntervention* **3**:142–148.

38. Pappone C, Augello G, Gugliotta F, & Santinelli V (2007) Robotic and magnetic navigation for atrial fibrillation ablation. How and why? *Expert Rev Med Devices* **4**:885–894.

39. Mediguide. MPS first in human MediGuide started its clinical trials in Regensburg University Hospital in Germany. http://www.mediguide.co.il/news/news.asp?newID=43&newsCatID=2.

40. Beyar R, Gruberg L, Deleanu D, *et al.* (2006) Remote-control percutaneous coronary interventions: concept, validation, and first-in-humans pilot clinical trial. *J Am Coll Cardiol* **47**:296–300.

43 Arterial Revascularization of Coronary Artery Disease

Hans-Joachim Schäfers & Takashi Kunihara

University Hospital of Saarland, Homburg, Germany

Historical background

Arterial conduits, i.e. the internal thoracic artery (ITA), have been used for construction of coronary artery bypass grafts (CABGs) since the early 1960s [1,2]. However, they were rapidly replaced by saphenous vein grafts (SVGs) because of the latter's availability, versatility, and ease of harvest [3], and SVGs were continuously used until the reports of Loop et al. [4] and Grondin et al. [5]. They demonstrated clearly superior mid-term patency and mid-term survival for the left ITA (LITA) grafted to the left anterior descending coronary artery (LAD) compared with SVGs.

Subsequently, the LITA anastomosed to the LAD became routine in coronary artery bypass surgery and remains the standard of care today. The superiority of the LITA also initiated increased interest in the use of the right ITA (RITA) or other arterial conduits for coronary artery bypass surgery. These included the radial artery, the right gastroepiploic artery (RGEA), and the inferior epigastric artery (IEA). All these arterial grafts have been extensively explored for ease of harvesting, propensity of complications at the donor site, diameter in relation to the target vessels, and propensity of spasm.

The radial artery was first used as a bypass graft by Carpentier et al. in 1971 to avoid the problems of graft degeneration seen in vein conduits [6]. The initial patency was disappointing, and its use was discontinued. It was only later that Acar and coworkers demonstrated acceptable long-term angiographic patency after some technical refinements, leading to a revival of this graft [7]. Subsequently, the radial artery became a standard option in CABG and the clinical results led to its use in many institutions. In the early 1990s, the IEA was investigated as an option for clinical use [8]. Although patency (80%) of the IEA was acceptable [9], it was suboptimal, and the IEA never gained widespread use because of its limited length, cumbersome preparation [10], and functional results.

Cardiovascular Interventions in Clinical Practice. Edited by Jürgen Haase, Hans-Joachim Schäfers, Horst Sievert and Ron Waksman. © 2010 Blackwell Publishing.

The use of the RGEA for CABG was first reported by Suma et al. [11] and Pym et al. [12] in 1987. In the subsequent years it was increasingly utilized as a third arterial graft, in addition to both ITAs (BITA), mostly in Japan [13–17]. *In situ* RGEA has been primarily used for grafting of the distal right coronary artery (RCA) or the distal circumflex territory because of its anatomical position. The relative invasiveness of the laparotomy required for its preparation and concerns over vasospasm made surgeons in most countries reluctant to use this graft routinely [18].

The superior results of the LITA grafted to the LAD prompted several groups to improve the clinical durability of a coronary bypass operation by using the RITA for a second coronary territory [19–25]. Initially, the results with BITA grafting were discussed controversially. Sergeant and colleagues found no superiority of BITA grafting over single ITA (SITA) with regard to survival [26] and return of angina [27]. Several other groups, however, demonstrated a clear advantage of BITA grafting over SITA with regard to survival and freedom from reintervention [21,28,29]. This evidence was further confirmed in 2004 with follow-up reaching up to 20 years [20]. The increased operative time required for the dissection of the second ITA and concern over an increased risk of sternal complications still makes many cardiac surgeons reluctant to use multiple arterial conduits in their routine practice. According to the Society of Thoracic Surgeon database, the BITA were used in only 2.8% of isolated CABG during 2002 and 2004 [30,31]. Only 15% of UK cardiac surgeons used more than one arterial graft for first time isolated multivessel CABG procedures between 1999 and 2000 [32].

Combining BITA with a third arterial graft for complete arterial revascularization was the final logical step. Initially, BITA was preferably combined with the RGEA, making complete arterial bypass surgery a long and cumbersome procedure reserved only for few young patients [33]. More widespread use of arterial revascularization became possible only after the introduction of aggressive use of sequential anastomoses by different groups in the mid-1980s [34–36]. Their approach allowed revascularization of three-vessel disease using composite BITA with sequential anastomoses. Tector et al. [37]

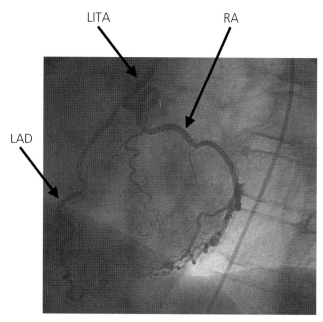

Figure 43.1 Angiographic finding of T-graft consisting of LITA and RA.

extended this technique, and complete arterial revascularization became one of the surgeon's options, both in routine coronary surgery and especially in patients with severe atherosclerosis of the ascending aorta. Owing to the apparent advantages of complete arterial revascularization, its proportion as part of coronary surgery is increasing over time both in the UK [38] and in other countries (Fig. 43.1).

Morphology and pathophysiology

The walls of the saphenous vein and arteries used as conduits in coronary artery surgery have similarities in their three-layered wall structure, but there are also major differences. The intima of the vein is thinner and more permeable than that of the artery, and thus more vulnerable to endothelial disruption by manipulation during harvesting. Endothelial damage, in turn, leads to accumulation of fibrin and platelet microemboli, increased neutrophil adherence, and a reduced production of tissue plasminogen activator [39–42]. Intimal fibrin and neutrophilic migration into intima and media can be observed in the early postoperative period [43,44]. Also, the extrinsic coagulation cascade mediated by tissue factor is activated by loss of endothelium. In addition, it has been demonstrated that harvesting of SVG attenuates thrombomodulin activity by up to 30% [45]. These prothrombotic conditions probably all contribute to the propensity for early SVG occlusion [46]. In addition, intimal thickening caused by phlebosclerosis exists before to grafting in up to 95% of SVG of patients over 60 years of age [47]. Variable degree of pre-existing medial fibrosis and smooth muscle cell hypertrophy may be responsible for differences of the compliance of implanted SVG [48,49].

In addition, there are marked differences in endothelial function between saphenous vein and arterial conduits. Production of prostacyclin and nitric oxide is less prominent in saphenous vein grafts than in the ITA, which may explain the differences in platelet aggregation [50,51]. The media of the saphenous vein contains less heparin sulfate than the internal thoracic as well as other arteries [40,46]. Endothelium of SVG stimulates medial smooth muscle cell contraction in response to thrombin, whereas thrombin-mediated vasorelaxation occurs in the internal thoracic artery [52–54]. Furthermore, sensitivity to vasoconstrictors such as endothelin-1 is higher in veins than in arteries. This tendency becomes more pronounced when the saphenous vein is denuded, most likely because the SVG wall is more dependent on vasa vasorum blood supply than the artery, and endothelin-1 is promoted by tissue hypoxia [41,46,55]. It has been pointed out also that the expression of endothelin-1 in SVG endothelium is increased and that the expression of nitric oxide synthase mRNA is decreased in the early phase of exposure of the SVG to arterial shear stress [56]. These characteristics of the saphenous vein make it more prone to platelet activation and susceptible to vasoconstriction, and may thus play a key role in postbypass remodeling of venous coronary bypass conduits.

Interestingly, there are also structural differences between different arterial conduits. The elastic laminae of the ITA consist of multilayer with multiple fenestrations, whereas those of the radial artery are monolayered with multiple fenestrations [57]. This may explain the higher susceptibility of the radial artery to atherosclerosis than the ITA. Clinically, however, this different tendency to develop atherosclerosis seems to have no impact on midterm patency [58], and two studies found no progress of atherosclerosis of the radial artery by intravascular ultrasound [59,60]. The media of the radial artery is approximately 1.7-fold thicker than that of the ITA. The former contains rich smooth muscle cells with several tight layers, whereas the latter consists of loose and unorganized myocytes [61,62]. Sympathetic and parasympathetic nerve fibers can be observed in the adventitia of the radial artery, but not in the adventitia of the ITA [63]. These differences may be responsible for the fact that spasm of the arterial graft is more frequently seen in the radial artery than the ITA [64–66].

Vasorelaxation of the radial artery and the ITA is considered to be similar both to endothelium-dependent (acetylcholine) and -independent (nitrates) agents, or via receptor- and nonreceptor-mediated (flow-mediated) mechanisms [67–72]. Arterial endothelium can produce relevant amounts of nitric oxide, and this is believed to be highest in the ITA [73,74]. On the other hand, it has been shown repeatedly that potency of vasoconstriction to various vasoconstrictors is more pronounced in the radial artery than in the ITA [30,71,75]. This is not only because of morphologic characteristics of the radial artery, but also because of different subtypes of receptors in their smooth muscle cells. Both arteries have a dominance of α-adrenoceptors ($\alpha_1 > \alpha_2$) with little β-adrenoceptor function. Endothelin-1-induced contraction, however, is endothelin A and B receptor-mediated in the ITA, whereas only endothelin A receptor-mediated contraction exists in the radial artery [76–78]. These structural and functional characteristics of the radial artery have been the basis for more aggressive antispasm prophylaxis with the use of the radial artery [75].

Prognosis of conduits

Vein grafts

Early bypass occlusion with a saphenous vein graft to a coronary artery occurs in up to 12% within the first month after CABG [46,79–81] and up to 15% in the first year [46,82,83]. Early SVG failure develops frequently in proximal or ostial lesions focally [83]. Between 1 and 6 years after CABG, SVGs become occluded at a rate of 1–2% per year and this increases to 4–5% per year in the following 5 years. Only 50–60% of SVGs are patent 10 years postoperatively, of which only half are angiographically intact [46,84–86]. As a clinical correlate, 20% of patients suffer from recurrent angina in the first year after CABG, using SVGs with an additional 4% per year in the following 5 years [46,87].

The underlying etiology of SVG disease consists of three distinct processes: thrombosis, intimal hyperplasia, and atherosclerosis [46,88]. Thrombosis occurs most frequently in the first month after saphenous vein grafting as a result of poor outflow, surgical error, or endothelial trauma during harvesting [39–42]. The prothrombotic characteristics of SVG as noted previously may accelerate thrombosis [46]. Neointimal hyperplasia occurs within the first year after implantation related to speculated mechanisms: increased cycling stretching by arterial pulse pressure [89], low flow velocity and low wall shear stress [90–92], turbulence of flow due to the mismatch in compliance [93], ischemic damage due to loss of vasa vasorum [94], and progression of preexisting medial fibrosis and smooth muscle cells hypertrophy [47]. Later, atherosclerosis with or without late thrombosis occurs. SVG atherosclerosis is characterized as more prominent and rapid accumulation of foam cells and inflammatory cells than common observation in the artery [40,46]. These findings resemble immune-mediated atherosclerosis, suggesting possible immunologic mechanisms in the pathogenesis of SVG atherosclerosis [95,96]. In addition, the nonphysiologic shear stress in conjunction with the characteristics of lipid metabolism may play an important role in the development of SVG atherosclerosis. Slower lipolysis, more rapid lipid uptake, and more active lipid synthesis are observed in SVG than in the artery [97–99].

The atherosclerotic degeneration of SVGs leads to repeat revascularization by surgery or percutaneous angioplasty in 4% of patients in the first 5 years after initial saphenous vein grafting, 19% until 10 years and 31% by 12 years [46,100]. Interestingly, both the interventional and the surgical approach carry an increased risk of periprocedural cardiac morbidity due to distal embolization from soft atherosclerotic debris found in the SVG [81,101–103]. Embolization is considered as an important factor in the increased risk of repeat bypass surgery [46,81]. Following percutaneous intervention of degenerated SVGs, a slow/no flow phenomenon is found in up to 15% and is associated with a high mortality and incidence of myocardial infarction [104,105], most likely a result of embolization of the soft atheromatous debris. In particular, SVGs older than 3 years are considered as being at high risk of this phenomenon [106]. Alternatives to prevent distal embolization (distal protection device, covered stent, or directional coronary atherectomy) have not been able to fully avoid this complication [88]. Spontaneous embolization of atheroma may also be the cause of the decrease in left ventricular function occasionally observed after conventional CABG [107]. Although percutaneous procedures can initially restore an adequate lumen of a degenerated SVG, they are associated with a higher frequency of restenosis/occlusion than similar procedures on the coronary arteries and lead to less freedom from recurrent angina. The process of SVG degeneration thus represents a therapeutic dilemma, and it most likely explains the limited therapeutic effect of conventional CABG in large trials [108,109].

Arterial grafts

Acute and long-term patency of arterial grafts is generally better than that of SVGs. It is, however, influenced by a number of factors, such as type of conduit (ITA, radial artery, GEA), territory or coronary vessel to be grafted, and the degree of stenosis in the native coronary artery. In addition, systemic factors may play a role, such as the presence of diabetes or renal failure. In general, atherosclerotic degeneration of arterial bypass grafts is very rare. On the contrary, arterial grafts remain viable and allow for remodeling over time to adapt to flow requirements, thus normalizing wall shear stress [110,111].

The ITA is currently the best studied conduit. While it generally has an excellent patency of >90% at 10 years it has been demonstrated that this is influenced by the degree of stenosis in the native coronary vessel (Fig. 43.2). Interestingly, the patency of the SVG is independent of the degree of coronary artery obstruction. One-year patency of the ITA is better than SVG patency for LAD, circumflex system, and also the posterior descending coronary artery (85–92%). ITA patency is actually worse than an SVG for grafts to the RCA (70–75%), if there is only a mild stenosis of that vessel. The influence of coronary artery stenosis diminishes over time, and 10-year patency of the ITA is superior to SVG with all degrees of coronary artery obstruction (Fig. 43.2) [85]. The reduced patency in the presence of less pronounced coronary artery stenosis has been attributed to spasm of arterial grafts when preserved resting blood flow in the native coronary leads to competing flow (Fig. 43.3).

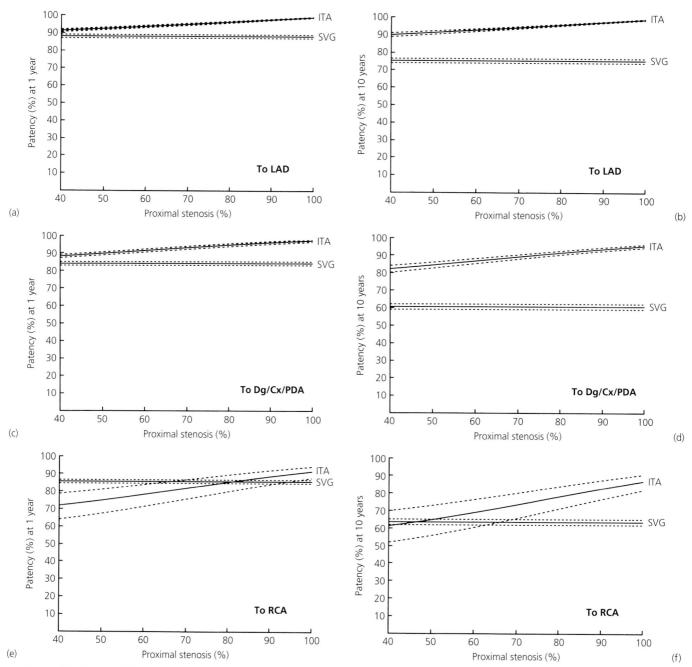

Figure 43.2 Patency of ITA versus SVG at 1 and 10 years analyzed by coronary territory and degree of stenosis in the native coronary artery. Reprint from Sabik *et al.* [85], with permission from Elsevier Science Inc.

Interestingly, the territory grafted by an artery seems to have an effect on arterial conduit patency, and this is consistent for all grafts. For the ITA, connection to the LAD diagonal system is associated with the best late patency followed by circumflex territory, and for both of them patency exceeds 90% after >5 years [112,113]. However, it is less than 90% when connected to RCA or distal circumflex arteries [114]. By contrast, the patency of the radial artery and the SVG seems less affected by the target vessel location [75,112,113].

Finally, there are differences between the different arterial conduits used. The LITA has the best patency (96–100%) in both the short and long term. Slightly inferior patency rates have been reported for the RITA, even though the reasons for its inferiority are not completely clear (Fig. 43.3). Excellent early (<0.5 year) patency rates have also been found for the radial artery (96–100%), which are similar to those of the ITA [75]. Midterm patency rates of the radial artery, however, vary between 83% and 95% and seem obviously inferior to

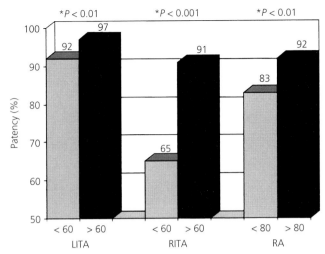

Figure 43.3 Influence of target vessel stenosis on graft patency. For LITA and RA, target vessel stenosis (criteria: 60% for LITA, 80% for RA) does not effect graft patency. Patency of RITA is greatly deteriorated when target vessel stenosis is less than 60%. Reprinted from Tatoulis *et al.* [113], with permission from Elsevier Science Inc.

those of the ITA (90–100%) but still superior to the SVG (63–92%) [75,115]. Although early patency of the RGEA grafts is excellent (97–98%) [13,14,116], late patency has been inferior to that of the ITA [117,118] and thus only similar to that of SVG [15,16]. In the latest report from Japan, the cumulative patency rate of the RGEA graft was only 66.5% at 10 years [13]. Any conclusions from this data have to be drawn carefully, as different factors interact in the endpoint of patency.

Competing flow and RCA territory in part explains the apparent inferiority of the RITA compared with the LITA, since the RITA is almost always anastomosed to the RCA. There may be additional factors related to the RITA, since its patency is somewhat inferior to that of the LITA, even when connected to branches of the left coronary system [113,119].

The radial artery is mostly grafted to non-LAD target vessels, and angiographies have been carried out usually only for symptomatic patients (3–47% of original grafts), thus not reflecting true patency [115]. Graft failure rates detected by symptom-directed angiography are approximately double of those by protocol-directed angiography [120]. A systematic angiographic study with follow-up of 92% of all conduits, regardless of symptoms, showed an 88% patency of the radial artery after 9 years, thus not significantly different from that of the ITA (96.3%) [60]. Two prospective, randomized, controlled trials specifically investigated the patency of the radial artery grafted to non-LAD target vessels with the RITA or the SVG [114,121–123]. One found superiority of radial artery patency (91.8%) over SVG patency (86.4%) at 1 year follow-up [121], whereas the second found no significant difference (radial artery: 87%, SVG: 94%) in older patients (age >70 years) at 5 years [123]. That study also found identical patency of

radial artery (95%) and RITA (100%) in young patients. Further investigations up to 10 years are awaited to draw a concrete conclusion.

Given the known effects of diabetes mellitus on endothelial function and life expectancy [28,124], it is not surprising that Sabik and colleagues identified diabetes as an independent predictor for late occlusion of both SVG and ITA [85]. Desai and associates [114] also found diabetes to be associated with SVG and radial artery occlusion at 1 year postoperatively. Buxton's group, however, failed to identify diabetes as a negative predictor of ITA patency [119]. On the other hand, the results of the Bypass Angioplasty Revascularization Investigation (BARI) randomized trial clearly showed that 10-year survival advantage of patients with diabetes mellitus receiving at least one arterial graft (64.3%) was significantly better than those receiving only vein grafts (39.4%) [125]. Thus, diabetes should not be a contraindication to the use of arterial grafts, but rather a reason for arterial revascularization [126].

Technical aspects

Choice of grafts

The choice of grafts used for the individual patient is influenced by the number of conduits required for complete revascularization, graft availability, and patient-related factors. The number of grafts required for complete revascularization depends on the number of territories to be supplied and the surgical strategy. The majority of patients referred for surgical revascularization suffer from triple-vessel coronary artery disease, and the second largest group will have stenosis of the left main coronary artery.

There is a considerable variation in revascularization strategies. Owing to concerns over limited bypass flow to more than one coronary artery, many surgeons still prefer one graft for each coronary branch to be connected. Two to five grafts will then be required for most revascularization procedures. Sequential anastomosing techniques can achieve the same extent of revascularization with fewer grafts. Dion [112] demonstrated identical patency of sequential anastomoses with an ITA compared with single ITAs. Sequential ITA anastomoses showed excellent patency rates of 95–96% to LAD and proximal circumflex system, but worse, 85% to the distal circumflex branches or distal RCA system [112]. These findings suggest that sequential grafting can be used safely for arterial conduits, maximizing the number of coronary arteries supplied by an arterial bypass. In addition, there are differences between *in situ* (connected to the subclavian artery, patency 96.3%) and free grafts (connected to aorta, patency 86.5%).

The T-graft technique carries the concept even further by anastomosing a second graft to the first graft, thus minimizing aortic manipulations and the length requirements for complete revascularization using only two grafts (Fig. 43.4). Thus the disadvantage of the free graft can be neutralized by connecting

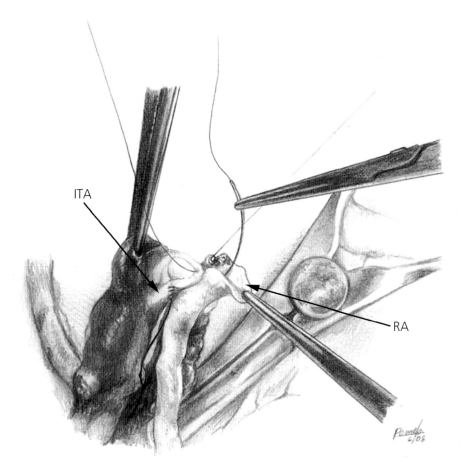

ITA

RA

Figure 43.4 Operating schema of
T-anastomosis between ITA and RA.

an ITA (e.g. RITA) to the LITA as T-graft. With this strategy the patency of RITA grafted to the RCA (93.5%) was similar to that to of the LAD and the circumflex artery (95.2% and 95.5%) [127]. In 2001, Tector and coworkers [128], who are the pioneers of this concept, published their results with BITA T-grafts in 897 patients, with a 5-year freedom from death of 86% and a freedom from reintervention rate of 94%. Similar data were published by Calafiore and associates [129]. Several retrospective studies [130–133] and one prospective randomized investigation [123], with a radial artery as second artery in T-grafts, showed similar mid-term survival benefit [134,135].

Off-pump CABG (OPCAB) surgery using composite arterial grafts can eliminate cannulation, cross-clamping, and side-biting of the aorta, and thus are indicated in selected candidates with a high risk of embolic stroke [136–138]. There are, however, still concerns that a composite arterial T-graft has less coronary flow reserve (CFR) than individual grafts in the early postoperative phase [139]. A CFR in T-grafts of less than 1.5 has been published if the T-graft was used only for left coronary system [139]. Our experience with T-graft that supplies all three coronary territories has shown a CFR of 1.8 early postoperatively, increasing up to 2.5 to 2.7 at 6 months postoperatively [140,141]. Recently further improvement of

CFR up to one year after CABG with a T-graft was found, similar to that using in situ BITA [142,143]. Thus, the T-graft configuration appears as a physiologically sound concept.

Today, the LITA continues to be the graft of primary choice because it is rarely affected by atherosclerosis, and its blood flow is almost always sufficient unless stenosis or occlusion of the left subclavian artery is present. The ideal second arterial conduit is probably the RITA because of its favorable vascular pathophysiology. There are, however, concerns regarding conduit length and an increased risk of deep sternal infection [144–148].

For many surgeons, including our group, the radial artery has emerged as the preferred second arterial conduit [123,130 –133]. When the radial artery is connected to the LITA, all coronary territories can be reached easily (Fig. 43.1). Harvesting of radial artery is simple, time-sparing, and rarely associated with complications [149,150]. In the presence of relevant chronic obstructive pulmonary disease (COPD) avoidance of RITA preparation minimizes postoperative pain, resulting in fewer pulmonary complications and avoiding the rare, but existing risk of phrenic nerve paralysis. The concern of spasm caused by competitive flow can be avoided by careful selection of target vessels with critical stenosis. A pathologic Allen's test, the presence of severe chronic renal insufficiency with need for dialysis access, severe peripheral vascular diseases including vasculitis or Raynaud's phenomenon, and the presence of carpal tunnel syndrome are considered as contraindications to radial artery harvesting [30]. It has been estimated that 5–12% of patients pose contraindications to radial artery harvesting due to pathological Allen's test, although this may include a fair amount of either false-positive or false-negative test results [151–153]. The presence of peripheral vascular disease or insulin-dependent diabetes is associated with an increased likelihood of radial artery atherosclerosis [119,154] resulting in stenosis (8.6%) or calcification (8.6%) [155]. The RGEA appears the last alternative as arterial graft and particularly important in patients undergoing redo CABG if other arterial conduits have already been used [156].

This approach may also be justified by two clinical studies from Italy that clarified similar mid-term clinical and angiographic results between the radial artery connected to the ascending aorta and the LITA [157,158]. Thus we have routinely been performing complete arterial revascularization using composite arterial grafts with an ITA/radial artery T-graft with regard to the balance between survival benefit and operative morbidity (Figs. 43.1 and 43.4) [159,160].

Pedicled or skeletonized

In the early days of coronary surgery the LITA was dissected without the accompanying veins and connective tissue, i.e. in a skeletonized fashion. Subsequently, the preparation with the surrounding tissue and structures became standard for its ease of dissection and somewhat less of a propensity to spasm. The advent of more extensive arterial grafting in CABG led to reassessment of the two techniques. Skeletonization of ITA was proposed by Sauvage in 1986 [34] and Keeley and associates in 1987 [161]. The apparent advantages of harvesting the ITA in skeletonized fashion are (1) increased conduit blood flow preventing hypoperfusion syndrome, (2) increased conduit length facilitating complete arterial revascularization, (3) reduced deep sternal wound infection by attenuating hypoperfusion of the sternum, and (4) reduced pain and sensory deficit. Possible concerns over skeletonization included compromise of the structural and functional integrity of the ITA resulting from mechanical damage to the vessel wall and loss of the vasa vasorum and draining vein. In fact, blood effusion in the adventitia and intraluminal microthrombus formation have been observed after skeletonization [162,163]. Several experimental and clinical studies revealed that skeletonization did not have detrimental effects on the structural and functional integrity of the ITA [163–168].

Some observational studies found superiority in blood flow of skeletonized ITAs compared with pedicled ITAs [169–172]. Skeletonized ITAs seem to have more vasodilation capacity after applying vasodilators than pedicled ITAs [172], a finding that is also confirmed by a randomized study [173]. Calafiore *et al.* [148] has already shown that significantly longer length in skeletonized LIMA than in pedicled LIMA both

before and after papaverine injection, thus enables significantly more sequential anastomoses, and total arterial myocardial revascularization. Two randomized studies have demonstrated that skeletonized technique in harvesting the ITA can reduce postoperative pain or dysesthesia [174,175].

Four randomized studies have confirmed that harvesting the ITA in skeletonized fashion is associated with less hypoperfusion of the sternum than by the pedicled technique [174,176–178]. Therefore, skeletonization of the ITA can reduce the incidence of deep sternal wound infection even when bilateral ITAs are harvested [148,179]. This beneficial effect is most evident in diabetic patients undergoing BITA revascularization [145–148]. As a consequence of the effects of skeletonization, BITA harvesting is not contraindicated, even for patients with diabetes, unless they are extremely obese. Indeed, since patients with diabetes who have more severe, diffuse, and distal disease potentially have most survival benefit from BITA, BITA should be aggressively used for them [144,147].

Pharmacological interventions

To prevent intraoperative arterial graft spasm, various vasodilators have been used such as phosphodiesterase inhibitors [180], including papaverine [159], calcium channel blockers [7], nitrates [67,68], phenoxybenzamine [181], and potassium channel openers [182]. However, to date no clinical studies have documented clinical benefits of calcium channel blockers or nitrates, even those of nifedipine that has a 31.6-fold more potent vasodilating effect than diltiazem [183–186]. In considering its use, one has to keep in mind that every pharmacologic intervention will have side-effects. The intraluminal use of papaverine carries the risk of endothelial injury because of its acidic pH [187]. Intravenous administration of calcium channel blockers is associated with hypotension and/or bradycardia [7]. Topical application of papaverine or nitroglycerin is relatively short-acting, whereas systemic infusion of nitroglycerin or phenoxybenzamine seems to be relatively long-acting [181,188–190].

Our routine approach

Our graft of first choice is the LITA, whenever the left coronary territory requires grafting, and second choice is the radial artery. The RITA is used only if the radial artery cannot be utilized because Allen's test is negative or calcifications are present. To increase length and facilitate sequential anastomoses, we employ a skeletonizing technique for all arterial grafts. Intraluminal application of papaverine (40 mg diluted with 20 mL of heparinized blood) has consistently prevented relevant spasm, and we have seen little need for postoperative spasmolytic treatment if the coronary anastomoses were intact. The mixture of papaverine with heparinized blood leads to a physiologic pH and avoids the problem of endothelial injury.

In the majority of patients we have employed the T-graft configuration without a negative impact on early morbidity or mortality (Figs. 43.1 and 43.4) [160]. We used to give calcium channel blockers topically to the radial artery but abandoned it and liberally leave it in warm condition (i.e. warm Ringer's lactate solution) after intraluminal injection of papaverine. Neither perioperative oral nor intravenous calcium channel blockers are given routinely in our practice. Only low doses of aspirin (100 mg/day) and clopidogrel (75 mg/day for 6–8 weeks) are given orally.

Indications for complete arterial revascularization

The indications for complete coronary revascularization are essentially those formulated in the current guidelines as for any coronary artery bypass operation [191]. Briefly, surgical revascularization carries a survival benefit in coronary multi-vessel disease and left main stem stenosis, particularly in the presence of impaired left ventricular function.

Owing to the superior durability of arterial bypass conduits, especially younger patient (<65 or <70 years of age) should benefit from complete arterial coronary revascularization [20,23,192]. Arterial revascularization may also be useful in older patients to decrease the risk of cerebrovascular complications of coronary surgery; it has also been beneficial in elderly patients (>70 years) by preventing recurrence of angina without increasing early postoperative risk [193]. OPCAB using the T-graft technique can completely eliminate aortic manipulations, even in triple-vessel coronary disease, and thus has the potential advantage of decreasing the likelihood of stroke in high-risk individuals [137,138,194].

Results

The superiority of CABG over percutaneous coronary interventional (PCI) treatment with regard to major adverse cardiac and cerebrovascular events (MACCEs) has been repeatedly demonstrated in multivessel coronary disease [195]. The latest meta-analysis with four randomized trials and a 5-year follow-up period demonstrated similar effectiveness between CABG and PCI with regard to death, stroke, and myocardial infarction, although CABG provided lower repeat revascularization rates [196]. However, bare metal stents were used for PCI in all four trials. The up-to-date results from currently on-going large scale randomized trials to compare CABG and PCI using drug-eluting stents (i.e. SYNTAX, Synergy between PCI with Taxus and Cardiac Surgery; CARDIA, Coronary Artery Revascularization in Diabetes) provided similar findings [197,198]. The SYNTAX study compared 1800 patients with three-vessel or left main coronary artery disease, whereas CARDIA investigated 510 patients with diabetes and coronary artery disease, except left main disease, who underwent CABG or PCI using drug-eluting stents. The studies found similar rates of death and myocardial infarction between the two groups at 1 year, although CABG was associated with lower repeat revascularization rates and higher stroke rates. The main question

remains whether and in whom complete arterial revascularization carries a benefit over conventional CABG with respect to survival and freedom from MACCE. As the concept of complete arterial coronary surgery is still relatively new, relevant information can be obtained from investigations looking at the effect of increasing the number of arterial grafts in CABG.

Survival: both versus single internal thoracic arteries

To date, there are no randomized clinical trials to comparing survival and freedom from MACCE of patients receiving BITA versus SITA. Using appropriate statistical strategies large observational studies have been thoroughly analyzed [19–25]. When BITA grafts are connected to the left side of the heart, clear survival benefits can be obtained [199]. This advantage and long-term patency are compromised if arteries are used as free grafts from the aorta (2-fold increased risk of graft failure compared with an *in situ* fashion) or to the RCA (83% vs. 90–95% in the left system at 82 months) [29,113,129,130,199,200]. Schmidt and coworkers [201] demonstrated superior survival of 93% at 9.6 years when the BITAs were connected to the left side of the heart (RITA–LAD plus LITA–circumflex), whereas survival fell by up to 70% when the RITA was anastomosed to the RCA system, in addition to LITA–LAD anastomosis. Endo and colleagues [23] reported that major adverse cardiac events (MACEs) were significantly reduced in BITA patients in a subgroup with an age below 71 years and an ejection fraction greater than 0.4. The Cleveland clinic experience clearly showed enhanced survival benefit of BITA in all generations regardless of left ventricular dysfunction or noncardiac risk factors, but it was maximal in younger patients (Fig. 43.5) [20].

Survival complete arterial revascularization

Numerous single-center publications, two recent randomized trials, and a large multicenter analysis ($n = 71\,470$) have shown that total arterial revascularization does not increase early postoperative morbidity or mortality [38,202–206]. Early mortality primarily depends on the risk profile of the patients, and arterial grafting has resulted in slightly lower but nonsignificant decrease in inhospital mortality compared with conventional CABG in some several studies [38,202–206]. A large multicenter analysis documented that total arterial revascularization provided lower observed inhospital mortality (2.04%) than predicted by the European System for Cardiac Operative Risk Evaluation (EuroScore; 2.31%), whereas standard CABG did not (3.00% vs. 2.98%, respectively) [38].

In addition, mid- to long-term survival has been good after arterial revascularization, with a 5-year survival of 91–96% [13,207,208] and freedom from cardiac death rate at 10 years of 87–94% [13,209,210]. In 1999, Tatoulis and Buxton [211] reported 5-year actual survival of 94% in 3220 patients who underwent complete arterial revascularization. Nine-year

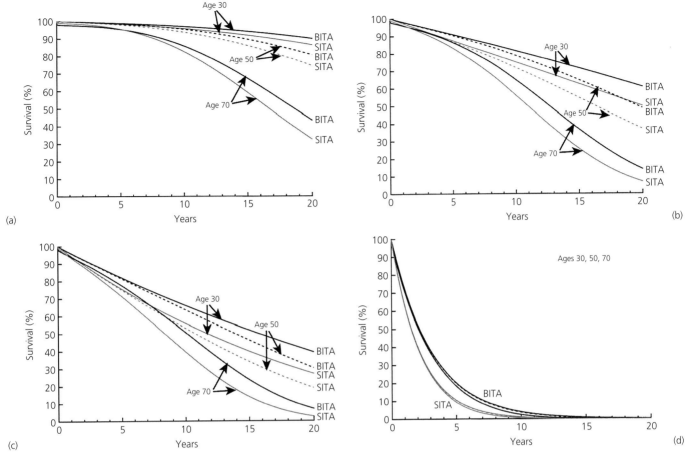

Figure 43.5 Enhanced survival benefit of BITA in all generations regardless of left ventricular dysfunction or noncardiac risk factors, but it was maximal in younger patients. (a) Patients with neither left ventricular dysfunction nor risk factors, (b) Patients with left ventricular dysfunction, (c) Patients with noncardiac risk factors, (d) Patients with both left ventricular dysfunction and noncardiac risk factors. Reprint from Lytle *et al.* [20], with permission from Elsevier Science Inc.

freedom from cardiac death among younger patients (mean age 56 years) further increased survival to 97.6% [212]. Calafiore and colleague reported that 42-month event-free survival was significantly better in total arterial revascularization (94%) than conventional CABG (86%) [213].

Despite these positive results there is still a controversial discussion regarding the value of an arterial graft for the RCA territory. Arterial bypass patency for this vessel has been lower than that of branches of the LCA [85,113,119]. Guru *et al.* [214] found no significant difference between CABG using two or three arterial grafts in terms of late death, repeat revascularization, and cardiac readmission. RGEA grafting to the RCA system—in combination with left-sided BITA grafting—has had no beneficial effect compared with SVG on mid-term survival and return of angina [33,202,215]. Furthermore, Pevni and associates [33] compared left-sided BITA with RCA grafting by free RITA, SVG, and RGEA, and without grafting, and reported similar absolute 6-year survival rates of 88%, 87%, 89.5%, and 85.5%, respectively, and return of angina rates of 10.8%, 6.3%, 10.6%, and 9.5%, respectively.

Freedom from clinical end points: major adverse cardiac events

While current data on survival after complete arterial revascularization is still limited, the evidence regarding MACE is more apparent. A prospective randomized study revealed significant superiority in 12-month freedom from cardiac events with complete arterial revascularization (96%) compared with conventional ones (67%) [204]. Long-term freedom from MACE after complete arterial revascularization has consistently been estimated at between 76% and 78% at 7–12 years after surgery [202,209,210,212]. As in patients receiving BITAs, this beneficial effect is especially increased in younger individuals. Twelve-year freedom form MACCE of patients younger than 65 years (82.6%) is 3.4-fold higher than that of patients over 65 years of age (65.8%) [210]. Also, the Toronto group found that patients receiving two or three arterial grafts had a significantly lower rate of cardiac readmission and MACEs compared with patients receiving only one arterial graft, which was confirmed by propensity-matched pair analysis [214].

By contrast, Sergeant and his group [216] found that the use of more than a single arterial graft provided no additional benefit in a population with unadjusted 1-month and 10-year freedom from infarction of 97% and 86%. Légaré and associates [205] documented that significant benefit of total arterial grafting on MACE was cancelled after risk adjustment. Thus, even though complete arterial revascularization appears as advantageous at this time, its effect on survival and freedom from MACE warrants further prospective, randomized investigations with large cohorts and long observation (>10 years).

Conclusion

Complete arterial revascularization of coronary artery disease has developed into a concept that can be applied on a routine basis without increasing morbidity or mortality. Using skeletonizing technique and economic use of conduits it can be applied to the majority of patients. It completely obviates the problem of SVG degeneration with all associated sequelae. Complete arterial revascularization should be considered as the primary option in CABG for younger patients (<70 years) and those at particularly high risk of embolic stroke from aortic atheroma.

References

1. Kolessov VI (1967) Mammary artery-coronary artery anastomosis as a method of treatment for angina pectoris. *J Thorac Cardiovasc Surg* **54**:535–544.

2. Spencer FC, Yong NK, & Prachuabmoh K (1964) Internal mammary-coronary artery anastomoses performed during cardiopulmonary bypass. *J Cardiovasc Surg (Torino)* **5**:292–297.

3. Favaloro RG (1968) Saphenous vein autograft replacement of severe segmental coronary artery occlusion: operative technique. *Ann Thorac Surg* **5**:334–339.

4. Loop FD, Lytle BW, Cosgrove DM, *et al.* (1986) Influence of the internal-mammary-artery graft on 10-year survival and other cardiac events. *N Engl J Med* **314**:1–6.

5. Grondin CM, Campeau L, Lesperance J, *et al.* (1984) Comparison of late changes in internal mammary artery and saphenous vein grafts in two consecutive series of patients 10 years after operation. *Circulation* **70**:I-208–212.

6. Carpentier A, Guermonprez JL, Deloche A, *et al.* (1973) The aorta-to-coronary radial artery bypass graft. A technique avoiding pathological changes in grafts. *Ann Thorac Surg* **16**:111–121.

7. Acar C, Jebara VA, Portoghese M, *et al.* (1992) Revival of the radial artery for coronary artery bypass grafting. *Ann Thorac Surg* **54**:652–659.

8. Perrault LP, Carrier M, Hebert Y, *et al.* (1993) Early experience with the inferior epigastric artery in coronary artery bypass grafting. A word of caution. *J Thorac Cardiovasc Surg* **106**:928–930.

9. Manapat AE, McCarthy PM, Lytle BW, *et al.* (1994) Gastroepiploic and inferior epigastric arteries for coronary artery bypass. Early results and evolving applications. *Circulation* **90**:II-144–147.

10. Buche M, Schoevaerdts JC, Louagie Y, *et al.* (1992) Use of the inferior epigastric artery for coronary bypass. *J Thorac Cardiovasc Surg* **103**:665–670.

11. Suma H, Fukumoto H, & Takeuchi A (1987) Coronary artery bypass grafting by utilizing in situ right gastroepiploic artery: basic study and clinical application. *Ann Thorac Surg* **44**:394–397.

12. Pym J, Brown PM, Charrette EJP, *et al.* (1987) Gastroepiploic coronary anastomosis: a viable alternative bypass graft. *J Thorac Cardiovasc Surg* **94**:256–259.

13. Suma H, Tanabe H, Takahashi A, *et al.* (2007) Twenty years experience with the gastroepiploic artery graft for CABG. *Circulation* **116**:I-188–191.

14. Kamiya H, Watanabe G, Takemura H, *et al.* (2004) Skeletonization of gastroepiploic artery graft in off-pump coronary artery bypass grafting: early clinical and angiographic assessment. *Ann Thorac Surg* **77**:2046–2050.

15. Hirose H, Amano A, Takanashi S, *et al.* (2002) Coronary artery bypass grafting using the gastroepiploic artery in 1 000 patients. *Ann Thorac Surg* **73**:1371–1379.

16. Hirose H, Amano A, & Takahashi A (2004) Bypass to the distal right coronary artery using in situ gastroepiploic artery. *J Card Surg* **19**:499–504.

17. Takahashi K, Daitoku K, Nakata S, *et al.* (2004) Early and mid-term outcome of anastomosis of gastroepiploic artery to left coronary artery. *Ann Thorac Surg* **78**:2033–2036.

18. Grandjean JG, Boonstra PW, den Heyer P, *et al.* (1994) Arterial revascularization with the right gastroepiploic artery and internal mammary arteries in 300 patients. *J Thorac Cardiovasc Surg* **107**:1309–1315.

19. Taggart DP, D'Amico R, & Altman DG (2001) Effect of arterial revascularisation on survival: a systematic review of studies comparing bilateral and single internal mammary arteries. *Lancet* **358**:870–875.

20. Lytle BW, Blackstone EH, Sabik JF, *et al.* (2004) The effect of bilateral internal thoracic artery grafting on survival during 20 postoperative years. *Ann Thorac Surg* **78**:2005–2012.

21. Buxton BF, Komeda M, Fuller JA, *et al.* (1998) Bilateral internal thoracic artery grafting may improve outcome of coronary artery surgery. Risk-adjusted survival. *Circulation* **98**:II-1–6.

22. Burfeind WR Jr, Glower DD, Wechsler AS, *et al.* (2004) Single versus multiple internal mammary artery grafting for coronary artery bypass: 15-year follow-up of a clinical practice trial. *Circulation* **110**:II-27–35.

23. Endo M, Nishida H, Tomizawa Y, *et al.* (2001) Benefit of bilateral over single internal mammary artery grafts for multiple coronary artery bypass grafting. *Circulation* **104**:2164–2170.

24. Rizzoli G, Schiavon L, & Bellini P (2002) Does the use of bilateral internal mammary artery (IMA) grafts provide incremental benefit relative to the use of a single IMA graft? A meta-analysis approach. *Eur J cardiothorac Surg* **22**:781–786.

25. Taggart DP (2002) Bilateral internal mammary artery grafting: are BIMA better? *Heart* **88**:7–9.

26. Sergeant P, Blackstone E, & Meyns B (1997) Validation and interdependence with patient-variables of the influence of procedural variables on early and late survival after CABG. K.U. Leuven Coronary Surgery Program. *Eur J Cardiothorac Surg* **12**:1–19.

27. Sergeant P, Blackstone E, & Meyns B (1998) Is return of angina after coronary artery bypass grafting immutable, can it be delayed, and is it important? *J Thorac Cardiovasc Surg* **116**:440–453.

28. Pick AW, Orszulak TA, Anderson BJ, *et al.* (1997) Single versus bilateral internal mammary artery grafts: 10-year outcome analysis. *Ann Thorac Surg* 1997;**64**:599–605.

29. Lytle BW, Blackstone EH, Loop FD, *et al.* (1999) Two internal thoracic artery grafts are better than one. *J Thorac Cardiovasc Surg* 1999;**117**:855–858.

30. Desai ND & Fremes SE (2007) Radial artery conduit for coronary revascularization: as good as an internal thoracic artery? *Curr Opin Cardiol* **22**:534–540.

31. Savage EB, Grab JD, O'Brien SM, *et al.* (2007) Use of both internal thoracic arteries in diabetic patients increases deep sternal wound infection. *Ann Thorac Surg* **83**:1002–1006.

32. Catarino PA, Black E, & Taggart DP (2002) Why do UK cardiac surgeons not perform their first choice operation for coronary artery bypass graft? *Heart* **88**:643–644.

33. Pevni D, Uretzky G, Yosef P, *et al.* (2005) Revascularization of the right coronary artery in bilateral internal thoracic artery grafting. *Ann Thorac Surg* **79**:564–569.

34. Sauvage LR, Wu HD, Kowalsky TE, *et al.* (1986) Healing basis and surgical techniques for complete revascularization of the left ventricle using only the internal mammary arteries. *Ann Thorac Surg* **42**:449–465.

35. Kamath ML, Matysik LS, Schmidt DH, *et al.* Sequential internal mammary artery grafts. Expanded utilization of an ideal conduit. *J Thorac Cardiovasc Surg* 1985;**89**:163–169.

36. Tector AJ, Schmahl TM, Canino VR, *et al.* (1984) The role of the sequential internal mammary artery graft in coronary surgery. *Circulation* **70**:I-222–225.

37. Tector AJ, Amundsen S, Schmahl TM, *et al.* (1994) Total revascularization with T grafts. *Ann Thorac Surg* **57**:33–38.

38. Baskett RJ, Cafferty FH, Powell SJ, *et al.* (2006) Total arterial revascularization is safe: multicenter ten-year analysis of 71 470 coronary procedures. *Ann Thorac Surg* **81**:1243–1248.

39. Simionescu M, Simionescu N, & Palade GE (1976) Segmental differentiations of cell junctions in the vascular endothelium. Arteries and veins. *J Cell Biol* **68**:705–723.

40. Cox JL, Chiasson DA, & Gotlieb AI (1991) Stranger in a strange land: the pathogenesis of saphenous vein graft stenosis with emphasis on structural and functional differences between veins and arteries. *Prog Cardiovasc Dis* **34**:45–68.

41. Verrier ED & Boyle EM Jr (1996) Endothelial cell injury in cardiovascular surgery. *Ann Thorac Surg* **62**:915–922.

42. Nachman RL & Silverstein R (1993) Hypercoagulable states. *Ann Intern Med* **119**:819–827.

43. Unni KK, Kottke BA, Titus JL, *et al.* (1974) Pathologic changes in aortocoronary saphenous vein grafts. *Am J Cardiol* **34**:526–532.

44. Bulkley BH & Hutchins GM (1977) Accelerated "atherosclerosis." A morphologic study of 97 saphenous vein coronary artery bypass grafts. *Circulation* **55**:163–169.

45. Cook JM, Cook CD, Marlar R, *et al.* (1991) Thrombomodulin activity on human saphenous vein grafts prepared for coronary artery bypass. *J Vasc Surg* **14**:147–151.

46. Motwani JG & Topol EJ (1998) Aortocoronary saphenous vein graft disease: pathogenesis, predisposition, and prevention. *Circulation* 97;916–931.

47. Stanley JC, Ernst CB, & Fry WJ (1973) Fate of 100 aortorenal vein grafts: characteristics of late graft expansion, aneurysmal dilatation, and stenosis. *Surgery* **74**:931–944.

48. Beard JD & Fairgrieve J (1986) Compliance changes in in-situ femoropopliteal bypass vein grafts. *Br J Surg* **73**:196–199.

49. Waddell WG, Vogelfanger IJ, Bosc M, *et al.* (1973) Changes in contractility, compliance and elasticity in experimental arterial vein-autografts. *Can J Surg* **16**:252–260.

50. Chaikhouni A, Crawford FA, Kochel PJ, *et al.* (1986) Human internal mammary artery produces more prostacyclin than saphenous vein. *J Thorac Cardiovasc Surg* **92**:88–91.

51. Angelini GD, Christie MI, Bryan AJ, *et al.* (1989) Surgical preparation impairs release of endothelium-derived relaxing factor from human saphenous vein. *Ann Thorac Surg* **48**:417–420.

52. Vanhoutte PM (1987) Endothelium-dependent contractions in arteries and veins. *Blood Vessels* **24**:141–144.

53. Lüscher TF, Diederich D, Siebenmann R, *et al.* (1988) Difference between endothelium-dependent relaxation in arterial and in venous coronary bypass grafts. *N Engl J Med* **319**:462–467.

54. Yang Z, Ruschitzka F, Rabelink TJ, *et al.* (1997) Different effects of thrombin receptor activation on endothelium and smooth muscle cells of human coronary bypass vessels. Implications for venous bypass graft failure. *Circulation* **95**:1870–1876.

55. Kourembanas S, Marsden PA, McQuillan LP, *et al.* (1991) Hypoxia induces endothelin gene expression and secretion in cultured human endothelium. *J Clin Invest* **88**:1054–1057.

56. Zhu ZG, Li HH, Zhang BR (1997) Expression of endothelin-1 and constitutional nitric oxide synthase messenger RNA in saphenous vein endothelial cells exposed to arterial flow shear stress. *Ann Thorac Surg* **64**:1333–1338.

57. Kaufer E, Factor SM, Frame R, *et al.* (1997) Pathology of the radial and internal thoracic arteries used as coronary artery bypass grafts. *Ann Thorac Surg* **63**:1118–1122.

58. Gaudino M, Tondi P, Serricchio M, *et al.* (2003) Atherosclerotic involvement of the radial artery in patients with coronary artery disease and its relation with midterm radial artery graft patency and endothelial function. *J Thorac Cardiovasc Surg* **126**:1968–1971.

59. Hagiwara H, Ito T, Kamiya H, *et al.* (2004) Mid-term structural change in the radial artery grafts after coronary artery bypass grafting. *Ann Thorac Surg* **77**:805–811.

60. Possati G, Gaudino M, Prati F, *et al.* (2003) Long-term results of the radial artery used for myocardial revascularization. *Circulation* **108**:1350–1354.

61. Van Son JA, Smedts F, Vincent JG, *et al.* (1990) Comparative anatomic studies of various arterial conduits for myocardial revascularization. *J Thorac Cardiovasc Surg* **99**:703–707.

62. Acar C, Jebara VA, Portoghese M, *et al.* (1991) Comparative anatomy and histology of the radial artery and the internal thoracic artery. Implication for coronary artery bypass. *Surg Radiol Anat* **13**:283–288.

63. Barry M, Touati G, Chardon K, *et al.* (2007) Histologic study of coronary, radial, ulnar, epigastric and internal thoracic arteries: application to coronary artery bypass grafts. *Surg Radiol Anat* **29**:297–302.

64. Lowe HC, Macina A, Torosoff M, *et al.* (2002) Recurrent spasm of radial artery graft mimicking fixed stenosis. *J Invasive Cardiol* **14**:640–641.

65. Merlo M, Terzi A, Tespili M, *et al.* (2003) Reversal of radial artery "string sign" at 6 months follow-up. *Eur J Cardiothorac Surg* **23**:432–434.

66. Kulkarni NM & Thomas MR (1999) Severe spasm of a radial artery coronary bypass graft during coronary intervention. *Catheter Cardiovasc Interv* **47**:331–335.

67. Wei W, Floten HS, & He GW (2002) Interaction between vasodilators and vasopressin in internal mammary artery and clinical significance. *Ann Thorac Surg* **73**:516–522.

68. Wei W, Chen ZW, Yang Q, *et al.* (2007) Vasorelaxation induced by vascular endothelial growth factor in the human internal mammary artery and radial artery. *Vascul Pharmacol* **46**:253–259.

69. Gaudino M, Glieca F, Trani C, *et al.* (2000) Midterm endothelial function and remodeling of radial artery grafts anastomosed to the aorta. *J Thorac Cardiovasc Surg* **120**:298–301.

70. Al-Bustami MH, Amrani M, Chester AH, *et al.* (2002) In vivo early and mid-term flow-mediated endothelial function of the radial artery used as a coronary bypass graft. *J Am Coll Cardiol* **39**:573–577.

71. He GW & Yang CQ (1997) Radial artery has higher receptor-mediated contractility but similar endothelial function compared with mammary artery. *Ann Thorac Surg* **63**:1346–1352.

72. Wei W, Chen ZW, Yang Q, *et al.* (2007) Vasorelaxation induced by vascular endothelial growth factor in the human internal mammary artery and radial artery. *Casvul Pharmacol* **46**:253–259.

73. He GW & Liu ZG (2001) Comparison of nitric oxide release and endothelium-derived hyperpolarizing factor-mediated hyperpolarization between human radial and internal mammary arteries. *Circulation* **104**:I-344–349.

74. Tadjkarimi S, O'Neil GS, Luu TN, *et al.* (1992) Comparison of cyclic GMP in human internal mammary artery and saphenous vein: implications for coronary artery bypass graft patency. *Cardiovasc Res* **26**:297–300.

75. Manabe S & Sunamori M (2006) Radial artery graft for coronary artery bypass surgery: biological characteristics and clinical outcome. *J Card Surg* **21**:102–114.

76. He GW & Yang CQ (1998) Characteristics of adrenoceptors in the human radial artery: clinical implications. *J Thorac Cardiovasc Surg* **115**:1136–1141.

77. Liu JJ, Chen JR, Buxton BF (1996) Unique response of human arteries to endothelin B receptor agonist and antagonist. *Clin Sci* **90**:91–96.

78. He GW & Yang CQ (1995) Comparison among arterial grafts and coronary artery: an attempt at functional classification. *J Thorac Cardiovasc Surg* **109**:707–715.

79. Goldman S, Copeland J, Moritz T, *et al.* (1988) Improvement in early saphenous vein graft patency after coronary artery bypass surgery with antiplatelet therapy: results of a Veterans Administration Cooperative Study. *Circulation* **77**:1324–1332.

80. Bourassa MG (1991) Fate of venous grafts: the past, the present and the future. *J Am Coll Cardiol* **5**:1081–1083.

81. Fitzgibbon GM, Kafka HP, Leach AJ, *et al.* (1996) Coronary bypass graft fate and patient outcome: angiographic follow-up of 5 065 grafts related to survival and reoperation in 1 388 patients during 25 years. *J Am Coll Cardiol* **28**:616–626.

82. Perrault LP, Jeanmart H, Bilodeau L, *et al.* (2004) Early quantitative coronary angiography of saphenous vein grafts for coronary artery bypass grafting harvested by means of open versus endoscopic saphenectomy: a prospective randomized trial. *J Thorac Cardiovasc Surg* **127**:1402–1407.

83. Caños DA, Mintz GS, Berzingi CO, *et al.* (2004) Clinical, angiographic, and intravascular ultrasound characteristics of early saphenous vein graft failure. *J Am Coll Cardiol* **44**:53–56.

84. Sabik JF & Blackstone EH (2008) Coronary artery bypass graft patency and competitive flow. *JACC* **51**:126–128.

85. Sabik JF 3rd, Lytle BW, Blackstone EH, *et al.* (2005) Comparison of saphenous vein and internal thoracic artery graft patency by coronary system. *Ann Thorac Surg* **79**:544–551.

86. Bourassa MG, Fisher LD, Campeau L, *et al.* (1985) Long-term fate of bypass grafts: the Coronary Artery Surgery Study (CASS) and Montreal Heart Institute experiences. *Circulation* **72**:V-71–78.

87. Cameron AA, Davis KB, & Rogers WJ (1995) Recurrence of angina after coronary artery bypass surgery: predictors and prognosis (CASS Registry). *J Am Coll Cardiol* **4**:895–899.

88. Peykar S, Angiolillo DJ, Bass TA, *et al.* (2004) Saphenous vein graft disease. *Minerva Cardioangiol* **52**:379–390.

89. Boerboom LE, Olinger GE, & Tie-Zhu L, *et al.* (1990) Histologic, morphometric and biochemical evolution of vein bypass grafts in a nonhuman primate model. III. Long-term changes and their modification by platelet inhibition with aspirin and dipyridamole. *J Thorac Cardiovasc Surg* **99**:426–432.

90. Allaire E & Clowes AW (1997) Endothelial cell injury in cardiovascular surgery: the intimal hyperplastic response. *Ann Thorac Surg* **63**:582–591.

91. Grondin CM, Lepage G, Castonguay YR, *et al.* (1971) Aortocoronary bypass graft: initial blood flow through the graft, and early postoperative patency. *Circulation* **44**:815–819.

92. LoGerfo FW, Soncrent T, & Tell T (1979) Boundary layer separation in models of side-to-end arterial anastomoses. *Arch Surg* **114**:1369–1373.

93. Clark RE, Apostoulou S, & Kardos JL (1976) Mismatch of mechanical properties as a cause of arterial prosthesis thrombosis. *Surg Forum* **27**:208–210.

94. Karayannacos PE, Hostetler JR, Bond MG, *et al.* (1978) Late failure in vein grafts: mediating factors in subendothelial fibromuscular hyperplasia. *Ann Surg* **187**:183–188.

95. Ratliff NB & Myles JL (1989) Rapidly progressive atherosclerosis in aortocoronary saphenous vein grafts: possible immune-mediated disease. *Arch Pathol Lab Med* **113**:772–776.

96. Brody JI, Pickering NJ, & Fink JB (1989) Immunocytochemical features of obstructed saphenous vein coronary artery bypass grafts. *J Clin Pathol* **42**:477–482.

97. Larson RM, Hagen P-O, & Fuchs JCA (1974) Lipid biosynthesis in arteries, veins, and venous grafts. *Circulation* **50**:III-139.

98. Shafi S, Palinski W, & Born GVR (1987) Comparison of uptake and degradation of low density lipoproteins by arteries and veins of rabbits. *Atherosclerosis* **66**:131–138.

99. Blankenhorn DH, Nessim SA, Johnson RL, *et al.* (1987) Beneficial effects of combined colestipolniacin therapy on coronary atherosclerosis and coronary venous bypass grafts. *JAMA* **257**:3233–3240.

100. Weintraub WS, Jones EL, Craver JM, *et al.* (1994) Frequency of repeat coronary bypass or coronary angioplasty after coronary artery bypass surgery using saphenous venous grafts. *Am J Cardiol* **73**:103–112.

101. Loop FD, Lytle BW, Cosgrove DM, *et al.* (1990) Reoperation for coronary atherosclerosis: changing practice in 2509 consecutive patients. *Ann Surg* **212**:378–386.

102. Cameron A, Kemp HG Jr, & Green GE (1988) Reoperation for coronary artery disease: 10 years of clinical follow-up. *Circulation* **78**:I-158–162.

103. Lefkovits J, Holmes DR, Califf RM, *et al.* (1995) Predictors and sequelae of distal embolization during saphenous vein graft

intervention from the CAVEAT-II trial: Coronary Angioplasty Versus Excisional Atherectomy Trial. *Circulation* **92**:734–740.

104. Abbo KM, Dooris M, Glazier S, *et al.* (1995) Features and outcome of no-reflow after percutaneous coronary intervention. *Am J Cardiol* **75**:778–782.

105. Kaplan BM, Benzuly KH, Kinn JW, *et al.* (1996) Treatment of no-reflow in degenerated saphenous vein graft interventions: comparison of intracoronary verapamil and nitroglycerin. *Cathet Cardiovasc Diagn* **39**:113–118.

106. Sdringola S, Assali AR, Ghani M, *et al.* (2001) Risk assessment of slow or no-reflow phenomenon in aortocoronary vein graft percutaneous intervention. *Catheter Cardiovasc Interv* **54**:318–324.

107. Keon WJ, Heggtveit HA, & Leduc J (1982) Perioperative myocardial infarction caused by atheroembolism. *J Thorac Cardiovasc Surg* **84**:849–855.

108. Kurbaan AS, Bowker TJ, Ilsley CD, *et al.* (2001) On behalf of the CABRI Investigators (Coronary Angioplasty versus Bypass Revascularization Investigation). Difference in the mortality of the CABRI diabetic and nondiabetic populations and its relation to coronary artery disease and the revascularization mode. *Am J Cardiol* **87**:947–950.

109. Henderson RA, Pocock SJ, Sharp SJ, *et al.* (1998) Long-term results of RITA-1 trial: clinical and cost comparisons of coronary angioplasty and coronary-artery bypass grafting. Randomised Intervention Treatment of Angina. *Lancet* **352**:1419–1425.

110. Fukui S, Fukuda H, Toda K, *et al.* (2007) Remodeling of the radial artery anastomosed to the internal thoracic artery as a composite straight graft. *J Thorac Cardiovasc Surg* **134**:1136–1142.

111. Girerd X, London G, Boutouyrie P, *et al.* (1996) Remodeling of the radial artery in response to a chronic increase in shear stress. *Hypertension* **27**:799–803.

112. Dion R, Glineur D, Derouck D, *et al.* (2000) Long-term clinical and angiographic follow-up of sequential internal thoracic artery grafting. *Eur J Cardiothorac Surg* **17**:407–414.

113. Tatoulis J, Buxton BF, & Fuller JA (2004) Patencies of 2127 arterial to coronary conduits over 15 years. *Ann Thorac Surg* **77**:93–101.

114. Desai ND, Naylor CD, Kiss A, *et al.* (2007) Radial Artery Patency Study Investigators. Impact of patient and target-vessel characteristics on arterial and venous bypass graft patency: insight from a randomized trial. *Circulation* **115**:684–691.

115. Mussa S, Choudhary BP, & Taggart DP (2005) Radial artery conduits for coronary artery bypass grafting: current perspective. *J Thorac Cardiovasc Surg* **129**:250–253.

116. Jegaden O, Eker A, Montagna P, *et al.* (1995) Technical aspects and late functional results of gastroepiploic bypass grafting (400 cases). *Eur J Cardiothorac Surg* **9**:575–580.

117. Suma H, Isomura T, Horii T, *et al.* (2000) Late angiographic result of using the right gastroepiploic artery as a graft. *J Thorac Cardiovasc Surg* **120**:496–498.

118. Voutilainen S, Verkkala K, Jarvinen A, *et al.* (1996) Angiographic 5-year follow-up study of right gastroepiploic artery grafts. *Ann Thorac Surg* **62**:501–505.

119. Shah PJ, Durairaj M, Gordon I, *et al.* (2004) Factors affecting patency of internal thoracic artery graft: clinical and angiographic study in 1434 symptomatic patients operated between 1982 and 2002. *Eur J Cardiothorac Surg* **26**:118–124.

120. Buxton BF, Durairaj M, Hare DL, *et al.* (2005) Do angiographic results from symptom-directed studies reflect true graft patency? *Ann Thorac Surg* **80**:896–900.

121. Desai ND, Cohen EA, Naylor CD, *et al.* (2004) Radial Artery Patency Study Investigators. A randomized comparison of radial-artery and saphenous-vein coronary bypass grafts. *N Engl J Med* **351**:2302–2309.

122. Hayward PA & Buxton BF (2007) Contemporary coronary graft patency: 5-year observational data from a randomized trial of conduits. *Ann Thorac Surg* **84**:795–799.

123. Buxton BF, Raman JS, Ruengsakulrach P, *et al.* (2003) Radial artery patency and clinical outcomes: five-year interim results of a randomized trial. *J Thorac Cardiovasc Surg* **125**:1363–1371.

124. Cho KR, Kim JS, Choi JS, *et al.* (2006) Serial angiographic follow-up of grafts one year and five years after coronary artery bypass surgery. *Eur J Cardiothorac Surg* **29**:511–516.

125. BARI Investigators (2007) The final 10-year follow-up results from the BARI randomized trial. *J Am Coll Cardiol* **49**:1600–1606.

126. Wendler O, Hennen B, Markwirth T, *et al.* (2001) Complete arterial revascularization in the diabetic patient—early postoperative results. *Thorac Cardiovasc Surg* **49**:5–9.

127. Dion R, Etienne PY, Verhelst R, *et al.* (1993) Bilateral mammary grafting. Clinical, functional and angiographic assessment in 400 consecutive patients. *Eur J Cardiothorac Surg* **7**:287–293.

128. Tector AJ, McDonald ML, Kress DC, *et al.* (2001) Purely internal thoracic artery grafts: outcomes. *Ann Thorac Surg* **72**:450–455.

129. Calafiore AM, Contini M, Vitolla G, *et al.* (2000) Bilateral internal thoracic artery grafting: long-term clinical and angiographic results of in situ versus Y grafts. *J Thorac Cardiovasc Surg* **120**:990–996.

130. Calafiore AM, Di Mauro M, D'Alessandro S, *et al.* (2002) Revascularization of the lateral wall: long-term angiographic and clinical results of radial artery versus right internal thoracic artery grafting. *J Thorac Cardiovasc Surg* **123**:225–231.

131. Lemma M, Gelpi G, Mangini A, *et al.* (2001) Myocardial revascularization with multiple arterial grafts: comparison between the radial artery and the right internal thoracic artery. *Ann Thorac Surg* **71**:1969–1973.

132. Caputo M, Reeves B, Marchetto G, *et al.* (2003) Radial versus right internal thoracic artery as a second arterial conduit for coronary surgery: early and midterm outcomes. *J Thorac Cardiovasc Surg* **126**:39–47.

133. Borger MA, Cohen G, Buth KJ, *et al.* (1998) Multiple arterial grafts. Radial versus right internal thoracic arteries. *Circulation* **98**:II-7–13.

134. Royse AG, Royse CF, & Raman JS (1999) Exclusive Y graft operation for multivessel coronary revascularization. *Ann Thorac Surg* **68**:1612–1618.

135. Barner HB, Sundt TM 3rd, Bailey M, *et al.* (2001) Midterm results of complete arterial revascularization in more than 1000 patients using an internal thoracic artery/radial artery T graft. *Ann Surg* **234**:447–452.

136. Taggart DP & Westaby S (2001) Neurological and cognitive disorders after coronary artery bypass grafting. *Curr Opin Cardiol* **16**:271–276.

137. Kim KB, Cho KR, Chang WI, *et al.* (2002) Bilateral skeletonized internal thoracic artery graftings in off-pump coronary artery bypass: early result of Y versus in situ grafts. *Ann Thorac Surg* **74**:S1371–1376.

138. Lev-Ran O, Braunstein R, Sharony R, *et al.* (2005) No-touch aorta off-pump coronary surgery: the effect on stroke. *J Thorac Cardiovasc Surg* **129**:307–313.

139. Sakaguchi G, Tadamura E, Ohnaka M, *et al.* (2002) Composite arterial Y graft has less coronary flow reserve than independent grafts. *Ann Thorac Surg* **74**:493–496.

140. Wendler O, Hennen B, Markwirth T, *et al.* (1999) T grafts with the right internal thoracic artery to left internal thoracic artery versus the left internal thoracic artery and radial artery: flow dynamics in the internal thoracic artery main stem. *J Thorac Cardiovasc Surg* **118**:841–8.

141. Markwirth T, Hennen B, Scheller B, *et al.* (2001) Flow wire measurements after complete arterial coronary revascularization with T-grafts. *Ann Thorac Surg* **71**:788–793.

142. Bonacchi M, Prifti E, Maiani M, *et al.* (2006) Perioperative and clinical-angiographic late outcome of total arterial myocardial revascularization according to different composite original graft techniques. *Heart Vessels* **21**:69–77.

143. Cho KR, Hwang HY, Kang WJ, *et al.* (2007) Progressive improvement of myocardial perfusion after off-pump revascularization with bilateral internal thoracic arteries: comparison of early versus 1-year postoperative myocardial single photon emission computed tomography. *J Thorac Cardiovasc Surg* **133**:52–57.

144. Stevens LM, Carrier M, Perrault LP, *et al.* (2005) Influence of diabetes and bilateral internal thoracic artery grafts on long-term outcome for multivessel coronary artery bypass grafting. *Eur J Cardiothorac Surg* **27**:281–288.

145. Hirose H, Amano A, Takanashi S, *et al.* (2003) Skeletonized bilateral internal mammary artery grafting for patients with diabetes. *Interact Cardiovasc Thorac Surg* **2**:287–292.

146. Peterson MD, Borger MA, Rao V, *et al.* (2003) Skeletonization of bilateral internal thoracic artery grafts lowers the risk of sternal infection in patients with diabetes. *J Thorac Cardiovasc Surg* **126**:1314–1319.

147. Matsa M, Paz Y, Gurevitch J, *et al.* (2001) Bilateral skeletonized internal thoracic artery grafts in patients with diabetes mellitus. *J Thorac Cardiovasc Surg* **121**:668–674.

148. Calafiore AM, Vitolla G, Iaco AL, *et al.* (1999) Bilateral internal mammary artery grafting: midterm results of pedicled versus skeletonized conduits. *Ann Thorac Surg* **67**:1637–1642.

149. Meharwal ZS & Trehan N (2001) Functional status of the hand after radial artery harvesting: results in 3977 cases. *Ann Thorac Surg* **72**:1557–1561.

150. Budillon AM, Nicolini F, Agostinelli A, *et al.* (2003) Complications after radial artery harvesting for coronary artery bypass grafting: our experience. *Surgery* **133**:283–287.

151. Barner HB (2002) Why total arterial revascularization? *Int J Angiol* **11**:129–131.

152. Abu-Omar Y, Mussa S, Anastasiadis K, *et al.* (2004) Duplex ultrasonography predicts safety of radial artery harvest in the presence of an abnormal Allen test. *Ann Thorac Surg* **77**:116–119.

153. Hirai M & Kawai S (1980) False positive and negative results in Allen test. *J Cardiovasc Surg* **21**:353–360.

154. Ruengsakulrach P, Brooks M, Sinclair R, *et al.* (2001) Prevalence and prediction of calcification and plaques in radial artery grafts by ultrasound. *J Thorac Cardiovasc Surg* **122**:398–399.

155. Oshima A, Takeshita S, Kozuma K, *et al.* (2005) Intravascular ultrasound analysis of the radial artery for coronary artery bypass grafting. *Ann Thorac Surg* **79**:99–103.

156. Takahashi K, Minakawa M, Kondo N, *et al.* (2002) Coronary artery bypass surgery by the transdiaphragmatic approach. *Ann Thorac Surg* **74**:700–703.

157. Iacò AL, Teodori G, Di Giammarco G, *et al.* (2001) Radial artery for myocardial revascularization: long-term clinical and angiographic results. *Ann Thorac Surg* **72**:464–468.

158. Lemma M, Mangini A, Gelpi G, *et al.* (2004) Is it better to use the radial artery as a composite graft? Clinical and angiographic results of aorto-coronary versus Y-graft. *Eur J Cardiothorac Surg* **26**:110–117.

159. Wendler O, Tscholl D, Huang Q, *et al.* (1999) Free flow capacity of skeletonized versus pedicled internal thoracic artery grafts in coronary artery bypass grafts. *Eur J Cardiothorac Surg* **15**:247–250.

160. Wendler O, Hennen B, Demertzis S, *et al.* (2000) Complete arterial revascularization in multivessel coronary artery disease with 2 conduits (skeletonized grafts and T grafts). *Circulation* **102**:III-79–83.

161. Keeley S (1987) The skeletonized internal mammary artery. *Ann Thorac Surg* **44**:324–325.

162. Noera G, Pensa P, Lodi R, *et al.* (1993) Influence of different harvesting techniques on the arterial wall of the internal mammary artery graft: microscopic analysis. *Thorac Cardiovasc Surg* **41**:16–20.

163. Gaudino M, Toesca A, Nori SL, *et al.* (1999) Effect of skeletonization of the internal thoracic artery on vessel wall integrity. *Ann Thorac Surg* **68**:1623–1627.

164. Ueda T, Taniguchi S, Kawata T, *et al.* (2003) Does skeletonization compromise the integrity of internal thoracic artery grafts? *Ann Thorac Surg* **75**:1429–1433.

165. Sasajima T, Wu MH, Shi Q, *et al.* (1998) Effect of skeletonizing dissection on the internal thoracic artery. *Ann Thorac Surg* **65**:1009–1013.

166. Yoshikai M, Ito T, Kamohara K, *et al.* (2004) Endothelial integrity of ultrasonically skeletonized internal thoracic artery: morphological analysis with scanning electron microscopy. *Eur J Cardiothorac Surg* **25**:208–211.

167. Higami T, Yamashita T, Nohara H, *et al.* (2001) Early results of coronary grafting using ultrasonically skeletonized internal thoracic arteries. *Ann Thorac Surg* **71**:1224–1228.

168. Gaudino M, Trani C, Glieca F, *et al.* (2003) Early vasoreactive profile of skeletonized versus pedicled internal thoracic artery grafts. *J Thorac Cardiovasc Surg* **125**:638–641.

169. Takami Y & Ina H (2002) Effects of skeletonization on intra-operative flow and anastomosis diameter of internal thoracic arteries in coronary artery bypass grafting. *Ann Thorac Surg* **73**:1441–1445.

170. Choi JB & Lee SY (1996) Skeletonized and pedicled internal thoracic artery grafts: effect on free flow during bypass. *Ann Thorac Surg* **61**:909–913.

171. Wendler O, Tscholl D, Huang Q, *et al.* (1999) Free flow capacity of skeletonized versus pedicled internal thoracic artery grafts in coronary artery bypass grafts. *Eur J Cardiothorac Surg* **15**:247–250.

172. Deja MA, Wos S, Golba KS, *et al.* (1999) Intraoperative and laboratory evaluation of skeletonized versus pedicled internal thoracic artery. *Ann Thorac Surg* **68**:2164–2168.

173. Castro GP, Dussin LH, Wender OB, *et al.* (2005) Comparative analysis of the flows of left internal thoracic artery grafts

dissected in the pedicled versus skeletonized manner for myocardial revascularization surgery. *Arq Bras Cardiol* **84**:261–266.

174. Boodhwani M, Lam BK, Nathan HJ, *et al.* (2006) Skeletonized internal thoracic artery harvest reduces pain and dysesthesia and improves sternal perfusion after coronary artery bypass surgery: a randomized, double-blinded, within-patient comparison. *Circulation* **114**:766–773.

175. Wimmer-Greinecker G, Yosseef-Hakimi M, Rinne T, *et al.* (1999) Effect of internal thoracic artery preparation on blood loss, lung function, and pain. *Ann Thorac Surg* **67**:1078–1082.

176. Cohen AJ, Lockman J, Lorberboym M, *et al.* (1999) Assessment of sternal vascularity with single photon emission tomography after harvesting of the internal thoracic artery. *J Thorac Cardiovasc Surg* **118**:496–502.

177. Kamiya H, Akhyari P, Martens A, *et al.* (2008) Sternal microcirculation after skeletonized versus pedicled harvesting of the internal thoracic artery: a randomized study. *J Thorac Cardiovasc Surg* **135**:32–37.

178. Lorberboym M, Medalion B, Bder O, *et al.* (2002) 99mTc-MDP bone SPECT for the evaluation of sternal ischaemia following internal mammary artery dissection. *Nucl Med Commun* **23**:47–52.

179. De Paulis R, de Notaris S, Scaffa R, *et al.* (2005) The effect of bilateral internal thoracic artery harvesting on superficial and deep sternal infection: the role of skeletonization. *J Thorac Cardiovasc Surg* **129**:536–543.

180. Na S, Oh YJ, Shim YH, *et al.* (2006) Effects of milrinone on blood flow of the Y-graft composed with the radial and the internal thoracic artery in patients with coronary artery disease. *Eur J Cardiothorac Surg* **30**:324–328.

181. Taggart DP, Dipp M, Mussa S, *et al.* (2000) Phenoxybenzamine prevents spasm in radial artery conduits for coronary artery bypass grafting. *J Thorac Cardiovasc Surg* **120**:815–817.

182. Sadaba JR, Mathew K, Munsch CM, *et al.* (2000) Vasorelaxant properties of nicorandil on human radial artery. *Eur J Cardiothorac Surg* **17**:319–324.

183. Kalus JS & Lober CA (2001) Calcium-channel antagonists and nitrates in coronary artery bypass patients receiving radial artery grafts. *Ann Pharmacother* **35**:631–635.

184. Patel A, Asopa S, & Dunning J (2006) Should patients receiving a radial artery conduit have post-operative calcium channel blockers? *Interact Cardiovasc Thorac Surg* **5**:251–257.

185. He GW & Yang CQ (2000) Comparative study on calcium channel antagonists in the human radial artery: clinical implications. *J Thorac Cardiovasc Surg* **119**:94–100.

186. Arena G & Abbate M (2000) Is calcium antagonist administration necessary after aortocoronary bypass with the radial artery? *Ital Heart J Suppl.* **1**:256–258.

187. Gao YJ, Yang H, Teoh K, *et al.* (2003) Detrimental effects of papaverine on the human internal thoracic artery. *J Thorac Cardiovasc Surg* **126**:179–185.

188. He G-W & Yang C-Q (1996) Use of verapamil and nitroglycerin solution in preparation of radial artery for coronary grafting. *Ann Thorac Surg* **61**:610–614.

189. Schulz E, Tsilimingas N, Rinze R, *et al.* (2002) Functional and biochemical analysis of endothelial (dys)function and NO/cGMP signaling in human blood vessels with and without nitroglycerin pretreatment. *Circulation* **105**:1170–1175.

190. Velez DA, Morris CD, Muraki S, *et al.* (2001) Brief pretreatment of radial artery conduits with phenoxybenzamine prevents vasoconstriction long term. *Ann Thorac Surg* **72**:1977–1984.

191. Eagle KA, Guyton RA, Davidoff R, *et al.* (2004) American College of Cardiology; American Heart Association. ACC/AHA 2004 guideline update for coronary artery bypass graft surgery: a report of the American College of Cardiology/American Heart Association Task Force on Practice Guidelines (Committee to Update the 1999 Guidelines for Coronary Artery Bypass Graft Surgery). *Circulation* **110**:e340–437.

192. Grandjean JG, Voors AA, Boonstra PW, *et al.* (1996) Exclusive use of arterial grafts in coronary artery bypass operations for three-vessel disease: use of both thoracic arteries and the gastroepiploic artery in 256 consecutive patients. *J Thorac Cardiovasc Surg* **112**:935–942.

193. Muneretto C, Bisleri G, Negri A, *et al.* (2003) Total arterial myocardial revascularization with composite grafts improves results of coronary surgery in elderly: a prospective randomized comparison with conventional coronary artery bypass surgery. *Circulation* **108**:II-29–33.

194. Matsuura K, Kobayashi J, Tagusari O, *et al.* (2001) Off-pump coronary artery bypass grafting using only arterial grafts in elderly patients. *Ann Thorac Surg* **80**:144–148.

195. Serruys PW, Ong AT, van Herwerden LA, *et al.* (2005) Five-year outcomes after coronary stenting versus bypass surgery for the treatment of multivessel disease: the final analysis of the Arterial Revascularization Therapies Study (ARTS) randomized trial. *J Am Coll Cardiol* **46**:575–581.

196. Daemen J, Boersma E, Flather M, *et al.* (2008) Long-term safety and efficacy of percutaneous coronary intervention with stenting and coronary artery bypass surgery for multivessel coronary artery disease: a meta-analysis with 5-year patient-level data from the ARTS, ERACI-II, MASS-II, and SoS trials. *Circulation* **118**:1146–1154.

197. Serruys PW, Morice MC, Kappetein AP, *et al.* (2009) SYNTAX Investigators. Percutaneous coronary intervention versus coronary-artery bypass grafting for severe coronary artery disease. *N Engl J Med* **360**:961–972.

198. Kapur A, Malik IS, Bagger JP, *et al.* (2005) The Coronary Artery Revascularisation in Diabetes (CARDia) trial: background, aims, and design. *Am Heart J* **149**:13–19.

199. Buxton BF, Ruengsakulrach P, Fuller J, *et al.* (2000) The right internal thoracic artery graft—benefits of grafting the left coronary system and native vessels with a high grade stenosis. *Eur J Cardiothorac Surg* **18**:255–261.

200. Verhelst R, Etienne PY, El Khoury G, *et al.* (1996) Free internal mammary artery graft in myocardial revascularization. *Cardiovasc Surg* **4**:212–216.

201. Schmidt SE, Jones JW, Thornby JI, *et al.* (1997) Improved survival with multiple left-sided bilateral internal thoracic artery grafts. *Ann Thorac Surg* **64**:9–14.

202. Esaki J, Koshiji T, Okamoto M, *et al.* (2007) Gastroepiploic artery grafting does not improve the late outcome in patients with bilateral internal thoracic artery grafting. *Ann Thorac Surg* **83**:1024–1029.

203. Damgaard S, Lund JT, Lilleør NB, *et al.* (2008) Comparable three months' outcome of total arterial revascularization versus conventional coronary surgery: Copenhagen Arterial Revascularization Randomized Patency and Outcome trial. *J Thorac Cardiovasc Surg* **135**:1069–1075.

204. Muneretto C, Negri A, Manfredi J, *et al.* (2003) Safety and usefulness of composite grafts for total arterial myocardial revascularization: a prospective randomized evaluation. *J Thorac Cardiovasc Surg* **125**:826–835.

205. Légaré JF, Hassan A, Buth KJ, *et al.* (2007) The effect of total arterial grafting on medium-term outcomes following coronary artery bypass grafting. *J Cardiothorac Surg* **2**:44.

206. Nishida H, Tomizawa Y, Endo M, *et al.* (2005) Survival benefit of exclusive use of in situ arterial conduits over combined use of arterial and vein grafts for multiple coronary artery bypass grafting. *Circulation* **112**:I-299–303.

207. Nishida H, Tomizawa Y, Endo M, *et al.* (2001) Coronary artery bypass with only in situ bilateral internal thoracic arteries and right gastroepiploic artery. *Circulation* **104**:I-76–80.

208. Grandjean JG, Voors AA, Boonstra PW, *et al.* (1996) Exclusive use of arterial grafts in coronary artery bypass operations for three-vessel disease: use of both thoracic arteries and the gastroepiploic artery in 256 consecutive patients. *J Thorac Cardiovasc Surg* **112**:935–942.

209. Tavilla G, Kappetein AP, Braun J, *et al.* (2004) Long-term follow-up of coronary artery bypass grafting in three-vessel disease using exclusively pedicled bilateral internal thoracic and right gastroepiploic arteries. *Ann Thorac Surg* **77**:794–799.

210. Veeger NJ, Panday GF, Voors AA, *et al.* (2008) Excellent long-term clinical outcome after coronary artery bypass surgery using three pedicled arterial grafts in patients with three-vessel disease. *Ann Thorac Surg* **85**:508–512.

211. Tatoulis J, Buxton BF, Fuller JA, *et al.* (1999) Total arterial coronary revascularization: techniques and results in 3 220 patients. *Ann Thorac Surg* 1999;**68**:2093–2099.

212. Formica F, Ferro O, Greco P, *et al.* (2004) Long-term follow-up of total arterial myocardial revascularization using exclusively pedicle bilateral internal thoracic artery and right gastroepiploic artery. *Eur J Cardiothorac Surg* **26**:1141–1148.

213. Calafiore AM & Di Giammarco G (1996) Complete revascularization with three or more arterial conduits. *Semin Thorac Cardiovasc Surg* **8**:15–23.

214. Guru V, Fremes SE, & Tu JV (2006) How many arterial grafts are enough? A population-based study of midterm outcomes. *J Thorac Cardiovasc Surg* **131**:1021–1028.

215. Lev-Ran O, Mohr R, Uretzky G, *et al.* (2003) Graft of choice to right coronary system in left-sided bilateral internal thoracic artery grafting. *Ann Thorac Surg* **75**:88–92.

216. Sergeant PT, Blackstone EH, & Meyns BP (1998) Does arterial revascularization decrease the risk of infarction after coronary artery bypass grafting? *Ann Thorac Surg* **66**:1–11.

44 Cell Therapy after Acute Myocardial Infarction

Birgit Assmus & Volker Schächinger
Goethe-Universität Frankfurt, Frankfurt, Germany

The concept of cardiac regeneration

Stem cells stand at the very beginning of life, and their multiplication and differentiation is the prerequisite for development of tissue and organs. With increasing differentiation the totipotency of stem cells is lost (Table 44.1). However, it is known that even in the adult organism there are niches of stem (progenitor) cells, capable of regenerating an organ. For example, dermatoblasts regenerate skin tissue and hemangioblasts are capable of renewing blood cells. Thereby, regenerative capacity of bone marrow progenitor cells is very large, being able to regenerate the whole bone marrow out of one single cell [1]. In hematology, this therapeutic principle has been used for decades to perform bone marrow transplantation in hemtatologic diseases. In nature, there are other examples of even more extensive regenerative capacities, e.g., complete regeneration of limbs in certain newts [2] or restitution of a complete body part in a worm [3].

Until recently, it was thought that the human heart did not possess any regenerative capacity, as adult cardiomyocytes are terminally differentiated and have lost their capacity to renew. The only response to an increased functional demand was seen to be hypertrophy of cardiomyocytes. However, this view has been challenged by findings in patients after heart transplantation with a sex mismatch [4,5]: in myocardial biopsies of male recipient patients receiving a female donor heart, Y-chromosomes were found, indicating that recipient cells were coming from outside the donor heart, migrating and integrating into the transplanted heart. Those Y-chromosomes containing cells were identified as both cardiomyocytes and as vascular cells (e.g., endothelium). There is evidence that these cells regenerating the heart are coming from the bone marrow—demonstrated in sex mismatch bone marrow transplant patients undergoing a myocardial biopsy [6]. Furthermore, recent findings indicate that the heart itself contains resident progenitor cells, which may contribute to regeneration of the heart [7]. Various groups have characterized different types of progenitor cells in the human myocardium [8].

Are progenitor cells a "fountain of youth"?

Recent evidence indicates that the plasticity of adult stem or progenitor cells (resulting in more differentiated stem cells) released from the bone marrow is much larger than previously suspected [9,10]. Traditionally, it has been thought that stem cells are committed to certain cell lines (tissue specificity) and, with increasing degree of maturation, loose their ability to dedifferentiate (return into a more immature form) or to transdifferentiate (changing the path to another cell line). However, plasticity of adult stem or progenitor cells is more extensive. Experimental data indicated that dedifferentiation as well as transdifferentiation of adult progenitor cells is possible. This culminated in the hypothesis that there is a continuous exchange of progenitor cells between the bone marrow, the blood and the organs [10]. The importance of this concept is underscored by additional findings, indicating that adult stem or progenitor cells have retained abilities, which were thought to be restricted to the embryonic stage, such as neovascularization [11,12], which means formation of new vessels (in contrast to extension of pre-existing vessels—arteriogenesis). Taken together, bone-marrow-derived progenitor cells released into the circulation may have capabilities which may be suitable to repair an injury of the vessel wall or to revascularize organs damaged by ischemia [13].

Based on the experimental findings described above, it was intriguing to speculate that progenitor cells circulating in the blood may be part of a physiologic repair system designed by nature to repair damaged organs [14]. However, this regenerative mechanism is most likely adjusted to a low-grade and slow injury, probably as a counterweight for degenerative or aging processes. However, in case of a "mass destruction," like an acute myocardial infarction, the physiologic repair capacity is obviously by no way sufficient.

In an attempt to therapeutically exaggerate the regenerating capabilities of progenitor cells, various animal studies [15–18] demonstrated that transplantation of progenitor cells in animals with experimental myocardial infarction reduces infarct

Cardiovascular Interventions in Clinical Practice. Edited by Jürgen Haase, Hans-Joachim Schäfers, Horst Sievert and Ron Waksman. © 2010 Blackwell Publishing.

Table 44.1 Glossary.

Stem cell	Cells that have the ability to self-replicate and give rise to specialized cells. Stem cells can be found at different stages of fetal development and are present in a wide range of adult tissues. Many of the terms used to distinguish stem cells are based on their origins and the cell types of their progeny. There are three basic types of stem cells: (1) totipotent stem cells, meaning their potential is total, have the capacity to give rise to every cell type of the body and to form an entire organism; (2) pluripotent stem cells, such as embryonic stem cells, are capable of generating virtually all cell types of the body but are unable to form a functioning organism; and (3) multipotent stem cells can give rise only to a limited number of cell types—for example, adult stem cells, also called organ- or tissue-specific stem cells, are multipotent stem cells found in specialized organs and tissues after birth. The primary function of multipotent stem cells is to replenish cells lost from normal turnover or disease in the specific organs and tissues in which they are found
Adult stem cell	Adult stem cells occur in mature tissues. Like all stem cells, adult stem cells can self-replicate. Their ability to self-renew can last throughout the lifetime of individual organisms. But unlike embryonic stem cells, it is usually difficult to expand adult stem cells in culture. Adult stem cells reside in specific organs and tissues, but account for a very small number of the cells in tissues. They are responsible for maintaining a stable state of the specialized tissues. To replace lost cells, stem cells typically generate intermediate cells called precursor or progenitor cells, which are no longer capable of self-renewal. However, they continue undergoing cell divisions, coupled with maturation, to yield fully specialized cells. Such stem cells have been identified in many types of adult tissues, including bone marrow, heart, blood, skin, gastrointestinal tract, dental pulp, retina of the eye, skeletal muscle, liver, pancreas, and brain. Adult stem cells are usually designated according to their source and their potential. Adult stem cells are multipotent because their potential is normally limited according to their source and their potential, and limited to one or more lineages of specialized cells. However, a special multipotent stem cell that can be found in bone marrow, called the mesenchymal stem cell, can produce all cell types of bone, cartilage, fat, blood, and connective tissues
Circulating progenitor cell	Circulating progenitor cells are mononuclear cells that can be isolated from peripheral blood. Under certain culture conditions they differentiate into a progenitor cell-like phenotype. If these freshly isolated mononuclear cells are cultured on fibronectin coated dishes with endothelial specific medium, they express endothelial marker proteins, surface markers, and improve neovascularization of ischemic tissue. These cells are so-called "endothelial progenitor cells"
Plasticity	Stem cell plasticity refers to the phenomenon of adult stem cells from one tissue generating the specialized cells of another tissue. The long-standing concept of adult organ-specific stem cells is that they are restricted to producing the cell types of their specific tissues. However, a series of studies have challenged the concept of tissue restriction of adult stem cells. Although the stem cells appear able to cross their tissue-specific boundaries, crossing occurs generally at a low frequency and mostly only under conditions of host organ damage. The finding of stem cell plasticity carries significant implications for potential cell therapy. For example, if differentiation can be redirected, stem cells of abundant source and easy access, such as blood stem cells in bone marrow or umbilical cord blood, could be used to substitute stem cells in tissues that are difficult to isolate, such as heart and nervous system tissue

size and improves vascularization of the myocardium and, importantly, ventricular function. However, there is an ongoing debate about the mechanisms of progenitor cell treatment, whether there is just *prevention* of myocardial deterioration owing to paracrine or other actions or whether there is actually a "regeneration" of cardiac myocytes [19,20]. Indeed, several studies did not find evidence of actual transdifferentiation of bone marrow cells into cardiomyocytes [21,22]; even in these studies there was improvement of myocardial function after bone marrow cell injection. The reasons for the discrepant findings are not explained, but may include different methods used. In addition, fusion of adult cardiomyocytes and progenitor cells are discussed. Nevertheless, there are various other potential mechanisms for how bone marrow cell therapy may beneficially affect myocardial function (Fig. 44.1; for review see reference 23):

Cytokine production
Progenitor cells release various cytokines and growth factors, which may interact with cardiac resident progenitor cells and/or increase neovascularization [24].

Neovascularization
Progenitor cells can promote neovascularization by differentiation into endothelial cells and/or incorporation into pre-existing vessels [25].

Interaction with extracellular matrix
Irrespective of the mechanism of progenitor cell therapy, clinical trials have already been performed, demonstrating the safety and feasibility of progenitor therapy and also giving a hint toward potential efficacy in acute myocardial infarction [26–28] and chronic ischemic heart disease [29–32]. It is

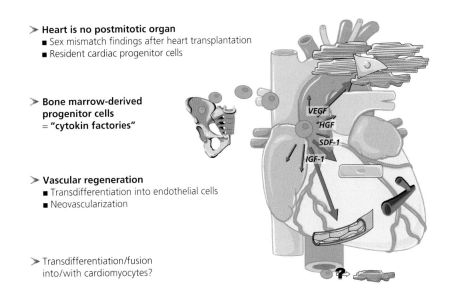

➤ **Heart is no postmitotic organ**
- Sex mismatch findings after heart transplantation
- Resident cardiac progenitor cells

➤ **Bone marrow-derived progenitor cells = "cytokin factories"**

VEGF
HGF
SDF-1
IGF-1

➤ **Vascular regeneration**
- Transdifferentiation into endothelial cells
- Neovascularization

➤ Transdifferentiation/fusion into/with cardiomyocytes?

Figure 44.1 Potential mechanisms of progenitor cell therapy on the heart.

important to understand that there is a large diversity of progenitor cells used in experimental and clinical trials, differing in origin, processing, and cell marker characteristics and function.

Clinical trials

Stamm *et al.* [33] delivered a selected fraction of bone marrow cells (CD133+ cells) to the heart by intramuscular injection during surgery, demonstrating the safety and feasibility of the approach.

In a first clinical trial using intracoronary injection of progenitor cells, Strauer *et al.* [26] treated 10 patients after an acute myocardial infarction by injecting progenitor cells aspirated from the bone marrow into the infarct coronary artery. A positive effect on myocardial perfusion as well as left ventricular function was seen.

In the Transplantation of Progenitor Cells and Regeneration Enhancement in Acute Myocardial Infarction (TOPCARE-AMI) trial, 59 patients were investigated 3–7 days after successful percutaneous revascularization via stent implantation of an infarct artery during acute myocardial infarction [34]. Patients were either treated with bone marrow derived progenitor cells or circulating progenitor cells given during low-pressure balloon insufflation directly into the lumen of the infarct artery. As previously described in a preliminary report of the first 20 patients [27], the study demonstrated that intracoronary infusion of progenitor cells with both types of cells was safe and feasible, as there were no unexpected adverse events and no evidence of inflammation or microembolization induced by the cell therapy. In addition, improvement of left ventricular ejection fraction was observed, associated with improved viability measured by positron emission tomography (PET) [27], and also a reduction of infarct size, assessed by MRI

(late enhancement) [35]. In addition, coronary flow reserve improved significantly in the infarct artery up to the level of the reference artery, indicating probable neovascularization and, therefore, increases in vascular conductance capacity might be associated with progenitor cell therapy [36].

These encouraging results were confirmed by the recently presented Bone Marrow Transfer to Enhance ST-Elevation Infarct Regeneration (BOOST) trial [28,37,38], which randomized 60 patients 1:1, with a control group and a group of those receiving intracoronary bone marrow-derived progenitor cell therapy after acute myocardial infarction. Whereas left ventricular ejection fraction improved by 6.7% in the bone marrow treated group, there was only a marginal change of left ventricular ejection fraction of 0.7% in the control group, which demonstrated a significant difference in favor of progenitor cell therapy. Nevertheless, further studies will have to formally establish this novel therapy and define the value within the current clinical scenario (Table 44.2).

REPAIR AMI and ASTAMI trial

The two largest clinical trials published so far are the Autologous Stem Cell Transplantation in Acute Myocardial Infarction (ASTAMI) and the REPAIR-AMI trial [39,40]. Both trials included patients with an acute myocardial infarction and successful stent-PCI for reperfusion. Bone marrow cells were obtained by aspiration of 50 mL bone marrow from the iliac crest under local anesthesia, and intracoronary infusion was performed using an over-the-wire balloon catheter, and the stop-flow technique. However, in the ASTAMI trial, in which 100 patients with anterior myocardial infarction were included and intracoronary infusion was applied at a median of 6 days after the acute myocardial infarction, no significant differences could be obtained with respect to left ventricular ejection fraction (LVEF) measured by different methods between the

Table 44.2 Overview of clinical trials.

Study	Patients/ design	Days post AMI	Cell type	Cell isolation procedure	Cell number	Safety	Myocardial function
Safety and feasibility studies							
Strauer et al. [26]	n = 20, 1:1 vs. control	8	BMC	40 mL Ficoll—overnight Teflon	28	+	Regional contractility ↑ (LVA)
							End-systolic volume ↓ (LVA)
TOPCARE–AMI [27,34,35]	n = 59	4.9	CPC BMC	250 mL/3 day culture	16	+	Perfusion ↑ (Szinti) Global contractility ↑ (LVA/MRI)
				50 mL/Ficoll—same day	213		End-systolic volume ↓ (LVA/MRI) Viability ↑ (MRI) Flow reserve ↑ (Doppler)
Fernandez-Aviles et al. [54]	n = 20	13.5	BMC	50 mL Ficoll—overnight Teflon	78	+	Global contractility ↑ (MRI)
							End-systolic volume ↓ (MRI)
Ruan et al. [55]	n = 20, 1:1 random/saline	0	BMC		MA	+	Global contractility ↑ (LVA)
Bartunek et al. [56]	n = 12	14	CD133+ BMC	Mouse antibody	12	Stenosis	Global contractility ↑ (LVA)
Chen et al. [57]	n = 69, 1:1 vs. control	18	B-MSC	10-day culture		+	Global contractility ↑ (LVA)
Single center/two centers, randomized							
BOOST [28,38]	n = 60 1:1 random	4.8	BMC vs. randomized control	Gelatine polysuccinate—same day infusion	2460	+	Global contractility ↑ (MRI) Infarkt size (LE) ↓ (NS) (MRI) Diastolic dysfunction ↓ (Echo)
Janssens et al. [41]	n = 67, 1:1 random/ placebo	< 24 h	BMC vs. i.c. placebo	Ficoll density gradient centrifugation—few hours after acute PCI	304	+	Global contractility ⇔ (no change) (MRI) Infarct size (LE) ↓ (MRI)
MAGIC Cell-3-DES (AMI) [58]		< 14	G-CSF mobilized CPC vs. control	COBE spectra apheresis system	56		Significantly greater improvement in LVEF and reduction in ESV in the cell infusion group
ASTAMI [40]	n = 100, 1:1 random	6	BMC vs. randomized control	Lymphoprep™ next day infusion	87	+	Global contractility ⇔ (no change) (MRI) (echocardiography/SPECT) Infarct size (LE) ⇔ (no change) (MRI)
Multicenter, double-blind, placebo-controlled, randomized							
REPAIR–AMI [39,46]	n = 204 1:1 random/ placebo	4	BMC vs. i.c. placebo	Ficol density gradient centrifugation—same or next day infusion	>230	+	Global contractility ↑ (LVA)
							Flow reserve ↑ (Doppler)

Methods used for functional assessment: LVA, left ventricular angiography; Szinti, szintigraphy; MRI, magnetic resonance imaging; Echo, echocardiography.

cell-infusion and the randomized control group not receiving an additional catheterization procedure after 6 months. In contrast, the REPAIR-AMI trial, which randomized 204 patients to receive either intracoronary infusion of bone marrow-derived progenitor cells (BMC) or intracoronary infusion of placebo at a median of 4 days after the acute myocardial infarction, demonstrated a significantly greater improvement in LVEF after 4 months in the BMC than in the placebo group. In detail, global LVEF increased from 47% ± 10% at baseline to 50% ± 13% at 4 months in the placebo group. In the BMC

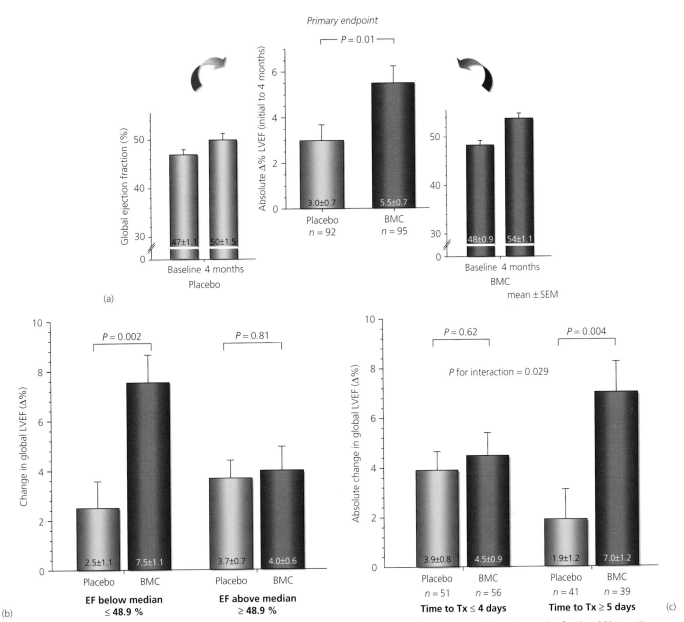

Figure 44.2 Results of the Repair-AMI trial: (a) improvement in left ventricular ejection fraction, (b) interaction with baseline ejection fraction, (c) interaction with time to treatment.

group, LVEF increased from 48% ± 9.1% to 54% ± 10%. At 4 months, LVEF was significantly higher in the BMC group than in the placebo group ($P = 0.021$), and the primary end point, the absolute increase in LVEF, was significantly greater in the BMC treated patients than in the placebo group ($P = 0.014$) (Fig. 44.2a). In addition, regional wall motion analysis demonstrated that recovery of contractile function was most pronounced in those left ventricular cords with the most severe impairment at baseline. Moreover, although end-diastolic volumes slightly increased in both groups, end-systolic left ventricular volumes remained constant in the BMC group, but increased in the placebo group. Taken together, the REPAIR-

AMI trial as a proof-of-concept trial met its primary end point and confirmed that patients with AMI treated with intra-coronary infusion of BMC have a greater recovery of left ventricular contractile function compared with standard treatment.

Subanalyses of the REPAIR-AMI trial revealed further interesting findings. First, there was a significant inverse relation between baseline left ventricular ejection fraction and absolute changes in LVEF at 4 months follow-up in the BMC group ($r = -0.21$; $P = 0.043$), but not in the placebo group ($r = +0.11$, $P = 0.31$). When the total patient population was dichotomized according to the median value of LVEF at baseline, there was

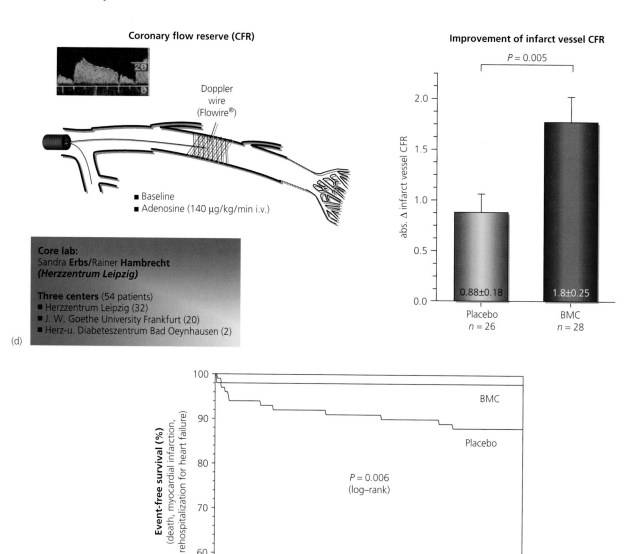

Figure 44.2 *(cont'd)* (d) Results of the Doppler substudy. For the Doppler procedure, the left or right coronary artery was cannulated with a 5F or 6F catheter. Before the assessment of coronary blood flow, 0.2 mg nitroglycerin was administered directly into the coronary circulation to achieve a maximal dilatation of the epicardial vessels without substantially affecting the microcirculation. Afterwards, a guidewire containing a 12-MHz pulsed Doppler ultrasound velocimeter (Flowire, Volcano Corp, Rancho Cordova, CA; Flow-MAP, Cardiometrics and Endosonics, Rancho Cordova, CA) was positioned in the infarct-related artery directly distal to the previously implanted stent. The average peak flow velocity (APV) measured by the Doppler velocimeter was continuously registered under baseline conditions and during intravenous adenosine infusion (140 μg/kg body weight). Subsequently, the Doppler wire was advanced into a noninfarcted reference vessel not undergoing percutaneous coronary intervention, and the measurements were repeated. The coronary flow reserve (CFR) of the infarct-related artery and the reverence vessel were computed as the ratio of adenosine-induced APV and APV at baseline. (e) Event-free survival.

a significant interaction between the treatment effect of BMC infusion and baseline ejection fraction, showing that patients with a baseline LVEF below the median value (48.9%) had a three-fold larger absolute increase in LVEF in the BMC receiving group than with placebo infusion (treatment effect 5.1 Δ%). These details demonstrate that patients with a large

AMI, who are at increased risk of developing adverse left ventricular remodeling and experiencing future cardiovascular events, derive most benefit from the BMC therapy, whereas patients with only a small myocardial infarction have no additional benefit from intracoronary BMC infusion (Fig. 44.2b).

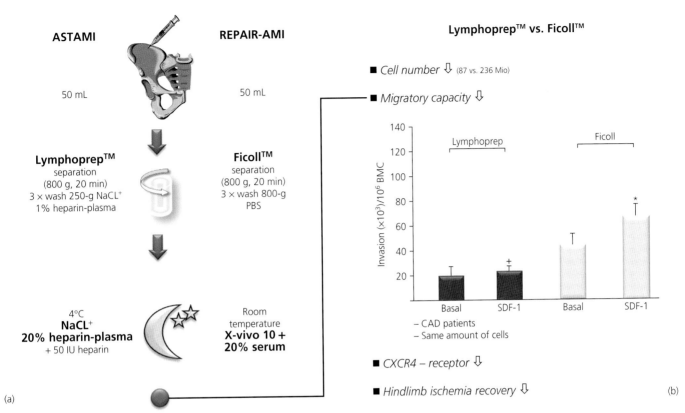

Figure 44.3 Comparison of cell isolation procedures of the REPAIR-AMI and the ASTAMI trial: (a) cell isolation procedures, (b) impact on *in vitro* invasion capacity.

Another interesting result of the REPAIR-AMI trial was that the beneficial effects on recovery of contractile function by infusing BMCs were confined to patients treated beyond 4 days after infarct reperfusion. Patients treated with intracoronary infusion of BMC earlier than day 4 had no advantage over the placebo group (Fig. 44.2c). These results correspond well to the results of the Janssens trial from Leuven, in which the intracoronary BMC therapy was performed within 24 h after the acute myocardial infarction [41]. There was no significant difference in contractile recovery (LVEF) between the BMC treated patients and the randomized control group. However, infarct size was smaller in the cell-treated group as shown by MRI detected reduction in late enhancement volume. A possible explanation for this small effect is that the microenvironment may be hostile still for the homing and survival of the infused cells owing to the increased oxidative stress following reperfusion.

The next question to be asked is why the ASTAMI trial was negative. Looking into the details of the REAPIR-AMI trial and the ASTAMI trial, it is evident that different methods of cell preparation were associated with different recovery and different numbers of infused cells, although both trials aspirated 50 mL of bone marrow [42,43] (Fig. 44.3a). It is well established that, in addition to patient-related differences, cell isolation procedures may significantly affect the function-ality of progenitor cells and, thus, determine the functional effects observed in patients after intracoronary administration. Indeed, Seeger *et al.* have previously demonstrated that even slight alterations in storage temperature, the choice of buffer solution, or the use of patients own plasma during cell isolation and processing profoundly impairs progenitor cell functionality, as measured by their CFU (colony forming units—forming colonies might be regarded as a cell-intrinsic functional property of progenitor cells) capacity, migratory capacity toward their chemoattractants, and neovascularization capacity of cells infused into a hind limb ischemia model [44] (Fig. 44.3b).

Mechanistic findings from the REPAIR-AMI trial

In animal experiments with acute myocardial infarction, increased capillary density and improved blood flow after ischemia are the most prominent mechanisms of action after progenitor cell infusion. To address this question and the potential impact of BMC therapy on neovascularization within the infarct area in humans, the "Doppler substudy" of the REPAIR-AMI trial investigated the effects of intracoronary BMC infusion on coronary blood flow regulation [45]. In 58 patients, coronary flow reserve (CFR) in the infarct artery and a reference vessel was assessed by intracoronary Doppler at the time of study therapy and at 4 months follow-up. Initial CFR was reduced in the infarct artery compared with the reference vessel in both groups (BMC: 2.0 ± 0.1 vs. 2.9 ± 0.2, $P < 0.05$; placebo: 1.9 ± 0.1 vs. 2.8 ± 0.2, $P < 0.05$). At 4 months' follow-up, CFR in the infarct artery had slightly improved in the placebo group ($+0.88 \pm 0.18$; $P < 0.001$ versus initial), but was markedly increased by 90% ($+1.80 \pm 0.25$; $P = 0.005$ vs. placebo) in BMC-treated patients resulting in complete normalization of CFR (3.8 ± 0.2, $P < 0.001$ vs. initial and placebo at 4 months). Moreover, in the infarct vessel, adenosine-induced minimal vascular resistance index declined only slightly in the placebo group, but considerably decreased by $-29 \pm 6\%$ in the BMC group, suggesting increased capillary density within the infarct area and improvement of maximal vascular conductance capacity (Fig. 44.2d).

In addition to improvement of neovascularization, attenuation or abolishment of progressive adverse left ventricular remodeling is another important mechanism for improved outcome after BMC therapy. As progressive adverse left ventricular remodeling after myocardial infarction is the pathomorphologic substrate of post-infarction heart failure and reduced survival, intracoronary infusion of BMC in patients with AMI is evolving as a new therapeutic strategy to recover impaired postinfarction left ventricular contractility and to attenuate end-systolic volume expansion. In the REPAIR-AMI trial, baseline LVEF was inversely correlated with end-systolic volume (ESV) expansion in the placebo, but not in the BMC group at 4 months. Likewise, end-diastolic volume (EDV) expansion was closely correlated with baseline LVEF in the placebo, but not in the BMC group. At 4 months, ESV increased in the placebo ($+6 \pm 22$ mL) but not in the BMC group (-0.6 ± 19 mL, $P = 0.04$ vs. placebo). Analyzing the interaction between convalescent LV contractile function and LV volumes revealed that the increase in LVEF did not occur at the expense of increases in ESV or EDV, respectively, in the BMC group. Thus, intracoronary administration of BMC eliminates the correlation between depressed LVEF after reperfusion therapy and left ventricular expansion during follow-up, and thereby abrogates early left ventricular remodeling after AMI.

Finally, convalescent left ventricular contractile function at 4 months was the single most important predictor of an improved subsequent clinical outcome at 2 years' follow-up. As it is well established from many pharmacologic therapies beneficially interfering with the left ventricular remodeling process after AMI, such as ACE-inhibitors or β-blockers that ameliorating adverse left ventricular remodeling is paralleled by substantial improvements in symptoms of heart failure and patients' prognosis after AMI, we further analyzed the impact of intracoronary BMC therapy on the prognosis of patients treated within the REPAIR-AMI trial. At 12 months, the prespecified cumulative end point of death, myocardial infarction, or necessity for revascularization was significantly reduced in the BMC group compared with the placebo group ($P = 0.009$) [46]. Likewise, the combined end point of death, recurrence of myocardial infarction and rehospitalization for heart failure was significantly reduced in patients receiving intracoronary BMC administration ($P = 0.006$; Fig. 44.2e). Intracoronary administration of BMC remained a significant predictor of a favorable clinical outcome by Cox regression analysis, adjusting for classical predictors of poor outcome after AMI. Thus, intracoronary administration of BMC is associated with a significant reduction of the occurrence of major adverse cardiovascular events after acute myocardial infarction. However, large-scale studies are warranted to confirm the effects of BMC administration on mortality and morbidity in patients with acute myocardial infarctions.

For this purpose, the REPAIR-AMI 2 trial is under preparation. The trial is a phase III clinical trial to investigate the efficacy of BMC in the treatment of acute myocardial infarction with failure of contractile recovery in more detail. In total, 1200 patients will be randomized during this multicenter, controlled study. Patients with a first acute STEMI with LVEF <40% and a significant regional wall motion abnormality will be included in the study if they have undergone successful acute reperfusion therapy within 12 h of symptom onset. They will be treated with autologous bone marrow-derived progenitor cells at days 5–7 post reperfusion. The combined primary end point will be death and rehospitalization for cardiovascular events, which is the universally accepted end point of large multicenter trials to investigate the effects of a given intervention on disease outcome in patients with acute myocardial infarction Secondary end points comprise, for example, cardiovascular death, hospitalization for any cause, nonfatal myocardial infarction, or stroke, as well as coronary revascularization.

Conclusion

Taken together, encouraging results for cardiac function improvement have been demonstrated for patients with acute myocardial infraction. However, further clinical outcome trials are warranted to establish this new therapeutic concept as an additional treatment to limit myocardial remodeling processes in patients surviving a heart attack.

In contrast, the results for patients suffering from ischemic cardiomyopathy are much more limited, although encouraging results from small trials suggest beneficial effects after intracoronary or intramyocardial application of bone marrow derived progenitor cells. Thus, it is evident that restoration of tissue vascularization and myocardial contraction many months and years after critical ischemia remains a major challenge in cardiovascular medicine.

To further optimize the cell therapy effects, specifically in patients with chronic ischemic heart failure, current enhancement strategies focus on modulation of homing factors and improvement of the functional capacities of the infused cells. As loss of cytokines or growth factors over time following myocardial infarction parallels negative remodeling and progression of heart failure, preconditioning of chronic ischemic tissue (e.g., by low-energy shock waves) might improve recruitment of circulating progenitor cells via enhanced expression of chemoattractant factors [47]. Low-energy shock wave-facilitated cell therapy may improve the efficacy of progenitor cell treatment in patients with chronic ischemia. Preliminary data from clinical investigations suggest that low-energy shock waves can also be applied as a stand alone therapy in patients for induction of endogenous angiogenesis [48]. However, a combined approach including shock wave application and intracoronary cell infusion may offer an increased therapeutic benefit. Another different future approach might be the combined intramyocardial gene therapy with growth factors preceding stem cell therapy.

Moreover, functional activation of the progenitor cells themselves may also lead to increased improvement after cell therapy. Previous studies have shown that cells from patients with ischemic cardiomyopathy are characterized by reduced neovascularization capacity and selective exhaustion of progenitor cell function in the bone marrow and in the peripheral blood, which may limit their therapeutic potential for clinical cell therapy [49–51].

By *ex vivo* stimulation using different drugs influencing signaling pathways involved in migration or homing of cells, the functional capacities might be enhanced before cells are re-administered to patients.

In this respect, incubation of isolated or cultured cells with drugs such as the nitric oxide synthase enhancer AVE9488 [52] or drugs that are capable to modulate differentiation or homing will be likely candidates to further optimize the efficacy of autologous cell therapeutics (for review see reference 53).

Finally, it is unlikely that a single administration of any dose of cells will completely reverse a disease process that has progressed over decades, therefore serial applications by catheter-based techniques will be necessary.

Taken together, for the future large randomized outcome trials for patients with acute myocardial infarction are essential, whereas for patients with ischemic cardiomyopathy smaller randomized trials investigating cell enhancements strategies and modulation of homing processes should be performed. In addition to these clinical approaches, basic research has to be intensified to provide further insights into the mechanisms of neovascularization enhancement and cardiac regeneration, as well as into the genetic control of stem cell differentiation for the final goal of developing a disease targeted regenerative therapeutic approach.

References

1. Engelhardt M, Deschler B, Müller CI, & Lübbert M (2003) Plastizität adulter Stammzellen: Wunschtraum oder Realität? Dt *Aerzteblatt* **100**:A3236–A3244.

2. Iten LB (1973) Forelimb regeneration from different levels of amputation in the newt, *N. viridescens*: Length, rate and stages. *Wilhelm Roux Arch Dev Biol* **173**:263–282.

3. Reddien PW, Bermange AL, Murfitt KJ, Jennings JR, & Sanchez Alvarado A (2005) Identification of genes needed for regeneration, stem cell function, and tissue homeostasis by systematic gene perturbation in planaria. *Dev Cell* **8**:635–649.

4. Quaini F, Urbanek K, Beltrami AP, *et al.* (2002) Chimerism of the transplanted heart. *N Engl J Med* **346**:5–15.

5. Muller P, Pfeiffer P, Koglin J, *et al.* (2002) Cardiomyocytes of noncardiac origin in myocardial biopsies of human transplanted hearts. *Circulation* **106**:31–35.

6. Deb A, Wang S, Skelding KA, Miller D, Simper D, & Caplice NM (2003) Bone marrow-derived cardiomyocytes are present in adult human heart: a study of gender-mismatched bone marrow transplantation patients. *Circulation* **107**:1247–1249.

7. Beltrami AP, Barlucchi L, Torella D, *et al.* (2003) Adult cardiac stem cells are multipotent and support myocardial regeneration. *Cell* **114**:763–776.

8. Parmacek MS & Epstein JA (2005) Pursuing cardiac progenitors: regeneration redux. *Cell* **120**:295–298.

9. Korbling M & Estrov Z (2003) Adult stem cells for tissue repair—a new therapeutic concept? *N Engl J Med* **349**:570–582.

10. Blau HM, Brazelton TR, & Weimann JM (2001) The evolving concept of a stem cell: entity or function? *Cell* **105**:829–841.

11. Asahara T, Masuda H, Takahashi T, *et al.* (1999) Bone marrow origin of endothelial progenitor cells responsible for postnatal vasculogenesis in physiological and pathological neovascularization. *Circ Res* **85**:221–228.

12. Takahashi T, Kalka C, Masuda H, *et al.* (1999) Ischemia- and cytokine-induced mobilization of bone marrow-derived endothelial progenitor cells for neovascularization. *Nat Med* **5**:434–438.

13. Isner JM & Asahara T (1999) Angiogenesis and vasculogenesis as therapeutic strategies for postnatal neovascularization. *J Clin Invest* **103**:1231–1236.

14. Isner JM, Kalka C, Kawamoto A, & Asahara T (2001) Bone marrow as a source of endothelial cells for natural and iatrogenic vascular repair. *Ann N Y Acad Sci* **953**:75–84.

15. Kawamoto A, Gwon HC, Iwaguro H, *et al.* (2001) Therapeutic potential of ex vivo expanded endothelial progenitor cells for myocardial ischemia. *Circulation* **103**:634–637.

16. Orlic D, Kajstura J, Chimenti S, *et al.* (2001) Bone marrow cells regenerate infarcted myocardium. *Nature* **410**:701–705.

17. Jackson KA, Majka SM, Wang H, *et al.* (2001) Regeneration of ischemic cardiac muscle and vascular endothelium by adult stem cells. *J Clin Invest* **107**:1395–1402.

18. Kocher AA, Schuster MD, Szabolcs MJ, *et al.* (2001) Neovascularization of ischemic myocardium by human bone-marrow-derived angioblasts prevents cardiomyocyte apoptosis, reduces remodeling and improves cardiac function. *Nat Med* **7**:430–436.

19. Leri A, Kajstura J, Nadal-Ginard B, & Anversa P (2004) Some like it plastic. *Circ Res* **94**:132–134.

20. Nygren JM, Jovinge S, Breitbach M, *et al.* (2004) Bone marrow-derived hematopoietic cells generate cardiomyocytes at a low frequency through cell fusion, but not transdifferentiation. *Nat Med* **10**:494–501.

21. Murry CE, Soonpaa MH, Reinecke H, *et al.* (2004) Haematopoietic stem cells do not transdifferentiate into cardiac myocytes in myocardial infarcts. *Nature* **428**:664–668.

22. Balsam LB, Wagers AJ, Christensen JL, Kofidis T, Weissman IL, & Robbins RC (2004) Haematopoietic stem cells adopt mature haematopoietic fates in ischaemic myocardium. *Nature* **428**: 668–673.

23. Dimmeler S, Burchfield J, & Zeiher AM (2008) Cell-based therapy of myocardial infarction. *Arterioscler Thromb Vasc Biol* **28**:208–216.

24. Urbich C, Aicher A, Heeschen C, *et al.* (2005) Soluble factors released by endothelial progenitor cells promote migration of endothelial cells and cardiac resident progenitor cells. *J Mol Cell Cardiol* **39**:733–742.

25. Urbich C, Heeschen C, Aicher A, Dernbach E, Zeiher AM, & Dimmeler S (2003) Relevance of monocytic features for neovascularization capacity of circulating endothelial progenitor cells. *Circulation* **108**:2511–2516.

26. Strauer BE, Brehm M, Zeus T, *et al.* (2002) Repair of infarcted myocardium by autologous intracoronary mononuclear bone marrow cell transplantation in humans. *Circulation* **106**:1913–1918.

27. Assmus B, Schächinger V, Teupe C, *et al.* (2002) Transplantation of Progenitor Cells and Regeneration Enhancement in Acute Myocardial Infarction (TOPCARE-AMI). *Circulation* **106**:3009–3017.

28. Wollert KC, Meyer GP, Lotz J, *et al.* (2004) Intracoronary autologous bone-marrow cell transfer after myocardial infarction: the BOOST randomised controlled clinical trial. *Lancet* **364**: 141–148.

29. Perin EC, Dohmann HF, Borojevic R, *et al.* (2003) Transendocardial, autologous bone marrow cell transplantation for severe, chronic ischemic heart failure. *Circulation* **107**:2294–2302.

30. Fuchs S, Satler LF, Kornowski R, *et al.* (2003) Catheter-based autologous bone marrow myocardial injection in no-option patients with advanced coronary artery disease: a feasibility study. *J Am Coll Cardiol* **41**:1721–1724.

31. Assmus B, Fischer-Rasokat U, Honold J, *et al.* (2007) Transcoronary transplantation of functionally competent BMCs is associated with a decrease in natriuretic peptide serum levels and improved survival of patients with chronic postinfarction heart failure: results of the TOPCARE-CHD Registry. *Circ Res* **100**:1234–1241.

32. Assmus B, Honold J, Schächinger V, *et al.* (2006) Transcoronary transplantation of progenitor cells after myocardial infarction. *N Engl J Med* **355**:1222–1232.

33. Stamm C, Westphal B, Kleine HD, *et al.* (2003) Autologous bone-marrow stem-cell transplantation for myocardial regeneration. *Lancet* **361**:45–46.

34. Schächinger V, Assmus B, Britten MB, *et al.* (2004) Transplantation of progenitor cells and regeneration enhancement in acute myocardial infarction. Final one-year results of the TOPCARE-AMI Trial. *J Am Coll Cardiol* **44**:1690–1699.

35. Britten MB, Abolmaali ND, Assmus B, *et al.* (2003) Infarct remodeling after intracoronary progenitor cell treatment in patients with acute myocardial infarction (TOPCARE-AMI): mechanistic insights from serial contrast-enhanced magnetic resonance imaging. *Circulation* **108**:2212–2218.

36. Schächinger V, Assmus B, Honold J, *et al.* (2006) Normalization of coronary blood flow in the infarct-related artery after intracoronary progenitor cell therapy: intracoronary Doppler substudy of the TOPCARE-AMI trial. *Clin Res Cardiol* **95**:13–22.

37. Hofmann M, Wollert KC, Meyer GP, *et al.* (2005) Monitoring of bone marrow cell homing into the infarcted human myocardium. *Circulation* **111**:2198–2202.

38. Meyer GP, Wollert KC, Lotz J, *et al.* (2006) Intracoronary bone marrow cell transfer after myocardial infarction: eighteen months' follow-up data from the randomized, controlled BOOST (BOne marrOw transfer to enhance ST-elevation infarct regeneration) trial. *Circulation* **113**:1287–1294.

39. Schächinger V, Erbs S, Elsässer A, *et al.* (2006) Intracoronary bone marrow-derived progenitor cells in acute myocardial infarction. *N Engl J Med* **355**:1210–1221.

40. Lunde K, Solheim S, Aakhus S, *et al.* (2006) Intracoronary injection of mononuclear bone marrow cells in acute myocardial infarction. *N Engl J Med* **355**:1199–1209.

41. Janssens S, Dubois C, Bogaert J, *et al.* (2006) Autologous bone marrow-derived stem-cell transfer in patients with ST-segment elevation myocardial infarction: double-blind, randomised controlled trial. *Lancet* **367**:113–121.

42. Lunde K, Solheim S, Aakhus S, Arnesen H, & Forfang K (2005) Effects on left ventricular function by intracoronary injections of autologous mononuclear bone marrow cells in acute anterior wall myocardial infarction: the ASTAMI randomized controlled trial. *Circulation* **112**:3364.

43. Schächinger V, Tonn T, Dimmeler S, & Zeiher AM (2006) Bone-marrow-derived progenitor cell therapy in need of proof of concept: design of the REPAIR-AMI trial. *Nat Clin Pract Cardiovasc Med* **3** (Suppl. 1):S23–28.

44. Seeger FH, Tonn T, Krzossok N, Zeiher AM, & Dimmeler S (2007) Cell isolation procedures matter: a comparison of different isolation protocols of bone marrow mononuclear cells used for cell therapy in patients with acute myocardial infarction. *Eur Heart J* **28**:766–772.

45. Erbs S, Linke A, Schachinger V, *et al.* (2007) Restoration of microvascular function in the infarct-related artery by intracoronary transplantation of bone marrow progenitor cells in patients with acute myocardial infarction: the Doppler Substudy of the Reinfusion of Enriched Progenitor Cells and Infarct Remodeling in Acute Myocardial Infarction (REPAIR-AMI) trial. *Circulation* **116**:366–374.

46. Schächinger V, Erbs S, Elsässer A, *et al.* (2006) Improved clinical outcome after intracoronary administration of bone-marrow-derived progenitor cells in acute myocardial infarction: final 1-year results of the REPAIR-AMI trial. *Eur Heart J* **27**:2775–2783.

47. Aicher A, Heeschen C, Sasaki K-i, Urbich C, Zeiher AM, & Dimmeler S (2006) Low-energy shock wave for enhancing recruitment of endothelial progenitor cells: a new modality to increase efficacy of cell therapy in chronic hind limb ischemia. *Circulation* **114**:2823–2830.

48. Fukumoto Y, Ito A, Uwatoku T, *et al.* (2006) Extracorporeal cardiac shock wave therapy ameliorates myocardial ischemia in patients with severe coronary artery disease. *Coron Artery Dis* **17**:63–70.

49. Heeschen C, Lehmann R, Honold J, *et al.* (2004) Profoundly reduced neovascularization capacity of bone marrow mononuclear cells derived from patients with chronic ischemic heart disease. *Circulation* **109**:1615–1622.

50. Tepper OM, Galiano RD, Capla JM, *et al.* (2002) Human endothelial progenitor cells from type II diabetics exhibit impaired proliferation, adhesion, and incorporation into vascular structures. *Circulation* **106**:2781–2786.

51. Walter DH, Haendeler J, Reinhold J, R *et al.* (2005) Impaired CXCR4 signaling contributes to the reduced neovascularization capacity of endothelial progenitor cells from patients with coronary artery disease. *Circ Res* **97**:1142–1151.

52. Sasaki K, Heeschen C, Aicher A, *et al.* (2006) Ex vivo pretreatment of bone marrow mononuclear cells with endothelial NO synthase enhancer AVE9488 enhances their functional activity for cell therapy. *Proc Natl Acad Sci USA* **103**:14537–14541.

53. Seeger FH, Zeiher AM, & Dimmeler S (2007) Cell-enhancement strategies for the treatment of ischemic heart disease. *Nat Clin Pract Cardiovasc Med* **4**(Suppl. 1):S110–113.

54. Fernandez-Aviles F, San Roman JA, Garcia-Frade J, *et al.* (2004) Experimental and clinical regenerative capability of human bone marrow cells after myocardial infarction. *Circ Res* **95**:742–748.

55. Ruan W, Pan CZ, Huang GQ, Li YL, Ge JB, & Shu XH (2005) Assessment of left ventricular segmental function after autologous bone marrow stem cells transplantation in patients with acute myocardial infarction by tissue tracking and strain imaging. *Chin Med J (Engl)* **118**:1175–1181.

56. Bartunek J, Vanderheyden M, Vandekerckhove B, *et al.* (2005) Intracoronary injection of CD133-positive enriched bone marrow progenitor cells promotes cardiac recovery after recent myocardial infarction: feasibility and safety. *Circulation* **112**:I178–183.

57. Chen SL, Fang WW, Ye F, *et al.* (2004) Effect on left ventricular function of intracoronary transplantation of autologous bone marrow mesenchymal stem cell in patients with acute myocardial infarction. *Am J Cardiol* **94**:92–95.

58. Kang HJ, Lee HY, Na SH, *et al.* (2006) Differential effect of intracoronary infusion of mobilized peripheral blood stem cells by granulocyte colony-stimulating factor on left ventricular function and remodeling in patients with acute myocardial infarction versus old myocardial infarction: the MAGIC Cell-3-DES randomized, controlled trial. *Circulation* **114**:I145–151.

3 Aortic Coarctation, Aneurysms, and Dissections

45 Pathology of Aortic Coarctation, Aneurysm, and Dissection

Faqian Li[1], Chi K. Lai[2] & Michael C. Fishbein[2]

[1]University of Rochester Medical Center, Rochester, NY, USA
[2]David Geffen School of Medicine at UCLA, Los Angeles, CA, USA

Introduction

The aorta is an elastic, pulsatile, high-pressure conduit that distends to buffer the impact of systole and recoils to ensure continuous blood flow during diastole. The aorta can be divided into thoracic and abdominal segments. The former is further subdivided into the ascending, transverse (aortic arch), isthmus, and descending aorta. The isthmus is a short segment between the origin of the left subclavian artery and the insertion of the ligamentum arteriosum to the descending aorta. In adults, normal aortic diameter has been estimated to be approximately 3 cm at the origin, 2.5 cm in the descending portion in the thorax, and 1.8–2 cm in the abdomen. However, these aortic dimensions vary according to body size and age. In children, normal aortic growth curves have been derived to assist in the determination of aortic developmental abnormalities [1]. Because the aorta endures continuous, pulsatile high pressure and shear stress, it is particularly prone to mechanical injury and various diseases. Congenital anomalies of the aorta are relatively uncommon and are often associated with other congenital cardiac defects.

Coarctation of the aorta

Definition

Coarctation of the aorta is typically a congenital, localized narrowing of any aortic segment. Acquired narrowing of the aorta may occur as a consequence of trauma, surgical procedures, fibromuscular dysplasia or inflammatory processes. Congenital aortic coarctation almost always occurs between the aortic isthmus and descending aorta in the region of the insertion of the ligamentum arteriosum or patent ductus arteriosus.

Prevalence and etiology

Morgagni first described aortic coarctation at autopsy in 1760 [2]. Coarctation of the aorta occurs in approximately 0.239

Cardiovascular Interventions in Clinical Practice. Edited by Jürgen Haase, Hans-Joachim Schäfers, Horst Sievert and Ron Waksman. © 2010 Blackwell Publishing.

per 1000 live births [3]. It accounts for 7% of all congenital heart diseases [4] and exhibits a slight male predominance of 1.5:1 [5]. In patients with Turner's syndrome (45,XO), the frequency of aortic coarctation can be 15% or higher [6].

The etiology of aortic coarctation remains elusive. Two main theories have been proposed. The flow hypothesis contends that decreased blood flow due to left-sided obstruction *in utero* leads to underdevelopment of the aorta at the level of the isthmus [7]. A second hypothesis, first suggested by Skoda in 1855, purports that ectopic ductal tissue within the aorta, or abnormal extension of ductal tissue from the ductus arteriosus to the aorta, is responsible for the constriction and coarctation of the aorta [8]. However, ductal tissue is not always observed at the coarctation site.

Pathologic findings

Aortic coarctation is classified according to its relationship to the insertion of the ductus or ligamentum arteriosum into the descending aorta [2]. The preductal type occurs immediately proximal to the insertion of the ductus arteriosus and distal to the left subclavian artery. In the postductal type, the constricted portion lies immediately distal to the site of insertion of the ductus or ligamentum arteriosum. Occasionally, the terms para- (Greek) or juxta- (Latin) ductal are used to describe coarctations that are directly opposite to the insertion of the ductus. This classification, however, is arbitrary because the coarctation site may shift from pre- to post ductal as the aortic arch grows during postnatal development. Therefore, the exact relationship of the coarctation to the ductus or ligamentum may not actually represent a true difference in the origin, but rather the stage of evolution of the aortic coarctation. This phenomenon may explain why coarctations in newborns are predominantly proximal to the ductus, while in older children the coarctations are often distal to the ligamentum.

Any type of coarctation may be associated with an open or closed ductus. Preductal coarctation is typically seen in infants and is often accompanied by a patent ductus that is in continuity with the descending aorta. Moreover, it is frequently associated with other congenital cardiac anomalies. One study in infants with congestive heart failure found an overall incidence of associated malformation to be approximately 70% [9]. In

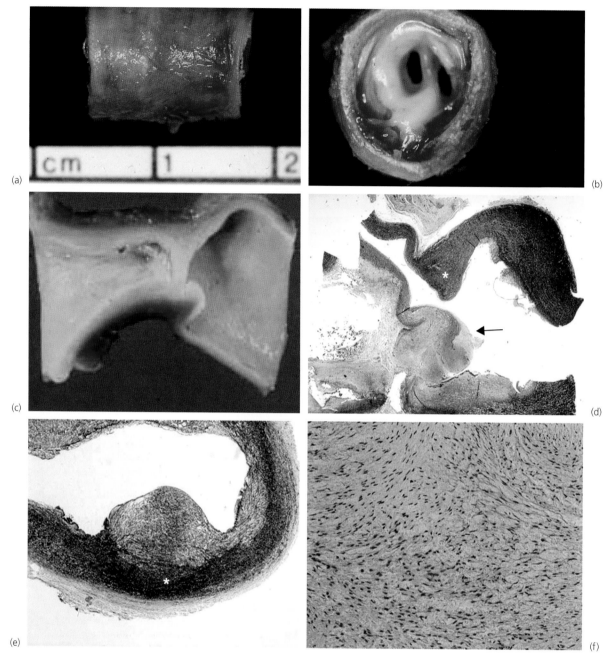

Figure 45.1 Coarctation of the aorta. (a) External view showing an aortic wall of normal caliber. (b) Internal view showing marked coarctation with white intimal proliferation at the site of the coarctation. (c) A different case showing the ridge-like projection of the aortic media at the site of coarctation. (d) Movat pentachrome stain showing thickening (asterisk) of the media and secondary intimal proliferation (arrow) at the site of the coarctation (×1.25). (e) Elastic tissue stain showing thickening of the media with disorganization (asterisk) of the elastic tissue at the site of coarctation (×1.25). (f) Hematoxylin and eosin stain showing thickening and disorganization of smooth muscle (×200).

another study, an even higher association with anomalies was found at autopsy. Hypoplasia of the aortic arch is the most common associated malformation, followed by ventricular septal defect, subaortic stenosis, and mitral valve anomalies [9]. In older children and adults, the postductal type is more common. The ductus is often closed with development of collateral circulation. This latter type is less commonly associated with other congenital cardiac anomalies, except for bicuspid aortic valve, which is common with both types of coarctation. Up to 10% of patients with aortic coarctations have detectable intracranial aneurysms, usually in the circle of Willis [10].

Grossly, the zone of greatest obstruction is often short and well defined (Fig. 45.1a–c). All sides of the aortic wall except the caudal aspect, where the ductus inserts, show constriction giving a concave outer contour. However, the luminal constriction is considerably more severe than what is apparent from the external surface of the aorta [2]. Hence, a cursory examination of only the outside of the aorta may miss the presence of a coarctation. The narrowed portion initially consists of an infolding from the aortic media that forms an obstructive ridge (Fig. 45.1b–d). Extending from this ridge is an additional shelf of tissue that further obstructs the lumen like a diaphragm. The size of the diaphragmatic opening determines the degree of blockage.

Microscopic features of aortic coarctation correlate with the gross appearance (Fig. 45.1c and d). The aortic media is significantly thickened with disorganization of the smooth muscle and elastic tissue components (Fig. 45.1d–f). In addition, cystic changes with fragmentation of elastin and increased collagen deposition may be observed in the aortic media [9]. Overlying the thickened media, there is intimal hyperplasia comprised largely of concentric layers of collagen (Fig. 45.1d), with variable amount of elastic tissue and smooth muscle cells present. The intimal thickening is believed to develop after infancy as this is minimal or absent in newborns. The aortic wall distal to the coarctation is often thinned and the luminal surface may show a corrugated patch due to fibrointimal thickening, resulting from a so-called "jet lesion."

Natural history

The prognosis for an unoperated aortic coarctation is poor. Patients may survive an average of 35 years with a mortality rate of 25% by the age of 20 years, 50% by 32 years, 75% by 46 years, and 90% by 58 years [11]. The most common cause of death is congestive heart failure, followed by aortic rupture, bacterial endocarditis, and intracranial hemorrhage. Aortic coarctation may recur after surgical repair or endovascular intervention, especially when correction is performed at a younger age.

Aortic aneurysms

The elasticity and tensile strength of the aorta are mainly determined by its medial layer, which is composed of smooth muscle cells, 40–70 layers of elastic fibers, and extracellular matrix proteins. Any disease or process that damages the aortic media can lead to abnormal dilation of the aorta. Terms used to describe enlargement of the aortic lumen, include dilation, ectasia, aneurysm, and pseudoaneurysm. Conventionally, an aneurysm is defined as a dilation of an aortic segment that exceeds 50% of its normal diameter [12]. A more stringent criterion requires dilation of >100% of the normal aortic size [13]. A true aneurysm contains all three aortic layers in its wall. In contrast, the wall of a pseudoaneurysm, which is actually a localized perforation, comprises only the adventitia and peri-aortic fibroconnective tissue. Aneurysms are further classified according to their etiology, gross morphology, and anatomic location. A fusiform aneurysm has a spindle-shaped

appearance and involves the entire circumference of the aorta. On the other hand, a saccular aneurysm only affects part of the aortic circumference, resulting in a spherical outpouching of the aortic wall (Fig. 45.2a). Moreover, aneurysms may involve the entire length of the aorta. During the early twentieth century, thoracic aortic aneurysms (TAAs) were twice as common as abdominal aortic aneurysms (AAAs) owing to an increased frequency of infectious TAAs, primarily syphilitic [14]. With the dramatic decline in the incidence of syphilitic aneurysms by the mid twentieth century, AAAs overtook and became much more common than TAAs. Although TAAs and AAAs share certain morphologic features in the aorta, there are differences in the underlying pathogenesis, etiology, molecular mechanism, genetic susceptibility, natural history, and clinical management between the two entities [15].

According to Laplace's law, which states that wall tension is proportional to the square of the radius, aortic aneurysms are prone to rupture or dissect. Without medical and surgical interventions, most patients with aneurysms eventually succumb to the fatal consequences of aortic rupture or dissection. Consequently, surveillance imaging of patients with aortic aneurysms is performed so that prophylactic repair of the aortic aneurysm can be performed before it reaches a critical diameter. Between 13 000 and 17 000 patients in the USA die annually from aortic aneurysm and/or dissection [16,17].

Thoracic aortic aneurysms

Thoracic aortic aneurysms are localized aortic dilations above the diaphragm. The normal diameter of the thoracic aorta gradually decreases along its length. "Normal" aortic diameter varies with age, sex, and body surface area [18,19]. Although absolute values have been used to predict the risk of aneurysm rupture, more recent studies have focused on criteria based on the aortic diameter normalized for body surface area [18]. The incidence of TAAs has been estimated at 6 per 100 000 per year in the early 1980s [20] and continues to increase dramatically [21]. The age-adjusted death rate for TAAs was about 2 per 100 000 per year in the 1980s and 1990s [16].

Thoracic aortic aneurysms may affect one or more thoracic aortic segments, with approximately 60% occurring in the ascending aorta (including the aortic root), 40% in the descending aorta, and 10% in the aortic arch [22]. Pathologically, ascending TAAs are frequently associated with cystic medial degeneration, whereas descending TAAs are usually due to atherosclerosis, similar to AAAs (discussed later).

Pathogenesis and risk factors

A variety of diseases can injure the aortic wall reducing its elasticity and tensile strength. These physical properties of the aorta are mainly determined by the aortic media, which can be weakened by physiologic and pathologic changes in the media, intima, adventitia, or the nourishing arteries of

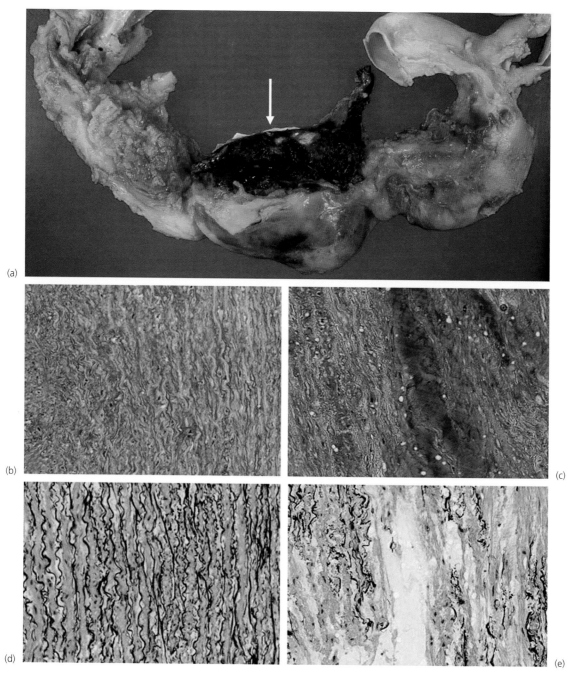

Figure 45.2 Aortic aneurysm. (a) Entire aorta showing multiple saccular aneurysms. The hemorrhagic appearing region (arrow) in the second aneurysm of the descending thoracic aorta corresponds to the site of rupture and fatal exsanguination. (b) Periodic acid-Schiff (PAS) stain of a normal appearing aortic wall. (c) PAS stain of aorta wall with cystic medial necrosis: note increased blue staining extracellular matrix. (d) Elastic tissue stain of a normal aorta. (e) Elastic tissue stain of an aorta with cystic medial degeneration, note the loss and fragmentation of elastic tissue (b–e, all ×200).

the aorta, the vasa vasorum. Among all the blood vessels, the thoracic aorta has the highest content of elastic fibers. Smooth muscle cells are arranged longitudinally among the concentric lamellae of elastic fibers with collagen and proteoglycans filling in the spaces between them. Fragmentation and/or loss of elastic fibers and smooth muscle cells are common findings in surgically resected and autopsied TAAs.

Age

There are significant age-related morphologic, biochemical, molecular, and biomechanical changes in the aorta. With increasing age, aortic length and circumference, as well as intimal thickness, increase; however, the medial thickness remains relatively stable. In addition, the aging aorta frequently exhibits medial degeneration, which is more commonly identified in TAAs and familial connective tissue disorders [23]. Fragmentation of elastin, with concomitant increase in collagen and proteoglycans, results in loss of distensibility and a decrease in tensile strength. These age-related changes are accelerated by hypertension and atherosclerosis [24].

Genetic factors

Inherited disorders with or without associated connective tissue diseases may affect the aorta [25]. These disorders may result in structural changes of the aortic media that predispose not only to the development of aneurysms, but also dissection.

Marfan's syndrome

Marfan's syndrome (MFS) is an autosomal dominant disorder of the connective tissue caused by genetic mutations in the fibrillin (FBN)-1 gene. One-quarter of patients with Marfan's syndrome have sporadic mutations with no known family history. FBN-1 is a large, cysteine-rich glycoprotein that is a major component of microfibrils surrounding the elastin protein core [26]. Interestingly, FBN-1 mutations have been identified in patients who do not meet the clinical criteria for the diagnosis of Marfan's syndrome, but have isolated presentations of related connective tissue disorders, such as skeletal abnormalities, aortic aneurysm, or ectopia lentis. Hundreds of mutations have been discovered in the FBN-1 gene.

Cardiovascular manifestations of Marfan's syndrome include mitral valve prolapse and insufficiency, aortic valve insufficiency, and thoracic aortic aneurysm and/or dissection. The histologic appearance of elastic tissue fragmentation and medial degeneration in the aorta of Marfan's syndrome patients suggest that elastin deficiency is the primary problem [22]. Recent studies, however, have discovered the regulatory role of FBN-1 protein on transforming growth factor (TGF)-β signaling. The cysteine-rich domains of FBN-1 share significant homology to the latent TGF-β binding protein and are able to bind TGF-β. The mutated FBN-1 protein loses its ability to interact with TGF-β, leading to enhanced TGF-β signaling [27]. In a murine Marfan's syndrome model, inhibition of TGF-β activation by losartan, an angiotensin II receptor and TGF-β antagonist, arrests aneurysm progression [28]. A randomized clinical trial has been designed to assess the efficacy of losartan in MFS patients [29].

Ehlers–Danlos syndrome

Ehlers–Danlos syndrome is a group of rare genetic connective tissue disorders with at least nine different forms. Vascular (type IV) Ehlers–Danlos syndrome is due to an autosomal dominant mutation in type III collagen, resulting in failure of amino-proteinases to cleave procollagen. Consequently, collagen synthesis is impaired, leading to vascular fragility, which manifests as aortic aneurysm and/or dissection [26].

Familial thoracic aortic aneurysm and dissection syndrome

A large database analysis revealed that 19% of patients with thoracic aortic aneurysm and/or dissection of this disease, and no other connective tissue disorders, had a family history [30]. The first locus for familial thoracic aortic aneurysm and dissection (TAAD) syndrome was mapped to the long arm of chromosome 5 (5q13–140) and termed the TAAD1 locus [31]. The same research group further linked two more loci (3p24–25 and 11q23–24) to this syndrome [32,33]. Therefore, genetic heterogeneity exists among patients with familial TAAD syndrome.

Turner's syndrome

Turner's syndrome may be associated with cardiovascular anomalies including aortic coarctation, bicuspid aortic valve, and aortic aneurysm and dissection. Approximately 40% of Turner's syndrome patients have aortic root dilation [34]. Since Turner's syndrome patients have short stature, their aortic diameters should be indexed to the body surface area. Aortic dissection occurs at an annual rate of 618 cases per 100 000 patients with Turner's syndrome [19].

Congenital cardiovascular anomalies

Aortic aneurysm and dissection can be associated with several congenital cardiovascular anomalies. Traditionally, hemodynamic disturbances in these conditions accounted for these associations. However, recent data revealed that medial degenerative changes were prevalent in patients with a variety of congenital heart diseases [35]. Bicuspid aortic valves have the highest association with aortic dilation. Even in young patients with normally functioning bicuspid aortic valves, 52% have aortic dilation [36]. Cystic medial degeneration has been identified in 75% of patients with bicuspid aortic valves [37].

Also commonly associated with other congenital cardiovascular anomalies, the sinus of Valsalva aneurysm is more often a congenital defect of fusion between the aortic media and the fibrous annulus of the aortic valve. Rare cases of acquired sinus of Valsalva aneurysms are caused by infectious endocarditis and syphilis. Weakness in the sinus wall results in focal dilation or formation of a blind pouch. The vast majority of these aneurysms are located in the right sinus [38]. Most patients are asymptomatic before rupture. Common sites of rupture include the right atrium and right ventricular outflow tract.

Infection

Infection was once the most common cause of TAAs, particularly syphilitic (or luetic) aneurysms, which are rarely seen in modern medical practice. Syphilitic infection primarily affects the vasa vasorum of the ascending thoracic aorta, causing obliterative endarteritis with concomitant ischemic injury of the aortic media (Fig. 45.3a–c). Destruction of elastin and smooth muscle

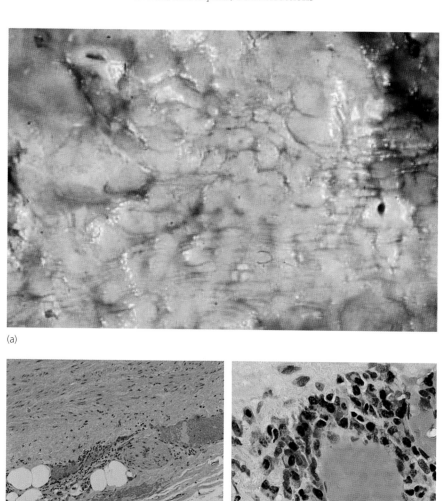

Figure 45.3 Examples of aortitis. (a) Typical tree barking appearance of an aorta with syphilitic aortitis; (b) Adventitia showing chronic inflammation and thickening of the vaso vasorum (H&E; hematoxylin and eosin ×00). (c) Higher power of (b) showing that many of the inflammatory cells are plasma cells, a typical finding in syphilitic aortitis (H&E, ×400). (d) An aorta with giant cell aortitis, note multinucleated giant cell (arrow) with surrounding inflammation (H&E, ×200). (e) Elastic stain of aorta with giant cell aortitis showing marked segmental loss (double head arrow) of elastic tissue with overlying intimal fibrosis (*; ×40).

cells leads to fibrosis and aortic dilation. Medial fibrosis and constriction result in longitudinal wrinkling of the intima giving a "tree-bark" gross appearance (Fig. 45.3a).

Mycotic aortic aneurysms result from bacterial or fungal infections of the aorta via implantation on the intimal surface, embolization into the vasa vasorum, contiguous extension of an adjacent infection, or traumatic inoculation [39].

Staphylococcus aureus is the most common pathogen. Recently, *Salmonella* spp. have emerged as frequent isolates in infected aortic aneurysms.

Aortitis

Two common vasculitides with aortic involvement are Takayasu arteritis in younger patients and giant cell arteritis in older patients. The former typically causes luminal narrowing, but up to 30% of cases develop aortic aneurysms [40], which may occur in the acute inflammatory or late sclerotic stages of the disease [22]; the latter typically involves the temporal or other cranial arteries. When the aorta is involved, the media shows focal granulomatous inflammation (Fig. 45.3d and e). In a 50-year follow-up study, 18% of patients with giant cell arteritis developed aortic aneurysm and/or dissection [41].

Chronic aortic dissection

A minority of patients may survive an aortic dissection. The destruction of the aortic wall by dissection and subsequent healing by fibrosis further undermine the structural integrity of the aorta. Consequently, patients with chronic aortic dissection are at high risk for aortic dilation and rupture.

Trauma and procedural injuries

Partial or complete transection of the aorta after penetrating or nonpenetrating traumatic injuries may affect the descending thoracic aorta just beyond the insertion site of the ligamentum arteriosum. This can lead to true or false aneurysms. Surgical and endovascular procedures may also injure the aortic wall, leading to aneurysmal dilation.

Pathologic findings

Multiple large series have detailed the pathologic findings of ascending TAAs. However, the pathology of descending TAAs has not been investigated on a large scale as they are presumed to be associated with atherosclerosis and have a similar pathogenesis and morphology to AAAs. The histologic appearance of ascending TAAs ranges from normal to complete loss of the media. The most common microscopic finding in ascending TAAs is medial degeneration, which is identified in 50–70% of cases [42–44]. Various terminologies such as cystic medial degeneration and cystic medial necrosis have been used to describe the histologic findings in TAAs. In fact, there are no true cysts, but rather, areas filled with basophilic, amorphous extracellular matrix consisting of proteoglycans (Fig. 45.2b and c). Whether true media necrosis is present is still debatable; however, histologic examination often demonstrates changes in smooth muscle cells, such as loss of nuclei and condensed, hypereosinophilic cytoplasm that are characteristic of coagulative-type necrosis. In addition, the aortic medial exhibits prominent fragmentation and loss of elastin and areas of fibrosis (Fig. 45.2d and e). In one study, collagen and elastin have been shown to be significantly reduced in aortas of patients with TAAs compared with that of controls [45]. Matrix metalloproteinases (MMPs), particularly MMP-2 and MMP-9, are increased at the leading edge of the medial degeneration, suggesting that they play a role in the remodeling of the extracellular matrix in TAAs [46]. The overall density of smooth muscle cells in the aortic media in patients with TAA remains controversial. He *et al.* [47] have found that smooth muscle cells in TAAs undergo apoptosis, leading

to a decrease in their density. However, other investigators have reported that the density is not reduced [46] or even increased [45]. Although inflammation is not apparent in medial degeneration by conventional histology, immunohistochemical stains have demonstrated an increase in cluster of differentiation CD3- and CD68-positive cells in the media of TAAs [47]. The degree of medial degeneration varies greatly and may not correlate with the severity of TAAs. A grading scheme was developed to compare medial degeneration between normal and diseased aortas [23,42] Medial degeneration is most severe in MFS patients; however, normal media may be seen as well. Consequently, there are no qualitative differences in medial degeneration between normal and diseased aortas [23].

Other pathologic findings in TAAs include aortic dissection (Fig. 45.4a and b), aortitis, syphilitic changes, and atherosclerosis. A recent study showed that up to 18% of aortas in patients with TAAs were normal [44]. Aneurysmal dilation of the ascending aorta can lead to aortic valve insufficiency. The term, annulo-aortic ectasia is often used by surgeons to denote this condition resulting from idiopathic or MFS-related medial degeneration.

Natural history

Most patients with TAAs are asymptomatic and identified by imaging studies performed for other unrelated clinical indications. Although the normal aorta may grow at a rate of 1 mm every 10 years, TAAs grow at a rate of 1 mm per year [48]. Larger and dissected aneurysms tend to enlarge at a faster rate [49]. Moreover, the rate of rupture and/or dissection is related to the size of the aneurysm. When a thoracic aneurysm exceeds 6 cm, the annual rate of rupture or dissection is over 6.9% and the mortality rate is at least 11.8% per year [48]. Elective surgical repair and endovascular stent placement restore the survival of TAA patients to near normal. For smaller aneurysms, clinical follow-up with radiologic imaging is recommended [13].

Abdominal aortic aneurysms

Abdominal aortic aneurysms can occur in any aortic segment below the diaphragm. As these aneurysms are so commonly present between the infrarenal aorta and the aortoiliac bifurcation, the term AAA is often clinically restricted to define an aneurysm at this site. The normal diameter of the infrarenal abdominal aorta is approximately 1.5–2.4 cm. By convention, an AAA is diagnosed when the infrarenal aorta dilates to 3.0 cm or more [50]. The prevalence of AAAs range from 1% to >10% and is dependent on age, sex, and race.

Pathogenesis and risk factors

Traditionally, AAAs are considered to be due to atherosclerosis, since they are invariably associated with severe atherosclerotic

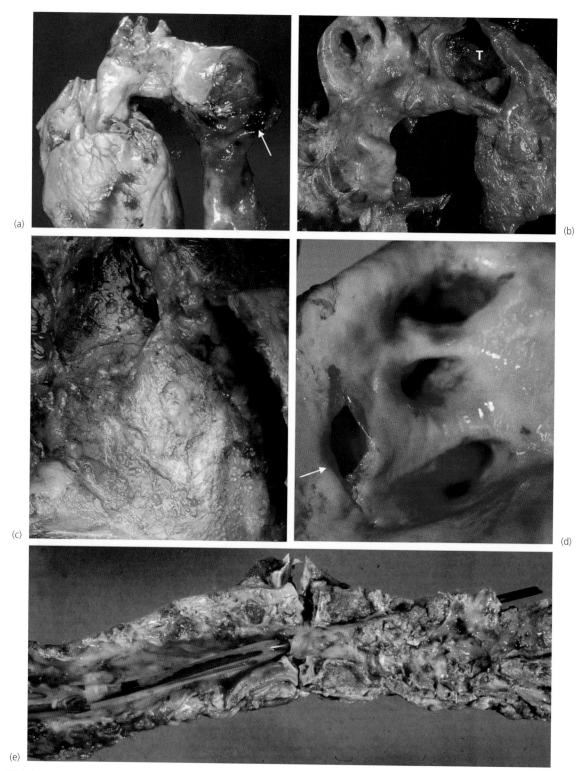

Figure 45.4 Aneurysms and dissection. (a) Unusual ruptured atherosclerotic saccular aneurysm (arrow) of the descending thoracic aorta just distal to the aortic arch. (b) Internal view of the aorta showing mural thrombus (T) within the aneurysm that has ruptured. (c) Distended pericardial sac that appears blue because of copious blood surrounding the heart in a patient with tamponade secondary to a ruptured type A dissection. (d) Type A dissection with intimal tear (arrow) just proximal to the great vessels. (e) Iatrogenic dissection due to placement of an intraaortic balloon pump in a severely atherosclerotic aorta.

damage of the aortic wall. However, recent clinical and basic research investigations have suggested that the pathogenesis of aneurysms differs at least in part from that responsible for occlusive atherosclerotic disease [15,50] First of all, only a small percentage of patients with abdominal atherosclerosis develop AAAs [15]. This suggests that even if atherosclerosis plays a pathogenetic role in the development of AAAs, it is only a prerequisite and additional factors are likely required for aneurysm formation. Second, proteinase inhibitors, such as TIMP-2 and PAI-1, are expressed at lower levels in AAAs than just atherosclerotic abdominal aortas alone, suggesting that there is differential remodeling of connective tissue between these two entities [51]. Finally, the inflammatory response in AAAs is usually transmural and primarily involves the outer medial and adventitial layers, compared with atherosclerosis, which tends to involve the intimal layer [15].

Proteolytic enzymes, mainly MMPs whose activity is inhibited by proteinase inhibitors, TIMP-2 and PAI-1, degrade elastic and collagen fibers. A shift in the balance of proteinases and their inhibitors toward proteolysis is likely involved in the weakening of the aortic wall during AAA formation [52]. Genetic manipulation in mice to overexpress or knockout MMPs and their inhibitors provide further evidence to support the role of proteolysis in the pathogenesis of AAA [12,15].

Genetic susceptibility

Familial clustering of AAAs indicates that genetic variation plays certain roles in AAA formation [25]. The underlying genetic defects and inheritance patterns of AAAs are not as well defined as that of TAAs. The frequency of AAAs in first-degree relatives is 15–19% compared with only 1–3% in the general population [50].

Smoking

Smoking is the strongest risk factor associated with the development of AAAs. The prevalence of AAAs in tobacco smokers is >4–8 times that of lifelong nonsmokers [50,53,54]. The rate of aneurysm expansion is also higher in current smokers than in nonsmokers (0.16 vs. 0.09 cm per year for small aneurysms; 0.28 vs. 0.25 cm per year for large aneurysms) [55,56].

Other risk factors

Besides tobacco smoking and genetic susceptibility, other important risk factors include age, sex, race, and hypertension [57]. AAAs are more common in Caucasians than in blacks, and more frequent in males than females. The prevalence of AAAs is about 4.0–8.9% in men and 1.0–2.2% in women between the ages of 50 and 80 years [58–60]. Of those in their eighth decade, the incidence of AAAs reached over 10% [61]. For hypertension, high diastolic blood pressure increases the prevalence of AAAs by 30–40% [54].

Pathologic findings

Abdominal aortic aneurysms are often single and frequently located between the renal arteries and the aorto-iliac bifurcation. Fusiform aneurysms that involve the entire aortic circumference are most common. A large laminated thrombus is frequently identified within the dilated lumen. Occasionally, AAAs can extend upward to the origin of the renal, superior, or inferior mesenteric arteries, or downward to involve the iliac arteries. When this occurs, narrowing or occlusion of these vessels by direct pressure or mural thrombi can lead to renal, intestinal, or limb ischemia. Severe atherosclerosis is generally present in the aorta adjacent to the aneurysm. The wall of an AAA generally contains atheromatous ulcers with calcification. The medial layer is often significantly thinned, with fragmentation and decreased concentration of elastic fibers [62]. There is also a slight increase in collagen deposition. Moreover, smooth muscle cells undergo apoptosis, resulting in decreased numbers of cells [63]. Inflammation is invariably present and mostly comprised CD4+ T-cells followed by B-cells. In contrast to the Th1-predominant immune response seen in atherosclerosis, AAAs exhibit a Th2-predominant immune response promoted by increased expression of interleukin (IL)-4, IL-5, and IL-10 [64]. MMP-1, MMP-2, MMP-3, and MMP-9 are increased in AAAs compared with normal aortic tissue, which accelerates the turnover of various extracellular matrix proteins, leading to progressive weakening of the aortic wall [65].

An inflammatory aneurysm of the abdominal aorta is most likely a variant of advanced AAAs rather than a distinct entity. It is characterized by dense adventitial fibrosis that extends and entraps adjacent adipose tissue, nerves, ganglia, and lymph nodes [66,67]. There is often a heavy inflammatory infiltrate with abundant lymphocytes and plasma cells. The inner surface of the aneurysmal wall consists of complex atherosclerotic plaques. The aortic media is often destroyed and replaced by fibrosis. The etiology of inflammatory AAA is unclear. One theory proposes that atherosclerotic involvement of the adventitia after complete medial destruction elicits an inflammatory reaction and fibrosis.

Natural history

Abdominal aortic aneurysms grow at an average rate of 0.26 cm per year [56]. Their expansion rate is not related to age or sex, but is strongly associated with the baseline diameter and smoking [56,68]. Aneurysms with a diameter of 2.8–3.9 cm and 4.0–4.5 cm grow 0.19 cm and 0.27 cm per year, respectively. When an aneurysm is greater than 4.5 cm, it grows at a much faster rate of 0.35 cm per year [56], or even at 0.7 cm per year [69]. The size of the aneurysm is also associated with the risk of rupture, which has a high mortality rate [69]. For aneurysms smaller than 5.0 cm, the annual risk of rupture is less than 1.5%. When aneurysms reach 5.0–5.9 cm they rupture at an annual rate of 6.5%. Larger aneurysms have a greater likelihood of rupture. When aneurysms rupture, 25% of patients die before reaching a hospital and 51% die at the hospital without any surgery [22]. For patients with surgery, the operative mortality rate is 46%. Therefore, the overall 30-day survival for ruptured aneurysms is only 11%. For an elective aneurysm repair, the mean 30-day mortality rate varies between 1.1% and 7.0% [50]. With advances in surgical techniques, the operative mortality rate is now well under 3%. The mortality rate for endovascular repair is even lower, at around 1.8%. Thus, the goal of clinical intervention is to have elective surgical or endovascular stent repair before patients have a significant risk of rupture.

Aortic dissection

Aortic dissection is the separation of the medial layer of the aortic wall. In classic aortic dissection, there is an intimal tear followed by antegrade and retrograde separation of the media, usually between the inner two-thirds and outer one-third. The extent of involvement is quite variable and can involve only a small aortic segment, or the entire aorta and its major branches, such as the coronary, carotid, subclavian, renal, iliofemoral, and anterior spinal arteries. Aortic dissection is an uncommon and fatal disease, if left untreated [14]. There is really no effective medical therapy or proven preventive measure [70]. Without surgical treatment, the mortality rate within the first 48 h increases 1% every hour and reaches 75% by the second week after the onset of symptoms. Despite new diagnostic tools and advancements in surgical treatment and endovascular interventions, the mortality rate remains high at 27% [71]. Each year, there are about two thousand new cases in the USA [72]. Aortic dissection diagnosed less than 2 weeks after the onset of symptoms is considered acute. When patients survive for >2 weeks without any corrective treatment, the process is then regarded as chronic.

Pathogenesis and risk factors

Currently, there is still considerable uncertainty regarding the pathogenesis of aortic dissection. One theory proposed >30 years ago considered the intimal tear to be the primary lesion, which provided an entry for blood under pressure to enter and split the aortic media [73]. Indeed, Larson and Edwards [74] reported that all of their 161 autopsied cases with aortic dissection demonstrated an intimal tear. Wilson and Hutchins [75], however, found that only 87% of their 204 cases with aortic dissection exhibited an intimal tear. They proposed that bleeding from the vasa vasorum caused an intramural hematoma and subsequent medial dissection, which could then rupture into the lumen to create an intimal tear. Clearly, damage to the vasa vasorum can cause medial necrosis of the aortic wall [76]. With modern imaging techniques, the entity of "intramural hematoma" without an associated intimal tear has been confirmed. Approximately 28–47% of patients who have only an intramural hematoma can progress into acute dissection, thus indicating that intramural hematomas may be precursor lesions to the classic aortic dissection [77].

Medial damage by a variety of causes has been advocated to be the structural basis of aortic dissection [77,78]. "Medial degeneration," consisting of loss of smooth muscle cells, medial fibrosis, loss and fragmentation of elastic fibers, and increased extracellular matrix, is a common histologic finding. However, severe medial degeneration is only identified in a minority of patients with aortic dissection. Moreover, structurally normal aortas may dissect [74]. When compared with the normal aging aorta, dissected aortas show similar structural changes [23]. Certainly, increased wall tension can induce aortic dilation and dissection. The ascending aorta endures the highest pressure, and thus the greatest wall tension according to Laplace's law, from cardiac systole owing to its proximity to the heart. Consequently, the ascending aorta is the most common site of dissection. In addition, certain connective tissue diseases predispose to dissection. In patients without such predisposing conditions, the majority will have systemic hypertension.

The incidence of aortic dissection is estimated to be 2.6–3.5 per 100 000 person-years [78]. Aortic dissection occurs twice as commonly in males than in females, with an average age at presentation of approximately 63 years [71]; the most common risk factor is hypertension [74]. However, other recognized predisposing factors include genetic susceptibility, congenital cardiac anomalies, atherosclerosis, previous cardiac or aortic surgery, aortitis, and a pre-existing aortic aneurysm.

Hypertension
Over 70% of patients with aortic dissection have a history of systemic hypertension [71,79]. However, only 34% of patients younger than 40 years of age have a history of hypertension. Medial degeneration is accelerated in hypertensive patients.

Genetic factors
Genetic disorders that contribute to TAAs are also applicable to aortic dissections. In particular, Marfan's syndrome accounts for 6–9% of all aortic dissections. About 50% of patients less than 40 years of age with aortic dissection will have Marfan's syndrome [80]. Aortic dissection is a major cause of mortality in patients with Marfan's syndrome, accounting for >40% of deaths [74].

Congenital anomalies
Approximately 9% of patients with aortic dissection have bicuspid aortic valves [80,81]. The relative risk of aortic dissection in patients with bicuspid aortic valves is nine times that of normal and further doubles in patients with unicuspid aortic valves. Aortic coarctation is associated with upper body hypertension and an increased risk of aortic dissection.

Trauma

Aortic dissection and rupture can occur with different types of trauma to the aorta, including iatrogenic trauma (Fig. 45.4e) due to catheters and intra-aortic balloon pumps [82].

Classification

The DeBakey classification subdivides aortic dissection into three types based on the origin of the intimal tear and the site of involvement [83]. A type I dissection exhibits an intimal tear (Fig. 45.4d) in the ascending aorta with dissection involving both the ascending and ascending aorta. A type II dissection also has an intimal tear in the ascending aorta, but the dissection is only limited to the descending aorta. A type III dissection demonstrates an intimal tear in the descending aorta and can be further subdivided into types IIIa and IIIb. Type IIIa involves only the descending aorta and/or aortic arch, whereas type IIIb extends to the ascending aorta. The simpler Stanford classification only considers the site of involvement, and divides aortic dissection into two types, A and B [84]. Any aortic dissection that involves the ascending aorta is classified as type A, and type B (Fig. 45.4a and b) signifies involvement that is limited to the descending aorta. Clinical management and prognosis is dependent on whether or not the proximal aorta is involved rather than the origin of the intimal tear. Consequently, the Stanford classification is more practical and used more often clinically.

Staging

Intramural hematomas and penetrating atherosclerotic ulcers are considered variants of aortic dissection [77,85]. However, whether these variants represent pathogenetically distinct entities, precursor lesions, or classic aortic dissections in the early stages of their evolution is unclear [85,86]. With modern imaging techniques, these variants are detected more frequently and have been observed to progress into classic aortic dissection [86–88]. A novel classification proposed by Svensson *et al.* [89] to denote five stages of aortic dissection has been adopted by the European Society of Cardiology task force on the diagnosis and management of aortic dissection [90]:

• class I classic dissection of the aortic wall with an intimal flap and false lumen;

• class II separation of the aortic wall with hematoma and without an intimal tear;

• class III limited dissection without hematoma and with an intimal tear and eccentric bulge of the aorta;

• class IV atherosclerotic ulcer, usually penetrating to the adventitia with a localized hematoma; and

• class V traumatic and iatrogenic dissection.

Pathologic findings

Type A dissection is far more common than type B. In a series of 161 necropsy cases of aortic dissection, Larson and Edwards [74] found that 121 (75%) were type A and 40 (25%) were type B. Furthermore, all cases exhibited an intimal tear. In

contrast, only 13% of patients in the autopsy series by Wilson and Hutchins [75] had no entry tear. Despite modern imaging studies, intimal tears are less frequently documented in clinical studies [88,91]. This may be a reflection of the relative insensitivity of the imaging modality to detect an intimal tear or a difference in severity and evolutionary stage of aortic dissection seen in clinical versus autopsy series. Patients with classic aortic dissection usually deteriorate rapidly and are more frequently seen at autopsy. In type A dissection, the tear may occur anywhere; however, the primary intimal tear (Fig. 45.4d) is usually located on the right anterior aspect of the ascending aorta over the right and noncoronary cusps, 1–3 cm above the sinotubular junction. In type B dissection, the primary intimal tear is commonly seen in the descending aorta distal to the left subclavian artery. It is usually transverse, 1–5 cm in length with sharp, jagged edges. It may also be diagonal or irregular, and, occasionally, it involves the entire circumference of the aorta. In addition, multiple tears and perforations of the aorta may be found. The dissection may propagate antegradely to the aorto-iliac bifurcation in the abdomen or extend in a retrograde fashion to involve the aortic root or the coronary ostia, which may block coronary blood flow leading to myocardial infarction. The thin-walled false lumen (Fig. 45.5b) created by the dissection may rupture into the pericardial cavity (Fig. 45.4c), mediastinum, pleural space, or retroperitoneal cavity, causing massive hemorrhage or cardiac tamponade. Occasionally, the blood re-ruptures into the aortic lumen, thus producing a second intimal tear and a communicating false vascular channel known as a "double-barreled aorta" (Fig. 45.5a) i.e., the aorta now has two patent lumens with blood flow, rather than just one.

Microscopically, various degrees of medial degeneration can be seen [81]; however, severe medial degeneration is only observed in 18% of cases [74]. Severe medial degeneration is more commonly present in younger patients with MFS or congenital cardiac anomalies. In chronic dissection, the hematoma is absorbed and replaced by granulation and fibrous tissue, resulting in a "healed" dissection that can be detected histologically (Fig. 45.5c).

Intramural hematoma

Aortic dissection without an intimal tear produces an intramural hematoma (Fig. 45.5d). An intramural hematoma may be initiated by infarction of the aortic media or caused by rupture of the vasa vasorum. The prevalence of an intramural hematoma varies from 10% to 30% [88,91]. Progression to classic aortic dissection occurs in 28–47% of the patients, and 21–47% of patients are associated with aortic rupture [77]. In about 10% of patients, the hematoma is reabsorbed, replaced by granulation tissue and healed by fibrosis.

Penetrating atherosclerotic ulcer

Rupture of an atherosclerotic plaque may produce a crater-like defect in the aortic media. It is usually located in the

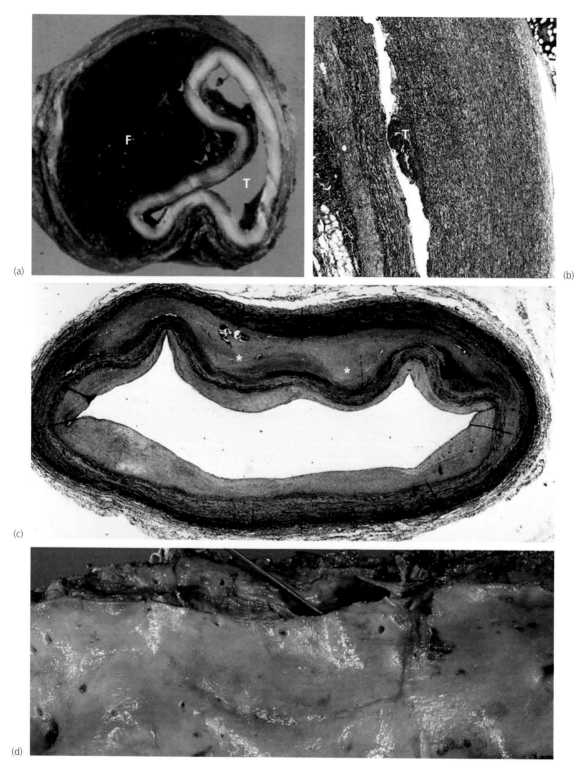

Figure 45.5 Aortic dissection. (a) Cross-section of a dissected aorta with marked narrowing of the true lumen (T) due to large hematoma in false lumen (F). (b) Trichrome stain of an aortic dissection showing hematoma (T) in the false lumen (×40). (c) Movat pentachrome stain showing healed dissection: note the scar tissue (*) within the media with associated intimal hyperplasia (×1.25). (d) A gross example of an intramural hematoma that has ruptured: note there is no intimal tear but there is a probe in the false lumen at the site of the intramural hematoma.

descending aorta in an area with severe atherosclerosis. The prevalence of penetrating atherosclerotic ulcer is approximately 6% [92]. Aortic rupture occurs in >38% of cases [93]. Another common complication is distal embolization of the atherosclerotic debris.

Natural history

Aortic dissection is difficult to clinically diagnose. Symptoms and physical findings vary greatly depending on the site and extent of arterial involvement. Misdiagnosis and inappropriate treatment of acute aortic dissection occur frequently, despite major advances in noninvasive imaging techniques [94]. Approximately 28% of aortic dissections were not diagnosed clinically before postmortem examination [79]. Many patients die before ever reaching the hospital. The overall in-hospital mortality for aortic dissection is approximately 27% (35% for type A and 15% for type B) [71]. The clinical management and outcome are dependent on whether or not the ascending aorta is involved. In type A dissection, >70% of patients are managed surgically with an operative mortality of approximately 26% [71,95,96]. The 1-year and 3-year survival rates for patients discharged alive is 96.1% and 90.5% with surgery and 88.6% and 68.7% without surgery, respectively [95]. Type B dissections are usually managed medically with a 10.7% mortality. Only about 20% of patients who develop complications undergo surgical repair with an operative mortality rate of 31.4% [71]. Whether type B dissection involves the aortic arch does not affect overall survival [97]. The 3-year survival for patients discharged alive is, respectively, 77.6%, 82.8%, and 76.2% for medical treatment, surgical repair, and endovascular therapy [98]. Clinical treatment, diagnosis, and outcomes are constantly changing and improving with modern imaging techniques and new endovascular stent therapy.

References

1. Aluquin VP, Shutte D, Nihill MR, *et al.* (2003) Normal aortic arch growth and comparison with isolated coarctation of the aorta. *Am J Cardiol* **91**:502–505.
2. Lindesmith GG, Stanton RE, Stiles QR, *et al.* (1971) Coarctation of the thoracic aorta. *Ann Thorac Surg* **11**:482–497.
3. Ferencz C, Rubin JD, McCarter RJ, *et al.* (1985) Congenital heart disease: prevalence at livebirth. The Baltimore–Washington Infant Study. *Am J Epidemiol* **121**:31–36.
4. Izukawa T, Mulholland HC, Rowe RD, *et al.* (1979) Structural heart disease in the newborn. Changing profile: comparison of 1975 with 1965. *Arch Dis Child* **54**(4):281–5.
5. Aboulhosn J & Child JS (2006) Left ventricular outflow obstruction: subaortic stenosis, bicuspid aortic valve, supravalvar aortic stenosis, and coarctation of the aorta. *Circulation* **114**:2412–2422.
6. Clark EB (1984) Neck web and congenital heart defects: a pathogenic association in 45 X-O Turner syndrome? *Teratology* **29**:355–361.
7. Hutchins GM (1971) Coarctation of the aorta explained as a branch-point of the ductus arteriosus. *Am J Pathol* **63**:203–214.
8. Brom AG (1965) Narrowing of the aortic isthmus and enlargement of the mind. *J Thorac Cardiovasc Surg* **50**:166–180.
9. Becker AE (1972) Congenital obstructive malformations of the aortic arch. *Cardiovasc Clin* **4**:1–18.
10. Connolly HM, Huston J 3rd, Brown RD Jr, *et al.* (2003) Intracranial aneurysms in patients with coarctation of the aorta: a prospective magnetic resonance angiographic study of 100 patients. *Mayo Clin Proc* **78**:1491–1499.
11. Campbell M (1970) Natural history of coarctation of the aorta. *Br Heart J* **32**:633–640.
12. Barbour JR, Spinale FG, & Ikonomidis JS (2007) Proteinase systems and thoracic aortic aneurysm progression. *J Surg Res* **139**:292–307.
13. Svensson LG, Kouchoukos NT, Miller DC, *et al.* (2008) Expert consensus document on the treatment of descending thoracic aortic disease using endovascular stent grafts. *Ann Thorac Surg* **85**(1, Supplement 1): S1–S41.
14. Kouchoukos NT & Dougenis D (1997) Surgery of the thoracic aorta. *N Engl J Med* **336**:1876–89.
15. Guo DC, Papke CL, He R, *et al.* (2006) Pathogenesis of thoracic and abdominal aortic aneurysms. *Ann N Y Acad Sci* **1085**:339–352.
16. Gillum RF (1995) Epidemiology of aortic aneurysm in the United States. *J Clin Epidemiol* **48**:1289–98.
17. Minino AM, Heron MP, Murphy SL, *et al.* (2007) Deaths: final data for (2004). *Natl Vital Stat Rep* **55**(19):1–119.
18. Davies RR, Gallo A, Coady MA, *et al.* (2006) Novel measurement of relative aortic size predicts rupture of thoracic aortic aneurysms. *Ann Thorac Surg* **81**:169–77.
19. Matura LA, Ho VB, Rosing DR, *et al.* (2007) Aortic dilatation and dissection in Turner syndrome. *Circulation* **116**:1663–1670.
20. Bickerstaff LK, Pairolero PC, Hollier LH, *et al.* (1982) Thoracic aortic aneurysms: a population-based study. *Surgery* **92**:1103–1108.
21. Olsson C, Thelin S, Stahle E, *et al.* (2006) Thoracic aortic aneurysm and dissection: increasing prevalence and improved outcomes reported in a nationwide population-based study of more than 14 000 cases from 1987 to 2002. *Circulation* **114**:2611–2618.
22. Isselbacher EM (2005) Thoracic and abdominal aortic aneurysms. *Circulation* **111**:816–828.
23. Schlatmann TJ & Becker AE (1977) Pathogenesis of dissecting aneurysm of aorta. Comparative histopathologic study of significance of medial changes. *Am J Cardiol* **39**:21–26.
24. Virmani R, Avolio AP, Mergner WJ, *et al.* (1991) Effect of aging on aortic morphology in populations with high and low prevalence of hypertension and atherosclerosis. Comparison between occidental and Chinese communities. *Am J Pathol* **139**:1119–1129.
25. Kuivaniemi H, Platsoucas CD, & Tilson MD 3rd (2008) Aortic aneurysms: an immune disease with a strong genetic component. *Circulation* **117**:242–252.
26. Hasham SN, Guo DC, & Milewicz DM (2002) Genetic basis of thoracic aortic aneurysms and dissections. *Curr Opin Cardiol* **17**:677–683.
27. Neptune ER, Frischmeyer PA, Arking DE, *et al.* (2003) Dysregulation of TGF-beta activation contributes to pathogenesis in Marfan syndrome. *Nat Genet* **33**:407–411.
28. Habashi JP, Judge DP, Holm TM, *et al.* (2006) Losartan, an AT1 antagonist, prevents aortic aneurysm in a mouse model of Marfan syndrome. *Science* **312**(5770):117–121.

29. Lacro RV, Dietz HC, Wruck LM, *et al.* (2007) Rationale and design of a randomized clinical trial of beta-blocker therapy (atenolol) versus angiotensin II receptor blocker therapy (losartan) in individuals with Marfan syndrome. *Am Heart J.* **154**:624–631.

30. Coady MA, Davies RR, Roberts M, *et al.* (1999) Familial patterns of thoracic aortic aneurysms. *Arch Surg* **134**:361–367.

31. Guo D, Hasham S, Kuang SQ, *et al.* (2001) Familial thoracic aortic aneurysms and dissections: genetic heterogeneity with a major locus mapping to 5q13–14. *Circulation* **103**:2461–1468.

32. Vaughan CJ, Casey M, He J, *et al.* (2001) Identification of a chromosome 11q23.2-q24 locus for familial aortic aneurysm disease, a genetically heterogeneous disorder. *Circulation* **103**:2469–2475.

33. Hasham SN, Willing MC, Guo DC, *et al.* (2003) Mapping a locus for familial thoracic aortic aneurysms and dissections (TAAD2) to 3p24–25. *Circulation* **107**:3184–3190.

34. Elsheikh M, Casadei B, Conway GS, *et al.* (2001) Hypertension is a major risk factor for aortic root dilatation in women with Turner's syndrome. *Clin Endocrinol (Oxf)* **54**:69–73.

35. Niwa K, Perloff JK, Bhuta SM, *et al.* (2001) Structural abnormalities of great arterial walls in congenital heart disease: light and electron microscopic analyses. *Circulation* **103**:393–400.

36. Nistri S, Sorbo MD, Marin M, *et al.* (1999) Aortic root dilatation in young men with normally functioning bicuspid aortic valves. *Heart* **82**:19–22.

37. de Sa M, Moshkovitz Y, Butany J, *et al.* (1999) Histologic abnormalities of the ascending aorta and pulmonary trunk in patients with bicuspid aortic valve disease: clinical relevance to the ross procedure. *J Thorac Cardiovasc Surg.* **118**:588–594.

38. Boutefeu JM, Moret PR, Hahn C, *et al.* (1978) Aneurysms of the sinus of Valsalva. Report of seven cases and review of the literature. *Am J Med.* **65**:18–24.

39. Worrell JT, Buja LM, & Reynolds RC (1988) Pneumococcal aortitis with rupture of the aorta. Report of a case and review of the literature. *Am J Clin Pathol.* **89**:565–568.

40. Matsumura K, Hirano T, Takeda K, *et al.* (1991) Incidence of aneurysms in Takayasu's arteritis. *Angiology* **42**:308–315.

41. Nuenninghoff DM, Hunder GG, Christianson TJ, *et al.* (2003) Incidence and predictors of large-artery complication (aortic aneurysm, aortic dissection, and/or large-artery stenosis) in patients with giant cell arteritis: a population-based study over 50 years. *Arthritis Rheum* **48**:3522–3531.

42. Pomerance A, Yacoub MH, & Gula G (1977) The surgical pathology of thoracic aortic aneurysms. *Histopathology* **1**:257–276.

43. Klima T, Spjut HJ, Coelho A, *et al.* (1983) The morphology of ascending aortic aneurysms. *Hum Pathol* **14**:810–817.

44. Homme JL, Aubry MC, Edwards WD, *et al.* (2006) Surgical pathology of the ascending aorta: a clinicopathologic study of 513 cases. *Am J Surg Pathol* **30**:1159–1168.

45. Tang PCY, Coady MA, Lovoulos C, *et al.* (2005) Hyperplastic cellular remodeling of the media in ascending thoracic aortic aneurysms. *Circulation* **112**:1098–1105.

46. Lesauskaite V, Tanganelli P, Sassi C, *et al.* (2001) Smooth muscle cells of the media in the dilatative pathology of ascending thoracic aorta: morphology, immunoreactivity for osteopontin, matrix metalloproteinases, and their inhibitors. *Hum Pathol* **32**:1003–1011.

47. He R, Guo DC, Estrera AL, *et al.* (2006) Characterization of the inflammatory and apoptotic cells in the aortas of patients with ascending thoracic aortic aneurysms and dissections. *J Thorac Cardiovasc Surg* **131**:671–678.

48. Davies RR, Goldstein LJ, Coady MA, *et al.* (2002) Yearly rupture or dissection rates for thoracic aortic aneurysms: simple prediction based on size. *Ann Thorac Surg* **73**:17–27, discussion 8.

49. Coady MA, Rizzo JA, Hammond GL, *et al.* (1997) What is the appropriate size criterion for resection of thoracic aortic aneurysms? *J Thorac Cardiovasc Surg* **113**:476–491, discussion 89–91.

50. Sakalihasan N, Limet R, & Defawe OD (2005) Abdominal aortic aneurysm. *Lancet* **365**(9470):1577–1589.

51. Defawe OD, Colige A, Lambert CA, *et al.* (2003) TIMP-2 and PAI-1 mRNA levels are lower in aneurysmal as compared to athero-occlusive abdominal aortas. *Cardiovasc Res* **60**:205–213.

52. Knox JB, Sukhova GK, Whittemore AD, *et al.* (1997) Evidence for altered balance between matrix metalloproteinases and their inhibitors in human aortic diseases. *Circulation* **95**:205–212.

53. Auerbach O & Garfinkel L (1980) Atherosclerosis and aneurysm of aorta in relation to smoking habits and age. *Chest* **78**:805–809.

54. Vardulaki KA, Walker NM, Day NE, *et al.* (2000) Quantifying the risks of hypertension, age, sex and smoking in patients with abdominal aortic aneurysm. *Br J Surg* **87**:195–200.

55. MacSweeney ST, Ellis M, Worrell PC, *et al.* (1994) Smoking and growth rate of small abdominal aortic aneurysms. *Lancet* **344**(8923):651–652.

56. Brady AR, Thompson SG, Fowkes FG, *et al.* (2004) Abdominal aortic aneurysm expansion: risk factors and time intervals for surveillance. *Circulation* **110**:16–21.

57. Lederle FA, Johnson GR, Wilson SE, *et al.* (2000) The Aneurysm Detection and Management Study Screening Program: validation cohort and final results. *Arch Intern Med* **160**:1425–1430.

58. Lindholt JS, Vammen S, Juul S, *et al.* (2000) Optimal interval screening and surveillance of abdominal aortic aneurysms. *Eur J Vasc Endovasc Surg* **20**:369–373.

59. Lederle FA, Johnson GR, & Wilson SE (2001) Abdominal aortic aneurysm in women. *J Vasc Surg* **34**:122–126.

60. Singh K, Bonaa KH, Jacobsen BK, *et al.* (2001) Prevalence of and risk factors for abdominal aortic aneurysms in a population-based study: the Tromso Study. *Am J Epidemiol* **154**:236–244.

61. Ogren M, Bengtsson H, Bergqvist D, *et al.* (1996) Prognosis in elderly men with screening-detected abdominal aortic aneurysm. *Eur J Vasc Endovasc Surg* **11**:42–47.

62. Campa JS, Greenhalgh RM, & Powell JT (1987) Elastin degradation in abdominal aortic aneurysms. *Atherosclerosis* **65**(1–2):13–21.

63. Henderson EL, Geng Y-J, Sukhova GK, *et al.* (1999) Death of smooth muscle cells and expression of mediators of apoptosis by T lymphocytes in human abdominal aortic aneurysms. *Circulation* **99**:96–104.

64. Shimizu K, Mitchell RN, & Libby P (2006) Inflammation and cellular immune responses in abdominal aortic aneurysms. *Arterioscler Thromb Vasc Biol* **26**:987–994.

65. Sangiorgi G, D'Averio R, Mauriello A, *et al.* (2001) Plasma levels of metalloproteinases-3 and -9 as markers of successful abdominal aortic aneurysm exclusion after endovascular graft treatment. *Circulation* **104**(12 Suppl. I):I288–295.

66. Walker DI, Bloor K, Williams G, *et al.* (1972) Inflammatory aneurysms of the abdominal aorta. *Br J Surg* **59**(8):609–614.

67. Feiner HD, Raghavendra BN, Phelps R, *et al.* (1984) Inflammatory abdominal aortic aneurysm: report of six cases. *Hum Pathol* **15**:454–459.

68. McCarthy RJ, Shaw E, Whyman MR, *et al.* (2003) Recommendations for screening intervals for small aortic aneurysms. *Br J Surg* **90**:821–826.

69. Brown PM, Pattenden R, Vernooy C, *et al.* (1996) Selective management of abdominal aortic aneurysms in a prospective measurement program. *J Vasc Surg* **23**:213–220, discussion 21–22.

70. Faivre L, Collod-Beroud G, Loeys BL, *et al.* (2007) Effect of mutation type and location on clinical outcome in 1013 probands with Marfan syndrome or related phenotypes and FBN1 mutations: an international study. *Am J Hum Genet* **81**:454–466.

71. Hagan PG, Nienaber CA, Isselbacher EM, *et al.* (2000) The International Registry of Acute Aortic Dissection (IRAD): new insights into an old disease. *JAMA* **283**:897–903.

72. Nienaber CA, Fattori R, Mehta RH, *et al.* (2004) Gender-related differences in acute aortic dissection. *Circulation* **109**:3014–3021.

73. Murray CA & Edwards JE (1973) Spontaneous laceration of ascending aorta. *Circulation* **47**:848–858.

74. Larson EW & Edwards WD (1984) Risk factors for aortic dissection: a necropsy study of 161 cases. *Am J Cardiol* **53**:849–855.

75. Wilson SK & Hutchins GM (1982) Aortic dissecting aneurysms: causative factors in 204 subjects. *Arch Pathol Lab Med* **106**:175–180.

76. Heistad DD, Marcus ML, Larsen GE, *et al.* (1981) Role of vasa vasorum in nourishment of the aortic wall. *Am J Physiol* **240**:H781–778.

77. Nienaber CA & Eagle KA (2003) Aortic dissection: new frontiers in diagnosis and management: Part I: from etiology to diagnostic strategies. *Circulation* **108**:628–635.

78. Tsai TT, Nienaber CA, & Eagle KA (2005) Acute aortic syndromes. *Circulation* **112**:3802–3813.

79. Spittell PC, Spittell JA Jr, Joyce JW, *et al.* (1993) Clinical features and differential diagnosis of aortic dissection: experience with 236 cases 1980 through 1990. *Mayo Clin Proc* **68**:642–651.

80. Januzzi JL, Isselbacher EM, Fattori R, *et al.* (2004) Characterizing the young patient with aortic dissection: results from the International Registry of Aortic Dissection (IRAD). *J Am Coll Cardiol* **43**:665–669.

81. Edwards WD, Leaf DS, & Edwards JE (1978) Dissecting aortic aneurysm associated with congenital bicuspid aortic valve. *Circulation* **57**:1022–1025.

82. Hurwitz LM & Goodman PC (2005) Intra-aortic balloon pump location and aortic dissection. *AJR Am J Roentgenol* **184**:1245–1246.

83. DeBakey ME, Beall AC Jr, Cooley DA, *et al.* (1966) Dissecting aneurysms of the aorta. *Surg Clin North Am* **46**:1045–1055.

84. Daily PO, Trueblood HW, Stinson EB, *et al.* (1970) Management of acute aortic dissections. *Ann Thorac Surg* **10**:237–247.

85. Coady MA, Rizzo JA, & Elefteriades JA (1999) Pathologic variants of thoracic aortic dissections. Penetrating atherosclerotic ulcers and intramural hematomas. *Cardiol Clin* **17**:637–657.

86. Ide K, Uchida H, Otsuji H, *et al.* (1996) Acute aortic dissection with intramural hematoma: possibility of transition to classic dissection or aneurysm. *J Thorac Imaging* **11**:46–52.

87. Vilacosta I, San Roman JA, Ferreiros J, *et al.* (1997) Natural history and serial morphology of aortic intramural hematoma: a novel variant of aortic dissection. *Am Heart J* **134**:495–507.

88. Nienaber CA, von Kodolitsch Y, Petersen B, *et al.* (1995) Intramural hemorrhage of the thoracic aorta. Diagnostic and therapeutic implications. *Circulation* **92**:1465–1472.

89. Svensson LG, Labib SB, Eisenhauer AC, *et al.* (1999) Intimal tear without hematoma: an important variant of aortic dissection that can elude current imaging techniques. *Circulation* **99**:1331–1336.

90. Erbel R, Alfonso F, Boileau C, *et al.* (2001) Diagnosis and management of aortic dissection: Task Force on Aortic Dissection, European Society of Cardiology. *Eur Heart J.* **22**:1642–1681.

91. Song JK, Kim HS, Kang DH, *et al.* (2001) Different clinical features of aortic intramural hematoma versus dissection involving the ascending aorta. *J Am Coll Cardiol.* **37**:1604–1610.

92. Vilacosta I, San Roman JA, Aragoncillo P, *et al.* (1998) Penetrating atherosclerotic aortic ulcer: documentation by transesophageal echocardiography. *J Am Coll Cardiol.* **32**:83–89.

93. Tittle SL, Lynch RJ, Cole PE, *et al.* (2002) Midterm follow-up of penetrating ulcer and intramural hematoma of the aorta. *J Thorac Cardiovasc Surg.* **123**:1051–1059.

94. Hansen MS, Nogareda GJ, & Hutchison SJ (2007) Frequency of and inappropriate treatment of misdiagnosis of acute aortic dissection. *Am J Cardiol.* **99**:852–856.

95. Tsai TT, Evangelista A, Nienaber CA, *et al.* (2006) Long-term survival in patients presenting with type A acute aortic dissection: insights from the International Registry of Acute Aortic Dissection (IRAD). *Circulation* **114**(1 Suppl.):I-350–356.

96. Fann JI, Smith JA, Miller DC, *et al.* (1995) Surgical management of aortic dissection during a 30-year period. *Circulation* **92**(9 Suppl.): II113–121.

97. Tsai TT, Isselbacher EM, Trimarchi S, *et al.* (2007) Acute type B aortic dissection: does aortic arch involvement affect management and outcomes? insights from the International Registry of Acute Aortic Dissection (IRAD). *Circulation* **116**(11 Suppl.): I-150–156.

98. Tsai TT, Fattori R, Trimarchi S, *et al.* (2006) Long-term survival in patients presenting with type B acute aortic dissection: insights from the International Registry of Acute Aortic Dissection. *Circulation* **114**(21):2226–2231.

46 Echocardiographic Assessment of Aortic Aneurysms and Dissections

Thomas Bartel

Medical University Innsbruck, Innsbruck, Austria

Introduction

Aortic aneurysms and dissections develop primarily as a consequence of aortic wall degeneration, for example in hypertension (overweight and cocaine use increase risk), atherosclerotic changes, and calcification. Less frequently, they can be caused by aortitis (giant cell arteritis, Takayasu's disease), metabolic connective tissue disorders (Marfan's syndrome, Turner's syndrome, Ehlers–Danlos syndrome), pregnancy (especially during the third trimester), or congenital heart disease (coarctation, bicuspid aortic valve). Traumatic (abrupt deceleration in an accident) or iatrogenic disruption (complication of cardiac catheterization) of one or more layers of the wall are also causative [1–4]. In particular, in acute type A aortic dissection, mortality escalates by the hour, making immediate diagnostics critical for survival. Since time is of essence in all cases of acute aortic syndrome, transthoracic echocardiography (TTE) is recommended as the initial diagnostic modality, because it can be used without preparation. The sensitivity of transesophageal echocardiography (TEE) in visualizing nearly the entire thoracic aorta is higher than that of TTE. However, in the superior segment of the ascending aorta, the aortic arch and the abdominal aorta, even TEE has "blind spots," which limit its diagnostic use. In addition to TTE and TEE combined, intraluminal phased array imaging (IPAI), also known as intracardiac echocardiography when used inside the heart, is a recently introduced diagnostic alternative, which has replaced aortic intravascular ultrasound (IVUS), a wire-guided technique without Doppler capabilities.

Transthoracic echocardiography

Different sound windows are required for optimal visualization of the ascending aorta and the aortic arch by TTE. The most proximal portion of the ascending aorta can be nicely displayed from the parasternal long-axis view. The basal parasternal short-axis view can be used for measuring the diameter of the aortic bulb, a measurement which is part of the routine check-up in patients with Marfan's syndrome and in other risk groups. Moreover, diameters of the aortic annulus, the sinotubular junction, and the adjacent proximal aorta can also be determined from parasternal views. Alternatively, the aortic root can be depicted in the apical three- and five-chamber views, and even in the transgastric long-axis and short-axis views, although with minor imaging quality [5]. TTE from the suprasternal notch is very useful for displaying the aortic arch and the very proximal part of the descending thoracic aorta, thereby compensating for the "blind spot" inherent to TEE. In many younger subjects, the aortic isthmus and the origins of left carotid artery and the left subclavian artery are visible. Color Doppler imaging may facilitate orientation. Spectral Doppler is routinely used to quantify possibly associated aortic regurgitation by qualitative assessment of the intra-aortic diastolic flow pattern: holodiastolic flow is indicative of severe aortic regurgitation. Continuous-wave Doppler is the non-invasive method of choice for measuring the systolic pressure gradient in aortic coarctation. In elderly patients, interposition of the lung frequently interferes with suprasternal echocardiographic viewing. In the presence of pleural effusion, the distal descending thoracic aorta can be sufficiently displayed from a paravertebral sound window. As known from epigastric sonography, the echocardiographic probe may be used to display the abdominal aorta in short-axis and long-axis views. Again, color Doppler facilitates detection of the abdominal aorta and differentiation between venous and arterial vessels. Aneurysms and dissections of the proximal abdominal aorta can be visualized. If the quality of TTE imaging is insufficient or if it is nondiagnostic, one should not hesitate to proceed with TEE, especially in acute aortic syndrome [6].

Acute aortic syndrome

Particularly in acute aortic syndrome, echocardiography is time saving compared with computed tomography (CT) or magnetic resonance imaging (MRI), and it can also be

Cardiovascular Interventions in Clinical Practice. Edited by Jürgen Haase, Hans-Joachim Schäfers, Horst Sievert and Ron Waksman. © 2010 Blackwell Publishing.

employed in critically ill patients as a bedside method that does not interrupt intensive care monitoring and management. Acute aortic syndrome occurs approximately 100 times less frequently than acute coronary syndrome. In addition to an aortic aneurysm presenting with increasing wall stress, classic aortic dissection as well as a variety of precursors and variants of dissection can initiate acute aortic syndrome [7]. The Svensson classification adds significantly to the well known Stanford classification and the classification according to DeBakey [8,9]. TEE is capable of adequately differentiating the following precursors and variants:

- class I classic dissection;
- class II intramural hematoma;
- class III local dissection;,
- class IV penetrating atherosclerotic aortic ulcer; and
- class V iatrogenic/traumatic transection/dissection.

All these precursors and variants are subdivided into lesions of type A and B according to the Stanford classification. This nomenclature describes any lesion with involvement of the ascending aorta (including DeBakey types I and II) as type A and lesions limited to the descending aorta as type B (DeBakey type III) [10].

Transesophageal echocardiography

Normal aortic dimensions and diagnostic standards

The normal diameter of the aorta varies depending on age, gender, body surface area, and distance to the aortic valve. Normal diameter ranges for the ascending and descending aorta are 1.4–2.1 cm/m^2 and 1.0–1.6 cm/m^2, respectively.

Ectasia of the aorta is defined as an ascending aortic diameter beyond 3.5 cm or a descending aortic diameter greater than 3.0 cm. An aortic aneurysm is defined as dilation exceeding 4.0 cm. Isolated dilation of the aortic bulb to >4.5 cm is called sinus of Valsalva aneurysm. All diameters should be measured in a plane perpendicular to the main flow, which can be difficult in cases of extensive kinking, as it occasionally occurs in the descending thoracic aorta. The following standard views are helpful for an adequate assessment of the ascending aorta and optimal positioning of the TEE probe:

- The aortic bulb and the very proximal part of the ascending aorta are best displayed in the midesophageal view at 120°.
- The full extent of the superior portion of the ascending aorta can be visualized in the upper longitudinal cut plane at 90° (also known as the "banana view").
- The transverse (orthogonal) view of the ascending aorta and its spatial relation to the right pulmonary artery and the superior vena cava are nicely visible in the upper cut plane at 0°.

Precise diameter measurements can be performed in the banana view by M-mode or in the upper transesophageal view at 0° by a two-dimensional display. Care is required when assessing the ascending aorta: artifacts also known as reverberations frequently occur in the banana view, mimicking a

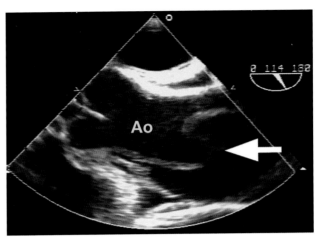

Figure 46.1 Type A dissection in a midesophageal view at 114°. Bright echoes and stochastic motion are indicative of a true dissection flap. The arrow indicates the dissection flap and the aorta. Ao, ascending aorta. Reprinted from Chapter 11 in *Echokardiographie*, Bartel T and Müller S (eds), with permission from Urban & Fischer by Elsevier.

dissection membrane. Reverberations can be discriminated from *true* echoes of intraluminal structures by analyzing their motion pattern (Fig. 46.1). M-mode and color-coded tissue Doppler M-mode (preferred) reveal that reverberations move in phase with the aortic wall. In contrast, dissection flaps are characterized by flotation. The stochastic motion of the flap is not related to the rhythmic motion of any neighboring structure. Confusion due to misinterpretation of reverberations and false-positive diagnosis of dissection in the ascending aorta has unfortunately caused surgical fatalities in the past.

The diameters of the aortic valve annulus and the aortic bulb are best determined from the midesophageal view. For assessing the descending thoracic aorta, the following standard views are recommended:

- transverse (orthogonal) cross-sectional views of the aorta at 0°, withdrawing the probe in steps of 5 cm from 40 to 25 cm of insertion length; and
- longitudinal (caudal to cranial) views at 90° using the same stepwise approach.

If the descending aorta is kinked, the angle of the TEE probe must be adjusted to depict adequate transverse and longitudinal views. Between 25 and 30 cm of insertion length, the origin of the left subclavian artery can be displayed. At the same level, a patent ductus Botalli can be demonstrated.

In case of aortic disease, TEE provides additional information about left and right ventricular function, wall motion abnormalities due to coronary involvement, pericardial effusion, and valve competence.

Aortic aneurysm

In most cases, a true aortic aneurysm can be considered the result of fusiform or saccular dilation of all aortic wall layers, most often due to atherosclerosis. Aneurysms of the ascending aorta often result from turbulent or regurgitant flow in severe aortic valve disease. Surgical therapy or endovascular stent implantation is indicated in symptomatic aneurysms and in aneurysms with a diameter exceeding 5.5 cm in the ascending aorta (in Marfan's syndrome, the recommended threshold is 4.5 cm) and 6.5 cm in the descending aorta (in Marfan's syndrome, the recommended threshold is 5.5 cm). If smaller and asymptomatic true aneurysms are detected, thrombus formation has to be ruled out. Spontaneous echo contrast is indicative of slow flow which predisposes to thrombus formation in the aneurysm sac. In these cases and in the presence of thrombotic material, the benefits of anticoagulant therapy should be weighed against the risk of hemorrhage. The absence of a dissection flap is an important factor in avoiding the false diagnosis of aortic dissection. On the other hand, a dissection flap may get overlooked. Especially in cases of false lumen thrombosis, a dissection flap must be ruled out by carefully rotating the probe and by completely scanning the entire region. Spontaneous dissection and wall rupture with concealed perforation or free hemorrhage into the chest are the most important complications, and they are clearly detectable by TEE.

Classic aortic dissection (class I)

Sensitivity and specificity of TEE were repeatedly shown to markedly exceed 95%. In addition to its bedside availability, the most important strength of TEE is its documented accuracy, which is similar to that of CT and MRI [11,12]. In the beginning of the TEE era, false-positive diagnoses occurred more frequently, because reverberations were misinterpreted. This led to lower specificities in some studies [11]. Today, more stringent criteria help to minimize the frequency of false-positive results. False-negative results can be effectively eliminated by the additional use of TTE with suprasternal notch views. Detection of pericardial effusion or severe aortic regurgitation is frequently the first clue of a type A dissection.

Transesophageal echocardiography-based diagnosis of aortic dissection relies on specific criteria. Identification of a mobile intimal flap displayed as a linear echo within the lumen of the aorta dividing it into a true and a false lumen is one, flow separation in both channels on either side of the flap is another highly sensitive feature of dissection. The size of the concave false lumen almost always exceeds that of the true lumen. The true lumen is convexly shaped and typically found at the inward curvature of the ascending aortic arch or the outward curvature of the descending aortic arch (Fig. 46.2). True and false lumen can also be distinguished by the pulsatile motion of the intimal flap toward the false lumen during systole. Depending on the flow in the false channel, the false lumen can completely or partially thrombose and therefore resemble a thickened aortic wall. Strict adherence to these criteria helps avoiding false-positive results and misinterpretation of artifacts [13]. This is of utmost importance in the differential diagnosis of other abnormal findings, which potentially underlie aortic dissection (i.e., wall thickening, plaque formation,

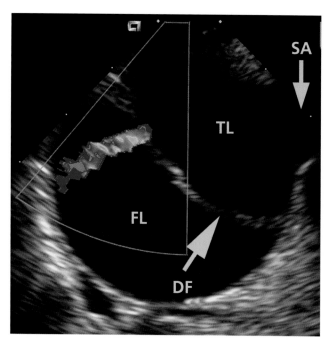

Figure 46.2 Transverse view of the descending aorta in class I type B dissection. A small intimal tear with flow from the smaller, convexly shaped true lumen into the larger concavely shaped false lumen. The left subclavian artery originates from the true lumen. DF, dissection flap; FL, false lumen; SA, subclavian artery (branching off); TL, true lumen.

previous surgical repair, and intraluminal masses). In type A aortic dissection, severity and mechanism of aortic regurgitation can also be reliably determined by TEE. This assessment influences decision-making about aortic valve replacement versus repair.

Color Doppler identifies forward systolic flow throughout the true lumen, which may be dwarfed by compression from the false lumen if re-entry is lacking. Flow in the false lumen is variable and depends on size, localization, and number of entries and re-entries. Two general types can be distinguished.

First, the flow in the false lumen with similar intensity and the same direction and timing as flow in the true lumen. This occurs due to large proximal entry tears if distal re-entries (exit sites) are also present. Continuous-wave Doppler readings demonstrate a comparatively low flow velocity and a low pressure gradient between true and false lumen (flow velocity <1.5 m/s). At the re-entry sites, late systolic reverse flow back into the true lumen can also be detected. This is described as aortic dissection with antegrade perfusion and without pressure separation. Spontaneous thrombus formation and subsequent healing are unlikely, since flow in the false lumen is quite high. Progression with extension of the false lumen must be expected due to pressure equalization between both channels [14].

Second, compared with true luminal flow, false luminal flow and pressure are significantly lower if the entries are smaller and more distally located. Depending on the distance between the beginning of the dissection and the first entry tear, retrograde flow can be observed in the proximal part of the false lumen. Peak flow in the false lumen may be delayed in comparison to peak flow in the true lumen. This represents delay of false luminal flow. At the entry tear, flow velocity is much higher, resulting in a significant pressure gradient between both channels. In contrast, flow inside the false lumen shows much lower intensity (best seen by color Doppler) than flow in the true lumen. Occasionally, there is swirling flow with spontaneous echo contrast. This is described as pressure-separated dissection with or without retrograde flow in the false lumen. There is a better chance of spontaneous thrombus formation in the false lumen and subsequent partial recovery. However, complete thrombosis of the false lumen must be differentiated from development of a pseudo-aneurysm, which can be difficult. Experience is needed to clearly ascertain that the hematoma is entirely located inside the vessel [15].

Multiple communications between both channels are often seen in the thoracic aorta, while communications can be missed in the abdominal portion. If both small and large entries are present, segments with slow flow tend to be remote from larger entry or re-entry tears, where high velocity flow prevents thrombus formation. All entry and re-entry sites should be reported in reference to the probe insertion length. These are important data for any surgical correction and for adequate endovascular placement of stent grafts. If the TEE report is incomplete, some communication sites between the true and false channel may not be adequately closed. Simple closure of only one entry tear can result in transformation of a more distally located re-entry site into an entry which will maintain significant flow in the distal part of the false lumen. Nevertheless, identification of the primary entry site is one of the major goals in TEE examination and is successfully accomplished in about 80% [16]. Diagnosing any concomitant coronary artery disease is another important issue. This also raises the question if preoperative coronary angiography is really mandatory, especially in emergencies. Potential benefits of addressing hemodynamically important coronary stenoses must be weighed against the risk of delaying life-saving treatment and the risk of disrupting aortic wall layers by catheter manipulation. In that respect, wall motion anomalies can be indicative of severe coronary artery disease and can provide good reason to proceed with coronary angiography before surgical treatment.

Complications of aortic dissection

To rapidly identify complications associated with aortic dissection, the combination of TEE and TTE is the method of choice. Acute aortic regurgitation resulting from annular dilation or disruption of leaflet suspension is a frequently seen complication of type A dissection. The diagnosis can be made easily by TTE, while TEE provides additional morphologic background information before surgical intervention. TTE is also a good tool for demonstrating pericardial effusion or tamponade. Presence of tamponade would be a reason to emergently move the patient to the operating room without further diagnostics. To identify the exact morphology of dissection, TEE can be performed in the operating room during induction of anesthesia. Free rupture of the aortic wall with immediate major hemorrhage into the mediastinum or pleural space causes sudden death. At other locations, ruptures may look different. Especially in type B dissection, contained rupture of the aortic wall can lead to pseudoaneurysm formation. Diagnostic goals include delineation of the intimal breach, the margins of the aortic wall, and the extent of the surrounding hematoma. Pleural effusion can be seen if the imaging depth is adequate and may be indicative of a concealed rupture. Transpulmonary echo contrast agents can also help to identify extravasation.

Life-threatening distal malperfusion results from a complete stop of antegrade perfusion due to increasing pressure in the false lumen and subsequent true luminal collapse, especially in type B dissection after primary stabilization of the patient. Immediate implantation of a covered stent graft to close the proximal entry tear is one therapeutic option. This will significantly lower the pressure in the false lumen. Stent graft implantation, however, requires close cooperation with other disciplines, which may be too time-consuming to arrange in an acute scenario. Another strategy is catheter-based fenestration of the distal dissection flap to decompress the false lumen and to restore antegrade flow in both channels. The alternative option, i.e. surgical fenestration, is known to be associated with mortality rates of up to 25% [8,18,19]. Mortality figures can even exceed 70% in patients with critical mesenteric or renal ischemia [20]. Immediate diagnosis and treatment within 2 h are mandatory to prevent irreversible bowel ischemia and to save the patient's life.

Involvement of a coronary ostium is another dangerous complication of type A dissection and can be detected in 80–90% of cases, especially if the dissection flap interferes with main stem coronary flow [17]. The left main stem including its bifurcation is best visualized in the orthogonal view of the ascending aorta in a transverse upper cut plane at 0°. Extension of type A dissection into the coronary arteries (coronary dissection) is more frequent than vessel obstruction [21].

Intramural hematoma (class II)

A minority of about 5% of all aortic dissections appear without a dissected membrane but with intramural bleeding into a degenerate media, typically due to rupture of the vasa vasorum [22]. Age and long-term hypertension are the main risk factors for this variant of aortic dissection. Focal distortion of the transverse circular configuration of the aorta and crescent-shaped or circular wall thickening of at least 7 mm is demonstrated by TEE. The longitudinal extension varies between 1 and 20 cm and there is no evidence of flow inside the hematoma. The hematoma's echo density depends on how quickly fibrosis progresses. In early stages, anechoic spots within the hematoma are indicative of a short history. Generally, sensitivity and specificity of TEE for class II dissection are similar to class I dissection [23]. According to recommendations for class I dissection, type A intramural hematoma requires immediate surgical intervention. About one–third of intramural hematomas progress to complete dissection, and in others (up to 25%) either contained or uncontained rupture occurs during follow-up and under antihypertensive treatment. Therefore, in cases of progressive wall thickening or an aortic diameter increase beyond 50 mm, elective surgical therapy or endovascular stent graft implantation should be considered. If a conservative strategy is preferred, short-term follow-up is always recommended to assess fibrotic transformation of the hematoma and subsequent healing [24]. For that purpose, TEE is again the method of choice, helping to avoid the repeated high radiation doses associated with CT angiography.

Penetrating atherosclerotic ulcer (class IV)

A penetrating atherosclerotic ulcer (PAU) may precede either class I or class II dissection and can rupture into the adventitia, leading to a pseudoaneurysm or free intrathoracic hemorrhage. PAU is defined as ulceration of an atheromatous plaque extending deeply through the intima and internal elastic lamina into the aortic media [25]. Similar to patients with class II dissection, patients presenting with a PAU are older than those with class I dissection. Main risk factors such as atherosclerosis and hypertension are evident in most of them. PAUs are predominantly found in the descending aorta (type B PAU), in which atherosclerosis tends to be more progressive than in the ascending segment. TEE reveals significant penetration adjacent to plaques that protrude into the vessel lumen. Penetration may appear as a crater-like outpouching of the aortic wall. Additionally, color Doppler might demonstrate some flow into broken up plaques as another equivalent of ongoing penetration. Asymptomatic patients presenting with PAU usually require aggressive antihypertensive treatment and short-term echocardiographic follow-up rather than surgical or interventional therapy [26].

Other variants of aortic dissection (classes III and V)

Local dissection (class III) is primarily located in the ascending aorta and may be overlooked by TEE if it is located in the "blind spot." In other words, TEE is significantly limited in type A—class III dissection. Thus, CT or angiography must be considered the diagnostic tools of choice in this subgroup. Fortunately, this variant is very rare, but it can progress into class I dissection at any time and therefore needs surgical repair. In contrast, type B—class III—dissection plays a minor role and can be managed conservatively if asymptomatic as spontaneous healing is likely.

Iatrogenic dissection and traumatic transection of the aorta (class V) occasionally occur as a result of catheter diagnostics,

interventional therapy, and a variety of severe traumas. Local and complete dissection can be created by manipulation with diagnostic coronary catheters. Intubation of coronary arteries, especially of the right coronary artery, can be challenging and lead to intimal injuries if the catheter is handled forcefully. In most cases, those lesions are only lacerations. However, if too much contrast agent is subsequently injected into such an intimal lesion and if the examiner is not adequately experienced, the result can be fatal rupture or a more or less extended type A dissection. Caution is also recommended when advancing an intra-aortic balloon pump through the aorta. This may mobilize plaques and cause type B dissection as a consequence. Aortic cannulation during cardiac surgery is another possible trigger for iatrogenic aortic dissection. TEE usually demonstrates partially thrombosed tissue protruding from the aortic wall and moving freely inside the lumen. Aortic transection typically occurs as a consequence of an accident, blunt trauma, or a deceleration injury (seat belt related trauma, fall from great heights). Transection must be considered an equivalent of contained rupture with hemorrhage into the pleural space, which can be depicted by TTE and even better by TEE. Patients with these injuries should be emergently transferred to surgery. In inoperable patients, endovascular stent graft implantation may be considered an alternative (Fig. 46.3).

Intraoperative and peri-interventional assessment

Intraoperative imaging from the epicardium and surface of the aorta is an option if one needs to carefully investigate the aortic root, the origins of the great vessels and suture lines after surgery, particularly in the area in which TEE has its "blind spot." Except for these cases, intraoperative TTE has been replaced by TEE, which can be used continuously during surgery. At the conclusion of cardiac surgery, TEE images confirm valve or prosthetic valve competency and allow prompt reinstitution of cardiopulmonary bypass if surgical revision is required. TEE also facilitates proper positioning of an intra-aortic balloon pump into the true lumen of the dissected aorta. In endovascular stent graft implantation, TEE is an ideal guiding tool and also allows to observe adequate opening and apposition of the stent and to check the result. Since angiography heavily depicts the proximal intimal tear, TEE is capable of securely demonstrating the entry flow into the false lumen. The TEE probe serves as a reference for stent deployment under fluoroscopic control (Fig. 46.3). In case of insufficient stent apposition, color Doppler TEE will nicely depict small endoleaks. After subsequent balloon post dilation, flow adjacent to the stent will disappear, indicating that the endoleak has been effectively treated. Functional imaging can assess if adequate antegrade flow has been restored, if at least the main intimal tear is closed and if flow in the false lumen has subsided. The same procedure can be used in localized aneurysms of the descending aorta, aiming to induce thrombus formation in the aneurysm sack and to prevent rupture of the aneurysm wall and embolization from the

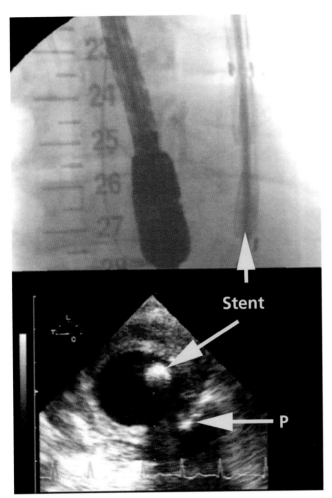

Figure 46.3 Status post defenestration: Contained perforation of the descending aorta is emergently treated by endovascular stent graft implantation guided by transesophageal echocardiography. P, perforation site.

aneurysm. As an alternative to TEE, IVUS has been proposed for effective guidance in endovascular stent graft implantation [27].

In distal malperfusion syndrome, percutaneous TEE-guided balloon fenestration of the dissection membrane is one therapeutic option for restoring antegrade flow if the true lumen collapse is located in the descending thoracic aorta. Movement of the puncture needle needs to be observed in longitudinal views, which help to avoid perforation of the aortic wall. After successful puncture of the dissection flap, a wire is introduced and a balloon inflated to widen the puncture site. Since fenestration is, in most cases, required in the abdominal portion of the aorta, TEE has a limited role in this respect. Alternatively, IVUS as well as IPAI may be employed [28].

Limitations of transesophageal echocardiography

Air in the lower respiratory tract between esophagus and ascending aorta creates a blind spot which does not only obscure parts of the ascending aorta and the superior transverse arch, but also the origins of the great vessels, except for the left subclavian artery take-off. This is not a great issue because involvement of these vessels does not necessarily change the surgical approach and can be assessed intraoperatively [29]. But type A dissection strictly limited to this area might be missed without an additional TTE and suprasternal notch views. False-negative results in type A dissection are extremely rare (e.g., in chronic dissection of the aortic arch) [30], but can be disastrous as the clinical management depends largely on any involvement of the proximal aorta. TEE is further limited by its restriction to the thoracic aorta. Epigastric views can partially compensate for this (abdominal blind spot of TEE). Extension of the dissection beyond the aortic bifurcation into the pelvic vessels cannot be displayed. IVUS and IPAI can be alternatively employed, but these diagnostic tools are invasive. Small entry tears can be difficult to detect with TEE if the flow through these communications is not aligned with the Doppler beam, so that not even color Doppler can detect jets. With the TEE probe fixed in the esophagus, the sound window and sound angle cannot be changed at will.

Near-field artifacts, also known as reverberations, may mimic a dissection flap if they run parallel to the aortic wall. Calcifications in the wall may be another cause of shadowing and reverberations. Aortic kinking and abrupt dilation may create a shelf-like structure in an echocardiographic cut plane and might be misinterpreted as an intimal flap. All these false-positive findings are characterized by moderate mobility of the structures in question. Reverberations move in phase with the aortic wall. In many cases, perpendicular imaging planes are extremely helpful in resolving these issues.

Although TEE is by now well established and provides exceptional high-resolution images of the aorta, the patient's supine position restricts the usefulness of TEE in percutaneous interventions. Continuous monitoring with TEE is, on the other hand, desirable for precise deployment of stent grafts and for achieving an optimal interventional result. On the other hand, patients do not tolerate the probe unless sedated or under general anesthesia. In acute aortic syndrome, insertion of a TEE probe may result in additional stress and blood pressure increase if sedation is insufficient or if the examination is unnecessarily prolonged. Caution is generally required to avoid any additional iatrogenic sympathicomimetic activation. In acute aortic syndromes, the TEE examination should have well-defined goals, be performed under intravenous sedation with 5–7 mg of midazolam, and should be completed by an experienced examiner with level three competence, according to the American Society of Echocardiography definition. Especially outside regular working hours, this method may not be useful in patients with acute aortic syndrome if no experienced examiner is available.

Intraluminal phased-array imaging

Miniaturized ultrasound-tipped catheter devices were primarily introduced for intravascular application. Although IVUS-based intraluminal imaging was also used for guiding intra-aortic interventions [27], it lacks Doppler capabilities and is further limited by poor ultrasound penetration. Thus, technical advances led from IVUS to the development of IPAI and to intracardiac echocardiography, its intracardiac imaging equivalent.

Technique and clinical use

Current devices (Acuson Inc., Mountain View, CA, USA) are multimodal, phased-array, transducer-tipped echocardiographic catheters. The 10F AcuNav™ catheter—the first intraluminal single plane probe on the market—has become the tool of choice for IPAI. Recently, a further miniaturized version of the catheter (8F AcuNav™ catheter) has facilitated IPAI, especially in the aorta, and probably increases safety and patient comfort. In addition to two-dimensional and M-mode imaging, the intraluminal echocardiographic catheter permits functional analysis. Its Doppler capabilities include pulsed wave, continuous wave, color flow, and tissue Doppler [20,31].

The disposable catheter can be navigated through the inferior vena cava (femoral venous access) or the superior vena cava (jugular venous access) to aim the probe at the adjacent abdominal aorta or the aortic arch. Special caution is required when navigating the intracardiac echocardiographic catheter through the pelvic veins. Adequate handling of the catheter device includes use of a long access sheath and fluoroscopy, two recommended precautions that enhance patient safety. The probe does not accommodate a guidewire and is therefore fundamentally different from IVUS catheters. These require guidewires and are therefore relatively safe to manipulate, but arbitrary views can be difficult to obtain, especially in the near field.

Diagnostic value in aortic dissection

Catheter-based echocardiographic equipment can also be employed to perform IPAI in type B aortic dissection. With respect to detection and localization of entries, IPAI was shown to be superior to IVUS and to TEE [32]. Although TEE has similar capabilities, it is still limited because its lower frequency results in poorer image resolution and its angle dependency makes it less sensitive to entry flow than IPAI. This is especially valid for dissection flaps aligned with the Doppler-beam, i.e., when the angle between Doppler-beam and entry flow is large. In this respect, IPAI does not only combine advantages of TEE and IVUS, but offers additional benefits.

In type B aortic dissection, detection and precise localization of tears in the intimal flap are important factors for therapeutic decision-making. In most cases, there are obviously more entries than demonstrable by angiography, IVUS, and TEE. However, the fact that such data form the basis for optimized stent–graft placement [33], which aims to close all entries into the false channel, mandates careful evaluation of the sensitivity of conventional diagnostic approaches. If over-

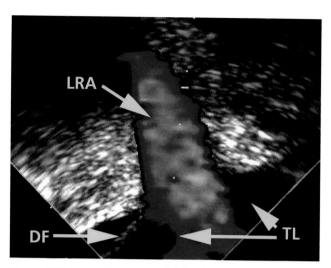

Figure 46.4 Intra-aortic phased-array imaging in type B aortic dissection. View from the true lumen to the dissection flap, which terminates next to the ostium of the left renal artery. DF, dissection flap; LRA, left renal artery; TL, true lumen. Reprinted from Bartel *et al.* [32], with permission.

looked or not properly closed by interventional treatment, even small tears can lead to significant flow into and inside the false lumen and subsequently impair the desired thrombus formation in the false lumen, thereby impeding healing of the dissection. Thus, measurement of interluminal gradients may also assist in clinical decision-making, as higher gradients are associated with lower pressures and flows in the false channel, making spontaneous thrombus formation more likely. Recently published results suggest that the effectiveness of aortic stent–graft placement may be improved by peri-interventional use of IPAI because this method identifies more entries and can also evaluate their hemodynamics [32,33].

With the IPAI-catheter positioned in the IVC, IPAI becomes an excellent tool to safely guide balloon fenestration of the dissection flap. One also needs to recall that false lumen puncture at a selected position may not be feasible, as the needle may simply slide over the surface of the very soft and compliant intimal flap. This can neither be demonstrated by fluoroscopy nor by IVUS. After IPAI identification of the optimal position for puncture, the fluoroscopic image of the tip of the IPAI-catheter serves as a marker for adequate needle orientation [28].

In contrast to TEE, IPAI has no blind spot, neither in the ascending aorta nor in the abdominal portion. IPAI can adequately show if the dissection membrane interferes with abdominal aortic side branches (Fig. 46.4). The necessity to navigate the IPAI-catheter within the aorta turns from a disadvantage into an advantage, as the Doppler-beam can be aligned with any particular flow between the true and false lumen and flow into any vessel that branches off. Thus, IPAI has great potential to become an effective guiding tool for aortic stent–graft implantation, especially in the abdominal portion.

References

1. Erbel R, Alfonso F, Boileau C, *et al.* (2001) Diagnosis and management of aortic dissection. *Eur Heart J* **22**:1642–1681.

2. Chauvel C, Cohen A, Alberto C, *et al.* (1994) Aortic dissection and cardiovascular syphilis: report of an observation with transesophageal echocardiography and anatomopathological findings. *J Am Soc Echocardiogr* **7**:419–421.

3. Evans JM, Bowles CA, Bjornsson J, *et al.* (1994) Thoracic aortic aneurysm and rupture in giant cell arteritis. A descriptive study of 41 cases. *Arthritis Rheum* **37**:1539–1547.

4. Marsalese DL, Moodie DS, Lytle BW, *et al.* (1990) Cystic medial necrosis of the aorta in patients without Marfan's syndrome: surgical outcome and long-term follow-up. *J Am Coll Cardiol* **16**:68–73.

5. Roman MJ, Devereux RB, Kramer-Fox R, *et al.* (1989) Two-dimensional echocardiographic aortic dimensions in children and adults. *Am J Cardiol* **64**:507–512.

6. Erbel R, Engberding R, Daniel W, *et al.* (1998) Echocardiography in diagnosis of aortic dissection. *Lancet* **1**:457–461.

7. Svensson LG, Labib SB, Eisenhauer AC, *et al.* (1999) Intimal tear without hematoma: an important variant of aortic dissection that can elude current imaging techniques. *Circulation* **99**:1331–1336.

8. DeBakey ME, McCollum CH, Crawford ES, *et al.* (1982) Dissection and dissecting aneurysms of the aorta: twenty-year follow-up of five hundred twenty seven patients treated surgically. *Surgery* **92**:1118–1134.

9. Erbel R, Oelert H, Meyer J, *et al.* (1993) Effect of medical and surgical therapy on aortic dissection evaluated by transesophageal echocardiography. Implications for prognosis and therapy. The European Cooperative study Group on Echocardiography. *Circulation* **87**:1604–1615.

10. DeSanctis RW, Doroghazi RM, Austen WG, *et al.* (1987) Aortic dissection. *N Engl J Med* **317**:1060–1067.

11. Nienaber CA, Spielmann RP, von Kodolitsch Y, *et al.* (1992) Diagnosis of thoracic aortic dissection: magnetic resonance imaging versus transesophageal echocardiography. *Circulation* **85**:434–447.

12. Nienaber CA, von Kodolitsch Y, Nicolas V, *et al.* (1993) The diagnosis of thoracic aortic dissection by noninvasive imaging procedures. *N Engl J Med* **328**:1–9.

13. Appelbe AF, Walker PG, Yeoh JK, *et al.* (1993) Clinical significance and origin of artefacts in transesophageal echocardiography of the thoracic aorta. *J Am Coll Cardiol* **21**:754–760.

14. Mohr-Kahaly S, Erbel R, Rennollet H, *et al.* (1989) Ambulatory follow-up of aortic dissection by transesophageal two-dimensional and color-coded Doppler echocardiography. *Circulation* **80**:24–33.

15. Erbel R, Mohr-Kahaly S, Renollet H, *et al.* (1987) Diagnosis of aortic dissection: the value of transesophageal echocardiography. *Thorac Cardiovasc Surg* **35**:126–133.

16. Adachy H, Kyo S, Takamoto S, *et al.* (1990) Early diagnosis and surgical intervention of acute aortic dissection by transesophageal color flow mapping. *Circulation* **82**(Suppl. 4):19–23.

17. Ballab RS, Nanda NC, Gatewood R, *et al.* (1991) Usefulness of transesophageal echocardiography in assessment of aortic dissection. *Circulation* **84**:1903–1914.

18. Laas J, Heinemann M, Schaefers HJ, *et al.* (1991) Management of thoracoabdominal malperfusion in aortic dissection. *Circulation* **84**(Suppl.): III20–III24.

19. Chavan A, Galanski M, & Pichlmair M (2000) Minimally invasive therapy options in aortic dissection. *Rofo* **172**:576–586.

20. Luxenberg DM, Silvestry FE, Herrmann HC, *et al.* (2005) Use of new 8 F intracardiac echocardiographic catheter to guide device closure of atrial septal defects and patent foramen ovale in small children and adults: initial clinical experience. *J Invasice Cardiol* **17**:540–545.

21. Penn MS, Smedira N, Lytle B, *et al.* (2000) Does coronary angiography before emergency aortic surgery affect in-hospital mortality? *J Am Coll Cardiol* **35**:889–894.

22. Eichelberger JP (1994) Aortic dissection without intimal tear. Case report and findings on transesophageal echocardiography. *J Am Soc Echocardiogr* **7**:82–86.

23. Willens HJ & Kessler KM (1999) Transesophageal echocardiography in the diagnosis of diseases of the thoracic aorta: part 1. Aortic dissection, aortic intramural hematoma, and penetrating atherosclerotic ulcer of the aorta. *Chest* **116**:1772–1779.

24. Song JK, Kim HS, Kang DH, *et al.* (2001) Different clinical features of aortic intramural hematoma versus dissection involving the ascending aorta. *J Am Coll Cardiol* **37**:1604–1610.

25. Stanson AW, Kazmier FJ, Hollier LH, *et al.* (1986) Penetrating atherosclerotic ulcers of the thoracic aorta: natural history and clinicopathologic correlations. *Ann Vasc Surg* **1**:15–23.

26. Harris JA, Bis KG, Glover JL, *et al.* (1994) Penetrating atherosclerotic ulcer of the aorta. *J Vasc Surg* **19**:90–98.

27. Koschyk DH, Meinertz T & Nienaber CA (2000) Images in cardiovascular medicine. Intravascular ultrasound for stent implantation in aortic dissection. *Circulation* **102**:480–481.

28. Bartel T, Eggebrecht H, Ebradlidze T, *et al.* (2003) Images in cardiovascular medicine. Optimal guidance for intimal flap fenestration in aortic dissection by transvenous two-dimensional and Doppler ultrasonography. *Circulation* **107**:e17–18.

29. Chan KL (1992) Impact of transesophageal echocardiography on the treatment of patients with aortic dissection. *Chest* **101**:406–410.

30. Grossman CM, Dagostino AN (1993) Advanced atherosclerosis in false channels of chronic aortic dissection. *Lancet* **342**:1428–1429.

31. Bartel T, Müller S, Caspari G, *et al.* (2002) Intracardiac and intraluminal echocardiography: indications and standard approaches. *Ultrasound Med Biol* **28**:997–1003.

32. Bartel T, Eggebrecht H, Müller S, *et al.* (2007) Comparison of diagnostic and therapeutic value of transesophageal echocardiography, intravascular ultrasonic imaging, and intraluminal phased-array imaging in aortic dissection with tear in the descending thoracic artery (type B). *Am J Cardiol* **99**:270–274.

33. Eggebrecht H, Herold U, Kuhnt O, *et al.* (2005) Endovascular stent graft treatment of aortic dissection: determinants of post-interventional outcome. *Eur Heart J* **26**:489–497.

47 MSCT for Assessment of Aortic Coarctation, Aneurysms, and Dissections

Leon D. Shturman & Suhny Abbara

Massachusetts General Hospital, Boston, MA, USA

Introduction

Like an elephant or a lion in the animal kingdom, the aorta certainly earns its undisputable respect among all the vessels, as it is the largest and strongest artery in the human body. The aorta is designed to carry approximately 200 million liters of blood throughout the body in an average lifetime [1]. Recently observed increased prevalence of aortic disease in the Western population is not only secondary to aging but also owing to increased clinical awareness. The modern clinician has to be familiar with the wide spectrum of aortic pathology.

The spectrum of clinical presentation of aortic disease varies from asymptomatic, clinically silent, to acute aortic syndromes with life-threatening complications. Therefore, indications for computed tomography (CT) scanning may derive from different clinical scenarios: symptomatic aortic disease, palpable pulsatile abdominal mass, or incidental findings on other imaging studies. Note that a thoracic aortic aneurysm may be completely undetectable clinically, as the aorta cannot be palpated there. What makes CT such a valuable diagnostic tool is its ability to obtain images in multiple planes with a wide field of view without acoustic window restrictions, as well as its high accuracy in evaluation of both thoracic and abdominal aorta with all its major branches.

In the early 1990s, slip ring technology allowed spiral- or single-detector CT (SDCT) to be introduced into clinical routine imaging in which it immediately demonstrated superiority over the conventional angiography by making visual assessment of the vessel from any angle possible [2–4]. However, the innovative modality had its own limitations: poor visualization of small aortic branches due to restrictive volume coverage, breathing and pulsation artifacts due to slow gantry rotation time in absence of cardiac gating, and limited coverage in z-dimension (~5 mm per rotation) [2–4]. Thankfully, technology was developing rapidly and in the late 1990s multidetector-row CT (MDCT) was introduced. MDCT signifi-

cantly improved image quality as a result of thinner collimation and improved resolution in the z-dimension, faster gantry rotation, larger detector arrays with more coverage in z-dimension, and increased table speed [5]. All those advances expanded clinical applications of CT as a noninvasive imaging tool. Modern 64 detector-row CT can be used as a single study to evaluate the entire aorta, including its smaller branches. Evaluation includes vessel lumen, wall, as well as extravascular structures making possible the diagnosis of ischemic bowel and renal infarcts [5]. Superior quality images are provided by MDCT by acquiring submillimeter isovolumetric voxels that allow two-dimensional (2-D) and three-dimensional (3-D) reconstructions with views from any angle in any plane [6].

Normal anatomy and normal variants

Anatomically, the entire aorta can be divided into thoracic and abdominal portions. The thoracic aorta extends from the aortic annulus to the diaphragmatic crura. The thoracic aorta consists of three parts: the ascending aorta, the aortic arch, and the descending thoracic aorta [7].

The ascending aorta is approximately 5 cm long and can be further divided into the aortic root and the tubular portion. The aortic root extends from annulus to the sinotubular junction (STJ) (Fig. 47.1a,b). It includes the right, left, and noncoronary sinus of Valsalva. The normal aortic root diameter is usually measured at ≤3.9 cm. The tubular portion of the ascending aorta lies between the STJ and the brachiocephalic trunk (BCT). The normal diameter of ascending aorta at the level of the right pulmonary artery is expected to be ≤3.5 cm (see Fig. 47.4a). There are only two branches of the ascending aorta, the right and left coronary arteries, arising from the corresponding sinus of Valsalva [7].

The aortic arch begins with the brachiocephalic trunk and extends to the origin of the left subclavian artery. The diameter of a normal aortic arch is ≤3 cm [7]. The arch is followed by the aortic isthmus that may be narrower than the proximal descending thoracic aorta. It is worthwhile mentioning that the isthmus is the most vulnerable portion of the aorta and is susceptible to tears from deceleration trauma due to the

Cardiovascular Interventions in Clinical Practice. Edited by Jürgen Haase, Hans-Joachim Schäfers, Horst Sievert and Ron Waksman. © 2010 Blackwell Publishing.

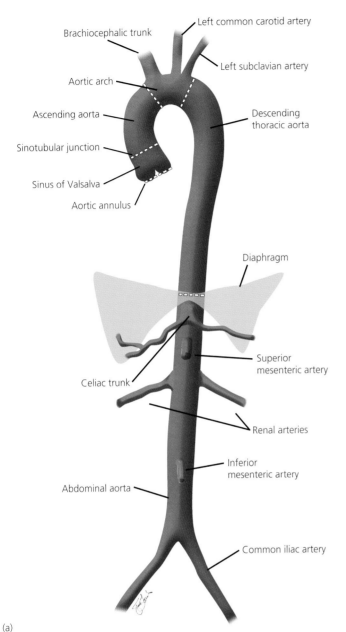

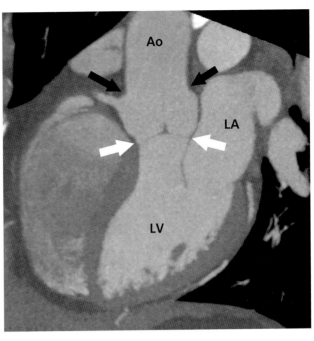

Figure 47.1 (a) Normal aortic anatomy. (b) Aortic annulus (white arrows), and sinotubular junction (black arrows).

(a)

transition of relatively immobile and more mobile aortic segments. The aortic arch gives rise to three branches: the brachiocephalic trunk (sometimes referred to as the innominate artery), the left common carotid artery (LCC), and the left subclavian artery. It is important to be aware of normal variants, such as the four-vessel arch in which the left vertebral artery originates directly from the arch (Fig. 47.1c). The bovine arch is another normal variant in which the brachiocephalic trunk and the LCC originate. Of note, this type of anatomy is not exactly as the arch anatomy of cattle; in cows the arch gives rise to a single trunk that subsequently divides into bilateral subclavian arteries and a bi-carotid trunk [8]. Finally, the ductus diverticulum (remnant of ductus arteriosus)

represents another normal variant which is nothing else but a smooth focal bulge with obtuse angles along the inner curvature of the isthmus. Opposite to normal variants, aortic transection is characterized by an acute angle with the aortic wall.

The descending thoracic aorta lies between the isthmus and the crura of the diaphragm. The diameter of the normal descending aorta is ≤2.5 cm [7]. There are multiple branches that originate from the descending thoracic aorta: bronchial, intercostal, spinal, and superior phrenic arteries, and a number of small-caliber mediastinal branches. The pseudocoarctation that usually is a product of a high arch with pseudo-kinking of the elongated aorta in which it is tethered by the ligamentum arteriosum is another rare normal variant.

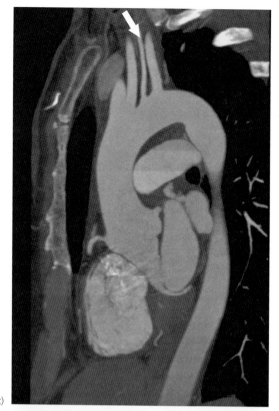

(c)

(d)

Figure 47.1 (cont'd) (c) Four-vessel arch. left vertebral artery (arrow) is arising directly from the aortic arch. Note: the normal descending thoracic aorta is weaving in and out of plane. (d) Volume-rendered reconstruction of the abdominal aorta with visceral branches.

The abdominal aorta (normal diameter 1.4–3 cm) begins where the descending thoracic aorta passes through the diaphragm and ends at the level of the forth lumbar vertebra in the bifurcation into the right and left common iliac arteries (Fig. 47.1d). Along its course, the abdominal aorta gives origin to the celiac trunk, superior, and inferior mesenteric and renal arteries.

Aortic dissection

Aortic dissection is part of the spectrum of acute aortic syndrome, which also includes intramural hematoma (IMH), penetrating atherosclerotic ulcer (PAU), ruptured aneurysms, and traumatic aortic injury. Aortic dissection is characterized by the formation of the intimal tear, including the inner layer of the aortic media that results in the formation of the false and true lumen separated by the intimal flap. Acute aortic dissection is a potentially life-threatening condition with a reported incidence of 2.9 per 100 000 persons per year with approximately 7000 cases per year in the USA [9]. There are multiple identifiable risk factors for aortic dissection, including pre-existent thoracic aneurysm, age, chronic hypertension, Marfan's syndrome, bicuspid aortic valve, and previous cardiovascular surgery. Frequency of aortic dissection varies between the regions of the aorta. Most commonly, intimal tears occur in the ascending aorta (65% of cases), 20% occur in the descending thoracic aorta, 10% in the aortic arch, and 5% in the abdominal aorta [10].

When time is of the essence, MDCT is an invaluable diagnostic tool which is easily accessible, with an ability of early and accurate detection of aortic dissection and with delineation of anatomic details, which allows early triage to appropriate treatment.

The two most common major classification systems are based on anatomical location and extension of the intimal flap: DeBakey types I, II, and III, and Stanford types A and B (Fig. 47.2a). DeBakey type I (the intimal flap involves both the ascending and descending thoracic aorta) and type II (the flap involves the ascending aorta only) correspond to the Stanford type A and constitute a surgical emergency (Fig. 47.2b,c). The DeBakey type III (the flap involves the descending aorta only) is equivalent to the Stanford type B (the flap does not involve the ascending thoracic aorta) (Fig. 47.2d). Type B is usually managed medically, with survival being greatest in the cases of noncommunicating and retrograde dissection [11]. Surgery in type B dissection is only reserved for patients with documented occlusion of major aortic branches, expansion of aorta or extension dissection (usually manifests as a recurrent pain), and aortic rupture, as well as an acute distal dissection in patients with Marfan's syndrome [12]. Timely diagnosis of acute aortic dissection is paramount, as dictated by the otherwise high mortality of untreated dissections in the acute phase (14 days from onset): mortality equals 1–2% per hour during the first 24 h and 80% over 2 weeks [13]. This is where MDCT is useful,

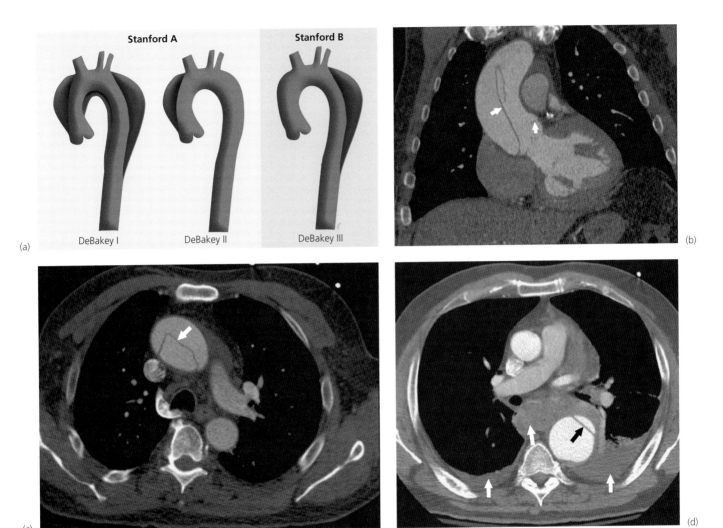

Figure 47.2 (a) Classification of aortic dissection. (b) Cardiac-gated MDCT shows a type A aortic dissection. Note: the fenestrated intimal flap (arrows) in the ascending aorta extending into the ostium of the left main coronary artery. (c) Axial MDCT image of the same patient demonstrates dissection flap in the dilated ascending aorta (arrow) and normal descending thoracic aorta. (d) Axial MDCT image of a different patient shows type B aortic dissection, as evident by an intimal flap in the descending thoracic aorta (black arrow) and normal ascending aorta. Note: bilateral hemothorax and mediastinal hematoma surrounding the descending thoracic aorta (white arrows), indicating rupture.

with early and accurate detection of this life-threatening condition, which in turn influences the type of treatment modality and its success rate and long-term outcome.

The goals of MDCT should not be limited only to the delineation of the intimal flap extension, although extension (involvement of iliac vessels) could be critical in patient selection for stent–graft repair. One should also not forget valuable information MDCT may provide in detection of the entry/re-entry site, relationships between true and false lumen, and flow in the aortic branches, as well as the presence of aortic insufficiency.

There are other imaging modalities available for the imaging of aortic dissection. Invasive aortography used to be the modality of choice for diagnosis of aortic dissection, with sensitivity and specificity rates of 77–90% and 90–100%, respectively [14]. However, the risk of catheter manipulation

and protocols requiring high-flow contrast injection make this modality less attractive. The arsenal of spiral CT includes utilization of axial and multiple plane reconstruction images of the intimal flap and adjacent great vessels, as well as 3-D volume-rendered reconstructions. Therefore, it is not surprising that, based on the results of the International Registry of Acute Aortic Dissection (IRAD), CT is found to be the most frequently used initial modality (66% of the cases). The sensitivity for spiral CT for detection of dissection is reported as 93% [15–17]. Transesophageal echocardiography (TEE), the second most frequently used modality, could compete as a bedside modality for unstable patients with a sensitivity of 87%. However, it has its own disadvantages, such as a presence of artifacts, "blind areas" (distal ascending aorta and proximal arch), and limitation to the thoracic aorta only, which may present serious drawbacks. TEE is followed by aortography and MRI with sensitivities of 88% and 100%, respectively [15–17]. When all imaging modalities have relatively high sensitivities, the frequency of its use would be predetermined by two factors: the safety and the availability.

Not too long ago there was a trend toward favoring MRI or TEE, which was based on comparisons with the older conventional spiral CT systems that were limited in aortic root visualization owing to pulsation artifact. At this point, there are no available data showing us head-to-head comparison between modern MDCT and MRI/TEE. Meanwhile, CT is probably the most rapidly advancing imaging diagnostic modality. Modern MDCT technology provides all necessary tools for successful diagnosis of aortic dissection: coverage of the entire aorta from supra-aortic branches to femoral arteries within a few seconds, increased temporal resolution with cardiac gating allowing for reduction of pulsation artifact (which otherwise could mimic type A dissections), and true volumetric imaging that allows for reconstruction of images in any plane [18]. Like no other imaging modality, unenhanced CT helps the clinician to visualize internal displacement of intimal calcifications. This finding should not be confused with aneurysms with calcified mural thrombus. The false lumen usually appears as a high-attenuation structure on unenhanced CT which helps to differentiate between these two conditions [19].

The major task in the diagnosis of suspected acute aortic dissection using CT is identification of an intimal flap, a thin linear luminal filling defect which separates the true lumen from the false one. Recent advances in endovascular repair emphasize the importance of accurate differentiation between false and true lumen. There are few pearls that may help clinicians to accomplish this task. Contrast-enhanced CT identifies true lumen by establishing its continuity with undissected portions of the aorta. The cross-sectional area of the false lumen is known to be notoriously larger than the area of the true lumen. Another finding that is specific for false lumen is known as a cobweb sign: thin linear areas of low attenuation, corresponding to remnants of the media. Finally, the beak sign is another helpful diagnostic hallmark of the false lumen. It represents the section of hematoma that cuts a space for the propagation of the false lumen [20–21].

The presence of identifiable flow in a patent false lumen is associated with certain prognostic findings. Slow flow in the false lumen eventually results in thrombus formation manifesting itself as a filling defect [20]. Based on IRAD data, patent false lumen resulted in a higher 3-year mortality (32%) than partially thrombosed lumen (14%) among the survivors of type B dissection [15]. Intimo-intimal intussusception is a rare and unusual type of aortic dissection that is characterized by a "circumferential dissection of intimal layer which invaginates like a wind sock." This may appear as a lumen wrapped around another lumen in the aortic arch with the inner lumen always being a true one [22].

Aortic aneurysm with intraluminal thrombus has to be differentiated from the aortic dissection with the thrombosed false lumen. There are few imaging findings that may help to solve this diagnostic dilemma: mural thrombus has smooth internal borders and maintains constant circumferential relationships with the aortic wall, whereas aortic dissection is a spiral-shaped process. Furthermore, CT can easily detect calcification in aneurysms, which are usually located at the periphery of the aorta [23] or within the center of the mural thrombus.

MDCT gained some edge in identifying early entry and re-entry sites in aortic dissection, which are difficult to detect with all other imaging modalities. High spatial and contrast resolution of MDCT enable clinicians to detect visceral as well as supra-aortic involvement, which always correspond to higher mortality, and, therefore, are not a trivial finding. Because of the ability of MDCT to acquire high-resolution submillimeter data with cardiac gating, it is now possible to reliably detect coronary involvement in the cases of aortic dissection.

However, there is no such thing as a perfect imaging modality. CT is not an exception and has its own pitfalls, which may even mimic aortic dissection. Most of them are linked to conventional spiral CT or MDCT in the absence of cardiac gating and related to wrongful timing or rate of contrast injection. Some of these pitfalls are streak artifacts, periaortic structures, pulsation artifacts, and aortic anomalies [24].

Intramural hematoma

Intramural hematoma (IMH), as well as penetrating atherosclerotic ulcer (PAU), is essentially considered to be an equivalent of aortic dissection for all prognostic and therapeutic purposes. Although, IMH was first described in the 1920s as "dissection without intimal tear," it became increasingly more recognized with advances of CT technology [25]. IMH may develop secondary to spontaneous rupture of the vasa vasorum of the medial aortic layer, PAU, or blunt trauma [26]. Hypertension is the most common identifiable predisposing risk factor. Rate of aortic rupture for IMH is reported to be higher (47.1%) than for type A (7.5%) or type B (4.1%) dissection [27].

As contrast within the vessel may obscure the diagnosis of IMH, unenhanced CT has proven to be an extremely valuable tool to show crescent-shaped hyperattenuation of circumferentially thickened aortic wall, which represents the hematoma within the medial layer with or without compression of aortic lumen [28]. The are few helpful findings to differentiate IMH from thrombosed false lumen: IMH remains unenhanced after the contrast injection, no intimal tear is seen, and finally IMH maintains constant circumferential relationships with aortic wall whereas the false lumen has longitudinal spiral geometry [29].

There are no clear cut imaging predictors for progression of IMH to dissection. Nevertheless, some findings, such as IMH type A, thick hematoma with compression of the true lumen, pericardial or pleural effusion, and an aortic diameter of > 5 cm, are reported to add some value in making this prediction [30–31].

Penetrating atherosclerotic ulcer

Penetrating atherosclerotic ulcer became a "younger sister" of IMH when it was first described in 1934 by Shennan [32] in the thoracic aorta as a focal contrast filled outpouching of aortic wall. Arterial hypertension and advanced age are the most common risk factors. The descending aorta is the most common location where PAU is found [33]. Morphologically, PAU could be described as an ulcerated atheroma disrupting the aortic intima [34]. Extension of the aortic ulcer into the medial layer often results in a formation of IMH, localized aortic dissection, saccular pseudoaneurysm, and even mediastinal hematoma in the cases of the breakthrough to the adventitia and its rupture [34].

Extensive aortic atherosclerosis in combination with IMH (often accompanied by the displaced intimal calcifications) is commonly shown with CT. CT features of PAU are strikingly similar to peptic ulcer: discrete contrast filled "collar button" [34]. One should not be surprised to find multiple lesions, considering the diffuse nature of atherosclerosis. PAU is more eccentric than irregular mural thrombus, with associated features such as thickened aortic wall, pseudoaneurysm, dissection, or even rupture [35].

Evaluation of aortic dissection after surgical repair

Although the current operative mortality for aortic dissection repair has been significantly reduced (5–7% vs. 40–50% in 1970s) survivors still remain at relatively high risk in the postoperative period, and therefore require lifetime monitoring [36]. New generations of MDCT offer thinner collimation, faster gantry rotation, 180° reconstruction algorithms, and submillimeter isovolumetric voxels (resolution in all three dimensions < 1 mm), which allows to minimize artifacts from metallic stents, surgical clips, and cardiac motion. Postoperative monitoring should focus on detection of dilation of the distal aorta, as it is a sign of a pending rupture. Other findings to be aware of are prosthetic graft degeneration, infection, malfunction of aortic valve prosthesis as well as possible aneurysm formation in locations remote from the previous repair. Based on the fact that aortic rupture is usually preceded by rapid expansion, Heinemann offered a postoperative schedule with a major goal to detect this expansion: CT was obtained at the time of discharge and was also performed once a year if the absolute aortic diameter was less than 5 cm, or was performed every 6 months if the absolute diameter was > 5 cm [37].

Aortic coarctation

Aortic coarctation in essence is a focal narrowing of the thoracic aorta, typically in the isthmus, often associated with chest wall collaterals (Fig. 47.3a,b). A fibrous ridge, the product of abnormal hyperplasia of tunica media, encircles the aorta and causes an obstructive lesion. Aortic coarctation is a relatively common malformation, responsible for 6–8% of all congenital heart defects affecting males (2–5 times more often than females) [38]. There are three known major anatomical types of stenotic segments causing an aortic arch obstruction: focal (aortic coarctation), diffuse (hypoplastic isthmus), and complete (aortic arch interruption) [39].

Before going deeper into the subject of aortic coarctation, it is important to mention a rare anomaly called pseudocoarctation, which is nothing else but abnormal kinking (without obstruction) of the elongated aortic arch and the first portion of the descending thoracic aorta, fixed by the ligamentum arteriosum but without chest wall collaterals, fibrous ridge, or gradient (Fig. 47.3d). This rare anomaly is explained by the failure of the 3rd to the 7th dorsal embryonic segments to fuse properly to form the normal aortic arch. Pseudocoarctation is not a completely benign condition and, with age, progressive dilation and even dissection may occur [40].

Most of the classifications of aortic coarctation are based on the anatomical location. Previously used classifications that divided an aortic coarctation on preductal (infantile) and postductal (adult) types could be misleading. Therefore, the contemporary approach is to use the left subclavian artery as a landmark, allowing the distinguishing between more common distal (juxtaductal) and less common proximal types [38].

The presence of aortic coarctation should alert the physician to search for associated abnormalities. There are data of increased familial risk of left ventricular outflow obstructions, including the left ventricle, aortic valve, and aortic arch [41]. The prevalence of aortic coarctation is increased in certain disorders, such as Turner's syndrome. There is a known association of aortic coarctation with the bicuspid aortic valve in 30–40% of patients with aortic coarctation, or more [42]. Other associated lesions include ventricular septum defect, patent ductus arteriosus, aortic stenosis, and mitral stenosis [43]. It is important to screen patients with aortic coarctation for the presence of intracerebral berry aneurysms which may cause subarachnoid or intracerebral hemorrhage even long after successful coarctation repair, and in normotensive patients [44]. Extensive collaterals are a compensatory response to coarctation that depends on the stenosis severity. Collaterals may compress the spinal cord or may rupture and produce the clinical picture of subarachnoid spinal hemorrhage [45].

In addition to the congenital variant, rare cases of acquired aortic coarctation are also reported; inflammatory aortitis (Takayasu) is the most common and usually affects the midthoracic or abdominal aorta (Fig. 47.3c). Severe atherosclerosis has also been reported but as a less common entity [46].

Although MRI is a modality of choice for the pediatric population secondary to lack of radiation and iodinated contrast, MDCT is rapidly improving. MDCT advances close the gap owing to easy availability. The faster scan acquisition time in CT (2–10 min vs. 30–45 min in MRI) allows decreasing of

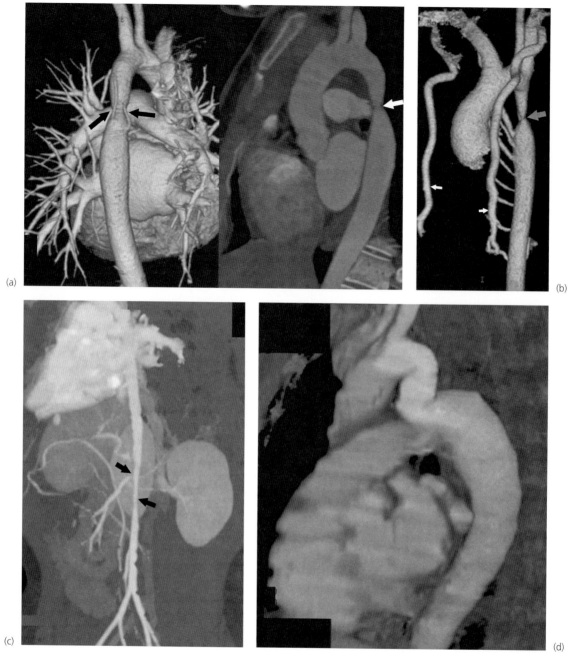

Figure 47.3 (a) Volume-rendered and multiplanar reconstructed CTA images of aortic coarctation demonstrate a mildly stenotic segment (arrows) and little collaterals. (b) Volume-rendered reconstruction of aortic coarctation in a different patient demonstrates high-grade coarctation (large arrow) and markedly enlarged left and right internal mammary arteries (small arrows) and intercostal collaterals. (c) Different patient with atypical coarctation of the abdominal aorta (arrows). (d) Aortic pseudocoarctation. Sagittal oblique volume-rendered 3-D projection shows an elongated proximal descending thoracic aorta with pseudo-kink.

the required sedation or anesthesia time, and the ability to adjust tube current, voltage, and pitch to the patients weight and age can result in drastic reduction of the radiation dose. Use of nonionic contrast with minimal iodine concentration helps to avoid nephrotoxicity [47].

Treatment of aortic coarctation largely depends on age, clinical presentation and severity. Early repair may prevent long-standing hypertension. Indications for repair include arterial hypertension, congestive heart failure, gradient more or equal to 30 mmHg, although extensive collaterals make resting gradient alone an unreliable indicator of severity [48]. Patients younger than 6 months are usually advised to have surgical repair rather than balloon angioplasty. There are multiple surgical techniques available, including resection with end-to-end anastomosis, subclavian flap aortoplasty in infants with long-segment coarctation, prosthetic patch (currently rarely used owing to increased occurrence of postoperative aneurysms and ruptures), and bypass graft across the coarctation, when the distance for end-to-end repair is too long [49]. Lifetime postoperative surveillance of these patients is necessary to monitor for residual coarctation (most common with resection and end-to-end anastomosis), aortic arch hypoplasia, aneurysm formation at the site of repair (most common with synthetic patch aortoplasty and subclavian flap arterioplasty), as well as restenosis, dissection, and pseudoaneurysm (most common with balloon angioplasty) [50]. Balloon angioplasty is an alternative to surgery and can be used in children and adults with native coarctation as well as restenosis after surgery [51–52].

Thoracic aortic aneurysm

A true aortic aneurysm is defined as a permanent pathologic, localized or diffuse dilation of the aorta, including all three layers (intima, media, and adventitia), to >50% of the normal or expected aortic diameter [53]. Aortic aneurysm is anything but a benign condition, being the 13th most common cause of death in USA. As life expectancy increases in the Western civilization, the incidence and prevalence of aortic aneurysms is also increasing and the incidence was reported as 10.9 cases/100 000 persons per year in 1998 [54]. Thoracic aneurysm is most commonly diagnosed between the age of 60 and 70 years and is 2–4 times more common in males than females. Hypertension is present in 60% of the cases. Thoracic aortic aneurysms are much less common than abdominal aortic aneurysms. Multiple aneurysms are present in up to 13% of all patients, but 25% of patients with thoracic aneurysm will also have an abdominal aortic aneurysm [55]. Although most thoracic aneurysms are atherosclerotic in nature, atherosclerosis has never been proven to be a direct cause of aneurysmal formation or growth, whereas cystic medial degeneration is a universal feature regardless the cause or location of thoracic aortic aneurysms. Cystic medial degeneration increases with age and arterial hypertension. In younger patients, cystic medial degeneration is commonly due to Marfan's or Ehlers–Danlos syndrome [56].

There are multiple classifications of thoracic aortic aneurysms based on extent and morphology. Thoracoabdominal aortic aneurysm refers to descending thoracic aneurysms that extend distally to involve the abdominal aorta. The Crawford classification distinguishes four types of thoracoabdominal aneurysms from proximal to distal extent [57] (Fig. 47.4c). Types I and II start at the left subclavian artery. Type I extends to the renal artery, and type II extends to the aortic bifurcation. Type II has been known to be associated with the worst postsurgical outcome, along with old age and renal insufficiency. Both types III and IV terminate distally at the aortic bifurcation. Type III starts at the mid thorax, whereas type IV starts at the level of the diaphragm. Morphologically, thoracic aneurysms are divided into fusiform (uniform in shape with

symmetrical dilation involving entire circumference of the aortic wall), saccular (localized outpouching of the aortic wall), and pseudoaneurysm (collection of blood and connective tissue outside of the aortic wall as the result of rupture of intima and media). Not all segments of the thoracic aorta are affected equally, in some cases aneurysms involve more than one segment: The aortic root and ascending aorta (aortic valve to innominate artery) are affected in 60% of cases, the arch in 10%, the descending thoracic aorta (distal to left subclavian artery) in 40%, and finally the thoracoabdominal in 10% [56]. CT goals are to define anatomical characteristics of thoracic aneurysms, including extent, location, and size, usually obtained strictly in the aortic short axis (orthogonal to the aortic segment long axis) (Fig. 47.4b,d). Size is the only proven risk factor predicting aortic rupture. Five-year risk of rupture is 0% for aneurysms less than 4 cm, 16% for 4–5.9 cm, and 31% for >6 cm in size [54].

In addition to size, CT can accurately detect the presence of complications such as rupture, mycotic aneurysms, and fistulas. CT provides necessary information for both postsurgical surveillance and the follow-up for the medically treated patients. CT can accurately detect the extent of the aneurysm and the involvement of aortic branches, which is essential for preoperative surgical evaluation [58].

Because of the tortuosity of the thoracic aorta, its size is better measured from double oblique tomograms perpendicular to the aortic flow lumen. All size-related prognostic information known today is based on transverse section measurements. The most sensitive measurement of the aneurysmal size is actually the aneurysm volume, not the aortic diameter or the cross-sectional area. Unfortunately, in the absence of advanced very specialized software, this method requires the manual drawing of regions of interest (ROIs) on each cross-section and, therefore, is very labor-consuming and not practical for everyday use.

Aortic root aneurysms may result in effacement of the sino-tubular junction in the setting of annuloaortic ectasia, which is usually diagnosed in patients with Marfan's and Ehlers–Danlos syndromes [59]. Aortic root aneurysm has also been associated with bicuspid aortic valve and familial thoracic aortic aneurysm syndrome (FTAAS). Most of the cases of tubular portion aneurysms of ascending aorta are idiopathic but may also be associated with bicuspid aortic valve, FTAAS, giant cell arteritis, and syphilis [60–63]. FTAAS became a real entity after it was discovered that up to 19% of the patients with thoracic aneurysms had a family history independent of Marfan's or Ehlers–Danlos syndromes [62].

Bicuspid aortic valves deserve special attention. Even normally functioning bicuspid aortic valves have been associated with enlargement of the aortic root and/or ascending aorta in 52% of the patients [60]. Bicuspid aortic valve is also known to be an independent predictor of ascending aortic aneurysm formation after surgical correction of coarctation [61].

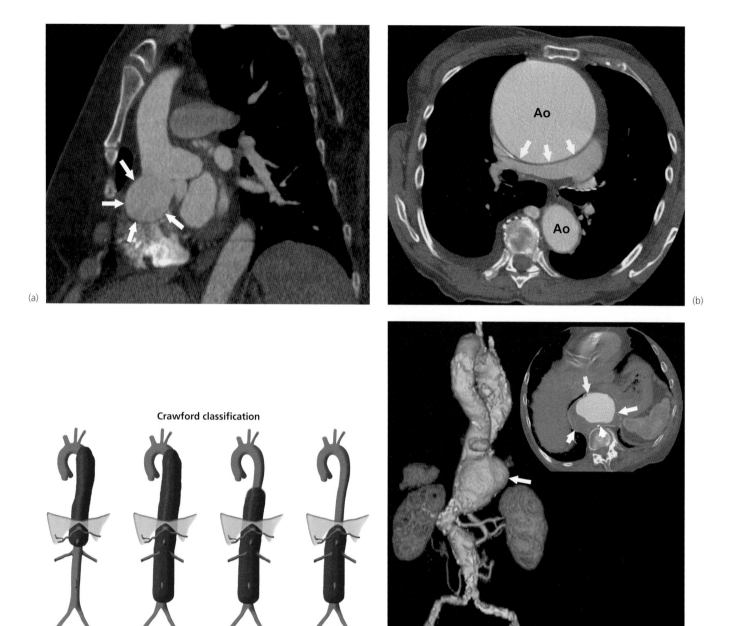

(a)

(b)

Crawford classification

I   II   III   IV

(c)

(d)

Figure 47.4 (a) Cardiac-gated CTA shows aneurysm of noncoronary sinus of Valsalva (arrows). (b) Axial image in a different patient with ascending aortic aneurysm shows compressing of right pulmonary artery (arrows). (c) Classification of thoracoabdominal aneurysm. (d) Thoracoabdominal aneurysm with mural thrombus (arrows).

Aneurysms of the ascending aorta or the aortic arch may result in mediastinal erosion and present with hoarseness (due to left vagus or left recurrent laryngeal nerve compression), hemidiaphragmatic paralysis due to compression of the phrenic nerve, tracheobronchial compression (wheezing, cough, and hemoptysis), esophageal compression (dysphagia), and superior vena cava syndrome. Aneurysmal compression of adjacent bones may cause chest or back pain. Other known thoracic aneurysm complications include thromboembolism, aorto-esophageal fistula, and finally dissection that may result

in pleural or pericardial effusions. Risk of dissection is also directly related to the size of the aneurysm. The dissection risk per year is only 2% for aneurysm <5 cm in size, but increases to 3% for 5–5.9 cm, and to >7% for aneurysms >6 cm in diameter, with 5-year survival of only 54% in the absence of surgery [64].

The average growth of thoracic aneurysms is 1–10 mm per year [65]. The rate of growth is related to the anatomical location as well as initial diameter of the aneurysm. Descending mid portion aortic aneurysms have the fastest growth rate, whereas ascending aneurysms have the slowest growth rate, despite larger initial diameter [65]. In general, larger aneurysms are growing faster: aneurysms >5 cm in diameter are growing on average 7.9 mm per year versus 1.7 mm per year for smaller size aneurysms [66].

Obvious indications for surgery include symptoms or evidence of dissection. Although optimal timing of surgical repair for thoracic aneurysm is uncertain, surgery is usually recommended for ascending aneurysm of 5–6 cm and descending aneurysm of 6–7 cm [67]. Some clinicians use aortic size index, calculated as the ratio of aortic diameter to body surface area in m², with the cut-off being ≥2.75 cm/m² [68]. Accelerated growth (>10 mm per year in aneurysms of <5 cm) is an additional indication for surgery [69]. Patients with Marfan's syndrome and bicuspid aortic valve belong to a special category. Aortic insufficiency of any severity in conjunction with aortic root or ascending aortic aneurysms, such as in Marfan's, requires aortic valve replacement plus aortic root repair, if the aneurysm is 5 cm or greater, some experts would even accept 4.5 cm or growth ≥0.5 cm per year [70,71]. A bicuspid aortic valve that requires aortic valve replacement (for aortic stenosis or insufficiency) should be accompanied by an aortic root replacement if the diameter of the aortic root or ascending aorta is >4.5 cm (smaller thresholds have been suggested for patients with smaller stature) [70]. In patients with a functional bicuspid aortic valve, aortic root repair or replacement of ascending aorta is indicated if root/ascending aorta is >5.0 cm in diameter or rate of growth is ≥0.5 cm per year [70]. Using the consistent technique is a paramount importance for follow-up imaging to monitor the growth of aortic aneurysm. One of the proposed follow-up schedules is to perform the first scan 6 months after the initial study, then yearly if no growth, or every 3–6 months (according to the size) if growth is rapid [56].

Sinus of Valsalva aneurysm

Aortic aneurysm of the sinuses of Valsalva is a rare congenital anomaly associated with the failure of proper development of elastic components of the aortic medial layer, resulting in its separation from the fibrous annulus of the aortic valve (Fig. 47.4a). The right coronary sinus of Valsalva is the most commonly affected, followed by the noncoronary sinus; the left coronary sinus is the least common site. Most cases are asymptomatic until rupture occurs, which is not uncommon in the young without previously established diagnosis. Sinus of Valsalva aneurysms usually rupture into right heart chambers (right atrium or right ventricle), causing left-to-right shunt with the symptoms of congestive heart failure. Another complication is protrusion into and obstruction of the right ventricular outflow tract (RVOT). In contrast to Marfan's disease, in which the aortic root is uniformly involved, the CT appearance of sinus of Valsalva aneurysm is that of an asymmetric sinus dilation. There are no clearly developed criteria for proper surgical timing; progressive increase in size rather than absolute measurement appear to be more frequently, clinically utilized [72,73].

Abdominal aortic aneurysm

The abdominal aorta is the number one site for arterial aneurysms, within which the most common site is between the renal artery and the inferior mesenteric artery. Abdominal aortic aneurysm (AAA) can be defined as a focal dilation of 1.5 times that of the diameter of the aorta measured at the level of the renal arteries. At the level of the renal artery the aortic diameter usually ranges from 1.4 to 3.0 cm; diameters of >3 cm are considered aneurysmal [74]. AAA is a diagnosis of middle-aged and elderly patients. Screening of patients older than 60 reveals AAA in 4–9% of the population, 56–88% of which are less than 3.5 cm in diameter. Clinically relevant aneurysms of >4 cm in size are detected only in 1% of men between the ages of 55 and 64 [75,76]. AAAs are responsible for 15 000 deaths per year in the USA [77]. Smoking is the most important risk factor affecting both formation and growth of AAAs. Other risk factors include family history, atherosclerosis, and hypertension [78–80]. Men are affected 4–5 times more frequently than women [75,78], but women have a higher risk of rupture than men [79].

Increasing detector rows of MDCT allowed reduction of scan acquisition times (>20 s to cover abdominal aorta with 4-row MDCT versus less than 10 s for 16-row MDCT). Today's MDCT can evaluate the entire thoracoabdominal aorta and iliac system in a single breath hold with high spatial resolution and higher luminal contrast concentration, and overall reduced contrast load to the patient [6]. In addition multiplanar and 3-D reconstruction capabilities improved the diagnostic quality [81,82]. Compared with MRI, the spatial resolution has become superior, and CT is far better for characterizing mural calcifications. MDCTs very well-known drawbacks are ionizing radiation and potential nephrotoxicity of iodinated contrast.

An AAA can be classified according to the cause, anatomical shape, and location. Based on the cause, AAAs can be divided into degenerative atherosclerotic, infectious, traumatic congenital, inflammatory, and, finally, postoperative [83]. Atherosclerotic penetrating ulcers have a potential of developing into small aneurysms with relatively high rupture rates in up to 40% of the cases [84]. According to anatomical shape, an AAA can be described as saccular, fusiform, and true or false [83]. Different anatomical location allows the distinguishing of thoracoabdominal aneurysm, suprarenal aneurysm, juxtarenal aneurysm (located at the level of the lowest renal artery or within 5 mm from the lowest main renal artery), and finally infrarenal aneurysm [83].

The responsibility for describing location, extent, diameter, length of the aneurysm neck, presence of mural thrombus, occlusion of branches (inferior mesenteric artery is commonly affected), as well as involvement of the iliac arteries, in addition to renal and other visceral vessels, lies with MDCT. CT should primarily focus on the diameter and expansion rate of AAA in the series of the follow-up images [85,86]. Clinicians should be aware that the diameter of AAA estimated by CT is usually 0.3–0.9 cm larger than the measurements obtained by ultrasound, and interobserver variability is 0.5 cm in up to 17% of cases [87,88]. Rupture risk of AAAs can be predicted not only from the maximum diameter, but also from the peak wall stress distribution (requires CT data plus the patient's blood pressure) [89]. Although the peak wall stress distribution concept requires further investigation, a maximum diameter of AAAs is still the most frequently used measurement in the routine practice to predict its risk of rupture. Annual risk of rupture of AAAs is markedly increased after reaching the diameter of 5.5 cm, being negligible for aneurysms of less than 4.0 cm in diameter. An AAA with a diameter of 4.0–4.9 cm has an annual risk of rupture of 0.5–5%, whereas 5.0–5.9 cm and 6.0–6.9 cm in size correspond to 3–15% and 10–20%, respectfully, of annual rupture risk [85,90]. In addition, an AAA expansion rate of >0.5 cm per 6 months (even for the small AAA), and symptomatic AAA can be considered a high-risk feature predictive of rupture [74]. Based on the size of AAA, it is proposed to follow AAAs with a diameter of 3–4 cm every 2–3 years, and 4.0–5.4 cm every 6–12 months [74]. Current guidelines recommend surgical intervention for tan asymptomatic AAA of ≥5.5 cm in diameter [74]. MDCT successfully eliminated invasive angiogram as a preoperative tool. Owing to its inability to visualize mural thrombus, an invasive angiogram provides inaccurate measurement of an AAA diameter. Furthermore, description of the aneurysm length, neck, and involvement of the iliac vessels is superior with MDCT, which is crucial in planning for endovascular aneurysm repair (EVAR) [91,92].

Endovascular aneurysm repair

The popularity of EVAR has been rising since early 1990s when it was used for the first time for infrarenal AAA repair, with the use of a stent graft (combination of metallic mesh-work and prosthetic graft material) delivered percutaneously through the femoral artery. The goal is to exclude the aneurysm from circulation to prevent its rupture [93,94]. It is impossible to overestimate the importance of accurate and detailed measurement of an AAA diameter before EVAR to select the proper size of the endovascular stent graft. Mismatch may result in stent migration, endoleak, rupture, and the need for open repair, which then in turn will be complicated by the presence of the stent graft [95].

Planning for EVAR demands detailed evaluation of the aneurysm neck including its length, tapering, degree of angulation and presence of mural thrombus [96]. The length of the aneurysm neck is measured from the most caudal renal artery to the beginning of the aneurysm. A sealing problem may occur if the length is less than 15 mm, requiring the use of the stent graft with suprarenal fixation via a fenestrated

stent portion [97,98]. Reverse tapering of >2 mm in the aneurysm neck within 1 cm below the renal artery will result in a problem with proximal fixation of the stent graft [96]. Angulation of the aneurysm neck (angle between longitudinal axis of the proximal neck of the aorta and longitudinal axis of the aneurysm) can be classified as mild (<40°), moderate (40–59°), and severe (>59°). Moderate and severe angulation may result in complications such as stent graft migration, kinking, and, finally, incomplete sealing, resulting in endoleaks and embolism [99]. The presence of mural thrombus in the neck of the aneurysm may be a contraindication for EVAR because it may prevent adequate sealing and result in endoleak or embolism [100]. Undetected accessory renal arteries originating from the aneurysm may cause endoleaks after EVAR and even result in renal infarcts if excluded from the circulation. As a preventive measure, if small, these accessory renal arteries could be embolized before EVAR. Another contraindication to EVAR due to risk of large bowel necrosis is the presence of bilateral common iliac aneurysms that would require exclusion of both internal iliac arteries [93,97]. Routine follow-up and monitoring for late complications after EVAR, which are much more common than after conventional surgical repair, are extremely important [101]. Clinicians should be actively looking for endoleaks, stent migration, kinking, thrombosis, aneurysm enragement, and infection with pseudoaneurysm formation. Triple-phase CT (unenhanced, arterial phase, and delayed phase for low-flow endoleaks) is usually utilized for routine follow-up. A baseline CT is usually performed before discharge (2–4 days after the procedure), the second CT in 6 months, and from then on annual CT imaging is necessary [102]. Presence of soft tissue stranding, fluid collections, and air around the aorta are signs of infection [103].

The proximal neck of the aneurysm may dilate after EVAR, and if dilation is severe it may result in stent migration and endoleaks [104]. Complications directly related to the procedure include perforation of the mural thrombus, shower embolism, aortic dissection, and hematoma or pseudoaneurysm at the arteriotomy site.

Expected early normal findings after EVAR should not be confused with endoleaks. It is not unusual to see early post-procedural air in the aneurysm sac, hyperattenuation around the stent graft (thrombosis of the previously patent lumen), and sometimes calcifications in the thrombus displaced from the aortic wall [105]. EVAR excludes the aneurysm sac from the circulation and, therefore, it is expected to observe a decrease in aneurysm sac diameter [106]. Although the maximum diameter of the aneurysm (measured in the short axis in two directions) is the most frequently used surveillance method, a volumetric approach is more precise. The reason is that endoleak or endotension may increase the volume of aneurysm without affecting its diameter [107,108].

Endoleak is a persistent blood flow into the aneurysm sac when the stent graft fails to exclude the aneurysm from the circulation [109]. Each of the four types of endoleak described below has its own clinical significance, in terms of the prognosis and the required treatment. Type I is an attachment site endoleak. It is subdivided into proximal (1a) and distal (1b) attachment site endoleaks. Intervention is always required if these types of endoleaks occur. Type II endoleak (the most frequent) is caused by the collateral flow from lumbar or inferior mesenteric arteries to the excluded aneurysm sac. Type II can be further characterized into "simple" type (2a) with one patent collateral branch and "complex" type (2b) with two or more collateral branches.

Fortunately, type II does not require any intervention unless the aneurysm demonstrates progressive expansion. Therefore, if more than four lumbar arteries arise from the aneurysm sac, its embolization before EVAR may be attempted to prevent type II endoleak [110]. Type III endoleak is attributed to structural stent graft failure, such as stent fracture or junctional separation, and always requires treatment. Type IV endoleak is usually identified at the time of the stent graft placement and caused by the porosity of the stent graft. Type IV occurs in fully anticoagulated patients and rarely requires intervention. Some experts argue that endotension should be called as a type V endoleak. Endotension refers to the expansion of the aneurysm in absence of an identifiable cause, even though some argue that some cases may be a result of an undetected type II endoleak [109,111]. Direct pressure measurement in the aneurysm sac is indicated if the sac does not appropriately decrease in size or volume and endotension is suspected. Intervention is required when an arterial pressure gradient is detected. Therefore, patients who underwent EVAR are in need of lifetime surveillance [111].

References

1. Isselbacher EM (2005) Diseases of the aorta: the normal aorta. In: Braunwald E, Zipes D, Libby P, Bonow R (eds). *Braunwald's Heart Disease: A Textbook of Cardiovascular Medicine*, 7th edn. Philadelphia: WB Saunders, pp. 1403–1404.

2. Van Hoe LS, Baert AL, Gryspeerdt S, *et al.* (1996) Supra and juxta renal aneurysms of the abdominal aorta: preoperative assessment with thin-section spiral CT. *Radiology* **198**:443–448.

3. Kaatee R, Van Leeuwen MS, DeLange EE, *et al.* (1998) Spiral CT angiography of the renal arteries: should a scan delay based on a test bolus injection or a fixed scan delay be used to obtain maximum enhancement of the vessel? *J Comput Assist Tomogr* **22**:541–547.

4. Armerding MD, Rubin GD, Beaulieu CF, *et al.* (2000) Aortic aneurysmal disease: assessment of stent graft treatment—CT versus conventional angiography. *Radiology* **215**:138–146.

5. Katz DS, Jorgensen MJ, & Rubin GD (1999) Detection and follow-up of important extraarterial lesions with helical CT angiography. *Clin Radiol* **54**:294–300.

6. Rubin GD (2003) MDCT imaging of the aorta and peripheral vessels. *Eur J Radiol.* **45**(Suppl. 1):S42–49. Review.

7. Hager A, Kaemmerer H, Rapp-Bernhardt U, *et al.* (2002) iameters of the thoracic aorta throughout life as measured with helical computed tomography. *J Thorac Cardiovasc Surg* **123**:1060–1066.

8. Layton KF, Kallmes DF, Cloft HJ, Lindell EP, & Cox VS (2006) Bovine aortic arch variant in humans: clarification of a common misnomer. *AJNR Am J Neuroradiol* **27**:1541–1542.

9. Mészáros I, Mórocz J, Szlávi J, *et al.* (2000) Epidemiology and clinicopathology of aortic dissection. *Chest* **117**:1271–1278.

10. Isselbacher EM (2005) Diseases of the aorta: aortic dissection. In: Braunwald E, Zipes D, Libby P, Bonow R (eds). *Braunwald's Heart Disease: A Textbook of Cardiovascular Medicine*, 7th edn. Philadelphia: WB Saunders, pp. 1415–1431.

11. Erbel, R, Oelert, H, Meyer, J, *et al.* (1993) Effect of medical and surgical therapy on aortic dissection evaluated by transesophageal echocardiography. Implications for prognosis and therapy. The European Cooperative Study Group on Echocardiography. *Circulation* **87**:1604.

12. DeSanctis RW, Doroghazi RM, Austen WG, & Buckley MJ (1987) Aortic dissection. *N Engl J Med* **317**:1060.

13. Coady MA, Rizzo JA, Goldstein LJ, & Elefteriades JA (1999) Natural history, pathogenesis, and etiology of thoracic aortic aneurysms and dissections. *Cardiol Clin* **17**:615–635.

14. Bansal RC, Chandrasekaran K, Ayala K, & Smith DC (1995) Frequency and explanation of false negative diagnosis of aortic dissection by aortography and transesophageal echocardiography. *J Am Coll Cardiol* **25**:1393–1401.

15. Moore AG, Eagle KA, Bruckman D, *et al.* (2002) Choice of computed tomography, transesophageal echocardiography, magnetic resonance imaging, and aortography in acute aortic dissection: International Registry of Acute Aortic Dissection (IRAD). *Am J Cardiol* **89**:1235–1238.

16. Cigarroa JE, Isselbacher EM, DeSanctis RW, *et al.* (1993) Diagnostic imaging in the evaluation of suspected aortic dissection. Old standards and new directions. *N Engl J Med* **328**:35–43.

17. Nienaber CA, von Kodolitsch Y, Nicolas V, *et al.* (1993) The diagnosis of thoracic aortic dissection by noninvasive imaging procedures. *N Engl J Med* **328**:1–9.

18. Morgan-Hughes GJ, Marshall AJ, & Roobottom CA (2003) Refined computed tomography of the thoracic aorta: the impact of electrocardiographic assistance. *Clin Radiol* **58**:581–588.

19. Greenberg RK, Secor JL, & Painter T (2004) Computed tomography assessment of thoracic aortic pathology. *Semin Vasc Surg* **17**:166–172.

20. Williams MP & Farrow R (1994) Atypical patterns in the CT diagnosis of aortic dissection. *Clin Radiol* **49**:686–689.

21. LePage MA, Quint LE, Sonnad SS, *et al.* (2001) Aortic dissection: CT features that distinguish true lumen from false lumen. *AJR Am J Roentgenol* **177**:207–211.

22. Nelsen KM, Spizarny DL, & Kastan DJ (1994) Intimointimal intussusception in aortic dissection: CT diagnosis. *AJR Am J Roentgenol* **162**:813–814.

23. Rubin GD (1997) Helical CT angiography of the thoracic aorta. *J Thorac Imaging* **12**:128–149.

24. Batra P, Bigoni B, Manning J, *et al.* (2000) Pitfalls in the diagnosis of thoracic aortic dissection at CT angiography. *Radiographics* **20**:309–320.

25. Krukenberg E (1920) Beitrage Zur Frage des Aneurysm a dissecans. *Beitr Pathol Anat Allg Pathol* **67**:329–351.

26. Fattori R, Bertaccini P, & Celletti F, *et al.* (1997) Intramural post-traumatic hematoma of the ascending aorta in a patient with a double aortic arch. *Eur Radiol* **7**:51–53.

27. Coady MA, Rizzo JA, & Elefteriades JA (1999) Pathologic variants of thoracic aortic dissections. Penetrating atherosclerotic ulcers and intramural hematomas. *Cardiol Clin* **17**:637–657.

28. Nienaber CA, von Kodolitsch Y, Petersen B, *et al.* (1995) Intramural hemorrhage of the thoracic aorta. Diagnostic and therapeutic implications. *Circulation* **92**:1465–1472.

29. Von Kodolitsch Y & Nienaber CA (1998) [Intramural hemorrhage of the thoracic aorta: diagnosis, therapy and prognosis of 209 in vivo diagnosed cases.] *Z Kardiol* **87**:797–807.

30. Von Kodolitsch Y, Csösz SK, Koschyk DH, *et al.* (2003) Intramural hematoma of the aorta: predictors of progression to dissection and rupture. *Circulation* **107**:1158–1163.

31. Kaji S, Nishigami K, Akasaka T, Hozumi T, *et al.* (1999) Prediction of progression or regression of type A aortic intramural hematoma by computed tomography. *Circulation* **100**(19 Suppl.):II281–286.

32. Shennan T (1934) Dissecting aneurysms. Medical Research Council Special Report series no. 193. London: Stationary Office.

33. Fattorri R & Russo V (2005) Magnetic resonance imaging and computed tomography of the thoracic aorta: aortic ulcers. In: Higgins CB, de Roos A. *MRI and CT of the Cardiovascular System*, 2nd edn. Philadelphia: Lippincott Williams & Wilkins, pp. 450–452.

34. Quint LE, Williams DM, Francis IR, *et al.* (2001) Ulcerlike lesions of the aorta: imaging features and natural history. *Radiology* **218**:719–723.

35. Kazerooni EA, Bree RL, & Williams DM (1992) Penetrating atherosclerotic ulcers of the descending thoracic aorta: evaluation with CT and distinction from aortic dissection. *Radiology* **183**:759–765.

36. Svensson LG & Crawford SE (1997) Statistical analyses of operative results. In: Svensson LG & Crawford SE (eds). *Cardiovascular and Vascular Disease of the Aorta*. Philadelphia: WB Saunders, pp. 432–455.

37. Heinemann M, Laas J, Karck M, & Borst HG (1990) Thoracic aortic aneurysms after acute type A aortic dissection: necessity for follow-up. *Ann Thorac Surg* **49**: 580–584.

38. Brickner ME, Hillis LD, & Lange RA (2000) Congenital heart disease in adults. First of two parts. *N Engl J Med* **342**:256.

39. Webb GD, Smallhorn JF, & Therrier J (2005) Congenital heart disease: coarctation of the aorta. In: Braunwald E, Zipes D, Libby P, Bonow R (eds). *Braunwald's Heart Disease: A Textbook of Cardiovascular Medicine*, 7th edn. Philadelphia: WB Saunders, pp. 1532–1535.

40. Fattorri R & Russo V (2005) Magnetic resonance imaging and computed tomography of the thoracic aorta: congenital aortic diseases. In: Higgins CB, de Roos A. *MRI and CT of the Cardiovascular System*, 2nd edn. Philadelphia: Lippincott Williams & Wilkins, pp. 462–468.

41. McBride KL, Pignatelli R, Lewin M, *et al.* (2005) Inheritance analysis of congenital left ventricular outflow tract obstruction malformations: segregation, multiplex relative risk, and heritability. *Am J Med Genet A* **134**:180–186.

42. Nihoyannopoulos P, Karas S, Sapsford RN, *et al.* (1987) Accuracy of two-dimensional echocardiography in the diagnosis of aortic arch obstruction. *J Am Coll Cardiol* **10**:1072–1077.

43. Levine JC, Sanders SP, Colan SD, *et al.* (2001) The risk of having additional obstructive lesions in neonatal coarctation of the aorta. *Cardiol Young* **11**:44–53.

44. Hodes HL, Steinfeld L, & Blumenthal S (1959) Congenital cerebral aneurysms and coarctation of the aorta. *Arch Pediatr* **76**:28–43.

45. Watson AB (1967) Spinal subarachnoid haemorrhage in patient with coarctation of aorta. *Br Med J* **4**:278–279.

46. Pagni S, Denatale RW, & Boltax RS (1996) Takayasu's arteritis: the middle aortic syndrome. *Am Surg* **62**:409–412.

47. Haramati LB, Glickstein JS, Issenberg HJ, *et al.* (2002) MR imaging and CT of vascular anomalies and connections in patients with congenital heart disease: significance in surgical planning. *Radiographics* **22**:337–347.

48. Attenhofer Jost CH, Schaff HV, Connolly HM, *et al.* (2002) Spectrum of reoperations after repair of aortic coarctation: importance of an individualized approach because of coexistent cardiovascular disease. *Mayo Clin Proc* **77**:646–653.

49. Parikh SR, Hurwitz RA, Hubbard JE, *et al.* (1991) Preoperative and postoperative "aneurysm" associated with coarctation of the aorta. *J Am Coll Cardiol* **17**:1367–1372.

50. Therrien J, Thorne SA, Wright A, *et al.* (2000) Repaired coarctation: a "cost-effective" approach to identify complications in adults. *J Am Coll Cardiol* **35**:997–1002.

51. Fawzy ME, Awad M, Hassan W, *et al.* (2004) Long-term outcome (up to 15 years) of balloon angioplasty of discrete native coarctation of the aorta in adolescents and adults. *J Am Coll Cardiol* **43**:1062–1067.

52. Hellenbrand WE, Allen HD, Golinko RJ, *et al.* (1990) Balloon angioplasty for aortic recoarctation: results of Valvuloplasty and Angioplasty of Congenital Anomalies Registry. *Am J Cardiol* **65**:793–797.

53. Johnston KW, Rutherford RB, Tilson MD, *et al.* (1991) Suggested standards for reporting on arterial aneurysms. Subcommittee on Reporting Standards for Arterial Aneurysms, Ad Hoc Committee on Reporting Standards, Society for Vascular Surgery and North American Chapter, International Society for Cardiovascular Surgery [see comments]. *J Vasc Surg* **13**:452–458.

54. Clouse WD, Hallett JW Jr, Schaff HV, *et al.* (1998) Improved prognosis of thoracic aortic aneurysms: a population-based study. *JAMA* **280**:1926–1929.

55. Crawford ES & Cohen ES (1982) Aortic aneurysm: a multifocal disease. *Arch Surg* **117**:1393.

56. Isselbacher EM (2005) Thoracic and abdominal aortic aneurysms. *Circulation* **111**:816–828.

57. Svensson LG, Crawford ES, Hess KR, *et al.* (1993) Experience with 1509 patients undergoing thoracoabdominal aortic operations. *J Vasc Surg* **17**:357–368.

58. Quint LE, Francis IR, Williams DM, *et al.* (1996) Evaluation of thoracic aortic disease with the use of helical CT and multiplanar reconstructions: comparison with surgical findings. *Radiology* **201**:37–41.

59. Adams JN & Trent RJ (1998) Aortic complications of Marfan's syndrome. *Lancet* **352**:1722–1723.

60. Nistri S, Sorbo MD, Marin M, *et al.* (1999) Aortic root dilatation in young men with normally functioning bicuspid aortic valves. *Heart* **82**:19–22.

61. von Kodolitsch Y, Aydin MA, Koschyk DH, *et al.* (2002) Predictors of aneurysmal formation after surgical correction of aortic coarctation. *J Am Coll Cardiol* **39**:617–624.

62. Coady MA, Davies RR, Roberts M, *et al.* (1999) Familial patterns of thoracic aortic aneurysms. *Arch Surg* **134**:361–367.

63. Nuenninghoff DM, Hunder GG, Christianson TJ, *et al.* (2003) Incidence and predictors of large-artery complication (aortic aneurysm, aortic dissection, and/or large-artery stenosis) in patients with giant cell arteritis: a population-based study over 50 years. *Arthritis Rheum* **48**:3522–3531.

64. Davies RR, Goldstein LJ, Coady MA, *et al.* (2002) Yearly rupture or dissection rates for thoracic aortic aneurysms: simple prediction based on size. *Ann Thorac Surg* **73**:17–27.

65. Bonser RS, Pagano D, Lewis ME, *et al.* (2000) Clinical and patho-anatomical factors affecting expansion of thoracic aortic aneurysms. *Heart* **84**:277–283.

66. Dapunt OE, Galla JD, Sageghi AM, *et al.* (1994) The natural history of thoracic aortic aneurysms. *J Thorac Cardiovasc Surg* **107**:1323.

67. Coady MA, Rizzo JA, Hammond GL, *et al.* (1999) Surgical intervention criteria for thoracic aortic aneurysms: a study of growth rates and complications. *Ann Thorac Surg* **67**:1922–1926.

68. Davies RR, Gallo A, Coady MA, *et al.* (2006) Novel measurement of relative aortic size predicts rupture of thoracic aortic aneurysms. *Ann Thorac Surg* **81**:169–77.

69. Lobato AC & Puech-Leao P (1998) Predictive factors for rupture of thoracoabdominal aortic aneurysm. *J Vasc Surg* **27**:446–453.

70. Bonow, RO, Carabello, BA, Chatterjee, K, *et al.* (2006) ACC/AHA 2006 guidelines for the management of patients with valvular heart disease. A report of the American College of Cardiology/American Heart Association Task Force on Practice Guidelines (Writing committee to revise the 1998 guidelines for the management of patients with valvular heart disease). *J Am Coll Cardiol* **48**:e1–148.

71. Gott VL, Pyeritz RE, Magovern GJ Jr, *et al.* (1986) Surgical treatment of aneurysms of the ascending aorta in the Marfan syndrome. Results of composite-graft repair in 50 patients. *N Engl J Med* **314**:1070–1074.

72. Webb GD, Smallhorn JF, & Therrier J (2005) Congenital heart disease: sinus of Valsalva aneurysm and fistula. In: Braunwald E, Zipes D, Libby P, Bonow R (eds). *Braunwald's Heart Disease: A Textbook of Cardiovascular Medicine*, 7th edn. Philadelphia: WB Saunders, pp. 1535–1536.

73. Abbara S, Kalva S, Cury RC, & Isselbacher EM (2007) Thoracic aortic disease: spectrum of multidetector computed tomography imaging findings. *J Cardiovasc Computed Tomogr* **1**:40–54.

74. Hirsch AT, Haskal ZJ, Hertzer NR, *et al.* (2006) ACC/AHA 2005 Practice Guidelines for the management of patients with peripheral arterial disease (lower extremity, renal, mesenteric, and abdominal aortic): a collaborative report from the American Association for Vascular Surgery/Society for Vascular Surgery, Society for Cardiovascular Angiography and Interventions, Society for Vascular Medicine and Biology, Society of Interventional Radiology, and the ACC/AHA Task Force on Practice Guidelines (Writing Committee to Develop Guidelines for the Management of Patients With Peripheral Arterial Disease): endorsed by the American Association of Cardiovascular and Pulmonary Rehabilitation; National Heart, Lung, and Blood Institute; Society for Vascular Nursing; TransAtlantic Inter-Society Consensus; and Vascular Disease Foundation. *Circulation* **113**: e463–654.

75. Singh K, Bønaa KH, Jacobsen BK, *et al.* (2001) Prevalence of and risk factors for abdominal aortic aneurysms in a population-based study: The Tromsø Study. *Am J Epidemiol* **154**:236–244.

76. Powell JT & Greenhalgh RM (2003) Small abdominal aortic aneurysms. *N Engl J Med* **348**:1895–1901.

77. Creager MA, Halperin JL, & Whittemore AD (1996) Aneurysmal disease of the aorta and its branches. In: Loscalzo J, Creager MA, Dzau VJ (ed.), *Vascular Medicine.* New York: Little, Brown, p. 901.

78. Lederle FA, Johnson GR, Wilson SE, *et al.* (1997) Prevalence and associations of abdominal aortic aneurysm detected through screening. *Ann Intern Med* **126**:441–449.

79. Norman PE & Powell JT (2007) Abdominal aortic aneurysm: the prognosis in women is worse than in men. *Circulation* **115**: 2865.

80. Lederle FA, Johnson GR, Wilson SE, *et al.* (2000) The aneurysm detection and management study screening program: validation cohort and final results. Aneurysm Detection and Management Veterans Affairs Cooperative Study Investigators. *Arch Intern Med* **160**:1425–1430.

81. Napoli A, Fleischmann D, Chan FP, *et al.* (2004) Computed tomography angiography: state-of-the-art imaging using multi-detector-row technology. *J Comput Assist Tomogr* **28**(Suppl. 1): S32–45.

82. Rydberg J, Buckwalter KA, Caldemeyer KS, *et al.* (2000) Multisection CT: scanning techniques and clinical applications. *Radiographics* **20**:1787–1806.

83. Chaikof EL, Blankensteijn JD, Harris PL, *et al.* (2002) Reporting standards for endovascular aortic aneurysm repair. *J Vasc Surg* **35**:1048–1060.

84. Eggebrecht H, Baumgart D, Schmermund A, *et al.* (2003) Penetrating atherosclerotic ulcer of the aorta: treatment by endovascular stent graft placement. *Curr Opin Cardiol* **18**: 431–435.

85. Nevitt MP, Ballard DJ, & Hallett JW Jr (1989) Prognosis of abdominal aortic aneurysms. A population-based study. *N Engl J Med* **321**:1009–1014.

86. Glimåker H, Holmberg L, Elvin A, *et al.* (1991) Natural history of patients with abdominal aortic aneurysm. *Eur J Vasc Surg* **5**:125–130.

87. Sprouse LR 2nd, Meier GH 3rd, Lesar CJ, *et al.* (2003) Comparison of abdominal aortic aneurysm diameter measurements obtained with ultrasound and computed tomography: is there a difference? *J Vasc Surg* **38**:466–471.

88. Lederle FA, Wilson SE, Johnson GR, *et al.* (1995) Variability in measurement of abdominal aortic aneurysms. Abdominal Aortic Aneurysm Detection and Management Veterans Administration Cooperative Study Group. *J Vasc Surg* **21**:945–952.

89. Fillinger MF, Marra SP, Raghavan ML, *et al.* (2003) Prediction of rupture risk in abdominal aortic aneurysm during observation: wall stress versus diameter. *J Vasc Surg* **37**:724–732.

90. Brewster DC, Cronenwett JL, Hallett JW Jr, *et al.* (2003) Guidelines for the treatment of abdominal aortic aneurysms. Report of a subcommittee of the Joint Council of the American Association for Vascular Surgery and Society for Vascular Surgery. *J Vasc Surg* **37**:1106–1117.

91. Diehm N, Herrmann P, & Dinkel HP (2004) Multidetector CT angiography versus digital subtraction angiography for aortoiliac length measurements prior to endovascular AAA repair. *J Endovasc Ther* **11**:527–534.

92. Blum U, Voshage G, Lammer J, *et al.* (1997) Endoluminal stent grafts for infrarenal abdominal aortic aneurysms. *N Engl J Med* **336**:13–20.

93. Rydberg J, Kopecky KK, Lalka SG, *et al.* (2001) Stent grafting of abdominal aortic aneurysms: pre- and postoperative evaluation with multislice helical CT. *J Comput Assist Tomogr* **25**:580–586.

94. Parodi JC, Palmaz JC, & Barone HD (1991) Transfemoral intraluminal graft implantation for abdominal aortic aneurysms. *Ann Vasc Surg* **5**:491–499.

95. Wyers MC, Fillinger MF, Schermerhorn ML, *et al.* (2003) Endovascular repair of abdominal aortic aneurysm without preoperative arteriography. *J Vasc Surg* **38**:730–738.

96. Dillavou ED, Muluk SC, Rhee RY, *et al.* (2003) Does hostile neck anatomy preclude successful endovascular aortic aneurysm repair? *J Vasc Surg* **38**:657–663.

97. Carpenter JP, Baum RA, Barker CF, *et al.* (2001) Impact of exclusion criteria on patient selection for endovascular abdominal aortic aneurysm repair. *J Vasc Surg* **34**:1050–1054.

98. Verhoeven EL, Prins TR, Tielliu IF, *et al.* (2004) Treatment of short-necked infrarenal aortic aneurysms with fenestrated stent grafts: short-term results. *Eur J Vasc Endovasc Surg* **27**:477–483.

99. Sternbergh WC 3rd, Carter G, York JW, Yoselevitz M, *et al.* (2002) Aortic neck angulation predicts adverse outcome with endovascular abdominal aortic aneurysm repair. *J Vasc Surg* **35**:482–486.

100. Gitlitz DB, Ramaswami G, Kaplan D, *et al.* (2001) Endovascular stent grafting in the presence of aortic neck filling defects: early clinical experience. *J Vasc Surg* **33**:340–344.

101. Lederle FA (2004) Abdominal aortic aneurysm—open versus endovascular repair. *N Engl J Med* **351**:1677–1679.

102. Armerding MD, Rubin GD, Beaulieu CF, *et al.* (2000) Aortic aneurysmal disease: assessment of stent graft treatment-CT versus conventional angiography. *Radiology* **215**:138–146.

103. Macedo TA, Stanson AW, Oderich GS, *et al.* (2004) Infected aortic aneurysms: imaging findings. *Radiology* **231**:250–257. Erratum in: *Radiology* 2006;**238**:1078.

104. Napoli V, Sardella SG, Bargellini I, *et al.* (2003) Evaluation of the proximal aortic neck enlargement following endovascular repair of abdominal aortic aneurysm: 3-years experience. *Eur Radiol* **13**:1962–1971.

105. Sawhney R, Kerlan RK, Wall SD, *et al.* (2001) Analysis of initial CT findings after endovascular repair of abdominal aortic aneurysm. *Radiology* **220**:157–160.

106. Farner MC, Carpenter JP, Baum RA, *et al.* (2003) Early changes in abdominal aortic aneurysm diameter after endovascular repair. *J Vasc Interv Radiol* **14**(2 Pt 1):205–210.

107. Kritpracha B, Beebe HG, & Comerota AJ (2004) Aortic diameter is an insensitive measurement of early aneurysm expansion after endografting. *J Endovasc Ther* **11**:184–190.

108. Pollock JG, Travis SJ, Whitaker SC, *et al.* (2002) Endovascular AAA repair: classification of aneurysm sac volumetric change using spiral computed tomographic angiography. *J Endovasc Ther* **9**:185–193.

109. Veith FJ, Baum RA, Ohki T, *et al.* (2002) Nature and significance of endoleaks and endotension: summary of opinions expressed at an international conference. *J Vasc Surg* **35**:1029–1035.

110. Görich J, Rilinger N, Sokiranski R, *et al.* (2001) Endoleaks after endovascular repair of aortic aneurysm: are they predictable?-initial results. *Radiology* **218**:477–480.

111. Stavropoulos SW & Baum RA (2004) Imaging modalities for the detection and management of endoleaks. *Semin Vasc Surg* **17**:154–160.

48 Percutaneous Treatment of Aortic Coarctation

John D.R. Thomson[1] & Shakeel A. Qureshi[2]

[1]Leeds General Infirmary, Leeds, UK
[2]Evelina Children's Hospital, London, UK

Introduction

Aortic coarctation is a common congenital cardiac defect, of which there are many anatomic variations. The morphologic spectrum varies from transverse arch and isthmal hypoplasia, seen most commonly in the newborn infant, to discrete stenosis distal to the left subclavian artery, the typical lesion in older patients. In rare cases, long segment tubular hypoplasia can affect a large segment of the thoracic or abdominal aorta. At the extreme end of severity is interruption of the aortic arch, which will not be dealt with in this chapter.

In those patients who survive infancy, the natural history of untreated coarctation is premature death from accelerated vascular disease, as a consequence of poorly controlled hypertension [1]. Relief of the stenosis improves blood pressure control and is indicated in all but the mildest form of obstruction in normotensive patients [2].

The treatment of aortic coarctation has evolved over the last 60 years. Initial surgical attempts described excision of the stenosis with end-to-end anastomotic repair. Subsequently, surgery for aortic arch obstruction developed to include a disparate group of operations, reflecting the highly variable anatomy and differing technical challenges. Despite the accumulated knowledge of the last 60 years, older patients in particular present significant technical challenges for operative repair, as evidenced by a consistent second peak in mortality during adult life reported in the surgical literature, the first being in early infancy [3]. Complications of surgical treatment include spinal cord damage, pleural effusion, paradoxical hypertension and infection [4,5]. In addition thoracotomy scars are particularly painful in older patients and the convalescent period may be prolonged.

It is against this background that percutaneous treatment for aortic coarctation in selected cases has found favor.

Cardiovascular Interventions in Clinical Practice. Edited by Jürgen Haase, Hans-Joachim Schäfers, Horst Sievert and Ron Waksman. © 2010 Blackwell Publishing.

Indications for treatment

The correct timing of intervention in many cases remains unclear, mainly because accurate predictors of outcome in these patients are incompletely understood. In infants with hemodynamic compromise, the indication for treatment is unequivocal. Because cardiovascular collapse outside of this age group is rare, in older patients an invasive gradient across the obstruction of 25 mmHg was traditionally taken as a cut-off value for treatment, although this is not universally accepted [6,7]. Furthermore, in older patients, the gradient across the site of the obstruction may be affected by the presence of longstanding arterial collateral vessels. Because the long-term outcome in these patients is influenced by arterial hypertension, many congenital cardiologists advocate treatment in those patients who have unequivocal systemic hypertension (usually above the 97th centile for age) along with evidence of important luminal obstruction, regardless of the gradient across the site of the coarctation [8].

Further work to refine our understanding of the risk factors, indications, and timing of treatment, particularly in adolescents and young adults with unrepaired coarctation, is required.

Balloon dilation

Early work on balloon dilation of experimental coarctation of the aorta in animal models together with later studies of postmortem and postsurgical specimens preceded the first balloon angioplasty in humans in 1982 [9,10]. Twenty-five years later, the technique remains controversial, because histologic data show that successful relief of stenosis is accompanied by damage to the aortic intima and media [9,11,12]. In addition, before treatment there is often evidence of thinning of the aortic wall and cystic medial necrosis at the site of the coarctation, making this segment of the aorta particularly vulnerable to aneurysm formation following balloon-induced trauma [13].

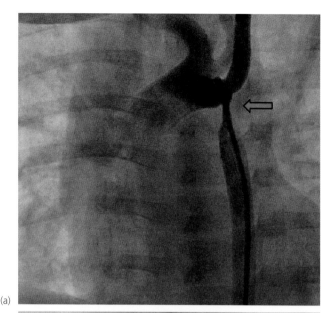

(a)

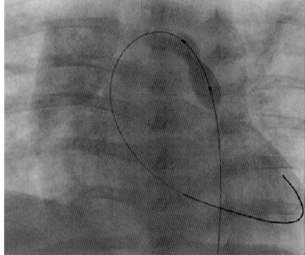

(b)

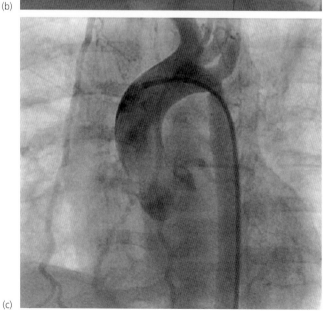

(c)

Equipment

A selection of balloons, appropriate for angioplasty of the aorta in patients of different ages, is required. Although each operator and each catheterizing laboratory will have its own preferences in the choice of equipment, examples of balloons currently utilized in our laboratories for this procedure in different age groups include the following:

• infants/smaller children—Tyshak®, Tyshak II®, Tyshak-Mini® (all NuMed Inc., Hopkinton, NY, USA), and Opta®/Powerflex® balloons (Boston Scientific, Natick, MA, USA);

• older children—Tyshak generation of balloons, Cristal (Merck, Whitehouse Station, NJ, USA);

• adults—Tyshak generation of balloons, Z-Med™ (NuMed), Cristal (Merck).

Other equipment needed for treatment includes:

• Perclose suture (Abbott, Abbott Park, IL, USA) for percutaneous closure of the access site;

• a selection of guidewires, including Terumo® or other super-floppy guidewires, for crossing tight stenoses;

• exchange length super stiff guidewires between 0.018 and 0.035 inches in diameter;

• high-flow pigtail catheters and Multitrack™ catheters (NuMed) for angiography and pressure measurements over a guidewire already in position.

Ideally a selection of covered Cheatham platinum stents (NuMed), or other covered stents or stent grafts, and appropriately sized balloon-in-balloon (BIB) delivery systems (NuMed) should be available in every laboratory carrying out balloon angioplasty of coarctation for use in the event of aortic dissection.

Technique

Balloon angioplasty of coarctation of the aorta may be a painful procedure and so it is best carried out under general anesthesia, although in experienced hands, the appropriate use of sedation and intravenous opiate in an awake patient is an alternative. Cross-matched blood should be available for immediate use in case of an emergency.

The technique for treatment of aortic coarctation is similar to other forms of balloon angioplasty(Fig. 48.1). Access is obtained via the femoral artery. Stability of the balloon is less of a concern in coarctation angioplasty than in placement of a stent, so femoral venous access for the placement of a temporary pacing wire in the right ventricle (see stent placement) is rarely required. The patient is heparinized (100 IU/kg) maintaining an activated clotting time of 200–300s in prolonged procedures. High-quality biplane angiography is an advantage, as accurate measurements of the aortic arch are

Figure 48.1 (*left*) Balloon angioplasty of recurrent coarctation at the site of end-to-end surgical repair in an infant of 3 months of age. Aortogram showing significant recoarctation (red arrow). Balloon inflation with a 10-mm Mini-Tyshak balloon, with waist formation. Aortogram (in this case with a pigtail catheter) following balloon angioplasty, showing improvement in luminal size, although some residual stenosis remains.

critical for correct selection of a balloon. Ascending aortograms are performed using a catheter (either a marker pigtail or a Multitrack monorail catheter), with radiopaque markings of known size in the left anterior oblique (LAO) and lateral projections. Occasionally additional projections are required. Once an acceptable image is obtained, a frame is stored and "road mapped" to guide positioning of the balloon, and, following this, every effort should be made to keep the table in the same position. The alternative is to insert an additional catheter into the ascending aorta, either using a radial or brachial artery approach or antegradely from the right heart and across to the ascending aorta via the atrial trans-septal route. This approach allows for repeated angiograms during balloon positioning.

Accurate measurements of the different segments of the aorta are essential. The diameter of the aorta at the isthmus above the coarctation, at mid-transverse arch level and at the level of the diaphragm are measured along with the minimum size at the level of the coarctation. A supportive exchange length guidewire (for example an Amplatz super stiff) is positioned either in the ascending aorta or right/left subclavian artery depending on the preference of the operator and the individual anatomy. In any case, positioning the guidewire in the carotid arteries should be avoided. Once the guidewire is in place, it should be left for the duration of the procedure, as repeated instrumentation of the aorta after balloon dilation is likely to extend aortic trauma, and may potentially be a risk factor for aneurysm formation.

There is no clear consensus on the selection of the balloon size for angioplasty. The diameter of the isthmus proximal to the coarctation, the transverse arch, and the descending aorta at the level of the diaphragm have all been used to determine the balloon diameter for dilation. Some operators suggest using a balloon diameter 2–3 times that of the coarctation segment itself, although this is illogical as the ratio bears no relation to the size of the adjacent normal aorta and could lead to significant and possibly dangerous overdilation of the normal aorta in patients with mild coarctation. In the data reported from the multicenter Valvuloplasty and Angioplasty of Congenital Anomalies (VACA) register, there was no relationship between the size of the selected balloon and the diameter of the coarctation in providing effective reduction of the gradient [14,15]. In addition, these data showed no clear relationship between the diameter of the balloon and formation of aneurysms, suggesting that the overall risk may relate to intrinsic wall characteristics rather than the size of the balloon. However, most experienced operators are careful not to overdilate the normal aorta proximal to the lesion. Our policy is to select a balloon exactly equal to the diameter of the adjacent proximal isthmus. In our experience, failure to achieve adequate relief of the gradient using a balloon of this size usually indicates elastic recoil of the aorta and the need for a stent rather than repeated dilation with progressively larger balloons, although there is some evidence of progressive remodeling of the aorta with time following balloon angioplasty [16].

Once the correctly sized balloon has been selected, it is carefully de-aired, passed over the guidewire through the sheath in the femoral artery, and advanced into position across the coarctation. In an anesthetized patient, the balloon can be accurately positioned using the road mapped image and the radiographic landmarks (e.g., in relation to the endotracheal tube). Inflation is performed with a pressure monitoring inflation device. In a successful angioplasty, a waist is seen on the balloon (Fig. 48.1b), which is abolished as the stenotic site is dilated. The process takes 10–15 s and the balloon is then deflated and removed. Further angiograms and pressure measurements are taken, generally using a Multitrack monorail catheter.

Balloon dilation of coarctation in the neonate and infant

Treatment of aortic coarctation by balloon angioplasty in neonates and infants is particularly controversial. Early attempts to treat this age group were limited by issues of vascular access, in which damage to the femoral arterial tree was a frequent and occasionally fatal complication [14]. Advances in balloon technology now mean that effective angioplasty can be achieved using balloons, which in some cases are small enough to be passed through a 3F sheath, whereas previously up to 7F or 8F sheaths were required. Although some of the technical problems have been addressed, follow-up data still show high rates of restenosis in neonates undergoing balloon angioplasty compared with older children and adults [17–20], and, in some studies, these patients appear to be at particular risk of aneurysm formation [21]. Although in some instances acceptable results can be achieved with angioplasty in this age group, the current consensus in the pediatric cardiology community is that these patients are on the whole best treated surgically [22]. The exception to this is the patient presenting with severe hemodynamic compromise after ductal closure unresponsive to high-dose intravenous prostaglandin infusion. Patients with ongoing acidosis are high-risk surgical candidates, and so balloon angioplasty may be indicated for initial palliation as a bridge to later surgical repair [23].

Results and complications of balloon angioplasty

A number of reports demonstrate that satisfactory reduction of gradient can be achieved immediately after balloon angioplasty [14–17,24,25]. Longer-term follow-up studies report variable results of sustained relief of the gradient, with important stenosis recurring in 7.5–50% of patients, most of whom require repeat procedures. As discussed above, the age of the patient at the time of balloon angioplasty appears to be an important risk factor for later restenosis [7,17,18,24–26].

Valuable data from the early era of balloon angioplasty (pre-1990) were reported to the VACA registry, which included 141 patients with native coarctation and 200 with recurrent or residual aortic arch obstruction after surgery [14,15]. These reports contain data on procedures performed in patients across all age ranges. In those undergoing treatment for aortic recoarctation, 5/200 (2.5%) died of complications related to the procedure (two vagal, one cerebral embolus, one aortic rupture, and one death due to shock in a patient presenting *in extremis*). Neurologic complications occurred in 3/200 (1.5%), and 17/200 (8.5%) experienced femoral artery complications, none of which resulted in permanent damage. Aortic intimal tears were evident in three (1.5%) patients on the postprocedural angiogram, one of which required surgical repair.

Data from the VACA registry on balloon dilation for native coarctation reported one death in a neonate (0.7% of the study population). The reasons for this are unclear but appear to relate to bleeding from the femoral arterial access site. Overall, complications occurred in 24/141 cases (17%), of which 14 were related to the femoral artery access. There were two aneurysms at the site of dilation, evident on post-procedural angiograms, in addition to late aneurysms in six patients, all of whom underwent later surgical repair. Thus, the overall rate of aneurysm formation was 5.6%.

The incidence of aneurysms following balloon dilation differs markedly in reports, from 0% to 35% [7,17,18,20,25,26,28]. Although rare, aneurysms can also occur late after balloon dilation. At a mean of 10.6 years after balloon angioplasty, Cowley *et al.* [28] detected a small number of new aneurysms >5 years after the initial intervention. However, most aneurysms appear to progress only rarely and so can be managed conservatively. Although their long-term clinical implications are questionable, avoiding aneurysm formation should be an aim of the treatment. In this regard, concerns remain about the longer-term results of balloon angioplasty.

Rates of complication in contemporary studies are much lower and, in particular, careful guide-wire positioning avoiding the head and neck vessels along with careful anticoagulation means that embolic neurologic complications are rarely reported in the modern era [20,26,27].

Acute aortic tears following balloon angioplasty remain a rare complication and, despite the lack of firm evidence, probably relate to overdilation of the normal aorta rather than rupture of the coarctation segment itself. Such events need early recognition and resuscitation of the patient by inflation of a balloon (under low pressure) to stabilize the aorta and prevent massive hemorrhage. Either emergency surgery in small babies or insertion of a covered stent across the tear in older patients is then required as a bail-out procedure.

Comparisons of surgical and balloon angioplasty

It is difficult to make meaningful comparisons of surgery and balloon angioplasty for coarctation of the aorta based on individual series, which are usually reported by units with a particular enthusiasm for one form of treatment or the other. In particular, surveillance protocols for the detection of aneurysms differ markedly between reported series.

With the uncertainties surrounding the best mode of treatment, several attempts have been made to compare surgery with balloon angioplasty. All the reported studies are limited by small numbers of patients. Three studies report retrospective comparisons, which raises concerns regarding bias and equivalence of groups [29–31]. A single randomized trial included only 36 patients undergoing treatment at ages ranging from 3 to 10 years [32]. Reduction in the gradient was similar between surgery and balloon angioplasty. Restenosis occurred more commonly in the angioplasty group, although this difference did not reach statistical significance. Neurologic complications occurred only in the surgical patients, and aneurysm formation only after angioplasty (20%). The authors restudied the original patient population over 10 years after the initial treatment [28]. Unfortunately only 55% of the balloon angioplasty group were available for long-term surveillance making interpretation of the data difficult. Late follow-up showed equivalence for the need for further intervention between the groups, but a higher rate of aneurysm formation (35% vs. 0%) was found in the angioplasty group, in which three aneurysms had developed late.

Balloon dilation of native versus residual or recurrent coarctation

In the opinion of some pediatric cardiologists, the risk of aortic disruption and aneurysm formation at the time of balloon angioplasty is lower in patients with restenosis after previous surgical repair compared with those with native coarctation. This is usually attributed to scar tissue at the site of the previous surgery protecting the aortic wall from rupture after dilation. Although aneurysm formation may be less of a concern in patients with recurrent arch obstruction, data from the VACA registry suggests that angioplasty of recurrent coarctation is actually a riskier procedure than angioplasty of native coarctation [14,15]. This is certainly the view of many experienced operators, who view dilation of recurrent arch obstruction, particularly many decades after surgical repair, with some trepidation. Although the aortic arch may be protected by scar tissue, the vessel itself is often rigid and relief of stenosis by balloon angioplasty is often accompanied by disruption of the vessel, as a consequence of stretching of the pre-existing suture or scar lines.

Stents

Having recognized the limitations of balloon dilation of aortic coarctation, stents were viewed as a potential solution to the problems of dissection, overdilation, and elastic recoil of the aorta. There is histologic data supporting the hypothesis that stenting results in less vascular injury than with angioplasty alone [33]. Stents also tack intimal flaps to the wall of the aorta, allowing healing to occur without causing intimal dissection along with reinforcing weakened areas of the aorta, which are potentially at risk of formation of false aneurysms.

The treatment of coarctation using stents dates back to 1991 [34], with the approach initially reserved for cases in which either surgery or angioplasty had failed. With time and increasing experience, in many cases stenting has become the procedure of choice for aortic coarctation in adolescents and adults in whom somatic growth is no longer an issue. Stents potentially offer an effective endovascular solution for complex arch problems, particularly those traditionally resistant to balloon dilation, such as transverse arch hypoplasia. Although complex arch anatomy may seem a less than ideal substrate for the insertion of a stent, it is important to remember the surgical challenges presented by these lesions, where often the only option is extraanatomic bypass of the obstruction using synthetic tube grafts.

Equipment

Stents

Stents that are currently available for use in the treatment of coarctation include the Palmaz (Cordis, Waterloo, Belgium), Intrastent Max™ large diameter (EV3 Inc., Plymouth, MN, USA), and Cheatham platinum (NuMed Inc., Hopkinton, NY, USA) stents.

The Palmaz stent is displayed in Fig. 48.2a. The Palmaz Johnson & Johnson series were the only stents available for the treatment of coarctation for many years. These stents are laser-cut from stainless steel so that, when fully expanded, the cells are diamond-shaped. The larger P10 series, available in 30, 40, and 50 mm lengths and dilatable to 26–28 mm are most suited to aortic stenting. These stents are rigid and have relatively sharp ends, making them less than ideal for inflation on a single large balloon, where flaring of the ends during deployment and hence exposure of the sharp tips of the stent to the vessel may damage the aortic wall. Shortening of the stent at larger diameters is significant. Despite these issues, the Palmaz stent has been used extensively for the treatment of coarctation and is effective even in the largest of adults.

In recent years, the Palmaz J & J series has been replaced by the Palmaz Genesis™ stent (Cordis). The architecture of these stents is complex, with a "sigmoid" connection between the cells, enhancing flexibility compared with the J & J range, in addition to removing the sharp ends. Palmaz Genesis stents are available in a variety of lengths and are both unmounted and premounted on balloons of up to 10 mm. At larger diameters, the radial strength of these stents is not as good as the original J & J, series and many operators have concerns about their use in the aorta.

The Intrastent Max™ large diameter stent is an open cell stent with rounded edges available in 16, 26, and 36 mm lengths (Fig. 48.2b). These stents do not shorten appreciably when fully expanded. At larger diameters (20–24 mm), this stent has a radial strength roughly equivalent to the Palmaz J & J series. Because of its open cell design, the stent is relatively flexible and the side of the stent can be crossed, allowing a guidewire, balloon, or even another stent to be inserted, making these stents particularly suitable for treating lesions in which there is a likelihood of covering an arterial side branch.

Cheatham-Platinum stents (NuMed) are made from Platinum wire with gold links creating large diamond shaped cells (each row of cells being termed a "ZIG") (Fig. 48.2c and d). The edges are rounded and so there is little or no risk of edge-related damage to the vessel wall during inflation. These stents have considerable radial strength and are available in 22, 28, 34, 39, and 45 mm lengths. Cheatham platinum stents are available not only as a bare metal implant, but also with a polytetrafluoroethylene covering for target vessel wall protection and the exclusion of aneurysms. Uncovered, these stents will easily expand to above 24 mm, but the polytetrafluoroethylene covering on the standard covered stent may be disrupted at an expansion diameter of approximately 22–24 mm. Larger covered stents capable of expanding beyond 24 mm can be ordered from the manufacturer but require larger delivery sheaths (>16F). Although relatively new, the Cheatham-Platinum stent was specifically designed for the needs of patients with congenital heart disease, and there is already considerable experience with its use in patients with coarctation of the aorta.

Other equipment

All of the above stents are balloon-expandable and need to be mounted on an appropriate balloon of the correct diameter. A selection of balloons including Opta/Powerflex (Cordis), Cristal (Merck) and Z-Med (NuMed) are required in diameters from 6 to 30 mm. Higher-pressure balloons such as the Mullins™ (NuMed) may be required also.

Many operators favor the use of the BIB® (NuMed) dilation catheter for the insertion of aortic stents (Fig. 48.2d). This balloon allows sequential inflation of the stent, with the inner balloon partially inflating the stent before the outer balloon is inflated to expand to the final diameter. This avoids or limits the so-called "Eiffel tower" effect, where one end of the balloon inflates before the middle, effectively "milking" the stent either forwards or backwards.

Long sheaths are necessary for the safe delivery and positioning of coarctation stents. The Cook Mullins Check-Flo® trans-septal sheath in lengths of up to 85 cm and internal diameters between 6F and 14F is currently the best available. This sheath is unbraided and so is prone to kinking in tortuous vessels; however, within the relatively straight distal aorta, its performance is good. Custom-made delivery systems are available in larger diameters.

Technique

The procedure is performed under general anesthesia. Femoral arterial access is obtained and, after an appropriate angiogram

(a)

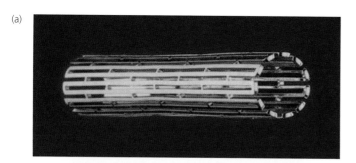

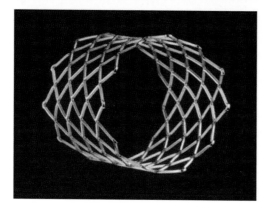

(b)

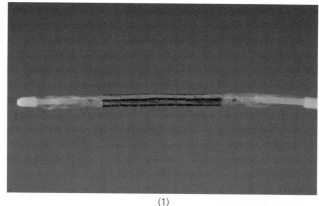

(1)

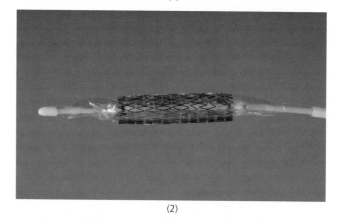

(2)

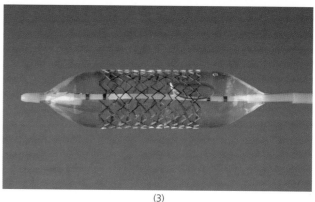

(3)

Figure 48.2 (a) Palmaz 4014 stent in unexpanded form (above) and after expansion (below). (b) Max large-diameter stent. Inflation sequence: (1) before inflation, mounted on a balloon-in-balloon (BIB) system, (2) after inflation of the inner balloon, (3) after full inflation (note that the "open architecture" of this stent which makes it particularly suitable for stenting across side vessels).

in the femoral artery, a Perclose suture (Abbott) is used to preclose the artery before the insertion of a larger delivery sheath. Femoral venous access is obtained if rapid right ventricular temporary pacing is to be used. This may be needed in patients at high risk of stent displacement or embolization such as those with aortic insufficiency with a high stroke volume and those with mild coarctation. Increasingly in our practice, a catheter is positioned above the coarctation from the radial artery both for angiography and to allow the coarctation, if necessary, to be crossed from above and an arterio-arterial circuit created in those stenoses that cannot be negotiated from below (Fig. 48.3). Once vascular access has been obtained the patient is heparinized, as for balloon angioplasty.

From the femoral arterial sheath, an end-hole catheter is passed through the coarctation and pressures are measured above and below the stenosis. The end-hole catheter is placed in either the ascending aorta or one of the subclavian arteries, depending on the preference of the operator and the anatomy of the patient. A superstiff exchange length guidewire is positioned, such that the floppy tip is well away from the site of the stenosis and the catheter is removed. During this maneuver every effort should be made to avoid instrumentation of head and neck vessels. A marker pigtail catheter or a Multitrack monorail catheter (NuMed) is used for angiography.

As in balloon angioplasty, accurate measurements of the various segments of the aorta are crucial. The diameter of the

(c)

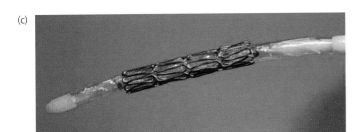

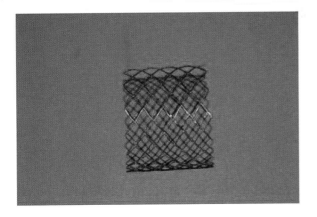

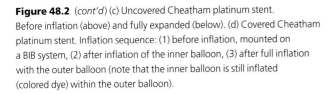

(d)

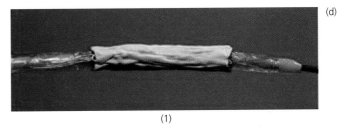

(1)

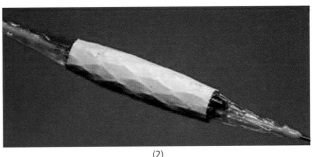

(2)

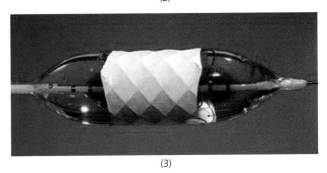

(3)

Figure 48.2 (*cont'd*) (c) Uncovered Cheatham platinum stent. Before inflation (above) and fully expanded (below). (d) Covered Cheatham platinum stent. Inflation sequence: (1) before inflation, mounted on a BIB system, (2) after inflation of the inner balloon, (3) after full inflation with the outer balloon (note that the inner balloon is still inflated (colored dye) within the outer balloon).

isthmal segment at maximum systolic expansion is used to select the balloon diameter, if there is no associated long segment hypoplasia. The length of the stent is based on the distance between the distal end of the left subclavian artery and approximately 15 mm beyond the site of the coarctation. The selected stent is mounted on the delivery balloon and firmly crimped manually. It is not our practice to de-air the delivery balloon but this is done by other operators, particularly for the delivery of lower profile stents or if there are particular concerns about balloon/stent stability.

At this point, an activated clotting time is checked and additional heparin given if required. The delivery sheath is prepared, flushed, and manually straightened with the introducer *in situ* to remove the normal trans-septal curve before insertion into the femoral artery. The sheath is advanced over the guidewire and, once across the coarctation site, the dilator is removed and the stent/balloon assembly passed over the guidewire and through the diaphragm of the sheath. It is important that a manually crimped stent is protected during the introduction through the hemostatic diaphragm of the sheath, using either a proprietary cover supplied with the stent or a manually cut short sheath, as a guard to prevent the stent slipping off the balloon. The stent/balloon assembly is advanced across the coarctation. The long sheath is retracted

backwards to expose the stent/balloon assembly and then further removed to take into account the shoulder of the balloon, which will protrude beyond the inflation marker, but still within 1–2 cm of the coarctation site. At this stage, either multiple hand injections of contrast/saline mix (50:50) through the side arm of the sheath or pump injections via a radial catheter are performed to check the position of the stent. This allows minor adjustments to the balloon/stent assembly position. Right ventricular pacing is then initiated and the balloon inflated using a pressure monitoring inflation device. If a BIB is used, two inflation devices and the correct number of assistants are required. With the BIB, the inner balloon is inflated first and, after checking the position of the stent, the outer balloon is inflated. The final expansion is achieved using slow adjustments of pressure on the inflator before deflation and careful removal of the balloon from within the stent and into the sheath. When a BIB has been used, the inner balloon is deflated first followed by the outer balloon.

A Multitrack catheter is inserted over the guidewire and angiograms and pressure measurements performed. If necessary, further dilation with a larger balloon is undertaken. We believe that flaring of the distal end of the stent is unnecessary.

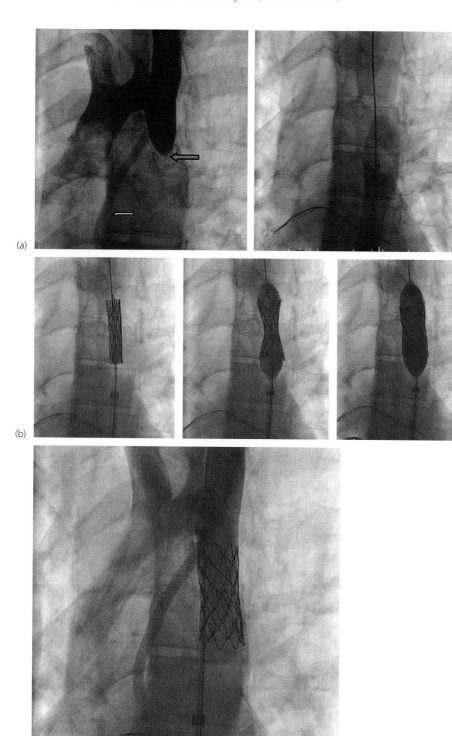

(a)

(b)

(c)

Figure 48.3 Very tight native coarctation in an adult patient. The lesion was crossed from above using a radial approach. (a) The left panel shows the aorta above the narrowing with an arrow marking a tiny connection with the descending aorta. The right panel shows a "blind" ending descending aortic segment. (b) After predilation with a small balloon to facilitate the passage of the delivery sheath a covered Cheatham platinum stent mounted on a balloon-in-balloon system was inserted and serially inflated. (c) Final result.

Once a satisfactory angiographic and hemodynamic result has been achieved, the guidewire is removed. It is advisable to perform fluoroscopy during removal to ensure that the wire is not caught on the stent struts. At this stage, a residual gradient is rare. In our experience, any gradient over 5–10 mmHg should be rectified, unless the stent is intentionally only partially inflated (see below). The arterial sheath is removed and the Perclose suture tightened to achieve hemostasis. If an arterial closure device has not been used, it is the preference of some operators to reverse heparin using protamine in preparation for manual pressure over the arterial access site. With large bore access, the operator should be prepared for a long period of digital pressure, and it is important to infiltrate the access site liberally with local anesthetic so that after reversal of general anesthesia the patient is comfortable and movement is minimized.

After insertion of the stent, some operators use low-molecular-weight heparin subcutaneously for 24–48 h. Aspirin 5 mg/kg or 75–150 mg daily in a normal-sized adult is given for up to 6 months following the procedure, although there is no clear evidence of its efficacy.

A follow-up protocol is necessary. The day after the procedure, a chest radiogram in the posterior–anterior and lateral projections should be taken as a baseline. Serial computed tomography scanning at 1–3 months and 12 months after stent insertion should be performed to exclude aneurysm formation, stent migration, or fracture. Repeat catheterization is indicated in persistently hypertensive patients, or if there is clinical evidence of re-coarctation or aneurysm formation at later follow-up.

Staged inflation of the stent

It is not known if there is any additional risk in fully dilating a tight coarctation with a stent in a single procedure. When using a bare metal stent in such a situation, it is the preference of many operators to partially inflate the stent to 60–70% of the final planned diameter, before redilating the stent fully 6–12 months after initial implantation. This practice evolved after acute aneurysms were observed when fully dilating stents at the initial implantation. In theory, staged dilation allows the disrupted aorta to heal and develop protective scarring, possibly reducing the likelihood of aneurysm formation [35,36]. Whether this is necessary, or even advisable, when implanting a covered stent is unknown, but until further data are available, it seems advisable to perform staged dilation in the most severe coarctations. The additional protection afforded by the polytetrafluoroethylene covering requires apposition against the aortic wall, and an underinflated covered stent has the potential to create a "tube within a tube" effect, which is undesirable. Further evaluation of this is needed.

Covering arterial branches

If possible, it is advisable to avoid placing a stent over any arterial branch arising from the aorta. In some situations, however, effective relief of the stenosis is dependent on stenting across a major arterial branch. If this is a potential risk, it is wise to delineate the anatomy of the vessel before insertion of the stent. In a "typical" coarctation, the vessel most commonly at risk is the left subclavian artery. Surgical data on procedures in which the subclavian artery is commonly sacrificed, and more recent experience with implantation of stent grafts for distal aortic disease, which by necessity excludes the left subclavian artery, suggest that complications relating to the exclusion of this artery, even in adult patients, are rare [37,38].

Arterial tributaries of the head and neck may be covered with a stent only after careful evaluation of the arterial circle of Willis. Aortic coarctation close to or involving head and neck vessels can be tackled percutaneously, but the procedure may require concomitant vascular surgical grafting.

Limitations of stenting

In smaller children, the main limitation of stenting is the requirement for repeated dilation in line with somatic growth. A prerequisite of successful redilation is a stent physically capable of achieving the required final diameter while maintaining sufficient radial strength. Such stents need relatively large delivery systems (>11F), and their safe insertion through the vasculature of smaller children is a potential problem. Therefore, in our opinion, stenting should be reserved for children above 10 years of age, except for exceptional cases in which surgery is inadvisable or carries unacceptable risks.

Results and complications

Although limited data are available, well over 1000 cases of stent implantation in both native and recurrent/residual coarctation have been reported in series to date [34–36,39–45]. Acute procedural results support the notion that stenting gives more predictable results than balloon angioplasty, although there are differences, such as improvements in technology in the study populations, which make a direct comparison unwise [34–36,39–45]. Deaths, although rare, are reported in 0–1.4% of cases after stenting. Neurologic damage, usually embolic stroke, occurs in 0–3.7% of patients, although the vast majority of studies report no neurologic damage after treatment. A single small outlying study of 27 patients reported by far the highest incidence in the literature [45]. Pooled data suggests that stenting of aortic coarctation is extremely effective and consistent in terms of acute and sustained reduction of the gradient across the coarctation. Important residual obstruction often relates to unmasked transverse arch hypoplasia rather than ineffective relief of the target stenosis [34,36,39–45].

Aneurysm formation occurs in 0–17% of cases after bare metal stenting [34,36,39–45]. Again, direct comparison of the relative risk with both angioplasty and surgical therapy is fraught with difficulty, not least because of the differences in post-treatment surveillance. Despite this, it seems highly likely that primary stenting of the aorta may be safer than angioplasty when evaluating the risk of aortic disruption and aneurysm formation.

By far the most frequent complications during insertion of stents relate to femoral vascular access, in which avulsion, stenosis, false aneurysm formation, and thrombosis can all occur. Reductions in the burden of arterial access complications have occurred over recent years, with improvements in the size and design of equipment for the procedure. Arterial access closure devices are an important adjunct for minimizing complications, but require experience before reliable results can be achieved and are not without complications themselves

[46]. Further improvements in technology are inevitable and may potentially make coarctation stenting a safer proposition in younger children. Stent migration occurs in approximately 5% of cases, and balloon rupture, paradoxical hypertension, and endocarditis are the other potential complications. Although neointimal proliferation is reported within aortic stents, it rarely translates to a significant problem [40].

There are two small series reporting results of covered stents as primary treatment for coarctation rather than for aneurysm formation [47,48]. Although published data currently exists in a small number of patients, it is encouraging that there are no reports of aneurysm at follow-up, making this an exciting therapeutic prospect for the future. Although there are some concerns about the risk of spinal cord injury relating to exclusion of vascular supply to the spine, the spinal cord vessels arise below the level of coarctation of the aorta, usually at the level of the T9–12 vertebrae. Any anxieties related to spinal cord injury with covered stents have not been borne out clinically, either in the reported experience with covered balloon-mounted stents or in the more extensive literature relating to stent grafting for distal aortic pathology, in which a considerable segment of the aorta is covered. In the latter group of patients, the risk of spinal cord damage appears to be 1–4% [49].

Transverse arch hypoplasia

Traditionally, percutaneous therapy has been aimed at patients with typical discrete coarctation. However, there are patients in whom gradients exist at multiple levels in the aorta, most commonly due to hypoplasia of the transverse arch. In addition to those patients presenting for the first time with newly diagnosed arch obstruction, there are many patients with a suboptimal surgical result, in whom residual transverse arch hypoplasia is the culprit [50].

Transverse hypoplasia can be treated surgically by performing an extended aortic arch repair. Technically this is a relatively easy procedure in a newborn infant with pliable tissues, but it is a more difficult operation in the older patient. Other surgical options include extensive patching of the hypoplastic area and extraanatomical grafting using a synthetic tube. All of these operations are a significant technical undertaking and are associated with risks related to both the degree of difficulty achieving a repair and the frequent need for cardiopulmonary bypass. Therefore, adequate relief of transverse arch hypoplasia using percutaneous stent implantation has potential benefits, although current clinical experience is limited.

Stent implantation in the transverse arch (Fig. 48.4) relies heavily on accurate measurement of the aortic arch and in particular the origins of the innominate, left common carotid and left subclavian arteries together with measurements of the length of the hypoplastic segment. Often multiple angiographic projections are required to delineate the exact

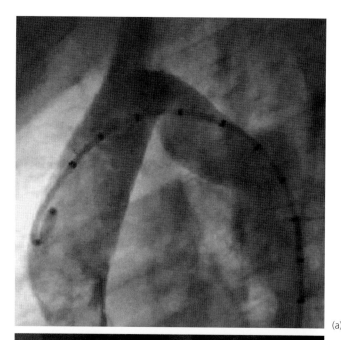

(a)

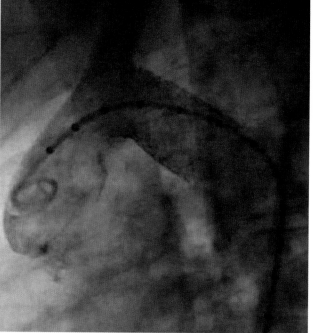

(b)

Figure 48.4 Transverse arch narrowing with a significant invasive gradient. (a) Before stenting. (b) After insertion of a Max large-diameter stent, with abolition of the gradient.

anatomy. Considerable information can be obtained by MRI scanning before angiography. Generally, these patients have a segment of the arch, which is of relatively normal size, and this area (often +1–2 mm) is used as a guide for selecting the balloon diameter for stent deployment in the hypoplastic segment. Selection of stents is particularly important when treating lesions in this area as the implications of stent migration are serious. For this reason, it is currently preferable to use the Mega or Max large-diameter (EV3) stent because of its open-cell design, flexibility, and relative lack of shortening. Particular care must be taken with covered stents, as there is little margin for error in accidentally covering head and neck vessels.

Because of the importance of stable and accurate positioning, BIB balloons and rapid right ventricular pacing are usually utilized. Delivery of the stent is through a Mullins sheath and the stent is positioned so that a small portion (usually around 3 mm) is protruding into origin of the left common carotid artery. With inflation, the stent will shorten and clear the origin of the carotid artery. After deployment, care must be taken not to dislodge the stent, while obtaining pressure measurements and performing angiography.

Conclusion

Percutaneous treatment for coarctation of the aorta is an important therapeutic option in correctly selected patients. Although balloon angioplasty is well studied and effective in terms of short-term reduction of gradient, it has limitations, and in many instances has been replaced by primary stenting.

With few exceptions, stent insertion should be reserved for patients over the age of 10 years because of growth potential and issues of femoral access. Although current experience with stents is mainly for the treatment of discrete native coarctation and recoarctation, they may also have a role in treating more complex arch morphologies, including transverse arch hypoplasia in correctly selected cases. In general, complication rates have improved over the years because of better equipment and understanding of the reasons for the complications. Although many of the critics of percutaneous treatment for aortic coarctation have concentrated on the risks of aneurysm formation, these complications have also decreased in frequency with technical improvements. Increasing experience will undoubtedly result in an increase in the role of covered stents in the future.

References

1. Campbell M (1970) Natural history of coarctation of the aorta. *Br Heart J* **32**:633–640.
2. English KM (2006) Stenting the mildly obstructive aortic arch: useful treatment or oculo-inflatory reflex? *Heart* **92**:1541–1543.
3. Cohen M, Fuster V, Steele PM, *et al.* (1989) Coarctation of the aorta. Long term follow up and prediction of outcome after surgical correction. *Circulation* **80**:840–845.
4. Connolly JE (1998) Hume memorial lecture. Prevention of spinal cord complications in aortic surgery. *Am J Surg* **176**:92–101.
5. Bouchart F, Dubar A, Tabley A, *et al.* (2000) Coarctation of the aorta in adults: surgical results and long term follow up. *Ann Thorac Surg* **70**:1483–1488.
6. Beekman RH, Rocchini AP, Dick MD, *et al.* (1987) Percutaneous balloon angioplasty for native coarctation of the aorta. *J Am Coll Cardiol* **10**:1078–1084.
7. Mendelsohn AM, Lloyd TR, Crowley DC, *et al.* (1994) Late follow-up of balloon angioplasty of coarctation of the aorta. *Am J Cardiol* **74**:696–700.
8. Rao PS & Solymar L (1988) Transductal balloon angioplasty or coarctation of the aorta in the neonate: preliminary observations. *Am Heart J* **116**:1558–1562.
9. Lock JE, Castaneda-Zuniga WR, Bass JL, *et al.* (1982) Balloon dilation of excised aortic coarctations. *Radiology* **143**:689–691.
10. Singer MI, Rowen M, & Dorsey TJ (1982) Transluminal aortic balloon angioplasty for coarctation of the aorta in the newborn. *Am Heart J* **103**:131–132.
11. Ino T, Kishiro M, Okubo M, *et al.* (1998) Dilatation mechanism of balloon angioplasty in children: assessment by angiography and intravascular ultrasound. *Cardiovasc Interven Radiol* **21**:102–108.
12. Sohn S, Rothman A, Shiota T, *et al.* (1994) Acute and follow-up intravascular ultrasound findings after balloon dilation of coarctation of the aorta. *Circulation* **90**:340–347.
13. Isner JM, Donaldson RF, Fulton D, *et al.* (1987) Cystic medial necrosis in coarctation of the aorta: a potential factor contributing to adverse consequences observed after percutaneous balloon angioplasty of coarctation sites. *Circulation* **75**:689–695.
14. Tynan M, Finley JP, Fontes V, *et al.* (1990) Balloon angioplasty for the treatment of native coarctation: results of valvuloplasty of congenital anomalies registry. *Am J Cardiol* **65**:790–792.
15. Hellenbrand WE, Allen HD, Golinko RJ, *et al.* (1990) Balloon angioplasty for aortic recoarctation: results of the Valvuloplasty and Angioplasty Congenital anomalies register. *Am J Cardiol* **65**:793–797.
16. Rao PS & Carey P (1989) Remodeling of the aorta following successful balloon coarctation angioplasty. *J Am Coll Cardiol* **14**:1312–1317.
17. Fletcher SE, Nihill MR, Grifka RG, *et al.* (1995) Balloon angioplasty of native coarctation of the aorta: midterm follow-up and prognostic factors. *J Am Coll Cardiol* **25**:730–734.
18. Redington AN, Booth P, Shore D, *et al.* (1990) Primary balloon dilation of coarctation of the aorta in neonates. *Heart* **64**:277–278.
19. Lock JE, Bass JL, Amplatz K, *et al.* (1983) Balloon dilation angioplasty of aortic coarctation in infants and children. *Circulation* **68**:109–116.
20. Rao PS, Galal O, Smith PA, *et al.* (1996) Five to nine year follow-up results of balloon angioplasty of native aortic coarctation in infants and children. *J Am Coll Cardiol* **27**:462–470.
21. Lee CL, Lin JF, Hsieh KS, *et al.* (2007) Balloon angioplasty of native coarctation and comparison of patients younger and older than 3 months. *Circ J* **71**:1781–1784.
22. Thomson JD, Mulpur A, Guerrero R, *et al.* (2006) Outcome after extended arch repair for aortic coarctation. *Heart* **92**:90–94.
23. Al-Ata J, Arfi AM, Hussain A, *et al.* (2007) Stent angioplasty: an effective alternative in selected infants with critical native aortic coarctation. *Pediatr Cardiol* **28**:183–192.
24. Morrow WR, Vick GW, Nihill MR, *et al.* (1988) Balloon dilation of unoperated coarctation of the aorta: short and intermediate term results. *J Am Coll Cardiol* **11**:133–138.
25. Anjos R, Qureshi SA, Rosenthal E, *et al.* (1992) Determinants of hemodynamic results of balloon dilation of aortic recoarctation. *Am J Cardiol* **66**:665–671.

26. Fawzy ME, Awad M, Hassan WH, *et al.* (2004) Long term outcome (up to 15 years) of balloon angioplasty of discrete native coarctation of the aorta in adolescents and adults. *J Am Coll Cardiol* **43**:1062–1067.

27. Walhout RJ, Lekkerkerker JC, Ernst SM, *et al.* (2002) Angioplasty for coarctation in different aged patients. *Am Heart J* **144**:180–186.

28. Cowley CG, Orsmond GS, Feola P, *et al.* (2005) Long-term, randomized comparison of balloon angioplasty and surgery for native coarctation of the aorta in childhood. *Circulation* **111**:3453–3456.

29. Fiore AC, Fischer LK, Schwartz T, *et al.* (2005) Comparison of angioplasty and surgery for neonatal aortic coarctation *Ann Thorac Surg* **80**:1659–1664.

30. Rodes-Cabau J, Miro J, Dancea A, *et al.* (2007) Comparison of surgical and transcatheter treatment for native coarctation of the aorta in patients > or = 1 year old. The Quebec native coarctation of the aorta study. *Am Heart J* **154**:186–192.

31. Walhout RJ, Lekkerkerker JC, Oron GH, *et al.* (2004) Comparison of surgical repair with balloon angioplasty for native coarctation in patients from 3 months to 16 years of age. *Eur J Cardiothorac Surg* **25**:722–727.

32. Shaddy RE, Boucek MM, Sturtevant JE, *et al.* (1993) Comparison of angioplasty and surgery for unoperated coarctation of the aorta. *Circulation* **87**:793–799.

33. Ohkubo M, Takahashi K, Kishiro M, *et al.* (2004) Histological findings after angioplasty using conventional balloon, radiofrequency thermal balloon and stent for experimental aortic coarctation. *Pediatr Int* **46**:39–47.

34. O'Laughlin MP, Perry SB, Lock JE, *et al.* (1991) Use of endovascular stents in congenital heart disease. *Circulation* **83**:1923–1939.

35. Magee AG, Brzezinska-Rajszys G, Qureshi SA, *et al.* (1999) Stent implantation for aortic coarctation and re-coarctation. *Heart* **82**:600–606.

36. Thanopoulos BD, Hadjinikolaou L, Konstadopoulou GN, *et al.* (2000) Stent treatment for coarctation of the aorta: intermediate-term follow-up and technical considerations. *Heart* **84**:65–70.

37. Caronno R, Piffaretti G, Tozzi M, *et al.* (2006) Intentional coverage of the left subclavian artery during endovascular stent graft repair for thoracic aortic disease. *Surg Endosc* **20**:915–918.

38. Rehders TC, Petzsch M, Ince H, *et al.* (2004) Intentional occlusion of the left subclavian artery during stent graft implantation in the thoracic aorta: risk and relevance. *J Endovasc Ther* **11**:659–666.

39. Suárez de Lezo J, Pan M, Romero M, *et al.* (2005) Percutaneous interventions on severe coarctation of the aorta: a 21-year experience. *Pediatr Cardiol* **26**:176–189.

40. Suárez de Lezo J, Pan M, Romero M, *et al.* (1999) Immediate and follow-up findings after stent treatment for severe coarctation of the aorta. *Am J Cardiol* **83**:400–406.

41. Forbes TJ, Garekar S, Amin Z, *et al.* (2007) Procedural results and acute complications in stenting native and recurrent coarctation of the aorta in patients over 4 years of age: a multi-institutional study. *Catheter Cardiovasc Interv* **70**:276–285.

42. Qureshi AM, McElhinney DB, Lock JE, *et al.* (2007) Acute and intermediate outcomes, and evaluation of injury to the aortic wall, as based on 15 years experience of implanting stents to treat aortic coarctation. *Cardiol Young* **17**:307–318.

43. Chessa M, Carrozza M, Butera G, *et al.* (2005) Results and mid-long-term follow-up of stent implantation for native and recurrent coarctation of the aorta. *Eur Heart J* **26**:2728–2732.

44. Mahadevan VS, Vondermuhll IF, & Mullen MJ (2006) Endovascular aortic coarctation stenting in adolescents and adults: angiographic and haemodynamic outcomes. *Catheter Cardiovasc Interv* **67**:268–275.

45. Harrison DA, McLaughlin PR, Lazzam C, *et al.* (2001) Endovascular stents in the management of coarctation of the aorta in the adolescent and adult: one year follow up. *Heart* **85**:561–566.

46. Derham C, Davies JF, Shahbazi R, *et al.* (2006) Iatrogenic limb ischemia caused by angiography closure devices. *Vasc Endovascular Surg* **40**:492–494.

47. Tzifa A, Ewert P, Brzezinska-Rajszys G, *et al.* (2006) Covered Cheatham-Platinum stents for aortic coarctation: early and intermediate-term results. *J Am Coll Cardiol* **47**:1457–1463.

48. Butera G, Piazza L, Chessa M, *et al.* (2007) Covered stents in patients with complex aortic coarctations. *Am Heart J* **154**:795–800.

49. Mitchell RS, Miller DC, & Dake MD (1997) Stent graft repair of thoracic aortic aneurysms. *Semin Vasc Surg* **10**:257–271.

50. Boshoff D, Budts W, Mertens L, *et al.* (2006) Stenting of hypoplastic aortic segments with mild pressure gradients and arterial hypertension. *Heart* **92**:1661–1666.

49   Surgical Treatment of Aortic Coarctation

Markus K. Heinemann

University Hospital, Johannes Gutenberg University, Mainz, Germany

Introduction

This chapter deals mainly with the surgical treatment of isolated aortic coarctation. A limited narrowing of the aorta is frequently associated with more complex forms of congenital heart disease. Brief comments on these combinations are made where relevant. Unusual forms of aortic obstruction caused by inflammatory or genetic disease (Takayasu's disease, Williams' syndrome) or located in the distal descending or abdominal aorta (midaortic syndrome) will not be discussed.

Historical background

Being an extracardiac vascular lesion, aortic coarctation was tackled surgically long before the advent of extracorporeal circulation. Gross [1,2] at Boston Children's Hospital, who had performed the first surgical correction of a congenital "heart" defect by ligating a patent ductus arteriosus in 1938, undertook a series of animal experiments investigating the effects of temporary occlusion of the descending aorta. The aim was to resect the stenotic segment of an aortic coarctation with reanastomosis of the aortic stumps—an operation he eventually did in a patient in June 1945. Independently, Crafoord in Sweden had already performed the same procedure on 19 October 1944 [3]. Both experiences were published in 1945 [1–3].

Blalock and Park [4] had suggested an extraanatomic mode of repair by turndown of the left subclavian artery onto the descending aorta based on animal experiments in 1944. Later alternative methods included the direct aortic enlargement as well as the patch aortoplasty by Vossschulte [5] and the subclavian flap technique by Waldhausen and Nahrwold [6].

Cardiovascular Interventions in Clinical Practice. Edited by Jürgen Haase, Hans-Joachim Schäfers, Horst Sievert and Ron Waksman. © 2010 Blackwell Publishing.

Morphology and pathophysiology

Coarctation of the aorta is commonly defined as a narrowing of the aortic isthmus, i.e., the segment between the take-off of the left subclavian artery and the junction with the ductus arteriosus. The degree of stenosis varies, with a cross-sectional area reduction below 50% becoming hemodynamically significant. Interrupted aortic arch is a completely different entity in which the aortic ends are separated and the vascular walls are not in continuity. Coarctation may be aggravated by hypoplasia of the aortic arch, which also complicates repair.

The development of aortic coarctation is influenced by two factors. In their classic fetal lamb experiments, Rudolph and Heymann [7] found that prenatal flow across the aortic isthmus into the lower body is only 10–15% of the combined fetal cardiac output compared with supply via the ductus arteriosus, which accounts for 50–60% of the combined cardiac output, rendering this segment an area of comparatively low flow. Any lesion compromising forward flow out of the fetal left ventricle also further contributes to isthmic flow reduction and predisposes inhibition of growth of the affected aortic segments. Thus, tubular hypoplasia of the aortic arch is encouraged.

The second etiologic factor is the atopical circumferential presence of ductal tissue in the aortic wall at the insertion site of the ductus arteriosus, leading to a shelf-like structure within the aortic lumen and an external indentation or formation of a "waist." Therefore, postnatally, a mild coarctation may be aggravated significantly by ductal constriction [8–10].

The clinical course of aortic coarctation is influenced by its severity, the status of the ductus arteriosus and the prevalence of associated intracardiac lesions. An isolated moderate aortic narrowing with a closed ductus will lead to proximal arterial hypertension with consecutive left ventricular hypertrophy and a pressure gradient between the upper and lower half of the body. If left untreated, impressive collateral vessels will enlarge over time and the pressure gradient may even decrease (see below). This form is usually tolerated astonishingly well and accounts for the cases of primary diagnosis in the adolescent or even in the adult. Symptoms are headaches, nosebleeds, cold feet, and claudication. Cerebral hemorrhage or the development and rupture of intracranial aneurysms are catastrophic late complications [11,12].

If the narrowing is severe, perfusion of the lower half of the body will be compromised at neonatal or infant age, leading to oliguria, metabolic acidosis, and even gut ischemia. This form is termed "critical coarctation" and represents an emergency. Severe narrowing may be temporarily overcome by persistence of an open ductus arteriosus. Perfusion of the lower half of the body will then be provided by the right ventricle, resulting in a more moderate pressure gradient and lower oxygen saturations below the obstruction. Ductal constriction or closure then provokes left ventricular decompensation.

Associated intracardiac lesions and coarctation influence each other, usually aggravating heart failure early in life. In the very common combination of coarctation with ventricular septal defect (VSD), the aortic obstruction leads to an increased left-to-right shunt across the VSD, boosting its significance and at the same time also diminishing left ventricular output and flow across the isthmus. The natural history very much depends on the size of the VSD. The association with more complex heart defects, a bicuspid aortic valve, or multiple left-sided obstructions (Shone's complex) shall not be discussed further.

The *collateral circulation* used by the body to provide blood supply across the level of the aortic obstruction is an impressive feature, especially in long-standing coarctation. The inflow is provided by the two internal mammary arteries. These vessels come off the subclavian arteries and join with the inferior epigastric arteries rising from the external iliac arteries. Thus, the mammary arteries provide two additional longitudinal arterial axes bridging from the upper to the lower half of the body. In coarctation, outflow is usually into the descending aorta via the intercostal arteries below the stenosis. Flow in these vessels is reversed and they can become greatly enlarged. If coarctation persists over years to decades, the enlarged, tortuous intercostal arteries cause permanent impressions in the undersurface of the ribs above them, the so-called rib-notching on plain chest X-ray. The thyrocervical trunks as well as the scapular and subscapular arteries are also part of the collateral network. It is understandable that a lateral thoracotomy under these circumstances can lead to significant blood loss.

Upon occlusion of the descending aorta, spinal cord blood supply heavily depends on proximal collateral feeding of the anterior spinal artery via the vertebral vessels. In the setting of an aberrant right subclavian artery coming off the descending aorta as the fourth branch and usually behind the coarctation, it is a technical necessity to temporarily clamp both subclavian arteries. Consequently, the risk of paraplegia is higher in these patients [13–15].

Indications

In principle, the diagnosis of coarctation of the aorta represents an indication for therapy. A reduction of aortic diameter approaching 50% indicates hemodynamic significance. The actual pressure gradient may be misleading because it is dependent on the status of the ductus arteriosus in the neonate and the degree of collateral vessel formation in the older patient. Nonetheless, a resting gradient of 20 mmHg or more is generally agreed upon as an indication for surgery, both in native and in recurrent coarctation [16].

Critical coarctation with compromised perfusion of the lower body requires urgent treatment. Emergency surgery was associated with a high mortality until it was realized that the ductal tissue could be influenced by the application of prostaglandin E_1 [17–19]. Consequently, surgery nowadays is routinely undertaken after a period of metabolic stabilization with a "re-opened" ductus and/or aorta.

When associated with a VSD, the operative strategy is determined by the significance of the intracardiac defect. The decision, however, can be difficult, because the two lesions influence each other hemodynamically. In smaller defects, coarctation repair is usually done first, with the development of the VSD followed closely. Large VSDs often require early concomitant closure. The aortic obstruction can then be corrected via the sternotomy on extracorporeal circulation, especially when tubular arch hypoplasia is present, or separately "off-pump" through a lateral incision [16,20–26].

Technical aspects

Access and circulatory support

Access to the descending aorta and aortic isthmus is generally through a left posterolateral thoracotomy in the fourth intercostal space. In long-segment arch hypoplasia the third intercostal space may facilitate exposure of the arch branches and the ascending aorta. In neonates and small children, incision of the trapezius muscle can usually be avoided owing to the flexibility of the tissue. Nonetheless, completely muscle-sparing extrapleural approaches have been described [27]. The recurrent laryngeal, vagus, and phrenic nerves must be identified to avoid damage during dissection or clamping. Keeping the plane of dissection close to the aortic adventitia should help to spare major lymphatic vessels.

The aortic arch can also be well exposed through a midline sternotomy. This incision is usually chosen when concomitant repair of intracardiac lesions or extensive arch reconstructions are to be done on extracorporal circulation. With the help of suction retractors, as used for off-pump coronary surgery or with the beating heart emptied on-pump, even the distal descending aorta can be reached from the front through

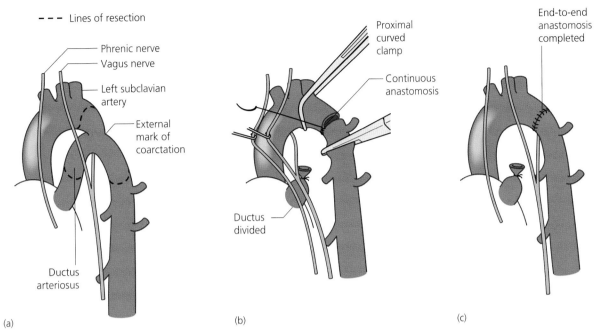

- - - Lines of resection

Phrenic nerve
Vagus nerve
Left subclavian artery
External mark of coarctation
Ductus arteriosus

(a)

Proximal curved clamp
Continuous anastomosis
Ductus divided

(b)

End-to-end anastomosis completed

(c)

Figure 49.1 Resection of coarctation with (end-to-end) anastomosis.

the posterior pericardium, for instance for insertion of an extraanatomic conduit in adults.

Coarctation surgery in children usually requires no supportive adjuncts. Prolonged cross-clamping time of the descending aorta, however, inflicts considerable ischemic injury on the lower body organs and the spinal cord. In cases of poor collateralization and basically in all adults, perfusion of the lower body half is required. These operations are done under monitoring of the right radial and one femoral arterial pressure. Partial cardiopulmonary bypass, for instance from the left atrium to the distal descending aorta or a femoral artery, can be established, decompressing the heart and deviating oxygenated blood downstream [28]. In complicated cases in which induction of hypothermia with the possibility of circulatory arrest is required, full extracorporeal circulation with an oxygenator and cannulation of the pulmonary artery can also be achieved through a lateral incision.

Resection and anastomosis

Resection is favored by most groups for the surgical treatment of discrete coarctation of the aorta. The descending aorta is approached posteriorly at the level of the ductal insertion site. Ligation and severing of the hemiazygous vein is usually necessary. The left subclavian artery, the distal arch, the ductus arteriosus, and the descending aorta are dissected and completely mobilized. One has to take care not to injure collateral branches, such as intercostal, esophageal, or bronchial arteries, which can be quite prominent and vulnerable even in a neonate. The presumed length of resection is envisaged

and, by moving the aorta in the field, it is checked if a tension-free anastomosis can be achieved. In case of doubt, further mobilization is mandatory. The aortic arch is clamped with a curved vascular clamp, usually between the left carotid and left subclavian artery, also occluding the latter. An angled clamp occludes the downstream descending aorta one or two intercostal spaces below the ductus. Intercostal arteries can be temporarily closed with liga clips. The ductus arteriosus is then ligated toward its pulmonary arterial end with a non-absorbable, monofilament fixation suture and divided. The aorta is transected below the ductal insertion site, and the wall structure as well as the endothelial aspect are inspected. Care is taken to resect all tissue suggesting ductal origin. In general, this is of a yellowish rather than white color, an onion-skin-like wall structure, and has a surface rougher than normal arterial intima. The cuff, finally resected, will universally be considerably longer than suggested by the preoperative imaging. The aortic stumps are then assessed for congruence of their diameters. Longitudinal incisions into the lower wall of the arch or along the posterior aspect of the distal aorta facilitate alignment if needed (Fig. 49.1).

Both aortic ends are then brought together by approximating the vascular clamps held by the first assistant. In case of tension, further mobilization is required. The end-to-end anastomosis is then begun at the point farthest from the surgeon, i.e., at the frontal aspect toward the mediastinum. Most surgeons prefer absorbable monofilament material (polydioxanone) with its theoretical advantages in the growing vessel [29–33]. The suturing begins from the outside-in on the distal segment, continued by inside-out on the proximal

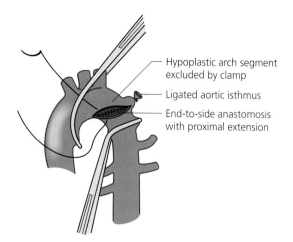

Figure 49.2 End-to-side anastomosis with proximal extension in arch hypoplasia.

- Hypoplastic arch segment excluded by clamp
- Ligated aortic isthmus
- End-to-side anastomosis with proximal extension

one, and so forth. The first stitches have to be done with utmost precision, as additional sutures to stop bleeding from this awkward corner can compromise the lumen of the anastomosed vessel. Most groups favor one continuous suture starting with the posterior aspect and continuing with the second needle at the anterior aspect. (Fig. 49.1b) Some surgeons choose interrupted stitches for the posterior and then a running suture for the anterior row [20]. The vessel is de-aired by partial opening of the distal clamp. The knot is tied and the clamps are released slowly with the anesthesiologist prepared to supply volume if necessary. A lack of drop in pressure of the right radial artery upon clamp release suggests a significant residual gradient.

In cases of tubular hypoplasia of the aortic arch, a so-called "extended" end-to-end anastomosis is applied. For this, the aortic arch and all its branch vessels are completely and extensively mobilized. The distal part of the ascending aorta before the take-off of the innominate artery is also part of the dissection. Distally, the aorta is freed over a length of at least four intercostal spaces. A specially formed curved clamp allows

proximal occlusion of the arch, including the left carotid and left subclavian artery as well as partial occlusion of the innominate artery [34,35]. Right radial pressure monitoring documents satisfactory flow to the right side of the brain. Thus, a long incision can be made into the concavity of the arch. With the distal aortic end being transected obliquely, a very long anastomosis augmenting the arch circumference can be accomplished. Another option is to ligate the aorta at the isthmus and to reimplant the distal end into a wide incision in the concavity of the arch [16,36–38]. Regardless of the technique, the arch incision must proximally be extended to the level of the innominate artery take-off (Figs. 49.1c and 49.2). If the radical dissection necessary to perform this anastomosis cannot be achieved, or the clamps cannot be safely applied without compromising perfusion of the right carotid artery, it may become necessary to switch to arch reconstruction with the help of extracorporeal circulation and circulatory arrest (through a sternotomy) [39].

Subclavian flap techniques

The subclavian flap technique as first described by Waldhausen [6] utilizes the proximal part of the left subclavian artery for augmentation of the stenotic aortic segment. The vessel is ligated and divided. A longitudinal incision is carried on the posterior aspect of the proximal subclavian stump across its aortic origin, through the isthmus and the stenosis, and onto the proximal descending aorta. The intra-aortic shelf is excised and the vascular flap turned down for enlargement of the aorta. As this technique compromises the blood supply of the left arm, it is usually reserved for special indications such as reoperations (Fig. 49.3).

A "reverse" subclavian flap can be used to augment a hypoplastic distal arch segment between the left carotid and left subclavian artery. The incision is made out of the anterior aspect of the subclavian stump, along the roof of the arch and into the carotid root. The actual coarctation, which lies distally, must be dealt with separately by resection and end-to-end anastomosis.

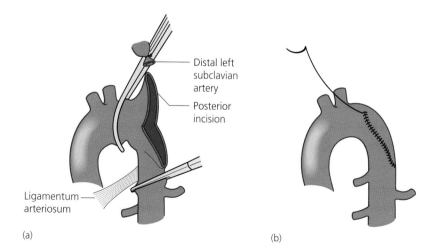

- Distal left subclavian artery
- Posterior incision

Ligamentum arteriosum

(a)

(b)

Figure 49.3 Classic subclavian flap technique.

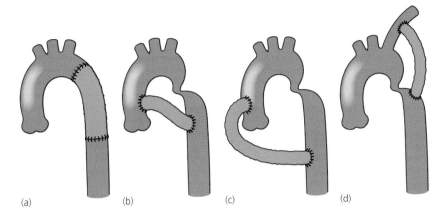

Figure 49.4 Bypass graft techniques.
(a) interposition graft, (b) ascending to descending aorta bypass, lateral approach, (c) ascending to descending aorta bypass, anterior approach, (d) Blalock–Park modification: graft from left subclavian artery to descending aorta.

(a)   (b)   (c)   (d)

Grafts and patches

Aortoplasty with a patch, as inaugurated by Vossschulte [5] in the 1950s, is technically relatively easy. Only the dorsal part of the isthmic region is dissected and a side-biting clamp is applied, including the subclavian take-off. The aorta is then incised longitudinally across the coarctation. The shelf can be partially resected. An oval or diamond-shaped prosthetic patch is used to close and augment the aortotomy. Dismal long-term results (see below) have rendered this approach obsolete.

In adults, the stenotic segment to be resected can be quite long, even in a seemingly discrete coarctation. With the tissues becoming less elastic with age, a tension-free direct anastomosis may not be possible. Implantation of a tube graft then is indicated. As this necessitates two suture lines and prolongs cross-clamping time, the supportive techniques used for replacement of the descending thoracic aorta in aneurysmatic disease or aortic dissection must be applied (see Chapter 53). In children in whom vascular growth is still an issue, graft replacement must be considered a last resort. In small diameters of 16 mm or less, polytetrafluoroethylene (PTFE) grafts are to be preferred over Dacron tubes because of their much more favorable patency.

Extraanatomic bypass grafts

The first extraanatomic bypass developed for repair of coarctation was described in the experimental work of Blalock and Park [4] (see above). Several other techniques followed later, mainly after prosthetic grafts had become available. Today certain forms of complex and/or recurrent coarctation can still be indications for a bypass procedure. Depending upon the anatomy, the length and location of the stenosis, and, if applicable, the kind of primary operation, various extraanatomic bypass techniques can be chosen from. The Blalock–Park turndown, or rather its modification with insertion of a prosthetic tube graft leaving the integrity of the subclavian artery intact, is relatively uninvasive. A sufficiently large feeding vessel is a prerequisite. Most other bypasses divert blood from the ascending to the descending aorta. They can be inserted via sternotomy, lateral, or anteroaxillary thoracotomy, with or without extracorporeal circulatory support, depending on history and pathology (Fig. 49.4). Knowledge of these historic techniques and their modifications utilizing modern technology provide the surgeon with a large and versatile armamentarium to deal with even the most complicated conditions expediently and very effectively [40–48].

Results

Hospital mortality for repair of isolated coarctation is low, being in the 2–10% range in neonates, depending on associated pathology, and as low as 1% in older infants, children, and adults. Similar risks have been reported both for end-to-end anastomosis and for the subclavian flap technique. Nowadays, however, the former is the universally preferred method in the great majority of centers. Its "extended" modification is liberally applied in small babies to facilitate an appropriate width of the anastomosis [35–39,49–54]. Diminutive absolute arch dimensions and very young age rather than low body weight have repeatedly been identified as risk factors for recurrence of coarctation with growth [16,20,55–57]. Recoarctation, commonly defined as a recurrent (or persistent) pressure gradient of 20 mmHg or more at rest, is the most frequent complication after repair. Its prevalence has been used to compare the different surgical techniques and suture materials, as well as to identify independent risk factors. It is universally accepted that remnants of ductal tissue and small arch diameters not primarily corrected carry the most significant risk. This puts the symptomatic neonate into focus, in whom tubular hypoplasia of the arch often complicates the anatomy of straightforward coarctation. A discrete shelf-like stenosis operated upon beyond the age of three months carries a very low risk of recurrence.

Presentation with cardiogenic shock and organ failure is still seen in association with constriction of the ductus in primarily asymptomatic neonates. Stabilization by administration of prostaglandins has significantly decreased the mortality in this formerly high-risk patient group [17–19,58].

With the standard subclavian flap technique, concerns about appropriate growth of the left arm remain [53,59,60]. Thus, only a few groups use it routinely today, the majority reserving it or its "reverse" variant for special situations.

Patch aortoplasty was abandoned after an unacceptably high incidence of late aneurysm formation with its associated morbidity and the necessity for complicated reoperations became known [61,62].

Regardless of the operative technique, it was found that repair later in life predisposes persistence of arterial hypertension, even if a good anatomical result has been achieved. Many patients need chronic antihypertensive medication. It must be assumed that the autoregulatory mechanisms of the kidneys, which are unsatisfactorily perfused before repair, do not recover to their full functionality afterwards [63,64]. Rigidity of vascular tissue may also play a role.

As with any operation involving clamping of the descending aorta, the most devastating complication after coarctation repair is paraplegia. It continues to be the subject of lawsuits and therefore should be addressed when obtaining informed consent. Underdevelopment of the collateral circulation, additional vascular abnormalities, such as anomalous right subclavian artery origin, or prolonged cross-clamping times significantly increase the risk [13–15,20]. In neonates and infants this is partially compensated by a better tolerance of ischemia. Supportive measures remain an exception for isolated coarctation repair in this age group. In older children and adolescents, distal perfusion pressure must me measured carefully, and partial or total cardiopulmonary bypass techniques applied liberally. In adults, in whom longer ischemic times are to be expected and in whom peripheral vascular or cardiac access is relatively easy, routine distal perfusion methods are recommended.

The introduction and refinement of interventional catheter techniques seemed to open a new and much less invasive treatment modality for aortic coarctation. Not surprisingly, the first and up to now still the majority of studies were undertaken in adults, adolescents and older children in whom concerns regarding the size of the vascular approach vessel or the implantation of intravascular stent material were less of an issue [65–70]. With the sometimes comparatively unsatisfactory results achieved by surgery in neonates, this patient group also became a target group for balloon dilation or even implantation of so-called growing stents [71–73]. The incipient enthusiasm fuelled by promising early results was soon put into perspective when intermediate-term follow-up data became available. It came as no surprise that chronic problems known from surgical treatment, such as persistent hypertension or recurrence of stenosis, showed a similar prevalence after interventional treatment. Other complications, such as aneurysm formation or aortic dissection, were observed with a markedly higher frequency.

Current indications and techniques for interventional treatment of aortic coarctation are extensively discussed in Chapter 48. From the surgical point of view, interventional techniques are the preferred treatment for recurrent coarctation, regardless of age. If they fail, surgical methods such as extraanatomic bypass grafts remain a further option. In the adult with a primary uncomplicated short-segment stenosis, catheter-based techniques are an alternative to surgery to be discussed with the patient, even though their true long-term results still remain uncertain. In smaller children, the controversial debate will continue, as studies published tend to be biased by the standpoint of the investigator [73–76]. Surgically thinking, it should be borne in mind that interventional techniques leave the original pathology of primary coarctation, i.e. aberrant ductal tissue, in place, merely changing its physical properties by partially destroying it. This will always run the risk of permanently damaging the already diseased aortic wall, providing an unstable situation for the future. The dangers of injuring a primarily unaffected segment of the aorta or the access vessel must also be taken into account. Implanting foreign material into a growing body which determines a vascular diameter is avoided by surgeons whenever possible and should not be dealt with too liberally.

Conclusion

Six decades of experience have provided the surgeons with a wide armamentarium of techniques for the treatment of aortic coarctation in its isolated or complicated form. With the appropriate method chosen and expeditiously performed, results are unequivocally very good, both in the short and also in the long term. Complete resection of the aberrant ductal tissue and reanastomosis of the aorta has become the established treatment modality for primary coarctation regardless of age or weight. If restenosis occurs, it can generally be dealt with permanently by interventional techniques.

References

1. Gross RE (1945) Surgical correction for coarctation of the aorta. *Surgery* **18**:673–678.
2. Gross RE & Hufnagel CA (1945) Coarctation of the aorta. Experimental studies regarding its surgical correction. *N Engl J Med* **233**:287–293.
3. Crafoord C & Nylin G (1945) Congenital coarctation of the aorta and its surgical treatment. *J Thorac Surg* **14**:347–361.
4. Blalock A & Park EA (1944) Surgical treatment of experimental coarctation (atresia) of aorta. *Ann Surg* **119**:445–456.
5. Vossschulte K (1961) Surgical correction of coarctation of the aorta by an "isthmusplastic" operation. *Thorax* **16**:338–345.
6. Waldhausen JA & Nahrwold DL (1966) Repair of coarctation of the aorta with a subclavian flap. *J Thorac Cardiovasc Surg* **51**:532–533.

7. Rudolph AM, Heymann MA, & Spitznas U (1972) Haemodynamic considerations in the development of narrowing of the aorta. *Am J Cardiol* **30**:514–525.

8. Brom AG (1965) Narrowing of the aortic isthmus and enlargement of the mind. *J Thorac Cardiovasc Surg* **50**:166–180.

9. Ho SY & Anderson RH (1979) Coarctation, tubular hypoplasia and the ductus arteriosus. Histological study of 35 specimens. *Br Heart J* **41**:268–274.

10. Pellegrino A, Deverall PB, Anderson RH, *et al.* (1985) Aortic coarctation in the first three months of life. An anatomopathological study with respect to treatment. *J Thorac Cardiovasc Surg* **89**:121–127.

11. Shearer WT, Turman JY, Weinberg WA, *et al.* (1970) Coarctation of the aorta and cerebrovascular accident. A proposal for early corrective surgery. *J Pediatr* **77**:1004–1009.

12. Liberthson RR, Pennington DG, Jacobs MC, *et al.* (1979) Coarctation of the aorta: review of 234 patients and clarification of management problems. *Am J Cardiol* **43**:835–840.

13. Brewer LA, Fosburg RA, Mulder GA, *et al.* (1972) Spinal cord complications following surgery for coarctation of the aorta—a study of 66 cases. *J Thorac Cardiovasc Surg* **64**:368–381.

14. Krieger KH & Spencer FC (1985) Is paraplegia after repair of coarctation of the aorta due principally to distal hypotension during aortic cross-clamping? *Surgery* **97**:2–7.

15. Hjortdal VE, Khambadkone S, deLeval MR, *et al.* (2003) Implications of anomalous right subclavian artery in the repair of neonatal aortic coarctation. *Ann Thorac Surg* **76**:572–575.

16. Castaneda AR, Jonas RA, Mayer JE, & Hanley FL (1994) *Cardiac surgery of the neonate and infant*, 1st edn. Philadelphia, PA: WB Saunders.

17. Olley PM, Coceani F, & Bodach E (1976) E-type prostaglandins: a new emergency therapy for certain cyanotic congenital heart malformations. *Circulation* **53**:728–731.

18. Elliott RB, Starling MB, & Neutze JM (1975) Medical manipulation of the ductus. *Lancet* **1**(7899):140–142.

19. Calder AL, Kirker JA, Neutze JM, *et al.* (1984) Pathology of the ductus arteriosus treated with prostaglandins. Comparison with untreated cases. *Pediatr Cardiol* **5**:85–92.

20. Kirklin JW & Barratt-Boyes BG (1993) *Cardiac Surgery*, 2nd edn. New York, NY: Churchill Livingstone.

21. Heinemann M, Ziemer G, Luhmer I, *et al.* (1990) Coarctation of the aorta in complex congenital heart disease: simultaneous repair via sternotomy. *Eur J Cardiothorac Surg* **4**:482–486.

22. Gaynor JW, Wernovsky G, Rychik J, *et al.* (2000) Outcome following single-stage repair of coarctation with ventricular septal defect. *Eur J Cardiothorac Surg* **18**:62–67.

23. Gaynor JW (2003) Management strategies for infants with coarctation and an associated ventricular septal defect. *J Thorac Cardiovasc Surg* **125**:887–889.

24. Massey R & Shore DF (2004) Surgery for complex coarctation of the aorta. *Int J Cardiol* **97**(Suppl. 1):67–73.

25. Alsoufi B, Cai S, Coles JG, *et al.* (2007) Outcomes of different surgical strategies in the treatment of neonates with aortic coarctation and associated ventricular septal defects. *Ann Thorac Surg* **84**:1331–1337.

26. Kanter KR, Mahle WT, Kogon BE, *et al.* (2007) What is the optimal management of infants with coarctation and ventricular septal defect? *Ann Thorac Surg* **84**:612–618.

27. Dave HH, Buechel ER, & Prêtre R (2006) Muscle-sparing extra-pleural approach for the repair of aortic coarctation. *Ann Thorac Surg* **81**:243–248.

28. Backer CL, Stewart RD, Kelle AM, *et al.* (2006) Use of partial cardiopulmonary bypass for coarctation repair through a left thoracotomy in children without collaterals. *Ann Thorac Surg* **82**:964–972.

29. Myers JL, Campbell DB, & Waldhausen JA (1986) The use of absorbable monofilament polydioxanone suture in pediatric cardiovascular operations. *J Thorac Cardiovasc Surg* **92**:771–775.

30. Friberg LG, Mellgren GW, Eriksson BO, *et al.* (1987) Subclavian flap angioplasty with absorbable suture polydioxanone (PDS). An experimental study in growing piglets. *Scand J Thorac Cardiovasc Surg* **21**:9–14.

31. Haluck RS, Richenbacher WE, Myers JL, *et al.* (1990) Results of aortic anastomoses made under tension using polydioxanone suture. *Ann Thorac Surg* **50**:392–395.

32. Arenas JD, Myers JL, Gleason MM, *et al.* (1991) End-to-end repair of aortic coarctation using absorbable polydioxanone suture. *Ann Thorac Surg* **51**:413–417.

33. Chang SH, Weng ZC, Yang AH, *et al.* (1998) Absorbable PDS-II suture and nonabsorbable polypropylene suture in aortic anastomoses in growing piglets. *J Formos Med Assoc* **97**:165–169.

34. Elliott MJ (1987) Coarctation of the aorta with arch hypoplasia: improvements on a new technique. *Ann Thorac Surg* **44**:321–323.

35. van Heurn LW, Wong CM, Spiegelhalter DJ, *et al.* (1994) Surgical treatment of aortic coarctation in infants younger than three months: 1985 to 1990. Success of extended end-to-end arch aortoplasty. *J Thorac Cardiovasc Surg* **107**:74–86.

36. Rajasinghe HA, Reddy VM, van Son JA, *et al.* (1996) Coarctation repair using end-to-side anastomosis of descending aorta to proximal aortic arch. *Ann Thorac Surg* **61**:840–844.

37. Younoszai AK, Reddy VM, Hanley FL, *et al.* (2002) Intermediate term follow-up of the end-to-side aortic anastomosis for coarctation of the aorta. *Ann Thorac Surg* **74**:1631–1634.

38. Deleon SY, Desikacharlu A, Dorotan JG, *et al.* (2007) Modified extended end-to-end repair of coarctation in neonates and infants. *Pediatr Cardiol* **28**:355–357.

39. Wright GE, Nowak CA, Goldberg CS, *et al.* (2005) Extended resection and end-to-end anastomosis for aortic coarctation in infants: results of a tailored approach. *Ann Thorac Surg* **80**:1453–1459.

40. Morris GC Jr, Cooley DA, deBakey ME, *et al.* (1960) Coarctation of the aorta with particular emphasis upon improved techniques of surgical repair. *J Thorac Cardiovasc Surg* **40**:705–722.

41. Goor DA & Lillehei CW (1975) *Congenital Malformations of the Heart. Embryology, Anatomy and Operative Considerations.* New York, NY: Grune & Stratton.

42. Robicsek F, Hess PJ, & Vajtai P (1984) Ascending-distal abdominal aorta bypass for treatment of hypoplastic aortic arch and atypical coarctation in the adult. *Ann Thorac Surg* **37**:261–263.

43. Sweeney MS, Walker WE, Duncan JM, *et al.* (1985) Reoperation for aortic coarctation: techniques, results, and indications for various approaches. *Ann Thorac Surg* **40**:46–49.

44. Robicsek F (1992) "Very long" aortic grafts. *Eur J Cardiothorac Surg* **6**:536–541.

45. Heinemann MK, Ziemer G, Wahlers T, *et al.* (1997) Extraanatomic thoracic aortic bypass grafts: indications, techniques, results. *Eur J Cardiothorac Surg* **11**:169–175.

46. Kanter KR, Erez E, Williams WH, *et al.* (2000) Extra-anatomic aortic bypass via sternotomy for complex aortic arch stenosis in children. *J Thorac Cardiovasc Surg* **120**:885–890.

47. Connolly HM, Schaff HV, Izhar U, *et al.* (2001) Posterior pericardial ascending-to-descending aortic bypass. An alternative surgical approach for complex coarctation of the aorta. *Circulation* **104**(Suppl. 1):I-133–137.

48. Schoenhoff FS, Berdat PA, Pavlovic M, *et al.* (2008) Off-pump extraanatomic aortic bypass for the treatment of complex aortic coarctation and hypoplastic aortic arch. *Ann Thorac Surg* **85**:460–464.

49. Ziemer G, Jonas RA, Perry SB, *et al.* (1986) Surgery for coarctation in the neonate. *Circulation* **74**(Suppl. 1):I-25–31.

50. Backer CL, Mavroudis C, Zias EA, *et al.* (1998) Repair of coarctation with resection and extended end-to-end anastomosis. *Ann Thorac Surg* **66**:1365–1371.

51. Pfammatter JP, Ziemer G, Kaulitz R, *et al.* (1996) Isolated aortic coarctation in neonates and infants: results of resection and end-to-end anastomosis. *Ann Thorac Surg* **62**:778–783.

52. Thomson JD, Mulpur A, Guerrero R, *et al.* (2006) Outcome after extended arch repair for aortic coarctation. *Heart* **92**:90–94.

53. Pandey R, Jackson M, & Ajab S (2006) Subclavian flap repair: review of 399 patients at median follow-up of fourteen years. *Ann Thorac Surg* **81**: 420–1428.

54. Barreiro CJ, Ellison TA, Williams JA, *et al.* (2007) Subclavian flap aortoplasty: still a safe, reproducible, and effective treatment for infant coarctation. *Eur J Cardiothorac Surg* **31**:649–653.

55. Bacha EA, Almodovar M, Wessel DL, *et al.* (2001) Surgery for coarctation of the aorta in infants weighing less than 2 kg. *Ann Thorac Surg* **71**:1260–1264.

56. Sudarshan CD, Cochrane AD, Jun ZH, *et al.* (2006) Repair of coarctation of the aorta in infants weighing less than 2 kilograms. *Ann Thorac Surg* **82**:158–163.

57. Mc Elhinney DB, Yang SG, Hogarty AN, *et al.* (2001) Recurrent arch obstruction after repair of isolated coarctation of the aorta in neonates and young infants: is low weight a risk factor? *J Thorac Cardiovasc Surg* **122**:883–890.

58. Fesseha AK, Eidem BW, Dibardino DJ, *et al.* (2005) Neonates with aortic coarctation and cardiogenic shock: presentation and outcomes. *Ann Thorac Surg* **79**:1650–1655.

59. Todd PJ, Dangerfield PH, Hamilton DI, *et al.* (1983) Late effect on the left upper limb of subclavian flap aortoplasty. *J Thorac Cardiovasc Surg* **85**:678–681.

60. van Son JAM, van Asten WNJC, van Lier HJJ, *et al.* (1990) Detrimental sequelae on the hemodynamics of the upper left limb after subclavian flap angioplasty in infancy. *Circulation* **81**:996–1004.

61. Aebert H, Laas J, Bednarski P, *et al.* (1993) High incidence of aneurysm formation following patch plasty repair of coarctation. *Eur J Cardiothorac Surg* **7**:200–205.

62. Knyshov GV, Sitar LL, Glagola MD, *et al.* (1996) Aortic aneurysms at the site of the repair of coarctation of the aorta: a review of 48 patients. *Ann Thorac Surg* **61**:935–939.

63. Hager A, Kanz S, Kaemmerer H, *et al.* (2007) Coarctation Long-term Assessment (COALA): significance of arterial hypertension in a cohort of 404 patients up to 27 years after surgical repair of isolated coarctation of the aorta, even in the absence of restenosis and prosthetic material. *J Thorac Cardiovasc Surg* **134**:738–745.

64. Duara R, Theodore S, Sarma PS, *et al.* (2008) Correction of coarctation of the aorta in adult patients—impact of corrective procedure on long-term recoarctation and systolic hypertension. *Thorac Cardiovasc Surg* **56**:83–86.

65. Carr JA (2006) The results of catheter-based therapy compared with surgical repair of adult aortic coarctation. *J Am Coll Cardiol* **47**:1101–1107.

66. Forbes TJ, Garekar S, Amin Z, *et al.* (2007) Procedural results and acute complications in stenting native and recurrent coarctation of the aorta in patients over 4 years of age: a multi-institutional study. *Catheter Cardiovasc Interv* **70**:276–285.

67. Forbes TJ, Moore P, Pedra CA, *et al.* (2007) Intermediate follow-up following intravascular stenting for treatment of coarctation of the aorta. *Catheter Cardiovasc Interv* **70**:569–577.

68. Rodés-Cabau J, Miró J, & Dancea A (2007) Comparison of surgical and transcatheter treatment for native coarctation of the aorta in patients > or = 1 year old, The Quebec Native Coarctation of the Aorta Study. *Am Heart J* **154**:186–192.

69. Musto C, Cifarelli A, Pucci E, *et al.* (2008) Endovascular treatment of aortic coarctation: long-term effects on hypertension. *Int J Cardiol* **130**:420–425.

70. Walhout RJ, Lekkerkerker JC, Oron GH, *et al.* (2004) Comparison of surgical repair with balloon angioplasty for native coarctation in patients from 3 months to 16 years of age. *Eur J Cardiothorac Surg* **25**:722–727.

71. Schaeffler R, Kolax T, Hesse C, *et al.* (2007) Implantation of stents for treatment of recurrent and native coarctation in children weighing less than 20 kilograms. *Cardiol Young* **17**:617–622.

72. Lee CL, Lin JF, Hsieh KS, *et al.* (2007) Balloon angioplasty of native coarctation and comparison of patients younger and older than 3 months. *Circ J* **71**:1781–1784.

73. Ewert P, Peters B, Nagdyman N, *et al.* (2008) Early and mid-term results with the Growth-Stent—a possible concept for transcatheter treatment of aortic coarctation from infancy to adulthood by stent implantation? *Catheter Cardiovasc Interv* **71**:120–126.

74. Karl TR (2007) Surgery is the best treatment for primary coarctation in the majority of cases. *J Cardiovasc Med* **8**:50–56.

75. Ebels T, Maruszewski B, & Blackstone EH (2008) What is the preferred therapy for patients with aortic coarctation? The standard gamble and decision analysis versus real results. *Cardiol Young* **18**:18–21.

76. Wong D, Benson LN, van Arsdell GS, *et al.* (2008) Balloon angioplasty is preferred to surgery for aortic coarctation. *Cardiol Young* **18**:79–88.

50 Endovascular Repair of Thoracic Aortic Aneurysms

Ibrahim Akin, Tim C. Rehders, Stephan Kische, Hüseyin Ince & Christoph A. Nienaber

University Hospital Rostock, Rostock School of Medicine, Rostock, Germany

Epidemiology

Over the past 30 years, the reported incidence of thoracic aortic aneurysms (TAAs) has increased as a result of better diagnostics and more people living to advanced age. Little is known, however, about the true prevalence and mortality rate of TAAs in a particular population [1–5]. Thoracic and thoracoabdominal aortic aneurysms (TAAs and TAAAs) are less common than infrarenal abdominal aortic aneurysms (AAAs), accounting for no more than 2–5% of the spectrum of degenerative aortic aneurysms. Lilienfeld and colleagues [6] reported an incidence of death in white males of TAA of 0.7/100 000 per year and for dissecting aneurysms of 1.5/100 000 per year. Accordingly, a population-based study in Rochester, Minnesota, reported an age- and gender-adjusted incidence of 5.9 new aneurysms per 100 000 person-years in a Midwestern community over a 30-year period, with median ages of 65 years for men and 77 years for women. The distribution of aortic segments was as follows: the ascending aorta was involved in 51%, the arch in 11%, and the descending thoracic aorta in 38% [7–9]. In contrast to abdominal aneurysms with male predominance, one-quarter to one-half of the TAAs was identified in women [10]. Moreover, one-quarter of the patients had concomitant infrarenal aneurysmal aortic disease and up to 13% had multiple aneurysms, whereas the risk of having a TAA, when AAA was diagnosed, was between 3.5% and 12% [11,13].

Etiology and pathogenesis

The pathogenesis of aortic aneurysms has not been established to its full extent, but it is believed to be multifactorial and to include atherosclerosis, increased tissue protease activity, antiprotease deficiency, mechanical factors, inflammatory

Cardiovascular Interventions in Clinical Practice. Edited by Jürgen Haase, Hans-Joachim Schäfers, Horst Sievert and Ron Waksman. © 2010 Blackwell Publishing.

disorders, infection, and genetic collagen defects, such as Marfan's syndrome and type IV Ehlers–Danlos syndrome. Up to 20% of patients with an aneurysm have a first-degree relative with the same disorder, suggestive of a genetic link [14]. The etiology of TAA is most often aortic dissection in 53%, arteriosclerosis in 29%, aortitis in 8%, cystic medial necrosis in 6%, and syphilis in 4% [15,16]. Aneurysms of the ascending thoracic aorta are often associated with cystic medial degeneration, which appears histologically as smooth muscle cell dropout and elastic fiber degeneration. Medial degeneration leads to weakening of the aortic wall, which in turn results in aortic dilation and aneurysm formation. The occurrence of cystic medial degeneration in young patients classically occurs with Marfan's syndrome, which is a heritable autosomal dominant disorder caused by mutations in one of the genes for fibrillin-1, or less commonly with connective tissue disorders, such as Ehlers–Danlos syndrome [17]. Cystic medial degeneration is also seen in patients with ascending thoracic aneurysms who do not have overt connective tissue disorders. Moreover, it is now recognized that, although cases of thoracic aortic aneurysms in the absence of overt connective tissue disorders may be sporadic, they are often familial and are now referred to the familial thoracic aortic aneurysm syndrome. A recent database analysis revealed at least 19% of affected patients with a family history of a thoracic aortic aneurysm presenting at a significantly younger age than patients with sporadic aneurysms [18].

A mutation on 3p24.2–25 explains both isolated and familial thoracic aortic aneurysms, with histologic evidence of cystic medial degeneration [19]. Mutations have also been mapped to two other chromosomal loci (5q13–14 and 11q23.2–q24) [20]. Considering that the medial layer of the aorta is composed of both vascular smooth muscle cells and extracellular matrix (ECM) proteins, primarily elastin and collagen, a balanced composition of vascular smooth muscle cells and ECM proteins appears critical for preserving functional properties of the aorta, and especially for its mechanical compliance with pulsatile blood flow. Disturbance of metabolic balance resulting in excessive ECM degradation may be key to progressive aortic wall deterioration with subsequent expansion or rupture [21]. Another mechanism relates to matrix metalloproteinases (MMP—family of >20 zinc-dependent proteolytic enzymes) instrumental for ECM metabolism and aortic wall remodeling, and potentially relevant for development of aneurysms or dissection [22,23]. Recent studies have shown excessive activation of MMP-9 in abdominal aortic aneurysms, with subsequent rapid expansion and rupture [24]. Some cases of ascending thoracic aortic aneurysms are associated with an underlying bicuspid aortic valve. Nistri *et al.* [25] used echocardiography to evaluate young people with normally functioning bicuspid aortic valves and found that 52% had aortic dilation (44% at the level of the tubular portion of the ascending aorta and 20% at the level of the sinuses) [25]. Cystic medial degeneration has been found to be the underlying cause of the aortic dilation associated with a bicuspid aortic valve. In one study, 75% of those with a bicuspid aortic valve undergoing aortic valve replacement surgery had biopsy-proven cystic medial necrosis of the ascending aorta, compared with only 14% of those with tricuspid aortic valves undergoing similar surgery [26].

Definition and classification

Aneurysmal degeneration can involve every part of the aortic vessel. The segment above the cusp of the aortic valve extending to the sinotubular ridge is known as the sinus of Valsalva. The proper ascending aorta extends from the sinotubular ridge to a line drawn at a right angle to the origin on the innominate artery. The aortic arch extends from the line drawn at a right angle proximal to the innominate artery origin to a line drawn in a right angle distal to the origin of the left subclavian artery. The descending thoracic aorta extends from the left subclavian artery to the aortic hiatus in the diaphragm, followed by the abdominal aorta extending to the bifurcation of the aorta, and is further divided into its subsegments. The diameter of normal aorta was measured and found to be approximately 30 mm at the aortic root, and 25 mm at the level of the diaphragm is certainly normal. Any

influence of anthropometric data on the aortic diameters was not apparent in the study of Hager and associates [27] (Fig. 50.1). The analyses of variance revealed no influence of weight, height, or body surface area, but it did reveal influence of sex and age [27]. Concerning the influence of age, this study matches with the study of Aronberg and associates, who showed that aortic diameters increase about 1 mm per decade during adulthood [28]. On the basis of these data, dilation of aortic segments should be defined as a deviation of >2 SD from the normal value. Therefore, localized aneurysm should continue to be defined as >50% dilation compared with the diameter of the adhering normal vessel [29]. The aneurysms below the origin of the left subclavian artery are classified according to the Crawford classification (TAA type I to type IV), recently adapted by Safi (TAA type V) [30,31] (Fig. 50.2).

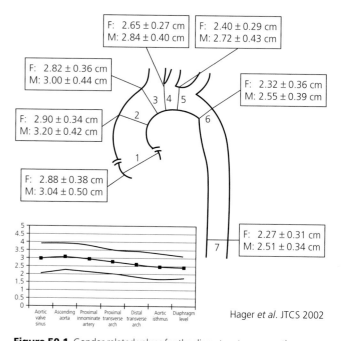

Figure 50.1 Gender related values for the diameter at seven aortic segments. Mean values ± standard deviation [27].

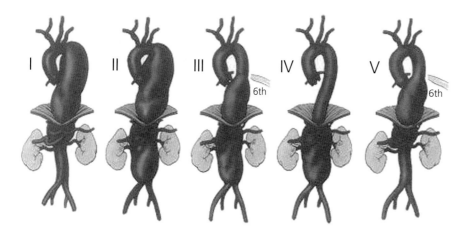

Figure 50.2 Classification of the thoracic aortic aneurysm [30,31].

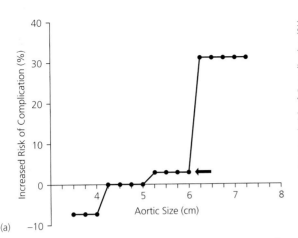

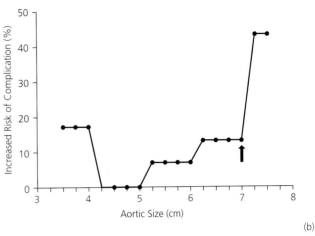

Figure 50.3 Influence of aortic size on cumulative lifetime incidence of natural complications of aortic aneurysm: y-axis, incidence of natural complications (rupture/dissection); x-axis, aortic size. (a) Ascending aorta, hinge point at 6 cm. (b) Descending aorta, hinge point at 7 cm [34].

Natural history

The natural history of TAAs has not been sufficiently defined. One reason for this is that both the etiology and location of an aneurysm may affect its rate of growth and propensity for dissection or rupture. The Yale group showed in their longitudinal data that the mean rate of growth for all thoracic aneurysms was significantly lower (0.1 cm/year) than of abdominal aneurysms (0.2–0.5 cm/year). The rate of growth, however, was greater for aneurysms of the descending aorta versus the ascending aorta, was greater for dissected versus nondissected aneurysms, and most pronounced in Marfan's syndrome [6,7]. Initial size can also be an important predictor of the rate of thoracic aneurysm growth; a study based on 721 patients supported the fact that TAA size had a profound impact on risk for rupture, with an annual rate of 2% in aneurysms <5 cm, 3% in aneurysms 5–5.9 cm, and 7% for aneurysms ≥6 cm in diameter. Therefore, the risk appears to rise abruptly as thoracic aneurysms reach a size of 6 cm [32–34] (Fig. 50.3). In several series aneurysm rupture occurred in 32–68% of medically treated patients, and rupture accounted for 32–47% of deaths; thus the 1-, 3-, and 5-year survival rate of thoracic aneurysms left without repair was 65%, 36%, and 20%, respectively [35]. Beyond this dimensional view, nondimensional variables with impact on expansion rate and risk of rupture should also be evaluated. The Mount Sinai group identified older age, the presence of even uncharacteristic pain, and the history of chronic obstructive pulmonary disease (COPD) as independent risk factors for rupture of TAA in a multivariate regression analysis [36], although symptomatic thoracic aneurysms have a 27% 5-year survival rate compared with 58% in asymptomatic patients [37]. For patients with TAAAs who are unfit for or who refused surgery, Crawford and DeNatale report a survival rate of only 24% at 2 years [4]. According to the natural history in 76 patients with arteriosclerotic aneurysms of the thoracic aorta, of whom 63 did not undergo surgery for aneurysms, 25 (40%) eventually died of rupture and 27% of unrelated cardiovascular conditions [38].

Therapy

To justify elective repair of TAA and prevent rupture, the overall mortality rate of the procedure must be lower than that without surgery. Numerous publications dealing with surgical treatment of TAAs suggest that rates of morbidity and mortality with repair of TAAs and TAAAs are well known; however, these are mostly from centers of excellence. To estimate the natural course of TAA and the risk of rupture, additional factors influencing the expansion rate and the risk of rupture should also be taken into consideration. A relationship between increasing aneurysm size, progressive expansion, the risk of rupture, and reduced survival has been demonstrated for abdominal aortic aneurysm [39,40], but not as clearly for TAA yet.

Medical management

Medical treatment serves the purpose of slowing the growth of thoracic aortic aneurysms, and reducing their risk of dissection or rupture. Patients should of course all be treated with β-blockers to reduce dP/dt (change in pressure/change in time). In a randomized study of adults with Marfan's syndrome, Shores *et al.* [41] found that treatment with propranolol over 10 years resulted in a slightly slower rate of aortic dilation, fewer aortic events, and a lower mortality in children [41]. Moreover, patients should be counseled to avoid heavy lifting or straining, because isometric exercise may abruptly increase intrathoracic pressure and blood pressure. As detailed earlier, several etiologies of thoracic aortic aneurysms, including a bicuspid

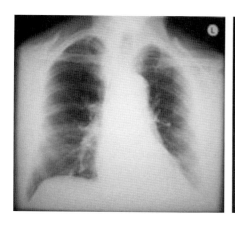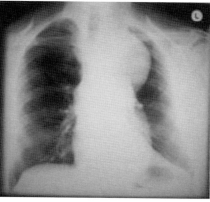

Figure 50.4 Serial chest radiograph of a patient with a true aortic aneurysm. **Left**: Baseline study demonstrates a normal anteroposterior chest film despite an enlarged aortic diameter. **Right**: Follow-up chest radiograph upon admission reveals a remarkable enlargement of the aortic knob and the descending thoracic aorta with an aortic diameter of 9 cm.

aortic valve, have a genetic component. Because thoracic aortic aneurysms are typically asymptomatic, the only way to detect their presence among other potentially affected familial members is with formal screening by noninvasive imaging (Fig. 50.4).

Surgical management

Surgical and/or interventional repair of aortic aneurysm serves two reasons: the prevention of rupture and the elimination of compression symptoms related to the mass effect of the aneurysm itself, such as pain, pulmonary, or nerval compression or dysphagia. Although there have been remarkable improvements of both procedures as a result of technical advances and refined prosthetic grafts, open surgical procedures are associated with substantial morbidity related to major thoracotomy, use of cardiopulmonary bypass, and postoperative complications, including bleeding, paraplegia, stroke, renal insufficiency, and the necessity for prolonged ventilatory support [42,43]. Comorbidities and increasing age account for mortality rates between 5% and 20% for surgical repair of descending TAAs, even at centers with considerable experience in the treatment of patients with TAA [44,45].

In the retrospective analysis of 1220 consecutive patients, predictors of operative mortality were renal insufficiency, increasing age, symptomatic aneurysms, and type II aneurysms, according to the Crawford classification. In terms of paraplegia, predictors were type II TAAs and diabetes. In patients with acute aortic dissection complicated by impending rupture of the thoracoabdominal segment, the incidence of postoperative paraplegia approaches 20% [10], and gastrointestinal complications manifest in 7% of patients. For patients presenting with ischemic end-organ complications of acute Stanford type B aortic dissection, mortality may exceed 50%. Kidney failure occurred in 18% of patients after thoracoabdominal aortic operations, requiring dialysis in approximately half of these patients. In contrast to the gradually improving results of elective operation, the surgical mortality once rupture has occurred remains dismal: in a recent study, the overall mortality rate associated with ruptured TAAs was 97%, even though 41% of patients reached the hospital alive [46].

Endovascular repair

In view of collateral morbidity and mortality associated with open surgical repair of descending TAAs, a totally endovascular approach would be less invasive and potentially safer, and would minimize paraplegia secondary to traumatizing blood supply to the spinal cord. A number of methods have been introduced to reduce the likelihood of paraplegia with open surgery; these include regional hypothermic protection of the spinal cord by epidural cooling during surgery, cerebrospinal fluid drainage, reimplantation of patient critical intercostal arteries, the use of intraoperative somatosensory evoked potential monitoring, and maintenance of distal aortic perfusion during surgery with the use of atriofemoral bypass to the distal aorta. With the use of these adjuncts, the incidence of paraplegia decreased slightly from a historical rate of 13–17% to a rate of 8–10% in most modern series [47–49]. Endovascular treatment of thoracic aortic aneurysms is achieved by transluminal placement of one or more stent-graft devices across the longitudinal extent of the lesion. The prosthesis bridges the aneurysmal sac to exclude it from high-pressure aortic blood flow, thereby allowing for sac thrombosis around the endograft and for possible remodeling of the aortic wall (Fig. 50.5). Thoracotomy, aortic cross-clamping, left-heart bypass, and single-lung ventilation are all avoided with an endovascular aortic procedure.

The use of stent-grafts was first reported by *Volodos et al.* in 1986 in a patient with post-traumatic pseudoaneurism of the thoracic aorta [50]. With technology proceeding at a fast pace, both custom-designed and commercially available stent grafts are available for treating thoracic aortic disease. By now, several institutions have substantiated both safety and effectiveness of stent-grafts for the repair of thoracic aortic aneurysms [51–54]. With increasing endovascular experience, numerous other aortic diseases, such as aortic dissection, penetrating atherosclerotic ulcers, aortopulmonary fistulas, and acute aortic rupture from blunt chest trauma, or mycotic aneurysms were investigated as a potential indication for endovascular treatment (Table 50.1).

Table 50.1 Current indications for endovascular treatment of thoracic aortic disease.

Disease etiology
Aortic aneurysms
    Atherosclerotic/degenerative
    Post-traumatic
    Mycotic
    Anastomotic
    Cystic medial necrosis
    Aortitis
Stanford type B aortic dissection
    Acute
    Chronic
Giant penetrating ulcer
Traumatic aortic tear
Aortopulmonary fistula
Marfan's syndrome

Aneurysm morphology
Aneurysm of the descending aorta
    Proximal neck length ≥ 2 cm
        < 2 cm if supra-aortic vessels have been transposed prior stent
graft placement
    Distal neck length ≥ 2 cm
    Diameter ≥ 6 cm

Patient's condition
Preferentially older age
Unfit for open surgical repair or high-risk patients
    Chronic obstructive pulmonary disease
    Severe coronary heart disease
    Severe carotid artery disease
    Renal insufficiency
    Suitable vascular access site
    Life expectancy of more than 6 months

Technique

Currently, there is ongoing controversy on which patients should be treated by endovascular means. The long-term durability of aortic-stent grafts is not yet known, and therefore cautious patient selection is advocated. The suitability of a given patient for endovascular repair is based on both clinical and anatomical considerations. At present, stent grafts are routinely used to treat patients with thoracic aneurysms distal to the aortic arch, and infrarenal abdominal aorta (Fig. 50.6). Inoue *et al.* [47] have performed aortic arch reconstructions using transluminally placed endovascular branched stent-grafts to treat aneurysms involving the aortic arch. This concept, however, was a failure with many complications and was not embraced in the community. Successful TAA exclusion requires normal segments of native aorta at both ends of the lesion of at least 15–25 mm to ensure adequate launching and contact between the endoprosthesis and the aortic wall with a tight circumferential seal. Devices are oversized by 10% in diameter to provide sufficient radial force for adequate fixation [48,55]. The preferred and most common site (41–58%) of vascular access is the common femoral artery [49,56]. Less frequently, access to the iliac artery (9–44%) via an extraperitoneal approach is required. Retroperitoneal exposure to the abdominal aorta is necessary in 14–30% of cases, especially in small elderly women [49,56]. In patients with multiple aortic aneurysms involving both the thoracic and abdominal aorta or aortic and descending aorta, a combination of conventional abdominal aortic replacement with endovascular stent-graft placement into the thoracic aorta under fluoroscopic guidance is feasible [57]. In patients with a very tortuous iliac artery and aorta, a stiff guidewire passing from a brachial entry point through the aorta and out at the femoral arteriotomy site may allow extra support for insertion of the delivery system. In highly selected patients,

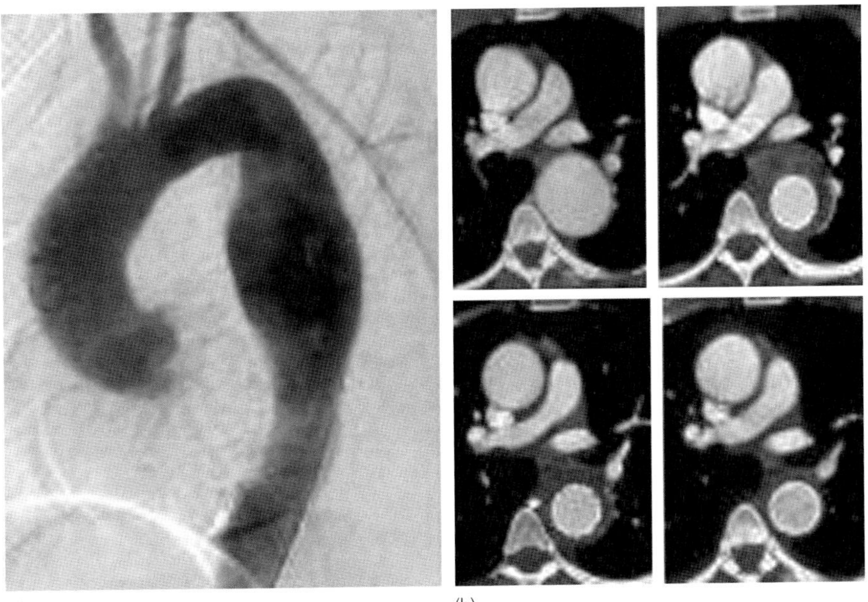

Figure 50.5 (a) CT-angiogram showing a circumspect aneurysm of the descending thoracic aorta in a middle-aged male patient selected for endografting. (b) 1-year follow-up after successful endovascular exclusion of the aneurysm by stent-graft placement demonstrates marked shrinkage of periprothetic aneurysm and optimal wall apposition of the stent-graft.

(a)

(b)

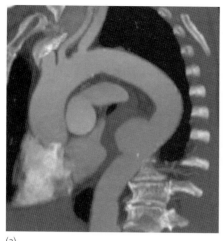
(a)

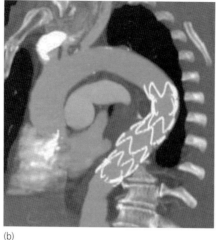
(b)

Figure 50.6 Descending aortic aneurysm. (a) Preoperative angiography in a 52 year-old man with a thoracic aortic descending aneurysm. (b) Serial computed tomography scans after successful stent-graft exclusion of the aneurysm demonstrate continued shrinkage of the periprosthetic thrombus mass.

without appropriate access through iliac or femoral arteries, endograft repair may be performed using an alternative approach for device delivery through a Dacron funnel sewn on an access vessel [58].

Based on diagnosed measurements obtained during angiography, transesophageal echocardiography, tomographic spiral CT, or MRI, the procedure is best performed in a hybrid laboratory with catheterization and imaging capabilities including digital angiography under general anesthesia. Preanasthetic midazolam (0.1 mg kg^{-1}) is administered 2 min before induction with etomidate (0.3 mg/kg), sufentanil (0.5 μg/kg), and then maintained with propofol (80–120 μg/kg/min). Neuromuscular blockade is achieved by rocuronium (0.65 mg/kg) and patients are ventilated to normocapnia monitored by endotidal carbon dioxide ($P_{ET}CO_2$) with fractional oxygen of 0.3 to 0.4. The right radial artery is used for continuous recordings of arterial pressure. After anesthesia 5000 units of heparin are administered. Using a percutaneous left brachial artery approach, a pigtail catheter is inserted into the ascending aorta over a guidewire for intraoperative angiographic evaluation via the left or right arm. The femoral or distal iliac artery is usually exposed surgically to accommodate a 24F stent graft system. Using the Seldinger technique, a stiff wire is placed over a pigtail catheter navigated with a soft wire in the aortic lumen under both fluoroscopic and transesophageal ultrasound guidance. Carefully advanced over the stiff wire, the stent graft is launched under rapid right ventricular pacing to avoid the windsock effect and misplacement. The endoprosthesis should extend at least 2 cm into "healthy" launching zone of normal aorta. Care must be taken not to occlude major arterial branches or to bypass them before stent graft placement. After deployment, short inflation of a latex balloon improves apposition of the stent struts to the aortic wall. Following the procedure, Doppler ultrasound and contrast fluoroscopy are performed for documenting the immediate result. After removing the sheath and guidewire the access sites are closed in standard surgical fashion.

Hybrid procedures for aortic arch pathologies

The aortic arch morphology is challenging because of angulation and the proximity of the supra-aortic branches that need to be preserved. Traditional open arch reconstruction using hypothermic cardiac arrest, extracorporeal circulation, and selective cerebral perfusion has been demonstrated to effectively manage aortic arch pathologies. However, this current standard procedure for any arch pathology carries significant mortality (2–9%) and risk of paraplegia and cerebral stroke in 4–13% of cases [59,61]. Therefore, open repair is often reserved for low-risk patients. Hybrid arch procedures (HAP) are a combination of debranching bypass (supra-aortic vessel transposition) to establish cerebral perfusion and subsequent thoracic endografting to provide patient-centered solutions for complex aortic arch lesions (Fig. 50.7). HAP is performed without hypothermic circulatory arrest and extracorporeal circulation and could expand the treatment group to older patients with severe comorbidities and redo surgery currently ineligible for open surgical intervention. There are two different hybrid approaches, with either extraanatomic or intrathoracic supra-aortic vessel transposition. To treat distal arch aneurysms involving both the left subclavian and the left common carotid artery, those vessels can be translocated upstream to the right common carotid artery approached via cervical access (hemiarch debranching) [62,63]. For arch aneurysms extending to the innominate artery the ascending aorta can be used, via sternotomy, as a donor site to revascularize all three supra-aortic arteries (total arch debranching) [64,65]. The key to success is the quality of the unimpaired ascending aorta as a donor site for the debranching bypass and proximal landing zone for the endografts.

Follow-up

When a thoracic aortic aneurysm is first detected its growth rate is not yet known. It is, therefore, appropriate to obtain a repeated imaging study 6 months after the initial study (Fig. 50.4). If the aneurysm is unchanged in size, it is then reasonable to obtain an imaging study on an annual basis in

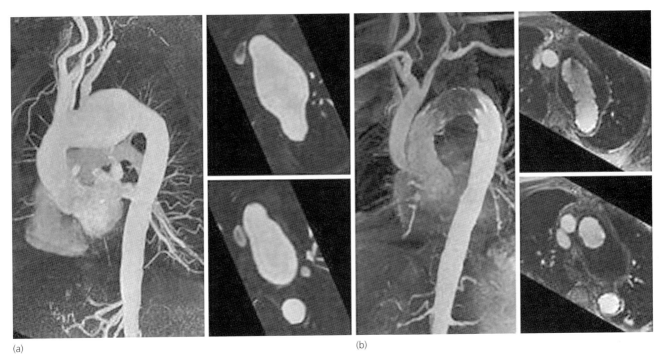

(a)

(b)

Figure 50.7 Contrast-medium enhanced MR-angiography of the aorta in a case of an aortic arch aneurysm. (a) Aneurysm of the aortic arch involving the supraaortic branches. (b) Postinterventional/surgical result after hybrid procedure with debranching of the supraaortic vessels and stent-graft implantation in the aortic arch.

most cases. In non-Marfan's patients and in the absence of acute aortitis, thoracic aortic aneurysms tend to grow slowly, and annual imaging is sufficient for surveillance. However, should there be a significant increase in aortic size per year (>0.5 cm per year), action is required or at least shorter imaging follow-up. Follow-up examinations should be performed at discharge, at 6 months, and at 12 months, and annually thereafter. Imaging studies include helical computed tomography (CT) and three-dimensional (3-D) reconstruction, or if endotension is suspected, MR angiography is the preferred method of evaluation [66].

Results from the literature

Primary technical success is generally defined as complete exclusion of the TAA, endograft patency, and restoration of normal blood flow immediately after endovascular repair (EVR). Secondary technical success is defined as complete TAA exclusion, graft patency, and restoration of blood flow within 30 days of endograft placement. Endoleak is defined as perigraft leakage of contrast medium into the TAA sac, as demonstrated by imaging either postinterventionally or during follow-up examinations. Endoleaks result from incomplete exclusion of the aneurysm. None of the studies provided a comparison of EVR with medical therapies or standard open repair of TAA or TAD. Several studies reported high success rates with 85–100% of procedures in successful deployment and functional exclusion of the aneurysm. Major complications occurred in 14–18% of patients, depending upon the acuity at presentation with very low incidence of paraplegia. Early and late mortality rate ranged from 0% to 14% and is usually attributable to the preoperative status of the patients. Most studies showed a patient survival rate of 70–80% at 1, 3, and 5 years (Table 50.2). The collective experiences of the European Collaborators on Stent graft Techniques for Abdominal Aortic Aneurysm Repair (EUROSTAR) and United Kingdom Thoracic Endograft registries with 249 patients demonstrate successful deployment in 87% of cases, a 30-day mortality rate of 5% for elective cases, and paraplegia and endoleak rates of 4% each [67]. The US Food and Drug Administration (FDA) phase II trial data from exclusive deployment of the Gore TAG endograft in 142 patients with TAA revealed similar results: technical success in 98%, a 30-day mortality rate of 1.5%, paraplegia in 3.5%, and endoleak in 8.8% [68].

Data from 457 patients treated with stent grafts and collected in a registry (113 emergency and 344 elective cases) revealed that, among 422 patients who survived the interventional procedure (inhospital mortality 5%), mortality during follow-up was 8.5% (36 patients), of whom 11 had died from the aortic disease; persistent endoleak was reported in 64 cases, of which 44 were primary (9.6%) and 21 occurred during follow-up (4.9%). Kaplan–Meier overall survival estimate at 1, 3 and 5 years were 90.9%, 85.4%, and 77.5% [68]. At the same intervals, freedom from a second procedure (either open conversion or endovascular) was 92.5%, 81.3%, and 70.0%, respectively [69].

Table 50.2 Overview of the published data.

Author, year [reference]	n	Follow-up (months)	Technical success (%)	30-Day mortality (%)	Paraplegia (%)	Endoleak (%)	Long-term survival (%)	Devices
Dake, 1998 [56]	103	22	83	9	3	24	73 (2 years)	Homemade
Ehrlich, 1998 [80]	10	NA	80	10	0	20	NA	Talent
Cartes-Zumelzu, 2000 [81]	32	16	90.6	9.4	3.1	15.4	90.2 (32 month)	Excluder, Talent
Grabenwoger, 2000 [71]	21	NA	100	9.5	0	14.3	NA	Talent, Prograft
Najibi, 2002 [79]	24	12	94.7	5.3	0	0	89.5 (1 year)	Excluder, Talent
Heijmen, 2002 [82]	28	21	96.4	0	0	28.6	96.4 (21 month)	Talent, Excluder
Schoder, 2003 [83]	28	22.7	100	0	0	25	80.2 (3 years)	Excluder
Bell, 2003 [84]	67	17	NA	2	4	4.8	89 (1 year)	Gore, Talent
Lepore, 2003 [85]	21	12	100	9.5	4.8	19	76.2 (1 year)	Excluder, Talent
Ouriel, 2003 [86]	31	6	NA	12.9	6.5	32.3	81.6	Excluder, Talent
Czerny, 2004 [87]	54	38	94.4	9.3	0	27.8	63 (3 years)	Excluder, Talent
Makaroun, 2004 [68]	142	29.6	97.9	1.5	3.5	8.8	75 (2 years)	TAG
Leurs, 2004 [67]	249	1–60	87	10.4	4	4.2	80.1 (1 year)	Excluder, Talent, Zenith, Endofit
Glade, 2005 [88]	42	15	NA	NA	2	NA	NA	Gore, Talent
Greenberg, 2005 [89]	100	14	NA	NA	1	6	83 (1 year)	Zenith
Riesenmann, 2005 [90]	50	9	96	NA	0	10	79.4 (1 year)	Talent
Ricco, 2006 [91]	166	NA	NA	5	3.6	16.2	NA	Gore, Talent
Wheatley, 2006 [92]	156	21.5	98.7	3.8	0.6	11.5	76.6 (1 year)	Gore
Bavaria, 2007 [93]	140	24	98	2.1	2.9	10	NA	Gore

At Stanford University first-generation thoracic aortic grafting was performed in 103 patients from 1992 to 1997. Of these patients, 60% were deemed unsuitable for open standard aortic replacement. The average diameter of the aneurysm was 6 cm (range 4–11 cm), and the length varied between 1 cm in post-traumatic aneurysm to 22 cm. In eight patients, a preoperative subclavian-to-carotid bypass or transposition was performed to allow the orifice of the subclavian artery to be covered with the stent graft without obstructing flow to the arm. The mortality rate in this pioneering study was 9%, with a 3% incidence of paraplegia. Complete exclusion of the aneurysm occurred in 84% of patients, and endoleaks were observed in 25 patients (24%), which was subsequently successfully treated in 11 patients by a combination of either overstenting or coiling. The survival rate was 81% at 1 year and 73% at 2 years. Late rupture occurred in 2% of patients at a 22-month average follow-up [70]. In another survey, Grabenwöger et al. [71] reported about 43 patients (32 TAA and 11 type B dissections) from 1996 to 2000. The median diameter and length of the aneurysms were 63 and 103 mm, respectively. For aneurysmal exclusion, one to six commercially available stent grafts per patient were necessary (mean

two stents). A subclavian-to-carotid artery transposition was performed in 12 out of 32 patients before endovascular repair of a TAA (38%). The technical success was 91%, as defined by total exclusion of the aneurysm from arterial circulation and the absence of an endoleak. The 30-day-mortality rate was 9.4%. In one patient, the device dislodged and perforated the aneurysm with subsequent fatal hemorrhage. In an other patient the celiac trunk was inadvertently covered with the device, resulting in ischemic necrosis of both the liver and spleen. One patient had a paraplegia, another one had a dissection of the iliac artery. The 32-month survival rate was 91% [71]. Dake et al. [56] reported a survival rate of 81% ± 4% at 1 year and 74% ± 5% at 2 years. In a 5-year clinical trial with the "first-generation" devices, 53% of 103 patients were free from treatment failure at 3.7 years [56].

In the study of Ishida et al. [72], survival rate was of 84.2% ± 6.6% at both 1 year and 2 years. Taylor et al. [73] completed a prospective case series of 37 patients. They concluded that EVR was an effective alternative that could be successfully deployed in 97% of patients. The sample, however, was heterogeneous (included both TAA and TAD) and half the patients required urgent surgery. The overall complication rate was 16%. The study protocol, however, was not homogeneous and the type of device used and follow-up was variable and relatively short (17.5 months on the average) [73].

A 6-year prospective case series involving 84 patients was completed by Ellozy et al. [74]. Primary technical success was achieved in 90%, and successful exclusion of the aneurysm was achieved in 82%. However, major procedure-related or device-related complications occurred in 38%, including proximal attachment failure (8%), distal attachment failure (6%), mechanical device failure (3%), periprocedural death (6%), and late aneurysm rupture (6%). More encouraging was the fact that only 3% suffered persistent neurologic complications [74].

Recently, periprocedural stroke rates of 0–7% have been reported [56,76], with the incidence of paraplegia ranging between 0% and 5% [56,75–77]. Although low, these rates remain significant, especially because it is impossible to reimplant intercostal arteries in this setting. Endoleak is the Achilles' heel of endovascular stent graft procedures. The rate of endoleak immediately after TAA stent graft placement has been reported to be between 4% and 24% [77,78].

Conclusion

For aneurysmic disease encompassing the descending thoracic aorta and, in selected cases, the distal aortic arch, use of endovascular stent grafts for repair of suitable anatomical conditions is a promising, nonsurgical alternative; however, morphology and graft sizing are paramount in case selection.

References

1. Ricotta JJ (2004) What's new in vascular surgery. *Am J Surg* **198**:600–625.
2. Davies RR, Goldstein KJ, Coady MA, *et al.* (2002) Yearly rupture or dissection rates for thoracic aortic aneurysms: simple prediction based on size. *Ann Thorac Surg* **73**:17–28.
3. DeBakey ME, McCollum CH, & Graham JM (1998) Surgical treatment of aneurysms of the descending thoracic aorta: long-term results in 500 patients. *J Cardiovasc Surg (Torino)* **19**:571–576.
4. Crawford ES & DeNatale RW (1986) Thoracoabdominal aortic aneurysms: observations regarding the natural course of the disease. *J Vasc Surg* **3**:578–582.
5. Pressler V & McNamara JJ (1980) Thoracic aortic aneurysm: natural history and treatment. *J Cardiovasc Surg* **79**:489–498.
6. Lilienfeld DE, Gunderson PD, Sprafka JM, *et al.* (1987) Epidemiology of aortic aneurysms. Mortality trends in the United States: 1951 to 1981. *Arteriosclerosis* **7**:637–643.
7. Bickerstaff LK, Pairolero PC, Hollier LH, *et al.* (1982) Thoracic aortic aneurysms: a population-based study. *Surgery* **92**:1103–1108.
8. Clouse WD, Hallett JW, Schaff HV, *et al.* (1998) Improved prognosis of thoracic aortic aneurysms: a population-based study. *JAMA* **280**:1926–1929.
9. Svenjo S, Bengtsson H, & Bergqvist D (1996) Thoracic and thoracoabdominal aortic aneurysm and dissection: an investigation based on autopsy. *Br J Surg* **83**:68–71.
10. Svensson LG, Crawford ES, Hess KR, *et al.* (1993) Experience with 1509 patients undergoing thoracoabdominal aortic operations. *J Vasc Surg* **17**:357–368.
11. Gloviczki P, Pairolero P, Welch T, *et al.* (1990) Multiple aortic aneurysms: the results of surgical management. *J Vasc Surg* **11**:19–27.
12. Crawford ES & Cohen ES (1982) Aortic aneurysm: a multifocal disease. Presidential address. *Arch Surg* **117**:1393–1400.
13. Olsson C, Thelin S, Stähle E, *et al.* (2006) Thoracic aortic aneurysm and dissection: increasing prevalence and improved outcomes reported in a nationwide population-based study of more than 14 000 cases from 1987 to 2002. *Circulation* **114**:2611–2618.
14. Thomson mm & Bell PR (2000) ABC of arterial and venous disease: arterial aneurysms. *BMJ* **320**:1193–1196.
15. Panneton JM & Hollier LH (1995) Nondissecting thoracoabdominal aortic aneurysms: Part I. *Ann Vasc Surg* **9**:503–514.
16. Cambria RP, Davison JK, Zannetti S, *et al.* (1997) Thoracoabdominal aneurysm repair: perspectives over a decade with the clamp-and-sew-technique. *Ann Surg* **226**:294–303.
17. Guo D, Hasham S, Kuang S-Q, *et al.* (2001) Familial thoracic aortic aneurysms and dissection. *Circulation* **103**:2461–2468.
18. Coady MA, Davies RR, Roberts M, *et al.* (1999) Familial patterns of thoracic aortic aneurysms. *Arch Surg* **134**:361–367.
19. Hasham SN, Willing MC, Guo DC, *et al.* (2003) Mapping a locus for familial thoracic aortic aneurysms and dissection (TAAD2) to 3p24–25. *Circulation* **107**:3184–3190.
20. Vaughan CJ, Casey M, He J, *et al.* (2001) Identification of a chromosome 11q23.2-q24 locus for familial aortic aneurysm disease, a genetically heterogeneous disorder. *Circulation* **103**:2469–2475.
21. Sinha I, Bethi S, Cronin P, *et al.* (2006) A biologic basis for asymmetric growth in descending thoracic aortic aneurysms: a role for matrix metalloproteinase 9 and 2. *J Vasc Surg* **43**:342–348.
22. Galis ZS & Khatri JJ (2002) Matrix metalloproteinases in vascular remodeling and atherogenesis. The good, the bad, and the ugly. *Circ Res* **90**:251–262.
23. Visse R & Nagase H (2003) Matrix metalloproteinases and tissue inhibitors of metalloproteinases. Structure, function, and biochemistry. *Circ Res* **92**:827–839.
24. Wilson WR, Anderton M, Schwalbe EC, *et al.* (2006) Matrix metalloproteinase-8 and -9 are increased at the site of abdominal aortic aneurysm rupture. *Circulation* **113**:438–445.
25. Nistri S, Sorbo MD, Marin M, *et al.* (1999) Aortic root dilatation in young men with normally functioning bicuspid aortic valves. *Heart* **82**:19–22.
26. de Sa M, Moshkovitz Y, Butany J, *et al.* (1999) Histologic abnormalities of the ascending aorta and pulmonary trunk in patients with bicuspid aortic valve disease: clinical relevance of the Ross procedure. *J Thorac Cardiovasc Surg* **118**:588–596.
27. Hager A, Kaemmerer H, Rapp-Bernhardt U, *et al.* (2002) Diameters of the thoracic aorta throughout life as measured with helical computed tomography. *J Thorac Cardiovasc Surg* **123**:1060–1066.
28. Aronberg DJ, Glazer HS, Madsen K, *et al.* (1984) Normal thoracic aortic diameters by computed tomography. *J Comput Assist Tomogr* **8**:247–250.

29. Johnston KW, Rutherford RB, Tilson MD, *et al.* (1991) Suggested standards for reporting on arterial aneurysms. Subcommittee on Reporting Standards for Arterial Aneurysms. Ad Hoc Committee on Reporting Standards, Society for Vascular Surgery and North American Chapter, International Society for Cardiovascular Surgery. *J Vasc Surg* **13**:452–458.

30. Crawford ES, Crawford JL, Safi HJ, *et al.* (1986) Thoracoabdominal aortic aneurysms: preoperative and intraoperative factors determining immediate and long-term results of operations in 605 patients. *J Vasc Surg* **3**:389–404.

31. Safi HJ & Miller CC (1999) Spinal cord protection in descending thoracic and thoracoabdominal aortic repair. *Ann Thorac Surg* **67**:1937–1939.

32. Sterpetti AV, Schultz RD, Feldhaus RJ, *et al.* (1985) Abdominal aortic aneurysm in elderly patients: selective management based on clinical status and aneurysmal expansion rate. *Am J Surg* **150**:772–776.

33. Davies RR, Goldstein LJ, Coady MA, *et al.* (2002) Yearly rupture or dissections rate for thoracic aortic aneurysms: simple prediction based on size. *Ann Thorac Surg* **73**:17–27.

34. Elefteriades JA (2002) Natural history of thoracic aneurysms: indications for surgery, and surgical versus nonsurgical risks. *Ann Thorac Surg* **74**:S1877–S1880.

35. Coady MA, Rizzo JA, Goldstein LJ, *et al.* (1999) Natural history, pathogenesis, and etiology of thoracic aortic aneurysms and dissection. *Cardiol Clin* **17**:615–635.

36. Juvonen T, Ergin MA, Galla JD, *et al.* (1997) Prospective study of the natural history of thoracic aortic aneurysms. *Ann Thorac Surg* **63**:1533–1545.

37. Joyce JW, Fairbrain JF II, & Kincaid OW (1964) Aneurysms of the thoracic aorta: a clinical study with special reference to prognosis. *Circulation* **29**:176–181.

38. McNamara JJ & Pressler V (1978) Natural history of arteriosclerotic thoracic aortic aneurysms. *Ann Thorac Surg* **26**:468–473.

39. Szilagyi DE, Smith RF, DeRusso FJ, *et al.* (1966) Contribution of abdominal aortic aneurysmectomy to prolongation of life. *Ann Surg* **164**:678–699.

40. Cronenwett JL, Murphy TF, Zelenock GB, *et al.* (1985) Actuarial analysis of variables associated with rupture of small abdominal aortic aneurysms. *Surgery* **98**:472–483.

41. Shores J, Berger KR, Murphy EA, *et al.* (1994) Progression of aortic dilatation and the benefit of long-term β-adrenergic blockade in Marfan's syndrome. *N Engl J Med* **330**:1335–1341.

42. Deeb MG, Jenkins E, Bolling SF, *et al.* (1995) Retrograde cerebral perfusion during hypothermic circulatory arrest reduces neurologic morbidity. *J Thorac Cardiovasc Surg* **109**:259–268.

43. Grabenwoger M, Ehrlich M, Cartez-Zumelzu F, *et al.* (1997) Surgical treatment of aortic arch aneurysms in profound hypothermic and circulatory arrest. *Ann Thorac Surg* **64**:1067–1071.

44. Cooley DA (1999) Aortic aneurysm operations: past, present, and future. *Ann Thorac Surg* **67**:1959–1962.

45. Safi H, Canobell MP, Miller CC 3rd, *et al.* (1997) Cerebral spinal fluid drainage and distal aortic perfusion decrease the incidence of neurological deficits: the results of 343 descending and thoracoabdominal aortic aneurysm repairs. *Eur J Vasc Surg* **14**:118–124.

46. Johansson G, Markstrom U, & Swedenborg J (1995) Ruptured thoracic aortic aneurysms: a study of incidence and mortality rates. *J Vasc Surg* **21**:985–988.

47. Inoue K, Hosokawa H, Iwase T, *et al.* (1999) Aortic arch reconstruction by transluminally placed endovascular branched stent graft. *Circulation* **100**:316–321.

48. Rousseeau H, Otal P, Colombier D, *et al.* (1999) Diagnosis and endovascular treatment of thoracic aortic diseases. *J Radiol* **80**:1064–1079.

49. Fann JI & Miller DC (1999) Endovascular treatment of descending thoracic aortic aneurysms and dissections. *Surg Clin North Am* **79**:551–574.

50. Volodos NL, Shekhanin VE, Karpovich IP, *et al.* (1986) A self-fixing synthetic blood vessel endoprosthesis. *Vestn Khir Im I I Grek* **137**:123–125.

51. Dake MD, Miller DC, Semba CP, *et al.* (1994) Transluminal placement of endovascular stent grafts for the treatment of descending thoracic aneurysms. *N Engl J Med* **33**:1729–1734.

52. Mitchell RS, Dake MD, Sembra CP, *et al.* (1996) Endovascular stent graft repair of thoracic aortic aneurysms. *J Thorac Cardiovasc Surg* **111**:1054–1062.

53. Kato M, Ohnishi K, Kaneko M, *et al.* (1996) A new graft-implanting method for thoracic aortic aneurysm or dissection with a stent graft. *Circulation* **94**:188–193.

54. Pavcnik D, Keller FS, Cobanoglu A, *et al.* (1995) Transfemoral intraluminal stent graft implanted for thoracic aortic aneurysm. *Thorac Cardiovasc Surg* **43**:208–211.

55. Fillinger MF (2000) Imaging of the thoracic and thoracoabdominal aorta. *Semin Vasc Surg* **13**:247–263.

56. Dake MD, Miller DC, Mitchell RS, *et al.* (1998) The "first generation" of endovascular stent grafts for patients with aneurysms of the descending thoracic aorta. *J Thorac Cardiovasc Surg* **116**:689–703.

57. Moon MR, Mitchell RS, Dake MD, *et al.* (1997) Simultaneous abdominal aortic replacement and thoracic stent graft placement for multilevel aortic disease. *J Vasc Surg* **25**:332–340.

58. Estes JM, Halin N, Kwoun M, *et al.* (2001) The carotid artery as alternative access for endoluminal aortic aneurysm repair. *J Vasc Surg* **33**:650–653.

59. Thurnsher SA & Grabenwöger M (2002) Endovascular treatment of thoracic aortic aneurysm: a review. *Eur Radiol* **12**:1370–1387.

60. Kazui T, Washiyama N, Muhammad BA, *et al.* (2001) Improved results of atherosclerotic arch aneurysm operations with a refined technique. *J Thorac Cardiovasc Surg* **121**:491–499.

61. Nakai M, Shimamoto M, Yamazaki F, *et al.* (2002) Long-term results after surgery for aortic nondissection aneurysm. *Kyobu Geka* **55**:280–284.

62. Czerny M, Zimpfer D, Fleck T, *et al.* (2004) Initial results after combined repair of aortic arch aneurysms by sequential transposition of the supra-aortic branches and consecutive endovascular stent graft placement. *Ann Thorac Surg* **78**:1256–1260.

63. Schumacher H, Von Tengg-Kobligk H, Ostovic M, *et al.* (2006) Hybrid aortic procedures for endoluminal arch replacement in thoracic aneurysms and type B dissections. *J Cardiovasc Surg* **47**:509–517.

64. Saleh HM & Inglese L (2006) Combined surgical and endovascular treatment of aortic arch aneurysms. *J Vasc Surg* **44**:460–466.

65. Czerny M, Gottardi R, Zimpfer D, *et al.* (2006) Transposition of the supraaortic branches for extended endovascular arch repair. *Eur J Cardiothorac Surg* **29**:709–713.

66. Cesare ED, Giordano AV, Cerone G, *et al.* (2000) Comparative evaluation of TEE, conventional MRI and contrast-enhanced 3D

breath-hold MRA in the post-operative follow-up of dissecting aneurysms. *Int J Cardioc Imaging* **16**:135–147.

67. Leurs LJ, Bell R, Degrieck Y, *et al.* (2004) Endovascular treatment of thoracic aortic disease: combined experience from the EUROSTAR and United Kingdom Thoracic Endograft registries. *J Vasc Surg* **40**:670–679.

68. Makaroun MS, Dillavou ED, Kee ST, *et al.* (2005) Endovascular treatment of thoracic aortic aneurysms: results of the phase II multicenter trial of the GORE TAG thoracic endoprosthesis. *J Vasc Surg* **41**:1–9.

69. Fattori R, Nienaber CA, Rousseau H, *et al.* (2006) Talent Thoracic Retrospective Registry. Results of endovascular repair of the thoracic aorta with the Talent Thoracic stent graft: the Talent Thoracic Retrospective Registry. *J Thorac Cardiovasc Surg* **132**: 332–339.

70. Mitchell RS, Miller DC, Dake MD, *et al.* (1999) Thoracic aortic aneurysm repair with an endovascular stent graft: the "first generation." *Ann Thorac Surg* **67**:1971–1974.

71. Grabenwöger M, Hutschala D, Ehrlich MP, *et al.* (2000) Thoracic aortic aneurysm: treatment with endovascular self-expandable stent grafts. *Ann Thorac Surg* **692**:441–445.

72. Ishida M, Kato N, Hirano T, *et al.* (2004) Endovascular stent graft treatment for thoracic aortic aneurysms: short- to midterm results. *J Vasc Interv Radiol* **15**:361–367.

73. Taylor PR, Gaines PA, McGuinness CL, *et al.* (2001) Thoracic aortic stent grafts—early experience from two centres using commercially available devices. *Eur J Vadc Endovasc Surg* **22**:70–76.

74. Ellozy SH, Carroccio A, Minor M, *et al.* (2003) Challenges of endovascular tube graft repair of thoracic aortic aneurysm: midterm follow-up and lesson learned. *J Vasc Surg* **38**:676–683.

75. Fattori R, Napoli G, Lovato L, *et al.* (2003) Descending thoracic aortic diseases: stent graft repair. *Radiology* **229**:176–183.

76. Cambria RP, Brewster DC, Lauterbach SR, *et al.* (2002) Evolving experience with thoracic aortic stent graft repair. *J Vasc Surg* **35**:1129–1136.

77. White RA, Donayre CE, Walot I, *et al.* (2001) Endovascular exclusion of descending thoracic aortic aneurysms and chronic dissections: initial clinical results with the AneuRx device. *J Vasc Surg* **33**:972–934.

78. Greenberg R, Resh T, Nyman U, *et al.* (2000) Endovascular aortic repair of descending thoracic aortic aneurysms: an early experience with intermediate-term follow-up. *J Vasc Surg* **31**: 147–156.

79. Najibi S, Terramani TT, Weiss VJ, *et al.* (2002) Endoluminal versus open treatment of descending thoracic aortic aneurysms. *J Vasc Surg* **36**:732–737.

80. Ehrlich M, Grabenwoeger M, Cartes-Zumelzu F, *et al.* (1998) Endovascular stent graft repair for aneurysms on the descending thoracic aorta. *Ann Thorac Surg* **66**:19–24.

81. Cartes-Zumelzu F, Lammer J, Kretschmer G, *et al.* (2000) Endovascular repair of thoracic aortic aneurysms. *Semin Interv Cardiol* **5**:53–57.

82. Heijmen RH, Deblier IG, Moll FL, *et al.* (2002) Endovascular stent grafting for descending thoracic aortic aneurysms. *Eur J Cardiothorac Surg* **21**:5–9.

83. Schoder M, Cartes-Zumelzu F, Grabenwoger M, *et al.* (2003) Elective endovascular stent graft repair of atherosclerotic thoracic aortic aneurysms: clinical results and midterm follow-up. *Am J Roentgenol* **180**:709–715.

84. Bell RE, Taylor PR, Aukett M, *et al.* (2003) Mid-term results for second-generation thoracic stent grafts. *Br J Surg* **90**:811–817.

85. Lepore V, Lonn L, Delle M, *et al.* (2003) Treatment of descending thoracic aneurysms by endovascular stent grafting. *J Card Surg* **18**:416–423.

86. Ouriel K & Greenberg RK (2003) Endovascular treatment of thoracic aortic aneurysms. *J Card Surg* **18**:455–463.

87. Czerny M, Cejna M, Hutschala D, *et al.* (2004) Stent graft placement in atherosclerotic descending thoracic aortic aneurysms: midterm results. *J Endovasc Ther* **11**:26–32.

88. Glade GJ, Vahl AC, Wisselink W, *et al.* (2005) Mid-term survival and cost of treatment of patients with descending thoracic aortic aneurysms; endovascular versus open repair: a case–control study. *Eur J Vasc Endovasc Surg* **29**:28–34.

89. Greenberg RK, O`Neill S, Walker E, *et al.* (2005) Endovascular repair of thoracic aortic lesions with the Zenith TX1 and TX2 thoracic grafts; intermediate-term results. *J Vasc Surg* **41**:589–596.

90. Riesenman PJ, Farber MA, Mendes RR, *et al.* (2005) Endovascular repair of lesions involving the descending thoracic aorta. *J Vasc Surg* **42**:1063–1074.

91. Ricco JB, Cau J, Marchand C, *et al.* (2006) Stent graft repair for thoracic aortic disease: results of an independent nationwide study in France from 1999 to 2001. *J Thorac Cardiovasc Surg* **131**:131–137.

92. Wheatley GH III, Gurbuz AT, Rodriguez-Lopez JA, *et al.* (2006) Midterm outcome in 158 consecutive Gore TAG thoracic endoprostheses: single center experience. *Ann Thorac Surg* **81**: 1570–1577.

93. Bavaria JE, Appoo JJ, Makaroun MS, *et al.* Endovascular stent grafting versus open surgical repair of descending thoracic aortic aneurysms in low-risk patients: a multicenter comparative trial. *J Thorac Cardiovasc Surg* **1333**:369–377.

51   Endovascular Repair of Abdominal Aortic Aneurysm

Richard R. Heuser[1] & Ramil Goel[2]

[1]St. Luke's Medical Center, Phoenix; and University of Arizona, College of Medicine, Tuscon, AZ, USA
[2]Banner Good Samaritan Medical Center, Phoenix, AZ, USA

Introduction

Aneurysm in the abdominal aorta is an abnormal dilation of the aortic lumen resulting from a focal weakness in the vessel wall. It is defined as an enlargement of the aorta to a size one and half times normal. Since the average diameter of the abdominal aorta is about 2 cm, the usual aortic diameter defining an aneurysm is 3 cm. The prevalence of abdominal aortic aneurysm of diameters between 2.9 and 4.9 cm is 1.3% for men aged 45–54 years and 12.5% for men aged 75–85 years. The corresponding figures for women are considerably lower at 0% and 5.2% [1]. It is also a significant contributor to mortality with about 15 000 deaths reported in the USA alone, as reported in 1996 [2]. It is seen in association with other atherosclerotic disease processes such as coronary artery disease and cerebrovascular disease. As the life expectancy from coronary artery disease improves, the incidence of abdominal aortic aneurysms (AAAs) and related mortality can be expected to rise.

The development of arterial aneurysms in general is a result of medial degeneration of arterial wall, which in itself is a result of complex biologic mechanisms which are not in the scope of this chapter [1]. The presence of abdominal aortic aneurysm is strongly associated with atherosclerosis, although it is still disputed if atherosclerosis is a causative factor in the pathogenesis of aortic aneurysm or if it is an epiphenomenon.

The risk factors for developing abdominal aortic aneurysm are similar to other risk factors for atherosclerosis, including smoking, male sex, family history, hypertension, presence of coronary artery disease (CAD), and peripheral artery disease (PAD). Although atherosclerosis is the most commonly associated factor with an abdominal aortic aneurysm, there are a number of nonatherosclerotic causes, which include cystic medial necrosis, and infections such as *Salmonella* and syphilis. In

one study, up to one-quarter of the patients with AAA did not have atherosclerosis in other vascular beds, suggesting that atherosclerosis might not be a significant causative factor in at least a fair proportion of patients; the etiology in some of the cases is hereditary in nature [3].

The majority of deaths from AAA are due to rupture of the aneurysmal wall, which is usually an acute event leading to exsanguination, hypotension, and eventual death. The results with surgical management in emergency settings have been dismal, with mortality rates approaching 50% [4]. This further underlines the need for prophylactic management of existing aneurysms.

Indications for elective repair

The risk of rupture rises exponentially as the size of the aneurysm increases. This is a function of the Laplace's law, which implies that the vessel wall tension is a product of the luminal pressure and the diameter of the vessel. As AAAs, by their natural history, usually expand and the risk of their rupture becomes imminent after a certain diameter, the risk of corrective surgery becomes justifiable. Other factors to help determine the risk of rupture of an AAA unfortunately have not been studied adequately. Based upon the best available current evidence, an aneurysmal diameter of 5.5 cm is regarded as the threshold for repair in an "average" patient [5]. This is also an American College of Cardiology/American Heart Association (ACC/AHA) class I recommendation [1].

The rate of growth of aneurysms also might be an important determinant of their risk of rupture [6]. This is related to the size of aneurysm, in that a larger aneurysm would expand more rapidly. Rapidly growing aneurysm might also identify increased inflammatory activity with increased collagenolysis and elastolysis within the aneurysm walls making it inherently unstable [7]. Average aneurysms expand at a rate of 0.3–0.4 cm per year, and aneurysms that increase by a rate of >1 cm per year have been treated surgically with good results [8], although ACC/AHA does not have a specific recommendation for treating rapidly growing aneurysms.

Cardiovascular Interventions in Clinical Practice. Edited by Jürgen Haase, Hans-Joachim Schäfers, Horst Sievert and Ron Waksman. © 2010 Blackwell Publishing.

Patients with symptoms of abdominal aortic aneurysm, including abdominal and/or back pain, are also indicated for repair; this is an ACC/AHA class I recommendation [1].

Endovascular repair of abdominal aortic aneurysms

The first successful placement of an intraluminal Dacron prosthetic graft using retrograde cannulation of the femoral artery was demonstrated by Parodi *et al.* in 1991 [9]. Over the course of the years the stent grafts and delivery systems have become increasingly sophisticated. This is reflected in their increased use at least in certain geographical regions [10]. Still the basic premise on which they all work remains the same; that of excluding the aneurysm from the circulation and allowing blood flow through the graft lumen.

The short-term risk of mortality from open surgical repair can vary between 2.7% for aneurysms <5.5 cm to 5% for bigger aneurysms [8,11]. The actual risk of mortality varies with the presence of various conditions, such as advanced age, renal insufficiency, cirrhosis, or cardiopulmonary disease. It is also affected by the volume of surgeries done in a particular center as well as the surgeon's expertise [12,13].

The performance of an endovascular procedure eliminates the need for a major transabdominal surgery and can be done under regional or even local anesthesia. This makes the procedure preferable in patients at high risk for open surgical repair of abdominal aortic aneurysms. This is an ACC class IIb recommendation [1].

The patients who fit into this group include those with severe cardiopulmonary disease, morbid obesity, and those with a history of multiple previous abdominal surgeries making another open abdominal surgery technically challenging. As the experience and operator comfort level with these devices grows, they are being used even for low to average risk patients who don't have any particular contraindication to open surgical repair. The data supporting the use of endovascular devices in this setting, however, is less strong and is discussed in detail below.

Technical considerations

Device description

Each endograft device consists of three essential components:
- The *delivery system* allows placement via a femoral artery approach. This usually would consist of an introducer sheath, a trocar, a deployment capsule, and a retractable cover. An ideal introducer sheath should be flexible enough to navigate the angulations in the iliac arteries, but at the same time being rigid enough to resist kinking.
- The *attachment system* seals the graft ends with the aortic luminal wall; the vascular attachment systems are always metallic, made of stainless steel, elgiloy, tantalum or nitinol.

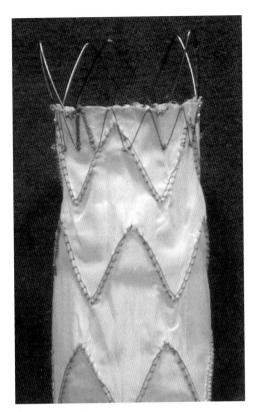

Figure 51.1 The Talent™ device.

The usual mechanism of attachment is friction, but barbs, hooks, and anchors can be used additionally for better anchorage.
- The *graft conduit* forms the new artificial lumen diverting blood from the aneurysmal segment of the aorta. The initial graft fabric was polyester, which has the advantage of being very strong, but fabrics made of polytetrafluoroethylene (PTFE) are increasingly gaining ground and are less thrombogenic.

Device types

The stent graft devices are termed "supported" when they contain a metallic framework throughout its length, providing support to the entire length of the endograft. The Talent™ (Medtronic AVE, Santa Clara, CA, USA) and the Gore Excluder™ device (W.L. Gore and Associates, Flagstaff, AZ, USA), shown in Figures 51.1 and 51.2, respectively, are examples of a supported device.

Unsupported devices have also been developed, in which the metallic support is present only at the sites where the device actually anchors to the aorta. They are exemplified by another device, the EVT Ancure™ (EVT Inc., Menlo Park, CA, USA). These devices, being more flexible, can adapt to changes in the aneurysm configuration, but are more prone to kinking and subsequent thrombosis. These problems may have contributed to the Ancure™ device being removed from the market. A clear-cut superiority of one type of device over another, however, is yet to be established.

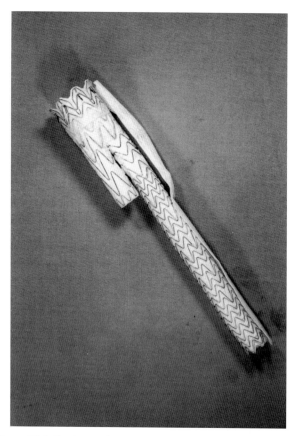

Figure 51.2 The Gore Excluder™ device.

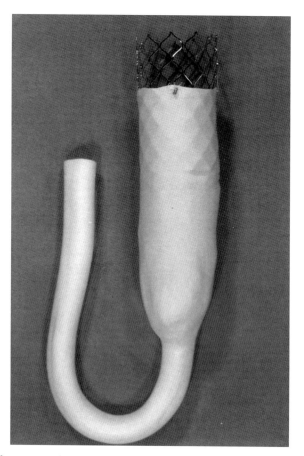

Figure 51.3 The bare proximal Palmaz stent.

Bifurcated forms of stent graft devices can also be categorized between those having a unibody, which afford better stent graft stability and less risk of dislodgement of components, and the modular types of device, which allow for greater customization.

Stent configuration and deployment

Almost 90% of the abdominal aortic aneurysms are infrarenal in location. This means that, for endovascular correction, an ideal aortic aneurysm should have an adequately long proximal neck, which is the distance between the origins of the renal arteries and the superior extent of the aneurysm. This allows for good anchorage of the superior end of the endograft, and a 1.5 to 2.0 cm length is required to provide successful fixation and prevent proximal endoleak [14]. This makes it a very strict criterion to meet for most aneurysms, which would than be excluded from consideration for endovascular repair. A solution in the form of a bare proximal stent, which allows for placement across the origins of the renal arteries without significantly obstructing blood flow through its interstices, has been developed. An example of such a device is the Palmaz stent, shown in Figure 51.3.

There is an understandable theoretical concern that such a device would cause obstruction of renal blood flow and limit future renal vascular interventions by narrowing access to the renal arteries through the interstices of the bare portion of the stent. These fears about the potential renal adverse effects of transrenal bare proximal stent in studies so far have not been found to be true [15].

The other obvious concern is that of having an adequate distal neck, which is the length of the aortic segment between the inferior margin of the aneurysm and the aortic bifurcation, permitting a distal attachment site in the aorta itself. A distal neck length of at least 12 mm is preferred [16]. This is rare as most aneurysms don't have suitably long distal necks. The solution in such cases is to have the distal attachment site not in the aorta but in one or both the iliac arteries, which is done by adding one or two limbs to the aortic graft, respectively. When attachment to both the iliac arteries is done, bifurcated endografts with two limbs extending into both the iliac arteries are chosen.

The bifurcated stents are assembled *in vivo*; a unibody device is placed as one piece and the contralateral limb is pulled from the opposite femoral artery approach. In a modular device, the main body is inserted from one side and the second limb is inserted and assembled through the contralateral side.

Other anatomic considerations

Unlike the open surgical technique, the endovascular approach requires the anatomic configuration of the infrarenal aorta to be studied in great detail with various sophisticated imaging techniques, such as computed tomography (CT) or magnetic resonance imaging (MRI), before the undertaking of the actual procedure.

Proximal and distal necks

Apart from evaluation of the lengths of proximal and distal necks of the aneurysm, there are other important anatomical aspects that need to be evaluated properly before undertaking endovascular correction of the aneurysm. A proximal neck diameter of more than 28–29 mm and a distal neck wider than 26 mm also interfere with proper anchorage [16]. The diameters of the proximal and distal neck also have to be assessed properly so that the correct size of endograft might be chosen. The stent diameter, in general, should be 10–20% greater than the proximal neck diameter. Selecting an oversized endograft runs the risk of kinking, with subsequent leak or thrombus formation. On the other hand, choosing an undersized device can also lead to leakage. The neck lumen wall should preferably be free of heavy calcification or thrombus formation. Thrombus in the neck lumen predisposes to endoleak and stent graft failure, whereas excessive calcification can increase the risk of stent graft migration.

Aneurysm diameter

An aneurysm diameter >6.5 cm is associated with a higher rate of postoperative complications [17]. In our experience, however, the actual size of the aneurysm has neither been a contraindication for endoluminal exclusion nor the source of any postoperative complications.

Angulation

Angulation between the long axis of either the neck or the aneurysm and the vertical plane, if >60°, can lead to difficulties in implantation, kinking, leakage, and an increased risk of downward migration of the device. In these cases, consideration of open repair should be entertained.

Iliac artery

As noted above, in the case of a short distal neck segment, attachment at the common iliac site is chosen, this artery, if short and/or wide, might be unsuitable for graft attachment. If the common iliac artery is not suitable, the external iliac artery might be used for attachment. If the hypogastric artery, which takes origin from the external iliac artery, is patent, it might retrogradely fill the aneurysmal sac, resulting in ineffective exclusion of the aneurysm from the circulation. The embolization of the hypogastric artery before the procedure will usually prevent such a situation.

Access artery

As opposed to coronary interventions, the introducer sheath for insertion of the stent graft for aneurysmal repair is fairly large, at 16–28F, and the size of the access artery is of greater significance. The femoral artery diameter has to be adequately wide to accommodate the delivery system insertion, and when the device fails to pass an iliac conduit created through a retroperitoneal incision can allow device insertion and implantation.

Accessory renal arteries

Accessory renal arteries are present in up to 30% of the population as an anatomical variation; obstruction of these arteries by the endograft can cause partial renal infarction in the distribution of the accessory renal artery.

Inferior mesenteric artery

A similar obstruction of the inferior mesenteric artery usually is of no significant clinical consequence, owing to the extensive collateral blood supply to the lower gastrointestinal tract. This, however, can be an important issue if the circulation through the celiac trunk and the superior mesenteric artery is already compromised due to reasons such as atherosclerotic stenosis. In such cases the lower gastrointestinal tract would be at risk for ischemia and the endograft procedure is contraindicated.

Apart from the hypogastric artery, the accessory renal, the lumbar, and the inferior mesenteric arteries also pose the risk of causing retrograde circulation and graft failure.

Complications

Perioperative complications

Access artery injuries

Injury to the access artery is a relatively common occurrence due to large bore catheters that are inserted in tortuous and calcified arteries. This mandates the use of fluoroscopic visualization throughout the procedure.

Postimplantation syndrome

An acute inflammatory syndrome develops immediately postoperatively in about 50% of the patients [18,19]. It is characterized by fever, leukocytosis, general malaise, back pain, and perigraft air on CT scan. The syndrome may last 4–10 days; the etiology is not clear but infection does not seem to be the underlying cause. In our experience, pre- and postimplantation treatment with indomethacin appears to mitigate this reaction. In fact, it is also thought of as a sign of a thrombosing aneurysm and, thus, it actually may be regarded as a confirmation of successful graft placement.

Embolization

Clinical as well as angiographically detectable macroembolization to the peripheral arterial system are known complications. When clinically significant ischemia is present it can be dealt with using local thrombolysis, Fogarty™ catheter extraction and aspiration thrombectomy [18]. Microembolization is very common and can be clinically manifest as renal failure and toe ischemia.

Postoperative outcomes

The immediate postoperative success rates are fairly high, ranging from 87% to 100% [18,20]. Postoperatively mortality is usually defined as death within 30 days of the procedure [21]. In the European Collaborators on Stent graft Techniques for Abdominal Aortic Aneurysm Repair (EUROSTAR) registry, the postoperative mortality in a sample size of 5612 patients was noted to be about 1.56% [21]. In much smaller sample sizes of patients, the 30-day mortality has ranged from 0% to 23% [20,22]. The average rates of postoperative mortality are significantly lower than similar statistics for open surgical repair. The operative mortality rates seen by the Dutch Randomized Endovascular Aneurysm Management (DREAM) trial group reveal a 30-day mortality rate of 1.2% for the endovascular repair group compared with 4.6% for the open surgery group [23]. Similar results were seen in the endovascular aneurysm repair (EVAR) trial 1 in which the 30-day mortality rate was 1.6% for patients undergoing endovascular repair versus 4.6% for those undergoing open surgery [24]. In this study, however, the group undergoing endovascular repair was also more prone to receive secondary interventions at a rate of 9.8%; the corresponding rate for the open surgical group was 5.8%.

The difference in postoperative mortality becomes even more apparent in patients with a higher risk profile. In a separate study of patients at the highest American Society of Anesthesiologists class (class IV), subgroup analysis revealed an inhospital postoperative mortality rate for endovascular repair of 4.7% compared with the corresponding figure for open repair, which was 19.2% [25].

Late complications

Endoleaks

This represents angiographically demonstrable blood flow into the aneurysmal sac after device placement, reflecting the failure of the device to completely exclude the aneurysm from circulation. If this is not addressed, it poses the risk of continued aneurysmal expansion and rupture. The endoleak, if developing within 30 days of the procedure, is termed as "primary" and a detection beyond that is defined as "secondary."

Endoleaks are also defined on the basis of their formation.
• Type I. This occurs around the proximal attachment site, distal attachment site, or in devices with a mono-iliac prosthesis around the iliac occluder device. This can happen if an undersized stent graft is chosen or if the proximal attachment site happens to fall into a diseased segment of aorta that dilates after device placement. Calcification and thrombus over the attachment site would also cause poor device attachment.
• Type II. This is the most common type of endoleak, which is caused by retrograde flow into the aneurysmal sac from the

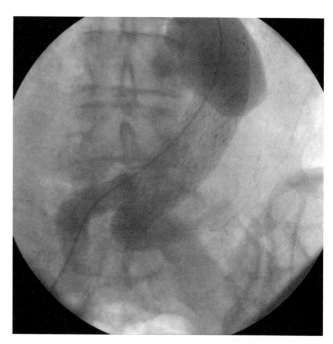

Figure 51.4 This angiogram shows a 1-year status postplacement of the AneuRx™ device in an 83-year-old asymptomatic female. The device had migrated down resulting in a significant endoleak. The patient underwent successful open repair.

aortic branches covered by the graft. Usually, there is an artery of origin through which the blood flows into the aneurysm and an outflow artery through which it flows out. The most common arteries involved are the lumbar arteries, but the inferior mesenteric artery, hypogastric artery and the accessory renal arteries can also be the culprit vessels.
• Type III. This type happens as a result of equipment malfunction, in the form of fabric tear, or separation between the modules in a modular system and is fairly uncommon.
• Type IV. This is due to diffusion of blood across the pores of an otherwise intact graft fabric. This leak is usually seen as a blush on angiography immediately following the procedure. In most cases these pores seal off within a month.

Device migration

This is one of the major long term complications of endovascular treatment of aortic aneurysms and can eventually lead to endoleak, aneurysm expansion, and subsequent rupture. The angiographic appearance of this complication is depicted in Figure 51.4.

Graft limb thrombosis

Thrombosis inside the lumen of the graft can be predisposed by kinking, which is more common in unsupported grafts; this, ironically, can also be caused by a successful graft placement, when a reduction in size of the aneurysm would lead to bending of the previously straight graft. X-ray studies in the anteroposterior and lateral planes at regular intervals can

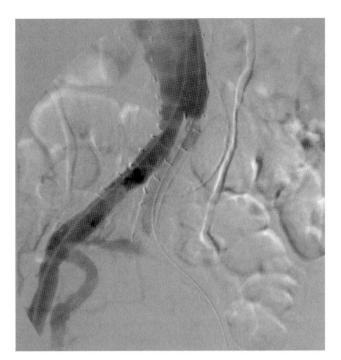

Figure 51.5 This angiogram was performed on a 73-year-old man who presented with acute left leg ischemia 18 months after placement of an ANCURE™ device. We successfully recanalized the left limb of the device.

help identify early kinks. The angiographic appearance of graft limb thrombosis is shown in Figure 51.5.

Long-term outcomes

The impressive improvement in mortality in the immediate postoperative period seen in patients undergoing endovascular repair of their aortic aneurysms over open surgical repair has so far not been shown to improve long-term survival. However, data on this issue are fairly limited, and the few trials done so far do not have an adequately long follow-up.

The DREAM Trial showed no difference in cumulative survival, with rates of 89.7% with endovascular repair versus 89.6% with surgical repair at the end of 1 year after the procedure [26]. Moreover, the rate of reintervention at 9 months was significantly higher, with endovascular repair at 11% for the endovascular group versus 4% with surgical group. It is to be noted that this trial was not designed to look at long term mortality and complication which were secondary outcomes.

The EVAR 1 Trial, which followed the patients up to 4 years postoperatively, found that the all-cause mortality at 4 years after randomization was similar in the two groups (around 28%), and the survival curves to 4 years showed no difference between the groups [27]. By 4 years, the proportion of patients with at least one complication following AAA repair was 41% in the EVAR group compared with 9% in the open repair group. The rate of aneurysm related mortality was, however, significantly lower at 4% in the EVAR group compared with 7% in the open surgical group.

Another trial that has reached a similar conclusion showed that the early gains in survival made in the endovascular repair group disappear after 2 years. It goes on to conclude that "for AAA > / = 5.5 cm, EVAR has not been shown to improve long-term survival or health status over open surgical repair (OSR) though peri-operative outcomes are improved." [28].

The cost advantages from a shorter hospital stay in patients receiving endovascular repair becomes more than offset by high device costs in the short term and by the need for reintervention and monitoring in the long term [27,28].

Again, adequate data on the long-term effects of endovascular devices in aortic aneurysms are still being obtained. With further developments in device, technique, and operator experience, the potential for improved long-term outcomes exists [29].

Conclusion

The immediate postoperative outcome for patients undergoing endovascular procedures is significantly better over those undergoing open surgical procedures. This difference is even more dramatic for the high-risk patients with multiple comorbidities. The long-term data are still incomplete, and early studies have raised questions about endovascular devices with respect to total costs, need for reintervention, and mortality. As more data are awaited, it is reasonable to keep in mind the ACC/AHA guidelines for infrarenal aortic aneurysms, which advise open surgical repair for good or average surgical candidates as a class I recommendation [1]. Endovascular repair for high-risk patients with cardiopulmonary and other associated diseases is a class IIa recommendation, and for low to average risk patients is a class IIb recommendation.

References

1. Hirsch AT, Haskal ZJ, Hertzer NR, *et al.* (2006) ACC/AHA 2005 guidelines for the management of patients with peripheral arterial disease (lower extremity, renal, mesenteric, and abdominal aortic): executive summary a collaborative report from the American Association for Vascular Surgery/Society for Vascular Surgery, Society for Cardiovascular Angiography and Interventions, Society for Vascular Medicine and Biology, Society of Interventional Radiology, and the ACC/AHA Task Force on Practice Guidelines (Writing Committee to Develop Guidelines for the Management of Patients With Peripheral Arterial Disease) endorsed by the American Association of Cardiovascular and Pulmonary Rehabilitation; National Heart, Lung, and Blood Institute; Society for Vascular Nursing; TransAtlantic Inter-Society Consensus; and Vascular Disease Foundation. *J Am Coll Cardiol* **47**:1239–1312.
2. Creager MA, Halperin JL, & Whittemore AD (1996) Aneurysmal disease of the aorta and its branches. In: Loscalzo J, Creager MA, & Dzau VJ (eds). *Vascular Medicine*. New York: Little Brown, p. 901.

3. Sterpetti AV, Feldhaus RJ, Schultz RD, *et al.* (1988) Identification of abdominal aortic aneurysm patients with different clinical features and clinical outcomes. *Am J Surg* **156**:466–469.

4. Dimick JB, Stanley JC, Axelrod DA, *et al.* (2002) Variation in death rate after abdominal aortic aneurysmectomy in the United States: impact of hospital volume, gender, and age. *Ann Surg* **235**:579–585.

5. Brewster DC, Cronenwett JL, Hallett JW Jr, *et al.* (2003) Guidelines for the treatment of abdominal aortic aneurysms. Report of a subcommittee of the Joint Council of the American Association for Vascular Surgery and Society for Vascular Surgery. *J Vasc Surg* **37**:1106–1117.

6. Bengtsson H, Bergqvist D, Ekberg O, *et al.* (1993) Expansion pattern and risk of rupture of abdominal aortic aneurysms that were not operated on. *Eur J Surg* **159**(9):461–467.

7. Anidjar S, Dobrin PB, Chejfec G, *et al.* (1994) Experimental study of determinants of aneurysmal expansion of the abdominal aorta. *Ann Vasc Surg* **8**:127–136.

8. Ashton HA, Buxton MJ, Day NE, *et al.* (2002) The Multicentre Aneurysm Screening Study (MASS) into the effect of abdominal aortic aneurysm screening on mortality in men: a randomised controlled trial. *Lancet* **360**(9345):1531–1539.

9. Parodi JC, Palmaz JC, Barone HD, *et al.* (1991) Transfemoral intraluminal graft implantation for abdominal aortic aneurysms. *Ann Vasc Surg* **5**:491–499.

10. Anderson PL, Arons RR, Moskowitz AJ, *et al.* (2004) A statewide experience with endovascular abdominal aortic aneurysm repair: rapid diffusion with excellent early results. *J Vasc Surg* **39**:10–19.

11. Lederle FA, Wilson SE, Johnson GR, *et al.* (2002) Immediate repair compared with surveillance of small abdominal aortic aneurysms. *N Engl J Med* **346**:1437–1444.

12. Birkmeyer JD, Siewers AE, Finlayson EV, *et al.* (2002) Hospital volume and surgical mortality in the United States. *N Engl J Med* **346**:1128–1137.

13. Dimick JB, Cowan JA Jr, Stanley JC, *et al.* (2003) Surgeon specialty and provider volumes are related to outcome of intact abdominal aortic aneurysm repair in the United States. *J Vasc Surg* **38**:739–744.

14. Zarins CK, White RA, Schwarten D, *et al.* (1999) AneuRx stent graft versus open surgical repair of abdominal aortic aneurysms: multicenter prospective clinical trial. *J Vasc Surg* **29**:292–308.

15. Forbes TL, Harding GE, Lawlor DK, *et al.* (2006) Comparison of renal function after endovascular aneurysm repair with different transrenally fixated endografts. *J Vasc Surg* **44**:938–942.

16. Guidant product manual (2000) Guidant corporation, Cardiac and Vascular Surgery Group, Menlo Park, California.

17. Peppelenbosch N, Buth J, Harris PL, *et al.* (2004) Diameter of abdominal aortic aneurysm and outcome of endovascular aneurysm repair: does size matter? A report from EUROSTAR. *J Vasc Surg* **39**:288–297.

18. Blum U, Voshage G, Lammer J, *et al.* (1997) Endoluminal stent grafts for infrarenal abdominal aortic aneurysms. *N Engl J Med* **336**:13–20.

19. Velázquez OC, Carpenter JP, Baum RA, *et al.* (1999) Perigraft air, fever, and leukocytosis after endovascular repair of abdominal aortic aneurysms. *Am J Surg* **178**:185–189.

20. Kubin K, Sodeck GH, Teufelsbauer H, *et al.* (2008) Endovascular therapy of ruptured abdominal aortic aneurysm: mid- and long-term results. *Cardiovasc Intervent Radiol* **31**:495–503.

21. Konig GG, Vallabhneni SR, Van Marrewijk CJ, *et al.* (2007) Procedure-related mortality of endovascular abdominal aortic aneurysm repair using revised reporting standards. *Rev Bras Cir Cardiovasc* **22**:7–13.

22. Brewster DC, Geller SC, Kaufman JA, *et al.* (1998) Initial experience with endovascular aneurysm repair: comparison of early results with outcome of conventional open repair. *J Vasc Surg* **27**:992–1003.

23. Prinssen M, Verhoeven EL, Buth J, *et al.* (2004) A randomized trial comparing conventional and endovascular repair of abdominal aortic aneurysms. *N Engl J Med* **351**:1607–1618.

24. Greenhalgh RM, Brown LC, Kwong GP, *et al.* (2004) Comparison of endovascular aneurysm repair with open repair in patients with abdominal aortic aneurysm (EVAR trial 1): 30-day operative mortality results: randomised controlled trial. *Lancet* **364**:843–848.

25. Teufelsbauer H, Prusa AM, Wolff K, *et al.* (2002) Endovascular stent grafting versus open surgical operation in patients with infrarenal aortic aneurysms: a propensity score-adjusted analysis. *Circulation* **106**:782–787.

26. Blankensteijn JD, de Jong SE, Prinssen M, *et al.* (2005) Two-year outcomes after conventional or endovascular repair of abdominal aortic aneurysms. *N Engl J Med* **9**(352):2398–2405.

27. EVAR trial participants (2005) Endovascular aneurysm repair versus open repair in patients with abdominal aortic aneurysm (EVAR trial 1): randomised controlled trial. *Lancet* **365**(9478):2179–2186.

28. Wilt TJ, Lederle FA, Macdonald R, *et al.* (2006) Comparison of endovascular and open surgical repairs for abdominal aortic aneurysm. *Evid Rep Technol Assess* (Full Rep) (144):1–113. Review.

29. Brooks MJ, Brown LC, & Greenhalgh RM (2006) Defining the role of endovascular therapy in the treatment of abdominal aortic aneurysm: results of a prospective randomized trial. *Adv Surg* **40**:191–204.

52   Acute Aortic Dissection

Sean O'Donnell & Shawn McMahon

Washington Hospital Center, Center for Vascular Care, Washington, DC, USA

Introduction

One of the earliest reports of aortic dissection dates back to 25 October 1760; King George II of England was 76 years old when he collapsed and died. An autopsy was performed the next day by physician to the late king, Dr. Nichols, who found that the pericardium was distended with a pint of blood. A transverse fissure on the inner side of the ascending aorta through which blood had recently passed in its external coat to form a raised area of ecchymosis which was interpreted as an aneurysm of the aorta. This early description and that of Morgagni, as well as others through the nineteenth century contributed to the current confusion between aortic dissection and an aortic aneurysm. One of the first accurate descriptions of aortic dissection was by Shekelton in the 1800s when he described the findings of an obliterated false lumen in a healed dissection. Laennec then described this entity as a dissecting aneurysm, which continues to be a misnomer as previously noted. Although an aortic aneurysm can be a complication of a chronic aortic dissection, the two are distinct entities. Intramural hematoma and penetrating aortic ulcers are other aortic pathologies in which relationship to the development of acute aortic dissection is not clearly understood. Acute aortic dissection is one of the most common emergencies of the aorta [1]. It presents one of the most challenging clinical catastrophes for physicians throughout the history of medicine to the present. Its incidence varies with age and risk factors but ranges from 5 to 30 cases per million per year [2,3]. Despite the advances in diagnosis and treatment, the inhospital mortality for aortic dissections remains high, at 27.4%, as reported by the International Registry of Acute Aortic Dissection (IRAD) [3].

Cardiovascular Interventions in Clinical Practice. Edited by Jürgen Haase, Hans-Joachim Schäfers, Horst Sievert and Ron Waksman. © 2010 Blackwell Publishing.

Classification

The classification of acute aortic dissection (AAD) can be confusing in the light of multiple classifications and its confusion with aneurysms. The two predominant classifications are shown in Figure 52.1 and are defined by the anatomical extent of the dissection. Probably the best known and most utilized classification is the Stanford classification, which divides aortic dissections into type A, which involve the ascending aorta, and type B, which consist of dissections limited to the aorta distal to the subclavian artery [4]. The second is the Debakey classification which more precisely describes the extent of the dissection, with type I involving both the ascending and descending aorta, type II limited to the ascending aorta, and type III involving only the aorta distal to the subclavian artery [5]. Type III is further divided into type IIIa, which is limited to the descending thoracic aorta proximal to the diaphragm, and type IIIb, including the abdominal aorta below the diaphragm. The distinction between acute and chronic aortic dissections is also important. The IRAD authors have define AAD as occurring within 14 days of the onset of symptoms and chronic aortic dissection as beyond that time period. This distinction is based primarily on the increased risk of morbidity and mortality during the acute period [3].

Current classifications have some limitations as modern imaging techniques can demonstrate. Often noted on current generation computed tomography angiography (CTA), magnetic resonance angiography (MRA), and intravascular ultrasound (IVUS), scanning aortic dissections can be very complex and can defy simple classifications. For example, type B dissections can have extension into the subclavian artery and the arch. Precise identification of the extent of the dissection can have important implications on treatment and prognosis as will be later discussed in this chapter.

Etiology and risk factor for acute aortic dissection

Age, gender, associated medical conditions, time of the year, and day have all been shown to influence the occurrence of

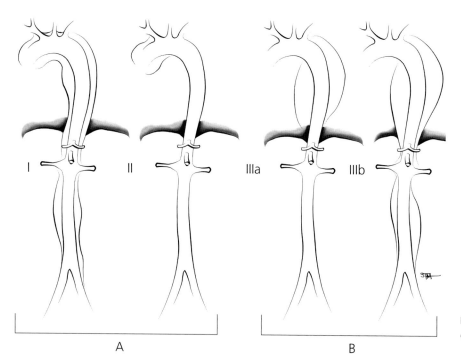

Figure 52.1 Classification for acute aortic dissection.

Table 52.1 Risk factors associated with acute aortic dissection.

Hypertension
Marfan's syndrome
Bicuspid aortic valve
Pre-eclampsia
Cocaine
Ehlers–Danlos syndrom
Turner's syndrome
Prior cardiac surgery
Syphilis

AAD (Table 52.1). Type A dissections occur more commonly in patients <60 years of age but type B dissections occur more frequently in patients >60 years old [3]. Dissections in patients under 40 years of age occur in patients with connective tissue disorders such as Marfan's syndrome and Ehlers–Danlos syndrome, as well as in pregnant women [3,6]. Among other medical conditions associated with AAD to include prior dissection, known aneurysm, atherosclerosis, and arteritis, hypertension tops the list, with 72.1% of patients in the IRAD database reported to have this disorder [3]. Cocaine use is another interesting risk factor which we have frequently seen in our experience and has been reported by others as a contributing factor in the development of AAD [7,8]. This appears to be related to the acute increase in blood pressure caused by a sympathetic discharge after ingestion. Time of onset of AAD associated with cocaine is usually <24 h after use.

An intimal and medial tear is the essential feature of AADs which leads to the pathologic symptoms. Although the exact cause of such tears is unknown, there is significant evidence, owing to the location of the initial tear or entry site, that the increased stresses from changes in the aortic wall during the cardiac cycle, change in pressure (dP)/change in time (dt), seen with untreated or poorly controlled hypertension are to blame. Those locations of the aorta experiencing the most stress have the highest frequency of developing a tear, with the entry site located in the ascending aorta in 65% and the descending aorta in 25% of AADs. The arch and abdominal aorta account for the other 10% [2,9]. Medial degeneration of the aortic wall, as seen in Ehlers–Danlos syndrome and Marfan's syndrome, also has a substantial role to play in the development of AAD [10]. It is highly probable that defects in the metabolism of medial collagen and elastin lead to medial degeneration contributing to AAD in patients without defined hereditary disease [11]. The role of atherosclerosis or previously existing degenerative aneurysms is unknown but not generally considered a significant factor in the etiology of AAD. It may, however, alter the outcome of patients with AAD, as preexisting atherosclerotic plaques tend to limit the progression of the dissection plane [9]. And the presence of a prior aortic aneurysm may predispose the patient to rupture.

Presenting signs and symptoms

The reports from the International Registry of Acute Aortic Dissection (IRAD) give us many insights into the presentation of AAD. Although it is not always the classic tearing pain that is described in many texts, severe chest, back or abdominal pain was reported in 95.5% of patients [3]. Chest pain (72.7%)

Table 52.2 Symptoms and signs of acute aortic dissection.

Symptoms
Chest pain
Back pain
Abdominal pain
Extremity pain
Pain that migrates from chest to abdomen
Cerebrovascular symptoms associated with stroke
Syncope

Signs
Absent or weak pulse in one or multiple extremities
Extremity weakness or paralysis
Cardiac murmur of aortic insufficiency
Signs of pericardial tamponade
Congestive heart failure
Widened mediastinum, loss of aortic knob or pleural effusion on CXR

was seen more commonly than back or abdominal pain, with type A dissections more frequently causing anterior chest pain and type B posterior chest pain. Most patients state the pain is the worst they have ever had, and some describe the pain as radiating or migrating. It is important also to note that 9.4% of patients in the IRAD report presented with syncope (Table 52.2). Hypertension at presentation was noted most frequently in patients with type B dissections (70.1%) while type A dissection patients were hypertensive 34.6% of the time. The presence of a cardiac murmur consistent with aortic valvular insufficiency was more common with type A dissections (44%). Pulse deficits, neurologic findings, and congestive heart failure were less common signs at presentation.

Complications

Acute aortic dissections can cause rupture of the adventitia into the pericardium, chest, or abdomen, resulting in hypotension and death. They can also extend into the root of the ascending aorta, leading to acute aortic valvular insufficiency and congestive heart failure. But it is the syndromes of malperfusion that make the diagnosis of AAD most vexing. Malperfusion results from the anatomic consequences of the intimal tear at the entry site, with the resulting extension of the tear in a subadventitial plane creating true and false channels or lumens in the aorta separated by a septum consisting of the intima and media. The dynamic interplay between the pressures in the true and false lumens account for the pathologic condition referred to as malperfusion. There are two distinct types of obstruction that result from the dissection and lead to malperfusion (Fig. 52.2). The first and easiest to understand is a static obstruction. This occurs when the dissection extends into a significant branch of the aorta, such as the superior mesenteric artery, and circumferentially dissects

into the branch and completely collapses the true lumen, with resulting ischemia. The second is a more subtle form of malperfusion, referred to as a dynamic obstruction, resulting from either collapse of the aortic true lumen during systole or intermittent obstruction of a major arterial orifice during systole. We have witnessed both dramatically while performing IVUS during the course of treating symptomatic AADs. This has also been demonstrated in *ex vivo* and phantom models of AAD [12–14]. Chung *et al.* [12,13] were able to demonstrate in their models that true lumen collapse was intimately dependent on the ratios of inflow capacity to outflow capacity in the true and false lumens. Therefore, increases in the entry tear to the false lumen and decreases in false lumen outflow by a lack of a re-entry tear or communication with a major visceral branch both lead to increasing collapse of the true lumen. This explains why one of the most lethal anatomical situations in type IIIb dissections results from the condition in which all major visceral branches come off the true lumen in the absence of a major re-entry tear (Fig. 52.3). A thorough understanding of this pathophysiology is essential to form effective treatment strategies for AAD.

The complications of AAD involving the ascending aorta (types I and II) are far more overt, frequently resulting in sudden death, whereas complications of AAD extending down the descending thoracic aorta and into the abdominal aorta can be far more insidious, but lethal nonetheless. Collapse of the true lumen above the diaphragm can result in malperfusion of both the abdominal viscera and the lower extremities. On the other hand, dynamic or static obstruction of visceral branches individually or in any combination may result in visceral ischemia, renal ischemia, or difficult to manage hypertension. Likewise, dynamic or static obstruction of the distal aorta or iliacs can result in lower extremity ischemia as an isolated presentation or in combination with visceral ischemia. Although less frequent, the supra-aortic trunks are not exempt from these forms of obstruction, resulting in cerebrovascular compromise. So one can see that AAD must be viewed with a deep respect for the diversity of presentations and complications that it is capable of causing.

Diagnosis and imaging

Owing to the variety of presentations depending on the extent of the AAD and its anatomy, as noted above, the diagnosis can be very challenging, even to the most experienced clinician. A good history and physical examination will most often narrow the diagnosis down to acute coronary syndrome versus AAD. Abdominal catastrophes, pulmonary pathologies, and musculoskeletal disorders can generally be excluded by a careful history and physical examination. Particularly in the appropriate clinical setting such as poorly controlled hypertension, recent cocaine ingestion or Marfan's syndrome would give one a high index of suspicion for AAD. Although

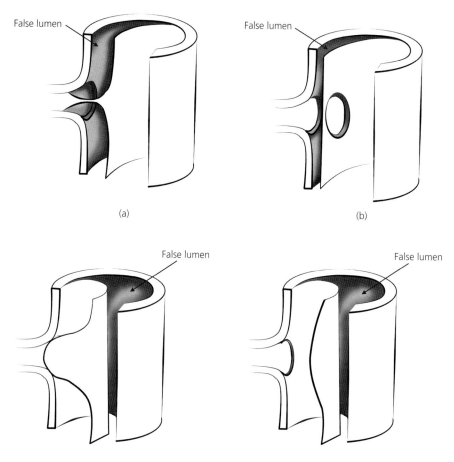

(a)

(b)

(c)

Figure 52.2 How side branches are affected by AAD. (a) Static obstruction. (b) Fenistration. (c) Dynamic obstruction.

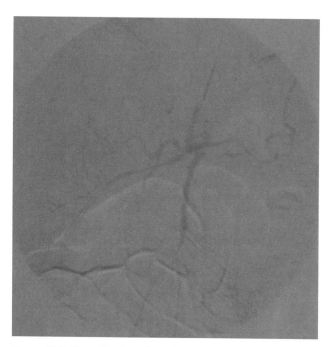

Figure 52.3 Visceral braches off completely collapsed true lumen.

a chest X-ray may suggest the presence of AAD by a widened mediastinum, enlargement of the aortic knob, or left pleural effusion, once suspected, one of three imaging modalities—CT angiography (CTA), MR angiography (MRA), and Trans-esophageal echocardiography (TEE)—can secure the diagnosis of AAD [15].

The most commonly utilized initial imaging test in the IRAD database was the CT scan with intravenous contrast [3]. CTA has the advantages of being widely available, identifying true and false lumens and the extent of side-branch involvement (Fig. 52.4). Its major disadvantage is the requirement for intravenous contrast which, in the setting of malperfusion, can be a major concern.

However, MRA, although perhaps the most accurate, is often not as readily available as CTA, and if used with contrast can have similar concerns as those for CTA. It can detect valvular insufficiency when associated with type I and II AAD and can demonstrate entry tears and extent of the dissection. It may be most suitable for long-term follow-up.

TEE, when available in the acute setting, can be extremely useful, especially for the rapid diagnosis of type I and II AAD in which the need for rapid diagnosis, identification of aortic valvular insufficiency, and need for surgical repair is critical.

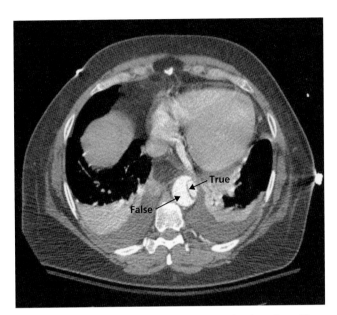

Figure 52.4 Computerized tomographic angiography of a patient with an acute type B aortic dissection with compression of the smaller true lumen by the pressurized larger false prior to endovascular repair.

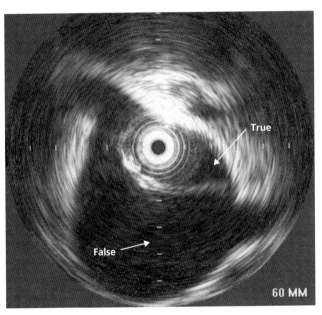

Figure 52.5 Intravascular ultrasound in a patient with an acute type B aortic dissection demonstrating collapse of the true lumen around the 8.2 french catheter at the level of the renal arteries prior to endograft coverage of the entry tear.

It is also particularly suited for patients with evidence of renal insufficiency. The major drawback to this modality is the dependency on a skilled technician and its limitations in detecting extension into the transverse aortic arch.

Intravascular ultrasound also warrants mention. It also is extremely accurate and can identify the extent of the dissection as well as the dynamic effect of the true lumen and its branches (Fig. 52.5). Used in combination with TEE, it can guide the treatment of complicated patients with malperfusion and help limit the need for intravenous contrast that may be better utilized for treatment. Of course the major disadvantage to IVUS is that it is invasive and should be reserved for complicated AAD requiring intervention.

Management

The major decision point in the management of AAD is the distinction between type A (types I and II) and type B (types IIIa,b), as all surgical candidates with type A dissections should be managed urgently with ascending aortic arch repair with or without aortic valvular replacement, depending on the presence or absence of aortic valvular insufficiency [16]. Principles of surgical management for type A dissections include replacement of the ascending thoracic aorta, reconstitution of the true lumen, maintenance of valvular competency, and coronary circulation, thus preventing ascending thoracic aortic rupture, pericardial tamponade and aortic valvular insufficiency. Type A dissections extending into the aortic arch and descending thoracic aorta may require circulatory arrest and aortic arch repair. With the advent of endovascular management of the descending and abdominal aorta, proximal repairs should take into account the potential need for distal endovascular repair, leaving an appropriate landing zone for future endograft repair of the more distal component (Fig. 52.6).

The majority of type B dissections, however, are managed medically [9]. In the IRAD database, patients with type B dissections initially treated medically had a mortality of 10.7% compared with patients undergoing surgery (31%). The major goal of medical management is to reduce the shear stress on the aortic wall, preventing enlargement of the aortic entry tear, further true lumen collapse with malperfusion, and possible rupture. Management benchmarks include a blood pressure of <135/80 mmHg and a heart rate <60 beats/min. This is accomplished by initial beta blockage followed by additional blood pressure control with antihypertensives. Our initial drug of choice is labetalol, which accomplishes both goals. Esmolol is an alternative supplemented by nitroprusside as needed. One must be careful not to use vasodilators in the absence of beta blockade, as this may increase the shear force on the aortic wall. Pain control with judicious use of narcotics is helpful, remembering that pain is often a good indicator of inadequate medical management. Once the patient is stable on intravenous medical management oral agents may be slowly substituted (Table 52.3). Care should be taken when using ACE inhibitors in patients with a rising creatinine and known renal artery involvement with the dissection.

In our practice, endovascular management has widely replaced the surgical management of complicated type B dissections. It is of paramount importance to have early and accurate imaging and a high index for the recognition of malperfusion syndromes to proceed with endovascular

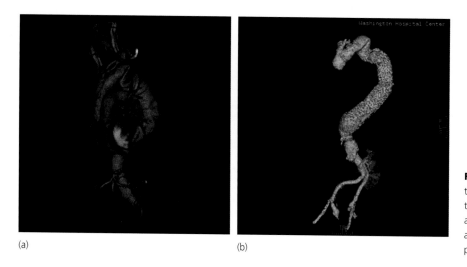

(a)   (b)

Figure 52.6 (a) Patient with prior type I repair to include the aortic arch leaving an "elephant trunk" extending into the descending thoracic aorta. (b) Subsequent endograft repair of a resulting thoracic aneurysm in the same patient.

Table 52.3 Agents used for medical treatment of acute aortic dissection.

Intravenous
Nitroprusside
Esmolol
Labetalol

Oral
Beta blockers
Alpha blockers
Calcium channel blockers
Central acting medications

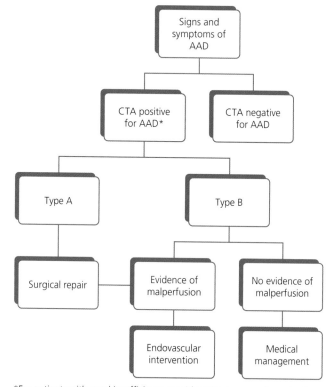

*For patients with renal insufficiency consider MRI, transesophageal echo or intravascular ultrasound for initial diagnosis.

Figure 52.7 Management algorithm for AAD.

management before end organ injury. Malperfusion resulting in renal failure, hypotension, and visceral and limb ischemia have been identified as independent risk factors for early mortality [17]. Although the role for endovascular treatment of uncomplicated type B AAD may be controversial, the use of endovascular therapies for patients with malperfusion syndromes has been promising [18–22]. The principal goals of endovascular management are (1) to establish access to the true lumen, (2) to cover the entry tear with an endograft, and (3) to correct any static or dynamic obstruction to the aortic true lumen, visceral, renal and lower extremity arteries (Fig. 52.7). Frequently, after accomplishing the first and second goals of covering the aortic entry tear, the third goal is fulfilled. Identifying the anatomy and gaining access to the true lumen is aided by the use of IVUS. It is essential to assure wire access in the true lumen from the femoral artery to the ascending thoracic aorta as placement of an endograft in the false lumen will not prove helpful. Multiple tears and re-entry sites are traps for the inexperienced operator; to think he/she has access in the true lumen only to find that partway up the aorta the wire has gone through a secondary tear and into the false lumen. The length of aorta to be covered initially and the need to treat secondary tears and re-entry sites has not been well defined. We have abandoned using bare metal stents to re-establish

the aortic true lumen after the initial entry tear is covered with an endograft as this has proved problematic for future reinterventions. Regardless of medical, endovascular, or surgical treatment, adherence to control of hypertension, cessation of cocaine use, and strict follow-up is essential to successful outcomes.

One particularly difficult patient population is the type A dissection patients who present with distal extension (type I) along with visceral and lower extremity ischemia. This particular constellation of clinical presentation and anatomy requires careful prioritizing of treatment goals. It has been demonstrated by Deeb *et al.* [23] that the conventional wisdom of initial surgical repair of the ascending thoracic aorta before correction of the visceral and/or lower extremity malperfusion may not be wise at all. They found a decrease in mortality from 89%, in patients who underwent immediate ascending thoracic aortic surgical repair, to 15%, in patients who had an endovascular repair of their malperfusion before their surgical repair.

Debates on aortic fenestration versus endograft coverage of the entry tear exist; however, *in vitro* models have demonstrated that only coverage of the entry tear reliably restores true lumen collapse [13]. Clinically, endograft coverage has been shown to be more effective in inducing false lumen thrombosis compared with fenestration [19].

Conclusion

Acute aortic dissection remains a lethal disease that affects a diverse population in their peak productive period of life. It is often associated with poorly controlled hypertension, congenital aortic diseases, and cocaine use. Diagnosis can prove difficult; however, careful history and physical examination along with the use of CTA and TEE can accurately make the diagnosis, define the anatomy, and determine the treatment strategy. The major determinant in the immediate management is the distinction between proximal type A (type I, II), treated with urgent surgical repair, and distal type B (IIIa,b) dissections, treated medically reserving endovascular therapies for complicated presentations with malperfusion syndromes. Regardless of the initial treatment, AAD is a diffuse aortic disease prone to progressive aneurysmal dilation, recurrent dissection, and rupture. Lifelong follow-up with serial imaging and control of hypertension is essential to successful outcomes.

References

1. Pretre R & von Segesser LK (1997) Aortic dissection. *Lancet* **349**(9063):1461–1464.
2. Black JH & Cambria RP (2008) Aortic dissections: perspectives for the vascular/endovascular surgery. In: K. Wayne Johnston (ed.) *Vascular Surgery*. 6th edn. Elsevier, pp. 1512–1533.
3. Hagan PG, Nienaber CA, Isselbacher EM *et al.* (2000) The International Registry of Acute Aortic Dissection (IRAD): new insights into an old disease. *JAMA* **283**:897–903.
4. Daily PO, Trueblood HW, Stinson EB *et al.* (1970) Management of acute aortic dissections. *Ann Thorac Surg* **10**:237–247.
5. DeBakey ME, Henly WS, Cooley DA *et al.* (1965) Surgical management of dissecting aneurysms of the aorta. *J Thorac Cardiovasc Surg* **49**:130–49.
6. Katz NM, Collea JV, Moront MG *et al.* (1984) Aortic dissection during pregnancy: treatment by emergency cesarean section

7. immediately followed by operative repair of the aortic dissection. *Am J Cardiol* **54**:699–701.
7. Eagle KA, Isselbacher EM, & DeSanctis RW (2002) Cocaine-related aortic dissection in perspective. *Circulation* **105**:1529–1530.
8. Hsue PY, Salinas CL, Bolger AF *et al.* (2002) Acute aortic dissection related to crack cocaine. *Circulation* **105**:1592–1595.
9. O'gara PT & DeSanctis RW (1995) Acute aortic dissection and its variants. Toward a common diagnostic and therapeutic approach. *Circulation* **92**:1376–1378.
10. Marsalese DL, Moodie DS, Lytle BW *et al.* (1990) Cystic medial necrosis of the aorta in patients without Marfan's syndrome: surgical outcome and long-term follow-up. *J Am Coll Cardiol* **16**:68–73.
11. Cambria RP, Brewster DC, Moncure AC *et al.* (1988) Spontaneous aortic dissection in the presence of coexistent or previously repaired atherosclerotic aortic aneurysm. *Ann Surg* **208**:619–624.
12. Chung JW, Elkins C, Sakai T *et al.* (2000) True-lumen collapse in aortic dissection: part I. Evaluation of causative factors in phantoms with pulsatile flow. *Radiology* **214**:87–98.
13. Chung JW, Elkins C, Sakai T *et al.* (2000) True-lumen collapse in aortic dissection: part II. Evaluation of treatment methods in phantoms with pulsatile flow. *Radiology* **214**:99–106.
14. Williams DM, LePage MA, & Lee DY (1997) The dissected aorta: part I. Early anatomic changes in an in vitro model. *Radiology* **203**:23–31.
15. Moore AG, Eagle KA, Bruckman D *et al.* (2002) Choice of computed tomography, transesophageal echocardiography, magnetic resonance imaging, and aortography in acute aortic dissection: International Registry of Acute Aortic Dissection (IRAD). *Am J Cardiol* **89**:1235–1238.
16. Erbel R, Alfonso F, Boileau C *et al.* (2001) Diagnosis and management of aortic dissection. *Eur Heart J* **22**:1642–1681.
17. Suzuki T, Mehta RH, Ince H *et al.* (2003) Clinical profiles and outcomes of acute type B aortic dissection in the current era: lessons from the International Registry of Aortic Dissection (IRAD). *Circulation* **108**(Suppl. 1): II312–II317.
18. Nienaber CA, Zannetli S, Barbieri B *et al.* (2005) INvestigation of STEnt grafts in patients with type B Aortic Dissection: design of the INSTEAD trial—a prospective, multicenter, European randomized trial. *Am Heart J* **149**:592–599.
19. Beregi JP, Haulon S, Otal P *et al.* (2003) Endovascular treatment of acute complications associated with aortic dissection: midterm results from a multicenter study. *J Endovasc Ther* **10**: 486–493.
20. Dake MD, Miller DC, Semba CP *et al.* (1994) Transluminal placement of endovascular stent grafts for the treatment of descending thoracic aortic aneurysms. *N Engl J Med* **331**:1729–1734.
21. Dake MD, Kato N, Mitchell RS *et al.* (1999) Endovascular stent graft placement for the treatment of acute aortic dissection. *N Engl J Med* **340**:1546–1552.
22. Greenberg R (2002) Treatment of aortic dissections with endovascular stent grafts. *Semin Vasc Surg* **15**:122–127.
23. Deeb GM, Williams DM, Bolling SF *et al.* (1997) Surgical delay for acute type A dissection with malperfusion. *Ann Thorac Surg* **64**:1669–1675.

53 Surgical Approaches to the Treatment of Aortic Aneurysms and Dissections

Kourosh Keyhani, Anthony L. Estrera, Charles C. Miller III & Hazim J. Safi

The University of Texas Medical School at Houston, Memorial Hermann Heart and Vascular Institute, Houston, TX, USA

Introduction

The most common disease of the aorta is aneurysm and dissection. The ascending aorta consists of two segments: the aortic root, which encompasses the aortic valve, the coronary arteries and the sinuses, and the tubular portion, which is from the supracoronary ascending aorta just proximal to the innominate artery. The transverse arch is between the innominate and left subclavian arteries and gives rise to the brachiocephalic arteries. The descending thoracic aorta extends from distal to the left subclavian artery to the 12th intercostal space. The abdominal aorta begins at the abdominal hiatus and gives rise to the celiac trunk, the superior mesenteric artery, inferior mesenteric artery, and both renal arteries.

Classifications

Dissection

It remains important to differentiate the classification of aneurysms from aortic dissection. Aortic dissections have been classified in several ways. Stanford type A classification involves the ascending aorta and transverse arch. DeBakey type I involves the ascending, transverse arch, descending, and abdominal aorta. DeBakey type II involves only the ascending aorta. Dissections distal to the left subclavian are classified as Stanford type B or DeBakey III. DeBakey III is classified further as "A" when it involves only the descending thoracic aorta and "B" involving the thoracoabdominal aorta (Fig. 53.1). With regard to the chronicity of dissection, acute is considered when the onset of pain to presentation is <14 days. The dissection is considered chronic when pain onset is >14 days.

Cardiovascular Interventions in Clinical Practice. Edited by Jürgen Haase, Hans-Joachim Schäfers, Horst Sievert and Ron Waksman. © 2010 Blackwell Publishing.

Descending thoracic aortic aneurysms

In the era of thoracic endovascular repair, the distinction between descending thoracic aortic aneurysms from thoracoabdominal aortic aneurysms became important. We discovered that replacement of the entire descending thoracic aorta was a risk factor for neurologic injury [1]. Thus, descending thoracic aortic aneurysm is classified based on the sixth intercostal space. In Figure 53.2, extent (a) is from the left subclavian to the sixth intercostal space, extent (b) is from the sixth intercostal space to T12, and extent (c) extends along the entire thoracic aorta.

Thoracoabdominal aortic aneurysms

Thoracoabdominal aortic aneurysms are classified based on our experience. In Figure 53.3, extent I is distal to the left subclavian to just above the renal arteries, extent II is distal to the left subclavian to below the renal arteries, extent III is from the sixth intercostal space to below the renal arteries, extent IV is from the 12th intercostal space to above the iliac bifurcation, and extent V is below the sixth intercostal space to just above the renal arteries. Different from the Crawford classification, the extent V was added to further distinguish those aneurysms of the mid-thoracoabdominal region. By further specifying the extent V from those that would have been previously classified as either extent I or III, the extent III aneurysms became a risk factor for neurologic injury [2].

Although there are many differing associations when considering the etiology of thoracic aneurysms and dissection, the underlying disease process is medial degeneration. There are genetic susceptibilities to this degeneration. Marfan's syndrome occurs in 1 in 5000 worldwide with associated skeletal, ocular, and cardiovascular complications [3]. Before the era of open-heart surgery, the majority of patients with MFS died prematurely of rupture of the aorta, with an average life expectancy of 45 years [4]. Aortic dilation is the result of genetic defects in a specific component of an elastic fibrin known as fibrillin-1 located on chromosome 15. It is inherited in an autosomal dominant manner. Interestingly, one-quarter of the patients do not have a family history and acquire the syndrome due to new mutation. Other genetic disorders that

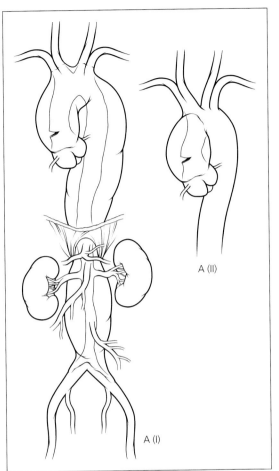

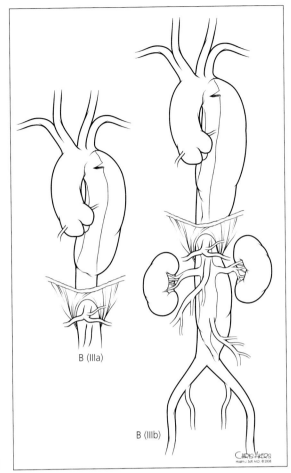

Figure 53.1 Stanford (letters) and DeBakey (Roman numerals) classification systems.

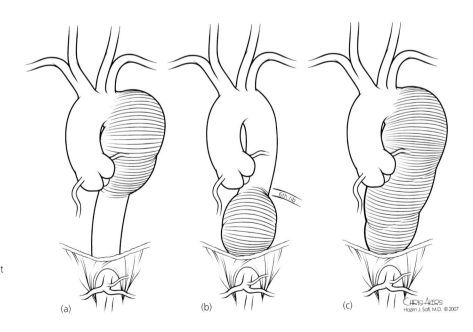

Figure 53.2 Descending thoracic aortic aneurysm is classified based on the sixth intercostal space. Extent (a) is from the left subclavian to the 6th intercostal space, extent (b) is from the sixth intercostal space to T-12, and extent (c) extends along the entire thoracic aorta.

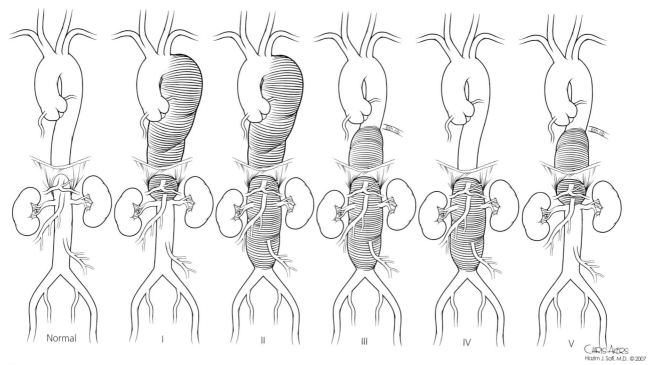

Figure 53.3 Classification of thoracoabdominal aortic aneurysms: Extent I is distal to left subclavian to just above the renal arteries, extent II is distal to the left subclavian to below the renal arteries, extent III is from the 6th intercostal space to below the renal arteries, extent IV is from the 12th intercostal space to above the iliac bifurcation, and Extent V is below the 6th intercostal space to just above the renal arteries.

predispose patients to aortic pathology are Turner's syndrome, Ehler–Danlos syndrome, and polycystic kidney disease. In patients with fibrillin-2 or postcongenital contraction, contractual arachnodactyly syndrome is supposedly related to Marfan's syndrome. Twenty percent of patients with thoracic aneurysms and dissections are due to familial disease, having been associated with mutations in chromosomes 3 and 5 [5,6]. It is also thought that genetic mutational factors predispose individuals to thoracic aortic aneurysms via the transformation of growth factor beta-2 receptors with thoracic aortic aneurysms and dissections [7]. TGF-β has also been the associated defect in Loeys–Dietz syndrome.

Historical background

Accurate figures on the population incidence, and therefore the natural history, of thoracic aortic aneurysms are difficult to estimate. The use of computed tomography (CT) for screening purposes would be the most sensitive and specific imaging technique, but radiation exposure and cost prohibit its use. In the well-described population studies of Rochester, Minnesota, the population historical cohort study from records collected between 1951 to 1980 shows that 11% underwent surgical therapy [8]. The reported incidence of thoracic aortic aneurysm was 5.9 person-years per 100 000 in 1980. A follow-up done by Bickerstaff and associates [8] showed that, in 1994, the estimated incidence increased to 10.4 per 100 000 [9]. This probably related to improved diagnosis by the ubiquitous use of the CT scans after 1985.

Evaluation of thoracic and thoracoabdominal aneurysms reveals lifetime probability of rupture of 75–80% [8,10], with 5-year untreated survival to be in the 10–20% range. In non-dissecting aneurysms, the median time to rupture has been reported to be in the range of 2–3 years [8,10–12]. Aneurysm size significantly influences the time elapsed, with a 43% risk of rupture within 1 year for aneurysms with diameters ≥6 cm, 80% with diameters of ≥8 cm and greater, and 4% with diameters <5 cm [13]. For acute dissecting aneurysms of the ascending aorta, the median time to rupture is approximately three days [10]. Patients with aneurysm ≥5 cm or documented aneurysm enlargement, or chest or back pain indicating expansion are considered for elective surgery. Acute type A dissection often requires urgent surgical repair. Type B dissection is treated medically and observed unless life-threatening complications occur.

Diagnostic imaging

The modality of choice to diagnose patients with aneurysms currently is the use of the CT scan. It is fast and ubiquitously available in many US emergency rooms. It can show the condition of the aortic wall, the extension of aneurysms and dissections, and allows the differentiation between true and false lumen as well as clots. In the diagnostics of aortic aneurysms and dissections, CT scanning has replaced the use of aortography. Spiral CT scanning supplements conventional CT scanning with the addition of three-dimensional reconstruction of the image, CT is indispensable for follow-up and tracking aneurysmal growth. In contrast to CT, magnetic resonance imaging (MRI) offers the potential advantage to allow imaging of aortic aneurysms and dissections without using contrast media, which may be of special advantage in patients with impaired renal function. The images are deducted by radiofrequency signals when the body hydrogen atoms react to strong magnetic fields. Relative contraindications for MRI consist of the presence of pacemakers and claustrophobia. Transesophageal echocardiography is the modality of choice in detecting acute dissection, whether in the descending or ascending aorta. The drawback is that it is invasive and, on occasion, requires the use of anesthesia. Another limitation of transesophageal echocardiography is that it does not show the transverse arch well. In contrast to the above mentioned diagnostic approaches, an intravascular ultrasound probe provides a view of the intraluminal aspect of the artery, especially with dissection.

Clinical presentation

The clinical manifestation of thoracic aortic aneurysm is variable. In most patients, it is an incidental finding without any specific symptoms. Usually, a large aneurysm will put pressure on adjacent structures. It can appear as back pain, vocal hoarseness due to paralysis of the recurrent laryngeal nerve, dyspnea caused by compression of the airway, dysphagia caused by compression on the esophagus, and pulmonary hypertension caused by pressure on the pulmonary artery, eventually causing a fistula or bleeding. Thoracoabdominal aortic aneurysms may press against the stomach causing weight loss. They can also be associated with atherosclerotic disease of the viscera and the renal arteries, causing intestinal angina or arterial hypertension, respectively. In patients with aortic insufficiency, a wide pulse pressure and a diastolic murmur may be present.

Indications for operation

In patients diagnosed with aneurysms of >5 cm enlargement, surgical therapy is indicated [13]. In addition, sudden changes in condition, such as pain, rapid increase in size of aneurysm, expansion, leakage of the aneurysm, or rupture, are considered mandatory for operation. Patients with Marfan's syndrome or inherited collagen disorders usually require operation in aneurysms <5 cm; 90% of the deaths in Marfan's syndrome are due to dissection or rupture. Patients with transforming

growth factor β2 mutations will require surgery earlier (even if the aneurysm is 4.5 cm) because they tend to dissect and rupture. In patients presenting with acute type A or DeBakey I or II dissection, surgical therapy is initiated after the patient is stabilized. The natural history of a patient with type A or DeBakey I or II is lethal, with a mortality rate increasing 1% per hour in the first 48 h; a rate of 75% in 2 weeks and 90% at 1 year. With type B aortic dissection, medical therapy is indicated and surgery is reserved for patients with impending rupture, aneurysm diameter of >5 cm, malperfusion to the viscera or lower extremities, or retrograde dissection to the ascending aorta. The goal of medical management is to keep systolic blood pressure below 120 mmHg. This is initiated by antihypertensive agents, including beta-blockers and/or calcium channel blockers. Additional agents may be added, such as nitroglycerin and, on rare occasions, nitroprusside, to help control systolic blood pressure.

Surgical treatment of ascending and aortic arch

The choice of repair for ascending aorta is determined by several factors, including anatomy, etiology, and age. In patients with large sinuses of Valsalva or Marfan's syndrome, we use the button technique and a composite valve graft prosthesis. In elderly patients or those in whom the sinuses of Valsalva are not enlarged, we replace only the aortic valve and the tubular portion of the ascending aorta. Our current surgical approach is based on the work of Griepp et al. [14] with the use of cardiopulmonary bypass, profound hypothermia, and circulatory arrest. In the past, circulatory arrest time >40 min increased the incidence of stroke, and arrest time >65 min increased the mortality rate [15]. Currently, we add the adjunct of retrograde cerebral perfusion to prevent stroke and death, first used continuously during aortic arch repairs by Ueda et al. [16], but first described by Mills and Ochsner [17].

The patient is placed in the supine position and a median sternotomy is performed. If the ascending aorta is aneurysmal and devoid of any atheromatous plaque, we cannulate the ascending aorta using a bi-caval cannulation and cool the patient until the electroencephalogram is isoelectric and the pupils are fixed and dilated with a nasopharyngeal temperature of <20°C. Subsequently, the ascending aorta and transverse arch are resected. A prefabricated graft with a side arm composed of woven Dacron impregnated with either collagen or gelatin is used for the reconstruction. After completing the proximal portion of the transverse arch, the sidearm is used to restore cerebral and systemic flow, which allows for rewarming. The head is elevated to allow for de-airing of the reconstruction. Attention is then turned to the ascending aorta. If the ascending aorta is aneurysmal, it will be resected above the supracoronary ascending aorta. If the valve is abnormal or the sinuses are dilated with severe aortic insufficiency, then the aortic root is replaced using the button technique in which the left and right main coronary arteries are reattached to a prefabricated aortic composite valve prosthesis. Currently, we also like to repair the aortic valve if it is minimally diseased using the Tirone David technique. In this procedure, the sinuses of Valsalva are excised, and the aortic valve is reattached into the aortic graft, followed by reattachment of the left and right main coronary arteries as a button into the main graft. At the end of the proximal reconstruction, the patient is rewarmed to a nasopharyngeal temperature of 36°C, and the patient is weaned from cardiopulmonary bypass.

In acute dissection of the ascending aorta (type A or DeBakey I or II), the same technique is used with one exception: we always use the open technique and cannulate the right or left femoral artery and, on rare occasions, the axillary artery. Once the patient's temperature is below 20°C and the electroencephalogram is isoelectric, we then excise most of the ascending aorta. The transverse arch is inspected and it is not resected unless it is totally disintegrated, ruptured, or has a large amount of hematoma. Most of the transverse arch is resected from the lesser curvature to the lateral wall, and the innominate and left common carotid arteries are reattached into a beveled graft. After completing this stage of the repair, the patient's cerebral and systemic circulation is rewarmed. Next, the ascending aorta and aortic valve are evaluated. The aortic valve is resuspended if it is free of disease. The aortic root is reconstructed using pledgeted 4–0 polypropylene sutures and the rest of the procedure is similar to that described earlier.

Results

In our experience of 994 patients with ascending and arch repair, glomerular filtration rate is a predictor of 30-day mortality. When the glomerular filtration rate is above $100\,mL/min/1.73\,m^2$ the mortality rate is 4.7%. The mortality rate increases with decreasing glomerular filtration rate such that at rates $<55\,mL/min/1.73\,m^2$, the mortality rate is 19.6% [18].

In our practice, the use of retrograde cerebral perfusion has been associated with a reduction in mortality and stroke. Our overall stroke rate is 2.8% in a series of 1107 repairs of the ascending and transverse aortic arch [19].

Surgical treatment of descending thoracic aorta

The method of treatment for a descending thoracic aortic aneurysm (DTAA) is similar to thoracoabdominal aortic aneurysm (TAAA) except that the incision is less invasive. We use the adjuncts of distal aortic perfusion, cerebrospinal fluid (CSF) drainage, and moderate hypothermia for both DTAA and TAAA repairs (Fig. 53.4). The incision is made in the bed of the sixth intercostal space with the removal of the rib on occasion to allow for better exposure. The patient is placed on distal aortic perfusion via the lower pulmonary vein and

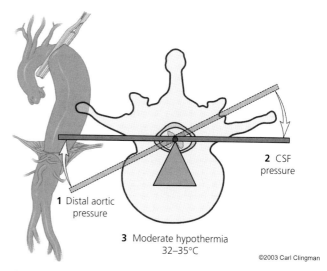

Figure 53.4 Spinal cord protection adjuncts. Distal aortic pressure is increased for perfusion, and CSF pressure is kept low to avoid neurological damage.

the left femoral artery or the left atrial appendage with a centrifugal pump and an in-line heat exchanger. The modified thoracoabdominal incision includes an incision of the costal cartilage without extension into the abdomen to allow for exposure of the entire thoracic aorta. Repair depends on the extent of the aneurysm. Proximally, we like to excise the descending thoracic aorta distal to the left subclavian and, lifting it off the esophagus to prevent a dreaded complication, esophageal graft fistula. We select a Dacron graft that is woven and impregnated with collagen and perform the anastomosis using either a 2–0 or 3–0 polypropylene suture. Once the proximal anastomosis is done, we use pledgeted interrupted sutures to control any bleeding. Lower intercostals (T8 to T12) and intercostal artery 6 are reattached, or bypassed when feasible. The distal anastomosis is performed in a similar fashion using 2–0 or 3–0 polypropylene sutures. The patient is then rewarmed to a nasopharyngeal temperature of 36°C.

Results

In our experience with descending thoracic aortic aneurysm, we performed 355 repairs between 1991 and 2004. Patients who received adjunct protection with distal aortic perfusion and CSF drainage had an overall neurologic deficit rate of 1.3%. Comparing the same group without any adjunct, the neurologic deficit increased to 6.5%. The immediate neurologic deficit was 0.8% for the adjunct and 4.8% for the nonadjunct group [1].

Surgical treatment of thoracoabdominal aortic aneurysm

The patient is taken to the operating room, where the anesthesiologist inserts a thermodilution balloon-tip catheter to measure pulmonary artery pressure and oxygenation, and a double-lumen endotracheal tube to isolate the left lung. Following this, the patient is placed in the right decubitus position and the anesthesiologist inserts a lumbar drain in the third and fourth lumbar spaces to keep the CSF pressure at 10 mmHg intraoperatively and postoperatively for 3 days. Next, the patient is positioned such that the left groin is tilted up 60° to gain access to the left femoral artery, while the shoulder blade is at right angle to the edge of the table. Once the chest and abdomen are prepared and draped, a thoracoabdominal incision is made extending toward the shoulder blade following the curve of the rib. The extent of the thoracoabdominal incision depends on the extent of the aneurysm; extent II, III and IV will require an incision extending below the umbilicus to allow access to the entire abdominal aorta, but for extent I and V we stay above the umbilicus.

The patient is then anticoagulated with sodium heparin (1 mg/kg of body weight) followed by cannulation of the left lower pulmonary vein. This is attached to the centrifugal pump with an online heat exchanger, and the femoral artery is used either directly or using a graft, to establish arterial inflow. The proximal descending thoracic aorta is isolated and lifted off the esophagus. We clamp sequentially starting at the mid-descending thoracic aorta distal or proximal to the left subclavian artery. We suture an appropriately sized Dacron tube graft impregnated with collagen or gelatin and use 2–0 or 3–0 polypropylene sutures to perform the anastomosis in a running fashion. The distal clamp is then placed above the celiac axis if possible and the remainder of the thoracic aorta is opened. The walls of the aorta are retracted using #2 silk retraction sutures. The lower intercostal arteries (8, 9, 10, 11, and 12) are identified and, if any are patent, then an oblique side hole is created in the graft to reattach the thoracic aorta containing the intercostal orifices to the graft. On rare occasions, we bypass to the individual intercostal arteries using 12 mm Dacron grafts. The graft is then passed into the aortic hiatus and into the abdominal portion. If feasible, we clamp the infrarenal aorta, the iliac, or the common femoral artery. The remainder of the aorta is opened and the walls retracted laterally using #2 silk retraction sutures. The celiac, superior mesenteric and the right and left renal arteries are inspected, and if atheromatous debris is present, endarterectomy is performed. We perfuse the celiac and superior mesenteric artery as well as the renal arteries with tepid blood and cold crystalloid solution to keep the kidney temperature below 15°C. A side hole is made opposite the visceral vessels and anastomosed to the graft using a 2–0 or 3–0 polypropylene suture. At the completion of the anastomosis, the patient is placed in the Trendelenburg position, the aorta is flushed of all air and debris, and pulsatile flow is re-established.

In patients with Marfan's syndrome, redo operation, or visceral artery dilation, a prefabricated graft with side arms (known as STAG) is used for reconstruction of the visceral arteries. The graft is stretched to the appropriate length and is cut and sutured to the abdominal aorta above the aortic bifurcation. Again, we place the patient in a Trendelenburg position to flush the graft and remove all air and debris. Once the anastomosis is complete, pulsatile flow is re-established to the lower extremities. The patient's nasopharyngeal temperature is allowed to reach above 36°C before being weaned from the distal aortic perfusion. The diaphragm is repaired using #1 polypropylene sutures. The muscular fascia of the abdomen is approximated using #1 polypropylene followed by intercostal closure using #1 nonabsorbable sutures. Next, the muscular fascia of the chest is closed with #2 polydioxanone monofilament synthetic absorbable suture (PDS) followed by #3 PDS running sutures. The patient is repositioned in the supine position and the bifurcation tube is replaced with a single endotracheal tube unless there is edema or coagulopathy. If the patient requires a large amount of blood, the availability of the Rapid Infusion System (RIS) and Cell-Saver (Hemonetics Corp., Braintree, MA, USA) is critical for rapid replenishment of blood volume.

The patient is moved to the intensive care unit, where the neurologic status is monitored closely, and the CSF pressure is maintained below 10 mmHg for 3 days. The CSF catheter should be watched diligently to prevent any kink or malfunction and replaced accordingly as this can be associated with delayed paraplegia [20,21]. When the patient is stable, extubated and is able to move his or her extremities, the CSF catheter is removed on the third postoperative day. The patient is transferred to regular care floor for another few days and then discharged home. It is important to keep the mean arterial pressure under control and above 80 mmHg. The hemoglobin is kept above 10 g/dL as the low hemoglobin is shown to be a risk factor for delayed paraplegia [20]. Preoperative and postoperative states are depicted in Figure 53.5.

Results

Neurologic deficit

Postoperative neurologic deficit has dramatically declined since the days of cross-clamp and sew technique. In our current practice, we cannot overemphasize the importance of adjuncts along with meticulous surgical detail, including reimplantation of intercostal arteries. Currently, the incidence of neurologic deficit is reduced to 2.4% for all TAAA and 3.3% for extent II TAAA. Looking at the extent breakdown, there was a correlation between aortic clamp time and immediate neurologic deficit. Patients with neurologic deficits have a decreased overall survival. The overall incidence of neurologic deficit in the last 5 years decreased to <2%, compared with 16% in the era of the clamp-and-sew technique. For extent II, which had the highest incidence of neurologic deficit, the incidence dropped to <3.3%.

Renal failure

We define acute postoperative renal failure as an increase in serum creatinine of 1 mg/dL per day for two consecutive

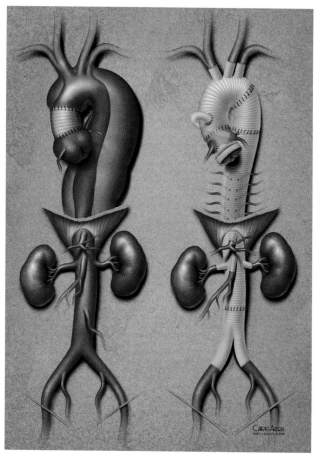

Figure 53.5 Left: extensive aortic aneurysm and chronic dissection, with initial repair of ascending aorta. Right: postoperative image with graft replacement of the ascending/arch, reimplantation of the great vessels, and completion of the elephant trunk repair.

Conclusion

In the current era of aortic surgery, much advancement has been made in treatment of aortic dissection and aneurysm. With the initiation of adjunct therapy, including distal aortic perfusion, moderate hypothermia, and CSF drainage, neurologic deficits have declined dramatically. However, renal failure continues to be a real issue that we are continuing to address with additional protective measures.

Acknowledgments

We wish to thank G. Ken Goodrick for editing, and Chris Akers for illustrations.

References

1. Estrera AL, Miller CC 3rd, Chen EP, *et al.* (2005) Descending thoracic aortic aneurysm repair: 12-year experience using distal aortic perfusion and cerebrospinal fluid drainage. *Ann Thorac Surg* **80**:1290–1296.
2. Estrera AL, Miller CC 3rd, Huynh TT, Porat E, & Safi HJ (2001) Neurologic outcome after thoracic and thoracoabdominal aortic aneurysm repair. *Ann Thorac Surg* **72**:1225–1230.
3. Dietz HC & Pyeritz RE (1995) Mutations in the human gene for fibrillin-1 (FBN1) in the Marfan syndrome and related disorders. *Hum Mol Genet* **4**(Spec No):1799–17809.
4. Murdoch JL, Walker BA, Halpern BL, Kuzma JW, & McKusick VA (1972) Life expectancy and causes of death in the Marfan syndrome. *N Engl J Med* **286**:804–808.
5. Guo D, Hasham S, Kuang SQ, *et al.* (2001) Familial thoracic aortic aneurysms and dissections: genetic heterogeneity with a major locus mapping to 5q13–14. *Circulation* **103**:2461–2468.
6. Hasham SN, Willing MC, Guo DC, *et al.* (2003) Mapping a locus for familial thoracic aortic aneurysms and dissections (TAAD2) to 3p24–25. *Circulation* **107**:3184–3190.
7. Pannu H, Fadulu VT, Chang J, *et al.* (2005) Mutations in transforming growth factor-beta receptor type II cause familial thoracic aortic aneurysms and dissections. *Circulation* **112**:513–520.
8. Bickerstaff LK, Pairolero PC, Hollier LH, *et al.* (1982) Thoracic aortic aneurysms: a population-based study. *Surgery* **92**:1103–1108.
9. Clouse WD, Hallett JW Jr, Schaff HV, Gayari mm, Ilstrup DM, & Melton LJ 3rd (1998) Improved prognosis of thoracic aortic aneurysms: a population-based study. *JAMA* **280**:1926–1929.
10. Pressler V & McNamara JJ (1980) Thoracic aortic aneurysm: natural history and treatment. *J Thorac Cardiovasc Surg* **79**:489–98.
11. Crawford ES & DeNatale RW (1986) Thoracoabdominal aortic aneurysm: observations regarding the natural course of the disease. *J Vasc Surg* **3**:578–582.
12. Perko MJ, Norgaard M, Herzog TM, Olsen PS, Schroeder TV, & Pettersson G. Unoperated aortic aneurysm: a survey of 170 patients. *Ann Thorac Surg* **59**:1204–1209.

days, or the need for hemodialysis. For patients who develop postoperative renal failure, we initiate early continuous venovenous hemodialysis or daily intermittent hemodialysis. Approximately one-third of our patients who develop acute renal failure remain on hemodialysis, and these patients have a prolonged length of hospital stay. Long-term survival for patients on hemodialysis is dismal.

The goals of perioperative renal protection are to maintain adequate renal oxygen delivery, reduce renal oxygen utilization and reduce direct renal tubular injury. The benefit of cold temperatures for metabolic suppression in organ protection is well known. Local hypothermia has been shown to protect against renal ischemia and reperfusion injury in laboratory animals. However, although there is some evidence that patients with cold visceral perfusion have superior survival and recovery rates, this strategy has not decreased the incidence of acute renal failure. The incidence of postoperative renal failure remains troublesome, and the pursuit for the optimal method of renal protection continues to be one of our top priorities.

13. Szilagyi DE, Elliott JP & Smith RF (1972) Clinical fate of the patient with asymptomatic abdominal aortic aneurysm and unfit for surgical treatment. *Arch Surg* **104**:600–606.

14. Griepp RB, Stinson EB, Hollingsworth JF, & Buehler D (1975) Prosthetic replacement of the aortic arch. *J Thorac Cardiovasc Surg* **70**:1051–1063.

15. Svensson LG, Crawford ES, Hess KR, *et al.* (1993) Deep hypothermia with circulatory arrest. Determinants of stroke and early mortality in 656 patients. *J Thorac Cardiovasc Surg* **106**:19–28.

16. Ueda Y, Miki S, Kusuhara K, Okita Y, Tahata T, & Yamanaka K (1990) Surgical treatment of aneurysm or dissection involving the ascending aorta and aortic arch, utilizing circulatory arrest and retrograde cerebral perfusion. *J Cardiovasc Surg* **31**:553–558.

17. Mills NL & Ochsner JL (1980) Massive air embolism during cardiopulmonary bypass. Causes, prevention, and management. *J Thorac Cardiovasc Surg* **80**:708–717.

18. Estrera AL, Miller CC 3rd, Madisetty J, *et al.* (2008) Ascending and transverse aortic arch repair: the impact of glomerular filtration rate on mortality. *Ann Surg* **247**:524–529.

19. Estrera A, Miller C, Lee T-Y, Shah P, & Safi H (2008) Ascending and transverse aortic arch repair: the impact of retrograde cerebral perfusion. *Circulation* **118**:S160–S106.

20. Azizzadeh A, Huynh TT, Miller CC 3rd, *et al.* (2003) Postoperative risk factors for delayed neurologic deficit after thoracic and thoracoabdominal aortic aneurysm repair: a case-control study. *J Vasc Surg* **37**:750–754.

21. Estrera AL, Miller CC 3rd, Huynh TT, *et al.* (2003) Preoperative and operative predictors of delayed neurologic deficit following repair of thoracoabdominal aortic aneurysm. *J Thorac Cardiovasc Surg* **126**:1288–1294.

4 Carotid and Cerebral Artery Disease

54   Pathology of Ischemic Stroke

Wolfgang Roggendorf
University of Würzburg, Würzburg, Germany

Introduction

The energy metabolism of the brain and their disturbances are reflected in the abundance of cerebrovascular diseases. Stroke is the main cause of adult neurologic disability and is third most common cause of death. This chapter focuses on brain ischemia, including stroke and focal ischemia and the counterpart global ischemia. Not included are basic information like anatomy and structure of brain vessels, brain vessel diseases, pathophysiology of brain or brain edema. This general information is given in the literature [1–6].

This chapter has been composed in the following manner: After a short general description of ischemia there is emphasis on (1) global ischemia and (2) regional ischemia (ischemic stroke), followed by (3) special forms of infarct and secondary effects. Clinical features and risks are then addressed, and the chapter finishes with aspects of pathogenetics and etiology.

Circulatory disorders of the brain are caused by interruption of the regular blood flow of the brain e.g., cardiac arrest, thromboembolic occlusion as a local factor. Autopsy studies have shown almost every brain infarct being assigned to one of the four causes: arteriothrombotic, embolic, lacunar, and hemodynamic or hypotensive. Other causes of circulatory disturbances are intracranial hemorrhages and increased intracranial pressure.

The condition in which the blood flow is sufficiently decreased as to result in either temporary or permanent loss of organ function is called ischemia. Ischemia can be subdivided into various forms, most important complete irreversible ischemia, global ischemia and regional ischemia. Table 54.1 shows the types of ischemia and the (neuro)pathologic findings.

The interpretation of cellular abnormalities induced by ischemia may be blurred by artifacts. There are postmortem alterations of the structural features. These artificial changes may be the result of one or more of the following: (1) prolonged agonal state, (2) excessive handling of the unfixed organ, and

Cardiovascular Interventions in Clinical Practice. Edited by Jürgen Haase, Hans-Joachim Schäfers, Horst Sievert and Ron Waksman. © 2010 Blackwell Publishing.

(3) prolonged delays in tissue fixation. Thus the postmortem interval (pm-delay) could produce difficulties in finding interpretation. At room temperature, there will be no major changes in structure and biochemical substances for up to 2 h. Recent studies on pH measurements and protein analyses revealed that there are only minimal changes in morphologic and biochemical structures up to 48 h if the brain is stored at 4–8°C [7,8].

Global (incomplete) ischemia

Global (incomplete) ischemia is a disorder of systemic circulation which may either reduce the entire cerebral blood flow (CBF) below the level of autoregulatory mechanisms or interrupt the CBF transitionally completely.

Clinical symptoms show a broad spectrum depending on factors such as duration of the circulatory crisis, age of the patient, body temperature, and anatomic condition of the vasculature. The characteristics of cardiac arrest, resuscitation, and environmental factors during the first hours or days after cardiac arrest are the most important factors influencing the outcome in the clinical situation [9].

Structural alterations secondary to global brain ischemia

Macroscopically you will find diffuse swelling with increased weight, narrowing of sulci and ventricles, an incomplete penetration of fixative, a decreased consistency of brain parenchyma and sometimes necrosis in the cortical areas, resulting in lamellation (Fig. 54.1).

Regarding microscopic changes, you will find an elective parenchymal necrosis which means that cerebral and cerebellar neurons are altered in volume and stainability. A unique feature of global ischemia is selective vulnerability of specific cell types and brain regions. There is a vacuolation of the neuropil and occasionally migration of the polynuclear leukocytes, and there is marked capillary dilation in some areas (Fig. 54.1).

Within a few days the above mentioned conditions could lead to the development of profound structural abnormalities, occasionally designed as "respirator brain." More common is

Table 54.1 Types of ischemic injury and their anatomic counterpart (modified from Garcia and Anderson [3]).

Ischemic injury	Anatomic counterpart
Complete irreversible ischemia	Somatic death: ischemic cellular changes precede autolysis by several hours
Global ischemia with various degrees of either reperfusion or incomplete ischemia	Brain death, elective parenchymal necrosis, nerve cell loss
Regional (arterial) ischemia: thrombotic, embolic	Brain infarction: ischemic or hemorrhagic
Regional (venous) ischemia	Brain infarction: hemorrhagic
Regional (arteriolar) ischemia	Brain infarction: lacunes and other microinfarctions

Table 54.2 Summary of cerebral infarction and sequential organization (modified from Petito [12]).

Time	Morphologic changes
24 h	Well-circumscribed area of necrosis and discoloration in an arterial territory
	Circumscribed pallor and acute neuronal necrosis, often at edge of infarct ("penumbral zone")
Days 1–2	Minimal polymorphonuclear leukocyte infiltrate
Days 2–5	Blood–brain barrier breakdown and cerebral edema
Days 3–5	Axonal retraction balls at edge of infarct, usually in white matter
Days 5–7	Appearance of lipid-laden macrophages, capillary hypertrophy, and hyperplasia
Day 14	Sheets of lipid-laden macrophages
Day 10–20	Surrounding rim of reactive astrocytes
≥3 months	Cystic space surrounded by reactive astrocytes

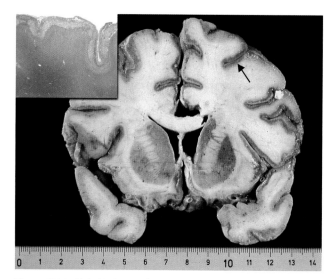

Figure 54.1 Global ischemia after cardiac arrest with severe hypoxic changes in the cortical areas and in part on the basal nuclei (arrow). The basal nuclei on the left side as well as the cortical areas from the temporal lobe are spared. Inset: Lamina necrosis with predilection of the third and fifth lamina.

the definition *brain death*, a situation in which the brain tissue disintegrates in a patient whose other tissues are relatively intact. These brains show a maceration which is sometimes difficult to differentiate from autolytic changes. For clinical criterion of brain death see established criterion by the advisory board of the German Medical Association [10].

Regional ischemia

Regional ischemia (e.g., *brain infarction*) is a well-circumscribed area of necrosis in specific vascular territory resulting from occlusion or severe hypoperfusion in the feeding artery [11]. *Atherosclerosis* is the most common cause of cerebral infarcts (ischemic stroke). Ischemic stroke is the clinical description of a localized neurologic deficit, which becomes manifest. As opposed to ischemic stroke, transient ischemic attacks (TIAs) are deficits which disappear before 24 h, usually within 30 min, so TIAs can be considered as incomplete infarction as opposed to a complete infarction (Table 54.2).

We divide the macroscopic and microscopic description of regional brain infarcts into three stages, according to Cervós-Navarro (1980) [1]. *Stage 1* comprises the acute (early) stage of an infarct. *Stage 2* comprises the destruction of the brain also designated encephalomalacia (*brain softening*); it starts during the first 3–7 days and reaches the maximum during the second week. *Stage 3* comprises the resorption and organization of the destroyed tissue which results in a cystic structure.

Gross features of regional ischemia include brain infarcts of arterial origin, which may appear pale (ischemic) or red (hemorrhagic). Especially brain infarcts in a very early stage are difficult to visualize. The difference between fresh brain infarcts and surrounding nonischemic tissue include the blurring of the cortical white matter boundary and the decreased consistency. Large infarcts are accompanied by

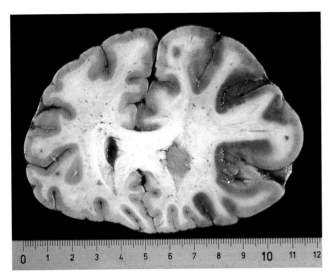

Figure 54.2 Early stage of an ischemic infarct in the territory of the right middle cerebral artery (MCA). There is a mild hemorrhagic component and a moderate brain edema with shifting of the midline from right to left.

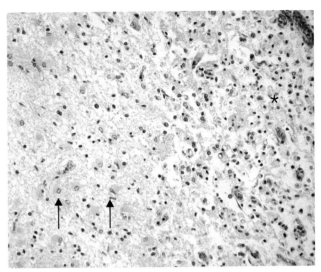

Figure 54.3 Border zone of an encephalomalacia with abundant lipid-laden macrophages in a brain infarct (*) about 5 weeks old. There is a gliosis in the penumbra shown on the left side (arrows) (×350).

displacement of the midline structures, deformity of the ventricles and prominent herniation at the uncus parahippocampalis. This swelling of the infarct hemisphere manifested by shift of the midline structures continues to develop for the first 2–5 days (Fig. 54.2). Hemisphere swelling disappears after about 2 weeks.

Red (hemorrhagic) infarcts of arterial origin differ from pale ones only by the petechiae, usually confined to the gray matter, especially in the cortex. There is no explanation for the selective localization of these petechiae to the gray matter. There is a second variety of hemorrhagic infarcts that develops in areas in which arteries are occluded by emboli. These hemorrhagic components of arterial brain infarction are ascribed to the effect of reperfusion, since CBF studies strongly support the view that cerebral arterial occlusions are transient and followed by reperfusion. This reperfusion finds destroyed vascular walls, which results in a hemorrhagic component of the brain infarct.

Microscopic feature of regional brain infarcts, the neuronal injury, is prominent in stage 1, starting at 12 h and reaching up to 3 days. The acute ischemic nerve cell loss shows an extreme eosinophilic structure of cytocoplasm, while other cellular elements are not much altered during this stage. The cellular infiltration is most prominent in stage 2, encephalomalacia. The microglia reaction, starting already after 24 h, reaches a maximum until the second week. There is also a leukocytic infiltration, which starts at day 2, and an increasing number of monocytes, which are transformed to lipid-laden macrophages (grid cells) to ingest fragments of necrotic cells (Fig. 54.3). Other prominent features are swollen axons and an increase of capillaries. Stage 3 is characterized by a very active astrogliosis. Larger brain infarcts are not covered by a network of astrocytic fibers, there are cysts with small bundles of astrocytic

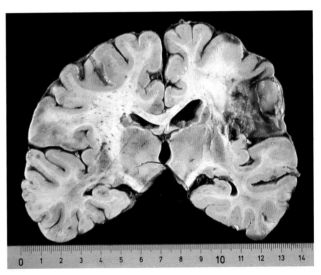

Figure 54.4 Typical appearance of a healed infarct in the territory of the middle cerebral artery (MCA) branch. This cystic lesion is covered by the meninges.

fibers surrounded by cerebrospinal fluid (Fig. 54.4). The time elapsed between the stroke and the final stage of healing of the infarction is directly proportional to the volume and tissue destroyed by the regional ischemia. Oligodendroglial cells, which are most vulnerable to the effect of ischemia, begin to disintegrate during the first stage. The specific role of microglia is described in detail by Kato and Walz [13].

There is a special variety of infarcts. One is the lacunar infarct (lacune), which is a brain lesion, presumed to be of ischemic origin. Lacunes occur mainly in the location of basal ganglia, internal capsule, thalamic nuclei, base of the pons and subcortical white matter. Lacunes are defined by their small size, about 15–35 mm. They are subject to the same tissue changes as normal necrosis. If the process of healing is completed lacunes become visible in the form of cavities with sharply circumscribed edges and a roughly spherical shape. Lacunes are associated with occlusive disease of the penetrating small arterioles [14] and they are especially frequent in brains with hypertensive vasculopathy but their etiology is more heterogeneous than originally proposed [15].

Another form of brain infarctions are hemorrhagic infarctions secondary to venous occlusions. The topography of brain softening secondary to venous (sinus) occlusion corresponds to that of one of the major venous territories. In the cerebral hemispheres the lesions show two patterns of distribution. Softenings are deeply bilateral, close to the midline and secondary to occlusions involving the internal cerebral veins and the vein of Galen or their tributaries. Softenings of cortical and subcortical structures are due to superficial veins or the sagittal superior sinus.

Numerous predisposing factors for intracranial venous thrombosis have been reported, among which infections and dehydration are most prominent.

Secondary effects

The most serious complications of severe infarcts are cerebral edema, hydrocephalus, and Wallerian degeneration. Vasogenic edema develops between the first and the second day; consequently, a transtentorial herniation and transforaminal herniation occurs, which may be followed by one-time bleedings in the upper pons, which is most life-threatening. An obstructive hydrocephalus develops acutely when edematous brain compresses the cerebrospinal fluid outflow. Wallerian degeneration can be seen after 2 weeks if there is a large hemispheric infarct, resulting in degeneration of axons distal to the infarct.

Clinical features and risk factors

The overall age-adjusted stroke incidence rate ranges between 100 and 300 per 100 000 population per year, and depends on methodology, population demographics, and country of origin. These numbers are based on the Oxford Study, the Framingham Study, and the Oslo Statistics. In the USA stroke mortality has been decreasing, whereas data from Oslo show an increase [16–19].

Risk factors

In addition to epidemiologic risk factors predisposing to the occurrence of stroke as listed in Table 54.3, there are modifiable risk factors the most important of which is hypertension. Other factors include atrial fibrillation, elevated serum lipids, cigarette smoking, and obesity.

Behavioral and neurologic abnormalities are common among patients subjected to open heart surgery or carotid

Table 54.3 Risk factors and effects on ischemic stroke incidence.

Risk factors	Effect on stroke incidence
Age	Doubles per decade over age 55
Sex	24%–30% greater in men
Race ethnicity	2.4-fold increase for African Americans
	2.0-fold increase for Hispanics
	Increased among Asians
Heredity	1.9-fold increase among first-degree relatives

Data from Sacco *et al.* [20].

intervention in the immediate postoperative period as well as a long time period after the intervention. There are recent studies on the longitudinal assessment of their neurocognitive function [21,22].

Stroke risk is increased among patients with carotid artery disease. The prevalence of asymptomatic carotid stenosis increases with age and may be observed in > 50% of individuals older than 65 years [23]. Although a symptomatic internal carotid stenosis > 70–80% is a clear indication for surgical or endovascular intervention, such an approach for asymptomatic lesions is more controversial. There are some recent results on cognitive functions after carotid artery revascularization [21] and also with MRI-studies on cerebral ischemia after carotid intervention [24]. However, histopathologic investigations on brain morphology following carotid stenting or endatherectomy are missing. There is one retrospective study over six years with neuropathologic findings after cardiac surgery [25]. Therefore, further studies are needed to elucidate structural long-term changes in the brain after carotid surgical intervention.

Etiology and pathogenesis

Selective vulnerability

Various brain components react in different or selective ways to the same ischemic injury. This traditional concept of selective vulnerability may be applied to different situations. There are sites in the brain where lesions of global ischemia are more likely to develop; these areas are unpredictable in a given individual but as a general rule the most distal arterial territories, so-called boundary zones or water-shed areas, are more susceptible to global ischemia than the rest of the brain. Similar areas are the pyramidal cell layer of the hippocampus and the Purkinje cell layer of the cerebellum. Neurons as a group are more susceptible to the same degree of ischemia than oligodendrocytes, and these are more vulnerable than astrocytes. The reasons for selective vulnerability are not completely understood; current theories focus on glutamate-induced neurotoxicity and disturbances of the protein synthesis [26]. There are calcium-dependent mechanisms and differential neuronal receptors or receptor modulation that may render certain neurons more sensitive or resistant to the effect of cerebral ischemia [27,28].

Ischemic penumbra

The term penumbra is borrowed from astronomy, where it refers to the vaguely shaded annulus that encompasses the moon during a total solar eclipse. In analogous fashion, a dense area of brain ischemia is surrounded by more or less concentric bands of hyperperfused tissue [3]. The severity of ischemia progressively diminishes with distance from the infarct core. The penumbra concept of focal ischemia is of considerable interest for stroke pathophysiology because it is the conceptual basis not only for understanding of infarct evolution, but also for therapeutic reversal of the acute neurologic symptomatology arising from stroke [4,29]. Hakim [30] defined the penumbra as fundamentally reversible, but he stressed that this reversibility is time-limited. In the context of therapeutic approach, the recently coined terms "neuroprotection" and "preconditioning" are in the focus of research.

Neuroprotection

In the wider sense neuroprotection is the preservation of structure and functional integrity of the brain by any kind of intervention that interferes with the deleterious effects of ischemia. However, as the penumbra can be effectively protected by improvement of blood flow alone, neuroprotective interventions are mediated not only by interferences with molecular *injury* cascades, but also by reducing the mismatch between blood flow and metabolism [4].

Ischemic preconditioning

The term "ischemic preconditioning" describes the phenomenon of a short, by definition harmless, ischemic period that provides protection against a subsequent ordinary (ischemic) injury. Ischemic injury is not restricted to the brain, it has also been observed in many other organs [31]. This topic is attracting much attention because preconditioning-induced ischemic tolerance is an effective experimental probe to understand how the brain protects itself. For details see the review by Obrenovitch [32]. This review is focusing on the molecular and related functional changes that are associated with and may contribute to brain ischemic tolerance. Postischemic structural changes in the brain as cell loss and tissue damage, neurogenesis, glial response, and altered abundance of neurotransmitter receptor density in the context of ischemic preconditioning are described in detail by Sommer [31].

Further aspects in the pathogenesis of ischemia are summarized under the topic 'The role of glial cells in cerebral ischemia and stroke-induced immune depression' [33,34].

Acknowledgments

We wish to thank Ms. U. Ahmad and Ms. M. Apfelbacher for expert assistance preparing the manuscript.

References

1. Cervós-Navarro J (1980) Gefäßerkrankungen und Durchblutungsstörungen des Gehirns. In: Doerr W and Seifert G (eds). *Spezielle pathologische Anatomie.* Berlin: Springer, pp. 1–412.
2. Roggendorf W (2002) Kreislaufstörungen des ZNS. In: Peiffer J, Schröder JM and Paulus W. *Neuropathologie.* Berlin: Springer Verlag, pp. 113–166.
3. Garcia JH & Anderson ML (1991) Circulatory disorders and their effects on the brain. In: Davis RL & Robertson DM (eds). *Textbook of Neuropathology.* Baltimore: Williams & Wilkins, pp. 621–719.
4. Hossmann KA (2005) Pathophysiology of focal brain ischemia. In: Kalimo H, Cerebrovascular diseases. Allen Press Inc., Lawrence, Kan, United States. pp. 201–214.
5. Kalimo H, Kaste M, & Haltia M (2002) Vascular diseases. In: Graham DI & Lantos PL (eds). *Greenfield's Neuropathology.* London: Hodder Arnold, pp. 281–357.
6. Roggendorf W & Cervós-Navarro J (1984) Normal and pathologic ultrastructure of human cerebral venules. In: Kapp JP & Schmidek HH (eds). Cerebral venous system and its disorders. Orlando: Grune & Stratton, pp. 37–60.
7. Ferrer I, Santpere G, Arzberger T, *et al.* (2007) Brain protein preservation largely depends on the postmortem storage temperature: implications for study of proteins in human neurologic diseases and management of brain banks: a BrainNet Europe Study. *J Neuropathol Exp Neurol* **66**:35–46.
8. Schmidt M, Monoranu C, Riederer P, *et al.* (2008) Quality control of human post mortem brain tissue: pH measurement useful as quality marker? *Clin Neuropathol* **27**:150.
9. Roine RO (2005) Global brain ischemia. In: Kalimo H, *Cerebrovascular Diseases.* Lawrence, KA: Allen Press Inc., pp. 238–243.
10. Wissenschaftlicher Beirat der Bundesärztekammer (1982) Kriterien des Hirntodes. *Dtsch Ärztebl* **79**:45–55. Fortschreibungen: *Dtsch Ärztebl* 1987;**83**:2940–2946, 1991;**88**:2855–2860, 1997;**94**:1032–1039. Ergänzungen gemäß Transplantations-gesetz: *Dtsch Ärztebl* 1998;**95**:1509–1516.
11. Garcia JH (1992) The evolution of brain infarcts: a review. *J Neuropathol Exp Neurol* **51**:387–93.
12. Petito CK (1993) Cerebrovascular Diseases, In: Nelson J, Parisi J & Schochet SS Jr (eds). *Principles and Practice of Neuropathology.* St. Louis: Mosby Year Book, Inc., pp. 436–458.
13. Kato H & Walz W (2000) The initiation of the microglial response. *Brain Pathol* **10**:137–143.
14. Fisher CM (1982) Lacunar strokes and infarcts: a review. *Neurology* **32**:871–876.
15. Tuszynski MH, Petito CK & Levy DE (1989) Risk factors and clinical manifestations of pathologically verified lacunar infarctions. *Stroke* **20**:990–999.
16. Bamford J, Sandercock P, Dennis M, *et al.* (1990) A prospective study of acute cerebrovascular disease in the community: the Oxfordshire Community Stroke Project 1981–86. 2. Incidence,

case fatality rates and overall outcome at one year of cerebral infarction, primary intracerebral and subarachnoid haemorrhage. *J Neurol Neurosurg Psychiatry* **53**:16–22.

17. Jorgensen HS, Plesner AM, Hubbe P, *et al.* (1992) Marked increase of stroke incidence in men between 1972 and 1990 in Frederiksberg, Denmark. *Stroke* **23**:1701–1704.

18. Jorgensen L & Torvik A (1969) Ischaemic cerebrovascular diseases in an autopsy series. 2. Prevalence, location, pathogenesis, and clinical course of cerebral infarcts. *J Neurol Sci* **9**:285–320.

19. Marquardsen J (1986) Epidemiology of strokes in Europe. In: Barnett HJM, Mohr JP, Steim FM and Yatsu FM. *Stroke, pathophysiology, Diagnosis and Management.* Churchill Livingstone, Edinburgh. pp. 31–43.

20. Sacco RL, Boden-Albala B, Abel G, *et al.* (2001) Race–ethnic disparities in the impact of stroke risk factors: the northern Manhattan stroke study. *Stroke* **32**:1725–1731.

21. Lal BK (2007) Cognitive function after carotid artery revascularization. *Vasc Endovascular Surg* **41**:5–13.

22. Newman MF, Kirchner JL, Phillips-Bute B, *et al.* (2001) Longitudinal assessment of neurocognitive function after coronary-artery bypass surgery. *N Engl J Med* **344**:395–402.

23. Pujia A, Rubba P, & Spencer MP (1992) Prevalence of extracranial carotid artery disease detectable by echo-Doppler in an elderly population. *Stroke* **23**:818–822.

24. Flach HZ, Ouhlous M, Hendriks JM, *et al.* (2004) Cerebral ischemia after carotid intervention. *J Endovasc Ther* **11**:251–257.

25. Emmrich P, Hahn J, Ogunlade V, *et al.* (2003) [Neuropathological findings after cardiac surgery-retrospective study over 6 years]. *Z Kardiol* **92**:925–937.

26. Sommer C, Gass P, & Kiessling M (1995) Selective c-JUN expression in CA1 neurons of the gerbil hippocampus during and after acquisition of an ischemia-tolerant state. *Brain Pathol* **5**:135–144.

27. Grishin AA, Gee CE, Gerber U, *et al.* (2004) Differential calcium-dependent modulation of NMDA currents in CA1 and CA3 hippocampal pyramidal cells. *J Neurosci* **24**:350–355.

28. Torres-Muñoz JE, Van Waveren C, Keegan MG, *et al.* (2004) Gene expression profiles in microdissected neurons from human hippocampal subregions. *Brain Res Mol Brain Res* **127**(1–2):105–114.

29. Heiss WD (2000) Ischemic penumbra: evidence from functional imaging in man. *J Cereb Blood Flow Metab* **20**:1276–1293.

30. Hakim AM (1987) The cerebral ischemic penumbra. *Can J Neurol Sci* **14**:557–559.

31. Sommer C (2008) Ischemic preconditioning: postischemic structural changes in the brain. *J Neuropathol Exp Neurol* **67**:85–92.

32. Obrenovitch TP (2008) Molecular physiology of preconditioning-induced brain tolerance to ischemia. *Physiol Rev* **88**:211–247.

33. Dirnagl U, Klehmet J, Braun JS, *et al.* (2007) Stroke-induced immunodepression: experimental evidence and clinical relevance. *Stroke* **38**(2 Suppl):770–773.

34. Nedergaard M & Dirnagl U (2005) Role of glial cells in cerebral ischemia. *Glia* **50**:281–286.

55 Interventional Treatment of Carotid Artery Disease

Jennifer Franke & Horst Sievert

CardioVascular Center Frankfurt, Frankfurt, Germany, and Washington, DC, USA

Introduction

Thirty years after its initial introduction in 1977, carotid artery stenting has developed into an endovascular technique to prevent ischemic stroke in patients with carotid artery disease. Although still under debate, it has received worldwide acceptance as an alternative to carotid endarterectomy. This chapter discusses the present indications and contraindications of carotid stenting, basic technical aspects of this procedure, as well as the technical management of challenging situations. Furthermore, the current status of clinical series and randomized trials is reviewed.

Historical background

Stroke is the third most frequent cause of death in developed countries. Nearly 50% of the patients show significant intellectual or physical disorders after suffering a stroke.

Ischemic events are the cause of the vast majority of strokes (80–85%). Nearly one-third of all ischemic strokes are caused by carotid artery disease. In carotid stenoses, >80% of clinical symptoms are due to embolism originating from arteriosclerotic plaques. In 20% the strokes occur because of hemodynamic impairment of the cerebral circulation [1,2]. The intention of interventional or surgical treatment of the carotid artery is therefore focused on removing debris that is likely to cause distal embolization or a hemodynamic significant vessel lumen narrowing.

In the past several years, carotid stenting has rapidly developed into an alternative to surgery and is increasingly the preferred method in surgically high-risk patients [3–6]. Many patients tend to favor stenting over surgery, because it is less invasive, does not cause a scar and requires only a short hospital stay <24 h. Other advantages of the interventional approach over carotid surgery include the ability to diagnose

Cardiovascular Interventions in Clinical Practice. Edited by Jürgen Haase, Hans-Joachim Schäfers, Horst Sievert and Ron Waksman. © 2010 Blackwell Publishing.

and treat embolic complications immediately. Furthermore, the fact that the patient can be awake during the procedure allows close neurologic monitoring. Complications like distal embolization can therefore be recognized and treated immediately.

Several large randomized trials of carotid surgery have proven the advantage of surgery in symptomatic patients compared with medical treatment alone. In 1991, the North American and European carotid surgical trials (NASCET and ECST trial) demonstrated the long-term benefit for symptomatic patients who experienced a stroke or TIA within the last 6 months and had a degree of carotid stenosis exceeding 50% [7–9].

However, among patients who suffered from carotid artery disease without any neurologic symptoms, the balance between surgical or interventional risk and long-term benefits of the procedure was indistinct and remained controversial for many years.

Results from the Veterans Affairs Asymptomatic Carotid Endarterectomy Trial (VA-trial) in 1993 and Asymptomatic Carotid Atherosclerosis Study (ACAS) in 1995 were promising, showing a significant reduction in the incidence of transient ischemic attack (TIA) and minor stroke. However, the reduction of the incidence of fatal or major stroke was not significantly reduced compared with medical treatment [10,11].

In 2004, the ACST trial examined asymptomatic patients and established beneficial results when the patient was younger than 75 years and had a stenosis exceeding 70% measured in duplex scan [12]. The risk of stroke or death within 30 days after surgery was 3.1%. Immediate carotid endarterectomy could lower the net 5 year stroke risk of 12% by half to only 6%. Half of this 5 year benefit involved disabling or fatal strokes. It was proven that surgery of asymptomatic lesions is justified because the risk of suffering a stroke in patients with adequate history under medical treatment alone was higher than the operative risk. The more comorbidities, the higher were the stroke and death rates but the greater the benefit from surgery within mid- and long-term course. The results of the Asymptomatic Carotid Surgery Trial (ACST) are an important extension of the results of earlier trials of asymptomatic carotid artery disease, because they had also proven the prevention of disabling and fatal strokes in women.

Morphology and pathophysiology

Atherosclerosis is known to be a systemic disease. In the majority of cases it is not limited to a specific vascular bed, instead it affects all arteries throughout the body. Patients who suffer from symptomatic atherosclerotic disease in one vascular bed, e.g., coronary heart disease are not only at risk of myocardial infarction, but are also at risk of atherosclerotic disease of supraaortal and cerebral arteries leading to stroke, as well as atherosclerotic disease of peripheral arteries leading to limb ischemia [13–15].

Atherosclerotic disease in the internal carotid artery begins as vessel wall thickening. When the intima–media complex measures >1mm the term plaque is used. Significant narrowing of the internal carotid artery or plaque rupture may lead to an ischemic occlusion of cerebral arteries. Or, in the case of unstable atherosclerotic lesions, thrombus formations can be released leading to cerebral embolism. These situations mostly result in a stroke. In 2004, Biasi *et al.* [16] reported on the index of echogenicity and named the grayscale median a risk indicator of stroke during carotid stenting. They concluded that carotid plaque echolucency, as measured by grayscale median ≤25, increases the risk of stroke in carotid artery stenting.

Knowledge of the extra- and intracerebral anatomy is fundamental. The left common carotid artery arises from the aortic arch, while the right arises from the bifurcation of the brachiocephalic trunk. Neither common carotid artery has side branches, but each divides into the internal and external carotid artery at the level of the upper boarder of the thyroid cartilage. The external carotid artery starts at the bifurcation of the common carotid artery supplying the jaw, face, neck, and meninges. The two terminal branches of the external carotid artery are the superficial temporal artery and maxillary artery. These two branches, in addition to the occipital artery, can serve as collateral channels for blood supply to the brain if the internal carotid artery or the vertebral artery is occluded. Vertebral arteries provide the brain with only a small amount of blood but can become more important if the carotid arteries are narrowed or blocked. The internal carotid artery ascends laterally behind the hypopharynx where it can be palpated. It bifurcates into the anterior cerebral artery and the larger middle cerebral artery. The extracranial segment of the internal carotid artery does not have significant branches visible. The first major intracranial branch is the ophthalmic artery.

In young adults and children the aortic arch is symmetrically curved and the origins of the brachiocephalic arteries are aligned in straight lines and courses superiorly [17]. The aging and arteriosclerotic process elongate and distend the aortic arch. The ostia of the brachiocephalic arteries are shifted—the aortic knob becomes more superior and posterior. It becomes more difficult to selectively catheterize these vessels. Furthermore, the internal carotid arteries themselves develop tortuosities during the aging process. This has to be considered during the intervention, as it can render cannulation of the artery as well as filter and stent placement challenging.

The most important intracranial collateral pathway is the circle of Willis, connecting through the anterior and posterior communicating arteries, the anterior, middle, and posterior cerebral arteries. In situations in which the atherosclerotic process develops gradually, this circle can compensate for an occluded internal carotid artery. Yet it is essential to know that the circle of Willis is not complete in all patients. In these patients, even a short, temporary occlusion of the internal carotid artery can result in a disabling stroke.

Indications for carotid stenting

Currently, the indications for intervention with carotid stenting are considered to be similar to those for carotid surgery. Therefore, the guidelines for surgery are applied to carotid stenting as well. Carotid stenting is recommended for symptomatic lesions of ≥50% and asymptomatic lesions ≥70%. Additionally, patients may favor a percutaneous approach, since the intervention is performed with the patient fully alert, allowing close monitoring of possible neurologic complications. Furthermore, it is less traumatic than endarterectomy, thus avoiding local wound problems, cranial nerve palsy, and scars. Patients can expect to leave the hospital within 24h and return to work after 72h. Another crucial aspect is that the majority of patients suffering from carotid artery stenosis have coexisting coronary heart disease and other comorbidities. Avoiding general anesthesia is beneficial concerning the risk of periprocedural myocardial infarction in this patient population (between 4% and 18%) [18].

Patients at high risk of surgical endarterectomy seem to benefit the most from percutaneous carotid stenting. A number of patient subgroups are considered to have higher surgical risk: patients with significant comorbidities, carotid restenosis, high-grade carotid stenosis with contralateral occlusion, radiation-induced carotid stenosis, and high cervical or intracranial carotid stenosis.

Patients with significant comorbidities
As this subgroup of patients was excluded from most endarterectomy trials, the indications and results of surgery are not well established. Myocardial infarction was the leading long-term cause of death after endarterectomy in patients with concomitant clinically important coronary artery disease [19]. Patients with significant carotid disease undergoing coronary artery bypass grafting have a risk of stroke from hypotension

during general anesthesia [20]. Published reports on combined endarterectomy and coronary artery bypass grafting suggest that the risk of stroke or death ranges from 7.4% to 9.4%, 1.5–2.0 times the risk of each operation alone [21].

Carotid restenosis

This situation is technically challenging because of scar tissue surrounding the carotid bifurcation. The complication rate of redo-endarterectomy is approximately 10% [22–24]. Early results indicate that carotid angioplasty and stenting can safely be achieved and is a valid alternative to carotid re-endarterectomy in this high-risk group [25–27].

High-grade carotid stenosis with contralateral occlusion

The perioperative risk of stroke or death in the presence of contralateral carotid occlusion was 14.3% in the North American Symptomatic Carotid Endarterectomy Trial (NASCET) [28]. To date there is no evidence that carotid shunting reduces the perioperative risk of stroke.

Radiation-induced carotid stenosis

This situation is a surgical challenge because of involvement of the distal common carotid artery as well as extensive scarring and fibrosis. Increased rates of postoperative infections and wound complications are seen after previous radiation [29].

High cervical or intracranial carotid stenosis

Very distal cervical lesions in patients with short, corpulent necks or intracranial stenosis are difficult or impossible to treat surgically. However, contraindications of carotid stenting exist as well. Severely tortuous, calcified and atherosclerotic aortic arch, and distal vessels leading to access difficulties, fresh thrombus at the lesion site, severe renal insufficiency precluding safe application of contrast medium, and intolerance of antiplatelet agents are all considered to be contraindications of carotid stenting. Patients with advanced age, unstable neurologic symptoms, coexistent proximal common carotid lesions, or severe kinking directly distal to the bifurcation are also considered to be at high-risk for carotid stenting procedures. These contraindications, however, are relative and less important if the patient needs treatment and has high surgical risk.

In the Carotid and Vertebral Artery Transluminal Angioplasty Study (CAVATAS) [5], it was clearly shown that the results of stenting are strongly dependent on a steep learning curve. This can be reduced if physicians undergo a formal training program, as was shown in the Carotid Artery Stenting with Emboli Protection Surveillance-Post-Marketing Study (CASES-PMS) [30]. Precautions such as selection of patients with favorable anatomical and clinical factors will help inexperienced operators to gain high success and low complication rates during his or her learning curve.

Technical aspects

Patient preparation

Before the carotid artery stenting procedure, aspirin (100–325 mg) and clopidogrel are administered (75 mg once a day if application is started at least 5 days before the procedure or 300 mg if administered immediately before the procedure). During the procedure, heparin (70/100 IU/kg) is administered, maintaining activated clotting time (ACT) between 250 and 300 s. At the end of the procedure it is advisable to repeat an ACT evaluation, particularly in elderly patients, in patients with high blood pressure and in patients in whom flow in the internal carotid artery was impaired before the procedure. These patients have been identified to have an increased risk of hyperperfusion syndrome [31].

Continuous electrocardiogram (ECG) monitoring is mandatory to control potential bradycardia. Blood pressure monitoring through the guiding catheter or through the introducer sheath is recommended to observe the patient's hemodynamics. Intravenous administration of 1 mg atropine 2–3 min before stent implantation prevents or attenuates possible bradycardia or asystole. In case of prolonged hypotension, administration of fluids often helps. Occasionally, an infusion pump of dopamine may be needed.

After the procedure, lifelong aspirin therapy is continued. Adjunctive clopidogrel is continued for 1 month. The use of glycoprotein IIb/IIIa receptor blockers is not recommended during carotid artery stenting [32,33].

Vascular access

A secure carotid access is essential to keep the complication rate of carotid stenting as low as possible. Femoral arterial access is the preferred, recommended approach because the aortic arch is physiologic, symmetrically curved, and the origins of the brachiocephalic arteries are aligned in straight lines superiorly. In these cases the common femoral artery is punctured with a Seldinger needle, and a 5–6F, 12-cm-long arterial sheath is placed. The sheath will be exchanged for a long carotid sheath during the procedure. If a guiding catheter is planned to be used instead of a carotid sheath, an 8 or 9F, 12-cm-long sheath is needed. Only if the femoral arteries are occluded, if they are highly diseased, or if access to the common carotid artery from the femoral artery is unsuccessful a brachial or radial access is preferred. The right brachial artery is favorable for the treatment of both the right and the left carotid artery. If specific situations, such as very tortuous arteries or occluded iliac arteries, prevent both types of access, a direct cervical percutaneous access or short cut-down can be considered.

Cannulation of the common carotid artery

To cannulate the common carotid artery, a 5F diagnostic catheter (Berenstein, Boston Scientific, Natick, MA, USA; right Judkins, Cordis, Miami Lakes, FL, USA; Head Hunter,

Terumo, Tokyo, Japan) is advanced over a 0.035-inch guide-wire or a glide wire into the ascending aorta in an over-the-wire technique. Afterwards, an angiogram of the aortic arch should be performed to reveal difficult or anomalous anatomy as this would require an exchange of the catheter [e.g., for a Sidewinder (Cordis, Miami Lakes, FL, USA), or Vitek catheter, (Cook Inc., Bloomington, IN, USA)].

When placed in the lower aortic arch, the tip of one of the above mentioned diagnostic catheters should point inferiorly or be placed over a guidewire. This prevents traumatic injury of the intima of the aortic arch and prevents the catheter from being trapped in vessel ostia.

When reaching the ascending aorta, the catheter is turned around 180°, which places the tip in a vertical upright position. The catheter is gently pulled back until it slips into the brachiocephalic trunk. Thereafter, the hydrophilic wire is advanced into the right common carotid artery. Keeping the wire in position, the catheter is advanced into the common carotid artery over the wire.

To enter the left common carotid artery, the catheter is pulled back very slowly from the ostium of the brachio-cephalic trunk. It should be turned 20° counter clockwise to have the tip of the catheter pointing slightly anteriorly. In elongated aortic arches the origin of the left common carotid artery migrates posteriorly. In this case the catheter may have to be rotated posteriorly instead of anteriorly.

Immediately after engaging the left common carotid artery, the catheter should be turned 20° clockwise to point the tip vertically or slightly posteriorly again. The position of the catheter can be confirmed by a small injection of contrast agent. It should be excluded that there is a subintimal entry of contrast agent or reduced blood flow. Thereafter, the hydro-philic wire is advanced up to the distal common carotid artery, followed by the catheter.

Cannulation the common carotid artery in difficult anatomy

If cannulation of the common carotid artery is unsuccessful with one of these simple catheters, we usually switch to a Sidewinder catheter. Such catheters form a loop in the ascending aorta. By pulling the catheter slightly backward, the tip engages the brachiocephalic trunk, thereafter the left common carotid artery and finally the left subclavian artery. In contrast, with the Vitek or Mani catheter (Cook Inc., Bloomington, IN, USA), a loop is formed in the descending aorta. By pushing this type of catheter, again the tip engages the vessels of the aortic arch (left subclavian first).

The wire is manipulated to enter the artery, followed by the catheter. To change the direction of the guidewire, the catheter can be rotated, advanced further, or be retracted slightly. Advancement of the catheter is performed slowly, taking advantage of the pulsating blood flow. At the same time the wire is withdrawn, so it does not change the position. The advancement of the catheter and withdrawal of the wire is performed alternately several times until the catheter is placed securely in the artery (push and pull technique). During this maneuver the wire should be kept in a firm position deep inside the common carotid artery, if possible inside the external carotid artery.

Visualization of the vessels

Injections of contrast agents in all brachiocephalic arteries should be performed by hand or a low-volume low-flow injector and with only small amounts of contrast (no more than 6 cc per injection). Larger volumes create a mixture of arterial, intermediate, and venous phases, thus obscuring early filling veins and other pathologies.

After entering the ostium of the target vessel (primarily the external carotid artery), a guidewire with hydrophilic coating is advanced, followed by the catheter to exchange the diagnostic catheter for an introducer sheath.

Some operators perform a four-vessel angiogram to check collaterals for interventions and rescue when needed. As it adds an additional risk to the procedure, the necessity can be questioned at least if a magnetic resonance angiography was obtained before the procedure. The absence of collaterals may cause seizures during balloon dilation, with transient closure of the internal carotid artery. However, this reaction is reversible after balloon deflation and therefore does not influence the proceedings of the procedure. To display the origin of the external carotid artery, we use bony landmarks as orientation instead of road mapping illustration.

Tortuosity of the vessel

If there is tortuosity, the vessel can be straightened with the wire. Asking patients to take a deep breath and to hold their breath can also help to straighten the vessels. To reduce a curve in the arch and to prevent stiffer wires from prolapsing the catheter down into the ascending aorta, it should be gently "eased back" on the catheter curve in the arch during advancement of the wires.

A sharp angle at the distal end of the catheter owing to vessel kinking can be reduced by rotating the catheter gently while holding the wire fixed, until the catheter can be placed at the desired position. If the advancement is still unsuccessful, a Simmons III catheter (Cordis, Miami Lakes, FL, USA) should be chosen to advance the glide wire into the external carotid artery. A 0.035-inch wire might be preferable to a 0.038-inch wire. Eventually, rapid torque of the wire might help advancement. Afterwards, the Simmons III catheter can be exchanged with a 4F multipurpose catheter. Thereafter, the hydrophilic wire or a moveable core wire is exchanged for a 0.035-inch Amplatz wire or a softer wire. Finally, the 4F catheter can be replaced for a 5F catheter.

Guiding catheter placement

An 8F guide (usually a right coronary guide) is advanced into the ascending aorta over a hydrophilic 0.035-inch wire. For difficult or anomalous anatomy, an aortogram of the arch vessels can be done and used as an assistance for selective cannulation. After angiography of the aortic arch and assessment of the anatomy, the guide is advanced into the common carotid artery. Before cannulation of the common carotid, careful aspiration and flush of saline should be performed to clear any debris or thrombus.

Carotid sheath placement

Cannulation of the common carotid artery is performed with a 5F diagnostic catheter, usually with a right coronary or a Headhunter catheter. Access to the external carotid artery is achieved with an angled hydrophilic guidewire. The diagnostic catheter is then advanced into the external carotid artery. The current wire is replaced by an exchange length 0.035-inch wire. Usually, a stiff Amplatz-type wire is used. The diagnostic guide is exchanged over the wire for a 6F, 90-cm sheath that is then advanced into the common carotid artery below the bifurcation. The sheath should be manipulated very gently during engagement because it can cause a tear at the ostium of the common carotid artery or dislodge atherosclerotic debris. Aspiration and flushing must be done meticulously to eliminate possible air within.

Carotid access if the external carotid artery is occluded or the common carotid artery is stenosed

Placing the 6F, 90-cm access sheath into the common carotid artery can be quite challenging when the external carotid artery is occluded, a critical lesion is situated below the bifurcation, or in situations where there is a critical ostial common carotid lesion. If possible, crossing the lesion with a stiff 0.038-inch wire should be avoided, as this is more likely to disrupt necrotic plaque material and cause distal embolization. If necessary, the 5F diagnostic catheter should be advanced over a 0.035-inch or 0.038-inch glide wire to be placed more distally just proximal to the lesion. Thereafter it can be exchanged over a 0.035-inch Amplatz Extra Stiff guidewire.

In the presence of a common carotid ostial lesion, it may be necessary to stent this first to allow sheath access. However, if the ostial lesion is not too tight, the bifurcation lesion should be treated first, then the ostial lesion on the "way out."

Predilation

Some operators predilate the stenosis with a small angioplasty balloon with a short inflation time of 5–10s to allow a better stent passage and positioning. We predilate only if primary stenting failed, as we believe that primary stenting may prevent distal embolization by fixing debris to the vessel wall.

Embolic protection

A major limitation of carotid angioplasty is peri-interventional distal embolization. Balloon dilation, stenting, and manipulation of the vessels through catheters and wires are likely to release debris that can cause severe cerebral damage. Therefore, in most centers, embolic protection devices are used routinely. Currently, there are three different approaches to cerebral protection: filters, distal occlusion balloons, and proximal occlusion balloons, which occlude the common and external carotid artery.

Distal occlusion balloons

Distal occlusive balloons were the first system of protection commercially available and therefore used on a large scale. They consist of a 0.014-inch guide with a balloon mounted on the distal portion that is inflated and deflated through a very small channel contained in the guide itself (Guardwire®, Temporary Occlusion and Aspiration System, Medtronic, Minneapolis, MN, USA; Medtronic Vascular: TriActiv® ProGuard™ Embolic Protection System, Kensey Nash, Exton, PA, USA; Kensey Nash). The lesion is crossed with the guide thereby positioning the balloon distally to the stenosis where it is inflated until the blood flow in the internal carotid artery is blocked. Following this, the angioplasty and stenting procedure is carried out. On completion of the procedure, a catheter is advanced up to the distal balloon and the column of blood contained in the occluded internal carotid artery is aspirated. In this way debris dislodged during the stent procedure can be eliminated. Afterwards, the balloon is deflated and the guide is removed. The advantages of distal occlusion balloons are their small diameter (2.2F) and their good maneuverability and flexibility. Possible disadvantages are that internal carotid artery occlusion is not tolerated by 6–10% of patients [34,35] and that it is not possible to image the vessel distal to the occlusion balloon with contrast medium during inflation.

Filters

Most filters consist of a metallic structure coated by a membrane of polyethylene or a nitinol net containing holes of 80–200μm in diameter. The filters are usually positioned at the distal portion of a 0.014-inch guide. At the beginning of the procedure, the filters are enclosed in a delivery catheter with which they are advanced distal to the stenosis. After the lesion is crossed, the filter is opened by removing the delivery sheath. At the end of the stenting procedure, the filter is closed into the distal tip of a retrieval catheter and removed from the carotid artery.

A large number of second or third generation filters are currently available. The technical characteristics of a good filter consists of a low profile (<3F), an adequate torque ability to cross tortuous vessels, and, when opened, an adequate apposition to the wall to assure the best possible embolic protection.

The FiberNet® device (Lumen Biomedical, Plymouth, MN, USA) (Fig. 55.1) is the first embolic protection device which combines features of a filter and of a distal occlusion device in one system. It consists of a three-dimensional polyethylene terephthalate (PET) fiber-based filter which has the ability to capture particles as small as 40μm, mounted onto a

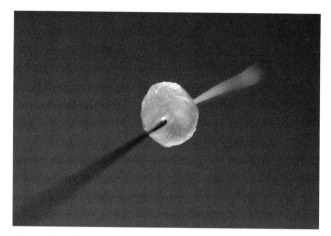

Figure 55.1 FiberNet distal embolic protection device (Lumen Biomedical).

0.014-inch, 190-cm wire and focal suction is provided through a retrieval catheter.

Proximal protection

Distal protection devices, both occlusive balloons and filters, have the disadvantage that it is mandatory to cross the lesion before they are inflated or opened. This unavoidable step carries the risk of embolization during this "unprotected" phase of the procedure. Proximal protection systems, such as the Gore Neuro Protection System (W.L. Gore & Associates, Inc., Newark, DE, USA) and MO.MA system (Invatec, Roncadelle, Italy) (Fig. 55.2), provide cerebral protection before passing any type of device through the stenosis. This is especially important in lesions which contain fresh thrombus. The operator can use the wire of his or her choice which helps to cross difficult lesions. These systems consist of a long introducer sheath with a balloon that is inflated in the common carotid artery. A second balloon, inflated in the external carotid artery, assures the total blockade of the antegrade blood flow in the internal carotid artery. The proximal protection systems facilitate the cerebral vascular connections of the circle of Willis. After the occlusion of the common and external carotid artery, the collateral flow through the circle of Willis creates so-called "backpressure" which prevents antegrade flow in the internal carotid artery. After stent positioning, and before deflation of the balloons in the common and external carotid artery, the blood in the internal carotid artery—possibly containing dislodged debris—is aspirated and removed. Intolerance of balloon occlusion seen in some patients is an ongoing disadvantage of proximal protection systems [36].

Stent implantation

Usually, a self-expandable stent is implanted. Balloon-expandable stents are recommended in ostial lesions of the common carotid artery, in extremely distal stenoses, and occasionally in very calcified, recoiling lesions. The disadvantage of the balloon-expandable stents is the difficulty to

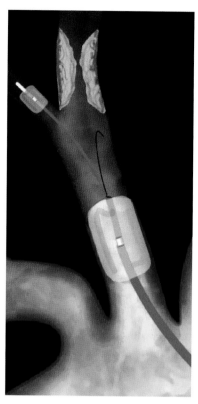

Figure 55.2 MO.MA proximal embolic protection device (Invatec).

adequately shape the stent to the vessel diameter as several balloon dilations may be needed in the internal and common carotid artery. Also stent compression has been described during follow-up.

In elongated arteries, self-expanding nitinol stents are the best choice. Their design allows them to adjust to the shape of the vessel, i.e., they do not tend to straighten the artery. Stents with low flexibility may cause severe kinking distal to the stent by straightening the vessel. This may produce a new stenosis distal to the stent. To treat severely calcified lesions, a stent with a high radial force is recommended. In general, closed-cell design stents have a higher radial force. Closed-cell stents provide better scaffolding to treat lesions with high emboligenic potential. However, the clinical impact of open cell design versus closed cell design, or probably more important of cell size and pore size, is still unclear.

The new hybrid design of the Cristallo Ideale Stent (Invatec) combines the advantages of both closed and open cell design (Fig. 55.3). It has open cell design in the proximal and distal sections to enhance conformability and to reduce radial force in healthy vessel segments, and closed cell design in the central part to secure appropriate scaffolding and to prevent plaque prolapse.

We recommend that the diameter of the stent should be 1–2 mm larger than the widest diameter to be covered. The most commonly used stents have a diameter of 6–8 mm if the stent is placed only in the internal carotid artery, or of

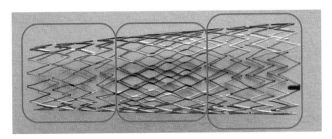

Figure 55.3 Cristallo Ideale stent (Invatec).

8–10 mm if it is deployed over the bifurcation. Overstenting the external carotid artery is safe and rarely causes an occlusion. The stent should cover the entire lesion. Most often 20- to 30-mm-long stents are used, in tandem stenoses, 40-mm-long stents are needed.

Postdilation

Postdilation is normally done with a 5- to 6-mm-diameter balloon to match the diameter of the internal carotid artery. Larger diameters might squeeze the debris through the stent mesh. To prevent dissections postdilation should be performed at nominal pressure. A residual stenosis of ≤30% is acceptable as this provides sufficient flow, and atherosclerotic debris is compressed enough to induce transformation into scar tissue. The stent will also extend further within the following hours. If there are segments of contrast-filled ulcerations outside of the stent struts, they do not have to be obliterated. Post dilation of the stent segment placed in the common carotid artery is not necessary and not recommended. If the external carotid artery becomes significantly stenosed or occluded after post dilation, there is no need to treat this.

After stent dilation, final angiograms of the carotid artery, including intracranial vessels, are performed. The cine run of the intracerebral arteries should always include the venous phase to objectively compare the preprocedure status with the final results after stenting. For these comparison purposes and to be prepared for further intracranial rescue procedures in case of stenting induced embolism, the angiography of the intracranial vessels should be performed in lateral and anteroposterior-30° cranial projection.

Results

Clinical series of carotid stenting

A summary of carotid stenting results, containing the data of 12 392 procedures involving 11 243 patients from 53 centers, was published in 2003 by Wholey *et al.* [37]. The incidence of complications occurring during the 30 days post implant was TIAs 3.1%, minor strokes 2.1%, major strokes 1.2%, and death 0.6%.

In 2001, Roubin *et al.* [38] reported a series of 528 consecutive patients undergoing carotid stenting. The major stroke rate was 1% (*n* = 6) and the minor stroke rate was 4.8% (*n* = 29). The overall stroke and death rate within 30 days was 7.4%.

In 2003 Cremonesi *et al.* [39] published a series of 442 consecutive patients treated with carotid stenting under embolic protection. Within 30 days, 1.1% of the patients experienced either a stroke or death.

Randomized trials

The CAVATAS was the first large study in which carotid angioplasty was compared with carotid endarterectomy [5]. The incidence of major adverse neurological events (MANEs) was 10% in both the carotid angioplasty and carotid endarterectomy groups.

The Protected Carotid Artery Stenting Versus Endarterectomy in High-risk Patients study compared carotid stenting with carotid endarterectomy using a randomized study design but also a registry study [6]. The incidence of MANEs was 4.5% for the stented patients and 6.6% for the carotid endarterectomy patients in the randomized study; this study enrolled high-risk patients for carotid endarterectomy. In the registry study, for which all patients could be entered, the incidence of MANEs was 6.9% in the stented patients.

The Endarterectomy Versus Angioplasty in Patients with Symptomatic Severe Carotid Stenosis (EVA-3S) compared carotid stenting to endarterectomy in patients with a symptomatic carotid stenosis of at least 60% [40]. The entrance criteria for participating interventionalists was set very low. A participating interventionalist was required to have performed only 12 previous carotid stenting procedures. The 30-day incidence of stroke or death was lower in the group of patients in whom the procedure was performed under embolic protection compared with those patients in whom carotid stenting was performed without embolic protection (18/227 [7.9%] versus 5/20 [25%], respectively, *P* = 0.03). For this reason the stenting arm of the trial without the use of an embolic protection device was stopped prematurely by the safety committee. The 30-day risk of any stroke or death was significantly higher after stenting (9.6%) than after endarterectomy (3.9%), which resulted in a relative risk of 2.5.

In the Stent-protected Percutaneous Angioplasty of the Carotid versus Endarterectomy trial (SPACE), patients with symptomatic carotid stenosis of >70% in duplex ultrasound or over 50% according to the NASCET measurement were included [41]. The use of embolic protection was optional. Many interventional centers had problems fulfilling the entrance criteria (>25 carotid stent procedures previously performed), which meant many centers had only very limited experience in this procedure. The rate of death or ipsilateral ischemic stroke was 6.84% in the group of patients treated with stent implantation compared with 6.34% in the group of patients treated with endarterectomy. Although embolic protection devices have become standard in most centers around the world, 73% of all interventions were performed without them. Complications such as myocardial infarction, contralateral stroke, or cranial nerve palsy—some of them more common to or only occurring during surgery—were not considered by the study. The trial was a noninferiority rather than a superiority trial, with a noninferiority margin defined as <2.5%, based on an event rate of 5%—the one-sided *P*-value for noninferiority was 0.09. The trial was halted prematurely owing to low recruitment and lack of further funding, after including only 1200 patients, while the analysis of >2500 patients would have been necessary to reach a statistical power of merely 80%. According to the investigators of the trial, the results failed to prove noninferiority of carotid stenting compared with endarterectomy.

Conclusion

In all major randomized trials so far, the differences between surgery and stenting have been very small. Future developments in the field of carotid intervention will include new stents with higher flexibility which can be introduced through smaller sheaths. We will have improved cerebral protection devices with better wall apposition and without need for a retrieval catheter. All these new developments will help carotid stenting to become the new gold standard for treatment of carotid atherosclerotic disease within the next few years.

References

1. American Heart Association. Heart Disease and Stroke Statistics–2004 Update. Available at: http://americanheart.org.
2. Wolf PA, Kannel WB, & McGee PC (1986) Epidemiology of strokes in North America. In: Barnet HJM, Stein BM, Mohr JP, Yatsu FM (eds). *Stroke: Pathophysiology, Diagnosis and Management*, Vol. 1, New York: Churchill Livingstone, p. 1929.
3. Mathias K (1981) Perkutane transluminale Katheterbehandlung supraaortaler Arterienobstruktionen. *Angio* **3**:47–50.
4. Roubin SG, New G, Iyer SS, *et al.* (2001) Immediate and late clinical outcomes of carotid artery stenting in patients with symptomatic and asymptomatic carotid artery stenosis. A 5-year prospective analysis. *Circulation* **103**:532–537.
5. (2001) Endovascular versus surgical treatment in patients with carotid stenosis in the carotid and vertebral artery transluminal angioplasty study (CAVATAS): a randomised trial. *Lancet* **357**: 1729–1737.
6. Yadav JS, Wholey MH, Kuntz RE, *et al.* (2004) Protected carotid-artery stenting versus endarterectomy in high-risk patients (the SAPPHIRE study). *N Engl J Med* **351**:1493–1501.
7. North American Symptomatic Carotid Endarterectomy Trial Collaborators (1991) Beneficial effect of carotid endarterectomy in symptomatic patients with high grade carotid stenosis. *N Engl J Med* **32**:445–453.
8. European Carotid Surgery Trialists' Collaborative Group (1998) Randomised trial of endarterectomy for recently symptomatic

carotid stenosis: final results of the MRC European Carotid Surgery Trial (ECST). *Lancet* **351**:1379–1387.
9. Mayberg MR, Wilson SE, Yatsu F, *et al.* (1991) Carotid endarterectomy and prevention of cerebral ischemia in symptomatic carotid stenosis. Veterans Affairs Cooperative Studies Program 309 Trialist Group. *JAMA* **266**:3289–3294.
10. Executive Committee for the asymptomatic carotid arteriosclerosis study (1995) Endarterectomy for the asymptomatic carotid artery stenosis. *JAMA* **273**:1421–1428.
11. Hobson RW, Weiss DG, Fields ES, *et al.* (1993) Efficacy of carotid endarterectomy for asymptomatic stenosis: the veterans affairs cooperative study group. *N Engl J Med* **328**:221–227.
12. MRC Asymptomatic Carotid Surgery Trial (ACST) Collaborative Group (2004) Prevention of disabling and fatal strokes by successful carotid endarterectomy in patients without recent neurological symptoms: randomised controlled trial. *Lancet* **363**:1491–1502.
13. Kannel WN (1994) Risk factors for atherosclerotic cardiovascular outcomes in different arterial territories. *Cardiovasc Risk* **1**:333–339.
14. Wilterdink JL & Easton JD (1992) Vascular event rates in patients with atherosclerotic cerebrovascular disease. *Arch Neurol* **49**:857–863.
15. Criqui MH, Langer RD, Fronek A, *et al.* (1992) Mortality over a period of 10 years in patients with peripheral arterial disease. *N Engl J Med* **326**:381–386.
16. Biasi G, Froio A, Diethrich E, *et al.* (2004) Carotid plaque echolucency increases the risk of stroke in carotid stenting: the Imaging in Carotid Angioplasty and Risk of Stroke (ICAROS) Study. *Circulation* **110**:756–762.
17. Heuser RR (ed.) (1999) Peripheral vascular stenting for cardiologists. London: Martin Dunitz, pp. 67–117.
18. Abrams J (1993) Preoperative cardiac risk assessment and management. *Curr Opin Gen Surg* **13**:8.
19. Yashon D, Jane JA, & Javid H (1966) Long-term results of carotid bifurcation endarterectomy. *Surg Gynecol Obstet* **122**:517–523.
20. Faggioli GL, Curl R, & Ricotta JJ (1990) The role of carotid screening before coronary artery bypass. *J Vasc Surg* **12**:724–731.
21. Loftus CM, Biller J, Hart MN, *et al.* (1987) Management of radiation-induced accelerated carotid atherosclerosis. *Arch Neurol* **44**:711–714.
22. Bergeron P, Chambran P, Benichou H, *et al.* (1996) Recurrent carotid artery disease: will stents be an alternative to surgery? *J Endovasc Surg* **3**:76–79.
23. Gray WA, DuBroff RJ, & White HJ (1997) A common clinical conundrum. *N Engl J Med* **336**:1008–1011.
24. Meyer FB, Piepgras DG, & Fode NC (1994) Surgical treatment of recurrent carotid artery stenosis. *J Neurosurg* **80**:781–787.
25. Theron J, Raymond J, Casasco A, *et al.* (1987) Percutaneous angioplasty of atherosclerotic and postsurgical stenosis of carotid arteries. *Am J Neuroradiol* **8**(Suppl. 3):495–500.
26. Yadav SS, Roubin GS, King P, *et al.* (1996) Angioplasty and stenting for restenosis after carotid endarterectomy: initial experience. *Stroke* **27**: 2075–2079.
27. Vitek JJ, Roubin GS, New G, *et al.* (2001) Carotid angioplasty with stenting in postcarotid endarterectomy restenosis. *J Invasive Cardiol* **13**:123–125.
28. Gasecki AP, Eliasziw M, Ferguson GG, *et al.* for the North American Symptomatic Carotid Endarterectomy Trial (NASCET) Group (1995) Long-term prognosis and effect of endarterectomy

in patients with symptomatic severe carotid stenosis and contralateral carotid stenosis or occlusion: Results from NASCET. *J Neurosurg* **83**:778–782.

29. Gerlock A & Mirfakhraee M (1985) Difficulty in catheterization of the left common carotid arteries. In: Gerlock A, Mirfakhraee M (eds). *Essentials of Diagnostic and Interventional Angiographic Techniques*. Philadelphia: WB Saunders, pp 106–119.

30. Katzen BT, Criado FJ, Ramee SR, *et al.* (2007) Carotid artery stenting with emboli protection surveillance study: thirty-day results of the CASES-PMS study. *Catheter Cardiovasc Interv* **70**:316–323.

31. Abou-Chebl A, Yadav JS, Reginelli JP, *et al.* (2004) Intracranial hemorrhage and hyperperfusion syndrome following carotid artery stenting: risk factors, prevention, and treatment. *J Am Coll Cardiol* **43**:1596–1601.

32. Hofmann R, Kerschner K, Steinwender C, *et al.* (2002) Abciximab bolus injection does not reduce cerebral ischemic complications of elective carotid artery stenting: a randomized study. *Stroke* **33**:725–7.

33. Qureshi AI, Saad M, Zaidat OO, *et al.* (2002) Intracerebral hemorrhages associated with neurointerventional procedures using a combination of antithrombotic agents including abciximab. *Stroke* **33**:1916–1919.

34. Al-Mubarak N, Roubin GS, Vitek JJ, *et al.* (2001) Effect of the distal-balloon protection system on microembolization during carotid stenting. *Circulation* **104**:1999–2002.

35. Tübler T, Schlüter M, Dirsch O, *et al.* (2001) Balloon-protected carotid artery stenting: relationship of periprocedural neurological complications with the size of particulate debris. *Circulation* **104**:2791–2796.

36. Rabe K, Sugita J, Sievert H, *et al.* (2006) Flow-reversal device for cerebral protection during carotid artery stenting—acute and long-term results. *J Interv Cardiol* **19**:55–62.

37. Wholey MH & Al-Mubarek N (2003) Updated Review of the Global Carotid Artery Stent Registry. *Catheter Cardiovasc Interv* **60**:259–266.

38. Roubin GS, New G, Iyer SS, *et al.* (2001) Immediate and late clinical outcomes of carotid artery stenting in patients with symptomatic and asymptomatic carotid artery stenosis: a 5 year prospective analysis. *Circulation* **103**:532–537.

39. Cremonesi A, Manetti R, Setacci F, *et al.* (2003) Protected carotid stenting: clinical advantages and complications of embolic protection devices in 442 consecutive patients. *Stroke* **34**:1936–1941.

40. Mas JL, Chatellier G, Beyssen B, *et al.* (2006) Endarterectomy versus stenting in patients with symptomatic severe carotid stenosis. *N Engl J Med* **355**:1660–1671.

41. SPACE Collaborative Group (2006) 30 day results from the SPACE trial of stent-protected angioplasty versus carotid endarterectomy in symptomatic patients: a randomised non-inferiority trial. *Lancet.* **368**:1239–1247.

56   Surgical Treatment of Carotid Artery Disease

Marc Bosiers[1], Christos Lioupis[1], Koen Deloose[1], Jurgen Verbist[2] & Patrick Peeters[2]

[1]Department of Vascular Surgery, AZ St-Blasius, Dendermonde, Belgium
[2]Imelda Hospital, Bonheiden, Belgium

Historical background

Eastcott *et al.* [1] in 1954 reported the first successful carotid operation for prevention of stroke. Many years later, DeBakey [2] claimed that he had performed a successful carotid endarterectomy (CEA) even earlier in 1953. An alternative technique, the so-called "eversion endarterectomy" was first described by DeBakey and colleagues [3] in 1959, while in 1985 Kieny [4] was the first to perform an eversion endarterectomy on the internal carotid artery (ICA). The technique of CEA has evolved over a period of 50 years and has been established as the time-honored, "gold standard" procedure for managing both symptomatic and asymptomatic carotid disease.

Morphology and pathophysiology

Atherosclerosis is the primary pathologic entity, accounting for 90% of lesions in the extracranial cerebrovascular system. The carotid bifurcation and especially the carotid bulb are particularly prone to atherosclerotic plaque formation. This predilection of the carotid bifurcation for atherosclerotic disease has been associated with arterial geometry, velocity characteristics, and wall shear stress [5]. There is a change in geometry, from a circular cross-section at the common carotid to an elliptical one at the level of the carotid sinus. This unique anatomy, found only in carotid bifurcation, disturbs the flow patterns. Along the outer wall of the internal carotid sinus, the velocity profile is flat and there is an area of flow separation with very low flow velocities and very low wall shear stress. Intimal thickening and atherosclerosis develop largely in such regions of relatively low and oscillating wall shear stress, flow separation and deviation from axially aligned, unidirectional flow [6]. As the atherosclerotic plaques enlarge, a parallel enlargement of the affected artery segment tends to limit the stenotic effect of the plaque [7,8]. However,

enlargement of the carotid sinus at the outer wall modifies the flow patterns, favoring plaque formation at the other sides of the arterial wall. Finally, atherosclerotic disease involves the entire circumference of the carotid, but even then plaques remain largest and most complicated at the outer wall of the carotid sinus.

Based on the adverse hemodynamic events in the normal carotid bifurcation, the optimal carotid reconstruction after a complete endarterectomy should eliminate the bulb and result in a smooth, gradually *tapered transition* from the larger diameter of the bifurcation to the smaller diameter internal carotid artery (ICA) [9]. Flow disturbances in general and wall shear stress gradients in particular are markedly reduced in carotid artery bifurcations that are smooth and gradually tapered and do not have a bulb, and they may minimize the hemodynamically induced component of early myointimal hyperplasia, thrombosis, and late atherosclerotic restenosis. Consequently patches, when used, should not simply widen the bulb and proximal ICA but rather should aid in the construction of a tapered transition (Fig. 56.1).

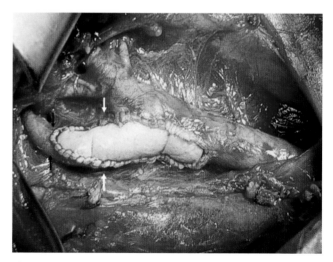

Figure 56.1 Completed endarterectomy with thin-walled polytetrafluoroethylene patch. Gradually *tapered transition* has been accomplished, from the larger diameter of the bifurcation (white arrows), to the smaller diameter of the internal carotid artery (black arrows).

Cardiovascular Interventions in Clinical Practice. Edited by Jürgen Haase, Hans-Joachim Schäfers, Horst Sievert and Ron Waksman. © 2010 Blackwell Publishing.

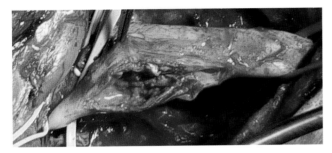

Figure 56.2 Arteriotomy from the common carotid artery to the internal carotid artery. *Soft vulnerable type* lesion in a symptomatic patient, with predominant lipid content and atheromatous grumous material.

In general, the clinical sequelae of atherosclerotic lesions are caused by their complications rather than the simple presence of hemodynamically significant stenosis. But the disruptive processes that underlie plaque instability appear to be closely associated with plaque size and stenosis [10]. Turbulence that develops in association with stenosis may compromise integrity of carotid plaques and contribute to erosion and ulceration [11]. Subsequent plaque disruption may result in embolization of plaque material. Secondary platelet or thrombus aggregations may also occur within the irregularities or ulcerations on the surface of the plaque that may be dislodged into the cerebral circulation.

Vulnerability of atherosclerotic plaques has been associated with their structure, composition, and consistency [12]. The various types of plaques have been classified according to their cell and lipid contents [13,14]. The *vulnerable type* lesion, with intermixed lipids and fibrous tissue, and the lesion with a large lipid core, intense inflammatory cell infiltration—covered by a thin or ruptured fibrous cap—are the most relevant to acute ischemic lesions [6]. Moreover, soft plaques with predominant atheromatous grumous material and hemorrhage are associated more often with symptoms [15]. Repeated intraplaque hemorrhages may result in gradual degeneration and formation of encysted atheromatous debris [16–18]. These plaques can be susceptible to mechanical stress and can ulcerate and discharge its contents as embolic material to the blood flow or enlarge and cause total occlusion of the vessel (Fig. 56.2) [19,20].

On the basis of these data, consistency of atherosclerotic carotid plaques should be assessed and considered as an important element in the therapeutic decision. Several invasive and noninvasive techniques have been used to identify *in vivo* high-risk plaques. Using the B-mode ultrasound, symptomatic plaques have been found to be more echolucent and less calcified than asymptomatic plaques. Ultrasound echolucency has been quantitated using computerized techniques for grayscale median (GSM) analysis, and it has been suggested that the GSM score should be considered in the decision-making algorithm when selecting patients with high-grade asymptomatic carotid stenosis for intervention [21]. In

the Asymptomatic Carotid Stenosis and Risk of Stroke (ACSRS) study, patients with a 70–99% stenosis and an echogenic plaque, had a 7-year cumulative risk of stroke of 1%, compared with a 14% risk of stroke at 7 years in patients with echolucent plaques [22]. However, corroborative data from similar studies are required before concluding that plaque echogenicity can be definitively used to select patients for carotid intervention. Another approach to identify plaque instability by means of duplex is the pixel distribution analysis (PDA) that can localize and quantify the amount of intraplaque hemorrhage, lipid, fibromuscular tissue, and calcium in the plaque. Using the PDA technique, significant differences were found between plaques in symptomatic and asymptomatic patients [23,24]. Recent data show that magnetic resonance imaging (MRI)-based computational analysis hold the best promise identification of vulnerable plaques *in vivo* [25]. MRI features of plaque instability, including a thin fibrous cap, a large necrotic core, and marked intraplaque hemorrhage, have been associated with an increased risk of ischemic events [26,27]. Finally, a number of studies have correlated elevated circulating concentrations of a range of proteins, *biomarkers,* to high-risk atherosclerotic plaque. Currently, none of these markers is highly specific and sensitive for predicting stroke, and findings have not been tested prospectively in carefully defined patient subgroups, e.g., asymptomatic patients.

Indications

The indications for carotid endarterectomy in symptomatic patients have been accrued from the two most influential randomized trials, the European Carotid Surgery Trial (ECST) and the North American Symptomatic Carotid Endarterectomy Trial (NASCET) [28,29]. Studies included patients who suffered a carotid territory hemispheric transient ischemic attack (TIA), a transient episode of monocular blindness (amaurosis fugax), or a nondisabling stroke. Different methods to measure the degree of stenosis were used; the NASCET measured the smallest lumen at the level of the stenosis and compared it with the lumen of the carotid artery distally to the carotid bulb, while ECST measured the residual ICA lumen compared with the local estimated diameter of the carotid bulb. Analysis of the pooled data from the two trials, after remeasuring ECST angiograms using the NASCET criteria, showed that patients with hemispheric or monocular TIAs or prior mild stroke, with a 70% or greater stenosis, have clear benefit after following CEA in avoiding any ipsilateral stroke or ipsilateral disabling stroke (five operations needed to prevent one stroke in 5 years) [30]. Surgery was of no benefit in patients with near occlusion. Another analysis of the pooled data from ECST and NASCET showed that benefit from surgery was greater in men than women and in those >75 years old [31]. Importantly, the subgroup analysis showed that patients operated on within 2 weeks had the maximal benefit, with benefit reduction 12 weeks after the presenting event. Especially for symptomatic females, the current evidence does not support that CEA provides any significant benefit, unless patients are treated within 2–4 weeks of their symptoms. A marginal benefit from CEA was reported in patients with a moderate stenosis 50–69% (15 operations needed to prevent one stroke in 5 years). On the basis of these data, surgery cannot be justified in this category of patients. Several morphologic factors have also been associated with increased benefit from CEA, including ulcerated plaques [32], contralateral occlusion [33], and tandem intracranial disease [34].

Patients considered for CEA may present with a variety of different symptoms from those included in the ECST and the NASCET, such as crescendo TIAs (TIAs with increase in frequency, duration, or severity), stroke in evolution (stroke with neurologic worsening during the ensuing hours or days after onset), global ischemia or progressive intellectual dysfunction. There are no data coming from randomized trials for managing these categories of neurologically impaired patients. For crescendo TIAs, early surgical intervention has been characterized as a "surgical imperative"—with no neurologic deficits in a subgroup analysis of the Veterans Administration Symptomatic Carotid Endarterectomy trial [35]; though, in a more recent retrospective study, a high risk of combined neurologic and cardiac complications after urgent carotid surgery for crescendo TIAs was reported [36]. Stroke in evolution presents high mortality and poor neurologic recovery with medical management, and it has been suggested that, compared with the natural history of this entity, immediate operative intervention by surgeons with considerable experience results in better salvage [37,38]. In patients with a minor stroke, CEA must be performed as rapidly as possible following the presenting event, since the benefit is significantly reduced if it takes place more than 12 weeks after the event. In contrast, for patients who present acutely with a major stroke or with radiologic evidence of hemorrhage or massive infarcts, operation during the acute phase should be avoided. In these cases, endarterectomy before neurologic recovery may result in neurologic deterioration owing to cerebral edema or hemorrhagic conversion of an initially ischemic infarction [39,40]. Moreover, CEA is not advisable in patients with devastating strokes and little neurologic function to loose, multiple comorbidities, and a short expectancy of life. In general, results from randomized trials should not be extrapolated to nonhemispheric symptoms or vertebrobasilar ischemia, which should not be considered an indication for endarterectomy. Similarly, impairment of cognitive functions as a result of carotid disease, although it is a new area of research, should not be included with CEA indications presently.

Patients with severe coronary artery disease and symptomatic or severely stenotic carotid disease require particular consideration. Two approaches are available: a *synchronous* procedure combining coronary artery bypass graft (CABG) and CEA and a *staged* approach intending to operate on the more threatening procedure first. A recent review of 97 published studies showed that mortality and combined death and stroke rates were highest in patients undergoing synchronous procedures. Reverse staged procedures (CABG-CEA) were associated with the highest risk of ipsilateral stroke, while staged procedures (CEA-CABG) were associated with the highest risk of perioperative myocardial infarction [41]. To further clarify the proper management of these patients, a need for randomized clinical trials of synchronous versus staged procedures has already been emphasized [42].

The two most important studies in asymptomatic patients are the Asymptomatic Carotid Atherosclerosis Study (ACAS) and the Asymptomatic Carotid Surgery Trial (ACST) [43,44]. ACAS showed that immediate CEA in asymptomatic patients with a 60–99% stenosis confers significant reduction in ipsilateral stroke at 5 years compared with best medical treatment (54% relative risk reduction—1% absolute risk reduction per annum). However, the data of ACAS have been challenged in terms of high surgeon selection and data projection from 2.7 years of follow-up to 5 years by actuarial analysis [34,45]. Moreover, ACAS demonstrated that immediate CEA do not prevent disabling or fatal stroke, do not confer benefit to women, and patients have to live at least 5 years to have any benefit [32]. The second study, the ACST, demonstrated that immediate CEA can confer a 50% reduction in disabling or fatal stroke, this benefit was recorded in patients up to 75 years of age. On the basis of these data, only younger asymptomatic patients with high-grade stenosis may gain a benefit from CEA, providing that the operative stroke and death rate remains <3%. Neither ACAS nor ACST showed significant benefit in asymptomatic females [31,46,47].

The role of best medical treatment, including statins, beta-blockers, angiotensin-converting enzyme inhibitor therapy, and dual antiplatelet therapy, has not been evaluated adequately. Taking into consideration the new advances in best medical treatment, it is evident that there is a need for more randomized studies to define asymptomatic patient subgroups that can benefit from CEA.

Technical aspects

Anesthetic management

Either general anesthesia or local anesthesia can be used for CEA. With general anesthesia the patient is quiet and stable, there is no difficulty in prolonging the procedure or extending the operation proximally or distally, and there is a satisfactory environment for training junior surgeons. It has also been suggested that some general anesthesia agents may reduce cerebral metabolic oxygen requirements and increase cerebral blood flow, while conferring a degree of neuroprotection [48]. Advocates of general anesthesia have reasoned that, local anesthesia may cause stress to both patient and surgeon and result in hurried and technically imperfect surgery, while factors that make cooperation and communication difficult (neurologic disorders, language barriers) add more difficulties. However, there is increasing evidence that CEA under local anesthesia does not increase anxiety, is tolerated by the majority of patients and is associated with a better perception of recovery [49]. Preservation of cerebral autoregulation, reduced need for shunting, and a probable reduction in cardiac morbidity and mortality have posed the hypothesis that CEA under local anesthesia may be associated with lower stroke and death rates. Local anesthesia preserves autoregulation and improves cerebral oxygenation during carotid clamping, which induces a reflex rise in systemic blood pressure [50]. However, to date the evidence related to changes in blood pressure and cardiac rhythm that may precipitate myocardial ischemia appear contradictory and no firm conclusions can be drawn [51,52]. With regional anesthesia, the need for shunting can be most accurately assessed (*awake testing*). Manifestations of intraoperative cerebral ischemia can be treated immediately, and use of a prophylactic shunt can be avoided in some anatomically difficult cases when not absolutely necessary. The assessment of the neurologic status of the patient after surgery and in the recovery room is also simplified without the after-effects of general anesthesia.

Overall, there is no convincing evidence at this time to enable the choice of an optimal anesthetic method. The only evidence to guide the choice of anesthesia comes from a systematic review [53], in which the metaanalysis of the data of the randomized studies showed that carotid endarterectomy under local anesthesia might be associated with lower risks of postoperative local hemorrhage than surgery under general anesthesia, but no evidence of a reduction in the odds of perioperative stroke or reductions in myocardial infarction, stroke, or death rates was found. The results of the General Anaesthesia Versus Local Anaesthesia for Carotid Surgery (GALA) trial (the randomization of which has now been completed) may provide many answers to the above questions.

Surgical technique

Conventional endarterectomy through a longitudinal arteriotomy is the most widely used technique of CEA. Eversion endarterectomy, which obviates the need of a longitudinal incision, and patching has been supported by a minority of surgeons. Interposition grafting is reserved for revisional operations or in cases of inadequate eversion endarterectomy, perhaps with a distal intimal flap. For the latter, although it gives an appropriate hemodynamic result, there are no large series documenting its long-term outcome for primary CEA.

Two incisions can be used for exposure of the carotid bifurcation: the vertical and the oblique incision. The majority of surgeons prefer the vertical incision because it can be extended easily. The incision is deepened through the platysma to gain access to the investing fascia. After incising the fascia the underlying carotid sheath is exposed. The carotid sheath is incised and the jugular vein is retracted laterally to expose the carotid artery. The facial vein is a constant landmark for the carotid bifurcation, and after its ligation and division the carotid artery can be visualized. Undue manipulation and palpation of the carotid bifurcation and the bulb of the internal carotid artery should be avoided (*no touch technique*), to reduce the risk of embolism. If a sinus bradycardia occurs, 1–2 mL of 1% lidocaine may be injected into the tissues between the external and internal carotid arteries to block the nerves and the carotid sinus. Mobilization of internal carotid artery continues to a point well above the atheromatous lesion. A usual approach is to expose the ICA approximately 1 cm distal to the highest identifiable disease. Early clamping of the ICA in patients likely to have unstable plaques should be pursued. Heparin (5000 IU) is administered intravenously before clamping of the carotid. An arteriotomy is performed from the common carotid artery to the internal carotid, beyond the end of the lesion. The appropriate plane of endarterectomy lies between the intima and the media layers at the level of the internal elastic lamina. Circumferential dissection using the Watson–Cheyne dissector is completed with a right-angle clamp, and the atheromatous plaque is sharply divided at the proximal limit in the common carotid artery. The atheromatous lesion is gently removed from the external carotid artery after dissection by eversion. Finally, the dissection proceeds up the internal carotid artery.

Achieving an optimal flow surface and distal end-point following carotid endarterectomy is of paramount importance. Residual disease and technical defects after completion of CEA have been associated with increased rates of perioperative stroke, restenosis, and late stroke [54,55]. Residual defects may include, intimal dissection and/or flaps at the internal carotid end point, a proximal end-point common carotid step, kinking of the carotid artery at the distal end of the arteriotomy, or a clamp injury to the CCA and ICA. Defects at the ICA end point—either intimal dissection, flaps or residual atheroma—can be secured with end point *tack sutures*. It has been suggested that when an adequate feathered endarterectomy is conducted, through an arteriotomy extending well beyond all macroscopic disease, tacking should be required only occasionally (approximately 2%) [56]. In case in which a tongue of plaque extends up the posterior inferior wall (sometimes spiral), the endarterectomy can be carefully carried into the internal carotid until the plaque thins. But if the tongue extends to the highest point of the obtainable arteriotomy, it is better to sharply transect it and secure it using tack sutures. Common carotid steps at the proximal end of endarterectomy >2 mm in depth have also been associated with postoperative emboli production and late restenosis [57]. Smoothing out of this residual step can

Table 56.1 Eversion endarterectomy: pro and contra.

Benefits of eversion endarterectomy	Drawbacks of eversion endarterectomy
Correction of elongated (tortuous or kinked) ICA, without using synthetic or venous patch material	More technically demanding procedure
	Suitable for plaques extending <2 cm in the ICA
	Not indicated in small caliber ICA
Shortened carotid clamp time	Potential difficulty of visualizing the distal limit of the endarterectomy and placing tacking sutures if required
Lower restenosis and late occlusion rate	
Lower risk of late stroke	Difficult shunt insertion/retention when required
No risk of patch infection	Requires completion imaging

ICA, internal carotid artery.

be accomplished with sharp beveling of the step or *eversion plication*, which also serves to cover the thrombogenic media and intima [58]. Redundancy of the carotid bifurcation after removal of the atheromatic plaque or natural kinking of the ICA are among the problems that can arise in a number of cases. The endarterectomized carotid artery can be shortened, either by resecting a part of the ICA and then re-anastomosing it or by performing an eversion plication. In cases in which there is marked coiling of the ICA, this can be managed by resecting the looped segment and re-anastomosing the two ends or, when this is not possible, to shorten the ICA by using a formal vein bypass. In general, a carotid bypass, preferably using a reversed long saphenous vein obtained from the upper thigh, should be performed only when there is inappropriate tension following plication or the endarterectomized surface is in a poor condition. Interposition grafting is also another way to manage a retained tongue of plaque in the ICA [56].

During eversion endarterectomy an incision is made parallel to the axis of the external carotid artery (ECA), and the ICA is completely transected. Downward traction of ICA permits straightening of ICA and better exposure. Endarterectomy is started at the proximal end of ICA stump and progresses circumferentially using fine atraumatic forceps. The atheromatous lesion is removed with gentle traction, trying to achieve a clean, smooth distal intimal step. Residual fragments can be removed by circumferential stripping using fine Adson forceps (Aesculap AG & Co KG, Tuttlingen, Germany) and copious heparin saline irrigation. Endarterectomy of the common carotid artery (CCA) and ECA follows through the initial incision. Reimplantation of the endarterectomized ICA to its normal anatomic position is performed. The operation should be carried out applying final control, either by intraoperative angiography or angioscopy. Routine use of eversion carotid endarterectomy has been considered by some surgeons. Potential benefits and drawbacks of eversion carotid endarterectomy, according to proponents and critics of the method are shown in Table 56.1.

A systematic review of randomized trials of eversion endarterectomy versus standard endarterectomy found five randomized trials [59]; the largest of which was the Eversion Carotid Endarterectomy Versus Standard Trial (EVEREST) [60]. The main findings of this review were that there were no significant differences between the two techniques in terms of the major clinical outcome events (perioperative or late stroke). A significant decrease in the risk of late carotid restenosis and occlusion during follow-up in patients undergoing eversion CEA when compared with conventional CEA was observed. However, upon critical appraisal of the summarized literature, there appear to be methodologic flaws, conceptual contradictions, and an increased potential of bias, and in view of this the generalizability of the conclusions is open to question. It remains also unclear whether carotid restenosis or occlusion increase the risk of clinical neurologic events, and no definite conclusions can be drawn on the impact of the eversion technique on the risk of restenosis-related stroke. Until better evidence is available, the choice of the surgical technique for CEA in patients who are suitable for both techniques should depend on the experience and preference of the operating surgeon.

Use of patch

Primary closure of carotid arteriotomy or patch angioplasty may be employed following completion of CEA. During primary closure a suture is used to approximate the adjacent arterial walls, while with patch angioplasty, closure of the arterial defect may be accomplished by the use of a patch (either autogenous vein or synthetic material). The principal advantages of primary arterial closure are a shortened closure time, simplicity, and lower potential for infectious and aneurysmal complications. However, it has been postulated that patch angioplasty may reduce both the risks of early thrombosis and late restenosis, reducing the rates of early and long-term strokes. The main concerns regarding patch closure include prolonged carotid occlusion time and some complications directly related to patch material itself, including prosthetic graft infection, pseudoaneurysm formation and rupture.

A recent metaanalysis of the available randomized trials showed that patch closure of the carotid artery is superior to primary closure in terms of perioperative and long-term risk of stroke and death, occlusion, or restenosis [61]. Data analysis from seven randomized trials showed that carotid patching can prevent 30 ipsilateral perioperative strokes and 75 strokes and deaths per 1000 patients treated. Nevertheless, the results of this metaanalysis must be interpreted with caution owing to the varying methodology of the randomized trials, the small number of important outcome events, and the incomplete follow-up of patients. The hypothesis that the potential benefit of patching may be restricted to small arteries cannot be tested because the results of the trials were not reported according to the degree of the narrowing. It is also unclear how narrow an artery should be before it can be decided that it should be patched. Two studies excluded arteries of 5 mm and 3.5 mm on the grounds that they were too narrow and they should be patched [62,63]. At this time no clear indications for selective patching can be given and, until more conclusive evidence is available, routine patching seems to offer the best outcomes.

The choice of patch material is a controversial issue. Use of autologous vein is associated with several advantages, including a less thrombogenic endothelialized surface, greater resistance against infections and better hemostasis. Central vein patch rupture occurring in the first postoperative week is the main drawback of vein patches. Saphenous vein harvested from the ankle carries a higher risk of rupture compared with vein harvested from the groin. Wound healing problems at the harvesting site is another concern. An updated metaanalysis shows that there are no obvious differences in the risks of stroke or death suffered by patients receiving venous or synthetic patches and no evidence supports the belief that synthetic patching is associated with a lower risk of patch rupture [61]. However, the incidence of major arterial complications such as rupture or infection after carotid patching is very low and any trials designed to reliably detect such differences should be of enormous size. It has been claimed that the use of polytetrafluoroethylene (PTFE) may increase the operation time, mainly because of increased bleeding through the suture holes; but, a well designed recent randomized trial that compared the use of PTFE and Dacron® (Unifi, Inc., Greensboro, NC, USA), found no significant benefit of PTFE over Hemoshield Dacron in terms of 30-day stroke rate and postoperative restenosis and similar mean hemostasis time [64]. On the basis of the available evidence, it seems reasonable that the choice of patch material be left to the surgeon's preference.

High carotid lesions

High disease can be encountered during the CEA, classically described as lesions cephalad to a line drawn between the tip of the mastoid process and the angle of the mandible. Preoperative identification of these patients allow for adjustments to operative and anesthetic technique. When duplex ultrasound suggests a high extending carotid lesion and cerebral angiography confirms this location, certain adjunctive measures may be planned, including nasotracheal intubation and temporary ipsilateral mandibular condyle subluxation (in conjunction with a maxillofacial specialist) [65,66]. In the case of an unexpected high lesion is encountered, a course of maneuvers may enable the procedure to be completed. Gently pulling the bifurcation downward, using an elastic loop placed around the ECA, may improve mobilization. Mobilization of the hypoglossal nerve by dividing the descending branch and the sternomastoid artery and careful elevation using a rubber sling placed around the nerve enhances distal access. The digastric muscle can be divided when necessary, the styloid process can be fractured using surgeon's finger and moved aside, and the styloid musculature and ligament can be divided as well. Use of a Pruitt–Inahara shunt facilitates distal dissection of ICA and, by avoiding application of a clamp, the length of the vessel available for suturing can be increased altogether. The sequence of mandibular condyle subluxation, digastric division and styloid fracture provides exposure to the distal-most 1 cm of extracranial ICA.

Avoiding cranial nerve injuries

Cranial nerve injuries following CEA result in substantial morbidity. Meticulous surgical technique can avoid many of them. The vagus nerve sometimes takes a more lateral or even anterior course along the common carotid artery, where it can be injured during cutting of the carotid sheath. Careful circumferential dissection of the CCA at the site of intended proximal clamping may avoid entrapment of the nerve by the tips of the clamp. Avoiding injudicious use of monopolar electrocautery close to the vagal trunk and paying attention not to place self-retaining retractors in the tracheoesophageal groove can avoid injury of recurrent laryngeal nerve. Careful isolation of the superior thyroid artery is needed to avoid incorporation or damage of the superior laryngeal nerve that passes directly posteriorly.

Dissection confined only to the plane adjacent to the ICA, and ECA if distal exposure is required, may avoid nerve injuries. Careful circumferential dissection of the facial vein and posterior inspection before ligation and division may avoid a hypoglossal nerve injury. The latter is also at risk during distal dissection of the ICA, which has always to take place under direct vision in a bloodless field without applying traction on it and avoiding using monopolar diathermy in close proximity to it. To avoid an injury of the glossopharyngeal nerve one should be very careful when mobilizing distally the ICA. When division of the stylohyoid muscle or resection of the styloid process has been decided upon, it should be performed after a mandibular subluxation. Finally, injudicious retraction of the upper edge of the incision should be avoided to minimize a marginal mandibular nerve injury.

Use of shunt intraoperative monitoring

Most patients have sufficient cerebral collateral flow from the other extracranial vessels via the circle of Willis to permit clamping of the carotid artery during CEA. However, in some patients the circle of Willis may be congenitally incomplete or atherosclerotic disease may affect contralateral, collateral, and intracerebral vessels, and cross-clamping the carotid artery during CEA may cause cerebral ischemia. Areas of recent or previous cerebral infarction have an increased risk of ischemia [67]. Advocates of *routine shunting* argue that use of an intraluminal shunt can retain adequate ipsilateral cerebral blood flow, reducing thereby the risk of ischemic stroke. Numerous shunt designs have been used, including simple tubes, tapered shunts held in position with special clamps [e.g., the Javid shunt (C.R. Bard, Inc., Karlsruhe, Germany)], and shunts with inflatable balloons at each end to hold it in position [e.g., the Pruitt-Inahara shunt (Le Maitre Vascular, Sulzbach/Ts. Germany)]. Routine use of a shunt can ensure adequate time for thorough endarterectomy, patching, or training a doctor. However, shunting may be associated with scuffing of the distal arterial intima, embolization of atheromatous debris or air, arterial dissection, and late restenosis. To avoid these risks, many surgeons have adopted a *selective shunting* policy of only those patients who are at most risk of developing cerebral ischemia during carotid cross-clamping. Overall, the evidence on the use of routine shunting from randomized controlled trials is limited [68]. A clinically important benefit from routine shunting, in both deaths and strokes, cannot be excluded. The potential of restenosis or late recurrent stroke also has not been substantiated. In the case of selective shunting in patients under general anesthesia, there is again little evidence to support the use of one form of monitoring over another [68].

Several methods for detecting preoperative cerebral ischemia have been employed, including stump pressure measurements, transcranial Doppler (TCD) monitoring of middle cerebral artery velocity, awake testing (during local anesthesia), electroencephalography (EEG), somatosensory evoked potentials (SSEP), and measurement of cerebral perfusion by intraarterial xenon or near-infrared spectroscopy. Choice of the best monitoring technique based on available evidence is not possible. All have their strengths and weaknesses. EEG is a well standardized method and seems also reliable in identifying a malpositioned or kinked shunt [69]; however, it is poor in the detection of subcortical or brainstem ischemia and requires significant expertise [70]. Testing of carotid artery stump pressure is not highly sensitive or specific; patients may be ischemic with pressures well above the accepted threshold of 25 mmHg and not be ischemic with pressures below the this level [71]. TCD is a reliable method overall; it can also detect

emboli, and is useful for both intraoperative and postoperative monitoring. But the indications for shunt placement have been variously stated; the method needs expensive equipment and expertise for signal interpretation, and it is not applicable in 10% of patients who do not have an acoustic window [72]. The awake testing appears to be accurate in identifying patients who need a shunt, it is inexpensive and does not require a special technician or expertise; however, it is not uniformly applicable because some patients cannot tolerate CEA under local anesthesia. Finally, measurement of SSEP is a comparatively easy technique of continuous monitoring of cerebral function, but a better study of the factors that affect responses is needed before this can be applied broadly.

Perioperative antithrombotic therapy

In general, all patients are prescribed antiplatelet therapy preoperatively, and this should not be discontinued before surgery. The benefit of reducing the risk of perioperative thromboembolic events outweighs any potential risk of increased bleeding complications [73]. Maintenance of heparin anticoagulation during the time of carotid clamping is universally used. A dose of 70 IU/kg is usually administered as a bolus dose 2 min before carotid clamping, although the administered dose varies considerably. A controversy still exists regarding heparin reversal with heparin at the end of operation. Two retrospective studies suggested that carotid endarterectomy without reversal of heparin anticoagulation is associated with a reduced postoperative stroke rate without a significant increase in morbidity rates [74,75], but in one of them the administration of protamine significantly reduced the incidence of postoperative hematoma [75]. The value of these data is limited and it seems that protamine administration can be applied, especially in the presence of excessive coagulopathic intraoperative bleeding.

Antiplatelet therapy (aspirin 80–325 mg/day) should be continued after the operation to prevent new neurologic events and reduce cardiovascular morbidity.

Results

Strong evidence has been accrued from randomized trials for patients with symptomatic disease. The NASCET study provided considerable support in favor of treating symptomatic patients with important stenosis (70–99%) with CEA [29]. The 30-day major stroke and death rates were 2.1% in the surgical group and 0.9% in the medical group. The cumulative risk of an ipsilateral stroke at 2 years was 9% for surgically treated patients and 26% in the medical treatment group (relative risk reduction of 65%, $P < 0.001$); however, the corresponding risk of major or fatal ipsilateral stroke was 2.5% (surgical group) and 13.1% (medical group) ($P < 0.001$). It was also demonstrated that there is a correlation between absolute risk reduction and severity of stenosis, with maximum benefit in patients with 90–99% ICA stenosis [76]. In patients with moderate ICA stenosis, there was a significant 39% relative-risk reduction for any stroke, but no reduction in major or fatal stroke. In the ECST trial, there was a much higher 30-day major stroke and death rate of 7.5%, but, despite this, the results favored surgical treatment in patients with high-grade stenosis (70–99%) [28]. The cumulative risk of an ipsilateral stroke at 3 years was 12.3% in surgical patients compared with 21.9% in the medical treatment group (*P* < 0.01); although the risk of major or fatal ipsilateral stroke at 3 years was 6% (surgical group) and 11% (medical group). In agreement with the NASCET, the same trend of increasing benefit with increasing grade of stenosis was noticed. All in all, it seems that CEA can reduce significantly the risk of stroke in symptomatic patients with a high grade of stenosis (70–99%) when conducted by experienced surgeons, with a rate of complications below the maximum acceptable 30-day combined mortality and neurologic deficit rates of <5% for TIAs and <7% for ischemic strokes [77]. The higher risk for stroke and death is overcome at 3 months and persists thereafter.

In asymptomatic patients, the ACAS trial showed a 30-day death and stroke rate of 2.3% [43]. Using Kaplan–Meier projections, the primary outcome of ipsilateral stroke was 5.1 for the surgical group and 11% for the medical group (5.9% absolute risk reduction in patients with 60–99% stenosis, *P* = 0.006). In accordance to these data, ACST demonstrated a 30-day death and stroke rate of 2.8% in patients with an asymptomatic 60–99% stenosis, and conferred a 5.4% absolute reduction in the risk of any stroke at 5 years [44]. These are probably the most convincing up-to-date data and provide evidence that surgical intervention in addition to medical therapy and risk factor modification offer benefit in at least some groups of patients with ICA asymptomatic stenosis >60%, providing that the operation is performed by experienced surgeons with a 30-day combined mortality and neurologic deficit rate <3%.

Mortality and stroke rates were the two end points in the randomized trials. Death as a result of CEA is fortunately rare, with the overall death rate approaching 1.3% in asymptomatic patients and 1.8% in symptomatic patients [78]. Myocardial infarction is the most common cause of non-stroke deaths, while death secondary to a stroke is much more usual in symptomatic patients compared with the asymptomatic patients. In the NASCET trial the rate or perioperative cardiac deaths was 0.4% and the rate of nonfatal myocardial infarctions was 0.8% [79]. In the ACAS trial the rates reported were 0.1% (cardiac death) and 0.4% (myocardial infarction) [80]. This demonstrated that symptomatic patients are at higher risk of perioperative cardiac events than asymptomatic patients.

Several different mechanisms of perioperative stroke have been reported, including ischemia during carotid artery clamping, postoperative thrombosis, and embolism, intracerebral hemorrhage, strokes from other mechanisms associated with the surgery, and stroke unrelated to the reconstructed artery [81]. Thrombosis and embolism is the most common cause of postoperative stroke. Postoperative thrombosis and embolization occur usually during the first 12 h after the procedure and are the result of technical imperfection. Problems identified commonly on re-exploration in these patients are intimal flap elevation, vessel stricture or fibrin-platelet aggregates [82]. The second most usual cause of postoperative stroke is that of intracerebral hemorrhage. CEA on patients with severely stenotic or pre-occlusive lesions, especially if combined with intraoperative or postoperative hypertension, increases the risk of intracranial hemorrhage [83]. Loss of intracranial vessel autoregulation in these patients may result in increased intracapillary pressure, cerebral edema, and hemorrhage (*hyperperfusion syndrome*), following correction of carotid artery stenosis [84]. Contrary to this, hypoperfusion may be a cause of perioperative stroke during carotid artery clamping. This is more common in patients with contralateral occlusion or hypotension and bradycardia and prompt shunt placement. Finally, a small number of strokes may be simply due to mechanisms related to surgery.

Alterations of blood pressure, in the form of hypertension or hypotension are common after CEA. Bradycardic hypotension is associated with overreactive response of carotid sinus baroreceptors due to changes in the compliance of the endarterectomized wall, and rarely persists over 24 h. Postoperative hypertension is more worrisome because it predisposes the patients to hyperperfusion syndrome and intracerebral hemorrhage. Therefore, prompt treatment of blood pressure alterations is mandatory.

The reported incidences of cranial nerve injuries associated with CEA show great discrepancies in different series. Higher incidences have been reported when routine pharyngeal function studies and laryngoscopy are performed. In the NASCET trial the incidence of cranial nerve injury was 8.6% (hypoglossal 3.7%, vagus 2.5%, marginal mandibular 2.2%), whereas the cranial nerve injury rate in ACAS was 4.9% [80,85]. Most of these injuries are transient, related to blunt injury rather than to division of the nerves, and in over 90% patients recover completely. Nerves at risk during CEA and clinical consequences are shown in Table 56.2.

Restenosis following CEA occurs with an incidence that varies from 3% to 25%, and is divided somewhat artificially into myointimal hyperplasia, usually discovered 6 months to 2 years after operation, recurrent atherosclerosis occurring beyond this period [86,87]. Early postoperative recurrence due to intimal hyperplasia rarely proceeds to occlusion and is less frequently associated with symptoms (low embolic potential) [88,89], whereas recurrent atherosclerosis has a higher stroke risk [90]. High-grade recurrent stenosis in

Table 56.2 Overview of nerves at risk during CEA.

Nerve	Injury	Clinical symptoms
Cervical plexus branches (transverse cervical nerve—greater auricular)	Incision	Insensate area medial to the incision/paresthesia—hyperesthesia over the ear lobe and angle of the jaw
Cranial nerve VII (cervical branch—marginal mandibular nerve)	Retraction	Drooping at the ipsilateral corner of the mouth–drooling
Cranial nerve IX	Incision dissection Clamping	Hemiparalysis and discoordination of pharyngeal musculature, significant dysphagia, postoperative blood pressure instability
Cranial nerve X (main vagus trunk—superior laryngeal nerve, recurrent laryngeal nerve)	Clamping Dissection	Fatigability & difficulty achieving high pitch (superior laryngeal nerve), vocal cord paralysis, hoarseness of voice, mild swallowing difficulties (recurrent laryngeal nerve)—acute airway obstruction (bilateral injury)
Cranial nerve XI	Dissection Incision	Winged scapula, difficulty in raising the shoulder, shoulder drop (paralysis of the serratus anterior muscle and the trapezius muscle)
Cranial nerve XII	Retraction Ligation Incision	Paralysis of ipsilateral myoglossus muscle, difficulty masticating, slurred speech
Sympathetic chain	Dissection Incision	Horner's syndrome

symptomatic patients or good-risk asymptomatic patients should be treated. Many studies have reported very good results with surgical management of high-grade asymptomatic or symptomatic restenosis with excellent protection from stroke and long-term durability [91–93]. Carotid angioplasty and stenting has also been proposed as an effective alternative method or even a preferred option owing to the increased risk of nerve injury with redo operations [94,95].

Carotid artery stenting (CAS) has emerged as an alternative to CEA, and a number of randomized trials have compared these two treatment modalities. Two recent nationally-based trials, the Endarterectomy Versus Angioplasty in Patients with Symptomatic Severe Carotid Stenosis (EVA-3S) and Stent-protected Percutaneous Angioplasty of the Carotid versus Endarterectomy (SPACE) trials, failed to show superiority of CAS over CEA [96,97]. SPACE demonstrated a 30-day death and stroke rate of 6.8% after CAS compared with 6.3% following CEA (*P* = 0.09), failing to prove that CAS was not inferior to CEA. EVA-3S suspended early after the stroke and death rate at 30 days was found to be 9.6% after CAS and 3.9% after CEA, challenging the opinion that cerebral protection devices can significantly improve outcomes after CAS. A concept in the methodology of carotid trials is randomization of patients considered "high-risk" to prove superiority of CAS over CEA in this category of patients [98]. The high-risk eligibility criteria included significant cardiac disease, severe pulmonary disease, contralateral occlusion, contralateral recurrent laryngeal nerve palsy, previous neck surgery, radiation arteritis, recurrent stenosis after CEA, and age >80 years. However, current evidence suggests that the risk of complications after CEA is not increased in most of the above categories. In a retrospective study, stroke and death risk was stratified according to inclusion and exclusion criteria for "high-risk" of the Stenting and Angioplasty with Protection in Patients at High Risk for Endarterectomy (SAPPHIRE) trial, and it was concluded that CEA can be performed in patients at high risk, with stroke and death rates well within accepted standards [99]. Previous studies have demonstrated that presence of severe medical comorbidities, such as cardiac dysfunction, pulmonary dysfunction, renal insufficiency, or particular anatomic features (i.e., contralateral carotid occlusion, ipsilateral carotid restenosis, and "high" carotid bifurcation), do not increase the rate of complications after CEA [100–102]. It has also been shown that octogenarians can undergo CEA with no more perioperative risks than younger patients [103]. Anatomic risk factors such as contralateral occlusion or lesion above C(2), or requirement of digastric division, were not found to increase complications, with the possible exception of reoperation and radiated neck [104]. On the basis of these data, the definition of "high risk" patient should not be used as a reason to abandon CEA in favor of CAS, although CAS is likely to be advantageous in reoperations and radiated necks or in reducing nonstroke morbidity in patients with many comorbidities.

Data from the completed randomized controlled trials cannot support clear indications for all the subgroups of patients with symptomatic and asymptomatic carotid disease. For the last six decades CEA has been used for managing carotid disease and is considered to be the gold standard method of treatment, with which every different treatment modality should be compared. There is currently no significant evidence that CAS provides better results compared with

CEA, and even in the so-called "high risk" patients CEA has proven to be a safe procedure with very low morbidity and mortality in centers with a high operative volume and experience. In future, any changes in clinical practice will come from new evidence, based on currently running randomized trials, and it seem that CEA and CAS would have a complementary role.

References

1. Eastcott HH, Pickering GW, & Rob CG (1954) Reconstruction of internal carotid artery in a patient with intermittent attacks of hemiplegia. *Lancet* **267**(6846):994–996.

2. DeBakey ME (1996) Carotid endarterectomy revisited. *J Endovasc Surg* **3**:4.

3. De Bakey ME, Crawford ES, Cooley DA, & Morris GC Jr (1959) Surgical considerations of occlusive disease of innominate, carotid, subclavian, and vertebral arteries. *Ann Surg* **149**:690–710.

4. Kieny R, Hirsch D, Seiller C, Thiranos JC, & Petit H (1993) Does carotid eversion endarterectomy and reimplantation reduce the risk of restenosis? *Ann Vasc Surg* **7**:407–413.

5. Zarins CK, Giddens DP, Bharadvaj BK, Sottiurai VS, Mabon RF, & Glagov S (1983) Carotid bifurcation atherosclerosis. Quantitative correlation of plaque localization with flow velocity profiles and wall shear stress. *Circ Res* **53**:502–514.

6. Bassiouny HS, Sakaguchi Y, Mikucki SA, *et al.* (1997) Juxtaluminal location of plaque necrosis and neoformation in symptomatic carotid stenosis. *J Vasc Surg* **26**:585–594.

7. Bonithon-Kopp C, Touboul PJ, Berr C, Magne C, & Ducimetiere P (1996) Factors of carotid arterial enlargement in a population aged 59 to 71 years: the EVA study. *Stroke* **27**:654–660.

8. Crouse JR, Goldbourt U, Evans G, *et al.* Risk factors and segment-specific carotid arterial enlargement in the Atherosclerosis Risk in Communities (ARIC) cohort. *Stroke* (1996) **27**:69–75.

9. Archie J (2000) How can I achieve the optimal flow surface and distal end-point following carotid endarterectomy? In: Naylor RA & Mackey WC (eds). *Carotid Artery Surgery: A Problem-based Approach,* London: WB Saunders, p 432.

10. Bassiouny HS, Davis H, Massawa N, Gewertz BL, Glagov S, & Zarins CK (1989) Critical carotid stenoses: morphologic and chemical similarity between symptomatic and asymptomatic plaques. *J Vasc Surg* **9**:202–212.

11. Zarins CKX, C. Glagov S (2005) Artery wall pathology in atherosclerosis. In: Rutherford RB (ed.) *Vascular Surgery,* 6th edn. Philadelphia: Elsevier Saunders.

12. Glagov S, Bassiouny HS, Sakaguchi Y, Goudet CA, & Vito RP (1997) Mechanical determinants of plaque modeling, remodeling and disruption. *Atherosclerosis* **131**(Suppl.):S13–S14.

13. Stary HC, Chandler AB, Dinsmore RE, *et al.* (1995) A definition of advanced types of atherosclerotic lesions and a histological classification of atherosclerosis. A report from the Committee on Vascular Lesions of the Council on Arteriosclerosis, American Heart Association. *Circulation* **92**:1355–1374.

14. Stary HC, Chandler AB, Glagov S, *et al.* (1994) A definition of initial, fatty streak, and intermediate lesions of atherosclerosis. A report from the Committee on Vascular Lesions of the Council

on Arteriosclerosis, American Heart Association. *Circulation* **89**: 2462–2478.

15. Avril G, Batt M, Guidoin R, Marois M, *et al.* (1991) Carotid endarterectomy plaques: correlations of clinical and anatomic findings. *Ann Vasc Surg* **5**:50–54.

16. Imparato AM, Riles TS, Mintzer R, & Baumann FG (1983) The importance of hemorrhage in the relationship between gross morphologic characteristics and cerebral symptoms in 376 carotid artery plaques. *Ann Surg* **197**:195–203.

17. Lusby RJ, Ferrell LD, Ehrenfeld WK, Stoney RJ, & Wylie EJ (1982) Carotid plaque hemorrhage. Its role in production of cerebral ischemia. *Arch Surg* **117**:1479–1488.

18. Ammar AD, Ernst RL, Lin JJ, & Travers H (1986) The influence of repeated carotid plaque hemorrhages on the production of cerebrovascular symptoms. *J Vasc Surg* **3**:857–859.

19. Ogata J, Masuda J, Yutani C, & Yamaguchi T (1990) Rupture of atheromatous plaque as a cause of thrombotic occlusion of stenotic internal carotid artery. *Stroke* **21**:1740–1745.

20. Torvik A, Svindland A, & Lindboe CF (1989) Pathogenesis of carotid thrombosis. *Stroke* **20**:1477–1483.

21. Grogan JK, Shaalan WE, Cheng H, *et al.* (2005) B-mode ultrasonographic characterization of carotid atherosclerotic plaques in symptomatic and asymptomatic patients. *J Vasc Surg* **42**:435–441.

22. Nicolaides AN, Kakkos SK, Griffin M, *et al.* (2005) Effect of image normalization on carotid plaque classification and the risk of ipsilateral hemispheric ischemic events: results from the asymptomatic carotid stenosis and risk of stroke study. *Vascular* **13**:211–221.

23. Lal BK, Hobson RW 2nd, Hameed M, *et al.* (2006) Noninvasive identification of the unstable carotid plaque. *Ann Vasc Surg* **20**:167–174.

24. Lal BK, Hobson RW 2nd, Pappas PJ, *et al.* (2002) Pixel distribution analysis of B-mode ultrasound scan images predicts histologic features of atherosclerotic carotid plaques. *J Vasc Surg* **35**:1210–1217.

25. Trivedi RA, Li ZY, U-King-Im J, Graves MJ, Kirkpatrick PJ, & Gillard JH (2007) Identifying vulnerable carotid plaques in vivo using high resolution magnetic resonance imaging-based finite element analysis. *J Neurosurg* **107**:536–542.

26. Takaya N, Yuan C, Chu B, Saam T, Underhill H, Cai J, *et al.* (2006) Association between carotid plaque characteristics and subsequent ischemic cerebrovascular events: a prospective assessment with MRI—initial results. *Stroke* **37**:818–823.

27. Altaf N, MacSweeney ST, Gladman J, & Auer DP (2007) Carotid intraplaque hemorrhage predicts recurrent symptoms in patients with high-grade carotid stenosis. *Stroke* **38**:1633–1635.

28. MRC European Carotid Surgery Trial (1991) Interim results for symptomatic patients with severe (70–99%) or with mild (0–29%) carotid stenosis. European Carotid Surgery Trialists' Collaborative Group. *Lancet* **337**:1235–1243.

29. (1991) Beneficial effect of carotid endarterectomy in symptomatic patients with high-grade carotid stenosis. North American Symptomatic Carotid Endarterectomy Trial Collaborators. *N Engl J Med* **325**:445–453.

30. Rothwell PM, Gutnikov SA, & Warlow CP (2003) Reanalysis of the final results of the European Carotid Surgery Trial. *Stroke* **34**:514–523.

31. Rothwell PM, Eliasziw M, Gutnikov SA, Warlow CP, & Barnett HJ (2004) Endarterectomy for symptomatic carotid stenosis in relation to clinical subgroups and timing of surgery. *Lancet* **363**:915–924.

32. Naylor AR (2004) Does the modern concept of "best medical therapy" render carotid surgery obsolete? *Eur J Vasc Endovasc Surg* **28**:457–461.

33. (1998) Randomised trial of endarterectomy for recently symptomatic carotid stenosis: final results of the MRC European Carotid Surgery Trial (ECST). *Lancet* **351**(9113):1379–1387.

34. Barnett HJ, Taylor DW, Eliasziw M, *et al.* (1998) Benefit of carotid endarterectomy in patients with symptomatic moderate or severe stenosis. North American Symptomatic Carotid Endarterectomy Trial Collaborators. *N Engl J Med* **339**:1415–1425.

35. Wilson SE, Mayberg MR, Yatsu F, & Weiss DG (1993) Crescendo transient ischemic attacks: a surgical imperative. Veterans Affairs trialists. *J Vasc Surg* **17**:249–255; discussion 55–56.

36. Karkos CD, McMahon G, McCarthy MJ, *et al.* (2007) The value of urgent carotid surgery for crescendo transient ischemic attacks. *J Vasc Surg* **45**:1148–1154.

37. Mentzer RM Jr, Finkelmeier BA, Crosby IK, & Wellons HA Jr (1981) Emergency carotid endarterectomy for fluctuating neurologic deficits. *Surgery* **89**:60–66.

38. Goldstone J & Moore WS (1976) Emergency carotid artery surgery in neurologically unstable patients. *Arch Surg* **111**:1284–1291.

39. Piotrowski JJ, Bernhard VM, Rubin JR, *et al.* (1990) Timing of carotid endarterectomy after acute stroke. *J Vasc Surg* **11**:45–51; discussion 51–52.

40. Solomon RA, Loftus CM, Quest DO, & Correll JW (1986) Incidence and etiology of intracerebral hemorrhage following carotid endarterectomy. *J Neurosurg* **64**:29–34.

41. Naylor AR, Cuffe RL, Rothwell PM, & Bell PR (2003) A systematic review of outcomes following staged and synchronous carotid endarterectomy and coronary artery bypass. *Eur J Vasc Endovasc Surg* **25**:380–389.

42. Ricotta JJ, Char DJ, Cuadra SA, *et al.* (2003) Modeling stroke risk after coronary artery bypass and combined coronary artery bypass and carotid endarterectomy. *Stroke* **34**:1212–1217.

43. (1995) Endarterectomy for asymptomatic carotid artery stenosis. Executive Committee for the Asymptomatic Carotid Atherosclerosis Study. *JAMA* **273**:1421–1428.

44. Halliday A, Mansfield A, Marro J, *et al.* (2004) Prevention of disabling and fatal strokes by successful carotid endarterectomy in patients without recent neurological symptoms: randomised controlled trial. *Lancet* **363**(9420):1491–1502.

45. Rothwell PM, Eliasziw M, Gutnikov SA, *et al.* (2003) Analysis of pooled data from the randomised controlled trials of endarterectomy for symptomatic carotid stenosis. *Lancet* **361**(9352):107–116.

46. Rothwell PM (2004) ACST: which subgroups will benefit most from carotid endarterectomy? *Lancet* **364**:1122–1123; author reply 1125–1126.

47. Kumar S & Sinha B (2004) ACST: which subgroups will benefit most from carotid endarterectomy? *Lancet* **364**:1125 author reply 1125–1126.

48. Campkin TV & Turner JM (1986) Anesthesia for the surgery of cerebral arterial insufficiency. London: Butterworths.

49. J McCarthy R, Trigg R, John C, Gough MJ, & Horrocks M (2004) Patient satisfaction for carotid endarterectomy performed under local anaesthesia. *Eur J Vasc Endovasc Surg* **27**:654–659.

50. McCleary AJ, Dearden NM, Dickson DH, Watson A, & Gough MJ (1996) The differing effects of regional and general anaesthesia on cerebral metabolism during carotid endarterectomy. *Eur J Vasc Endovasc Surg* **12**:173–181.

51. Prough DS, Scuderi PE, McWhorter JM, Balestrieri FJ, Davis CH Jr, & Stullken EH (1989) Hemodynamic status following regional and general anesthesia for carotid endarterectomy. *J Neurosurg Anesthesiol* **1**:35–40.

52. Bhattathiri PS, Ramakrishnan Y, Vivar RA, *et al.* (2005) Effect of awake Carotid Endarterectomy under local anaesthesia on peri-operative blood pressure: blood pressure is normalised when carotid stenosis is treated under local anaesthesia. *Acta Neurochir* (*Wien*) **147**:839–845.

53. Rerkasem K, Bond R, & Rothwell PM (2004) Local versus general anaesthesia for carotid endarterectomy. *Cochrane Database Syst Rev* (2):CD000126.

54. Jackson MR, D'Addio VJ, Gillespie DL, & O'Donnell SD (1996) The fate of residual defects following carotid endarterectomy detected by early postoperative duplex ultrasound. *Am J Surg* **172**:184–187.

55. Reilly LM, Okuhn SP, Rapp JH, *et al.* (1990) Recurrent carotid stenosis: a consequence of local or systemic factors? The influence of unrepaired technical defects. *J Vasc Surg* **11**:448–459; discussion 459–460.

56. Archie JP Jr (1993) Carotid endarterectomy with reconstruction techniques tailored to operative findings. *J Vasc Surg* **17**:141–149; discussion 149–151.

57. Archie JP (1996) The endarterectomy-produced common carotid artery step: a harbinger of early emboli and late restenosis. *J Vasc Surg* **23**:932–939.

58. Stoney RJ (1997) Regarding "The endarterectomy-produced common carotid artery step: a harbinger of early emboli and late restenosis." *J Vasc Surg* **25**:958–959.

59. Cao PG, de Rango P, Zannetti S, Giordano G, Ricci S, & Celani MG (2001) Eversion versus conventional carotid endarterectomy for preventing stroke. *Cochrane Database Syst Rev* (1):CD001921.

60. Cao P, Giordano G, De Rango P, *et al.* (1998) A randomized study on eversion versus standard carotid endarterectomy: study design and preliminary results: the Everest Trial. *J Vasc Surg* **27**:595–605.

61. Bond R, Rerkasem K, Naylor R, & Rothwell PM (2004) Patches of different types for carotid patch angioplasty. *Cochrane Database Syst Rev* (2):CD000071.

62. Myers SI, Valentine RJ, Chervu A, Bowers BL, & Clagett GP (1994) Saphenous vein patch versus primary closure for carotid endarterectomy: long-term assessment of a randomized prospective study. *J Vasc Surg* **19**:15–22.

63. Katz D, Snyder SO, Gandhi RH, *et al.* (1994) Long-term follow-up for recurrent stenosis: a prospective randomized study of expanded polytetrafluoroethylene patch angioplasty versus primary closure after carotid endarterectomy. *J Vasc Surg* **19**:198–203; discussion 204–205.

64. AbuRahma AF, Stone PA, Flaherty SK, & AbuRahma Z (2007) Prospective randomized trial of ACUSEAL (Gore-Tex) versus Hemashield-Finesse patching during carotid endarterectomy: early results. *J Vasc Surg* **45**:881–884.

65. Dossa C, Shepard AD, Wolford DG, Reddy DJ, & Ernst CB (1990) Distal internal carotid exposure: a simplified technique for temporary mandibular subluxation. *J Vasc Surg* **12**:319–325.

66. Shaha A, Phillips T, Scalea T, *et al.* (1988) Exposure of the internal carotid artery near the skull base: the posterolateral anatomic approach. *J Vasc Surg* **8**:618–622.

67. Fieschi C, Agnoli A, Battistini N, Bozzao L, & Prencipe M (1968) Derangement of regional cerebral blood flow and of its regulatory mechanisms in acute cerebrovascular lesions. *Neurology* **18**:1166–1179.

68. Bond R, Rerkasem K, Counsell C, *et al.* (2002) Routine or selective carotid artery shunting for carotid endarterectomy (and different methods of monitoring in selective shunting). *Cochrane Database Syst Rev* (2):CD000190.

69. Whittemore AD, Kauffman JL, Kohler TR, & Mannick JA (1983) Routine electroencephalographic (EEG) monitoring during carotid endarterectomy. *Ann Surg* **197**:707–713.

70. Evans WE, Hayes JP, Waltke EA, & Vermilion BD (1985) Optimal cerebral monitoring during carotid endarterectomy: neurologic response under local anesthesia. *J Vasc Surg* **2**:775–777.

71. Harada RN, Comerota AJ, Good GM, Hashemi HA, & Hulihan JF (1995) Stump pressure, electroencephalographic changes, and the contralateral carotid artery: another look at selective shunting. *Am J Surg* **170**:148–153.

72. Jorgensen LG & Schroeder TV (1996) Transcranial Doppler for carotid endarterectomy. *Eur J Vasc Endovasc Surg* **12**:1–2.

73. Kresowik TF, Bratzler D, Karp HR, *et al.* (2001) Multistate utilization, processes, and outcomes of carotid endarterectomy. *J Vasc Surg* **33**:227–234; discussion 234–235.

74. Mauney MC, Buchanan SA, Lawrence WA, *et al.* (1995) Stroke rate is markedly reduced after carotid endarterectomy by avoidance of protamine. *J Vasc Surg* **22**:264–269; discussion 269–270.

75. Levison JA, Faust GR, Halpern VJ, *et al.* (1999) Relationship of protamine dosing with postoperative complications of carotid endarterectomy. *Ann Vasc Surg* **13**:67–72.

76. Morgenstern LB, Fox AJ, Sharpe BL, Eliasziw M, Barnett HJ, & Grotta JC (1997) The risks and benefits of carotid endarterectomy in patients with near occlusion of the carotid artery. North American Symptomatic Carotid Endarterectomy Trial (NASCET) Group. *Neurology* **48**:911–915.

77. Moore WS, Barnett HJ, Beebe HG, *et al.* (1995) Guidelines for carotid endarterectomy. A multidisciplinary consensus statement from the Ad Hoc Committee, American Heart Association. *Circulation* **91**:566–579.

78. Rothwell PM, Slattery J, & Warlow CP (1996) A systematic comparison of the risks of stroke and death due to carotid endarterectomy for symptomatic and asymptomatic stenosis. *Stroke* **27**:266–269.

79. Paciaroni M, Eliasziw M, Kappelle LJ, Finan JW, Ferguson GG, & Barnett HJ (1999) Medical complications associated with carotid endarterectomy. North American Symptomatic Carotid Endarterectomy Trial (NASCET). *Stroke* **30**:1759–1763.

80. Young B, Moore WS, Robertson JT, *et al.* (1996) An analysis of perioperative surgical mortality and morbidity in the asymptomatic carotid atherosclerosis study. ACAS Investigators. Asymptomatic Carotid Artheriosclerosis Study. *Stroke* **27**:2216–2224.

81. Riles TS, Imparato AM, Jacobowitz GR, *et al.* (1994) The cause of perioperative stroke after carotid endarterectomy. *J Vasc Surg* **19**:206–214; discussion 215–216.

82. Bandyk DF, Kaebnick HW, Adams MB, & Towne JB (1988) Turbulence occurring after carotid bifurcation endarterectomy: a harbinger of residual and recurrent carotid stenosis. *J Vasc Surg* **7**:261–274.

83. Pomposelli FB, Lamparello PJ, Riles TS, Craighead CC, Giangola G, & Imparato AM (1988) Intracranial hemorrhage after carotid endarterectomy. *J Vasc Surg* **7**:248–255.

84. Reigelmm, Hollier LH, Sundt TM Jr, Piepgras DG, Sharbrough FW, & Cherry KJ (1987) Cerebral hyperperfusion syndrome: a cause of neurologic dysfunction after carotid endarterectomy. *J Vasc Surg* **5**:628–634.

85. Ferguson GG, Eliasziw M, Barr HW, *et al.* (1999) The North American Symptomatic Carotid Endarterectomy Trial: surgical results in 1415 patients. *Stroke* **30**:1751–1758.

86. Stoney RJ & String ST (1976) Recurrent carotid stenosis. *Surgery* **80**:705–710.

87. Imparato AM & Weinstein GS (1986) Clinicopathologic correlation in postendarterectomy recurrent stenosis. A case report and bibliographic review. *J Vasc Surg* **3**:657–662.

88. O'Donnell TF Jr, Callow AD, Scott G, Shepard AD, Heggerick P, & Mackey WC (1985) Ultrasound characteristics of recurrent carotid disease: hypothesis explaining the low incidence of symptomatic recurrence. *J Vasc Surg* **2**:26–41.

89. Samson RH, Showalter DP, Yunis JP, Dorsay DA, Kulman HI, & Silverman SR (1999) Hemodynamically significant early recurrent carotid stenosis: an often self-limiting and self-reversing condition. *J Vasc Surg* **30**:446–452.

90. Frericks H, Kievit J, van Baalen JM, & van Bockel JH (1998) Carotid recurrent stenosis and risk of ipsilateral stroke: a systematic review of the literature. *Stroke* **29**:244–250.

91. Jain S, Jain KM, Kumar SD, Munn JS, & Rummel MC (2007) Operative intervention for carotid restenosis is safe and effective. *Eur J Vasc Endovasc Surg* **34**:561–568.

92. Cho JS, Pandurangi K, Conrad MF, *et al.* (2004) Safety and durability of redo carotid operation: an 11-year experience. *J Vasc Surg* **39**:155–161.

93. O'Hara PJ, Hertzer NR, Karafa MT, Mascha EJ, Krajewski LP, & Beven EG (2001) Reoperation for recurrent carotid stenosis: early results and late outcome in 199 patients. *J Vasc Surg* **34**:5–12.

94. Kadkhodayan Y, Moran CJ, Derdeyn CP, & Cross DT 3rd (2007) Carotid angioplasty and stent placement for restenosis after endarterectomy. *Neuroradiology* **49**:357–364.

95. Hobson RW 2nd, Goldstein JE, Jamil Z, *et al.* (1999) Carotid restenosis: operative and endovascular management. *J Vasc Surg* **29**:228–235; discussion 235–238.

96. Mas JL, Chatellier G, & Beyssen B (2004) Carotid angioplasty and stenting with and without cerebral protection: clinical alert from the Endarterectomy Versus Angioplasty in Patients With Symptomatic Severe Carotid Stenosis (EVA-3S) trial. *Stroke* **35**:e18–20.

97. Ringleb PA, Allenberg J, Bruckmann H, *et al.* (2006) 30 day results from the SPACE trial of stent-protected angioplasty versus carotid endarterectomy in symptomatic patients: a randomised non-inferiority trial. *Lancet* **368**(9543):1239–1247.

98. Yadav JS, Wholey MH, Kuntz RE, *et al.* (2004) Protected carotid-artery stenting versus endarterectomy in high-risk patients. *N Engl J Med* **351**:1493–1501.

99. Mozes G, Sullivan TM, Torres-Russotto DR, *et al.* (2004) Carotid endarterectomy in SAPPHIRE-eligible high-risk patients: implications for selecting patients for carotid angioplasty and stenting. *J Vasc Surg* **39**:958–965 discussion 965–966.

100. Ballotta E, Da Giau G, Baracchini C, & Manara R (2004) Carotid endarterectomy in high-risk patients: a challenge for endovascular procedure protocols. *Surgery* **135**:74–80.

101. Pulli R, Dorigo W, Barbanti E, *et al.* (2005) Does the high-risk patient for carotid endarterectomy really exist? *Am J Surg* **189**:714–719.

102. Illig KA, Zhang R, Tanski W, Benesch C, Sternbach Y, & Green RM (2003) Is the rationale for carotid angioplasty and stenting in patients excluded from NASCET/ACAS or eligible for ARCHeR justified? *J Vasc Surg* **37**:575–581.

103. Ballotta E, Da Giau G, Militello C, *et al.* (2006) High-grade symptomatic and asymptomatic carotid stenosis in the very elderly. A challenge for proponents of carotid angioplasty and stenting. *BMC Cardiovasc Disord* **6**:12.

104. Gasparis AP, Ricotta L, Cuadra SA, *et al.* (2003) High-risk carotid endarterectomy: fact or fiction. *J Vasc Surg* **37**:40–46.

57 Interventional Management of Acute Ischemic Stroke

Sabareesh K. Natarajan, Kenneth V. Snyder, Adnan H. Siddiqui, Elad I. Levy & L. Nelson Hopkins

Millard Fillmore Gates Hospital, Kaleida Health, Buffalo, NY, USA

Introduction

Stroke remains the third most common cause of death in industrialized nations, and the single most common reason for permanent adult disability [1]. The World Health Organization (WHO) estimated in 2002 that there were 15.3 million strokes per year and 5.5 of the 57 million deaths worldwide every year are attributed to stroke [2]. Figure 57.1 shows the mortality and the loss of disability-associated life years (DALY) worldwide owing to stroke as published by the WHO in 2002 [2,3]. Each year, approximately 795 000 Americans experience a new or recurrent stroke [4]. Moreover, 30–50% of stroke survivors do not regain functional independence, 15–30% of all stroke survivors are permanently disabled, and 25% die within 1 year of the initial stroke. This means that every 40 s someone in the USA has a stroke, and every 3–4 min someone dies from a stroke. The direct and indirect costs of stroke for 2009 are estimated at $68.9 billion [4]. The incidence of new or recurrent stroke per year is projected to rise to 1.2 million per year by 2025 (Fig. 57.2) [5].

Treatment goals

To protect patients from the high rates of morbidity and mortality associated with stroke, various systemic and local treatment options have been advocated. Despite different approaches in the treatment strategy, all studies have underlined the crucial determinants for neurologic outcome after acute ischemic stroke [6–11] (Table 57.1). Hence, fast and sufficient reperfusion in combination with a low rate of symptomatic intracranial hemorrhage (sICH) is key to successful stroke treatment.

Cardiovascular Interventions in Clinical Practice. Edited by Jürgen Haase, Hans-Joachim Schäfers, Horst Sievert and Ron Waksman. © 2010 Blackwell Publishing.

Table 57.1 Determinants of neurologic outcome after ischemic stroke.

Size of the ischemic brain area perfused by the occluded vessel
Time window between onset of symptoms and revascularization
Recanalization rate associated with a specific treatment
Occurrence of symptomatic intracranial hemorrhage

Intravenous thrombolysis

Subsequent to the publication of the results of the National Institute of Neurological Disorders and Stroke (NINDS) study [6], the US Food and Drug Administration (FDA) in 1996 approved intravenous (i.v.) recombinant tissue plasminogen activator (rt-PA) administered within 3 h of symptom onset for acute stroke. The advantages of this strategy are that it is relatively easy and rapid to initiate and it does not require highly specialized equipment or technical expertise. However, a reanalysis of the NINDS study [12] revealed the limited effect of intravenous thrombolysis (IVT) in patients with severe stroke (National Institute of Health Stroke Scale [NIHSS] score > 16). The NIHSS score increases with the size of the vessel occluded. An NIHSS score of > 12 suggests an occlusion of a proximal large vessel (such as the basilar artery, internal carotid artery [ICA], and middle cerebral artery [MCA]—M1 and M2 segments) and, therefore, a high thrombus burden [13]. The recanalization rates of intravenous rt-PA for proximal large-vessel arterial occlusion are poor and range from only 10% for ICA occlusion to 30% for MCA occlusion [14].

Evidence for increasing the time window

Despite the approval of intravenous rt-PA as the sole pharmacologic treatment for acute stroke in the USA, < 1% of acute ischemic stroke patients in the USA receive intravenous rt-PA within the 3-h window, primarily because of a delay in hospital presentation [15]. The European Cooperative Acute

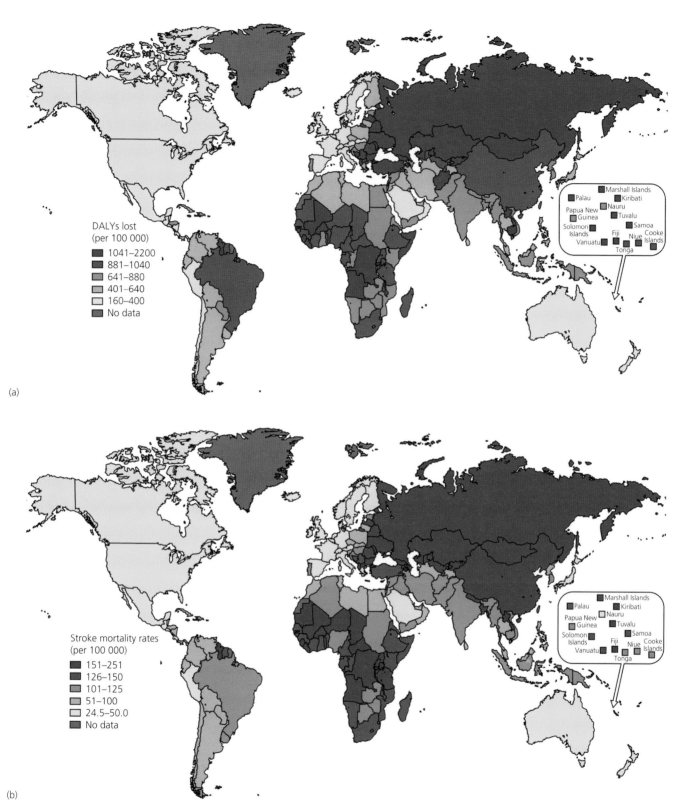

(a)

(b)

Figure 57.1 (a) Age-adjusted and sex-adjusted stroke mortalities in 2002. (b) Age-adjusted and sex-adjusted DALY loss due to stroke in 2002. From the WHO [2] and modified in Johnston *et al.* [3], reproduced with permission from Elsevier Ltd.

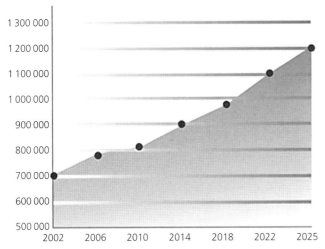

Figure 57.2 Projected number of strokes in the USA from 2002 to 2025. Modified from Broderick *et al.* [5].

Stroke Study (ECASS) III trial has extended the time window for intravenous rt-PA to 4.5 h, albeit in a somewhat narrower subgroup of patients than those for whom intravenous rt-PA is approved [16]. The pooled analysis by Hacke *et al.* [17] demonstrates better outcomes at 3 months with IVT up to 4.5 h after stroke onset. A recent metaanalysis by Lansberg *et al.* [10] estimated that the number of patients needed to treat (NNT) to benefit one patient after intravenous rt-PA were 3.6 for patients treated between 0 and 90 min, 4.3 with treatment between 91 and 180 min, 5.9 with treatment between 181 and 270 min, and 19.3 with treatment between 271 and 360 min. The NNT for harm estimates for the corresponding time intervals are 65, 38, 30, and 14. Thus, this metaanalysis confirmed more benefit than harm up to 4.5 h. The metaanalysis by Wardlaw *et al.* [18] demonstrates higher benefit when compared with the risk of being dead or disabled up to 6 h after IVT, thus formally providing level 1 evidence, even in patients selected by "only" noncontrast computed tomographic imaging.

There is increasing evidence that identification of potentially salvageable brain tissue with advanced magnetic resonance (MR) and computed tomography (CT) imaging may allow the selection of patients who can be effectively and safely treated with IVT for up to 9 h postictus [19–25]. Although MR-based perfusion imaging is a useful imaging modality for determining salvageable tissue, CT perfusion has been shown to be comparable [26, 27] and is widely available. Although the evidence for a longer time window for treatment is increasing, the NNT increases with the time window and the outcome is better if the treatment is initiated earlier [10]. Recent mechanical revascularization strategies re-establish flow faster than thrombolytics and thus may increase the benefit of treatment even when there is a delay.

Evidence for aggressive recanalization

Rha and Saver [11] reviewed recanalization and outcome data from all articles published from 1985 to 2002 that evaluated vessel recanalization in acute stroke. Fifty-three studies encompassing 2066 patients were included. Good functional outcomes (modified Rankin Scale [mRS] score ≤2) at 3 months were more frequent in recanalized versus nonrecanalized patients (odds ratio [OR], 4.43; 95% confidence interval [CI], 3.32–5.91). The 3-month mortality rate was reduced in recanalized patients (OR, 0.24; 95% CI, 0.16–0.35). Recanalization rates according to method of intervention were: spontaneous, 24.1%; IVT, 46.2%; intraarterial thrombolysis (IAT), 63.2%; combined IVT and IAT, 67.5%; and mechanical treatment, 83.6%. Thus, endovascular methods can achieve higher recanalization rates and, hence, better outcomes. In the Mechanical Embolus Removal in Cerebral Ischemia (MERCI) trial [28], multi-MERCI trial [29], and the combined analysis of Interventional Management of Stroke (IMS) I and II data [30], the outcome, as measured by mRS score of <2 at 3 months, was significantly better and the 3-month mortality was significantly lower in patients who had thrombolysis in myocardial infarction (TIMI) 2 or 3 recanalization (partial or complete recanalization, respectively) after therapy than in patients in whom vessels failed to recanalize.

Endovascular stroke therapy

Compared with systemic IVT, local intraarterial techniques expand the time window for treatment and may increase the recanalization rate. The local approach is promising to reduce or eliminate exposure to thrombolytic drugs and, therefore, to reduce the risk of accompanying hemorrhage. Early reocclusion after thrombolysis has been shown by transcranial Doppler (TCD) to occur in 34% of patients receiving intravenous rt-PA, and may result in neurologic worsening in many of these patients [31–33]. Various endovascular treatment options, including a range of pharmacological and mechanical approaches, have been advocated.

Intracerebral hemorrhage after reperfusion

Intracerebral hemorrhage occurs in the vast majority of patients in the core of the infarction [34]. sICH usually occurs within 24–36 h of reperfusion [34]. The mortality rate after sICH in the NINDS trial was 47% [34]. The IVT trials—NINDS, Alteplase Thrombolysis for Acute Noninterventional Therapy in Ischemic Stroke (ATLANTIS), and ECASS II—show an increased hemorrhage rate of 6–8% with intravenous thrombolytics, compared with 1% with placebo [17]. The higher the dose of thrombolytics [35] and higher the initial stroke severity [36], the higher the rate of sICH. In the NINDS trial [6], patients with NIHSS scores >20 at admission were 11 times more likely to endure as sICH than patients with NIHSS scores ≤5. In some countries, an NIHSS score >25 is a contraindication for any thrombolytic therapy. The patients in the Prolyse in Acute Cerebral Thrombolysis (PROACT) II trial [9] had an sICH rate of 10.9%, but they had higher mean NIHSS scores at presentation when compared with patients enrolled in the intravenous rt-PA trials, and they also had higher recanalization and, hence, higher reperfusion rates. Hypertension during the first 24 h after stroke revascularization [36] and pretherapeutic hyperglycemia [36] contribute to increased risk of sICH. In PROACT II [9], there was an increased risk of sICH in patients with a pretherapeutic glycemia value of >200 mg/dL. A glycemia value of >400 mg/dL represents a contraindication to cerebral thrombolysis.

The association of ICH after treatment with early ischemic changes and hyperdense MCA sign on baseline CT scan is controversial, not sensitive, and not reproducible. Attempts to increase the reliability and reproducibility of stroke diagnosis on noncontrast CT imaging have led to the development of the Alberta Stroke Programme Early CT Score (ASPECTS) [37], which provides a quantitative (10-point) assessment of MCA stroke burden on CT with high interobserver reliability in acute stroke. Lower ASPECT scores correlate well with more proximal occlusions [38] and have proven valuable for prognostication in acute stroke. When assessing dichotomized ASPECT scores, patients with low stroke burden (ASPECTS >7) on CT imaging incur less sICH after IVT and have a higher chance of gaining independence (mRS ≥2) [37]. The use of CT perfusion images rather than noncontrast CT increases prognostic accuracy of the ASPECT score, with final infarct mirroring cerebral blood volume (CBV) or cerebral blood flow (CBF) deficits when reperfusion is or is not achieved, respectively [39]. The Diffusion-weighted Imaging Evaluation For Understanding Stroke Evolution (DEFUSE) trial [40] was the first study that directly established a strong relationship between MR imaging (MRI), hemodynamic and tissue parameters, and sICH. In this study, early reperfusion was associated with fatal ICH in patients with the "malignant profile" (baseline diffusion-weighted imaging volume >100 mL and/or perfusion-weighted imaging deficit >100 mL with 8 s or longer of T_{max} [time to peak of the deconvoluted curve]).

Perfusion imaging-based patient selection

Despite better recanalization across all the major published ischemic stroke trials using IVT and endovascular interventions, the clinical outcome (mRS ≤2) at 3 months remains at approximately 40%. We believe that using perfusion imaging would allow us to better select patients with salvageable brain tissue who would benefit from revascularization, and thus lead to a higher percentage of patients having a better outcome. Perfusion imaging has also been shown to identify patients with increased risk of sICH, as described in the previous section.

Cerebral perfusion refers to tissue (capillary)-level blood flow. Brain tissue flow can be described by several parameters, including CBF, CBV, and mean transit time (MTT). CBV is defined as the total volume of flowing blood in a given volume in the brain, with units of milliliters of blood per 100 g of brain tissue. CBF is defined as the volume of blood moving through a given volume of brain per unit of time, with units of milliliters of blood per 100 g of brain tissue per min. MTT is defined as the average transit time of blood through a given brain region, measured in seconds. "Core" is typically operationally defined as the CBV lesion volume and "penumbra," as the MTT or CBF lesion volume [41]. "Mismatch" is typically defined, therefore, as the difference between these. We select our patients for revascularization if they have an ischemic penumbra more than half the territory of the occluded vessel and if the core is <30% of the occluded territory. In our experience, patients with even small ischemic cores in the basal ganglia or occupying >30% of the occluded vessel territory presage a higher rate of sICH and poor outcome.

Different institutions use different modalities to assess cerebral perfusion; these include MR, CT, single photon emission computed tomography, positron emission tomography, and xenon-CT. At our institution, because all stroke patients are usually first screened with an emergent noncontrast CT scan (to determine hemorrhagic versus ischemic stroke and/or eligibility for i.v. or intraarterial treatment), we have found it relatively simple to proceed with the extra 10 min and <130 mL of contrast material necessary to provide CT perfusion and CT angiography information that has significantly influenced our decision-making in stroke. Other groups [42–44] have similarly noted benefits of combined CT angiography and CT perfusion imaging in rapid assessment of acute stroke, and Smith *et al.* [45] have demonstrated the safety of this approach without previous determination of a serum creatinine level. The newer 320-slice CT perfusion scanner creates whole-brain perfusion maps comparable with MR perfusion imaging. In our experience, CT angiography has been found to be significantly better than MR angiography, with respect to resolution, detail, and avoidance of common MR artifacts, secondary to low-flow or turbulent flow phenomena, and vessel calcification.

Magnetic resonance imaging has several disadvantages. Concern for metal implants, increased susceptibility to motion artifact, difficulties with a relatively closed environment with respect to patients on mechanical ventilation or multiple intravenous drips, and FDA regulatory concerns regarding renal function in gadolinium-enhanced studies have all led to increased time screening for and then spent in the MRI suite, compared with CT imaging. MR perfusion imaging provides only relative estimates of CBF, CBV, and MTT, whereas CT perfusion provides absolute values that have been validated against xenon-CT and positron emission tomography [46]. There is dampened enthusiasm for accuracy of MR perfusion in predicting true penumbra [47,48], and diffusion-weighted imaging lesions may, at least in part, be reversible [49]. In some cases, MRI may even fail to show CT-documented hypoattenuation in lesions that are destined for infarction (the so-called "reverse discrepancy") [50].

Intraarterial thrombolysis

To perform IAT, a microcatheter is placed proximal to or directly into the thrombus. Technically, a long 6- or 7-French (F) sheath is placed into the femoral artery, and a 6F or 7F guiding catheter is advanced into the ICA or vertebral artery of the affected side. A microcatheter is then navigated to the occlusion site over a microwire. The theoretical advantages and disadvantages of IAT are presented in Table 57.2.

PROACT I

The Prolyse in Acute Cerebral Thromboembolism I (PROACT I) study [8] evaluated the safety and efficiency of intraarterial administration in the treatment of acute ischemic stroke. Results for the PROACT I study and other important stroke trials involving interventional treatment are summarized in Table 57.3 (the NINDS [6] and ECASS III [16] data have been summarized for comparison in the same table). Forty patients with an angiographically proven occlusion of the M1 or M2 segment of the MCA and a mean of 5.5h from symptom onset were included. Fourteen patients (mean NIHSS, 19) were randomized into the control placebo group, 26 patients (mean NIHSS, 17) were treated with local administration of prourokinase (6 mg) over the course of 120 min into the proximal thrombus surface. Any mechanical manipulation of the clot was not allowed. Partial or complete recanalization (TIMI 2 or 3) occurred in 57.7% of the patients treated

---

Table 57.2 Intraarterial thrombolysis.

Advantages

Angiographic evaluation reveals the precise occlusion site, the extent of collaterals, and assesses the grade of recanalization during treatment

A higher effective dosage of thrombolytic agent is delivered directly to the thrombus, thus reducing the systemic side effects

The approach facilitates combination with mechanical recanalization techniques

Disadvantages

Time-consuming procedure that delays the initiation of treatment compared with i.v. thrombolysis

Manipulation of cervical and cranial vessels with the risk of peri-interventional complications

Demands highly specialized centers with high human and financial resources

Direct endovascular access to the distal intracranial vasculature (e.g., distal M2 and M3 segments of the middle cerebral artery) is limited

---

with prourokinase compared with 14.3% in the control group. sICH within 24h occurred in 15.4% of the treatment group and 7.1% of the placebo group. The number of patients was too small to demonstrate a statistically significant benefit in terms of clinical outcomes or mortality at 90 days. Nevertheless, the absolute increase in favorable clinical neurologic outcome over the placebo group was 10–12%. The mortality rate was decreased from 42.9% in the placebo group to 26.9% in the prourokinase group. The results of the PROACT I study suggest an enhanced recanalization with prourokinase and a positive trend toward better neurologic outcome and survival rate.

In the prourokinase group, the rates of recanalization were dependent on the administered dose of heparin: 81.8% of the patients treated with high-dose heparin (100 IU/kg bolus followed by 1000 IU/h infusion for 4h) demonstrated recanalization, whereas only 40% in the low-dose heparin subgroup (2000 IU bolus followed by a 500 IU/h infusion for 4h) demonstrated recanalization. However, the rate of sICH at 24h was also higher in the high-dose heparin group (27.3% vs. 6.7%). All patients in the prourokinase group with early CT changes involving > 33% of the MCA territory had ICH.

PROACT II

The PROACT II trial [9] was a large-scale, multicenter, randomized (2:1), phase III trial that included 180 patients with angiographically confirmed M1 or M2 occlusion within the first 6h after symptom onset. In this trial, 121 patients (mean NIHSS, 17) received low-dose intravenous heparin (2000 IU bolus, 500 IU/h) and intraarterial prourokinase (9 mg infused over the course of 2h) proximally to the thrombus; again, any mechanical disruption of the thrombus was not allowed. Fifty-nine patients from the control group (mean NIHSS, 17) received only low-dose intravenous heparin. The median time to initiation of prourokinase treatment was 5.3h. The intraarterial treatment group showed a significantly (P < 0.001) higher rate of partial or complete recanalization in 66% of patients compared with 18% in the heparin-only group. Excellent neurologic outcome (mRS ≤2) was achieved in 40% of the treated patients compared with 25% in the control group (absolute benefit, 15%; relative benefit, 58%; NNT, 7; P = 0.043). The rate of sICH within 24h was elevated to 10% in the prourokinase group compared with 2% in the control group (P = 0.06), but no significant difference in the 90-day mortality rate was found (25% in the treatment group and 27% in the control group). This study was able to demonstrate the beneficial effect of IAT on the recanalization and clinical outcome of patients with M1 and M2 occlusions.

A pooled analysis of PROACT I and II data showed that the OR of better outcome with treatment was 2.49 (P = 0.022), greater than the OR (2.13) in the original PROACT II analysis [51]. The Japanese Middle Cerebral Artery Embolism Local Fibrinolytic Intervention Trial (MELT) [52] studied safety and clinical efficacy of intraarterial infusion of urokinase in patients

Table 57.3 Summary of important stroke trials.

Study	No. of patients	Type of study	Treatment	Time window from symptom onset (h)	Mean Presentation NIHSS	Recanalization rate (%)	sICH rate (%)	mRS ≤2 or ≤1* at 3 months (%)	Mortality at 3 months (%)	Main results
NINDS [6]	333 (168 vs. 165)	RCT	i.v. rt-PA (0.9 mg/kg) vs. placebo	0–3	14 vs. 15	NR	6.4 vs. 0.6	39 vs. 26*	21 vs. 24	No difference between groups at 24 h (trend in favor of treatment); Significant improvement in functional status at 90 days in treated group (P = 0.30)
ECASS III [16]	821 (418 vs. 403)	RCT	i.v. rt-PA (0.9 mg/kg) vs. placebo	3–4.5	10.7 vs. 11.6	NR	2.4% vs. 0.2%	52.4 vs. 45.2*	7.7 vs. 8.4	Significant difference in sICH rates (P < 0.001); Significant improvement in functional status at 3 months (P=0.04); Significant difference in sICH rates (P = 0.008); No difference in mortality (P = 0.68)
PROACT [8]	40 (26 vs. 14)	RCT	IA r-prourokinase (6 mg) + i.v. heparin (high or low dose) vs. i.v. heparin (high or low dose)	0–6	17 vs. 19	57.7 vs. 14.3	15.4 vs. 7.1	30.8 vs. 21.4*	26.9 vs. 42.9	Significant higher recanalization efficacy with IAT (P = 0.17); No significant difference in sICH (P = 0.64)
PROACT II [9]	180 (121 vs. 59)	RCT	IA r-prourokinase (9mg) + i.v. heparin (low dose) vs. i.v. heparin (low dose)	0–6	17 vs. 17	66 vs. 18	10 vs. 2	40 vs. 25	25 vs. 27	Significant better outcome at 3 months (P = 0.04) and significant higher recanalization rate (P < 0.001) in the treatment group; Difference in sICH not significant (P = 0.06)
IMS-I [121]	80 (IAT-62)	Prospective	i.v. rt-PA (0.6 mg/kg) + IA rt-PA (4 mg in clot+9mg/h) (if clot identified by angiography after IVT) + low-dose i.v. heparin	0–3	18	56	6.30	43, 30*	16%	Results compared with NINDS rt-PA and placebo arms; Significant better 3-month outcomes when compared with NINDS placebo Odds ratio >2; Difference in mortality or sICH not significant
IMS-II [81]	81 (IAT-55)	Prospective	i.v. rt-PA (0.6 mg/kg) + IA rt-PA (22 mg over 2 h using EKOS or normal catheter) (if clot identified by angiography after IVT) + low-dose i.v. heparin	0–3	19	58	9.90	46	16	Results compared with NINDS rt-PA and placebo arms; Significant better 3-month outcomes when compared to NINDS placebo OR >2.7; Better outcomes in the recanalized cohort when compared to non-recanalized (P = 0.046)
MERCI [122]	141	Prospective	IA Merci (I generation) + IAT, no IVT	0–8	20	60.3 (48 device alone)	7.80	36	34	Difference in mortality or sICH not significant; Better functional outcome at 3 months in recanalized patients when compared with nonrecanalized (P = 0.01)
Multi-MERCI [29]	164	Prospective	IA Merci (I & II generation) + IAT + IVT allowed	0–8	19	68 (55 device alone)	9.80	36	26	Higher rates of recanalization with second-generation devices
Penumbra [92]	125	Prospective	IA Penumbra + IAT	0–8	17	81.6 (device alone)	11.20	25	32.80	Higher rates of recanalization when compared with previous mechanical revascularization therapies

Note: results are presented for treatment group versus control group for randomized controlled trials.

ECASS, European Cooperative Acute Stroke Study; IA, intraarterial; IAT, intraarterial thrombolysis; IMS, Interventional Management of Stroke; IVT, intravenous thrombolysis; MERCI, Mechanical Embolus Removal in Cerebral Ischemia; mRS, modified Rankin scale; NINDS, National Institute of Neurological Disorders and Stroke; NR, not reported; PROACT, Prolyse in Acute Cerebral Thromboembolism; RCT, randomized controlled trial; rt-PA, recombinant tissue plasminogen activator; sICH, symptomatic intracranial hemorrhage.

with acute stroke treated within 6 h of symptom onset. As in PROACT I and II, patients displaying angiographic occlusions of the M1 or M2 MCA segments were randomized. Mechanical thrombus disruption was permitted only with a microguidewire. No other mechanical techniques were allowed. Intraarterial infusion of urokinase (120 000 IU for 5 min) was performed and repeated until the total dose reached 600 000 IU, 2 h had passed after starting the infusion, or complete recanalization was achieved. The trial was aborted prematurely by the steering committee after the approval of intravenous rt-PA in Japan. A metaanalysis of the PROACT I, PROACT II, and MELT trials, including 204 patients treated with IAT and 130 control patients, showed a lower rate of death or dependency at long-term follow-up with IAT compared with controls (58.5% vs. 69.2%; $P = 0.03$; OR 0.58; 95% CI 0.36–0.93) [53].

These studies established superiority of IAT within 6 h over antithrombotic therapy for MCA M1 and M2 occlusions. There is no level 1 data of the efficacy of IAT for distal ICA or posterior circulation occlusion. The superiority of IAT over IVT has not been demonstrated by randomized clinical studies. The FDA did not approve prourokinase, and it is currently not available for clinical use. Current American Heart Association/American Stroke Association (AHA/ASA) guidelines [54] recommend the use of IAT with rt-PA within 6 h from symptom onset for selected patients who have a major stroke due to MCA occlusion and who are not eligible for IVT. Therefore, at present, this approach should not preclude intravenous administration of rt-PA in all other eligible patients.

Special situations

Approximately 16–28% of ischemic stroke patients awaken with their deficits [55,56]. In these *wake-up strokes*, the onset of symptoms is defined as the "time last seen well." Because this is the time the patient went to sleep, these patients, unfortunately, are usually placed outside the window for thrombolysis or ineligible for entry into reperfusion clinical trials. Barreto *et al.* [57] reported that patients with wake-up stroke have a better outcome when they are treated. Adams *et al.* [58] in their post hoc analysis of wake-up stroke in the Abciximab in Emergency Stroke Treatment Trial-II (AbESTT-II) trial reported poorer outcomes after treatment. In our unpublished series Natarajan SK *et al.* [59] of 30 patients with stroke onset >8 h and wake-up stroke (mean presentation NIHSS, 13) selected for treatment on the basis of results of CT perfusion studies, a combination of endovascular revascularization strategies resulted in TIMI 2 or 3 recanalization in 67% of patients, with an sICH rate of 10%. At 3 months, 20% of patients improved to mRS <2, and the mortality was 33.3%.

Posterior circulation stroke differs in several aspects. The evolution of clinical symptoms is often gradual, making precise assessment of the onset of symptoms and of the time window for treatment difficult. Atherothrombosis (unstable plaque with thrombus) is more common. The risk of reocclusion after recanalization is therefore higher [60–63]. The natural history shows a poor outcome with a high mortality rate of 70–80%, unless recanalization is achieved [60,64]. A metaanalysis [65] of IAT in basilar artery occlusion shows a recanalization rate of 64% and a mortality rate of 87% in nonrecanalized patients, with a significant ($P < 0.001$) reduction in mortality to 37% in recanalized patients. Another metaanalysis [66] of IVT or IAT for basilar artery occlusion showed that the likelihood of a good outcome was 2% without recanalization. Recanalization was achieved more frequently with IAT (65% vs. 53%, $P = 0.05$), but the outcomes after IAT and IVT were similar. Levy *et al.* [67] performed a metaanalysis for predictors of outcome after IAT for vertebrobasilar artery occlusion and found failure to recanalize was associated with a higher mortality rate (relative risk, 2.34; 95% CI, 1.48–3.71). Studies have suggested extending the time window for treatment beyond or up to 24 h postictus [62,68,69].

Small retrospective case series [70,71] show the safety and efficacy of IAT with acceptable recanalization rates and outcomes in patients with *distal ICA occlusion*.

A metaanalysis [72] of 158 patients derived from eight different reports that had IAT for *central retinal artery occlusion* (CRAO) within 8.4 ± 4 h of symptom onset showed visual improvement in 93% of patients. The European Assessment Group for Lysis in the Eye (EAGLE) in 2002 started a randomized multicenter study comparing conservative management with IAT in patients with CRAO who presented within 20 h of symptom onset and with a visual acuity <0.32 [73,74].

For *periprocedural stroke* after major surgery, IAT may be considered and is proven to be relatively safe [75].

In the case of *failure of IVT* (e.g., lack of early improvement in neurologic status and NIHSS scores after the procedure), IAT may be considered [76].

Thrombolytic agents

These drugs are plasminogen activators and act by converting the inactive proenzyme, plasminogen, into the active enzyme, plasmin. Plasmin digests fibrinogen, fibrin monomers, and cross-linked fibrin (as found in a thrombus) into fibrin-degradation products. The plasminogen activators vary in stability, half-life, and fibrin selectivity. In general, the older nonfibrin-selective drugs (e.g., urokinase and streptokinase) can result in systemic hypofibrinogenemia and are not used now, whereas the fibrin-selective agents (e.g., rt-PA and r-prourokinase) are mostly active at the site of thrombosis (Table 57.4).

Antithrombotic therapy

The plasmin generated by thrombolysis leads to the production of thrombin, which is a potent platelet activator and converts fibrinogen to fibrin. Reocclusion after IVT (34%) and IAT (17%) has been shown [77]. Therefore, a strong

Table 57.4 Thrombolytics for stroke revascularization.

Alteplase (rt-PA) has a plasma half-life of 3.5 min and a high degree of fibrin affinity and specificity. The rt-PA dose used in cerebral IAT has ranged between 20 and 60 mg. The disadvantages of alteplase include its relatively short half-life and limited penetration into the clot matrix because of strong binding with surface fibrin and some neurotoxic properties, including activation of metalloproteinases leading to cerebral hemorrhage and edema and amplification of calcium currents through the *N*-methyl D-aspartate receptor, leading to excitotoxicity and neuronal death [123]

Prourokinase (r-prourokinase) is the proenzyme precursor of urokinase. It has a plasma half-life of 7 min and high fibrin specificity

Reteplase is a structurally modified form of alteplase, with a longer half-life (15–18 min). In addition, it does not bind as highly to fibrin; unbound reteplase can thus, theoretically, better penetrate the clot and potentially improve *in vivo* fibrinolytic activity

Tenecteplase is another modified form of rt-PA with a longer half-life (17 min), greater fibrin specificity, and greater resistance to plasminogen activator inhibitor-1

Desmoteplase is more potent and more selective for fibrin-bound plasminogen than any other known plasminogen activator. It is not activated by fibrinogen or β-amyloid proteins (factors that may exacerbate the risk for ICH) and inhibits rt-PA-induced potentiation of excitotoxic injury. The trials Desmoteplase in Acute Ischemic Stroke Trial (DIAS), Dose Escalation of Desmoteplase for Acute Ischemic Stroke (DEDAS), and DIAS-2 [19,20,25] evaluated the effect of i.v. administration of desmoteplase 3–9 h after symptom onset in patients with stroke who present with mismatch on magnetic resonance imaging or computed tomography perfusion

rationale exists for the adjuvant use of antithrombotic agents. Systemic anticoagulation with intravenous heparin is used in the periprocedural phase of IAT for augmentation of the thrombolytic effect, prevention of acute reocclusion, and reduction in the risk of catheter-related embolism. However, these benefits must be weighed against the potentially increased risk of ICH when heparin is combined with a thrombolytic agent.

Glycoprotein IIb/IIIa antagonists

The use of glycoprotein (GP) IIb/IIIa antagonists, such as abciximab (ReoPro, Eli Lilly, Indianapolis, IN, USA), eptifibatide (Integrilin, Millennium Pharmaceuticals/Schering-Plough, Kenilworth, NJ, USA), or tirofiban (Aggrastat, Merck & Company, Whitehouse Station, NJ, USA) in ischemic stroke remains investigational. The Combined Approach to Lysis Utilizing Eptifibatide and rt-PA in Acute Ischemic Stroke (CLEAR) trial [78] evaluated the combination of low-dose intravenous rt-PA and eptifibatide in patients with NIHSS scores of >5 who presented within 3 h from stroke onset.

The study enrolled a total of 94 subjects, with 69 patients receiving the combination therapy and 25 patients receiving intravenous rt-PA therapy. There was one (1.4%) sICH in the combination group and two (8.0%) in the standard treatment group (*P* = 0.17). There was a nonsignificant trend toward increased efficacy with the standard-dose rt-PA treatment arm. The ReoPro Retavase Reperfusion of Stroke Safety Study Imaging Evaluation (ROSIE) is an NIH-sponsored phase 2 trial that is evaluating the use of intravenous reteplase in combination with abciximab for the treatment of MRI-selected patients with stroke within 3–24 h from onset. Preliminary analysis of the first 21 patients enrolled has revealed no sICH or major hemorrhage [79]. Conversely, the AbESTT II trial, a phase 3 multicenter, randomized, double-blinded, and placebo-controlled study evaluating the safety and efficacy of abciximab in acute ischemic stroke treated within 6 h after stroke onset or within 3 h of awakening with stroke symptoms, was stopped early due to high rates of sICH or fatal ICH in the abciximab-treated patients (5.5% vs. 0.5%, *P* = 0.002) [80]. Data for the use of glycoprotein IIb/IIIa inhibitors in conjunction with IAT and mechanical revascularization are even more scant. We use these drugs at our center for reocclusion after reopening of the vessel to change the prothombotic state to an antithrombotic state. When we do so, we try to maintain the activated coagulation time at <200 s to minimize bleeding.

Augmented fibrinolysis

Intraarterial sonothrombolysis was shown to be of benefit in the IMS-II trial [81]. The MicroLysUS infusion catheter (EKOS, Bothell, WA, USA) is a 2.5F single-lumen end-hole design microcatheter with a 2-mm 2.1-MHz piezoelectric sonography element (average power, 0.21–0.45 W) at its distal tip, which creates a microenvironment of ultrasonic vibration to facilitate thrombolysis. The net result is enhanced clot dissolution without fragmentation of emboli. The device was used in 33 of the 81 patients enrolled in the IMS-II trial. A comparison of final angiographic outcomes between IMS-II subjects treated with the EKOS catheter and IMS-I subjects treated with the standard microcatheter demonstrated TIMI grade 2 or 3 recanalization rates at the specific site of arterial occlusion of 73% (24 of 33) in EKOS-treated patients versus 56% (33 of 59) in standard microcatheter-treated patients (*P* = 0.11) [81]. This device is being investigated further in the randomized IMS-III trial.

Intravenous and intraarterial thrombolysis— bridging therapy

At many centers, accessible occlusions in the anterior circulation are treated with IAT, either in patients in whom reperfusion did not occur after IVT or even as a first line of treatment. As mentioned, however, there is no randomized trial comparing clinical outcome after IVT and IAT. An NIHSS >12 suggests an occlusion of a proximal, large vessel and, therefore, a high thrombus burden [13]. Recanalization rates of IV rt-PA for proximal arterial occlusion are poor and range from only 10% for ICA occlusion to 30% for MCA occlusion [14]. In the NINDS trial [6], patients with NIHSS scores >20 had a <6% absolute risk reduction in achieving mRS <1 at 90 days. These patients with large vessel occlusions with a high clot burden are less likely to improve with IVT. PROACT II [9] gives proof of reperfusion and good outcomes after IAT in large vessel occlusion.

In the IMS-II trial [81], combination IV and IA therapy had a better outcome than placebo treatment in the NINDS trial [6]; and, if secondary outcome measures (mRS, NIHSS, and Barthel Index) were considered, a statistically better outcome was seen with combination therapy in IMS-II than with IV treatment in NINDS. Recanalization was achieved only after rescue IA therapy in most patients in the NINDS trial. A bridging strategy between IV and IA thrombolysis has the advantage of not delaying IV therapy, while identifying nonresponders with persisting large artery occlusion. This approach is being tested in IMS-III, with initial IV rt-PA followed by artery reopening by thrombolytics or clot retrieval if vessel occlusion is demonstrated [82]. A summary of the trials (IMS-I and IMS-II) using combination IVT and IAT is shown in Table 57.3.

Intraarterial versus intravenous thrombolysis

The outcome and morbidity of patients treated with IVT and IAT were compared at two different stroke treatment centers [83]. Patients were selected based on the presence of a hyperdense MCA sign on CT imaging, indicating an M1 occlusion. Fifty-five patients were treated with IAT using urokinase; 59 patients underwent IVT with rt-PA. Although the time to treatment was significantly ($P = 0.0001$) longer in the IAT group (mean 244 min) than in the IVT group (mean 156 min), the study revealed a more frequent favorable outcome for patients treated with intraarterial urokinase (53%) compared with patients treated with IVT (23%; $P = 0.001$). In addition, the mortality rate was reduced in the IAT group compared with the IVT group (4.7% vs. 23%; $P = 0.001$).

Mechanical recanalization techniques

Although thrombolysis is effective in some patients, the restricted improvement in outcomes, limited recanalization rate, and the rate of complications give room for further improvement in stroke treatment strategies. Recent developments have been focused on the possibilities of mechanical recanalization. All mechanical thrombectomy devices are delivered by endovascular access via a proximal approach to the occlusion site.

The mechanical recanalization systems can be divided into two major groups according to where they apply force on the thrombus: (1) *proximal devices* apply force to the proximal base of the thrombus (this group includes various aspiration catheters), and (2) *distal devices* approach the thrombus prox-

Table 57.5 Mechanical revascularization strategies.

Advantages
They lessen and may even preclude the use of chemical thrombolytics, thus reduce the incidence of symptomatic intracranial hemorrhage
They may extend the treatment window beyond the limit of 6–8h
Mechanical fragmentation of the clot increases the surface area of the clot available for endogenous and exogenous fibrinolysis
Recanalization time may be faster
They may be effective for thrombi or other material resistant to thrombolytics that occlude the vessel
They have emerged as the key option for patients who have contraindication for pharmacologic thrombolysis such as recent surgery or abnormal hemostasis [124], or have a late presentation [28,29]

Disadvantages
Technical difficulty of navigating these devices through the intracranial vasculature
Excessive trauma to the vasculature
Distal embolization from fragmented thrombus

imally but then are advanced by guide wire and microcatheter across the thrombus to be unsheathed distally, where force is applied to the distal base of the thrombus. This group includes snare-like, basket-like, or coil-like devices.

In an animal model [84], proximal devices were faster in application and associated with a low complication rate. The distal devices were more successful at removing thrombotic material, but their method of application and attendant thrombus compaction increased the risk of thromboembolic events and vasospasm [85,86].

Advantages and disadvantages of mechanical revascularization strategies overall are summarized in Table 57.5.

Distal devices

Compared with IAT and the use of proximal devices, the use of distal devices is technically more complex. Distal devices are regularly used in combination with proximal balloon occlusion in the ICA, in addition to aspiration from the guiding catheter, to reduce this risk of distal thromboembolism. In general, an 8–9F sheath and balloon catheter of similar size are used. After placement of the balloon catheter in the ICA, a microcatheter in combination with a microwire is navigated to the occlusion site. This catheter then has to be advanced beyond the thrombus. For some devices, an injection of contrast material is recommended distal to the thrombus to estimate the length of the occlusion and to illustrate the anatomy of the distal vessel. The device is then introduced into the microcatheter and unsheathed behind the thrombus. The balloon at the tip of the guiding catheter is inflated. During slow retraction of the device and mobilization of the thrombus, aspiration is applied at the guiding catheter. The device and

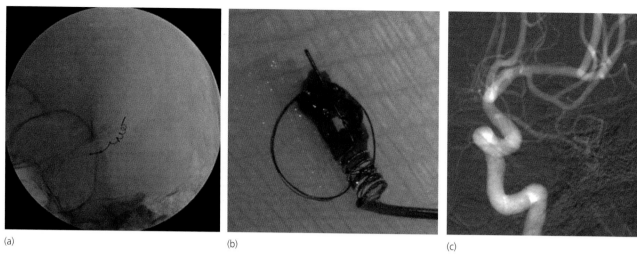

(a)   (b)   (c)

Figure 57.3 Merci clot retriever device (Concentric Medical) for a patient with an acute middle cerebral artery occlusion. (a) Plain film during angiogram showing a Merci device in the M1. (b) Clot removed with the Merci retriever. (c) Post-Merci recanalization angiogram showing TIMI 3 recanalization.

thrombus are retrieved into the guiding catheter, and the balloon is deflated. In clinical practice, the entire procedure often has to be repeated multiple times to recanalize the vessel. Furthermore, the application of the balloon catheter might be limited in cases of high-grade ICA stenosis. Although the approach is similar for all distal devices, the design and performance of the available device might differ significantly.

Merci device

The Merci Retrieval device (Concentric Medical, Inc., Mountain View, CA, USA) (Fig. 57.3) is a shaped wire constructed of nitinol. The flexible corkscrew-like tip can easily be delivered through a microcatheter into the vessel distal to the occlusion site. When deployed, it returns to its preformed coiled shape to ensnare the thrombus. The thrombus is bypassed and the retriever deployed from inside the catheter distal to the thrombus. The corkscrew-like tip is pulled back slowly to ensnare the clot as a corkscrew would ensnare a cork. The retriever is then retracted into the guide catheter under proximal flow arrest. Different versions of the device are available (Fig. 57.4); in the first-generation devices (X5 and X6), the nitinol wire was shaped in helical tapering coil loops. The second-generation devices (L4, L5, and L6) differ from the first generation X devices by the inclusion of a system of arcading filaments attached to a nontapering helical nitinol coil, which has a 90° angle in relation to the proximal wire component. The third-generation devices (V series) have variable pitch loops under a linear configuration with attached filaments. The retriever device is deployed through a 2.4F microcatheter (14X or 18L, Concentric Medical). The recent addition of a 4.3F distal access catheter has provided additional coaxial support to the system, resulting in improved deliverability with the potential for simultaneous thromboaspiration as well. The devices are available in various diameters, from 1.5 to 3 mm, depending on the caliber of the occluded vessel.

In 2004, the FDA approved the use of the Merci device for clot removal from intracranial vessels in patients with ischemic stroke. FDA approval was based on a review of data obtained in the multicenter MERCI trial that involved 141 patients (mean age 60 years; mean NIHSS score 20) ineligible for standard thrombolytic therapy [87]. The time window between onset of clinical symptoms and endovascular treatment was extended to 8 h, compared with the 6-hour window usually applied for IAT. This trial reported a recanalization rate (TIMI 2 or 3) using the X-type Merci retriever of 48%. sICH was found in 7.8% of the patients, mainly after treatment of ICA and MCA occlusions (90%). In the study, the number of attempts to retrieve the clot was limited to six; a mean of 2.9 attempts was performed for recanalization and the mean procedural time was 2.1 h. With respect to device-related complications, the study reported vessel perforations (4.2%), subarachnoid hemorrhages (2.1%), and embolization of thrombotic material (2.1%).

The recently published Multi MERCI trial [29] was a prospective, multi-center, single-arm registry that included 164 patients (mean age 68 years; mean NIHSS 19) treated with different Merci retrieval systems (X5, X6, and L5). Again, the time window between onset of clinical symptoms and endovascular treatment was extended to 8 h, and the majority of patients (92%) were treated for an ICA or MCA occlusion. Patients with persistent large vessel occlusion after IVT (with rt-PA) were also included in the study, and adjunctive IAT using rt-PA was allowed. In 55% of the interventions, mechanical thrombectomy led to recanalization (TIMI 2 and 3). After adjunctive IAT, 68% of the target vessels were recanalized. Clinically significant device-related complications occurred in 5.5%, and the rate of sICH was 9.8%. At

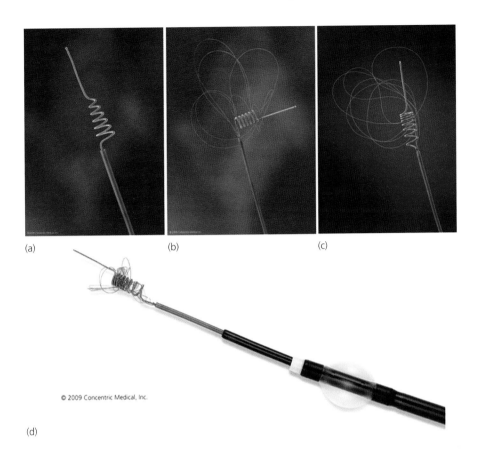

Figure 57.4 Types of Merci devices:
(a) Type X, (b) type L, (c) type V. (d) Catheter
system. Courtesy of Concentric Medical.
Mountain View, CA, USA.

© 2009 Concentric Medical, Inc.

90 days, 36% of the patients had a favorable outcome (mRS, 0–2) and the mortality rate was 34%. Two ongoing prospective randomized trials are using the device, the MR and Recanalization of Stroke Clots Using Embolectomy (MR RESCUE; NCT00389467) trial and the IMS-III trial [82].

The Merci device has also increased recanalization rates with intracranial ICA occlusion. Flint *et al.* [88] reported 80 patients (mean age, 67 years; mean NIHSS score, 20; mean time from stroke onset to treatment, 4.1 h) with angiographically proved intracranial ICA occlusion who were enrolled in the MERCI and Multi MERCI Part I trials. Eleven patients (14%) also received intravenous rt-PA. Recanalization of the intracranial ICA was achieved in 53% of patients with the Merci retriever alone (42 of 80) and in 63% (50 of 80) with the Merci retriever plus adjunctive endovascular treatment. Overall, 25% (20 of 79 patients) had a good neurologic outcome at 90 days (39% of recanalized patients vs. 3% of nonrecanalized patients, $P = 0.001$). The overall 90-day mortality rate was 46% (30% of recanalized patients vs. 73% of nonrecanalized patients, $P = 0.001$). The rate of sICH was 10% (8 of 80 patients).

Phenox clot retriever

The Phenox Clot Retriever (Phenox, Bochum, Germany) consists of a highly flexible nitinol–platinum alloy compound core wire surrounded by an attenuated palisade of perpendicularly oriented, stiff, polyamide microfilaments trimmed in a conical shape, which have an increasing diameter distally and are resistant to unraveling. This flexible design allows the use of two devices simultaneously (e.g., in bifurcations or larger vessels), and the microfilaments might be able to reduce distal emboli owing to a filter effect [89]. The device is molded to the body of a 0.010-inch microguidewire and is available in three sizes ranging from 1–3 mm proximally and from 2–5 mm distally. It is introduced into the target vessel through a 0.021- or 0.027-inch microcatheter deployed distal to the thrombus and slowly pulled back under continuous aspiration via the guiding catheter. The smallest version is capable of recanalizing vessels with diameters well below 2 mm, such as the distal MCA branches [90]. A second generation of the device (Phenox Clot Retriever CAGE) incorporates a nitinol cage into the previous design and was developed for the treatment of thrombi with firmer consistency.

Other distal devices like the Neuronet device (Guidant, Santa Clara, CA, USA), the Catch device (Balt, Montmorency, France), the Attractor-18 device (Boston Scientific/Target Therapeutics, Fremont, CA, USA), the Alligator Retrieval Device (Chestnut Medical Technology, Menlo Park, CA, USA), the In-Time Retriever (Boston Scientific, Natick, MA, USA), the Trispan device (Boston Scientific), and the Ensnare device (InterV, Gainesville, FL, USA) are being tried for embolectomy in stroke.

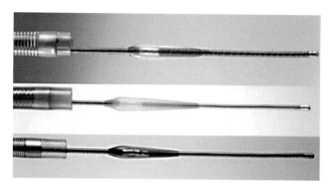

Figure 57.5 Penumbra device: sizes 026-inch, 032-inch and 041-inch, from bottom to top. Courtesy of Penumbra, Alameda, CA, USA.

Proximal devices

From the procedural point of view, proximal devices are comparable to IAT. Access is usually gained with a 6–8F sheath. After placement of the guiding catheter, the device is navigated to the proximal surface of the clot. This approach omits repetitive passing of the occlusion site.

Thromboaspiration devices

Penumbra device

The most remarkable and promising device of this group is the Penumbra system (Penumbra, Alameda, CA, USA) (Fig. 57.5). It has received FDA approval for use in the revascularization of patients with acute ischemic stroke. The Penumbra system consists of a microcatheter attached to continuous aspiration via a dedicated aspiration pump system. A microwire/separator with an olive-shaped tip is used to fragment the thrombus from proximal to distal. Direct thrombus extraction can also be attempted with a ring retriever while a balloon-guided catheter is used to temporarily arrest flow. Both microcatheter and separator are available in various sizes and diameters to adjust the device to different anatomic settings.

A prospective, single-arm, independently monitored trial was performed to assess the efficiency and safety of the system [91]. A total of 23 patients (mean age, 60 years; mean NIHSS score, 21) were enrolled within 8 h after the onset of symptoms. Most (43%) patients had occlusions in the posterior circulation. In nine patients, additional IAT was performed using rt-PA. The target vessel was recanalized (TIMI 2 or 3) in all patients. The high mortality rate (45%) was likely related to the patient population enrolled. sICH occurred in 15% of the patients. McDougall *et al.* [92] reported the results of a prospective multicenter single-arm trial of 125 patients with acute stroke who underwent revascularization with the Penumbra device. TIMI 2 or 3 recanalization was achieved in 81.6% patients with an sICH rate of 11.2%.

Angiojet system

The Angiojet (Possis Medical, Minneapolis, MN, USA) is a catheter designed to perform hemolytic thrombectomy based

on the Venturi effect (see also chapter 35, Fig. 35.5). In addition to the catheter, the system has a high-pressure water pump to pump a saline solution in a 0.5-mm metal tube to the catheter tip. The catheter lumen is located in a 4F catheter in which the main lumen is used to house the microwire and for aspiration. At the catheter tip, water can be sprayed in small jets backward into the catheter, thus creating negative pressure that sucks in the endovascular thrombotic material and conveys it in a backflow out of the catheter. The poor flexibility of the first Angiojet catheter limited its use to segments of the large vessels supplying the brain. Nevertheless, this method has been successfully used to treat some patients with ICA occlusions or basilar artery thromboses [93]. A safety study of a smaller version of the Angiojet, the NeuroJet (Possis Medical), which was designed to enable catheterization of the MCA, was terminated early owing to vessel dissections. Modifications of both the catheter and the study protocol are currently undergoing evaluation in a phase 1 trial, the Thrombectomy in Middle Cerebral Artery Embolism (TIME) study.

Mechanical thrombus disruption

Microguidewire manipulation and snare

The most common method for mechanical thrombus disruption is probing the thrombus with a microguidewire. This technique appears to be useful in facilitating pharmacologic thrombolysis [94]. Alternatively, a snare can be used for multiple passes through the occlusion to disrupt the thrombus [95,96]. A snare can also be used for clot retrieval, mostly in situations in which the clot has a firm consistency or contains solid material [97].

Balloon angioplasty

Percutaneous balloon angioplasty is a known angiologic–cardiologic procedure for the treatment of vessel occlusions. By omitting the repetitive retrieval attempts needed for mechanical thrombectomy, this approach may reduce severe complications and thromboembolic events. Nakano *et al.* [98] compared results for 36 patients with acute stroke who underwent intraarterial thrombolytic therapy alone and 34 patients who underwent angioplasty and subsequent intraarterial thrombolytic therapy. The rate of partial or complete recanalization (based on TIMI scores of 2 or 3), was 91.2% for the angioplasty group versus 63.9% for the thrombolytic group, and the incidence of ICH was 2.9% for the angioplasty group and 19.4% for the thrombolytic group. Independent outcome (scored by mRS at 3 months) was also better in the angioplasty group (in 73.5 vs. in 50% of the thrombolytic group). Although limited data exist regarding the rate of acute restenosis after intracranial angioplasty for stroke, concerns based on the cardiac literature persist; and the additional treatment of occlusive and atherosclerotic lesions with intracranial stent therapy is becoming more popular. In a multicenter randomized trial comparing stent placement with angioplasty for acute myocardial infarction, the mean minimal residual luminal diameter was larger after treatment with stent therapy than with angioplasty alone [99]. In addition, the need for target-vessel revascularization because of ischemia, as well as the occurrence of death and reinfarction, were lower with stenting. The trial concluded that in patients with acute myocardial infarction, implantation of a stent has clinical benefits beyond those of angioplasty alone.

Laser-assisted thrombolysis

Two devices (EPAR and LaTIS) that use different laser technologies have been used to disrupt intracranial clots. The EPAR (Endovasix, Belmont, CA, USA) is a mechanical clot-fragmentation device. However, the emulsification of the thrombus is a mechanical thrombolysis and not a direct laser-induced ablation. The LaTIS laser device (LaTIS, Minneapolis, MN, USA) uses the slow injection of contrast material as a "light pipe" to carry the energy from the catheter to the embolus. In a pilot study of 34 patients, vessel recanalization occurred in 11 of 18 patients (61.1%) in whom complete EPAR treatment (IAT in 13 patients) was possible [100]. EPAR treatment was not possible in the rest. One patient had a vessel rupture resulting in fatality. There were two sICHs (5.9% of 34 patients) and the overall mortality rate was 38.2%. The LaTIS device was evaluated in a safety and feasibility trial at two US centers [101]. A preliminary account reported that the device could not be deployed to the level of the occlusion in two of the first five patients, and enrollment was stopped at 12 patients [101].

Stent-assisted revascularization

Self-expanding stents designed specifically for the cerebrovasculature are available and can be delivered to target areas of intracranial stenosis with a success rate of >95%, with an increased safety profile as they are deployed at significantly lower pressures than balloon-mounted coronary stents [102]. Advantages and disadvantages of stent-assisted revascularization are summarized in Table 57.6. Studies of arterial reocclusion during IAT have shown rates of 17%, with a subsequent association with poor outcome [77].

Balloon-mounted coronary stents

Initial clinical experience with stents involved the use of coronary balloon-mounted stents to re-establish flow through acutely occluded vessels. Levy *et al.* [103] reported 19 patients with a median baseline NIHSS score of 16 in whom the average time-to-treatment was 210 ± 160 min with balloon-mounted stents. The overall recanalization rate (TIMI 2 or 3) was 79%, and there was no sICH. In another report [104], independent predictors for recanalization of occluded vessels included stenting (*P* < 0.001) and the use of intraarterial thrombolytics and, if there was extensive clot burden or if a stent was placed, administration of eptifibatide. These

Table 57.6 Stent-assisted revascularization.

Advantages
Immediate restoration of flow in the occluded vessel
High recanalization rates
Decreased chances of reocclusion after treatment
Stents with radial expansive force like Wingspan (Boston Scientific, Natick, MA) can be used in atherothrombotic lesions with proven safety.

Disadvantages
A large number of stokes are caused by emboli in a normal intracranial vessel and, hence, may need only embolectomy and not a permanent scaffold.
Stent navigability and deployment is possible only in the proximal vessels around the circle of Willis and not in the distal intracranial vasculature.
Patients need to be on dual antiplatelet therapy for 3 months after stent placement; this may potentially increase the intracranial hemorrhage rate.

studies established the concept of stents for acute stroke revascularization.

Self-expanding stents

A total of five intracranial self-expanding stents (SESs) are currently available: (1) the Neuroform stent (Boston Scientific), (2) the Enterprise stent (Cordis/Johnson & Johnson, Warren, NJ, USA), (3) the Leo stent (Balt Extrusion, Montmorency, France), (4) the Solitaire/Solo stent (ev3, Irvine, CA, USA), and (5) the Wingspan stent (Boston Scientific) (Fig. 57.6). The first four devices are currently marketed for stent-assisted coil embolization of wide-necked aneurysms, whereas the Wingspan stent is approved for the treatment of symptomatic intracranial atherosclerotic disease. Both the Neuroform and the Wingspan stents have an open-cell design, whereas the Enterprise, Leo, and Solitaire/Solo stents have a closed-cell design. The closed-cell design allows resheathing of the stent after partial deployment (70% for Enterprise; 90% for Leo) [105,106] or even full deployment (Solitaire/Solo) [107].

Higher rates of recanalization and lower rates of vasospasm and side-branch occlusion were noticed with SESs than with balloon-mounted stents in a canine model of vessels acutely occluded with thromboemboli [108]. As opposed to acute coronary syndromes in which plaque rupture in an underlying atheroma is the most frequent culprit, most cases of acute intracranial vascular occlusions are related to an embolus in the absence of any *in situ* vascular pathology. Therefore, balloon angioplasty with high-pressure balloons and balloon-expandable stents is typically not necessary to recanalize the vessel and may only increase the chance of serious complications, such as vessel rupture or dissection. Finally, SESs cause less endothelial damage and, therefore, may result in lower

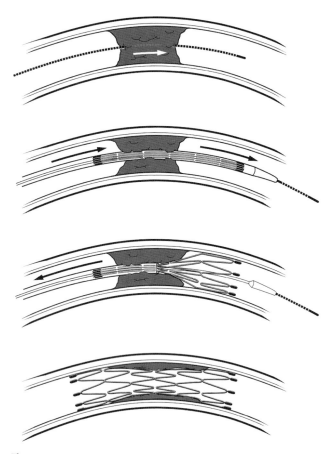

Figure 57.6 Wingspan stent (Boston Scientific, Natick, MA, USA) for recanalization. From top to bottom: occlusive clot crossed with a microwire; placement of stent across the occlusion; deployment of stent, thus trapping the occlusion; and recanalization. From Levy *et al.* [109], with permission from the American Society of Neuroradiology.

rates of early reocclusion or late stent stenosis. SESs with higher radial force (e.g., Wingspan) will likely play a key role in the management of patients with acute stroke related to intracranial atherosclerotic disease [102].

Levy *et al.* [109] described the use of SESs (Neuroform3 or Wingspan) to treat 18 patients with stroke (19 lesions) presenting with acute focal occlusions involving the MCA (9 lesions), the internal carotid artery terminus (ICAT-T) (7 lesions), or the vertebrobasilar system (3 lesions). Stent placement was the initial mechanical maneuver in six cases, whereas other cases involved a combination of pharmacologic and/or mechanical maneuvers prestenting, including 10 balloon angioplasties and nine clot retrieval attempts. Glycoprotein IIb/IIIa inhibitors were administered in 10 patients intra- or immediately postprocedurally to avoid acute in-stent thrombosis. TIMI 2 or 3 revascularization was achieved in 15 of 19 lesions (79%). There were no intraprocedural complications, but seven patients had ICH (either intraparenchymal or subarachnoid) on postprocedural CT imaging, two of which were fatal. One patient developed early stent rethrombosis. The inhospital mortality rate was 38.9% (7 of 18 patients).

Four patients had mRS scores of ≤3 at the 3-month follow-up evaluation.

Zaidat *et al.* [110] evaluated the use of Neuroform (four patients) or Wingspan (five patients) stents in nine patients with acute stroke with occlusions involving the MCA (six lesions), ICA (two lesions), or the vertebrobasilar junction (one lesion). Successful stent deployment across the clot occurred in eight of nine (89%) patients. In one patient, a Wingspan stent could not be tracked beyond the MCA–ICA junction and was deployed in the proximal clot. Complete (TIMI 3) and partial or complete (TIMI 2 or 3) recanalization occurred in 67% and 89% of the patients, respectively. There was one ICH (11%) and one acute in-stent thrombosis (successfully treated with abciximab and balloon angioplasty). The mortality rate was 33% (three of nine patients). All survivors achieved an mRS score of ≤2. Follow-up angiography was performed in four of the nine patients at a mean of 8 months (range 2–14 months) and showed no stent restenosis.

On the basis of these preliminary data, we received FDA approval for a pilot study, Stent-Assisted Recanalization in acute Ischemic Stroke (SARIS) [111], to evaluate the Wingspan stent for revascularization in patients who did not improve after IVT or had a contraindication for IVT. Mean time from stroke onset to intervention was 5 h 13 min. Total time from procedure onset to vessel recanalization was 45 min. Average presenting NIHSS score was 14. Seventeen patients presented with a TIMI score of 0 and three patients presented with a TIMI score of 1. Occluded vessels included the right MCA (11 patients), left MCA (five patients), basilar artery (three patients), and right carotid "T" (Terminus) (one patient). Self-expanding intracranial stents were placed in 19 of 20 enrolled patients. One patient experienced recanalization of the occluded vessel with positioning of the Wingspan stent delivery system prior to stent deployment. In two patients, the tortuous vessel did not allow tracking of the Wingspan stent. The more navigable Enterprise stent was used in both these cases. Twelve patients had other adjunctive therapies: IA eptifibatide (10 patients), IA rt-PA (two patients), angioplasty (eight patients), intravenous rt- PA (two patients). TIMI 2 or 3 recanalization was achieved in 100% of patients; 65% of patients improved >4 points in NIHSS score after treatment. One patient (5%) had sICH and two had asymptomatic ICH. At 1-month follow-up, 12 of 20 (60%) patients had an mRS ≤2, and nine (45%) had an mRS ≤1. Mortality at 1 month was 25%. None of these patients died due to any cause related to stent placement; all deaths were due to the severity of the initial stroke and associated comorbidities.

Temporary endovascular bypass

The need for an aggressive antithrombotic regimen after stent implantation remains one of the major limitations to its use in acute stroke. However, the advent of closed-cell stents has allowed resheathing–removal of the stent after recanalization is achieved, obviating the need for dual antiplatelet therapy, which could potentially increase the risk of hemorrhagic conversion of the infarct. In addition, this technique should eliminate the risk of delayed in-stent stenosis. Kelly *et al.* [112] and Hauck *et al.* [113] reported the use of the Enterprise stent as a temporary endovascular bypass in acute stroke. In both cases, the Enterprise stent was partially deployed for some time and retrieved with successful recanalization of the occluded vessel.

Stent platform-based thrombectomy device

The Solitaire™ FR Revascularization Device (ev3, Irvine, CA, USA) (Fig. 57.7) is a recoverable self-expanding thrombectomy device developed based on the Solitaire/Solo stent [107]. The advantages of this device are that it is a fully recoverable SES platform-based device that can be used as both a temporary endovascular bypass and a thrombectomy device. The device restores flow immediately and avoids the placement of a permanent stent and, thus, the necessary antithrombotic therapy and risk of in-stent stenosis. Moreover, it can be electrolytically detached like a coil in case a permanent stent is necessary, such as in the setting of an atherothrombotic lesion. We evaluated the safety and efficacy of this device in a canine stroke model with soft and firm clots [114]. The device could be easily deployed and recovered and restored TIMI 2 or 3 flow immediately in all cases. Minimal residual clot in two of four instances required a second pass for complete clot retrieval. Minimal vasospasm was observed in two of four cases.

Extracranial carotid revascularization

Acute strokes related to isolated proximal (extracranial) ICA occlusions typically have a better prognosis, given the compensatory collateral flow at the level of the external carotid artery—ICA anastomosis (e.g., ophthalmic artery) and/or circle of Willis. However, patients with an incomplete circle of Willis or with tandem occlusions of the intracranial ICA–MCA often present with severe strokes and are potential candidates for emergent revascularization. Stent placement in the proximal cervical vessels may also be required to gain access to the intracranial thrombus with other mechanical devices or catheters. Furthermore, brisk antegrade flow is essential for the maintenance of distal vascular patency, as is particularly evident in patients with severe proximal stenoses who commonly develop rethrombosis after vessel recanalization. Recent case series have shown success and good outcome after endovascular treatment of acute ischemic stroke due to proximal extracranial ICA occlusions [115–119]. The distal intracranial lesions seen after stenting of the extracranial lesion may be due to emboli caused by reopening of the occluded ICA. This could be prevented or at least minimized by using a balloon guide catheter, such as the Concentric guide (Concentric Medical), or a sheath, such as the Gore flow-reversal device (WL Gore & Associates, Flagstaff,

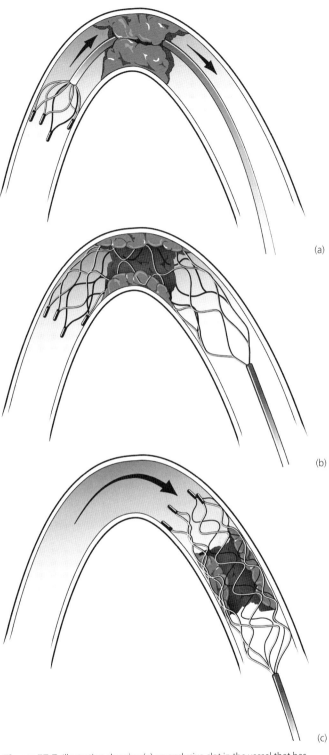

(a)

(b)

(c)

Figure 57.7 Illustration showing (a) an occlusive clot in the vessel that has been crossed by the Rebar microcatheter (ev3). The microwire has been exchanged with the Solitaire device (ev3) that is being deployed in the direction shown by the arrows. (b) The Solitaire device is completely deployed and pushes the clot to the side, restoring blood flow immediately in the occluded vessel. (c) The Solitaire with the clot and the Rebar are pulled with the clot into the guide catheter with constant syringe aspiration from the guide catheter.

Table 57.7 Our protocol for acute stroke revascularization.

- Patients with a diagnosis of stroke arriving at the emergency room within 3 h of symptom onset are given i.v. rt-PA unless they have a contraindication to i.v. rt-PA
- Patients who have contraindications for thrombolytic agents are evaluated for mechanical revascularization strategies, and patients who fail to improve by 4 points on the NIHSS after i.v. thrombolysis are evaluated for endovascular revascularization
- All patients who either arrive between 3 and 24 h of stroke onset, have wake-up strokes, or have an NIHSS score >8 at presentation are evaluated for endovascular revascularization
- The decision to perform a cerebral angiogram is done after assessing the following: premorbid status of the patient, CT angiogram from the heart to the head, CT perfusion studies to evaluate the ischemic penumbra, and a noncontrast cranial CT scan to rule out ICH
- A cerebral angiogram is performed and revascularization considered only if the patient had a premorbid mRS ≤1, CT perfusion studies show a penumbra of >50% of the volume of the territory of the occluded vessel, and CT does not show ICH
- Every patient considered for endovascular revascularization is given a bolus of i.v. heparin that is weight adjusted to maintain the activated coagulation time 250 s or greater. If the patient is not taking aspirin or clopidogrel (or ticlopidine) the patient will be treated with aspirin (enteric-coated, if necessary), 325 mg. Patients considered for stent placement will be given a loading dose of either clopidogrel (600 mg) or ticlopidine (1 g)
- Endovascular revascularization options—IAT with rt-PA, wire manipulation, Merci device, Penumbra—are chosen depending on the site and length of occlusion, ability to use thrombolytics in the patient, and nature of the clot. We prefer to use mechanical revascularization strategies as the first choice in preference to IAT whenever possible
- Intraaterial glycoprotein IIb/IIIa is used for situations in which reocclusion due to thrombus formation is seen after recanalization
- Wingspan stent placement is used as a bail out in patients who cannot be recanalized with current FDA-approved modalities and have an occlusion at a site that can be stented under Humanitarian Device Exemption and FDA-approved trials
- IAT and the mechanical revascularization methods are combined when appropriate
- The patients are observed in the intensive care unit for 6–12 h post treatment, and the blood pressure is kept around 150/90 mmHg to avoid reperfusion injury

CT, computed tomography; FDA, Food and Drug Administration; IAT, intraarterial thrombolysis; ICH, intracranial hemorrhage; NIHSS, National Institute of Health Stroke Scale; rt-PA, recombinant tissue plasminogen activator.

AZ, USA), for temporary flow arrest or flow reversal with aspiration, especially when antegrade flow is restored. The operator needs to check to make sure that the inner diameter of the balloon guide catheter is large enough to accommodate the chosen stent system.

In our series (EF Hauck *et al.*, unpublished data, 2009) of 22 patients with extracranial complete ICA occlusion, 21 patients had tandem intracranial occlusions (petrocavernous ICA 7; ICA-T 7; and MCA 7). The mean age was 62.5 years and mean presentation NIHSS score was 14.4. A single stent was used in six patients, and multiple stents were used in 12 patients (cervical only). Adjunctive therapy was used—intraarterial rt-PA (two patients), microwire manipulation (seven patients), Penumbra (two patients), Merci (eight patients), eptifibatide (15 patients), intracranial angioplasty (two patients). TIMI 2 or 3 recanalization was achieved in 77.3% of patients; 50% of patients had NIHSS score ≤3 at discharge. Recanalization was possible in 15 of 17 (88.2%) patients, with partial distal preservation of vessels, whereas it was not possible in all five patients who had complete occlusion at multiple segments of the ICA distal to the proximal occlusion. Thus, opening a complete occlusion of the extracranial ICA is possible and safe. The operator needs to assess for distal lesions, because they are common, with possibly CT or MR angiography before intervention as another complete distal occlusion may make the possibility of revascularization dismal. A recent report has recommended IAT through the posterior communicating or anterior communicating arteries to achieve higher recanalization rates and better outcomes [120].

The current protocol for selection of treatment strategies for revascularization of acute ischemic stroke patients at our institute is shown in Table 57.7.

Conclusion

Clinical outcome after acute ischemic stroke depends on the territory affected, the time span between onset of symptoms and revascularization, the recanalization rate of any specific revascularization strategy, and the occurrence of ICH or major procedure-related complications. At most centers, IVT or IAT are now the standard treatment, sometimes combined in a bridging concept. Although established, thrombolytic therapy is not effective in all patients, carries a risk of ICH, and has a limited time window for treatment. Current research therefore focuses on various mechanical revascularization techniques to achieve fast and sustained reperfusion. New-generation thrombolytic drugs are believed to reduce the incidence of sICH and prolong the time window for treatment. Initial clinical results for mechanical recanalization are encouraging, but more clinical data on the various different devices and approaches are necessary.

We should not forget the cardiac roadmap, on which IVT was first proven, then increasingly replaced by acute mechanical intervention after superiority was shown in clinical trials. Even now, some expert stroke centers, including our center, routinely use IAT in the setting of a highly organized system in partnership with an interventional team. Intraarterial thrombolysis in patients beyond standard clinical time windows and in wake-up strokes, if there is evidence of salvageable penumbral tissue on CT or MR imaging, is also being routinely practiced at these centers. However, this approach has not been licensed in the absence of a confirmatory trial. The future in the treatment of acute ischemic stroke is likely a combination of different mechanical and thrombolytic techniques, probably in a staged escalation fashion.

References

1. (1989) Report of the WHO Task Force on Stroke and other Cerebrovascular Disorders. Stroke—1989. Recommendations on stroke prevention, diagnosis, and therapy. *Stroke* **20**:1407–1431.

2. World Health Organization. The Atlas of Heart Disease and Stroke. [WWW Document] URL http://www.who.int/cardiovascular_diseases/resources/atlas/en/ [Accessed on 28 May 2009].

3. Johnston SC, Mendis S, & Mathers CD (2009) Global variation in stroke burden and mortality: estimates from monitoring, surveillance, and modelling. *Lancet Neurol* **8**:345–354.

4. Lloyd-Jones D, Adams R, Carnethon M, *et al.* (2009) Heart disease and stroke statistics—2009 update: a report from the American Heart Association Statistics Committee and Stroke Statistics Subcommittee. *Circulation* **119**:e21–181.

5. Broderick JP & William M (2004) Feinberg Lecture: stroke therapy in the year 2025: burden, breakthroughs, and barriers to progress. *Stroke* **35**:205–211.

6. National Institute of Neurological Disorders and Stroke rt-PA Stroke Study Group. (1995) Tissue plasminogen activator for acute ischemic stroke. *N Engl J Med* **333**:1581–1587.

7. Broderick JP (2009) Endovascular therapy for acute ischemic stroke. *Stroke* **40**:S103–S106.

8. del Zoppo GJ, Higashida RT, Furlan AJ, Pessin MS, Rowley HA, & Gent M (1998) PROACT: a phase II randomized trial of recombinant pro-urokinase by direct arterial delivery in acute middle cerebral artery stroke. PROACT Investigators. Prolyse in Acute Cerebral Thromboembolism. *Stroke* **29**:4–11.

9. Furlan A, Higashida R, Wechsler L, *et al.* (1999) Intraarterial prourokinase for acute ischemic stroke. The PROACT II study: a randomized controlled trial. Prolyse in Acute Cerebral Thromboembolism. *JAMA* **282**:2003–2011.

10. Lansberg MG, Schrooten M, Bluhmki E, Thijs VN, & Saver JL (2009) Treatment time-specific number needed to treat estimates for tissue plasminogen activator therapy in acute stroke based on shifts over the entire range of the modified Rankin Scale. *Stroke* **40**:2079–2784.

11. Rha JH & Saver JL (2007) The impact of recanalization on ischemic stroke outcome: a meta-analysis. *Stroke* **38**:967–973.

12. Ingall TJ, O'Fallon WM, Asplund K, *et al.* (2004) Findings from the reanalysis of the NINDS tissue plasminogen activator for acute ischemic stroke treatment trial. *Stroke* **35**:2418–2424.

13. Fischer U, Arnold M, Nedeltchev K, *et al.* (2005) NIHSS score and arteriographic findings in acute ischemic stroke. *Stroke* **36**:2121–2125.

14. Wolpert SM, Bruckmann H, Greenlee R, Wechsler L, Pessin MS, & del Zoppo GJ (1993) Neuroradiologic evaluation of patients with acute stroke treated with recombinant tissue plasminogen activator. The rt-PA Acute Stroke Study Group. *AJNR Am J Neuroradiol* **14**:3–13.

15. Barber PA, Zhang J, Demchuk AM, Hill MD, & Buchan AM (2001) Why are stroke patients excluded from TPA therapy? An analysis of patient eligibility. *Neurology* **56**:1015–1020.

16. Hacke W, Kaste M, Bluhmki E, *et al.* (2008) Thrombolysis with alteplase 3 to 4.5 hours after acute ischemic stroke. *N Engl J Med* **359**:1317–1329.

17. Hacke W, Donnan G, Fieschi C, *et al.* (2004) Association of outcome with early stroke treatment: pooled analysis of ATLANTIS, ECASS, and NINDS rt-PA stroke trials. *Lancet* **363**:768–774.

18. Wardlaw JM, Sandercock PA, & Berge E (2003) Thrombolytic therapy with recombinant tissue plasminogen activator for acute ischemic stroke: where do we go from here? A cumulative meta-analysis. *Stroke* **34**:1437–1442.

19. Hacke W, Albers G, Al-Rawi Y, *et al.* (2005) The Desmoteplase in Acute Ischemic Stroke Trial (DIAS): a phase II MRI-based 9-hour window acute stroke thrombolysis trial with intravenous desmoteplase. *Stroke* **36**:66–73.

20. Furlan AJ, Eyding D, Albers GW, *et al.* (2006) Dose Escalation of Desmoteplase for Acute Ischemic Stroke (DEDAS): evidence of safety and efficacy 3 to 9 hours after stroke onset. *Stroke* **37**:1227–1231.

21. Albers GW, Thijs VN, Wechsler L, *et al.* (2006) Magnetic resonance imaging profiles predict clinical response to early reperfusion: the diffusion and perfusion imaging evaluation for understanding stroke evolution (DEFUSE) study. *Ann Neurol* **60**:508–517.

22. Thomalla G, Schwark C, Sobesky J, *et al.* (2006) Outcome and symptomatic bleeding complications of intravenous thrombolysis within 6 hours in MRI-selected stroke patients: comparison of a German multicenter study with the pooled data of ATLANTIS, ECASS, and NINDS tPA trials. *Stroke* **37**:852–858.

23. Kohrmann M, Juttler E, Fiebach JB, *et al.* (2006) MRI versus CT-based thrombolysis treatment within and beyond the 3 h time window after stroke onset: a cohort study. *Lancet Neurol* **5**:661–667.

24. Davis SM, Donnan GA, Parsons MW, *et al.* (2008) Effects of alteplase beyond 3 h after stroke in the Echoplanar Imaging Thrombolytic Evaluation Trial (EPITHET): a placebo-controlled randomised trial. *Lancet Neurol* **7**:299–309.

25. Hacke W, Furlan AJ, Al-Rawi Y, *et al.* (2009) Intravenous desmoteplase in patients with acute ischaemic stroke selected by MRI perfusion-diffusion weighted imaging or perfusion CT (DIAS-2): a prospective, randomised, double-blind, placebo-controlled study. *Lancet Neurol* **8**:141–150.

26. Schaefer PW, Barak ER, Kamalian S, *et al.* (2008) Quantitative assessment of core/penumbra mismatch in acute stroke: CT and MR perfusion imaging are strongly correlated when sufficient brain volume is imaged. *Stroke* **39**:2986–2992.

27. Wintermark M, Meuli R, Browaeys P, *et al.* (2007) Comparison of CT perfusion and angiography and MRI in selecting stroke patients for acute treatment. *Neurology* **68**:694–697.

28. Smith WS, Sung G, Starkman S, *et al.* (2005) Safety and efficacy of mechanical embolectomy in acute ischemic stroke: results of the MERCI trial. *Stroke* **36**:1432–1438.

29. Smith WS, Sung G, Saver J, *et al.* (2008) Mechanical thrombectomy for acute ischemic stroke: final results of the Multi MERCI trial. *Stroke* **39**:1205–1212.

30. Tomsick T, Broderick J, Carrozella J, *et al.* (2008) Revascularization results in the Interventional Management of Stroke II trial. *AJNR Am J Neuroradiol* **29**:582–587.

31. Alexandrov AV & Grotta JC (2002) Arterial reocclusion in stroke patients treated with intravenous tissue plasminogen activator. *Neurology* **59**:862–867.

32. Janjua N, Alkawi A, Suri MF, & Qureshi AI (2008) Impact of arterial reocclusion and distal fragmentation during thrombolysis among patients with acute ischemic stroke. *AJNR Am J Neuroradiol* **29**:253–258.

33. Saqqur M, Molina CA, Salam A, *et al.* (2007) Clinical deterioration after intravenous recombinant tissue plasminogen activator treatment: a multicenter transcranial Doppler study. *Stroke* **38**:69–74.

34. The National Institute of Neurological Disorders and Stroke rt-PA Stroke Study Group (1995) Tissue plasminogen activator for acute ischemic stroke. *N Engl J Med* **333**:1581–1587.

35. Levy DE, Brott TG, Haley EC Jr, *et al.* (1994) Factors related to intracranial hematoma formation in patients receiving tissue-type plasminogen activator for acute ischemic stroke. *Stroke* **25**:291–297.

36. Derex L, Hermier M, Adeleine P, *et al.* (2005) Clinical and imaging predictors of intracerebral haemorrhage in stroke patients treated with intravenous tissue plasminogen activator. *J Neurol Neurosurg Psychiatry* **76**:70–75.

37. Barber PA, Demchuk AM, Zhang J & Buchan AM (2000) Validity and reliability of a quantitative computed tomography score in predicting outcome of hyperacute stroke before thrombolytic therapy. ASPECTS Study Group. Alberta Stroke Programme Early CT Score. *Lancet* **355**:1670–1674.

38. Hill MD, Demchuk AM, Tomsick TA, Palesch YY, & Broderick JP (2006) Using the baseline CT scan to select acute stroke patients for IV-IA therapy. *AJNR Am J Neuroradiol* **27**:1612–1616.

39. Parsons MW, Pepper EM, Chan V, *et al.* (2005) Perfusion computed tomography: prediction of final infarct extent and stroke outcome. *Ann Neurol* **58**:672–679.

40. Albers GW, Thijs VN, Wechsler L, *et al.* (2006) Magnetic resonance imaging profiles predict clinical response to early reperfusion: the diffusion and perfusion imaging evaluation for understanding stroke evolution (DEFUSE) study. *Ann Neurol* **60**:508–517.

41. Shetty SK & Lev MH (2005) CT perfusion in acute stroke. *Neuroimaging Clin N Am* **15**:481–501, ix.

42. Esteban JM & Cervera V (2004) Perfusion CT and angio CT in the assessment of acute stroke. *Neuroradiology* **46**:705–715.

43. Kloska SP, Nabavi DG, Gaus C, *et al.* (2004) Acute stroke assessment with CT: do we need multimodal evaluation? *Radiology* **233**:79–86.

44. Maruya J, Yamamoto K, Ozawa T, *et al.* (2005) Simultaneous multi-section perfusion CT and CT angiography for the assessment of acute ischemic stroke. *Acta Neurochir (Wien)* **147**:383–392.

45. Smith WS, Roberts HC, Chuang NA, *et al.* (2003) Safety and feasibility of a CT protocol for acute stroke: combined CT, CT angiography, and CT perfusion imaging in 53 consecutive patients. *AJNR Am J Neuroradiol* **24**:688–690.

46. Latchaw RE (2004) Cerebral perfusion imaging in acute stroke. *J Vasc Interv Radiol* **15**:S29–S46.

47. Fiehler J, Foth M, Kucinski T, *et al.* (2002) Severe ADC decreases do not predict irreversible tissue damage in humans. *Stroke* **33**:79–86.

48. Kucinski T, Naumann D, Knab R, *et al.* (2005) Tissue at risk is overestimated in perfusion-weighted imaging: MR imaging in acute stroke patients without vessel recanalization. *AJNR Am J Neuroradiol* **26**:815–819.

49. Schellinger PD, Fiebach JB, & Hacke W (2003) Imaging-based decision making in thrombolytic therapy for ischemic stroke: present status. *Stroke* **34**:575–583.

50. Kim EY, Ryoo JW, Roh HG, *et al.* (2006) Reversed discrepancy between CT and diffusion-weighted MR imaging in acute ischemic stroke. *AJNR Am J Neuroradiol* **27**:1990–1995.

51. Wechsler LR, Roberts R, Furlan AJ, *et al.* (2003) Factors influencing outcome and treatment effect in PROACT II. *Stroke* **34**:1224–1229.

52. Ogawa A, Mori E, Minematsu K, *et al.* (2007) Randomized trial of intraarterial infusion of urokinase within 6 hours of middle cerebral artery stroke: the middle cerebral artery embolism local fibrinolytic intervention trial (MELT) Japan. *Stroke* **38**:2633–2639.

53. Saver JL (2007) Intraarterial fibrinolysis for acute ischemic stroke: the message of MELT. *Stroke* **38**:2627–2628.

54. Adams HP Jr, del Zoppo G, Alberts MJ, *et al.* (2007) Guidelines for the early management of adults with ischemic stroke: a guideline from the American Heart Association/American Stroke Association Stroke Council, Clinical Cardiology Council, Cardiovascular Radiology and Intervention Council, and the Atherosclerotic Peripheral Vascular Disease and Quality of Care Outcomes in Research Interdisciplinary Working Groups: The American Academy of Neurology affirms the value of this guideline as an educational tool for neurologists. *Circulation* **115**:e478–534.

55. Fink JN, Kumar S, Horkan C, *et al.* (2002) The stroke patient who woke up: clinical and radiological features, including diffusion and perfusion MRI. *Stroke* **33**:988–993.

56. Serena J, Davalos A, Segura T, Mostacero E, & Castillo J (2003) Stroke on awakening: looking for a more rational management. *Cerebrovasc Dis* **16**:128–133.

57. Barreto AD, Martin-Schild S, Hallevi H, *et al.* (2009) Thrombolytic therapy for patients who wake-up with stroke. *Stroke* **40**:827–832.

58. Adams HP Jr, Leira EC, Torner JC, *et al.* (2008) Treating patients with 'wake-up' stroke: the experience of the AbESTT-II trial. *Stroke* **39**:3277–3282.

59. Natarajan SK, Snyder KV, Siddiqui AH, Ionita CC, Hopkins LN, & Levy EI (2009) Safety and effectiveness of endovascular therapy after 8 hours of acute ischemic stroke onset and wake-up strokes. *Stroke* **40**:3269–3274.

60. Zeumer H, Freitag HJ, Grzyska U, & Neunzig HP (1989) Local intraarterial fibrinolysis in acute vertebrobasilar occlusion. Technical developments and recent results. *Neuroradiology* **31**:336–340.

61. Hacke W, Zeumer H, Ferbert A, Bruckmann H, & del Zoppo GJ (1988) Intraarterial thrombolytic therapy improves outcome in patients with acute vertebrobasilar occlusive disease. *Stroke* **19**:1216–1222.

62. Becker KJ, Monsein LH, Ulatowski J, Mirski M, Williams M, & Hanley DF (1996) Intraarterial thrombolysis in vertebrobasilar occlusion. *AJNR Am J Neuroradiol* **17**:255–262.

63. Jahan R (2005) Hyperacute therapy of acute ischemic stroke: intraarterial thrombolysis and mechanical revascularization strategies. *Tech Vasc Interv Radiol* **8**:87–91.

64. Archer CR & Horenstein S (1977) Basilar artery occlusion: clinical and radiological correlation. *Stroke* **8**:383–390.

65. Smith WS (2007) Intraarterial thrombolytic therapy for acute basilar occlusion: pro. *Stroke* **38**:701–703.

66. Lindsberg PJ & Mattle HP (2006) Therapy of basilar artery occlusion: a systematic analysis comparing intraarterial and intravenous thrombolysis. *Stroke* **37**:922–928.

67. Levy EI, Firlik AD, Wisniewski S, Rubin G, Jungreis CA, Wechsler LR, *et al.* (1999) Factors affecting survival rates for acute vertebrobasilar artery occlusions treated with intraarterial thrombolytic therapy: a meta-analytical approach. *Neurosurgery* **45**:539–548.

68. Zeumer H, Hacke W, & Ringelstein EB (1983) Local intraarterial thrombolysis in vertebrobasilar thromboembolic disease. *AJNR Am J Neuroradiol* **4**:401–404.

69. Zeumer H, Freitag HJ, Zanella F, Thie A, & Arning C (1993) Local intraarterial fibrinolytic therapy in patients with stroke: urokinase versus recombinant tissue plasminogen activator (r-TPA). *Neuroradiology* **35**:159–162.

70. Arnold M, Nedeltchev K, Mattle HP, *et al.* (2003) Intraarterial thrombolysis in 24 consecutive patients with internal carotid artery T occlusions. *J Neurol Neurosurg Psychiatry* **74**:739–742.

71. Jansen O, von Kummer R, Forsting M, Hacke W, & Sartor K (1995) Thrombolytic therapy in acute occlusion of the intra-cranial internal carotid artery bifurcation. *AJNR Am J Neuroradiol* **16**:1977–1986.

72. Noble J, Weizblit N, Baerlocher MO, & Eng KT (2008) Intra-arterial thrombolysis for central retinal artery occlusion: a systematic review. *Br J Ophthalmol* **92**:588–593.

73. Feltgen N, Neubauer A, Jurklies B, *et al.* (2006) Multicenter study of the European Assessment Group for Lysis in the Eye (EAGLE) for the treatment of central retinal artery occlusion: design issues and implications. EAGLE Study report no. 1: EAGLE Study report no. 1. *Graefes Arch Clin Exp Ophthalmol* **244**:950–6.

74. Feltgen N, Reinhard T, Kampik A, Jurklies B, Bruckmann H, & Schumacher M (2006) [Lysis therapy vs. conservative therapy: randomised and prospective study on the treatment of acute central retinal artery occlusion (EAGLE study)]. *Ophthalmologe* **103**:898–900.

75. Chalela JA, Katzan I, Liebeskind DS, *et al.* (2001) Safety of intraarterial thrombolysis in the postoperative period. *Stroke* **32**:1365–1369.

76. Kim DJ, Kim DI, Kim SH, Lee KY, Heo JH, & Han SW (2005) Rescue localized intraarterial thrombolysis for hyperacute MCA ischemic stroke patients after early non-responsive intravenous tissue plasminogen activator therapy. *Neuroradiology* **47**:616–621.

77. Qureshi AI, Siddiqui AM, Kim SH, *et al.* (2004) Reocclusion of recanalized arteries during intraarterial thrombolysis for acute ischemic stroke. *AJNR Am J Neuroradiol* **25**:322–328.

78. Pancioli AM, Broderick J, Brott T, *et al.* (2008) The combined approach to lysis utilizing eptifibatide and rt-PA in acute ischemic stroke: the CLEAR stroke trial. *Stroke* **39**:3268–76.

79. Dunn B, Davis LA, Todd JW, Chalela JA, & Warach S (February 5, 2004) for the ROSIE Investigators. ReoPro Retavase Reperfusion of Stroke Safety Study—Imaging Evaluation (ROSIE). Presented at the 29th International Stroke Conference, San Diego, CA.

80. Adams HP Jr, Effron MB, Torner J, *et al.* (2008) Emergency administration of abciximab for treatment of patients with acute ischemic stroke: results of an international phase III trial: Abciximab in Emergency Treatment of Stroke Trial (AbESTT-II). *Stroke* **39**:87–99.

81. IMS Investigators (2007) The Interventional Management of Stroke (IMS) II Study. *Stroke* **38**:2127–2135.

82. Khatri P, Hill MD, Palesch YY, *et al.* (2008) Methodology of the Interventional Management of Stroke III Trial. *Int J Stroke* **3**:130–137.

83. Mattle HP, Arnold M, Georgiadis D, *et al.* (2008) Comparison of intraarterial and intravenous thrombolysis for ischemic stroke with hyperdense middle cerebral artery sign. *Stroke* **39**:379–383.

84. Gralla J, Schroth G, Remonda L, *et al.* (2006) A dedicated animal model for mechanical thrombectomy in acute stroke. *AJNR Am J Neuroradiol* **27**:1357–1361.

85. Gralla J, Burkhardt M, Schroth G, *et al.* (2008) Occlusion length is a crucial determinant of efficiency and complication rate in thrombectomy for acute ischemic stroke. *AJNR Am J Neuroradiol* **29**:247–52.

86. Gralla J, Schroth G, Remonda L, Nedeltchev K, Slotboom J, & Brekenfeld C (2006) Mechanical thrombectomy for acute ischemic stroke: thrombus-device interaction, efficiency, and complications in vivo. *Stroke* **37**:3019–3024.

87. Smith WS, Sung G, Starkman S, *et al.* (2005) Safety and efficacy of mechanical embolectomy in acute ischemic stroke: results of the MERCI trial. *Stroke* **36**:1432–8.

88. Flint AC, Duckwiler GR, Budzik RF, Liebeskind DS, & Smith WS (2007) Mechanical thrombectomy of intracranial internal carotid occlusion: pooled results of the MERCI and Multi MERCI Part I trials. *Stroke* **38**:1274–1280.

89. Liebig T, Reinartz J, Hannes R, Miloslavski E, & Henkes H (2008) Comparative in vitro study of five mechanical embolec-tomy systems: effectiveness of clot removal and risk of distal embolization. *Neuroradiology* **50**:43–52.

90. Henkes H, Reinartz J, Lowens S, *et al.* (2006) A device for fast mechanical clot retrieval from intracranial arteries (Phenox clot retriever). *Neurocrit Care* **5**:134–40.

91. Bose A, Henkes H, Alfke K, *et al.* (2008) The Penumbra System: a mechanical device for the treatment of acute stroke due to thromboembolism. *AJNR Am J Neuroradiol* **29**:1409–1413.

92. McDougall CG, Clark W, Mayer T, *et al.* For the Penumbra Stroke Trial Investigators (2008) The Penumbra Stroke Trial: safety and effectiveness of a new generation of mechanical devices for clot removal in acute ischemic stroke. *International Stroke Conference 2008.* New Orleans, LA, February 22.

93. Mayer TE, Hamann GF, Schulte-Altedorneburg G, & Bruckmann H (2005) Treatment of vertebrobasilar occlusion by using a coronary waterjet thrombectomy device: a pilot study. *AJNR Am J Neuroradiol* **26**:1389–1394.

94. Barnwell SL, Clark WM, Nguyen TT, O'Neill OR, Wynn ML, & Coull BM (1994) Safety and efficacy of delayed intraarterial urokinase therapy with mechanical clot disruption for throm-boembolic stroke. *AJNR Am J Neuroradiol* **15**:1817–1822.

95. Bergui M, Stura G, Daniele D, Cerrato P, Berardino M, & Bradac GB (2006) Mechanical thrombolysis in ischemic stroke attributable to basilar artery occlusion as first-line treatment. *Stroke* **37**:145–50.

96. Qureshi AI, Siddiqui AM, Suri MF, *et al.* (2002) Aggressive mechanical clot disruption and low-dose intraarterial third-generation thrombolytic agent for ischemic stroke: a prospective study. *Neurosurgery* **51**:1319–27; discussion 1327–9.

97. Kerber CW, Barr JD, Berger RM, & Chopko BW (2002) Snare retrieval of intracranial thrombus in patients with acute stroke. *J Vasc Interv Radiol* **13**:1269–1274.

98. Nakano S, Iseda T, Yoneyama T, Kawano H, & Wakisaka S (2002) Direct percutaneous transluminal angioplasty for acute middle cerebral artery trunk occlusion: an alternative option to intraarterial thrombolysis. *Stroke* **33**:2872–2876.

99. Grines CL, Cox DA, Stone GW, *et al.* (1999) Coronary angioplasty with or without stent implantation for acute myocardial infarction. Stent Primary Angioplasty in Myocardial Infarction Study Group. *N Engl J Med* **341**:1949–1956.

100. Berlis A, Lutsep H, Barnwell S, *et al.* (2004) Mechanical thrombolysis in acute ischemic stroke with endovascular photoacoustic recanalization. *Stroke* **35**:1112–1116.

101. Nesbit GM, Luh G, Tien R, & Barnwell SL (2004) New and future endovascular treatment strategies for acute ischemic stroke. *J Vasc Interv Radiol* **15**:S103–S110.

102. Henkes H, Miloslavski E, Lowens S, Reinartz J, Liebig T, & Kuhne D (2005) Treatment of intracranial atherosclerotic stenoses with balloon dilatation and self-expanding stent deployment (WingSpan). *Neuroradiology* **47**:222–228.

103. Levy EI, Ecker RD, Horowitz MB, *et al.* (2006) Stent-assisted intracranial recanalization for acute stroke: early results. *Neurosurgery* **58**:458–463.

104. Gupta R, Vora NA, Horowitz MB, *et al.* (2006) Multimodal reperfusion therapy for acute ischemic stroke: factors predicting vessel recanalization. *Stroke* **37**:986–990.

105. Peluso JP, van Rooij WJ, Sluzewski M, & Beute GN (2008) A new self-expandable nitinol stent for the treatment of wide-neck aneurysms: initial clinical experience. *AJNR Am J Neuroradiol* **29**:1405–1408.

106. Lubicz B, Leclerc X, Levivier M, *et al.* (2006) Retractable self-expandable stent for endovascular treatment of wide-necked intracranial aneurysms: preliminary experience. *Neurosurgery* **58**:451–457.

107. Yavuz K, Geyik S, Pamuk AG, Koc O, Saatci I, & Cekirge HS (2007) Immediate and midterm follow-up results of using an electrodetachable, fully retrievable SOLO stent system in the endovascular coil occlusion of wide-necked cerebral aneurysms. *J Neurosurg* **107**:49–55.

108. Levy EI, Sauvageau E, Hanel RA, Parikh R, & Hopkins LN (2006) Self-expanding versus balloon-mounted stents for vessel recanalization following embolic occlusion in the canine model: technical feasibility study. *AJNR Am J Neuroradiol* **27**:2069–2072.

109. Levy EI, Mehta R, Gupta R, Hanel RA, Chamczuk AJ, Fiorella D, *et al.* (2007) Self-expanding stents for recanalization of acute cerebrovascular occlusions. *AJNR Am J Neuroradiol* **28**:816–822.

110. Zaidat OO, Wolfe T, Hussain SI, *et al.* (2008) Interventional acute ischemic stroke therapy with intracranial self-expanding stent. *Stroke* **39**:2392–2395.

111. Levy EI, Siddiqui AH, Crumlish A, *et al.* (2009) First food and drug administration-approved prospective trial of primary intracranial stenting for acute stroke: SARIS (stent-assisted recanalization in acute ischemic stroke). *Stroke* **40**:3552–3556.

112. Kelly ME, Furlan AJ, & Fiorella D (2008) Recanalization of an acute middle cerebral artery occlusion using a self-expanding, reconstrainable, intracranial microstent as a temporary endovascular bypass. *Stroke* **39**:1770–1773.

113. Hauck EF, Mocco J, Snyder KV, & Levy EI (2009) Temporary endovascular bypass: a novel treatment for acute stroke. *AJNR Am J Neuroradiol* [Epub ahead of print].

114. Natarajan SK, Siddiqui AH, Hopkins LN, & Levy EI. Retrievable, detachable stent-platform-based clot-retrieval device (Solitaire™ FR) for acute stroke revascularization. *Vascular Disease Management* (in press).

115. Jovin TG, Gupta R, Uchino K, *et al.* (2005) Emergent stenting of extracranial internal carotid artery occlusion in acute stroke has a high revascularization rate. *Stroke* **36**:2426–2430.

116. Nikas D, Reimers B, Elisabetta M, *et al.* (2007) Percutaneous interventions in patients with acute ischemic stroke related to obstructive atherosclerotic disease or dissection of the extracranial carotid artery. *J Endovasc Ther* **14**:279–288.

117. Dabitz R, Triebe S, Leppmeier U, Ochs G, & Vorwerk D (2007) Percutaneous recanalization of acute internal carotid artery occlusions in patients with severe stroke. *Cardiovasc Intervent Radiol* **30**:34–41.

118. Lavallee PC, Mazighi M, Saint-Maurice JP, *et al.* (2007) Stent-assisted endovascular thrombolysis versus intravenous thrombolysis in internal carotid artery dissection with tandem internal carotid and middle cerebral artery occlusion. *Stroke* **38**:2270–2274.

119. Miyamoto N, Naito I, Takatama S, Shimizu T, Iwai T, & Shimaguchi H (2008) Urgent stenting for patients with acute stroke due to atherosclerotic occlusive lesions of the cervical internal carotid artery. *Neurol Med Chir (Tokyo)* **48**:49–56.

120. Ozdemir O, Bussiere M, Leung A *et al.* (2008) Intraarterial thrombolysis of occluded middle cerebral artery by use of collateral pathways in patients with tandem cervical carotid artery/middle cerebral artery occlusion. *AJNR Am J Neuroradiol* **29**:1596–1600.

121. IMS Investigators (2004) Combined intravenous and intra-arterial recanalization for acute ischemic stroke: the Interventional Management of Stroke Study. *Stroke* **35**:904–911.

122. Gobin YP, Starkman S, Duckwiler GR, *et al.* (2004) MERCI 1: a phase 1 study of Mechanical Embolus Removal in Cerebral Ischemia. *Stroke* **35**:2848–2854.

123. Yepes M, Roussel BD, Ali C, & Vivien D (2009) Tissue-type plasminogen activator in the ischemic brain: more than a thrombolytic. *Trends Neurosci* **32**:48–55.

124. Nogueira RG & Smith WS (2009) Safety and efficacy of endovascular thrombectomy in patients with abnormal hemostasis: pooled analysis of the MERCI and multi MERCI trials. *Stroke* **40**:516–522.

58 Interventional Treatment of Intracerebral Aneurysms

Pascal Jabbour[1], Adytia Pandey[2] & Erol Veznedaroglu[3]

[1]Department of Neurosurgery, Thomas Jefferson University Hospital, Jefferson Hospital for Neuroscience, Philadelphia, PA, USA
[2]Department of Neurosurgery, University of Michigan, Ann Arbor, MI, USA
[3]Department of Neurosurgery, Stroke and Cerebrovascular Center of New Jersey, Trenton, NJ, USA

Introduction

Intracranial aneurysms represent any outpouching from a cerebral vessel which does not represent its normal architecture. These aneurysms can be described as saccular ("berry"), fusiform, dissecting, pseudoaneurysms, or traumatic aneurysms. The most prevalent of these are the saccular aneurysms, which are present in approximately 0.2–8.9% of the population [1]. The goal of this chapter is to introduce the reader to the diagnosis, treatment, and follow-up of both ruptured and unruptured saccular aneurysms.

Cerebral aneurysms are thought to arise from weakness within the tunica media of the vessel, thus allowing for expansion of the vascular wall with time and introduction of inciting factors such as smoking and hypertension. Cerebral aneurysms form at regions where there is stress related to turbulent flow. Such stress is most commonly present at branching points within the Circle of Willis. More than 80% of aneurysms are present within the anterior circulation while 10–20% arise within the posterior circulation.

Risk factors that increase the probability of developing cerebral aneurysms are polycystic kidney disease, aortic coarctation, α_1-antitrypsin deficiency, Ehlers–Danlos syndrome type IV, fibromuscular dysplasia, and a family history of cerebral aneurysms [2–4]. Patients harboring cerebral aneurysms are usually diagnosed due to symptoms related to rupture and thus development of subarachnoid hemorrhage (SAH), or mass effect upon cerebral structures as the aneurysm expands, or cerebral ischemia from thrombus formation within the aneurysmal sac. Nonetheless, screening has led to the diagnosis of asymptomatic patients. There is a four time higher incidence of aneurysms within first degree relatives of patients presenting with SAH [5].

Cardiovascular Interventions in Clinical Practice. Edited by Jürgen Haase, Hans-Joachim Schäfers, Horst Sievert and Ron Waksman. © 2010 Blackwell Publishing.

Natural history of symptomatic and asymptomatic aneurysms

The International Study of Unruptured Intracranial Aneurysms (ISUIA) has defined the natural history of asymptomatic intracranial aneurysms [1]. The 5-year rupture rate based on size is as follows for anterior circulation aneurysms, not including posterior communicating artery aneurysms (PCOMs): 0% for <7 mm, 2.6% for 7–12 mm, 14.5% for 13–24 mm, and 40% for >25 mm. The same rates for PCOMs and posterior circulation aneurysms is as follows: 2.5% for <7 mm, 14.5% for 7–12 mm, 18.4% for 13–24 mm, and 50% for >25 mm [1].

The consensus has been that individuals 60 years of age or less harboring intracranial aneurysm of ≥7 mm should be offered treatment [6]. Within our own practice, the majority of patients presenting with SAH harbor aneurysms <10 mm and some even <5 mm. Individuals who have severe headaches, family history of SAH, or use tobacco are at a higher risk of rupture and thus are offered treatment of aneurysms at <7 mm.

Patients who present with SAH have a 15% immediate mortality and a 50% mortality at 6 months [7,8] (Fig. 58.1). Clinical outcome is related to the presenting clinical condition of the patient (Table 58.1) [9]. Such an outcome is

Table 58.1 Classification of the Hunt and Hess clinical grading scale in subarachnoid hemorrhage patients.

1 Asymptomatic or patient has a mild headache and possibly a stiff neck.
2 Moderate to severe headache, nuchal rigidity, can have oculomotor palsy—patient is fully awake and alert.
3 Drowsy patient is confused, frequently mild focal signs.
4 Stupor, moderate to severe hemiparesis, and early decerebrate posturing.
5 Coma, moribund, and/or extensor posturing. Patient will probably die within a few hours no matter what is done medically and/or surgically.

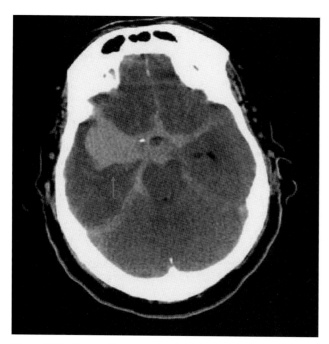

Figure 58.1 Computed tomography of the head showing diffuse SAH in bilateral Sylvian fissures and a right temporal hematoma (arrow).

related to rupture of the aneurysm as well as delayed neurologic deficits related to spasm of the intracranial vasculature [10–12]. Treatment of the ruptured aneurysm and the related vasospasm and hydrocephalus has led to better outcomes.

Endovascular treatment of cerebral aneurysms

The treatment paradigm for intracerebral aneurysms has been revolutionized over the past 10 years. The once "gold standard" of craniotomy for clip ligation of aneurysm has been challenged by the less invasive endovascular route. The explosion of new devices and technologies has made endovascular therapy more "user friendly," safer, and has allowed for better short- and long-term outcomes.

Endovascular embolization of cerebral aneurysms using platinum microcoils is a treatment made possible by the parallel evolution of several technologies, in particular, computerized imaging and flexible, hydrophilic micro catheterization systems. The development of the detachable type of microcoil by Guglielmi (Guglielmi Detachable Coil; GDC) took advantage of the newest developments in intravascular navigation to enable the percutaneous endovascular embolization of cerebral aneurysms. The first percutaneous coil embolization of an aneurysm in a living human using the GDC was reported in 1991 [10].

Neurosurgeons trained in both microsurgical clip ligation and endovascular coil embolization employ a multimodality

treatment strategy in our cerebrovascular division to treat cerebral aneurysms. Particular attention is paid to the architecture of the aneurysm itself in addition to the tortuosity of arteries that would require microcatheter navigation to gain access to the lesion. In general, the aneurysm with a relatively narrow inflow region (i.e. neck) is considered a more suitable lesion for coil embolization than one with a larger neck. However, aneurysms with large necks have been made more suitable for coil embolization using a series of technologic advancements, which progressed from balloon remodeling to the current stent technology. Similarly, tortuous arterial anatomy was a relative contraindication for coil embolization.

The susceptibility of a given aneurysm to embolization treatment was not entirely predictable despite the identification of key angiographic features. In particular, inflow zones that initially appeared wide on DSA were actually found to be narrow on three-dimensional (3-D) rotational angiography and lent themselves to coiling. Conversely, some lesions that appeared very suitable for embolization turned out to require clip ligation because the angle of the neck prevented microcatheterization or arterial/perforating branches could be observed by superselective angiography to be derived from the very fundus of the lesion, or the aneurysm orifice was unexpectedly wide. The addition of 3-D rotational angiography imaging capabilities has reduced the degree of uncertainty with preoperative diagnostic angiogram.

Technical procedure

Coil embolization procedures are performed under general endotracheal anesthesia in the Interventional Neurosurgical Suite. All subarachnoid hemorrhage patients with a Hunt and Hess grade III or higher are monitored with ventriculostomy catheters, central venous catheters, and radial arterial lines to better optimize the medical management of vasospasm. During the endovascular procedure, patients are monitored with hemodynamic parameters as well as continuous electroencephalography, somatosensory evoked potentials, and brainstem auditory evoked responses [13–15].

The essential characteristic and therapeutic goal of the coil procedure is the induction of thrombosis within the aneurysm by the deployment of platinum microcoils. Detailed cerebral angiography is performed to obtain the best projection angles for the demonstration of the aneurysm orifice and its relationship to neighboring blood vessels. Aneurysm size is then measured digitally to guide coil selection. All catheter systems are continuously flushed with pressurized heparinized saline and kept meticulously devoid of air bubbles. Once the aneurysm orifice has been engaged with the microcatheter, platinum microcoils of different shape, size, and stiffness are selected sequentially and passed through the microcatheter into the aneurysm. After each coil is introduced within the aneurysm, subtraction angiography is performed to assure that all afferent and efferent vessels are patent. A coil may be withdrawn without detachment if DSA results are unsuitable or if there appears to be a risk or manifestation of prolapse into the lumen of the parent artery, or compromise of distal circulation. For patients with subarachnoid hemorrhage, heparinization is started once the dome of the aneurysm is protected. For unruptured aneurysms, the patient is heparinized at the beginning of the procedure. The activated clotting time (ACT) is used as the index of the degree of anticoagulation and is considered satisfactory when it is twice that of the baseline. The end point of the intervention is complete angiographic elimination of the aneurysm fundus in multiple angiographic views under full anticoagulation. When this is achieved the microcatheter is withdrawn from the aneurysm and a final angiogram is performed to confirm absent fundus filling without the microcatheter. Postoperatively, heparinization is maintained for 24h, and in certain circumstances followed by Dextran-40 for an additional 24h.

Although the ultimate goal of aneurysm treatment is permanent obliteration of the aneurysm, this goal is not always achieved by either endovascular or microsurgical means. A protective effect of treatment that does not result in complete elimination may result from partial clipping or partial coil embolization, despite the measurable risk of regrowth and rupture of anerurysmal remnants [16,17]. This circumstance is more common in coil embolization than in clip ligation, because of the nature of the treatment itself in its current state of technology. Specifically, complete coil embolization of the aneurysm fundus, despite the persistence of a portion of the aneurysm neck, reduces the risk of aneurysm rupture or coil herniation into the parent vessel, with protection from rehemorrhage in the acute phase of neurologic recovery from subarachnoid hemorrhage. Our data suggest that the incidence of repeat SAH in such coiled patients is low (approximately 0.85%), and therefore coil embolization of the fundus may be protective, despite the presence of a neck remnant in nearly 20% of treated patients [15]. This protective effect of partial embolization is also supported by the International Subarachnoid Aneurysm Trial (ISAT) [18]. Our repeat subarachnoid hemorrhage is similar to the 0.9% reported by Lempert *et al.* [19] in their review of endovascular treatment of posterior circulation aneurysms. This is complemented by the less traumatic nature of the procedure compared with skilled microneurosurgery, which requires complex skull base exposures, dissection, and retraction of brain tissue, cranial nerve manipulation, and lengthier anesthetic requirements. Another circumstance in which coil embolization may be advantageous includes multiple aneurysms with an uncertain source of SAH.

Follow-up selective cerebral angiography is performed at 6 months, after which noninvasive imaging (magnetic resonance imaging, magnetic resonance angiography [MRI, MRA] and computed tomography [CT] angiography) is used. The duration of follow-up imaging is determined on a case-by-case basis, age being a prominent consideration. For a patient of advanced age. For example, it is less imperative to aggressively pursue follow-up angiography, in view of the relative risk for the older patient. Similarly, ambiguous or worrisome angiographic features at the time of or after treatment prompts earlier or more frequent angiographic follow-up.

Limitations of coil embolization and future developments

Although safe and effective and perhaps superior in the subarachnoid hemorrhage population, coil embolization has its limitations. Recurrence rates have historically been as high as 50%; however, with the use of modern coils, stent technology, and better imaging the recurrence rate is likely closer to 20% [14,15]. Giant aneurysms, thrombosed aneurysms, and fusiform lesions remain more suitable for open surgical clip ligation.

The once problematic "wide necked aneurysm" is now routinely being treated with both complex coils with "memory" and stent assistance. The advent of bioactive coils also has proved promising but long-term results remain to be seen [20,21]. The concept is to promote a robust inflammatory response within the aneurysmal sac to induce healing over a delayed period. The Hydrocoil is a coil that is coated with a polymer that swells after introduction to the blood stream, helping to increase volumetric occlusion [22]. The inability to achieve 100% occlusion with coil alone has led to the development of a glue or liquid polymer to occlude the small interstices of aneurysms. The Onyx 500 polymer (EV3, California, USA) is the first to be Food and Drug Administration (FDA) approved for use in humans [23]. The very early results are promising but this technique requires balloon assistance.

Technique and long-term follow up

Case examples

The following case examples have been taken from reference 24.

Internal carotid artery aneurysm embolized with Onyx

We report a case of an 83-year old woman, with past medical history of high blood pressure and smoking, who presented to us after having had the worst headache of her life with acute onset of left hemiparesis and lethargy. On admission, she had a Hunt and Hess grade of IV; she was intubated and densely hemiparetic on the left side. CT of the head (Fig. 58.1) showed diffuse subarachnoid hemorrhage and a right temporal intracerebral hemorrhage. Owing to the poor clinical grade and the comorbidities of the patient, it was decided to proceed with an endovascular approach.

Cerebral angiography revealed a right sided dysplastic aneurysm of the communicating segment of the carotid artery. The aneurysm was wide necked and thus required stent assistance. As that the patient had an intracerebral hematoma,

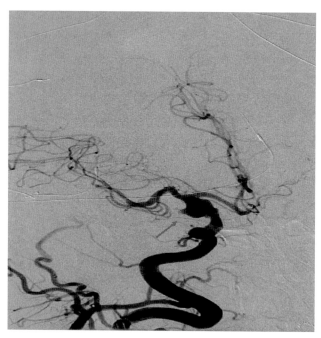

Figure 58.2 Right internal carotid artery injection—early arterial phase: anteroposterior projection.

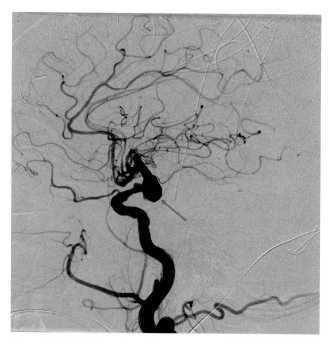

Figure 58.3 Right internal carotid artery injection—early arterial phase: lateral projection.

the required anticoagulation for stent placement would be detrimental to the patient's condition (Figs. 58.2, 58.3, and 58.4). Thus this was an ideal case for Onyx embolization of the aneurysm.

A 6F microcatheter was introduced into the affected internal carotid artery. An Onyx-compatible Hyperglide Balloon (Micro Therapeutics Inc., Irvine, CA, USA) was introduced and placed at the level of the neck of the aneurysm. Thereafter, the 6F guide system was used to introduce an Onyx HD 500 compatible microcatheter (Rebar, Titan; Micro Therapeutics) into the lumen of the aneurysm. With the balloon inflated (Fig. 58.5), a slow test injection with contrast material was done. A satisfactory seal test is achieved with stasis of contrast material within the aneurysm with no flow within the parent vessel.

For the injection techniques of Onyx, we followed the instructions for use from Micro Therapeutics. For each injection cycle, the internal carotid artery was occluded for a maximum of 5 min: 3 min for injection of the embolic material and 2 min to allow precipitation of the injected embolic material. After an injection cycle, the circulation was re-established for at least 3 min. At the end of the treatment the microcatheter—after aspiration and 10 min waiting time to allow for solidification of the embolic material—was withdrawn from the aneurysm under protection of the inflated balloon. After the aneurysm was secured (Figs. 58.6 and 58.7), the patient was taken to the operating room to evacuate her temporal hematoma. At the time of the hematoma evacuation, the embolized aneurysm was visualized and several digital images were obtained (Fig. 58.8).

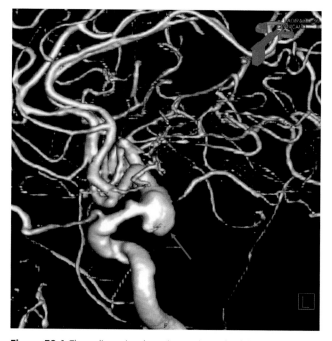

Figure 58.4 Three-dimensional rotation angiography delineating the angioarchitecture of the aneurysm.

Stent assisted coiling

A 57-year-old woman with a history of multiple aneurysms, treated previously with clipping and coiling, presented now for an elective treatment of a right sided PCOM with a wide neck (Figs. 58.9, 58.10).

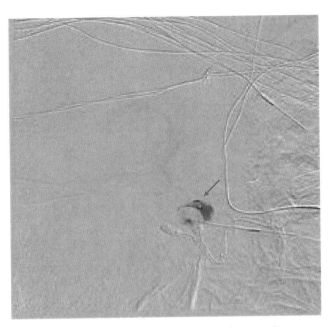

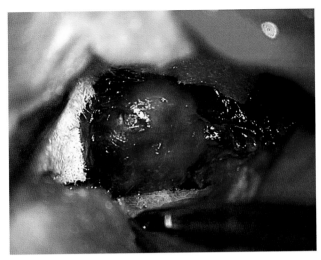

Figure 58.7 Intraoperative picture showing the aneurysm already embolized with Onyx.

Figure 58.5 Balloon is Inflated in the internal carotid artery and microinjection reveals the entire volume of the aneurysm with no contrast within the parent vessel.

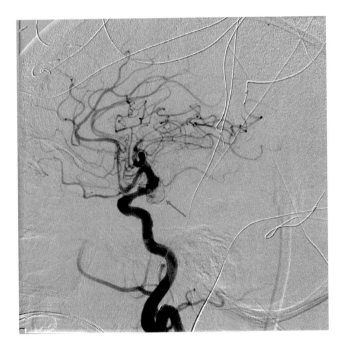

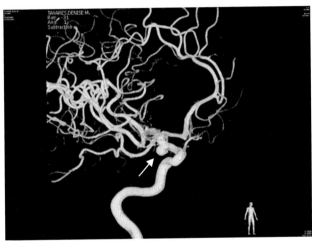

Figure 58.8 Three-dimensional angiography revealing a right posterior communicating artery aneurysm with a wide neck.

Figure 58.6 Right internal carotid artery injection early arterial phase with a lateral projection shows complete occlusion of the aneurysm with patency of the parent vessel.

Conclusion

Data from our clinical series and others support the idea that endovascular coil embolization is a reliable form of treatment

for both ruptured and unruptured cerebral aneurysms [15,25–28]. This form of treatment appears from preliminary data to be protective against subarachnoid hemorrhage [25,27]. Endovascular embolization in the current state of technologic advancement carries acceptable morbidity (3%) and mortality (<0.5%) when performed by experienced operators, and is similar to that observed by other authors [29]. We have recently reported our 10-year experience of treating posterior circulation aneurysms with coil embolization in 236 patients harboring ruptured and unruptured aneurysms. To date, this represents the largest series of posterior circulation aneurysms treated using coil embolization [19,25,28,30–32]. The ISAT has reported that the relative risk of death or significant disability at 1 year for patients treated with coils was 22.6% lower than in surgically-treated patients [27]. Treatment of cerebral aneurysms has to be determined on a case by case basis, with primary emphasis given to patient

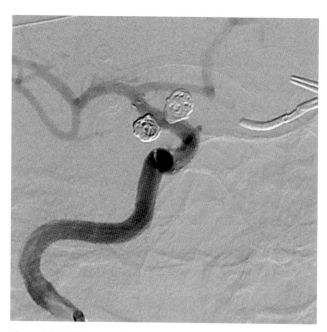

Figure 58.9 Right internal carotid artery injection in an anteroposterior projection showing complete occlusion of the right posterior communicating artery aneurysm.

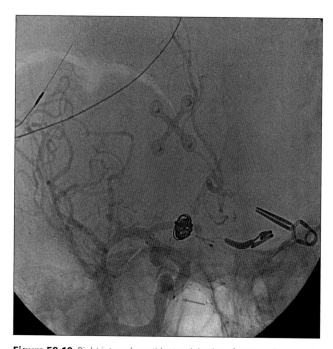

Figure 58.10 Right internal carotid artery injection after Neuroform stent placement. Arrows indicate the proximal and distal markers of one stent.

comorbidities as well as the angioarchitecture of the aneurysm. The phenomenon of delayed reopening of coiled aneurysms is characterized in our experience by a low incidence and a low rate of subsequent subarachnoid hemorrhage in patients followed up to 5 years [14,15].

Although not likely to replace open surgery, the continued advancements in technology and supportive clinical data will allow endovascular therapy to become a more durable mode of treatment. All patients should be evaluated by either a surgeon trained in both procedures or by an interventionalist and surgeon. The collaboration and amalgamation of this team approach benefits the patient and physician alike. Only future studies will delineate the long-term clinical and angiographic success of endosaccular therapy with the advent of covered stents, liquid embolic agents, and bioactive coils [21].

References

1. Wiebers DO, Whisnant JP, Huston J 3rd, *et al.* (2003) Unruptured intracranial aneurysms: natural history, clinical outcome, and risks of surgical and endovascular treatment. *Lancet* **362**:103–110.
2. Mettinger KL & Ericson K (1982) Fibromuscular dysplasia and the brain. I. Observations on angiographic, clinical and genetic characteristics. *Stroke* **13**:46–52.
3. Schievink WI, Katzmann JA, & Piepgras DG (1998) Alpha-1-antitrypsin deficiency in spontaneous intracranial arterial dissections. *Cerebrovasc Dis* **8**:42–44.
4. Schievink WI, Katzmann JA, Piepgras DG, & Schaid DJ (1996) Alpha-1-antitrypsin phenotypes among patients with intracranial aneurysms. *J Neurosurg* **84**:781–784.
5. Ruggieri PM, Poulos N, Masaryk TJ, *et al.* (1994) Occult intracranial aneurysms in polycystic kidney disease: screening with MR angiography. *Radiology* **191**:33–39.
6. Komotar RJ, Mocco J, & Solomon RA (2008) Guidelines for the surgical treatment of unruptured intracranial aneurysms: the first annual J. Lawrence pool memorial research symposium—controversies in the management of cerebral aneurysms. *Neurosurgery* **62**:183–193; discussion 193–184.
7. Ljunggren B, Saveland H, Brandt L, & Zygmunt S (1985) Early operation and overall outcome in aneurysmal subarachnoid hemorrhage. *J Neurosurg* **62**:547–551.
8. Whisnant JP, Sacco SE, O'Fallon WM, Fode NC, & Sundt TM Jr (1993) Referral bias in aneurysmal subarachnoid hemorrhage. *J Neurosurg* **78**:726–732.
9. Hunt WE & Hess RM (1968) Surgical risk as related to time of intervention in the repair of intracranial aneurysms. *J Neurosurg* **28**:14–20.
10. Guglielmi G, Vinuela F, Dion J, & Duckwiler G (1991) Electrothrombosis of saccular aneurysms via endovascular approach. Part 2: Preliminary clinical experience. *J Neurosurg* **75**:8–14.
11. Kassell NF, Torner JC, Haley EC Jr, Jane JA, Adams HP, & Kongable GL (1990) The International Cooperative Study on the Timing of Aneurysm Surgery. Part 1: Overall management results. *J Neurosurg* **73**:18–36.
12. Kassell NF, Torner JC, Jane JA, Haley EC Jr, & Adams HP (1990) The International Cooperative Study on the Timing of Aneurysm Surgery. Part 2: Surgical results. *J Neurosurg* **73**:37–47.
13. Birknes JK, Hwang SK, Pandey AS, *et al.* (2006) Feasibility and limitations of endovascular coil embolization of anterior communicating artery aneurysms: morphological considerations. *Neurosurgery* **59**:43–52; discussion 43–52.

14. Pandey A, Rosenwasser RH, & Veznedaroglu E (2007) Management of distal anterior cerebral artery aneurysms: a single institution retrospective analysis 1997–2005. *Neurosurgery* **61**:909–916; discussion 916–907.

15. Pandey AS, Koebbe C, Rosenwasser RH, & Veznedaroglu E (2007) Endovascular coil embolization of ruptured and unruptured posterior circulation aneurysms: review of a 10-year experience. *Neurosurgery* **60**:626–636; discussion 636–627.

16. David CA, Vishteh AG, Spetzler RF, Lemole M, Lawton MT, & Partovi S (1999) Late angiographic follow-up review of surgically treated aneurysms. *J Neurosurg* **91**:396–401.

17. Drake CG, Friedman AH, & Peerless SJ (1984) Failed aneurysm surgery. Reoperation in 115 cases. *J Neurosurg* **61**:848–856.

18. Leung CH, Poon WS, & Yu LM (2003) The ISAT trial. *Lancet* **361**:430–431; author reply 432.

19. Lempert TE, Malek AM, Halbach VV, *et al.* (2000) Endovascular treatment of ruptured posterior circulation cerebral aneurysms. Clinical and angiographic outcomes. *Stroke* **31**:100–110.

20. Deng J, Zhao Z, & Gao G (2007) Periprocedural complications associated with endovascular embolisation of intracranial ruptured aneurysms with matrix coils. *Singapore Med J* **48**:429–433.

21. Veznedaroglu E, Koebbe CJ, Siddiqui A, & Rosenwasser RH (2008) Initial experience with bioactive cerecyte detachable coils: impact on reducing recurrence rates. *Neurosurgery* **62**:799–805; discussion 805–796.

22. Gunnarsson T, Klurfan P, terBrugge KG, & Willinsky RA (2007) Treatment of intracranial aneurysms with hydrogel coated expandable coils. *Can J Neurol Sci* **34**:38–46.

23. Weber W, Siekmann R, Kis B, & Kuehne D (2005) Treatment and follow-up of 22 unruptured wide-necked intracranial aneurysms of the internal carotid artery with Onyx HD 500. *AJNR Am J Neuroradiol* **26**:1909–1915.

24. Nelson PK & Levy DI (2001) Balloon-assisted coil embolization of wide-necked aneurysms of the internal carotid artery: medium-term angiographic and clinical follow-up in 22 patients. *AJNR Am J Neuroradiol* **22**:19–26.

25. Eskridge JM & Song JK (1998) Endovascular embolization of 150 basilar tip aneurysms with Guglielmi detachable coils: results of the Food and Drug Administration multicenter clinical trial. *J Neurosurg* **89**:81–86.

26. Evans JJ, Sekhar LN, Rak R, & Stimac D (2004) Bypass grafting and revascularization in the management of posterior circulation aneurysms. *Neurosurgery* **55**:1036–1049.

27. Molyneux AJ, Kerr RS, Yu LM, *et al.* (2005) International subarachnoid aneurysm trial (ISAT) of neurosurgical clipping versus endovascular coiling in 2143 patients with ruptured intracranial aneurysms: a randomised comparison of effects on survival, dependency, seizures, rebleeding, subgroups, and aneurysm occlusion. *Lancet* **366**:809–817.

28. Pierot L, Boulin A, Castaings L, Rey A, Moret J (1996) Endovascular treatment of pericallosal artery aneurysms. *Neurol Res* **18**:49–53.

29. Leibowitz R, Do HM, Marcellus ML, Chang SD, Steinberg GK, & Marks MP (2003) Parent vessel occlusion for vertebrobasilar fusiform and dissecting aneurysms. *AJNR Am J Neuroradiol* **24**:902–907.

30. Bendok BR, Przybylo JH, Parkinson R, Hu Y, Awad IA, & Batjer HH (2005) Neuroendovascular interventions for intracranial posterior circulation disease via the transradial approach: technical case report. *Neurosurgery* **56**:E626; discussion E626.

31. Gruber DP, Zimmerman GA, Tomsick TA, van Loveren HR, Link MJ, & Tew JM Jr (1999) A comparison between endovascular and surgical management of basilar artery apex aneurysms. *J Neurosurg* **90**:868–874.

32. Raymond J & Roy D (1997) Safety and efficacy of endovascular treatment of acutely ruptured aneurysms. *Neurosurgery* **41**:1235–1245; discussion 1245–1236.

59 Surgical Treatment of Cerebral Aneurysms

Rabih G. Tawk, Adnan H. Siddiqui, Elad I. Levy & L. Nelson Hopkins

School of Medicine and Biomedical Sciences, University at Buffalo, State University of New York, Buffalo, NY, USA

Historical background

Historically, the treatment of cerebral aneurysms has traversed an indirect, somewhat serendipitous course. Surgical management of aneurysms dates back to the late 1800s, when large intracranial aneurysms were accidentally encountered during craniotomy for suspected brain tumor. The first planned ligation of a carotid artery for the treatment of a saccular aneurysm was performed in 1928 [1], and early cases had limited success given the association with cerebral infarction [2,3].

In 1931, Dott [4] performed the first planned direct treatment of an intracranial aneurysm, which was accomplished by wrapping a ruptured aneurysm with muscle. The following year, Olivecrona exposed a posterior fossa aneurysm, mistaking it for a tumor, and ligated it intracranially [5]. Since the mid 1930s, several authors [6,7] reported wrapping and packing of aneurysms of the circle of Willis, with varying degrees of success. Dandy [8] first used an intracranial clip to occlude an aneurysm in 1937, and reported several more intracranial procedures in 1941 [9]. At a national neurosurgical meeting in 1938, German [10] and other surgeons reported on the excision of aneurysms. During the 1940s, Dott [11] pioneered several intracranial procedures, including temporary clip occlusion and proximal intracranial vessel ligation. By the mid 1950s, several authors reported clipping and ligature of internal carotid artery (ICA) aneurysms [5,12–14]. In 1953, the first large series of intracranial occlusion was reported [14]. Of the 100 patients who underwent surgery after a 3-week "free interval quiescent period" subsequent to aneurysmal subarachnoid hemorrhage (SAH), mortality was approximately 3%. Owing to the morbidity of this disease, neurosurgeons were subsequently forced to justify not only optimal surgical techniques, but also the need for operative techniques (versus medical therapy or observation) in general and especially for cases of unruptured intracranial aneurysm (UIA). In the absence of scientific evidence,

the beliefs of surgeons often served to guide surgery and current state-of-the-art microsurgery. Yasargil in the late 1960s pioneered the usage of the operating microscope for surgical treatment of aneurysms [15]. With improved visualization and better designed microsurgical clips, the treatment of ruptured as well as incidentally discovered unruptured aneurysms gained momentum and widespread acceptance. Pioneers such as Drake [16] further accumulated a wealth of experience in treatment of the more formidable posterior circulation aneurysms, making microsurgical clip ligation a necessary element of a neurosurgeon's armamentarium. This resulted in a dramatic increase in surgical treatment for this disease with a consequential decline in surgical morbidity and mortality. It is only within the last 10 years that improved endovascular technologies and their testing against microsurgical clip ligation through trials such as the International Study of Unruptured Intracranial Aneurysms (ISUIA) [17,18] and the International Subarachnoid Aneurysm Trial [19,20] are making surgical clip ligation a more circumspect choice for the treatment of both ruptured and unruptured intracranial aneurysms.

Incidence of intracranial aneurysms and aneurysmal subarachnoid hemorrhage

The incidence of intracranial aneurysms is difficult to estimate. The prevalence is 5% and ranges from 0.2–7.9% in autopsy studies [21]; the variability largely depends on the use of microscopes for dissection, hospital referral patterns, autopsy protocols, and overall interest. The ratio of ruptured to unruptured aneurysms is 5:3 to 5:6, with a rough estimate of 1:1 (50% of these aneurysms rupture), with only 2% of aneurysms presenting during childhood [22]. On the other hand, the available data on the incidence of aneurysmal SAH suggests a range that depends on geography. For example, in the USA two large studies have been performed. The first was reported from Framingham, Massachusetts, and yielded a rate of 28 cases per 100 000 adults (30–88 years old) per year [23]. The second study was from Rochester, Minnesota, which gave a rate of 10.8 cases per 100 000 persons per year

Cardiovascular Interventions in Clinical Practice. Edited by Jürgen Haase, Hans-Joachim Schäfers, Horst Sievert and Ron Waksman. © 2010 Blackwell Publishing.

between 1945 and 1974 for all ages [24]. Among patients in Greenland, the incidence of SAH was 9.3 per 100 000 for all ages [25]. Moreover, the age-adjusted average annual rate of SAH may vary among different populations in the same geographic region. For instance, in Izumo, Japan, the incidence was 18.3 per 100 000 for the general population, and 92.3 per 100 000 persons per year for men in the eighth decade [26].

Natural history: ruptured versus unruptured aneurysms

Aneurysmal SAH carries a high fatality rate; therefore, ruptured and unruptured intracranial aneurysms are approached differently. On average, 60% of patients with SAH die or are severely disabled; among the remaining 40%, approximately one-half have significant neuropsychologic and cognitive deficits that prohibit their return to work [27–30]. Many patients with SAH may not receive medical care; furthermore, even with treatment, nearly half are dead within 30 days and two-thirds of these deaths occur within 48 h of aneurysm rupture [27,28,31]. Among survivors, only one-third make a full recovery.

Untreated patients remain at risk over the long term for rehemorrhage (annual rebleeding rate 3–5%) and death [32,33]. In the retrospective part of the ISUIA, 66% of the patients who had SAH from a previously unruptured aneurysm died [17]. Juvela and colleagues [34] reported 52% mortality in patients with ruptured aneurysms. Tsutsumi and colleagues [35] reported a mortality rate of 86% as a result of aneurysm rupture.

Although exhaustive literature reviews on UIA are available, there have been no prospective studies on the natural history of UIAs to date, and most reports are from patients with a history of SAH from a different aneurysm. Juvela [36] retrospectively examined the long-term natural history of UIAs and the risk factors for aneurysm rupture in 142 patients (131 with previous SAH) in Helsinki (Finland). These patients were observed from 1956 to 1978 (median follow-up of 19.7 years), when unruptured aneurysms were not treated in Helsinki. During 2575 person-years, 33 of the 142 patients (23%) had SAH, resulting in an annual incidence of 1.3%. The cumulative rates of SAH were 10.5% at 10 years, 23% at 20 years, and 30.3% at 30 years. Twenty-nine of 33 aneurysms that eventually ruptured were smaller than 10 mm in diameter at the time of the original diagnosis (18 were ≤6 mm). One important observation of this study is that aneurysms that ruptured had increased in size (≥1 mm) more than those aneurysms that did not rupture. The annual rupture rate was 1.3% and was similar to that in previous reports (1–2.3%) [21,37].

In another study, Tsutsumi and colleagues [35] observed 62 patients with UIAs detected incidentally on cerebral angiography performed for causes unrelated to their aneurysms. The 5- and 10-year cumulative risks of SAH from small

(<10 mm) aneurysms were 4.5% and 13.9%, respectively; the 5- and 10-year cumulative risks from large (>10 mm) aneurysms were 33.5% and 55.9%, respectively.

In 1998, the retrospective arm of the ISUIA was published [17]. The natural history of 1937 UIAs in 1449 patients was evaluated with respect to the risks of aneurysm rupture and surgical intervention. In group 1 (727 patients with no history of SAH from a different aneurysm), the cumulative rate of rupture of aneurysms <10 mm at diagnosis was <0.05% per year; in group 2 (722 patients with a history of SAH from a different aneurysm that had been repaired successfully), the rate was approximately 11 times higher (0.5% per year). The rupture rate of aneurysms larger than 10 mm was <1% per year in both groups; but in group 1, the rate was 6% in the first year for giant aneurysms (25 mm in diameter). The size and location of the aneurysm were independent predictors of rupture. Aneurysms 10 mm or more in diameter had a relative risk of rupture of 11.6. For posterior circulation aneurysms, the relative risk was 13.8 for basilar tip locations and 13.6 for vertebrobasilar locations. Because of the exceedingly low rupture rate among group 1 patients with aneurysms smaller than 10 mm and relatively higher morbidity and mortality rates associated with surgical repair, the question arose as to whether surgery would result in a reduction in the rates of disability and death in patients with UIAs smaller than 10 mm and no history of SAH. These findings became the subject of significant controversy and had an impact on neurosurgical practice in the management of UIA.

The results of the retrospective arm of the ISUIA indicated that the risk of rupture of an aneurysm smaller than 10 mm in a patient with no previous SAH (group 1) was 0.05% [17]. Furthermore, the combined morbidity and mortality rates associated with the surgical management of these lesions were 17.5% at 30 days and 15.7% at 1 year. With a risk of rupture 10 to 12 times lower than previously estimated and the risk associated with treatment approximately double that for historical controls, the recommendation was to manage patients expectantly when their aneurysms were smaller than 10 mm. This recommendation led to controversy, with prominent cerebrovascular surgeons noting that the ISUIA population was biased toward patients with low risk for rupture because those with particularly worrisome symptoms, aneurysm morphologic configuration, and family history of SAH were preferentially treated and not included in the study [38–41].

In 2003, the results of the prospective arm of the ISUIA [18] showed that the 5-year cumulative rupture rates for aneurysms in the anterior circulation in patients with no previous SAH (group 1) was 0% in lesions smaller than 7 mm and 2.5% in lesions of the posterior communicating artery or posterior cerebral circulation. Aneurysm size and location were significant predictors of rupture, and patient age combined with aneurysm size and location was a significant predictor of treatment outcome. Although significantly different from the retrospective data, the ISUIA prospective data underscores the need for individual counseling with respect to lesion size, site, patient age, and comorbidities in each patient who presents with a cerebral aneurysm.

Risk factors for aneurysm rupture

The patient-specific factors associated with an increased risk of SAH include female gender (particularly women with the onset of menarche at an earlier age, nulligravidity, or early pregnancy), smoking, increased age, hypertension, binge alcohol drinking, ischemic heart disease, autosomal dominant polycystic kidney disease, use of oral contraceptive drugs, and a family history of SAH [31,42–44]. Aneurysm-specific factors associated with an increased risk of SAH include increased size, irregular shape, posterior circulation, or anterior communicating artery location, symptomatic aneurysm, association with arteriovenous malformations, aneurysms that increase in size on follow-up imaging, dome to neck ratio >1.6, and previous SAH from another aneurysm [17,45–47]. The ISUIA investigators found that aneurysm size and posterior cerebral location outweighed all other factors [48]. Other factors associated with aneurysm rupture include an increase in or an elevated atmospheric pressure and a diurnal and seasonal variation with a peak in winter and a nadir in summer [49,50].

The influence of aneurysm size on aneurysm rupture is unclear. Aneurysm size >10mm is thought to be the strongest predictor of rupture. However, in many large clinical series of SAH, the vast majority of aneurysms are <10mm [51,52]. For example, in a retrospective database of 945 patients of whom 86% had ruptured aneurysms, Weir and colleagues [47] observed that 77% of the ruptured aneurysms were 10mm or smaller.

Experimental work at our laboratory has identified a strong correlation between aneurysm to parent vessel size ratio ("size ratio"; defined as maximum aneurysm height/average parent vessel diameter) and rupture risk, with a higher size ratio (>2), irrespective of aneurysm type and absolute aneurysm or vessel size, giving rise to flow patterns typically observed in ruptured intracranial aneurysms [53]. The potential of this new parameter for rupture risk assessment is under investigation in the clinical arena.

Management of ruptured aneurysms

The primary cause of death or disability after aneurysm rupture is the effect of the initial hemorrhage and subsequent rebleeding [27]. Consequently, the management of all patients with suspected SAH requires immediate evaluation, stabilization, and transfer to neurosurgical care. A growing body of evidence exists that supports the management of patients with cerebral aneurysms at specialized centers by experienced practitioners [54]. Management requires a dedicated multidisciplinary team that can offer both surgical and endovascular options at any time for aneurysm obliteration as

well as endovascular treatment of vasospasm, a major determinant of poor outcome in patients with SAH. The key to successful treatment is aneurysm obliteration to prevent rebleeding and facilitate management of associated conditions. Prominently, cerebral vasospasm, which results from a delayed vasoconstriction of major intracranial arteries in response to blood breakdown products in the cerebrospinal fluid (CSF), remains a major management hurdle. Additionally, hydrocephalus of a communicating variety frequently complicates the initial presentation after SAH and needs to be managed acutely with CSF flow diversion through either a ventriculostomy or the placement of lumbar drain. In almost 50% of patients with aneurysmal SAH, a permanent CSF flow diversion through either a ventriculoperitoneal or lumboperitoneal shunt is required. Although many factors can affect patient outcome, the clinical status or grade at admission is the best predictor of the clinical course and outcome. The most frequently used grading systems include the Hunt and Hess Scale [55] and the World Federation of Neurosurgical Societies Scale [56], which is based on the Glasgow Coma Scale (Table 59.1). In addition, a computed tomography (CT) grading system proposed by Fisher and colleagues [57] is often used to predict angiographic vasospasm (Table 59.1). The validity of the Fisher grading has been called into question in the modern era of vasospasm prophylaxis [58]. In general, patients with a good clinical grade (Hunt and Hess grade I, II, or III) are less likely to have severe SAH on CT imaging or other findings, such as intracranial hemorrhage (ICH), intraventricular hemorrhage (IVH), hydrocephalus, systemic complications, or vasospasm than are patients with a poor clinical grade (Hunt and Hess grade IV or V). Similarly, morbidity and mortality are significantly less in good-grade patients, and in the setting of aneurysm rupture, these result from the initial hemorrhage, subsequent rebleeding, and vasospasm [27,28,59].

Important surgical decisions include the timing of surgery to prevent rebleeding, use of endovascular and/or surgical treatment options, and management of associated factors such as ICH, IVH, hydrocephalus, or vasospasm, all of which can adversely affect the outcome. For example, ICH increases the likelihood of mortality in patients with SAH [60,61]. However, many poor grade patients (grade IV or V), including those with brainstem compression and large ICH, can have favorable outcomes if they are rapidly resuscitated and operated on [62]. Factors such as young age, better clinical grade, and small ICH volume (<25mL) are associated with better outcomes. For diagnosis and initiation of a management plan, CT angiography can be performed rapidly and can detect >90% of aneurysms larger than 3–5mm [63,64]. The loading dose of contrast material has to be considered carefully, especially in patients with renal failure. However, at many centers, surgical planning, including ICH evacuation and aneurysm occlusion, is often based solely on the findings on CT angiography. However, the gold standard for diagnosis

Table 59.1 Commonly used clinical and radiographic grading systems used after aneurysm rupture.

(a) Hunt and Hess Scale [55]

0	No SAH
I	Asymptomatic or mild headache, mild nuchal rigidity
II	Moderate to severe headache, nuchal rigidity, no neurologic deficit except cranial nerve palsy
III	Drowsiness, confusion, or mild focal deficit
IV	Stupor or mild to moderate hemiparesis, possible early decerebrate rigidity
V	Deep coma, decerebrate posturing, moribund

(b) World Federation of Neurosurgical Societies Scale [56]

Grade	Glasgow Coma Scale score	Motor deficit
0	15	Absent and no SAH
1	15	Absent
2	13–14	Absent
3	13–14	Present
4	7–12	Present or absent
5	3–6	Present or absent

(c) Fisher grade [57]

Grade	Computed tomography scan findings
1	No blood detected
2	Diffuse, thin layer of subarachnoid blood (vertical layers < 1-mm thickness)
3	Localized clot or thick layer of subarachnoid clot (vertical layers ≥ 1-mm thickness)
4	Intracerebral or intraventricular blood with diffuse or no subarachnoid blood

SAH, subarachnoid hemorrhage.

and subsequent management algorithms for patients with SAH remains conventional angiography using digital subtraction angiography (DSA) technology. DSA allows for confirmation of the diagnosis; in those cases in which an aneurysm is not found, it provides an excellent modality for evaluation of other vascular diseases, such as arteriovenous malformation, arteriovenous fistula, vasculitis, and even venous disease such as cortical venous or dural sinus thrombosis. Further, DSA allows for careful evaluation of morphologic features of the aneurysm, which bears a great impact on subsequent treatment modality selection.

For surgical treatment of ruptured aneurysm with ICH, large bone flaps are preferable to prevent brain herniation and strangulation, and they provide easy access to the hemorrhage. Mannitol, CSF drainage, and optimization of osmolarity and hypocarbia allow critical brain relaxation. If cerebral swelling persists, ventriculostomy, dural augmentation, and bone flap removal and placement in the abdominal wall, versus freezing for storage, can be very helpful. For patients with Hunt and Hess grade III or higher, ventriculostomy allows drainage of CSF and control of intracranial hypertension. In addition, it allows continuous monitoring of intracranial pressure and cerebral perfusion pressure. Clinical improvement within 24 h of ventriculostomy placement suggests a favorable outcome, but is not always associated with a favorable outcome [65–67]. Ventricular drainage should be performed carefully to avoid altering aneurysm transmural pressure and precipitate rebleeding. In patients with Hunt and Hess grade IV or V, clinical and radiographic findings on admission are often insufficient to predict outcome [62,68,69]. Prediction of outcome based only on admission findings may result in withholding treatment from

30% of the poor-grade patients, who subsequently experience favorable outcomes [62]. Hence, in the majority of poor-grade patients, continued observation with intracranial pressure monitoring and follow-up imaging may help in determining the outcome. In general, the majority of poor-grade patients who are able to follow commands within 5 days of an aneurysm rupture do well and those who die generally do so within the same time frame [68,69]. Patients who do not do well frequently develop elevated intracranial pressure, and progressive ischemic changes are seen on follow-up imaging [68].

Complications of ruptured aneurysms

Complications from aneurysm surgery revolve around the structures intimately involved with these lesions, namely, parent and adjacent vessels and cranial nerves. For example, clip ligation may result in compromise of primary vascular patency; as a result, neurologic symptoms may develop immediately or in a delayed fashion. Any evidence of a new neurologic deficit should be considered an emergency and managed accordingly. Visual deterioration after paraclinoid aneurysm surgery is usually attributed to excessive optic nerve manipulation without adequate detethering of the nerve within the optic canal or arterial perforator compromise during aneurysm exposure. Re-exploration and clip adjustment should be entertained when an intraoperative angiogram reveals a significant residual aneurysm or compromise of the parent vessel or a side branch, or if micro-Doppler intraoperative ultrasound studies reveal occlusion of the parent vessel or a side branch. Palsy of the oculomotor, trochlear, trigeminal, or abducens nerve, as well as ptosis and miosis secondary to sympathetic fiber disruption, generally result from surgical trauma during anterior clinoidectomy, clip blade advancement, cranial nerve manipulation, or cavernous sinus packing. These deficits are usually partial and transient in nature and are best avoided through careful widespread dissection and untethering and opening of arachnoid planes, thereby reducing the need for mechanical retraction of critical neurovascular structures. Overall, diligent arachnoidal dissection to relax the constraints on basal cisterns (which contain the vast majority of intracranial aneurysms) as well as to release large quantities of CSF, further increasing surgical working space and reducing the need for mechanical retraction of brain, form the cardinal principles of microsurgical clipping of aneurysms

Aneurysm regrowth and SAH after surgical clipping is also a known complication of aneurysm surgery. Lozier and colleagues [70] reported 0.18% annual rate of postoperative SAH for all clipped aneurysms and a 0% annual rate for completely clipped lesions over a 7.4 ± 3.7 year follow-up period. In a series of 1170 patients with 12 years of follow-up, Asgari and colleagues [71] reported a 0.4% rehemorrhage rate in completely clipped aneurysms. David and colleagues [72] reported a 1.5% recurrence rate in a series of 135 aneurysms

clipped without residual. In the acute phase, aneurysm rebleeding occurs in approximately 20–30% of ruptured aneurysms within 30 days and then at a rate of approximately 3% per year [33,73]. The highest risk of rebleeding is on SAH day 1 (4%) and occurs at a constant rate of 1–2% per day during the next 4 weeks [74,75]. Poor clinical grade, posterior circulation aneurysms, excess ventricular drainage, and abnormal hemostatic parameters are associated with an increased risk of rebleeding [76,77]. Aneurysm rebleeding has a dismal prognosis: >70% of patients who experience rerupture die.

Acute hydrocephalus is often observed after aneurysm rupture, particularly in poor-grade patients and those with thick subarachnoid blood on CT imaging. Several clinical series describe favorable results using external ventricular drainage for hydrocephalus or IVH after aneurysm rupture, provided early aneurysm occlusion is achieved [78–80]. Acute hydrocephalus is often associated with vasospasm [81]; ventricular drainage should therefore be accompanied by early aneurysm occlusion to allow effective use of hyperdynamic therapy and angioplasty. On the other hand, 20% of patients with SAH develop chronic hydrocephalus and approximately half of patients with acute hydrocephalus eventually require insertion of a permanent shunt [82]. Factors associated with hydrocephalus include increased ventricular size and IVH at admission, poor clinical grade, preexisting hypertension, alcoholism, female sex, increased aneurysm size, pneumonia, and meningitis [82]. The need for a permanent shunt can be reduced by external ventricular drainage, including long, tunneled catheters, serial lumbar punctures, and perhaps by performing a lamina terminalis fenestration at the time of craniotomy [83,84]. Whether an aneurysm is occluded using surgical or endovascular techniques does not influence the subsequent risk for hydrocephalus [85].

Management of unruptured aneurysms

The management of these patients is still controversial. The risk of a UIA is related to hemorrhage, with a 45–80% severe morbidity and mortality rate [17,27,29,30,34,35,40]. Prevention of this rupture is believed to be the most effective strategy for lowering these mortality rates. However, all treatment modalities carry some risks, and in formulating recommendations for treatment, the natural history of UIAs must be considered carefully along with the patient's life expectancy. Assessing life expectancy includes consideration of the patient's age, medical condition, and family history. This allows the counseling physician to make a calculated judgment about the lifetime risk of a UIA, compared with the risk of treatment. For example, a relatively benign natural history makes observation a reasonable or even a preferred choice, particularly in the older population, whereas a more malignant natural history in the younger patient makes treatment more urgent. Life expectancy tables can be helpful in providing an estimate of the patient's life expectancy. This complex assessment is further complicated by having different modes of therapy, and each mode has its own advantages, disadvantages, and complications.

Although the management of patients with unruptured aneurysms is a subject of ongoing debate, the prospective ISUIA [18] is frequently quoted when counseling these patients and managing UIAs (Table 59.2). In the series, 4060 patients were assessed and 1692 patients had conservative treatment of their aneurysm. Patients in group 1 (1077 patients) had no history of SAH, and patients in group 2 (615 patients) had a history of SAH from a separate aneurysm. Over a mean follow-up of 4.1 years, 3% (51 patients) in the nonoperated cohort had a confirmed aneurysm rupture. Larger aneurysm size was associated with greater risk of rupture in group 1 patients who did not have surgery, but not in group 2. The 5-year mortality rate was 12.7% in those patients with

Table 59.2 Yearly and 5-year cumulative rupture rates in unruptured aneurysms according to ISUIA.

Size (mm) and location	SAH rate (%)	
	Group 1	Group 2
Retrospective arm (1998)		
<10	0.05	0.5
≥10	1.0	1.0
≥25	6.0	Not reported
Prospective arm (2003)		
<7		
Cavernous	0	0
Anterior circulation[a]	0	1.5
Posterior circulation[b]	2.5	3.4
7–12		
Cavernous	0	0
Anterior circulation	2.6	2.6
Posterior circulation	14.5	14.5
13–24		
Cavernous	3.0	3.0
Anterior circulation	14.5	14.5
Posterior circulation	18.4	18.4
≥25		
Cavernous	6.4	6.4
Anterior circulation	40.0	40.0
Posterior circulation	50.0	50.0

Table based on Ecker and colleagues [112].
Group 1, patients with no history of SAH from a different aneurysm; group 2, patients with a history of SAH from a different aneurysm that had been repaired successfully.
[a]Includes anterior communicating artery, internal carotid artery, and middle cerebral artery.
[b]Includes posterior communicating artery, posterior cerebral artery, basilar artery, and vertebral artery.

unruptured aneurysms. Asymptomatic patients in group 1 with unruptured aneurysms <7 mm in diameter in the anterior circulation had the lowest-risk natural history. Among 4060 patients for whom surgery was planned, 1917 patients underwent open surgical repair and 451 had endovascular repair of their aneurysm. The morbidity and mortality rates at 1 year with open surgery were 12.6% for group 1 and 10.1% for group 2. Risk factors for poorer outcome included age older than 50 years, larger aneurysmal size and location in the posterior circulation, history of ischemic cerebrovascular disease, and symptoms other than rupture. In those patients undergoing endovascular repair, the initial morbidity and mortality rates were 9.1% and 9.5%, respectively. This endovascular group, however, had older patients with larger unruptured aneurysms and a higher proportion of aneurysms in the posterior circulation. Limitations of the study include the nonrandomized nature of the groups, >50% of all patients had follow-up for <5 years, and the small number of patients in the endovascular group.

In daily clinical practice, the decision-making process and management strategy are influenced by comorbidities, patient preferences, anatomical configuration, and endovascular techniques available at the particular institution. Among patient-related factors, neurologic grade and age are the most important factors to determine prognosis [86].

Surgical treatment

Aneurysm surgical clipping was introduced to neurosurgery several decades ago and is considered a well established modality for the treatment of aneurysms [87]. In patients with UIAs, the risks of the intervention must be thoroughly considered. As with other surgeries, high-volume centers and experienced surgeons offer better outcomes and fewer complications [88].

A systemic metaanalysis of surgical treatment for unruptured aneurysms identified 61 studies with a total of 2460 patients (57% female; mean age, 50 years) and at least 2568 unruptured aneurysms (27% >25 mm, 30% located in the posterior circulation) with a mean follow-up of 24 weeks [89]. Mortality was 2.6%, and permanent morbidity 10.9% in this cohort. Postoperative mortality and morbidity were significantly lower in later years for patients with nongiant and anterior circulation aneurysms. The lowest morbidity and mortality were found with small anterior circulation aneurysms (0.8% mortality, 1.9% morbidity) and the worst with large posterior fossa aneurysms (9.6% mortality, 37.9% morbidity).

In phase II of the ISUIA (prospective arm), surgery-related mortality was found at 1 year to be 2.7% in patients with no previous SAH and 0.6% in patients who had previously had an SAH. Morbidity rates were 9.9% and 9.8%, respectively [18]. Unlike most previous studies, cognitive impairment was considered a complication. The risk associated with surgical treatment was 13.7% at 30 days and 12.6% at 1 year in patients with unruptured aneurysms.

Preoperative preparation

Patients presenting with SAH are immediately admitted to the intensive care unit and generally treated within 1–2 days of admission. The preoperative assessment should include a complete neurologic examination and a comprehensive medical evaluation. The optimal treatment modality is selected in an individualized manner after completion of radiographic workup and stabilization of the patient. In cases of ruptured aneurysm, this typically requires the following: performance of a formal cerebral diagnostic angiogram; placement of an external ventriculostomy drain for patients with hydrocephalus or poor neurologic grade; placement of multiple large-bore intravenous lines and, often, a central venous line or even a Swan–Ganz catheter for optimal hydration; volume expansion; placement of an intraarterial line for continuous blood pressure monitoring to prevent a spike above 130–140 mmHg systolic blood pressure; and intubation and sedation for patients who are somnolent, lethargic, or comatose. In cases of UIAs, patients are evaluated and treated in an elective manner unless there is rapid progression of symptoms from mass effect or thromboembolic complications with neurologic decline.

Anesthesia and neurophysiologic monitoring

Prophylactic antibiotics, intravenous steroids and antiepileptic agents, mild hypothermia (i.e., hypothermic circulatory arrest to facilitate surgical treatment of complex aneurysms by providing brain ischemic protection), and an indwelling arterial line for blood pressure monitoring are routinely used during surgery. Continuous evoked potential and electroencephalographic monitoring is being used increasingly. Modest reduction of arterial carbon dioxide pressure, CSF drainage through a wide opening of the Sylvian fissure, and, in cases of ruptured aneurysms, intravenous administration of mannitol, are all utilized for brain relaxation. When temporary focal circulatory arrest is employed for complex aneurysms, mild hypertension is induced and helps with collateral flow to the ischemic territory, and intravenous barbiturates are titrated to induce electroencephalographic burst suppression and lower the metabolism to prolong the survival of nervous cells under ischemic circumstances. (Temporary focal circulatory arrest refers to occlusion of the vessel proximal to the aneurysm, which is a basic principle in aneurysm surgery in case there is rupture before clipping. Occasionally, it is used for complex aneurysms to facilitate and optimize clip placement. Hypertension helps with collateral perfusion, and barbiturates decrease the metabolism of cells and prolong their survival under ischemic circumstances.)

Pterional craniotomy

Surgical approaches and principles of clip application as well as alternatives for clipping have been well established. Options, including proximal vessel occlusion and flow reversal, bypass surgery with extracranial or intracranial donor vessel, aneurysm trapping, wrapping, and other microvascular techniques and approaches for complex aneurysms have also been described [90–92], and a detailed description is beyond the scope of this chapter. However, it is important to realize that with the increased popularity of endovascular techniques, the acquisition of surgical techniques is becoming increasingly difficult and requires further training with expert vascular neurosurgeons at centers with large case volumes; therefore, the pterional approach, popularized by Yasargil and colleagues [87,93,94], is most commonly used and will be discussed briefly. This approach provides optimal exposure to the anterior circulation as well as the upper basilar artery and its bifurcation.

The patient is placed supine on the operating table with a shoulder roll beneath the ipsilateral shoulder. The head is fixed in a radiolucent rigid fixation system (allowing intraoperative angiography), turned 45° toward the contralateral side, and elevated above the heart (to promote venous drainage). For all paraclinoid aneurysm cases, the patient's neck on the same side as the lesion is prepared and draped in the sterile field to allow access to the cervical carotid bifurcation for proximal ICA control, retrograde suction decompression, or saphenous vein bypass grafting as needed. Cervical ICA exposure has been shown to be effective in patients with clinoidal segment aneurysms and in patients harboring complex, giant, or ruptured ophthalmic aneurysms. In Yasargil's description, the vertex is lowered, thereby allowing gravity to retract the frontal and temporal lobes gently [87,93,94]. The neck is extended slightly so that the zygoma is positioned as the highest point in the field. A curvilinear incision is extended from the temporal process of the zygoma, about 1 cm anterior to the tragus of the ear, to the midforehead hairline. If a patient has a receding hairline, a better cosmetic result is achieved by extending the incision posteriorly and beyond the midline to avoid producing a visible scar. The skin flap is reflected anteriorly, along with the underlying temporalis muscle. A variation on this theme is the interfascial temporalis flap [95] to preserve the frontalis branch of the facial nerve, while maximizing exposure [95]. The scalp, including the galea, is reflected downward by opening the plane between the pericranium and the galea. The temporal fascia is incised just above the fat pad containing the branches of the facial nerve to the forehead so that the fat pad and facial branches can be reflected downward with the scalp flap. A cuff of pericranium and temporalis fascia is preserved along the anterior part of the temporal line to facilitate closure of the temporalis muscle and fascia. The temporalis muscle and its fascia are reflected inferiorly, and a free frontotemporal bone flap with the center of its base at the pterion is elevated and removed. This maneuver can be achieved with a single or several drill or burr holes to allow the craniotome footplate to be introduced into the correct plane. The anteromedial extent of the flap depends on the aneurysm, ranging from 1 cm anterior to the pterion for aneurysms of the middle cerebral artery to almost the midline for aneurysms of the anterior communicating complex. The size of the flap is individualized based on the degree of pneumatization of the frontal sinus, which in case of exposure, should be exenterated and sealed with a pericranial flap before closure. The remainder of the lateral wall of the sphenoid wing is removed. This maneuver is achieved with a high-speed drill or performed in a piecemeal fashion with a rongeur until the bone is flush with the floor of the anterior cranial fossa. The sphenoid wing can be drilled to varying extents, even beyond the superior orbital fissure and, when necessary, to the anterior clinoid process. The dura is opened in a curvilinear fashion based on the pterion and tacked to create flaps that serve as gutters and drain extradural bleeding. Meticulous attention to hemostasis during the opening phase of the operation greatly facilitates the intradural portion of the operation by preventing the surgical field from becoming obscured by blood. As a general rule, proximal control of blood flow should be obtained before dissecting the aneurysm. Dissection over the aneurysm dome should be delayed to prevent premature rupture. This will allow the application of proximal occlusion to facilitate aneurysm clipping. After aneurysm dissection, restoration of normal blood pressure, induction of a burst suppression electroencephalogram pattern with optimal rheology, and the selection of appropriate sites for clip application, temporary or final clips are applied. Clip application has to be performed carefully to ensure optimal aneurysm obliteration without causing narrowing or occlusion of afferent and efferent vessels. Aneurysm aspiration, Doppler ultrasound, or intraoperative angiography through a formal transfemoral route using C-arm imaging or through a fluorescence filter in the microscope to visualize intravascular indocyanine green (injected intravenously) is used to verify aneurysm obliteration.

Postoperative care

Postoperative care for patients with ruptured intracranial aneurysms depends on the grade and corresponding clinical status. Patients with SAH are monitored in the intensive care unit, utilizing standard protocols for the management of SAH, including aggressive hydration, avoidance of dehydration and hypotension, and monitoring for vasospasm during the window of risk. At our center, these patients have daily transcranial Doppler imaging studies for at least 21 days. CT angiography and CT perfusion imaging are useful diagnostic adjuncts and can be used to demonstrate vasospasm and resultant ischemia in the case of clinical suspicion of vasospasm. In the case of neurologic deterioration, a diagnostic angiogram with the injection of vasodilatory agents, such as papaverine, or calcium-channel blockers (e.g. verapamil or nicardipine), or balloon angioplasty is used for distal and diffuse or focal and proximal vasospasm, respectively. In the case of a UIA with no surgical complications, the patient is monitored generally in the intensive care unit for 1 to 2 days,

followed by early mobilization and normalization of diet and medications. Postoperative angiography is frequently performed to ensure obliteration of the aneurysm and guide the future follow-up plan.

Prognostic factors and surgical outcome

In addition to SAH grade, a variety of factors can be used as potential predictors of surgical outcome. These include the hospital case volume and the experience of the surgeons, patient age, and the location and size of the aneurysm [16,18]. According to the Nationwide Inpatient Sample hospital discharge database (1996 to 2002) [96], 3498 patients were treated at 463 hospitals; 2.1% died and 16.1% were discharged to facilities other than home after UIA repair surgery. Mortality was lower at high-volume hospitals (1.6% vs. 2.2%); discharge other than to home occurred in 15.6% of patients after surgery at high-volume hospitals (20 or more cases per year), compared with 23.8% at low-volume hospitals (fewer than four cases per year).

Patient age

In the ISUIA prospective arm, a 2.4 relative-risk increase was observed in patients 50 years of age and older [18]. Takahashi [97] found the worst surgical outcome to be in patients older than 80. Keeping aneurysm size and location constant, Khanna and colleagues [98] reported an association between poor outcome and older age, which, in addition to medical comorbidities in the older age group, could be due to an increased incidence of atherosclerosis and/or calcified aneurysm.

Aneurysm location

Aneurysm location within the posterior circulation was associated with an increased incidence of poor outcome in the ISUIA [17,18]. Solomon and colleagues [99] observed 50% morbidity and mortality with surgery for unruptured giant basilar aneurysms, compared with 13% for anterior circulation giant aneurysms. Drake [16] reported a 14.3% morbidity with surgical treatment of unruptured asymptomatic aneurysms in the posterior circulation compared with 0% morbidity for aneurysms of the anterior circulation. Aneurysms of the anterior communicating artery projecting superiorly and posteriorly and clinoidal and cavernous segment aneurysms are also associated with higher morbidity and mortality due to difficulty achieving safe exposure and proximal control [100,101].

Aneurysm size

According to Solomon and colleagues [99], the combined morbidity and mortality rates for unruptured aneurysms were 0% for aneurysms 10 mm or smaller, 6% for aneurysms between 10 and 25 mm and 20% for aneurysms larger than 25 mm. Drake [16] reported 15% morbidity and mortality for nongiant posterior circulation aneurysms, compared with

39% for giant posterior circulation aneurysms, although ruptured aneurysms were also included in his series. Aneurysms larger than 12 mm are associated with a relative risk of poor surgical outcome of 2.6 [18].

Timing of aneurysm surgery

In patients with ruptured aneurysms, several factors influence whether surgery should be early or delayed. In the early 1980s, the optimal timing of surgery for ruptured aneurysms was the subject of considerable controversy [102]. It was initially thought that the best results were obtained when the operation was delayed until the clinical condition was stable and the reactive brain swelling accompanying the initial hemorrhage had subsided. Subsequently, it was found that delaying surgery was associated with aneurysm rebleeding, and it was argued that early surgery could be performed with acceptable results [103]. Early aneurysm occlusion eliminates the risk of rebleeding and appears to be associated with improved outcome. Nonrandomized studies, describing concurrent cohorts or historical controls, and large clinical series [29,103,104] have observed a tendency for patients undergoing early surgery to experience better outcomes. A single randomized study examined surgical timing in patients with good clinical grades (Hunt and Hess grades I to III) with anterior circulation aneurysms [105]. At 3 months, independent outcomes were observed in 91.5% of patients undergoing surgery within 72 h of SAH, 78.6% of those undergoing surgery between 4 and 7 days after SAH, and 80% undergoing surgery >8 days after SAH. Some investigators have suggested that ultra-early surgery within 12 h of SAH may benefit patients because the risk of bleeding is greatest during this time period. Although this is feasible, there are no data to show that outcome is any better [106]. The international Cooperative Study on the Timing of Aneurysm Surgery [29] was a prospective nonrandomized study with 3251 patients. The study demonstrated that among patients who were alert at the time of admission, 78% experienced a favorable 6-month outcome when surgery was performed between 0 and 3 days after SAH. When surgery was delayed for >14 days, 69% of these patients experienced a favorable outcome. Among stuporous or comatose patients, timing of surgery was not associated with outcome. In a separate analysis of the 722 patients treated at 27 North American centers, early surgery was associated with better outcome; 70.9% of patients undergoing surgery between 0 and 3 days after SAH experienced a good recovery, whereas 62.9% of patients had a similar outcome if surgery was performed after 14 days [103]. These results suggest that surgery within 3 days of SAH offers the most reasonable chance of good outcome for ruptured anterior circulation aneurysms. Early medical and surgical interventions reduce the deleterious consequences of cerebral ischemia, particularly in the poor-grade patient. Although cerebral swelling is more frequent in poor-grade patients, the incidence of surgical complications during early surgery is similar in poor- and good-grade patients [107]. Alternatively, patients with significant swelling on admission are treated endovascularly to secure their aneurysm. Advanced age should not exclude the patient from early surgery, in part because elderly patients are more likely to have intracerebral hematomas and a decreased cerebrovascular reserve that increases their risk for delayed ischemia [108]. In patients at high risk for vasospasm, early surgery and aneurysm obliteration allows a safer hypervolemic, hypertensive therapy and angioplasty. For complex lesions such as giant aneurysms, those that require revascularization, or those with which prolonged periods of temporary occlusion are anticipated during surgery, delayed surgery may be preferable.

The timing of aneurysm occlusion for posterior circulation aneurysms is less well defined. The Cooperative Study on the Timing of Aneurysm Surgery included too few posterior circulation aneurysms to draw meaningful conclusions [29]. However, other studies suggest that early surgery may lead to a reduction in morbidity and mortality [109–111]. For example, Hillman and colleagues [110] prospectively reviewed 59 cases of ruptured posterior fossa aneurysms treated during a 1-year period. Fifty percent of 26 patients scheduled for late surgery made a good recovery, whereas 72% of the 23 patients scheduled for early surgery made a good recovery. Intraoperative complications were equally common in the early or delayed surgery groups.

Poor-grade patients

Between 20% and 40% of patients admitted to hospital after aneurysm rupture are in poor clinical condition (Hunt and Hess grades IV and V). The association between poor outcome and poor clinical grade after SAH has been well described. However, the published data suggest that an aggressive policy may provide these patients their best chance of recovery. Treatment includes rapid resuscitation and emergent placement of an external ventriculostomy drain to control intracranial pressure and hydrocephalus, early aneurysm occlusion, and prevention of vasospasm. The use of noninvasive physiologic assessment such as transcranial Doppler, and invasive monitoring of intracranial pressure and cardiac hemodynamics are critical to guide therapy.

Conclusion

The approach to the management of patients harboring cerebral aneurysms may be altered by a variety of special circumstances, especially when it comes to ruptured or unruptured, symptomatic or asymptomatic aneurysms. Surgical treatment of cerebral aneurysms remains challenging, and it is important to realize that, with the increased popularity of endovascular techniques, the acquisition of surgical techniques is becoming difficult and requires further training with expert vascular neurosurgeons at centers with large case volumes.

Illustrative case

A 52-year-old woman with a family history of cerebral aneurysms was found to have an incidental 4.6 × 5.7 mm left middle cerebral artery (MCA) aneurysm on angiography (Fig. 59.1a, anteroposterior view; Fig. 59.1b, lateral view). The aneurysm was not suitable for endovascular treatment, and the patient was admitted for surgery and clipping. Using the operative microscope, an adequate exposure of the MCA branches within the Sylvian fissure was performed,

and the aneurysm was identified (Fig. 59.1c, intraoperative photograph). The proximal MCA was identified along with the aneurysm neck and MCA branches. After temporary clipping of the proximal MCA, the aneurysm was rendered soft and was occluded with a combination of bayonet and right angle clips (Fig. 59.1d, intraoperative photograph). After removal of the temporary clip, Doppler ultrasonography was used to confirm occlusion of the aneurysm and patency of the MCA branches. After surgery, the patient had an unremarkable recovery and remained neurologically intact.

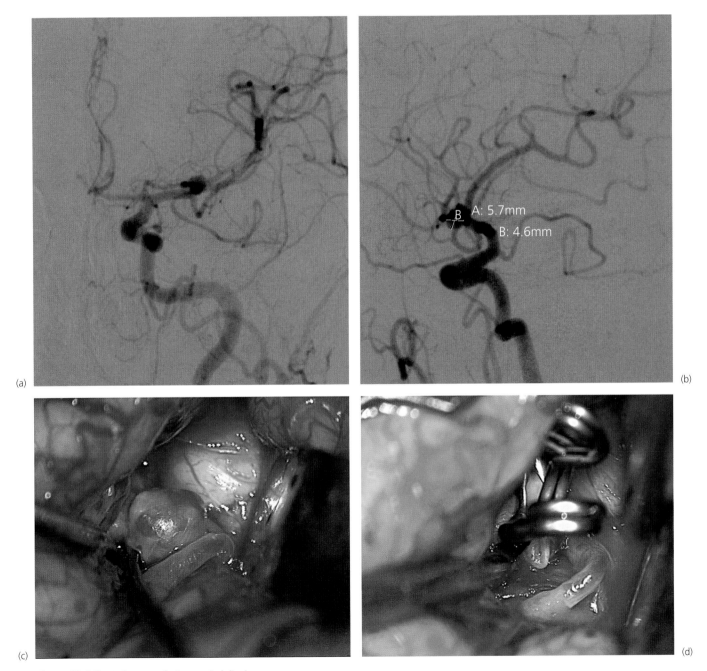

(a)

(b)

A: 5.7mm
B: 4.6mm

(c)

(d)

Figure 59.1 Illustrative case of microsurgical clipping.

References

1. Schorstein J (1940) Carotid ligation in saccular intracranial aneurysms. *Br J Surg* **28**:50–70.

2. Magnus V (1927) Aneurysms of the internal carotid artery. *JAMA* **88**:1712–1713.

3. Sossman MC & Vogt EC (1926) Aneurysms of the internal carotid artery and the circle of Willis, from a roentgenological viewpoint. *AJR Am J Roentgenol* **15**:122–134.

4. Dott NM (1933) Intracranial aneurysms: cerebral arterioradiography: surgical treatment. *Edinburgh Med J* **40**:219–240.

5. Norlen G, Falconer M, Jefferson G, & Johnson R (1952) The pathology, diagnosis and treatment of intracranial saccular aneurysms. *Proc R Soc Med* 45:291–302.

6. McConnell AA (1937) Subchiasmal aneurysm treated by implantation of muscle. *Zentralbl Neurochir* **2**:269–274.

7. Tőnnis W (1934) Traumatischer Aneurysma der linken Art. carotis int mit Embolie der linken Art. cerebri ant. und retinae. *Zentrabl f Chir* **61**:844–848.

8. Dandy WE (1938) Intracranial aneurysm of the internal carotid artery: cured by operation. *Ann Surg* 107:654–659.

9. Dandy WE (1941) The surgical treatment of intracranial aneurysms of the internal carotid artery. *Ann Surg* 114:336–340.

10. German WJ (1938) Intracranial aneurysms: a surgical problem. *Zentralbl Neurochir* **3**:352–354.

11. Dott NM (1969) Intracranial aneurysmal formations. *Clin Neurosurg* **16**:1–16.

12. Falconer MA (1951) The surgical treatment of bleeding intracranial aneurysms. *J Neurol Neurosurg Psychiatry* **14**:153–186.

13. Norlen G (1963) Some aspects of the surgical treatment of intracranial aneurysms. *Clin Neurosurg* **9**:214–222.

14. Norlen G & Olivecrona H (1953) The treatment of aneurysms of the circle of Willis. *J Neurosurg* **10**:404–415.

15. Al-Shatoury HA, Raja AI, & Ausman JI (2000) Timeline: pioneers in cerebral aneurysms. *Surg Neurol* **54**:465–470.

16. Drake CG (1981) Progress in cerebrovascular disease. Management of cerebral aneurysm. *Stroke* **12**:273–283.

17. International Study of Unruptured Intracranial Aneurysms Investigators (1998) Unruptured intracranial aneurysms—risk of rupture and risks of surgical intervention. *N Engl J Med* **339**:1725–1733.

18. Wiebers DO, Whisnant JP, Huston J 3rd, *et al.* (2003) Unruptured intracranial aneurysms: natural history, clinical outcome, and risks of surgical and endovascular treatment. *Lancet* **362**:103–110.

19. Molyneux A, Kerr R, Stratton I, *et al.* (2002) International Subarachnoid Aneurysm Trial (ISAT) of neurosurgical clipping versus endovascular coiling in 2143 patients with ruptured intracranial aneurysms: a randomised trial. *Lancet* **360**:1267–1274.

20. Molyneux AJ, Kerr RS, Yu LM, *et al.* (2005) International Subarachnoid Aneurysm Trial (ISAT) of neurosurgical clipping versus endovascular coiling in 2143 patients with ruptured intracranial aneurysms: a randomised comparison of effects on survival, dependency, seizures, rebleeding, subgroups, and aneurysm occlusion. *Lancet* **366**(9488):809–817.

21. Wiebers DO, Whisnant JP, Sundt TM Jr, & O'Fallon WM (1987) The significance of unruptured intracranial saccular aneurysms. *J Neurosurg* 66:23–29.

22. Almeida GM, Pindaro J, Plese P, Bianco E, & Shibata MK (1977) Intracranial arterial aneurysms in infancy and childhood. *Childs Brain* **3**:193–199.

23. Sacco RL, Wolf PA, Bharucha NE, *et al.* (1984) Subarachnoid and intracerebral hemorrhage: natural history, prognosis, and precursive factors in the Framingham Study. *Neurology* **34**:847–854.

24. Ingall TJ, Whisnant JP, Wiebers DO, & O'Fallon WM (1989) Has there been a decline in subarachnoid hemorrhage mortality? *Stroke* **20**:718–724.

25. Ostergaard Kristensen M (1983) Increased incidence of bleeding intracranial aneurysms in Greenlandic Eskimos. *Acta Neurochir (Wien)* **67**:37–43.

26. Inagawa T, Ishikawa S, Aoki H, Takahashi M, & Yoshimoto H (1988) Aneurysmal subarachnoid hemorrhage in Izumo City and Shimane Prefecture of Japan. Incidence. *Stroke* **19**:170–175.

27. Broderick JP, Brott TG, Duldner JE, Tomsick T, & Leach A (1994) Initial and recurrent bleeding are the major causes of death following subarachnoid hemorrhage. *Stroke* **25**:1342–1347.

28. Fogelholm R, Hernesniemi J, & Vapalahti M (1993) Impact of early surgery on outcome after aneurysmal subarachnoid hemorrhage. A population-based study. *Stroke* **24**:1649–1654.

29. Kassell NF, Torner JC, Haley EC Jr, Jane JA, Adams HP, & Kongable GL (1990) The International Cooperative Study on the Timing of Aneurysm Surgery. Part **1**: Overall management results. *J Neurosurg* **73**:18–36.

30. Ljunggren B, Saveland H, Brandt L, & Uski T (1984) Aneurysmal subarachnoid hemorrhage. Total annual outcome in a 1.46 million population. *Surg Neurol* **22**:435–438.

31. ACROSS Group (2000) Epidemiology of aneurysmal subarachnoid hemorrhage in Australia and New Zealand: incidence and case fatality from the Australasian Cooperative Research on Subarachnoid Hemorrhage Study (ACROSS). *Stroke* **31**:1843–1850.

32. Winn HR, Richardson AE, & Jane JA (1973) Late morbidity and mortality in cerebral aneurysms: a ten-year follow-up of 364 conservatively treated patients with a single cerebral aneurysm. *Trans Am Neurol Assoc* **98**:148–150.

33. Winn HR, Richardson AE, & Jane JA (1977) The long-term prognosis in untreated cerebral aneurysms: I. The incidence of late hemorrhage in cerebral aneurysm: a 10-year evaluation of 364 patients. *Ann Neurol* **1**:358–370.

34. Juvela S, Porras M, & Heiskanen O (1993) Natural history of unruptured intracranial aneurysms: a long-term follow-up study. *J Neurosurg* **79**:174–182.

35. Tsutsumi K, Ueki K, Morita A, & Kirino T (2000) Risk of rupture from incidental cerebral aneurysms. *J Neurosurg* **93**:550–553.

36. Juvela S (2002) Natural history of unruptured intracranial aneurysms: risks for aneurysm formation, growth, and rupture. *Acta Neurochir Suppl* **82**:27–30.

37. Yasui N, Suzuki A, Nishimura H, Suzuki K, & Abe T (1997) Long-term follow-up study of unruptured intracranial aneurysms. *Neurosurgery* **40**:1155–1160.

38. Brett A (1999) Unruptured intracranial aneurysms. *N Engl J Med* **340**:1441–1442.

39. Caplan LR (1998) Should intracranial aneurysms be treated before they rupture? *N Engl J Med* **339**:1774–1775.

40. Juvela S, Porras M, & Poussa K (2000) Natural history of unruptured intracranial aneurysms: probability of and risk factors for aneurysm rupture. *J Neurosurg* **93**:379–387.

41. Riina HA & Spetzler RF (2002) Unruptured aneurysms. *J Neurosurg* **96**:61–62.

42. Juvela S, Hillbom M, Numminen H, & Koskinen P (1993) Cigarette smoking and alcohol consumption as risk factors for aneurysmal subarachnoid hemorrhage. *Stroke* **24**:639–646.

43. Teunissen LL, Rinkel GJ, Algra A, & van Gijn J (1996) Risk factors for subarachnoid hemorrhage: a systematic review. *Stroke* **27**:544–549.

44. Okamoto K, Horisawa R, Kawamura T, *et al.* (2001) Menstrual and reproductive factors for subarachnoid hemorrhage risk in women: a case-control study in nagoya, Japan. *Stroke* **32**:2841–2844.

45. Brown RD Jr, Wiebers DO, & Forbes GS (1990) Unruptured intracranial aneurysms and arteriovenous malformations: frequency of intracranial hemorrhage and relationship of lesions. *J Neurosurg* **73**:859–863.

46. Juvela S, Poussa K, & Porras M (2001) Factors affecting formation and growth of intracranial aneurysms: a long-term follow-up study. *Stroke* **32**:485–491.

47. Weir B, Disney L, & Karrison T (2002) Sizes of ruptured and unruptured aneurysms in relation to their sites and the ages of patients. *J Neurosurg* **96**:64–70.

48. Mitchell P, Gholkar A, Vindlacheruvu RR, & Mendelow AD (2004) Unruptured intracranial aneurysms: benign curiosity or ticking bomb? *Lancet Neurol* **3**:85–92.

49. Buxton N, Liu C, Dasic D, Moody P, & Hope DT (2001) Relationship of aneurysmal subarachnoid hemorrhage to changes in atmospheric pressure: results of a prospective study. *J Neurosurg* **95**:391–392.

50. Nyquist PA, Brown RD Jr, Wiebers DO, Crowson CS, & O'Fallon WM (2001) Circadian and seasonal occurrence of subarachnoid and intracerebral hemorrhage. *Neurology* **56**:190–193.

51. Kassell NF & Torner JC (1983) Size of intracranial aneurysms. *Neurosurgery* **12**:291–297.

52. Rosenorn J & Eskesen V (1993) Does a safe size-limit exist for unruptured intracranial aneurysms? *Acta Neurochir* (*Wien*) **121**:113–118.

53. Dhar S, Tremmel M, Mocco J, *et al.* (2008) Morphology parameters for intracranial aneurysm rupture risk assessment. *Neurosurgery* **63**:185–196; discussion 196–197.

54. Fridriksson S, Hillman J, Landtblom AM, & Boive J (2001) Education of referring doctors about sudden onset headache in subarachnoid hemorrhage. A prospective study. *Acta Neurol Scand* **103**:238–242.

55. Hunt WE & Hess RM (1968) Surgical risk as related to time of intervention in the repair of intracranial aneurysms. *J Neurosurg* **28**:14–20.

56. Teasdale GM, Drake CG, Hunt W, *et al.* (1988) A universal subarachnoid hemorrhage scale: report of a committee of the World Federation of Neurosurgical Societies. *J Neurol Neurosurg Psychiatry* **51**:1457.

57. Fisher CM, Kistler JP, & Davis JM (1980) Relation of cerebral vasospasm to subarachnoid hemorrhage visualized by computerized tomographic scanning. *Neurosurgery* **6**:1–9.

58. Claassen J, Bernardini GL, Kreiter K, *et al.* (2001) Effect of cisternal and ventricular blood on risk of delayed cerebral ischemia after subarachnoid hemorrhage: the Fisher scale revisited. *Stroke* **32**:2012–2020.

59. Pakarinen S (1967) Incidence, aetiology, and prognosis of primary subarachnoid haemorrhage. A study based on 589 cases diagnosed in a defined urban population during a defined period. *Acta Neurol Scand* **43**(Suppl. 29):1–28.

60. Hauerberg J, Eskesen V, & Rosenorn J (1994) The prognostic significance of intracerebral haematoma as shown on CT scanning after aneurysmal subarachnoid haemorrhage. *Br J Neurosurg* **8**:333–339.

61. O'Sullivan MG, Sellar R, Statham PF, & Whittle IR (1996) Management of poor grade patients after subarachnoid haemorrhage: the importance of neuroradiological findings on clinical outcome. *Br J Neurosurg* **10**:445–452.

62. Le Roux PD, Dailey AT, Newell DW, Grady MS, & Winn HR (1993) Emergent aneurysm clipping without angiography in the moribund patient with intracerebral hemorrhage: the use of infusion computed tomography scans. *Neurosurgery* **33**:189–197.

63. Anderson GB, Steinke DE, Petruk KC, Ashforth R, & Findlay JM (1999) Computed tomographic angiography versus digital subtraction angiography for the diagnosis and early treatment of ruptured intracranial aneurysms. *Neurosurgery* **45**:1315–1322.

64. Murai Y, Takagi R, Ikeda Y, Yamamoto Y, & Teramoto A (1999) Three-dimensional computerized tomography angiography in patients with hyperacute intracerebral hemorrhage. *J Neurosurg* **91**:424–431.

65. Arnold H, Schwachenwald R, Nowak G, & Schwachenwald D (1994) Aneurysm surgery in poor grade patients. Results, and value of external ventricular drainage. *Neurol Res* **16**:45–48.

66. Nowak G, Schwachenwald R, & Arnold H (1994) Early management in poor grade aneurysm patients. *Acta Neurochir* (*Wien*) **126**:33–37.

67. Rajshekhar V & Harbaugh RE (1992) Results of routine ventriculostomy with external ventricular drainage for acute hydrocephalus following subarachnoid haemorrhage. *Acta Neurochir* (*Wien*) **115**(1–2):8–14.

68. Le Roux PD, Elliott JP, Newell DW, Grady MS, & Winn HR (1996) Predicting outcome in poor-grade patients with subarachnoid hemorrhage: a retrospective review of 159 aggressively managed cases. *J Neurosurg* **85**:39–49.

69. Bailes JE, Spetzler RF, Hadley MN, & Baldwin HZ (1990) Management morbidity and mortality of poor-grade aneurysm patients. *J Neurosurg* **72**:559–566.

70. Lozier AP, Kim GH, Sciacca RR, Connolly ES Jr, & Solomon RA (2004) Microsurgical treatment of basilar apex aneurysms: perioperative and long-term clinical outcome. *Neurosurgery* **54**:286–299.

71. Asgari S, Wanke I, Schoch B, & Stolke D (2003) Recurrent hemorrhage after initially complete occlusion of intracranial aneurysms. *Neurosurg Rev* **26**:269–274.

72. David CA, Vishteh AG, Spetzler RF, Lemole M, Lawton MT, & Partovi S (1999) Late angiographic follow-up review of surgically treated aneurysms. *J Neurosurg* **91**:396–401.

73. Alvord EC Jr, Loeser JD, Bailey WL, & Copass MK (1972) Subarachnoid hemorrhage due to ruptured aneurysms. A simple method of estimating prognosis. *Arch Neurol* **27**:273–284.

74. Kassell NF & Torner JC (1983) Aneurysmal rebleeding: a preliminary report from the Cooperative Aneurysm Study. *Neurosurgery* **13**:479–481.

75. Rosenorn J, Eskesen V, Schmidt K, & Ronde F (1987) The risk of rebleeding from ruptured intracranial aneurysms. *J Neurosurg* **67**:329–332.

76. Fujii Y, Takeuchi S, Sasaki O, Minakawa T, Koike T, & Tanaka R (1996) Ultra-early rebleeding in spontaneous subarachnoid hemorrhage. *J Neurosurg* **84**:35–42.

77. Pare L, Delfino R, & Leblanc R (1992) The relationship of ventricular drainage to aneurysmal rebleeding. *J Neurosurg* **76**:422–427.

78. Mohr G, Ferguson G, Khan M, *et al.* (1983) Intraventricular hemorrhage from ruptured aneurysm. Retrospective analysis of 91 cases. *J Neurosurg* **58**:482–487.

79. Shimoda M, Oda S, Shibata M, Tominaga J, Kittaka M, & Tsugane R (1999) Results of early surgical evacuation of packed intraventricular hemorrhage from aneurysm rupture in patients with poor-grade subarachnoid hemorrhage. *J Neurosurg* **91**:408–414.

80. Raimondi AJ & Torres H (1973) Acute hydrocephalus as a complication of subarachnoid hemorrhage. *Surg Neurol* **1**:23–26.

81. Black PM (1986) Hydrocephalus and vasospasm after subarachnoid hemorrhage from ruptured intracranial aneurysms. *Neurosurgery* **18**:12–16.

82. Sheehan JP, Polin RS, Sheehan JM, Baskaya MK, & Kassell NF (1999) Factors associated with hydrocephalus after aneurysmal subarachnoid hemorrhage. *Neurosurgery* **45**:1120–1128.

83. Tomasello F, d'Avella D, & de Divitiis O (1999) Does lamina terminalis fenestration reduce the incidence of chronic hydrocephalus after subarachnoid hemorrhage? *Neurosurgery* **45**:827–832.

84. Hasan D, Vermeulen M, Wijdicks EF, Hijdra A, & van Gijn J (1989) Management problems in acute hydrocephalus after subarachnoid hemorrhage. *Stroke* **20**:747–753.

85. Gruber A, Reinprecht A, Bavinzski G, Czech T, & Richling B (1999) Chronic shunt-dependent hydrocephalus after early surgical and early endovascular treatment of ruptured intracranial aneurysms. *Neurosurgery* **44**:503–512.

86. Le Roux PD & Winn HR (1999) Intracranial aneurysms and subarachnoid hemorrhage management of the poor grade patient. *Acta Neurochir Suppl* **72**:7–26.

87. Yasargil MG, Antic J, Laciga R, Jain KK, Hodosh RM, & Smith RD (1976) Microsurgical pterional approach to aneurysms of the basilar bifurcation. *Surg Neurol* **6**:83–91.

88. Hoh BL, Rabinov JD, Pryor JC, Carter BS, & Barker FG 2nd (2003) In-hospital morbidity and mortality after endovascular treatment of unruptured intracranial aneurysms in the United States:1996–2000: effect of hospital and physician volume. *AJNR Am J Neuroradiol* **24**:1409–1420.

89. Raaymakers TW, Rinkel GJ, Limburg M, & Algra A (1998) Mortality and morbidity of surgery for unruptured intracranial aneurysms: a meta-analysis. *Stroke* **29**:1531–1538.

90. Lawton MT, Quinones-Hinojosa A, Chang EF, & Yu T (2005) Thrombotic intracranial aneurysms: classification scheme and management strategies in 68 patients. *Neurosurgery* **56**:441–454.

91. Meyer FB, Friedman JA, Nichols DA, & Windschitl WL (2001) Surgical repair of clinoidal segment carotid artery aneurysms unsuitable for endovascular treatment. *Neurosurgery* **48**:476–486.

92. Veznedaroglu E, Benitez RP, & Rosenwasser RH (2004) Surgically treated aneurysms previously coiled: lessons learned. *Neurosurgery* **54**:300–305.

93. Yasargil MG, Gasser JC, Hodosh RM, & Rankin TV (1977) Carotid-ophthalmic aneurysms: direct microsurgical approach. *Surg Neurol* **8**:155–165.

94. Krayenbuhl HA, Yasargil MG, Flamm ES, & Tew JM Jr (1972) Microsurgical treatment of intracranial saccular aneurysms. *J Neurosurg* **37**:678–686.

95. Yasargil MG, Reichman MV, & Kubik S (1987) Preservation of the frontotemporal branch of the facial nerve using the interfascial temporalis flap for pterional craniotomy. Technical article. *J Neurosurg* **67**:463–466.

96. Barker FG 2nd, Amin-Hanjani S, Butler WE, Ogilvy CS, & Carter BS (2003) In-hospital mortality and morbidity after surgical treatment of unruptured intracranial aneurysms in the United States:1996–2000: the effect of hospital and surgeon volume. *Neurosurgery* **52**:995–1009.

97. Takahashi T (2002) The treatment of symptomatic unruptured aneurysms. *Acta Neurochir* Suppl. **82**:17–19.

98. Khanna RK, Malik GM, & Qureshi N (1996) Predicting outcome following surgical treatment of unruptured intracranial aneurysms: a proposed grading system. *J Neurosurg* **84**:49–54.

99. Solomon RA, Fink ME, & Pile-Spellman J (1994) Surgical management of unruptured intracranial aneurysms. *J Neurosurg* **80**:440–446.

100. Proust F, Debono B, Hannequin D, *et al.* (2003) Treatment of anterior communicating artery aneurysms: complementary aspects of microsurgical and endovascular procedures. *J Neurosurg* **99**: 3–14.

101. Guidetti B & La Torre E (1975) Management of carotid-ophthalmic aneurysms. *J Neurosurg* **42**:438–442.

102. Kassell NF & Drake CG (1982) Timing of aneurysm surgery. *Neurosurgery* **10**:514–519.

103. Haley EC Jr, Kassell NF, & Torner JC (1992) The International Cooperative Study on the Timing of Aneurysm Surgery. The North American experience. *Stroke* **23**:205–214.

104. Hernesniemi J, Vapalahti M, Niskanen M, *et al.* (1993) One-year outcome in early aneurysm surgery: a 14 years experience. *Acta Neurochir* (Wien) **122**(1–2):1–10.

105. Ohman J & Heiskanen O (1989) Timing of operation for ruptured supratentorial aneurysms: a prospective randomized study. *J Neurosurg* **70**:55–60.

106. Laidlaw JD & Siu KH (2002) Ultra-early surgery for aneurysmal subarachnoid hemorrhage: outcomes for a consecutive series of 391 patients not selected by grade or age. *J Neurosurg* **97**:250–259.

107. Le Roux PD, Elliot JP, Newell DW, Grady MS, & Winn HR (1996) The incidence of surgical complications is similar in good and poor grade patients undergoing repair of ruptured anterior circulation aneurysms: a retrospective review of 355 patients. *Neurosurgery* **38**:887–895.

108. Groden C, Kremer C, Regelsberger J, Hansen HC, & Zeumer H (2001) Comparison of operative and endovascular treatment of anterior circulation aneurysms in patients in poor grades. *Neuroradiology* **43**:778–783.

109. Hernesniemi J, Vapalahti M, Niskanen M, & Kari A (1992) Management outcome for vertebrobasilar artery aneurysms by early surgery. *Neurosurgery* **31**:857–862.

110. Hillman J, Saveland H, Jakobsson KE, *et al.* (1996) Overall management outcome of ruptured posterior fossa aneurysms. *J Neurosurg* **85**:33–38.

111. Peerless SJ, Hernesniemi JA, Gutman FB, & Drake CG (1994) Early surgery for ruptured vertebrobasilar aneurysms. *J Neurosurg* **80**:643–649.

112. Ecker RD & Hopkins LN (2004) Natural history of unruptured intracranial aneurysms. *Neurosurg Focus* **17**(5):E4.

5   Renal and Peripheral Artery Disease

60 Sonographic Assessment of Renal Artery Stenosis

Jörg Radermacher
Johannes Wesling Klinikum Minden, Minden, Germany

Introduction

Routine examination (screening) of the renal arteries to exclude stenosis should never be performed because the false-positive and false-negative rate would be too high in a disease as rare as renal artery stenosis (prevalence about 1–4% in the hypertensive population). Only selected hypertensive patients with features suggesting the presence of renal artery stenosis, such as the presence of an abdominal bruit, presence of atherosclerotic arterial disease in other vascular beds, use of three and more antihypertensive drugs without adequate control of blood pressure, or other clinical clues, should be examined [1]. This requires access to all the relevant clinical findings before the start of the investigation.

It is helpful for the examiner to be familiar with the various etiologic forms of stenosis found in the renal arteries, which have varying predilection points, and also with the various age-related and sex-related distributions.

Arteriosclerotic stenoses (80–90% of all forms of renovascular hypertension; high age at first manifestation; occurs in women significantly less often than in men) mainly arise near the origin of the renal artery, but areas of bifurcation of the main renal artery and intrarenal segments may also be affected. On the other hand, the often multiple fibromuscular stenoses are equally distributed between proximal, middle, and distal segments of the renal arteries (10–20% of all forms of renovascular hypertension; congenital; already symptomatic in children; first manifestation at a young age; occurs in women significantly more often than men) [2]. Possible rarer causes of renal artery stenosis are diseases of the aorta (dissecting aneurysm, syphilitic aortitis, congenital coarctation), renal arteritides (in obliterating endangiitis, periarteritis nodosa), injury, dissection, tumor or thrombosis of the renal arteries, intrarenal cysts, and extrinsic lesions with compression of the renal arteries (pheochromocytoma, perirenal hematoma, retroperitoneal fibrosis).

Cardiovascular Interventions in Clinical Practice. Edited by Jürgen Haase, Hans-Joachim Schäfers, Horst Sievert and Ron Waksman. © 2010 Blackwell Publishing.

Equipment

Duplex and color flow Doppler sonography are the usual techniques to delineate the renal arteries. Usually today, multifrequency sector or vector transducers with a B-mode frequency between 2 and 5 MHz are used. Multifrequency transducers—automatically or on demand—provide a lower transmission frequency around 2 MHz to increase the penetration depth in obese patients. Fixed frequency transducers of 3.5 MHz are still in use; however, in obese patients a switch to a 2-MHz sector transducer may be required, lengthening the overall examination time. A 5 MHz transmission frequency is not generally advised. Although the B-mode may give excellent pictures in lean patients, the physical limitations of this transducer do not allow measuring of the large frequency shifts which will be present in severe renal artery stenosis.

Three-dimensional reconstruction of two-dimensionally produced B-mode ultrasound sections or the delineation of extended vessels segments using B-mode or color-mode panoramic imaging (e.g., SieScape, Siemens Medical Systems, Deerfield, IL, USA) provide a more presentable documentation of the renal arteries that can be used when presenting the ultrasound findings to referring physicians or surgeons. Presently, however, these techniques do not improve the diagnostic accuracy of renal artery scanning.

Intravascular renal artery ultrasound may be helpful in selected cases to evaluate eccentric stenoses. However, the method requires the use of single-use-materials and is therefore too costly to be advised on a more general level. Transgastric ultrasonography has not been found to be of clinical value in the scanning of renal arteries outside an experimental setting [3].

Qualitative and especially quantitative evaluation of flow within the renal arteries requires continuous wave or pulse-wave Doppler modes. The pulsed-wave Doppler mode is used most frequently, because it allows obtaining Doppler signals from precisely defined renal artery segments located up to 10–15 cm distally from the transducer. On the other hand, the continuous-wave Doppler mode can measure the high flow velocities, associated with severe degrees of stenoses.

Some modern machines using velocity matched spectrum analysis from a pulsed-wave Doppler signal make it possible to delineate velocity waveforms with peak velocity up to several times the Nyquist limit [4].

B-mode alone is often used in examination of renal arteries to detect arteriosclerotic wall plaques or aneurysms.

Power Doppler (synonym: color power Doppler, color Doppler energy mode) and *ultrasound contrast agents* at present do not facilitate detection of renal artery stenosis. Although visualization of all abdominal arteries, including the renal arteries, is greatly improved by ultrasound contrast agents, no advantage could be shown regarding the accuracy of detection of renal artery stenosis [5].

A multitude of new ultrasound techniques may greatly improve the visualization of renal arteries and vessels: second harmonic imaging/tissue harmonic imaging [6,7]; noise/artifact suppression software (XRES, SonoCT, Philips ATL, DA Best, The Netherlands); daylight sonography (Photopic [8], Siemens Medical Systems, Deerfield, IL, USA); SieScape Color SieScape panorama imaging [9] (Siemens Medical Systems, Deerfield, IL, USA); 3-D power Doppler [10]; phase inversion ultrasonography [7]. However, none of these techniques has been evaluated in sufficient depth to predict their future role in evaluating the renal arteries.

Examination conditions

External influences are of decisive importance in precise Doppler sonographic studies and not only during complex investigations or in difficult examination conditions (extreme obesity, meteorism, emphysema, extreme shortness of breath). Assuming that the equipment has been optimally adjusted, it is still necessary to have a room that can be darkened to ensure good reproduction of the examination findings on the monitor. It is of equal importance to provide adequate room temperature and comfortable positions for both the patients and the examiner during the examination.

Calculating and allowing sufficient time for the examination is an absolute prerequisite. The time required is not only dependent on the examiner's experience and the individual examination conditions presented by the patient, but is also affected by the results of the examination. Pathologic results usually require further examinations.

The examination is usually carried out with the patient in the supine position. Under special circumstances (pregnancy, obesity), or to display proximal portions of the renal artery more vertically oriented to the transducer, it may be better to place the patient in a lateral position. The patient should always be in a relaxed position, as any tension in the abdominal muscles increases the distance from the transducer to the abdominal arteries. Elevating the upper body by about 30° not only makes the patient feel comfortable, but also displaces the intraabdominal organs more caudally, which usually improves the visual field. A suitable support placed under the knees may further help to relax the abdominal muscles.

Some investigators prefer a patient who has fasted for at least 8 h because they fear gas and food remnants in the stomach and intestines, which may complicate the investigation. In addition, carminative medications, taken on the day of or before the examination, are frequently advised. However, although meteorism may somewhat prolong the examination it hardly ever prevents the experienced investigator from performing a successful examination, and the patient will be grateful because he or she did not have to fast for yet another investigation. If the renal arteries are superimposed by gas in the intestine, continuous gentle pressure with the transducer for several minutes will almost certainly displace these structures.

Anatomy of renal arteries

Bilaterally, the *renal arteries* originate approximately 0.5–1.5 cm caudal to the superior mesenteric artery at the level of the first and second lumbar vertebrae, almost at a right angle to the abdominal aorta. In most cases, the right renal artery leaves the aorta in the 10 o'clock position, proceeds ventrally, and reaches the kidney in a convex, curving fashion. The left renal artery usually leaves the aorta at the 4–5 o'clock position [1]. In side-to-side comparisons, the somewhat longer right renal artery (3.5–9.0 cm; left renal artery 2.5–8.0 cm) proceeds dorsal and lateral to the inferior vena cava and the left renal artery proceeds dorsal to the left renal vein. In the hilum, the vessel divides into a dorsal and ventral main branch that usually divides into five *segmental arteries* in the renal sinus. After further subdivision in the parenchyma in first the *interlobar arteries*, which proceed between the medullary rays, and second the *arcuate arteries*, which run at a right angle on top of the medullary rays, the glomeruli are fed by the interlobular arteries and afferent vessels. Multiple renal arteries occur in about 20–30% of cases [1], in up to 8% of cases there are even three arteries or more to a single kidney [11].

Examining sequence

After conventional B-mode scanning of the kidneys, the origin of the renal arteries is estimated from the B-mode or color Doppler picture. Then color Doppler mode is used to detect flow abnormalities from ostial medial and distal parts within each renal artery, and, if flow abnormalities are detected, Doppler spectra are derived from these regions. Finally, the distal renal artery and intrarenal arteries are located with color Doppler mode, and two to three Doppler signals from proximal segmental arteries of each kidney are analyzed.

The routine examination of renal arteries in a time-saving way requires the use of color flow Doppler mode. It decreases the examination time because a deviation of flow velocity within a stenosis is clearly noticeable either by a lighter color or, more frequently, by an aliasing phenomenon. Doppler spectra can be selectively obtained from these specific regions of interest, which reduces the examination time. In addition, quantitative measurements of flow velocities in the renal arteries require angle-corrected measurements, and since renal arteries cannot be routinely seen in B-mode, angle-correction also requires the use of color flow Doppler. Precise flow rates (mL/min), however, are difficult to calculate because of the difficulty in obtaining a reliable measurement of the cross-sectional area of the renal artery.

B-mode sonography to detect renal arteries and size differences of kidneys

The main value of B-mode imaging of renal arteries is the evaluation of plaques and the imaging of vascular stents. Certain B-mode findings may help to make a specific diagnosis. One or two small kidneys combined with hypertension necessitate the definitive exclusion of renal artery stenosis.

Renal arteries

Under favorable examination conditions, the renal arteries can be followed distally, starting from their origin at the abdominal aorta for a varying distance. Their diameter is between 4 and 6 mm. Measurements of the arterial lumen of renal arteries are difficult to achieve because of the small size of the renal arteries and the location far apart from the ultrasound scanner. Using the M-mode procedure makes it easier to ascertain the precise boundaries between wall structures and the internal lumen, and the new technologies including second harmonic imaging and sono-CT will also facilitate the B-mode imaging of renal arterial walls.

When measuring the cross-section, the "leading edge method" should be used. This is always measured in a strictly sagittal plane and the true diameter of the lumen as well as the thickness of one wall need to be included in the defined cross-section. With careful examination, reliable size indications are possible for the renal artery, at least in the sagittal plane. It can be helpful to look at transverse sections of the

right renal artery underneath the caval vein to find multiple right renal arteries.

Renal size

It is frequently stated that the right kidney is somewhat smaller than the left one. This is only true for renal length [12] but not for renal volume. Most observers measure only kidney length because the measurement of this parameter is most reproducible [13], but renal length correlates only poorly with renal volume [14]. Renal volume, measured in 128 healthy volunteers by volume CT analysis, was not different between left and right kidneys [15]. We analyzed renal volume from renal ultrasound in 100 healthy living renal donors (Table 60.1). Although the overall length of the left kidney was slightly longer, no significant difference could be found in kidney volume. Body weight and body surface area are closely correlated to kidney volume (both $R^2 = 0.42$), and more so than body mass index ($R^2 = 0.11$; Radermacher, unpublished data). The correlation of kidney length to body weight ($R^2 = 0.24$), body surface area ($R^2 = 0.25$) or body mass index ($R^2 = 0.06$) is less tight than that to kidney volume. A simple formula to estimate whether a measured renal volume is normal is to multiply the body weight (measured in kg) by two. This number gives the approximate volume of one kidney.

Color flow Doppler mode

Evaluating the displayed color patterns can be rendered impossible by *unfavorable color adjustments*. Frequent potential errors include:

• specifying an inadequate low velocity (pulse repetition frequency) for the color adjustment, with resulting aliasing or multiple aliasing, especially when the renal artery is investigated for signs of renal artery stenosis;

• having almost a right angle between the color flow Doppler plane and the vascular axis, with resulting poor to absent color coding of the arterial lumen;

• incorrect color filter selection, with reduced color output;

• undercontrolled or overcontrolled color amplification, with poor color display or color noise.

Table 60.1 Sonographically measured kidney sizes from 100 healthy living renal donors.

	Right kidney				Left kidney			
	Length (mm)	Width (mm)	Depth (mm)	Volume (mL)	Length (mm)	Width (mm)	Depth (mm)	Volume (mL)
All ($n = 100$)	114 ± 8	50 ± 7	55 ± 6	151 ± 39	116 ± 8*	51 ± 6	52 ± 5*	154 ± 37
Men ($n = 44$)	116 ± 9	52 ± 7	55 ± 6	161 ± 42	118 ± 9	53 ± 6	53 ± 6	168 ± 39
Women ($n = 56$)	113 ± 7	49 ± 7	54 ± 6	143 ± 36	114 ± 7	50 ± 5	51 ± 50*	143 ± 31

Values are means ± SD.
*Significant difference between left and right kidneys.

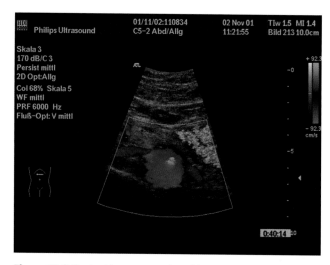

Figure 60.1 Proximal transverse section of the upper abdomen at the level of the origin of the renal arteries. With color flow Doppler sonography the proximal and medial part of the right renal artery and the proximal part of the left renal artery can be visualized in about 85–90% of cases.

The examination always starts with the transducer placed just distal to the xiphoid process, because here the liver may serve as a window into the renal arteries. Using color flow Doppler mode helps significantly to *identify* the renal arteries and to follow their course (Fig. 60.1). This becomes even more important when the examination conditions for B-mode sonography are poor. The renal arteries are examined along their longitudinal axis. Color is also beneficial in the middle and distal arterial segment in slim patients.

Imaging both main renal arteries, including registering several Doppler frequency spectra from the proximal and middle segment of the renal arteries, is possible in 84–100% of cases. In our own prospective investigations using color flow duplex sonography before angiography, with 536 arteries in 226 patients, the ability to evaluate the renal arteries in their proximal and middle vascular segments was found to be 84% overall (right renal artery 91%, left renal artery 85%). The imaging ability was higher in women (91%) than in men (77%), and higher in normal weight or slightly obese (body mass index <30: 87%) than in extremely obese patients (body mass index >30: 61%).

With the color flow Doppler mode, rapid visual identification of zones of elevated flow velocity, which are characteristically encountered near stenoses, or disturbed flow patterns near plaques or in the lumen of aneurysms are possible. It is important to choose the highest pulse repetition frequency possible when looking for renal artery stenoses. Artifacts due to air movement in overlying bowl segments will be less likely to occur and, more importantly, the specificity of the color findings improves. An experienced examiner with knowledge of the equipment-specific audio and color adjustments will be able to make a rough estimate of the degree of stenosis on the basis of the audio and color patterns. However,

this cannot replace the need to register and evaluate a frequency spectrum. Criteria indicating a pathologic finding with the color flow Doppler mode are changed color intensity (lightness); aliasing; color change (change direction); color band with a tapering width; and separation phenomena; turbulent flow (usually indicated by a separate (green) color).

Intrarenal color Doppler signals and frequency spectra can be registered without exception in all healthy individuals without renal artery occlusion. By visually displaying the course of intrarenal arteries, angle-corrected flow velocity measurement recordings of well-defined Doppler spectra for rapid and precise analysis of resistance index and acceleration time values are also possible in these vascular segments.

Accessory renal arteries cannot, with the available technique, be reliably found with color flow Doppler sonography. Even experienced investigators will find only about one-quarter of these supernumerary vessels.

A complete examination of both renal arteries with duplex sonography alone takes about 20–90 min [16], whereas the evaluation with color flow imaging can be done within 15–30 min [1].

Doppler sonography

Distal and medial portions of the renal arteries are best visualized through the kidney from a dorsolateral or, rarely, from a ventrolateral or dorsal approach. The latter approach also allows measurements of intrarenal velocity spectra, which are usually obtained from segmental renal arteries. The frequency spectra of the renal and intrarenal arteries typically show a low resistance flow, which is characterized by an antegrade blood flow even in end-diastole (Fig. 60.2). It is important to note that Doppler examinations have to be optimized and that reproducible measurements are only possible when the Doppler signal meets the vascular flow direction at the smallest possible incident angle. Without angle adjustments erroneously low flow velocities are measured; incorrectly large angle corrections produce a flow velocity that is too high. Doppler signals should never be obtained from vessels at angels >60° not only because flow velocity measurements become unreliable but because the quality of the Doppler signal is greatly reduced. Indirect sign of stenosis like acceleration time and even the so-called robust parameter resistance index can no longer be measured reliably.

This means that transducer positions need to be selected that allow imaging of the target arterial segment of the renal arteries at the most acute angle possible between the vascular axis and the transducer. If color flow mode suggests a stenosis—in atherosclerotic stenoses, usually in the ostial portion of the renal artery—this usually requires the transducer to be placed in either the left or right flank region to achieve an acute angle (Fig. 60.3).

Renal artery stenosis can be detected by direct visualization of the stenosis within the renal artery or by evaluating indirect (poststenotic) signs of stenoses in intrarenal arteries

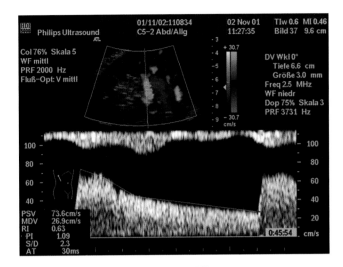

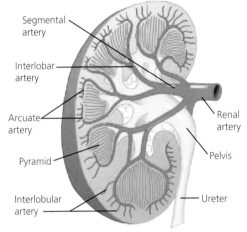

Figure 60.2 A Doppler sonogram of a normal segmental renal artery, using a dorsolumbar section. The arterial flow directed toward the transducer is coded red; while the opposite flow direction in the intrarenal veins is shown in blue. The pulse repetition rate is preselected at a relatively low level compared with the main renal artery setting, since relatively slow flow velocities predominate in both vascular systems. AT, acceleration time; MDV, end-diastolic velocity; PI, Pulsatility index; PSV, maximum systolic velocity; RI, resistance index; S/D, systolic–diastolic ratio.

(Fig. 60.4). The direct and indirect approach will be discussed separately.

In 85–90% of renal arteries and almost 100% of intrarenal arteries it is possible to register a Doppler frequency spectrum that is free of artifacts and which can be used to perform quantitative measurements. To improve the quality of the Doppler spectra further, it can be helpful to choose a fairly wide Doppler gate. There is a controversy over which intrarenal arterial segment gives the most reproducible results [17,18]; however, most investigators use segmental renal arteries.

Owing to its more precise local resolution capabilities, the pulsed-wave Doppler is preferable in the initial investigation of renal artery stenosis. If there are high-grade arterial narrowings, however, that cause a marked increase in the intrastenotic flow velocity, continuous-wave Doppler signal processing is useful. The pulsed-wave Doppler has limitations in relation to depth, owing to the Nyquist limit when attempting to detect very high frequencies or velocities. Precise measurement of these very high velocities is only possible with the continuous-wave Doppler mode. Modern ultrasound machines, however, use a trick which seemingly enables pulsed-wave Doppler ultrasound to measure flow velocities beyond its theoretical limitations.

Extremely high-grade flow obstructions that have only a thread-like fast flow jet or an intrastenotically decreased flow velocity can sometimes be clearly recognized with duplex sonography only after extensive and careful examination of the overall arterial caliber. In particular, filiform stenoses with a reduced maximum flow velocity can be inadvertently missed if the sensitivity of the Doppler frequencies during the examination is not preselected and evaluated for both the high-frequency and low-frequency ranges (high or low pulse repetition frequency). However, this preselection and testing of different Doppler frequencies is very time consuming and cannot, therefore, be generally advised. In extremely high-grade stenoses, the indirect intrarenal Doppler signs of stenosis will almost always be present (prolonged acceleration time, difference in left and right kidney resistance index [RI] values, and missing early systolic peak), and these stenoses will therefore be picked up by these indirect signs.

Although this hemodynamic situation can also be a problem, using the color flow Doppler mode in such cases provides visual support for the identification of the remaining narrow lumen of an extremely high-grade stenosis through which the blood is still flowing. These high-grade stenoses give off a bright "twinkle" at the site of stenosis, even though the remaining part of the renal artery may be missed because there is not sufficient color saturation.

Direct signs of stenosis

To confirm the presence and quantify the degree of a renal artery stenosis, spectral analyses from pulse wave or continuous wave frequency spectra have to be analyzed at the site of maximum flow velocity and as far distal to this location as possible. If the B-mode image shows pathologic findings (plaques or ultrasound shadows emanating from the vascular wall near the transducer, suddenly increased vascular calibre), then this region must be investigated with particular care to identify flow acceleration or flow disturbances with the assistance of the Doppler frequency curve. In most cases, however, a flow alteration as depicted by color flow Doppler mode (see above) will be the hallmark of a renal vascular stenosis. A stenosis >50% (diameter reduction) in the renal artery can be assumed qualitatively when spectral broadening appears [19] or can be assumed using the following quantitative flow parameters:

- elevated maximum systolic flow velocity (Fig. 60.4)—the angle-corrected maximum systolic flow velocity is locally

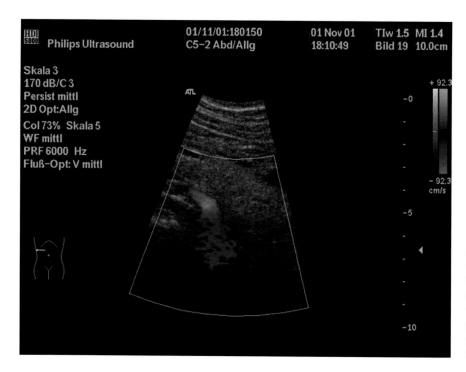

Figure 60.3 An oblique view of the right renal artery from a right subcostal midclavicular approach. The origin of the right renal artery is seen at an incident angle, allowing for reliable Doppler measurements. When the same investigation is performed in a subxiphoid transverse section through the upper abdomen (see Figs. 60.1 and 60.4) the origin of the right renal artery cannot be analyzed by Doppler ultrasound.

>140–180–198 cm/s [20,21]—the cut-off value of 180 cm/s has found the widest acceptance;

• increased ratio of intrastenotic compared with aortic maximum systolic flow velocity (renal–aortic ratio)—the angle-corrected flow velocity in the stenotic segment of the renal artery is >3.3–3.5 times faster than flow velocity in the aorta [16,21–23];

• increased ratio of intrastenotic compared with pre- or poststenotic blood flow (renal–renal ratio) [1].

If flow velocities from both an intrastenotic and a post- or prestenotic segment of the renal artery can be visualized (renal–renal ratio) more precise quantitation of stenosis is possible. A stenosis of >50% diameter reduction is present when the intrastenotic flow velocity is at least four times faster than the pre- or poststenotic velocity [1]. The exact degree of stenosis (%) can be calculated as 100(1 − [poststenotic velocity/intrastenotic velocity]). The correlation coefficient of Doppler-estimated degrees of stenoses compared with the gold standard (planimetric calculation using) intravascular ultrasound was 0.97 (own unpublished results).

Indirect signs of stenosis

Distal to a severe (>60% diameter reduction) renal artery stenosis, so-called tardus and parvus phenomena can be observed. Tardus means that the initial increase in flow velocity during early systole is delayed, and parvus means that the maximum systolic velocity is decreased. Prolonged acceleration time [24–26] (Fig. 60.4) and acceleration index [24] (tardus) as well as decreased pulsatility and resistance index (parvus) are the most frequently used parameters to detect these indirect signs of stenosis. Both a very low RI

value and an RI difference between right and left kidney of greater 5–10% are considered a sign of stenosis. Another indirect sign of stenosis is the missing early systolic peak [27] in a Doppler spectrum.

For abnormal values see Table 60.2. In direct comparison, tardus phenomena (prolonged acceleration time and acceleration index) are more accurate indices for renal artery stenosis than parvus phenomena (pulsatility and resistance index) [28–30]. According to our own data, a prolonged acceleration time is correlated more closely ($R^2 = 0.20$) to a severe degree of stenosis than is either the absolute RI value ($R^2 = 0.10$) or the RI difference ($R^2 = 0.15$). Furthermore, a prolonged acceleration time can be evaluated as an indirect sign of stenosis in patients with single kidneys, whereas the RI difference cannot.

Another sign suggesting renal artery stenosis or occlusion are renal cortical perforating vessels with flow toward the kidney [31]. All of these signs allow only a qualitative statement regarding stenosis, whereas quantitation is possible only using the direct signs mentioned above.

Occluded renal arteries are difficult to distinguish from severely stenosed renal arteries. An occlusion can be suspected if:

• there is no flow signal registered from the vascular lumen, although the renal arteries are clearly identified in B-mode;

• in side-to-side comparison, there is a clearly lower intrarenal flow velocity with a maximal systolic blood flow of <25 cm/s after angle correction;

• in side-to-side comparisons, a clearly lower value is calculated for the resistance index and the kidney is smaller (<9 cm), without other causes for this being present.

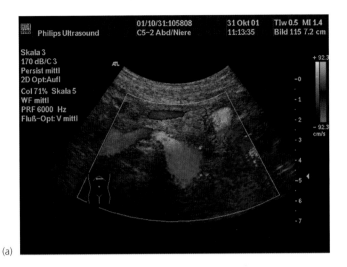

(a)

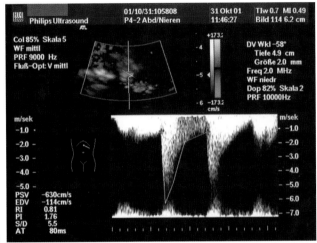

(b)

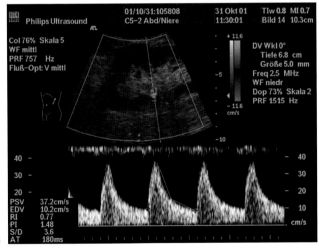

(c)

Figure 60.4 (a) A left renal artery stenosis after the origin from the aorta, demonstrated by color flow Doppler sonography through locally circumscribed aliasing, which reflects the elevated mean flow velocity in this segment. (b) The maximum systolic flow velocity in the stenosis was 630 cm/s. (c) Intrarenal segmental artery with a delayed acceleration time (AT > 70 ms) as an indirect sign of a renal artery stenosis in the proximal vascular bed.

Table 60.2 Pathologic values for Doppler indices derived from segmental renal arteries to suggest renal artery stenosis.

Index	Normal value
Parvus sign	
Resistance index	Either absolute resistance index value <0.45–0.5 [63] or difference between left and right kidney >5–10% [64–66]
Tardus sign	
Pulsatility index	<0.93 [28,67]
Acceleration time	>70 ms [1,24,25,68,69,70]
Acceleration index	<3.78 m/s [24,68]
Acceleration index ratio	Ratio of acceleration indices between the stenosed and nonstenosed kidney is >1.8 [70]
Early systolic peak	Peak lost [26,27]

V_{dias}, end-diastolic velocity; V_{max}, maximum systolic velocity; V_{mean}, mean velocity.

Failure to detect a Doppler or color flow Doppler signal alone, without being able to display the artery morphologically, is an uncertain sign of renal artery occlusion. If duplex sonography indicates possible renal artery occlusion, an attempt should be made to register the refilling of the renal artery or of intrarenal arteries, which frequently occurs despite total occlusion of the main renal artery through collateral vessels. In our own patients, intrarenal arterial flow signals could be registered in 25 of 35 patients with angiographically verified renal artery occlusions. In the 25 patients with detectable distal blood flow, the intrarenal Pourcelot resistance index was, on average, 0.57 ± 0.17 on the occluded side, with a maximum systolic flow velocity of 14 ± 5 cm/s (range 5–22 cm/s) on the occluded side as opposed to 42 ± 9 cm/s (range 31–62 cm/s) on the nonoccluded side. The resistance index was, on average, 17% lower than in the contralateral kidney (Radermacher, unpublished data). However, in five patients the resistance index was >0.80 and was not significantly different on the occluded than on the nonoccluded side. Similar findings (Delta RI 26% (13–36%) have been made by Karasch *et al.* [20]. A cut-off value of 20–25 cm/s maximum systolic blood flow in segmental renal arteries distinguished best between total renal artery occlusion and nonoccluded vessels.

Factors influencing resistance index

Resistance index is influenced by a variety of parameters, which should be kept in mind when using the resistance index. In a group of normotensive individuals, it was shown that the end-diastolic flow velocity in the renal arteries and intrarenal arteries decreases with advancing age, so that an age-dependent increase in the intrarenal resistance indices occurs

Table 60.3 Age-related normal values for the resistance index (RI) in the segmental renal artery in patients with normal blood pressure (BP) and hypertension. Values are given as the mean ± SD (Radermacher et al.) [67].

	Age (years)						
	21–30	31–40	41–50	51–60	61–70	71–80	≥
Normal BP							
Number of subjects	6	28	42	52	15	—	—
V_{max} (cm/s)	56 ± 10	65 ± 20	56 ± 14	50 ± 12	50 ± 10	—	—
V_{dias} (cm/s)	18 ± 7	24 ± 7	20 ± 5	17 ± 5	16 ± 3	—	—
RI	0.68 ± 0.06	0.63 ± 0.04	0.63 ± 0.04	0.66 ± 0.04	0.68 ± 0.05	—	—
Hypertensive subjects							
Number of subjects	130	258	339	532	548	279	40
V_{max} (cm/s)	43 ± 18	39 ± 17	40 ± 16	41 ± 18	39 ± 16	38 ± 14	37 ± 16
V_{dias} (cm/s)	15 ± 8	14 ± 7	14 ± 6	13 ± 7	10 ± 7	9 ± 6	6 ± 3
RI	0.64 ± 0.08	0.65 ± 0.08	0.66 ± 0.07	0.70 ± 0.07	0.74 ± 0.07	0.77 ± 0.07	0.83 ± 0.05

(Table 60.3) [32] after the age of 8–10 years; before that time renal vascular resistance continuously declines after birth [33]. This age dependant increase in resistance index is much more apparent in patients with hypertension than in patients with normal blood pressure. The increase in RI values is mainly due to a decrease in diastolic blood flow with advancing age.

Maximum systolic velocity, diastolic velocity, and resistance index decrease from the main renal artery to the segmental renal artery, the interlobar, the arcuate, and finally the interlobular artery [34]. Furthermore, these flow velocities are affected by respiratory, digestive [35], hormonal, and pharmacologic influences. For example, the RI in the renal arteries increases during inspiration, and increases even more during the Valsalva maneuver, which is frequently performed to position the kidneys more caudally [36]. Also, the cold pressor test, a test of the sympathetic nervous system, causes an increase of resistance index from 0.59 to 0.69 in healthy controls [32]. Renal resistance index values have been reported to increase 90–240 min postprandially [35]; however, also bivariate effects, with an increased renal vascular resistance after a protein meal in hypercapnic patients and a decrease of resistance in normal controls, have been observed [37]. Resistance index measured by Doppler ultrasound is correlated more closely to renal blood flow (RBF) than to the glomerular filtration rate (GFR) or, astonishingly, than to the renal vascular resistance calculated from RBF and GFR [38]. Renal resistance index is furthermore influenced by extrarenal factors associated with vascular stiffness, such as pulse pressure. Pulse rate has an influence on resistance index with bradycardia, leading to a lower end-diastolic flow and a higher resistance index, and tachycardia, causing the opposite. Schwerk et al. suggested a corrective formula to account for different pulse rates [39]; however, for pulse rates in the range of 50–70 beats per minute, there is little change in resistance index values. In kidney transplants that are usually located nonanatomically near the surface in the left or right iliac fossa, special care should be taken not to exert pressure on the transplant with the transducer because this can lead to decreased arterial inflow and elevated peripheral resistance.

Reproducibility

The intrarenal resistance indices only show slight differences, both in the kidney as a whole and in side-to-side comparisons. At least two to three measurements from a specific vessel site within each kidney are averaged. The intraobserver and interobserver coefficients of variation for the measurements of the resistance index were 2.0% for the evaluation of 14 patients and 3.2% for the evaluation of 420 patients, respectively; the coefficient of variation was 2.8% for the evaluation of 264 patients by the same observer on consecutive days [40]. The average side-to-side difference in 258 angiographically normal renal arteries was 2.6% (0.0–9%), measured intrarenally in segmental renal arteries.

Diagnostic accuracy

Experienced examiners (> 50 patients examined prospectively with findings compared with intraarterial angiography) are able to diagnose a renal artery stenosis with a sensitivity of 86–98% and a *specificity* of 83–98%. In our own investigations to detect atherosclerotic stenoses and occlusions of the renal arteries, we used a combination of direct and indirect parameters of renal artery stenosis and we were able to attain a sensitivity of 96.7% and a specificity of 98%, based on 536 renal arteries with 197 stenoses in comparison with the angiographic results [1]. The positive predictive value in this group was 96.7%; the negative predictive value was 98% (Table 60.4).

Table 60.4 Stenosis criteria and the associated sensitivities and specificities in detecting angiographically controlled stenoses of the renal arteries using duplex and color flow duplex sonography.

	Patient number	Stenosis criterion	Technical failure (%)	Degree of stenosis (%)	Sensitivity/ specificity (%)
Direct criteria					
Hansen et al. [71]	74	RAR > 3.5	8	≥60	93/98
Karasch et al. [72]	53	V_{max} > 180 cm/s	15	≥50	92/92
Olin et al. [73]	102	V_{max} > 200 cm/s or RAR > 3.5	10	≥60	98/98
Postma et al. [21]	61	Doppler frequency >4 kHz and broadened Doppler spectrum	25	≥50	63/86
Schäberle et al. [74]	76	V_{max} > 140 cm/s	N.A.	≥50	86/83
Nchimi et al. [75]	91	V_{max} > 180 cm/s	9	≥60	91/97
Indirect criteria (paravus–tardus)					
Baxter et al. [30]	73	AT > 70 ms	16	≥70	89/97
Kliewer et al. [24]	57	AT ≥ 70 ms	0	≥50	82/20
Riehl et al. [23]	214	RI < 0.45 or ΔRI ≥ 8%	0	≥70	93/96
Schwerk et al. [64]	72	ΔRI ≥ 5%	0	≥50	82/92
			0	≥60	100/94
Speckamp et al. [70]	123	ΔAI ≥ 80%	N.A.	≥70	100/94
Stavros et al. [26]	56	Loss of ESP	0	≥60	95/97
Strunk et al. [25]	50	AT ≥ 70 ms	4	≥50	77/46
Bardelli [44]	106	AI_{max} 9/s, AT > 80 ms	0	≥60	93/84
			0		93/65
Combination of direct and indirect criteria					
Krumme et al. [76]	135	V_{max} > 180 cm/s and/or ΔRI ≥ 5%	0	≥50	89/92
Radermacher et al. [1]	226	V_{max} > 180 cm/s and RRR >4 and/or AT ≥ 70 ms	0	≥50	97/98

Only publications with >50 patients investigated were considered. All Doppler sonographic studies had to be performed prospectively and had to be compared with intraarterial angiography as the established gold standard. Technical failure: the renal artery or intrarenal arteries could not be analyzed with Doppler ultrasonography. Degree of stenosis: cut-off value of stenosis (% diameter reduction) for which the test has been evaluated.
AI, acceleration index; AI_{max}, maximum acceleration index; AT, acceleration time; ESP, early systolic peak; N.A., data not available; RI, resistance index (= Pourcelot index); RRR, renal–renal ratio; V_{max}, maximum systolic velocity.

Direct parameter

A stenosis of 75% or more area reduction (i.e., about 50% diameter reduction) was diagnosed if the flow in the main renal artery exceeded the threshold value of 180 cm/s and if the maximum systolic flow distal to the stenotic site was less than one-quarter of the intrastenotic flow velocity (renal artery$_{intrastenotic}$/renal artery$_{pre-or\ poststenotic}$ ratio >4; see continuity equation). If 180 cm/s had been used as the sole diagnostic criterion, 13% false-positive stenoses >50% would have been diagnosed, which would have reduced the specificity and the positive predictive value.

Indirect parameter

If color Doppler flow mode was not able to find direct evidence of a stenosis we relied solely on an intrarenal indirect para-

meter, namely a prolonged acceleration time >70 ms (tardus phenomenon). The indirect parameters of stenosis have been found to provide good sensitivity and specificity, but, in general, a more severe degree of stenosis is required for these parameters to become positive. In stenoses of <60% diameter reduction, the diagnostic accuracy is fairly low (Table 60.4).

Our own experience with 33 patients (66 renal arteries) suffering from *fibromuscular dysplasia* shows that these stenoses, which are distributed evenly between proximal, medial, and distal segments of the renal arteries, can also be recognized by color flow Doppler sonography with a sensitivity of 100%, a specificity of 94%, and positive and negative predictive values of 94% and 100%, respectively. Studies to confirm this in larger patient groups are not yet available for this relatively rare disease.

Comparison of the different diagnostic parameters

A review and some authors compared different diagnostic parameters and found peak systolic velocity superior to the renal aortic ratio (RAR) and acceleration time [41,42]. The RI and the renal–renal ratio, however, were not included in that analysis. In another study, peak systolic velocity (PSV), RI difference and RAR were compared with angiographic and pressure wire estimation of stenosis. PSV and RAR correlated best whereas RI difference showed a low sensitivity of 31% but a high specificity of 97% [43]. Yet another study compared acceleration time, acceleration index, and RI and pulsatiliy index in 106 patients who subsequently underwent angiography and found the RI and pulsatility indices lacking in negative predictive value [44]. Relying on the difference in resistance indices as a criterion for renal artery stenosis will also not be possible in patients with bilateral renal artery stenosis, which occurs in about one-third of patients or in patients with transplant or single kidneys. The most reliable method to detect stenoses of 50% and more in all patients seems to be a combination of a direct stenosis criterion with an indirect intrarenal derived criterion.

Multiple and accessory renal arteries and pole arteries cannot be reliably detected with ultrasonography, even when the examiner carries out a targeted and systematic search for these vascular variants [45]. Only 0–28% of accessory renal arteries are found during a routine examination of the renal arterial system [1,30], which, at present, makes this method unsuitable as a sole imaging technique before living kidney donations.

Color Doppler sonography after treatment of renal artery stenosis or for follow-up of known stenoses

Percutaneous transluminal renal angioplasty with or without stent placement is a safe and effective treatment for arteriosclerotic nonostial renal artery stenoses, with good early and long-term results. In these patients, in particular, and also after reconstructive vascular surgery, duplex and color flow Doppler sonography are suitable for assessing the success of the procedure and carrying out follow-up observations in patients with native and transplant kidneys [46–48]. Angioplasty or angioplasty with stent placement do not protect from further stenoses. Restenosis or *de novo* stenosis rates of about 10% per year have been observed in both patient groups [49].

Progression of atherosclerotic renal artery stenosis is relatively common. In a patient group including 36 men and 40 women, with a mean follow-up of 32 months, Zierler et al. [50] report a cumulative incidence of progression from below 60% up to or above 60% stenosis of: 30% at 1 year, 44% at 2 years, and 48% at 3 years. Therefore, duplex scans should be performed regularly in patients with known renal artery stenosis.

Prognostic significance of Doppler sonography

The prognostic significance of the pre-interventional resistance index as a predictor of clinical success of percutaneous transluminal angioplasties or operations for renal artery stenosis is a topic of intense debate. Frauchiger et al. [51] investigated 32 patients who subsequently underwent correction of renal artery stenosis with Doppler ultrasound. They found a cortical diastolic–systolic (d/s) ratio of below 0.30 (corresponding to a resistance index above 0.70) to be prognostic of treatment failure. None of 11 clinically successful procedures had a diastolic–systolic ratio of <0.30 (RI > 0.70) compared with 7 of 24 patients with treatment failure. Cohn et al. [52], using the same cut-off value of d/s ratio had similar findings in 23 patients. In all patients who improved blood pressure and renal function, the diastolic–systolic ratio was above 0.30 (RI < 0.70), whereas all patients who failed to improve blood pressure or renal function had a decreased d/s ratio. More recently, we published a paper using a more strict cut-off value of resistance index of 0.80 [49]. The resistance index was measured prospectively in proximal segmental arteries of both kidneys. A resistance index value of >0.80 in either kidney was considered prognostic of treatment failure. Among the 35 patients with resistance index values of at least 0.80 before revascularization, mean ambulatory blood pressure failed to decrease in 34 and renal function declined in 28. Among the 96 patients with resistance index values below 0.80, mean blood pressure decreased in all but six and renal function worsened in only three. Garcia Criado confirmed these findings but found a much lower accuracy of RI to predict lack of improvement of blood pressure and renal function [53]. Zeller et al. [54] reported blood pressure improvement and improvement of renal function independent of an RI above or below 0.80, but simultaneously displayed data showing no significant improvement in blood pressure or renal function in patients with an RI > 0.80 and a significant improvement of both parameters in those with an RI < 0.80. Voiculescu found that a very low RI (<0.55) predicted treatment success [55]. Randomized trials on the predictive role of RI are under way.

Conclusion and comparison to other techniques to detect renal artery stenosis

Color Doppler ultrasonography has become the screening method of choice. Captopril scintigraphy shows poor performance when performed on outpatients and also in newer studies [56,57]. Magnetic resonance angiography and CT angiography (MRA and CTA) claim a higher diagnostic accuracy [56–59], especially when the studies are published by radiologists, whereas studies published by clinicians do not find such a difference [60,61]. Vasbinder first published a metaanalysis of published studies. That metaanalysis found MRA and CTA superior to ultrasonography and captopril scintigraphy. The same author later performed a large trial on the diagnostic accuracy of CTA and MRA in comparison with renal angiography. In that trial the diagnostic accuracy of CTA and MRA was quite low [62]. A large, multicenter study comparing color Doppler with MRA and CTA with predefined parameters to define stenosis is still missing. Studies from European countries where physicians perform the ultrasound investigation show a good diagnostic accuracy of color Doppler sonography more frequently than American studies, where only technicians perform the investigation.

The potentially nephrotoxic contrast agents in CT angiography and the occurrence of nephrogenic systemic sclerosis due to gadolinium containing agents in magnetic resonance investigations, which have led to guidelines suggesting not to investigate patients with a GFR < 30 mL/min, show that both MRA and CTA are not ideal screening methods.

Even though the majority of published studies would support a superior diagnostic accuracy of MRA and spiral CT, the good diagnostic accuracy of ultrasonography combined with its noninvasiveness, the lack of adverse effects, the lower cost and its greater acceptance by patients make it the primary investigation of choice in patients deemed likely to suffer from renal artery stenosis.

References

1. Radermacher J, Chavan A, Schaffer J, et al. (2000) Detection of significant renal artery stenosis with color Doppler sonography: combining extrarenal and intrarenal approaches to minimize technical failure. *Clin Nephrol* **53**:333–343.

2. Kaplan NM (1994) Renal vascular hypertension. In: Retford DC (ed.). *Clinical Hypertension*, 6th edn. Baltimore: Williams and Wilkins, pp. 319–341.

3. Keen RR, Yao JS, Astleford P, Blackburn D, & Frazin LJ (1996) Feasibility of transgastric ultrasonography of the abdominal aorta. *J Vasc Surg* **24**:834–842.

4. Torp H & Kristoffersen K (1995) Velocity matched spectrum analysis: a new method for suppressing velocity ambiguity in pulsed-wave Doppler. *Ultrasound Med Biol* **21**:937–944.

5. Claudon M, Plouin PF, Baxter GM, Rohban T, & Devos DM (2000) Renal arteries in patients at risk of renal arterial stenosis: multicenter evaluation of the echo-enhancer SH U 508A at color and spectral Doppler US. Levovist Renal Artery Stenosis Study Group. *Radiology* **214**:739–746.

6. Hancock J, Dittrich H, Jewitt DE, & Monaghan MJ (1999) Evaluation of myocardial, hepatic, and renal perfusion in a variety of clinical conditions using an intravenous ultrasound contrast agent (Optison) and second harmonic imaging. *Heart* **81**:636–641.

7. Kim AY, Choi BI, Kim TK, Kim KW, Lee JY, & Han JK (2001) Comparison of contrast-enhanced fundamental imaging, second-harmonic imaging, and pulse-inversion harmonic imaging. *Invest Radiol* **36**:582–588.

8. Bleck J, Gebel M, Witt B, et al. (1998) Sonography under Daylight Conditions. *Ultraschall Med* **6**:259–264.

9. Kroger K, Massalha K, Dobonici G, & Rudofsky G (1998) SieScape: a new sonographic dimension with fictive images. *Ultrasound Med Biol* **24**:1125–1129.

10. von Herbay A & Haussinger D (2001) Abdominal three-dimensional power Doppler imaging. *J Ultrasound Med* **20**:151–157.

11. Emamian SA, Nielsen MB, Pedersen JF, & Ytte L (1993) Kidney dimensions at sonography: correlation with age, sex, and habitus in 665 adult volunteers. *AJR Am J Roentgenol* **160**:83–86.

12. Emamian SA, Nielsen MB, & Pedersen JF (1995) Intraobserver and interobserver variations in sonographic measurements of kidney size in adult volunteers. A comparison of linear measurements and volumetric estimates. *Acta Radiol* **36**:399–401.

13. Thakur V, Watkins T, McCarthy K, et al. (1997) Is kidney length a good predictor of kidney volume? *Am J Med* Sci **313**:85–89.

14. Gremigni D, Todescan GC, Giannardi G, Villari N, Boddi V, & Brizzi E (1984) [Renal volume and human somatic type]. *Boll Soc Ital Biol Sper* **60**:887–893.

15. Rivolta R, Cardinale L, Lovaria A, & Di Palo FQ (2000) Variability of renal echo-Doppler measurements in healthy adults. *J Nephrol* **13**:110–115.

16. Taylor DC, Kettler MD, Moneta GL, et al. (1988) Duplex ultrasound scanning in the diagnosis of renal artery stenosis: a prospective evaluation. *J Vasc Surg* **7**:363–369.

17. Eibenberger K, Schima H, Trubel W, Scherer R, Dock W, & Grabenwoger F (1995) Intrarenal Doppler ultrasonography: which vessel should be investigated? *J Ultrasound Med* **14**:451–455.

18. Maresca G, Summaria V, De Gaetano AM, Danza FM, Valentini AL, & Marano P (1995) [Color Doppler echography in the tissue characterization of renal masses]. *Radiol Med* (Torino) **89**:470–480.

19. Kohler TR, Zierler RE, Martin RL, et al. (1986) Noninvasive diagnosis of renal artery stenosis by ultrasonic duplex scanning. *J Vasc Surg* **4**:450–456.

20. Karasch T, Neuerburg-Heusler D, Strauss A, & Rieger H (1994) Farbduplexsonographische Kriterien arteriosklerotischer Nierenarterienstenosen und–verschlüsse. In: Keller E & Krumme B (eds.). *Farbkodierte Duplexsonographie in der Nephrologie*. Berlin: Springer.

21. Postma CT, van Aalen J, de Boo T, Rosenbusch G, & Thien T (1992) Doppler ultrasound scanning in the detection of renal artery stenosis in hypertensive patients. *Br J Radiol* **65**(778):857–860.

22. Desberg AL, Paushter DM, Lammert GK, et al. (1990) Renal artery stenosis: evaluation with color Doppler flow imaging. *Radiology* **177**:749–753.

23. Riehl J, Schmitt H, Bongartz D, Bergmann D, & Sieberth HG (1997) Renal artery stenosis: evaluation with colour duplex ultrasonography. Nephrol Dial Transplant **12**:1608–1614.

24. Kliewer MA, Tupler RH, Carroll BA, et al. (1993) Renal artery stenosis: analysis of Doppler waveform parameters and tardus-parvus pattern. *Radiology* **189**:779–787.

25. Strunk H, Jaeger U, & Teifke A (1995) [Intrarenal color Doppler ultrasound for exclusion of renal artery stenosis in cases of multiple renal arteries. Analysis of the Doppler spectrum and tardus parvus phenomenon]. *Ultraschall Med* **16**:172–179.

26. Stavros AT, Parker SH, Yakes WF, *et al.* (1992) Segmental stenosis of the renal artery: pattern recognition of tardus and parvus abnormalities with duplex sonography. *Radiology* **184**:487–492.

27. Kliewer MA, Hertzberg BS, Keogan MT, *et al.* (1997) Early systole in the healthy kidney: variability of Doppler US waveform parameters. *Radiology* **205**:109–113.

28. Burdick L, Airoldi F, Marana I, *et al.* (1996) Superiority of acceleration and acceleration time over pulsatility and resistance indices as screening tests for renal artery stenosis. *J Hypertens* **14**:1229–1235.

29. Lucas P, Blome S, & Roche J (1996) Intra-renal Doppler waveform analysis as a screening test for renal artery stenosis. *Australas Radiol* **40**:276–282.

30. Baxter GM, Aitchison F, Sheppard D, *et al.* (1996) Colour Doppler ultrasound in renal artery stenosis: intrarenal waveform analysis. *Br J Radiol* **69**(825):810–815.

31. Bertolotto M, Quaia E, Galli G, Martinoli C, & Locatelli M (2000) Color Doppler sonographic appearance of renal perforating vessels in subjects with normal and impaired renal function. *J Clin Ultrasound* **28**:267–276.

32. Boddi M, Sacchi S, Lammel RM, Mohseni R, & Serneri GG (1996) Age-related and vasomotor stimuli-induced changes in renal vascular resistance detected by Doppler ultrasound. *Am J Hypertens* **9**:461–466.

33. Lin GJ & Cher TW (1997) Renal vascular resistance in normal children—a color Doppler study. *Pediatr Nephrol* **11**:182–185.

34. Martinoli C, Bertolotto M, Crespi G, Pretolesi F, Valle M, & Derchi LE (1998) Duplex Doppler analysis of interlobular arteries in transplanted kidneys. *Eur Radiol* **8**:765–769.

35. Avasthi PS, Greene ER, & Voyles WF (1987) Noninvasive Doppler assessment of human postprandial renal blood flow and cardiac output. *Am J Physiol* **252**(6 Pt 2):F1167–1174.

36. Takano R, Ando Y, Taniguchi N, Itoh K, & Asano Y (2001) Power Doppler sonography of the kidney: effect of Valsalva's maneuver. *J Clin Ultrasound* **29**(7):384–388.

37. Sharkey RA, Mulloy EM, Kilgallen IA, & O'Neill SJ (1997) Renal functional reserve in patients with severe chronic obstructive pulmonary disease. *Thorax* **52**:411–415.

38. Terry JD, Granger SH, Chen BC, *et al.* (1993) Adjusted resistive index: a method to estimate rapidly renal blood flow: preliminary validation in hypertensives. *J Ultrasound Med* **12**:751–756.

39. Schwerk WB, Restrepo IK, & Prinz H (1993) [Semiquantitative analysis of intrarenal arterial Doppler flow spectra in healthy adults]. *Ultraschall Med* **14**:117–122.

40. Grunert D, Schoning M, & Rosendahl W (1990) Renal blood flow and flow velocity in children and adolescents: duplex Doppler evaluation. *Eur J Pediatr* **149**:287–292.

41. Williams GJ, Macaskill P, Chan SF, *et al.* (2007) Comparative accuracy of renal duplex sonographic parameters in the diagnosis of renal artery stenosis: paired and unpaired analysis. *AJR Am J Roentgenol* **188**:798–811.

42. Kawarada O, Yokoi Y, Takemoto K, Morioka N, Nakata S, & Shiotani S (2006) The performance of renal duplex ultrasonography for the detection of hemodynamically significant renal artery stenosis. *Catheter Cardiovasc Interv* **68**:311–318.

43. Staub D, Canevascini R, Huegli RW, *et al.* (2007) Best duplex-sonographic criteria for the assessment of renal artery stenosis—correlation with intra-arterial pressure gradient. Ultraschall Med. **28**:45–51.

44. Bardelli M, Veglio F, Arosio E, Cataliotti A, Valvo E, & Morganti A (2006) New intrarenal echo-Doppler velocimetric indices for the diagnosis of renal artery stenosis. *Kidney Int* **69**:580–587.

45. el-Azab M, Mohsen T, el-Diasty T, & Shokeir AA (1996) Doppler ultrasonography in evaluation of potential live kidney donors: a prospective study. *J Urol* **156**:878–880.

46. Tullis MJ, Zierler RE, Glickerman DJ, Bergelin RO, Cantwell-Gab K, & Strandness DE Jr (1997) Results of percutaneous transluminal angioplasty for atherosclerotic renal artery stenosis: a follow-up study with duplex ultrasonography. *J Vasc Surg* **25**:46–54.

47. Ruggenenti P, Mosconi L, Bruno S, *et al.* (2001) Post-transplant renal artery stenosis: the hemodynamic response to revascularization. *Kidney Int* **60**:309–318.

48. Edwards JM, Zaccardi MJ, & Strandness DE Jr (1992) A preliminary study of the role of duplex scanning in defining the adequacy of treatment of patients with renal artery fibromuscular dysplasia. *J Vasc Surg* **15**:604–609; discussion 609–611.

49. Radermacher J, Chavan A, Bleck J, *et al.* (2001) Use of Doppler ultrasonography to predict the outcome of therapy for renal-artery stenosis. *N Engl J Med* **344**:410–417.

50. Zierler RE, Bergelin RO, Davidson RC, Cantwell Gab K, Polissar NL, & Strandness DE Jr (1996) A prospective study of disease progression in patients with atherosclerotic renal artery stenosis. *Am J Hypertens* **9**:1055–1061.

51. Frauchiger B, Zierler R, Bergelin RO, Isaacson JA, & Strandness DE Jr (1996) Prognostic significance of intrarenal resistance indices in patients with renal artery interventions: a preliminary duplex sonographic study. *Cardiovasc Surg* **4**:324–330.

52. Cohn EJ Jr, Benjamin ME, Sandager GP, Lilly MP, Killewich LA, & Flinn WR (1998) Can intrarenal duplex waveform analysis predict successful renal artery revascularization? *J Vasc Surg* **28**:471–80; discussion 480–1.

53. Garcia-Criado A, Gilabert R, Nicolau C, *et al.* (2005) Value of Doppler sonography for predicting clinical outcome after renal artery revascularization in atherosclerotic renal artery stenosis. *J Ultrasound Med* **24**:1641–1647.

54. Zeller T, Muller C, Frank U, *et al.* (2003) Stent angioplasty of severe atherosclerotic ostial renal artery stenosis in patients with diabetes mellitus and nephrosclerosis. *Catheter Cardiovasc Interv* **58**:510–515.

55. Voiculescu A, Schmitz M, Plum J, *et al.* (2006) Duplex ultrasound and renin ratio predict treatment failure after revascularization for renal artery stenosis. *Am J Hypertens* **19**:756–763.

56. Eklof H, Ahlstrom H, Magnusson A, *et al.* (2006) A prospective comparison of duplex ultrasonography, captopril renography, MRA, and CTA in assessing renal artery stenosis. *Acta Radiol* **47**:764–774.

57. Qanadli SD, Soulez G, Therasse E, *et al.* (2001) Detection of renal artery stenosis: prospective comparison of captopril-enhanced Doppler sonography, captopril-enhanced scintigraphy, and MR angiography. *AJR Am J Roentgenol* **177**:1123–1129.

58. Schoenberg SO, Rieger J, Weber CH, *et al.* (2005) High-spatial-resolution MR angiography of renal arteries with integrated parallel acquisitions: comparison with digital subtraction angiography and US. *Radiology* **235**:687–698.

59. Argalia G, Cacciamani L, Fazi R, Salera D, & Giuseppetti GM (2004) [Contrast-enhanced sonography in the diagnosis of renal artery stenosis: comparison with MR-angiography]. *Radiol Med (Torino)* **107**:208–217.

60. Cianci R, Coen G, Manfredini P, *et al.* (2006) Diagnosis and outcome of renal function in patients with renal artery stenosis: which role have color Doppler sonography and magnetic resonance angiography? *Minerva Cardioangiol* **54**:139–144.

61. Vasbinder GB, Nelemans PJ, Kessels AG, Kroon AA, de Leeuw PW, & van Engelshoven JM (2001) Diagnostic tests for renal artery stenosis in patients suspected of having renovascular hypertension: a meta-analysis. *Ann Intern Med* **135**:401–411.

62. Vasbinder GB, Nelemans PJ, Kessels AG, *et al.* (2004) Accuracy of computed tomographic angiography and magnetic resonance angiography for diagnosing renal artery stenosis. *Ann Intern Med* **141**:674–682; discussion 682.

63. Handa N, Fukunaga R, Uehara A, *et al.* (1986) Echo-Doppler velocimeter in the diagnosis of hypertensive patients: the renal artery Doppler technique. *Ultrasound Med Biol* **12**:945–952.

64. Schwerk WB, Restrepo IK, Stellwaag M, Klose KJ, & Schade BC (1994) Renal artery stenosis: grading with image-directed Doppler US evaluation of renal resistive index. *Radiology* **190**:785–790.

65. Patriquin HB, Lafortune M, Jequier JC, *et al.* (1992) Stenosis of the renal artery: assessment of slowed systole in the downstream circulation with Doppler sonography. *Radiology* **184**:479–485.

66. Bude RO, Rubin JM, Platt JF, Fechner KP, & Adler RS (1994) Pulsus tardus: its cause and potential limitations in detection of arterial stenosis. *Radiology* **190**:779–784.

67. Radermacher J (2000) *Bedeutung der fabkodierten Duplexsonographie für die Diagnose und Prognose von Nierenerkrankungen.* Hannover: Hannover Medical School.

68. Handa N, Fukunaga R, Etani H, Yoneda SK, K, & Kameda T (1988) Efficacy of echo-Doppler examination for the evaluation of renovascular disease. *Ultrasound Med Biol* **14**:1–5.

69. Ripolles T, Aliaga R, Morote V, *et al.* (2001) Utility of intrarenal Doppler ultrasound in the diagnosis of renal artery stenosis. *Eur J Radiol* **40**:54–63.

70. Speckamp F, Vorwerk D, Schurmann K, *et al.* (1995) Color-coded duplex ultrasonography in the diagnosis of renal artery stenosis. *Rofo Fortschr Geb Rontgenstr Neuen Bildgeb Verfahr* **162**:412–419.

71. Hansen KJ, Tribble RW, Reavis SW, *et al.* (1990) Renal duplex sonography: evaluation of clinical utility. *J Vasc Surg* **12**:227–236.

72. Karasch T, Strauss AL, Grun B, *et al.* (1993) [Color-coded duplex ultrasonography in the diagnosis of renal artery stenosis]. *Dtsch Med Wochenschr* **118**(40):1429–1436.

73. Olin JW, Piedmonte MR, Young JR, DeAnna S, Grubb M, & Childs MB (1995) The utility of duplex ultrasound scanning of the renal arteries for diagnosing significant renal artery stenosis. *Ann Intern Med* **122**:833–838.

74. Schaberle W, Strauss A, Neuerburg-Heusler D, & Roth FJ (1992) [Value of duplex sonography in diagnosis of renal artery stenosis and its value in follow-up after angioplasty (PTA)]. *Ultraschall Med* **13**:271–276.

75. Nchimi A, Biquet JF, Brisbois D, *et al.* (2003) Duplex ultrasound as first-line screening test for patients suspected of renal artery stenosis: prospective evaluation in high-risk group. *Eur Radiol* **13**:1413–1419.

76. Krumme B, Blum U, Schwertfeger E, *et al.* (1996) Diagnosis of renovascular disease by intra- and extrarenal Doppler scanning. *Kidney Int* **50**:1288–1292.

61 Interventional Treatment of Renal Artery Stenosis

Thomas Zeller

Heart Centre Bad Krozingen, Krozingen, Germany

Historical background

The first renal artery balloon angioplasties were performed by Felix Mahler in Berne and Andreas Grüntzig in Zürich in 1977 [1,2]. Until the beginning of the 1990s balloon angioplasty was the only method of percutaneous treatment of renal artery stenosis (RAS) with satisfying acute and long-term results for angioplasty of stenoses caused by fibromuscular dysplasia (FMD) and atherosclerotic RAS of the renal artery trunk with procedural success rates of 82–100% and restenosis rates of about 10% [3–7]. However, balloon angioplasty of ostial atherosclerotic lesions was limited by a low acute technical success rate of 50–62% and a high restenosis rate of up to 47% in the long term, owing to dissections, elastic recoil, and rigidity of the lesion [3,8].

The introduction of stenting has revolutionized percutaneous renal revascularization. Following promising single centre reports [8–15], two randomized studies proved the superiority of stenting over conventional balloon angioplasty [3,16] in the treatment of atherosclerotic ostial RAS, the most common manifestation of RAS. Now, using premounted low-profile stent devices, atherosclerotic RAS can be treated successfully in almost all cases with restenosis rates ranging from 0% to 23%, depending on the diameter of the renal artery [16–20].

Morphology and pathophysiology

Atherosclerosis accounts for approximately 90% of the cases of RAS, with increasing numbers resulting from the demographic development of the population. Atherosclerotic RAS is most often caused by plaque formation in the aortic wall, with progression into the renal artery origin resulting in the typical appearance of the eccentric ostial athero-sclerotic RAS (Fig. 61.1a). The prevalence of atherosclerotic RAS increases with age, particularly in patients with diabetes, hyperlipidemia, diffuse type of peripheral occlusive disease, coronary artery disease, or hypertension [21,22]. Atherosclerotic RAS is a progressive disease, even in initially unaffected arteries, with as much as an 18% occlusion rate within 1 year [23–26]. There is a close association between severity of RAS and kidney atrophy that may lead to ischemic nephropathy [27,28]. However, the loss of kidney filtration capacity in RAS is not only due to hypoperfusion, but also because of recurrent microembolism and other not yet completely known mechanisms. The exact etiology of the development of ischemic nephropathy is still uncertain [29].

The second frequent etiology of RAS (FMD) is a collection of vascular diseases that affects the three layers of the arterial vessel wall, intima, media, and adventitia, and is of unknown etiology. FMD accounts for < 10% of cases of RAS. FMD tends to affect mainly younger women, is located at the distal half of the renal artery trunk or the side branches, and is characterized by a beaded, aneurysm-like appearance on angiography (Fig. 61.1b). FMD rarely leads to vessel occlusion or ischemic nephropathy [29,30].

Clinical manifestation of renal artery stenosis

Arterial hypertension

Hypoperfusion of the kidney activates the renin–angiotensin–aldosterone system (Goldblatt phenomenon) causing classic renovascular hypertension, primarily in young patients with FMD [29–31]. However, in patients with atherosclerosis, RAS induces an acceleration of a pre-existing essential hypertension, usually in bilateral stenotic kidney disease and occasionally leading to the development of the typical recurrent flush pulmonary edema [29]. In atherosclerotic RAS, renal artery revascularization rarely cures hypertension but may improve blood pressure control. Uncontrolled hypertension may lead to organ failures, such as congestive heart failure, pulmonary edema, hypertensive encephalopathy, hypertensive intracerebral mass bleeding, end-stage kidney disease, and aneurysms [29,32].

Cardiovascular Interventions in Clinical Practice. Edited by Jürgen Haase, Hans-Joachim Schäfers, Horst Sievert and Ron Waksman. © 2010 Blackwell Publishing.

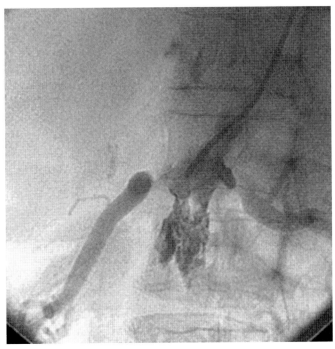
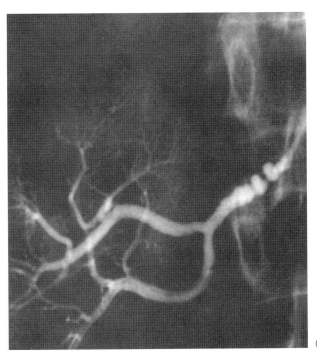

Figure 61.1 Bilateral atherosclerotic renal artery stenosis and total occlusion of the infrarenal aorta (a) right-sided renal artery stenosis of the due to fibromuscular dysplasia (b).

Left ventricular dysfunction

Left ventricular hypertrophy has a substantial impact on morbidity and mortality [33,34]. The most common cause of left ventricular hypertrophy and consecutive heart failure is hypertension [35,36]. Hypoperfusion of the kidney activates the renin–angiotensin–aldosterone system [29,31]. Aldosterone is not only a well-recognized promoter of hypertension [37], in patients with heart failure, it may be associated with myocardial fibrosis, left ventricular hypertrophy, and remodeling [38]. Left ventricular fibrosis and hypertrophy may primarily lead to diastolic dysfunction, and in the long run to systolic dysfunction.

Renal insufficiency

Ischemic kidney dysfunction may be caused by severe bilateral RAS or by unilateral stenosis in a functional single kidney [29]. If renal function is impaired in the case of unilateral RAS with two preserved kidneys, renal insufficiency is not only caused by hypoperfusion of the affected kidney, but also by structural (mostly bilateral) kidney disease, potentially induced by chronic hypertension and/or diabetes mellitus (nephrosclerosis) [29,39,40].

Indications

Every patient with an indication for endovascular revascularization of RAS should be hospitalized. Peri- and postprocedural supervision of blood pressure and renal function is mandatory; therefore, even if endovascular revascularization of RAS has become a relatively simple interventional procedure technically, it should not be performed as an outpatient procedure.

Indications for endovascular revascularization

In general, each decision for revascularization is an individual one that considers the overall patient constitution and prognosis.

1 uni- or bilateral RAS ≥70% with mild, moderate, or severe hypertension (according to the WHO criteria), especially in patients with a low compliance for taking the prescribed drugs, and with multiple cardiovascular risk factors;
2 uni- or bilateral RAS ≥70% with or without mild or moderately impaired renal function;
3 uni- or bilateral RAS ≥70% with recurrent pulmonary edema;
4 unstable angina without coronary revascularization options in patients with recurrent hypertensive crises and uni- or bilateral RAS ≥70%;
5 acute or subacute renal failure or anuria due to total occlusion or subtotal stenosis of one or both renal arteries;
6 RAS ≥70% in patients with single functional kidney.

Contraindications for endovascular revascularization

Absolute contraindications are (1) patients with chronic dialysis-dependent ischemic nephropathy who are not included in a clinical trial; and (2) limited life expectancy due to concomitant noncardiovascular or incurable disease. Relative contraindications include (1) severe contrast medium intolerance (alternative contrast media such as carbon dioxide or gadolinium using digital subtraction technique); and (2) impossible access to the renal artery due to iliac and subclavian artery occlusions.

Technical aspects

The following information on technical aspects of interventional treatment of RAS was found in reference 41.

Arterial access

Femoral approach
The femoral access site is the standard approach for renal interventions with few exceptions, such as untreated severe stenosis/occlusion of the pelvic arteries or abdominal aorta, severe kinking of the pelvic arteries or an acute angle of the renal artery.

Using the right femoral approach for right RAS and the left femoral approach for left RAS is often helpful, because the guiding catheter may perfectly adapt to the anatomy of the pelvic artery and aorta (Fig. 61.2a).

The "guiding catheter technique" is recommended (Fig. 61.2a–d), requiring a 6F or 7F sheath with a hemostatic valve. Normally, a standard sheath with a length of 11 cm is used (various manufacturers e.g. Avanti™; J & J Cordis Corp., Bridgewater, NJ, USA, or Terumo Corp.). In tortuous iliac arteries a longer sheath (23 cm, various manufacturers) for better manipulation of catheters and wires may be helpful. Following puncture of the artery with a Seldinger needle the sheath is introduced over a short introducer guidewire (Seldinger technique).

Alternatively, a guiding sheath (VistaBriteTip IG™, J & J Cordis Corp.) can be used. This device consists of a guiding catheter (renal double curved) with a brite tip and a hemostatic valve, and it replaces the conventional sheath. Hereby the outer device diameter is downsized by 1F (5F instead of 6F) and the risk of local complications at the access site may be reduced.

Brachial approach
Both a left and right brachial approach can be used. However, the left brachial access is safer because no brain providing artery except the left vertebral artery must be passed with a wire or catheter. Mostly a 6F, more seldomly a 7F, sheath is introduced into the brachial artery in the fossa antecubitalis using a micro puncture set. As for the femoral approach, the use of a guiding catheter (90 cm length) is recommended. Most-used catheter types are the "right Judkins 4," the "right Amplatz 1," and the "Multipurpose" catheters (various companies, Fig. 61.2e–g).

Alternatively, a 90-cm-long straight 6F sheath (Cook Corp., Bjaeverskov, Denmark) or a multipurpose shaped guiding-sheath (VistaBriteTip IG™) can be positioned proximal to the origin of the renal artery.

Renal artery angiography
In a nontortuous aorta, the origins of right and left renal arteries are identified best in a 20° left anterior oblique (LAO) projection (Fig. 61.3a and b). Semiselective and selective baseline angiogram should be performed to determine the optimal projection for the intervention. Before the first selective renal angiography, the guiding catheter tip should be cleaned from debris collected by catheter manipulation along the aortic wall by retrograde flushing of the catheter or aspiration of 10 cc of blood via a Y-connector ("proximal protection"). This technique reduces the risk of renal embolism.

Technique of renal artery stenting
The guiding catheter technique (Fig. 62.2) is the fastest technique with the lowest intervention and radiation time. Using the *femoral approach,* various guiding catheter configurations, such as "renal double curve" (RDC), "hockey stick," "right Amplatz" (AR-1), "right Judkins" (JR-4), or "internal mammarian artery" (IMA) are available to guarantee a stable position proximal to the renal artery origin.

After placing the guiding catheter close to the renal artery origin, a steerable stiff 0.014-inch guidewire with a flexible tip should be used to cross the lesion. Some authors, such as Feldman *et al.* [42], recommend a so-called "no-touch technique" (Fig. 61.4a–c).

Coming from the femoral access it can become difficult to introduce a guidewire in renal arteries with an acutely angled off-take. The telescoping technique may solve this access problem. The renal artery orifice is cannulated using a 5F SOS-Omni Soft-Vu-catheter™ (AngioDynamics Inc., Queensbury, NY, USA) inserted through the lumen of a 7F guiding catheter. After introduction of the guidewire through the SOS catheter, the guiding catheter can then be advanced over the diagnostic catheter close to the orifice of the renal artery and the diagnostic catheter pulled out thereafter (Fig. 61.4d–g).

For renal artery revascularization via the *brachial approach,* various shapes of 6F guiding catheters such as JR-4, AR-1, or "Multipurpose, are available (Fig. 61.2e–g). Several low profile renal stent devices (e.g. Palmaz blue™, J & J Cordis Corp.; RX Herculink plus™, Guidant/Abbott Vascular Corp., Brussels, Belgium; Radix™, Sorin Biomedica Corp., Saluggia, Italy; Hippocampus™, Invatec, Roucadelle, Italy/ev3 Corp., Paris, France) enable direct stenting in the vast majority of the cases.

Alternatively, a long 6F sheath (90 cm, e.g., Cook Corp.) can be positioned near the origin of the renal artery. Selective engagement of the renal artery has to be performed with a 4F or 5F diagnostic catheter of various shapes ("Multipurpose" or others) to introduce a long 0.014-inch guidewire (300 cm) through the lesion into the renal artery. After removal of the 5F diagnostic catheter the stent can be placed.

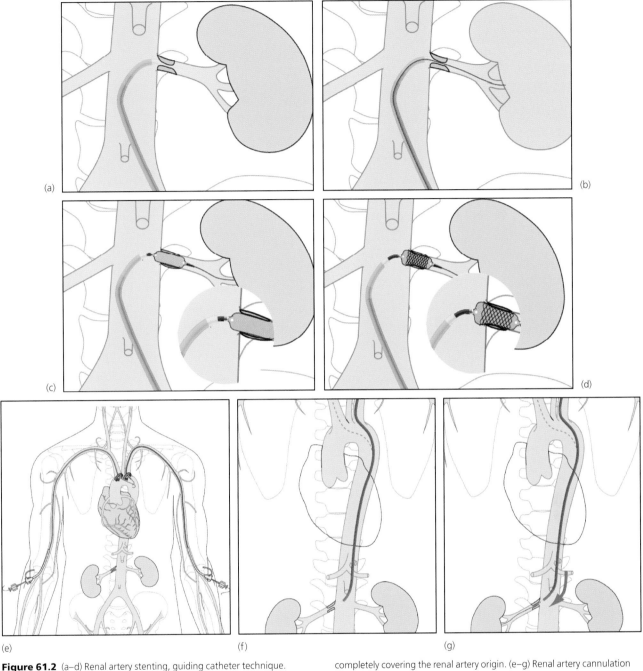

Figure 61.2 (a–d) Renal artery stenting, guiding catheter technique. (a) Selective catheterization of the renal artery with a guiding catheter (renal double curved [RDC] or RDC I). (b) The lesion is gently crossed with a 0.014-inch guidewire. (c) Predilation of the lesion (optional) with an undersized balloon (3 mm). (d) Stent deployment: the proximal stent struts should protrude 1–2 mm into the lumen of the aorta. Note: do not place the guiding catheter close to the renal artery origin; otherwise the stent could be dislocated too far distally into the renal artery not completely covering the renal artery origin. (e–g) Renal artery cannulation via the brachial approach. A 6F sheath is introduced into the brachial artery and a guiding catheter advanced over a 0.035-inch Terumo J-wire into the descending aorta (e). After the guidewire is advanced downstream into the abdominal aorta the guiding catheter is placed proximal to the renal artery origin (f). Finally, the guidewire (0.014-inch) is advanced into the renal artery and direct stenting or predilation can be performed (g).

Angioplasty technique

Usually a stiff 0.014-inch guidewire with a soft tip is used. In cases of highly calcified tight lesions, predilation should be performed starting with a 3-mm followed by a 5-mm monorail balloon. If the 5-mm balloon does not open up completely, a cutting balloon (Boston Scientific Corp., Natick, MA, USA) or a scoring balloon (AngioScore™, AngioSculpt, London, UK) has to be used for plaque modulation. Otherwise, full-stent

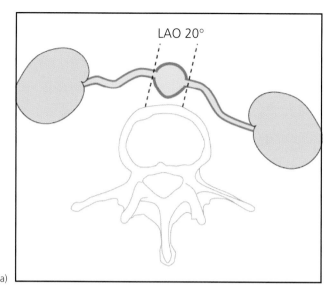

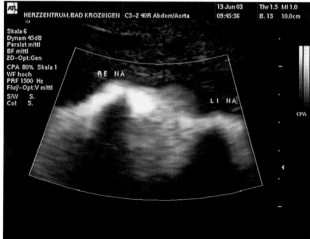

Figure 61.3 Drawing (a) and duplex image (power mode) (b) of the normal anatomy of renal artery orifices (broken line shows optimal angiographic view).

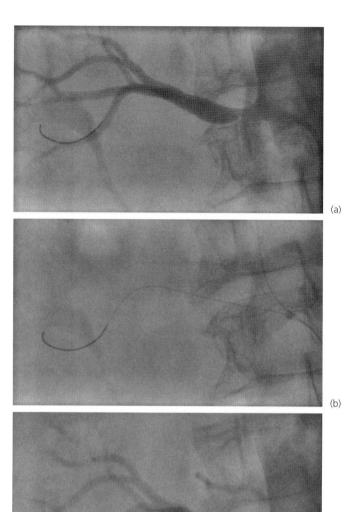

Figure 61.4 (a–c) Treatment of a right-sided renal artery stenosis using the "no-touch technique." Angiographic appearance before treatment (a); two 0.014-inch guidewires in place, one in the renal artery, one in the suprarenal position (b). Result after stenting, both guidewires still in place (c).

expansion would be impossible. Pre-interventional pressure gradient measurement is not recommended as routine procedure because a reliable determination of the gradient would need a pressure-wire, which is expensive and time-consuming. Moreover, a generally accepted definition of a hemodynamically relevant pressure gradient does not yet exist.

For ostial lesions, balloon-expandable stents are standard. For postostial lesions, short self-expanding nitinol stents can be used alternatively (4F shaft devices can be introduced via a 6F guiding catheter!). The balloon–vessel or the stent–vessel ratio should be 1:1. Overexpansion of the stent compared with the vessel diameter should not exceed 0.5 mm to avoid vessel perforation or dissection [41]. For full stent expansion, dilation time should be at least 20–30 s. Stent length should be kept as short as possible to completely cover the entire lesion. Especially in renal arteries providing hyper-mobile kidneys, stent fractures with consecutive acute thrombotic vessel occlusions have been reported recently.

The role of drug-eluting stents and covered stents in the treatment of RAS remains to be determined. Excellent results are reported for the management of in-stent restenoses [43,44]. Another possible indication for both devices might be small renal artery diameters (<5 mm) because of the higher risk for restenosis development in smaller renal arteries [17,18,20].

The indication for using *distal protection devices* during renal artery interventions is still a matter of debate. Until 2008, no dedicated protection device for renal application had been available [45]. Larger randomized trials comparing protected

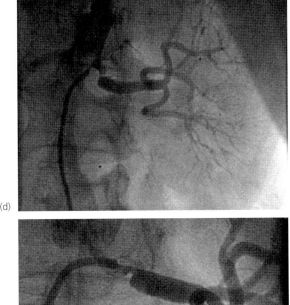

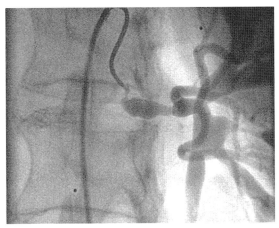

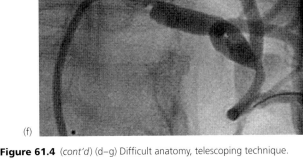

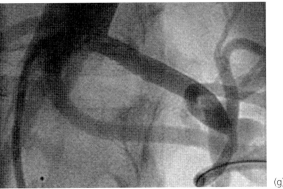

Figure 61.4 (*cont'd*) (d–g) Difficult anatomy, telescoping technique. (d) Nonselective angiography via a renal double curve guiding catheter; anatomy not suitable for insertion of a guidewire. (e) Engagement of the origin of the left renal artery with a 5F SOS-Omni-Soft-VU™ catheter introduced through the 7F guiding catheter.

(f) A stiff 0.018-inch guidewire was introduced through the 5F catheter and thereafter, the 7F guiding catheter was advanced over the SOS catheter close to the renal artery origin SOS catheter, which was then removed. (g) Left renal artery after implantation of a 6 × 20 mm stent.

renal artery stenting with unprotected intervention are still missing. A first small study (Prospective Randomized Study Comparing Renal Artery Stenting With or Without Distal Protection; RESIST trial) presented by C. Cooper at the TCT 2007 meeting could not prove any difference in renal functional outcome comparing protected (distal filter device) with unprotected renal artery stenting.

Postinterventional result documentation

After each intervention, selective and semiselective angiograms of the target lesion and the distal (intrarenal) arteries should be performed without a guidewire in place to document the final result and exclude peripheral embolism, dissection, or perforation. Intravascular ultrasound is only indicated for study purposes. Treatment success is achieved if the residual diameter stenosis after angioplasty is < 30%.

Postinterventional care

Antiplatelet medication after intervention routinely consists of 100 mg of acetylsalicylic acid (ASA) once a day for life and 75 mg clopidogrel once a day (alternatively 250 mg ticlopidine twice a day) for 4 weeks, although there is no evidence

based on comparative controlled data for this regimen. Additional heparin administration after intervention is not required. Short time intermediate care supervision might be indicated, especially in younger patients with a nonatherosclerotic RAS, in whom severe hypotension may occur following the revascularization procedure.

To prevent contrast-induced nephropathy, sufficient volume substitution with iso-osmolar saline infusion—depending on the patient's cardiac functional status—is recommended, especially in patients with already impaired renal function. Monitoring of renal function and blood pressure is mandatory before discharge. The time of bed rest after the intervention depends on the sheath size used, the access site and the application of closure devices.

Results

Effect of revascularization on arterial hypertension

Published studies of the outcome of revascularization of RAS have had numerous limitations. Hypertension has been classified as cured, improved, or unchanged, but the ability to make direct comparisons among studies is limited because of differences in medical therapy, target blood pressure, technique of blood pressure measurement, and criteria for improvement [29,32]. Conventional balloon angioplasty is the therapy of choice for RAS caused by fibromuscular dysplasia with cured or improved hypertension in 60–92% of the cases [4,7]. However, results are far less encouraging for atherosclerotic lesions with cured hypertension in <30% [9–11,29,32]. Two small randomized trials of conventional balloon angioplasty and medical therapy demonstrated a significant decrease in blood pressure and in the number of antihypertensive medication in the angioplasty group, but cure of hypertension was rare [3,46]. However, in the EMMA trial [3] there was a 27% cross-over rate in the medication group because of insufficient blood pressure control. The latest randomized trial comparing conventional balloon angioplasty with medical therapy failed to show a difference in outcomes (Dutch Renal Artery Stenosis Intervention Cooperative Study Group; DRASTIC [24]). But there are a number of methodologic limitations in this trial. The intention-to-treat analysis of this study is confounded by the fact that a high number of medically treated patients underwent angioplasty during a follow-up period (44%). In addition, the high restenosis rate of 48% in the angioplasty group equalizes the differences in the two groups after 12 months. Moreover, the patient population in this randomized trial included a significant number of patients without hemodynamically relevant RAS (40–70%). At the time this trial was performed, simple balloon angioplasty of atherosclerotic ostial RAS was common. This practice has now been essentially replaced by primary stent angioplasty because of much better acute and long-term results for this technique [9,10,29,32]. Although the authors did not find a difference in the outcome of renal function and blood pressure, it is encouraging that they have documented a significantly lower number of antihypertensive drugs in the angioplasty group.

Like other revascularization techniques, stenting of atherosclerotic RAS has been associated with a statistically significant decrease in blood pressure and in the need for medication during long-term follow-up [8–16]. The rates of cure of hypertension in atherosclerotic RAS after stenting are low and are comparable with surgery and conventional balloon angioplasty [29,47]. Currently, there is no randomized study available comparing stenting of severe, e.g. at least 70%, RAS with medication to prove the superiority of endovascular revascularization. However, it has to be considered that medical therapy has limitations in the treatment of hypertension in patients with RAS. These include limited patient compliance in taking the prescribed drugs with resultant inadequate blood pressure control. Moreover, ACE-inhibitors, diuretics and other antihypertensive drugs may lead to an acute ischemic nephropathy in patients with RAS [48,49]. Furthermore, under exclusive medical treatment, a progressive development of chronic ischemic nephropathy has been described [27,28].

Various predictors of improved blood pressure control after stent-angioplasty of at least 70% atherosclerotic RAS, such as the number of antihypertensive drugs taken before the intervention and bilateral renal disease, have been reported [10,15]. In contrast to the results of Radermacher et al. [50], who found nephrosclerosis to be predictive for treatment failure in terms of improved blood pressure control, other studies could not confirm this finding [13,51]. This difference in outcome may be due to the fact that Radermacher et al. included patients with hemodynamically not relevant stenoses of 50–70% in approximately one-third of their patients. Furthermore, their analysis was based on the inclusion of three different types of revascularization techniques, such as angioplasty with stenting, without stenting, and surgery. Sixty-two percent of the patients were treated with plain balloon angioplasty. The rate of restenosis and reintervention following plain balloon angioplasty is usually high (up to 48% [3]) and might have influenced the blood pressure outcome in their study.

Effect of revascularization on kidney function

According to recent American Heart Association guidelines, slowed decline in renal function suffices to claim a benefit from renal artery angioplasty [52]. Discrepant results on the effect of balloon angioplasty and stenting of RAS on renal function have been published; in patients with normal baseline creatinine level, renal function was mostly preserved [9–15]. In a study of mine including 456 patients with RAS and a mean follow-up of 34 ± 20 months, those with slight to moderate renal dysfunction at baseline had unchanged renal function (36%) and an improved function in 46%, respectively [15]. These results are similar to some previous data (van de Ven et al. [16], Rocha-Singh et al. [53] and Iannone et al. [54]). However, Blum et al. [9] found no significant change of creatinine independent of baseline renal function. White et al. [12] treated 100 patients and also found no significant change in creatinine level; however, in 9 of 44 (20%) patients with impaired renal function, creatinine normalized. The results show only a trend toward amelioration of renal function and may be a consequence of either the small sample size, or the inclusion of patients with a diameter stenosis of 50–70% in these studies [3,11,16,50,55]. Lesions of <70% diameter stenosis are not hemodynamically relevant and therefore do not cause hypoperfusion induced nephropathy [56]. There are few data on patients with severely impaired renal function: in our own patient cohort with severe renal dysfunction, renal function improved in 71%, was unchanged in 21%, and deteriorated in only 8% during long-term follow-up [15]. In seven patients (32%), a planned chronic hemodialysis could be deferred. These results are very similar to the results published by Korsakas et al. [57] and Taylor et al. [58]. In contrast, Pattynama et al. [59] who had analyzed 40 azotemic patients with 61 RAS treated interventionally, serum creatinine concentration was not improved after 1 year (2.4 mg% before intervention, 2.5 mg% after 1 year). In 60% of these patients, renal function was improved or preserved; in 40% it was deteriorated. There was no difference found between bilateral and unilateral disease.

Multivariate analysis of my own prospective cohort [58] identified baseline serum creatinine concentration, simultaneous bilateral intervention, diameter stenosis, and the absence of a coronary three-vessel disease as independent predictors for improvement of renal function after stenting [15]. Most other reports suggest that only treatment of bilateral severe renal artery stenosis should be beneficial in terms of improvement of renal function [10,54,60]. While Radermacher et al. [50] found no benefit for intervention in patients with severe nephrosclerosis as defined as intrarenal resistance index >0.8, in my own [58] study cohort this parameter was not predictive for the improvement of renal function nor was it the presence of diabetes mellitus [13,14,51].

Effect of revascularization on patient survival

Ischemic nephropathy is an important cause of end-stage disease [28,39,52,61], and among patients who are receiving dialysis, those with renovascular disease have the lowest survival rate, with a median survival of 25–34 months and a 5-year mortality rate exceeding 80% [6,28,52]. Thus it could be expected that survival of patients with renal dysfunction might be improved after successful revascularization. Disappointingly, two large series failed to proof a beneficial effect of revascularization on survival of patients with severe renal insufficiency pre-interventionally defined as a serum creatinine concentration >2.5 mg/dL [10,62]. Dorros et al. [10] found baseline creatinine concentration of >1.5 mg/dL and bilateral disease predictive for an increased mortality. In another study of mine [62], on patient survival, following renal artery, stent-angioplasty left ventricular cardiac dysfunction, age, and a baseline creatinine level of >2.5 mg/dL were independent predictors of mortality in multivariate analysis [62]. In this the cause of death was congestive heart failure or myocardial infarction (73%), stroke (13.5%), and malignant disease (13.5%).

Effect of revascularization on left ventricular hypertrophy

Former necropsy studies found a higher prevalence of left ventricular hypertrophy in patients with hypertension and RAS than in patients with essential hypertension [63]. My own echocardiographic findings confirm these results; 73% of the patients with RAS had left ventricular hypertrophy while it was present only in 56% of the patients with essential hypertension.

Results of a study investigating the impact of stent-supported percutaneous revascularization of severe RAS show a substantial reduction of the left ventricular mass index in patients who underwent stent-supported revascularization of atherosclerotic RAS, in particular when left ventricular

hypertrophy was present at baseline [64]. In contrast, patients with essential hypertension tended toward progression of left ventricular mass index and toward deterioration of hypertension control. The regression of left ventricular mass index in patients after stent-revascularization confirms the results of to two former small studies investigating the impact of balloon angioplasty and surgery of at least 50% RAS of different etiology [65,66]. In these two small studies, the reduction in blood pressure was assumed to be responsible for the regression of hypertrophy. However, multivariate analysis of the own study cohort resulted in stent revascularization as the only independent predictor for the regression of left ventricular hypertrophy.

Conclusion

In summary, stent-supported angioplasty of severe ostial RAS improves renal function and blood pressure control in a broader spectrum of patients than previously assumed. Diabetes mellitus, nephrosclerosis and unilateral involvement do not justify withholding renal stent-supported angioplasty in severe RAS. The greatest benefit with respect to renal function is found in patients whose renal function is already impaired or who have concomitant left ventricular dysfunction. Several small studies indicate an impact of revascularization on left ventricular hypertrophy leading to diastolic and systolic left ventricular dysfunction and being one of the major predictors for mortality. Thus, the aim must be to improve primary and secondary prevention, and to achieve an earlier diagnosis and, when indicated, treatment of renal, coronary, and cerebral occlusive disease. In patients with an advanced stage of renal failure the indication for stenting of atherosclerotic RAS should be determined individually for each patient, considering his or her overall prognosis.

References

1. Grüntzig A, Vetter W, Meier B, et al. (1978) Treatment of renovascular hypertension with percutaneous transluminal dilatation of a renal artery stenosis. *Lancet* **1**:801–802.
2. Mahler F, Krneta A, & Haertel M (1979) Treatment of renovascular hypertension by transluminal renal artery dilatation. *Ann Intern Med* **90**:56–57.
3. Plouin PF, Chatellier G, Darne B, et al. (1998) Blood pressure outcome of angioplasty in atherosclerotic renal artery stenosis: a randomized trail. The EMMA-study group. *Hypertension* **31**: 823–829.
4. Van Bockel JH & Weibull H (1994) Fibrodysplastic disease of renal arteries. *Eur J Vasc Surg* **8**:655–657.
5. Baert AL, Wilms G, Amery A, et al. (1990) Percutaneous transluminal renal angioplasty: initial results and long-term follow-up in 202 patients. *Cardiovasc Intervent Radiol* **13**:22–28.

6. Bonelli FS, McKusick A, Textor SC, *et al.* (1995) Renal artery angioplasty: technical results and clinical outcome in 320 patients. *Mayo Clin Proc* **70**:1041–1052.

7. Cluzel P, Raynaud A, Beyssen B *et al.* (1994) Stenoses of renal branch arteries in fibromuscular dysplasia: results of percutaneous transluminal angioplasty. *Radiology* **193**:227–232.

8. Dorros G, Prince C, & Mathiak L (1993) Stenting of renal artery stenosis achieves better relief of the obstructive lesion than balloon angioplasty. *Cath Cardiovasc Diagn* **29**:191–198.

9. Blum U, Krumme B, Flügel P, *et al.* (1997) Treatment of ostial renal-artery stenoses with vascular endoprostheses after unsuccessful balloon angioplasty. *N Engl J Med* **336**:459–465.

10. Dorros G, Jaff M, Mathiak L, *et al.* (1998) 4-year follow-up of Palmaz–Schatz stent revascularisation as treatment for atherosclerotic renal artery stenosis. *Circulation* **98**:642–647.

11. Henry M, Amor M, Henry I, *et al.* (1996) Stent placement in the renal artery: three-year experience with the Palmaz stent. *J Vasc Interven Radiol* **7**:343–350.

12. White CJ, Ramee SR, Collins TJ, *et al.* (1999) Renal artery stent placement: utility in lesions difficult to treat with balloon angioplasty. *J Am Coll Cardiol* **30**:1445–1450.

13. Zeller T, Müller C, Frank U, *et al.* (2003) Stent-angioplasty of severe atherosclerotic ostial renal artery stenosis in patients with diabetes mellitus and nephrosclerosis. *Cath Cardiovasc Interven* **58**:510–515.

14. Zeller T, Frank U, Müller C, *et al.* (2003) Predictors of improved renal function after primary stenting of severe atherosclerotic ostial renal artery stenosis. *Circulation* **108**:2244–2249.

15. Zeller T, Frank U, Müller C, *et al.* (2004) Stent-supported angioplasty of severe atherosclerotic renal artery stenosis preserves renal function and improves blood pressure control: Long-term results of a prospective registry with 456 lesions. *J Endovasc Ther* **11**:95–106.

16. Van de Ven PJG, Kaatee R, Beutler JJ, *et al.* (1999) Arterial stenting and balloon angioplasty in ostial atherosclerotic renovascular disease: a randomised trail. *Lancet* **353**:282–286.

17. Zeller T, Rastan A, Kliem M, *et al.* (2005) Impact of carbon coating on restenosis rate after stenting of atherosclerotic renal artery stenosis. *J Endovasc Ther* **12**:605–611.

18. Zeller T, Müller C, Frank U, *et al.* (2003) Gold coating and restenosis after primary stenting of ostial renal artery stenosis. *Cath Cardiovasc Intervent* **60**:1–6.

19. Sapoval M, Zähringer M, Pattynama P, *et al.* (2005) Low-profile stent system for treatment of atherosclerotic renal artery stenosis: The GREAT Trial. *J Vasc Interv Radiol* **16**:1195–1202.

20. Lederman RJ, Mendelsohn FO, Santos R, *et al.* (2001) Primary renal artery stenting: characteristics and outcomes after 363 procedures. *Am Heart J* **142**:314–323.

21. Harding MB, Smith LR, Himmelstein SI *et al.* (1992) Prevalence and associated risk factors in patients undergoing routine cardiac catheterization. *J Am Soc Nephrol* **2**:1608.

22. Missouris CG, Buckenham T, Cappuccio FP, *et al.* (1994) Renal artery stenosis: a common and important problem in patients with peripheral vascular disease. *Am J Med* **96**:10–14.

23. Zierler RE, Bergelin RO, Davidson CD, *et al.* (1996) A prospective study of disease progression in patients with atherosclerotic renal artery stenosis. *Am J Hypertens* **9**:1055–1061.

24. Van Jaarsveld BC, Krijnen P, Pieterman H, *et al.* For the Dutch Renal Artery Stenosis Intervention Cooperative Study Group. (2000) The effect of balloon angioplasty on hypertension in atherosclerotic renal-artery stenosis. *N Engl J Med* **342**:1007–1014.

25. Tollefson DFJ & Emst CB (1991) Natural history of atherosclerotic renal artery stenosis associated with aortic disease. *J Vasc Surg* **14**:327–331.

26. Schreiber MJ, Pohl MA, & Novick AC (1984) The natural history of atherosclerotic and fibrous renal artery disease. *Urol Clin North Am* **11**:383–392.

27. Rimmer JM & Gennari FJ (1993) Atherosclerotic renovascular disease and progressive renal failure. *Ann Intern Med* **118**:712–719.

28. Caps MT, Zierler RE, Polissar NL, *et al.* (1998) Risk of atrophy in kidneys with atherosclerotic renal artery stenosis. *Kidney Int* **53**:735–742.

29. Safian RD & Textor SC (2001) Renal-artery stenosis. *N Engl J Med* **344**:431–442.

30. Sang CN, Whelton PK, Hamper U, *et al.* (1989) Etiologic factors of renovascular fibromuscular dysplasia: a case-controlled study. *Hypertension* **14**:472–479.

31. Border WA & Noble NA (1998) Interactions of transforming growth factor-beta and angiotensin II in renal fibrosis. *Hypertension* **31**:161–188.

32. Zeller T (2005) Renal artery stenosis: Epidemiology, clinical manifestation and percutaneous endovascular therapy. *J Intervent Cardiol* **18**:497–506.

33. Levy D, Garrison RJ, Savage D, *et al.* (1989) Left ventricular mass and incidence of coronary heart disease in an elderly cohort: the Framingham Heart Study. *Ann Intern Med* **110**:101–107.

34. Levy D, Garrison RJ, Savage D, *et al.* (1990) Prognostic implications of echocardiographically determined left ventricular mass in the Framingham Heart Study. *N Engl J Med* **322**:1561–1566.

35. Levy D, Larson MG, Vasan RS, *et al.* (1996) The progression from hypertension to congestive heart failure. *JAMA* **275**:1557–1562.

36. Vasan RS & Levy D (1996) The role of hypertension in the pathogenesis of heart failure: a clinical mechanistic overview. *Arch Intern Med* **156**:1789–1796.

37. Vasan RS, Evans JC, Larson MG, *et al.* (2004) Serum aldosterone and the incidence of hypertension in nonhypertensive persons. *N Engl J Med* **351**:8–10.

38. Vasan RS, Evans JC, Benjamin EJ, *et al.* (2004) Relations of serum aldosterone to cardiac structure: gender-related differences in the Framingham Heart Study. *Hypertension* **43**:957–962.

39. Shanly PF (1996) The pathology of chronic renal ischemia. *Semin Nephrol* **16**:21–32.

40. Dean RH, Tribble RW, Hansen KJ, *et al.* (1991) Evolution of renal insufficiency in ischemic nephropathy. *Ann Surg* **213**:446–455.

41. Zeller T (2004) Endovascular treatment of renal artery stenosis. In: Marco J, Serruys P, Biamino G, Fajadet J, de Feyter P, Morice MC (eds). *The Paris Course on Revascularization.* Toulouse-Balma, France: Europa Edition, pp. 387–415.

42. Feldman RL, Wargovich TJ, & Bittl JA (1999) No-touch technique for reducing aortic wall trauma during renal artery stenting. *Cath Cardiovasc Interv* **46**:245–248.

43. Zeller T, Sixt S, Rastan A, *et al.* (2007) Treatment of recurring instent restenosis following reintervention after stent-supported renal artery angioplasty. *Cath Cardiovasc Intervent* **70**:296–300.

44. Zeller T, Schwarzwälder U, Rastan A, *et al.* (2007) Treatment of instent restenosis following stent-supported renal artery angioplasty. *Cath Cardiovasc Intervent* **70**:454–459.

45. Henry M, Klonaris C, Henry I, *et al.* (2001) Protected renal stenting with the PercuSurge GuardWire device: a pilot study. *J Endovasc Ther* **8**:227–237.

46. Webster J, Marshall F, Abdalla M, *et al.* (1998) Randomized comparison of percutaneous angioplasty vs continued medical therapy for hypertensive patients with atheromatous renal artery stenosis. *J Hum Hypertens* **12**:329–335.

47. Erdoes L, Berman SS, Hunter GC, *et al.* (1996) Comparative analysis of percutaneous transluminal angioplasty and operation for renal revascularization. *Am J Kidney Dis* **27**:496–503.

48. Hricik DE, Browning PJ, Kopelman R, *et al.* (1983) Captopril-induced functional renal insufficiency in patients with bilateral renal-artery stenoses or stenosis in a solitary kidney. *N Engl J Med* **308**:373–376.

49. Toto RD, Mitchell HC, Lee HC, *et al.* (1991) Reversible renal insufficiency due to angiotensin converting enzyme inhibitors in hypertensive nephrosclerosis. *Ann Intern Med* **115**:513–519.

50. Radermacher J, Chavan A, Bleck J, *et al.* (2001) Use of Doppler ultrasonography to predict the outcome of therapy for renal-artery stenosis. *N Engl J Med* **334**:410–417.

51. Voiculescu A, Schmitz M, Plum J, *et al.* (2006) Duplex ultrasound and rennin ratio predict treatment failure after revascularization for renal artery stenosis. *Am J Hypertens* **19**:756–763.

52. Rundback JH, Sacks D, Kent KC, *et al.* (2002) Guidelines for the reporting of renal artery revascularization in clinical trials. *Circulation* **106**:1572–1585.

53. Rocha-Singh KJ, Ahuja RK, Sung CH, *et al.* (2002) Long-term renal function preservation after renal artery stenting in patients with progressive ischemic nephropathy. *Catheter Cardiovasc Intervent* **57**:135–141.

54. Ianonne LA, Underwood PL, Nath A, *et al.* (1996) Effect of primary balloon expandable renal artery stents on long-term patency, renal function, and blood pressure in hypertensive and renal insufficient patients with renal artery stenosis. *Cath Cardiovasc Diagn* **37**:243–250.

55. Harden PN, MacLeod MJ, Rodger RSC, *et al.* (1997) Effect of renal-artery stenting on progression of renovascular renal failure. *Lancet* **349**:1133–1136.

56. Mustert BR, Williams DM, & Prince MR (1998) In vitro model of arterial stenosis: correlation of MR signal dephasing and trans-stenotic pressure gradients. *Magn Reson Imaging* **16**:301–310.

57. Korsakas S, Mohaupt MG, Dinkel HP, *et al.* (2004) Delay of dialysis in end-stage renal failure: prospective study on percutaneous renal artery interventions. *Kidney International* **65**:251–258.

58. Taylor A, Sheppard D, MacLeod MJ, *et al.* (1997) Renal artery stent placement in renal artery stenosis: technical and early clinical results. *Clin Radiology* **52**:451–457.

59. Pattynama P, Becker GJ, Brown J, *et al.* (1994) Percutaneous angioplasty for atherosclerotic renal artery disease: effect on renal function in azotemic patients. *Cardiovasc Intervent Radiol* **17**:143–146.

60. La Batide-Alanore A, Azizi M, Froissart M, *et al.* (2001) Split renal function outcome after renal angioplasty in patients with unilateral renal artery stenosis. *J Am Soc Nephrol* **12**:1235–1241.

61. Mailloux LU, Napolitano B, Bellucci AG, *et al.* (1994) Renal vascular disease causing end-stage renal disease, incidence, clinical correlates, and outcomes: A 20-year clinical experience. *Am J Kidney Diseases* **4**:622–629.

62. Zeller T, Müller C, Frank U, *et al.* (2003) Survival after stent-angioplasty of severe atherosclerotic ostial renal artery stenoses. *J Endovasc Ther* **10**:539–545.

63. Wright JR, Shurrab AE, Cooper A, *et al.* (2005) Left ventricular morphology and function in patients with atherosclerotic renovascular disease. *J Am Soc Nephrol* **16**:2746–2753.

64. Zeller T, Rastan A, Schwarzwälder U, *et al.* (2007) Regression of left ventricular hypertrophy following stenting of renal artery stenosis. *J Endovasc Ther* **14**:189–197.

65. Yoshitomi Y, Nishikimi T, Abe H, *et al.* (1996) Comparison of changes in cardiac structure after treatment in secondary hypertension. *Hypertension* **27**:319–323.

66. Symonides B, Chodakowska J, Januszewicz A, *et al.* (1999) Effects of the correction of renal artery stenosis on blood pressure, renal function and left ventricular morphology. *Blood Pressure* **8**:141–150.

62   Pathology of Iliac and Lower Extremity Artery Disease

Christian Ihling

Gemeinschaftspraxis für Pathologie, Frankfurt, Germany

Anatomy and age-related structural changes in the iliac artery and the lower extremity arteries

Macroscopic anatomy

The common iliac arteries are two large vessels which are about 4 cm in length and >1 cm in diameter. They originate from the aortic bifurcation and terminate when dividing into the external iliac artery and internal iliac artery. The right common iliac artery is slightly longer than the left. Both common iliac arteries are accompanied by the common iliac veins.

The internal iliac artery commonly divides into an anterior division and a posterior division, supplying the pelvic organs as well as the muscular and osseous components of the pelvic wall. The length of the internal iliac artery is variable and depends on its ending type. It varies between 20 and 90 mm with a mean value of 49 mm. The lengths of the common iliac and internal iliac arteries bear an inverse proportion to each other, the internal iliac artery being long when the common iliac artery is short, and vice versa [1]. There are no major differences between male and female nor between left and right. The vessel diameter ranges between 4 and 11 mm [2]. The ending of the internal iliac artery is quite variable.

At the level of the inguinal ligament the external iliac artery becomes the common femoral artery which bifurcates into the superficial and the deep femoral artery. The superficial femoral artery continues down the thigh medial to the femur, goes through the adductor hiatus and ends in the popliteal fossa. After the passage of the adductor hiatus the superficial femoral artery becomes the popliteal artery, which trifurcates below the knee.

The external iliac artery and the femoral arteries carry the blood to the lower limb and are accompanied by the external iliac vein, which is located posterior to the artery.

The deep femoral artery is the largest branch of the femoral artery and arises 3–5 cm below the inguinal ligament on the lateral side. It goes down the thigh close to the femur and does not leave the thigh.

Microscopic anatomy

The basic architecture and cellular composition of blood vessels are virtually the same throughout the whole vascular

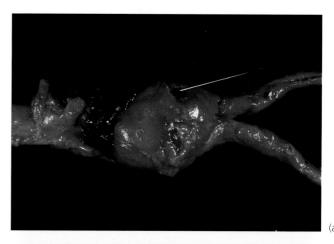

(a)

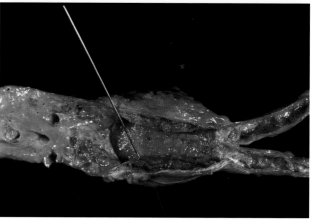

(b)

Figure 62.1 (a and b) Ruptured atherosclerotic aneurysm of the abdominal aorta with parietal thrombus and severe focally stenotic atherosclerosis of the iliac arteries. Findings at autopsy.

Cardiovascular Interventions in Clinical Practice. Edited by Jürgen Haase, Hans-Joachim Schäfers, Horst Sievert and Ron Waksman. © 2010 Blackwell Publishing.

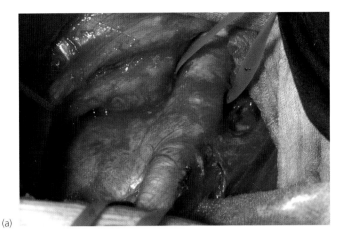

(a)

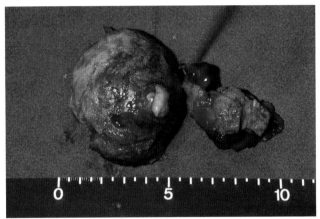

(b)

Figure 62.2 (a and b) Isolated atherosclerotic aneurysm of the iliac artery with parietal thrombus (b). Courtesy of Professor G. Fraedrich, Department of Vascular Surgery, University of Innsbruck, Austria.

system. However, certain features vary and reflect distinct local functional requirements. These structural changes are mainly in the media and in the extracellular matrix.

The common iliac artery is, in its proximal parts, an elastic artery rich in elastic fibers forming a network to protect the smooth muscle cells against the mechanical forces imposed on the vasculature during systole. However, the content of elastic fibers in the media diminishes gradually with growing distance to the aortic bifurcation and with the reduction of lumen diameter in its distal parts and in its branches.

The femoral arteries are muscular arteries. The media of muscular arteries is mainly composed of circularly and spirally oriented smooth muscle cells. Elastin is reduced to the internal and external elastic laminae. Blood flow is regulated by lumen size through smooth muscle cell contraction.

Age-related structural changes
In older individuals arteries of the elastic type often lose elasticity and become wider, the vessel wall being more stiff. Thus the arteries become more tortuous and dilated leading to the development of kinkings.

In addition, diffuse intimal thickening develops. This change is, however, more prominent in the femoral artery. Severe kinkings of the iliac arteries can make transfemoral cardiac, carotid, intracerebral or renal artery interventions more difficult. Limited kinkings in the iliac arteries may be straightened using long introducer sheaths. Extreme kinkings, however, may require the selection of alternative access sites (brachial or radial arteries).

Pathology

Pathology of peripheral arterial disease
Peripheral arterial disease often is the result of a systemic disease that affects multiple arteries. The systemic pathologic processes are diverse and include atherosclerosis, degenerative diseases, dysplastic disorders, vascular inflammations (arteritis), and *in situ* thrombosis, as well as thromboembolism.

By far the most common disease process affecting the iliac, the femoral, and the popliteal arteries is atherosclerosis. Therefore, the following text is focused mainly on atherosclerosis of the pelvic and limb arteries and its sequels. In addition, the main topics of the pathology of vascular interventions are discussed. Finally, rare entities associated with arterial dissection or rupture are reported.

Atherosclerosis of the iliac arteries and lower extremity arteries: etiology, risk factors, prevalence and prognosis
The epidemiology and the risk factors of iliac and lower extremity atherosclerosis are similar to that of classic atherosclerosis elsewhere [3–7], for example smoking [8–12], diabetes [13–15], hypertension [8], hyperlipidemia [4,6,12,14] family history, hyperhomocysteinemia [16], and elevated levels of C-reactive protein, a serum marker of systemic inflammation [5]. Lower extremity atherosclerosis is widespread and affects a large proportion of adults worldwide [7,17]. The incidence increases with age [18]. Since atherosclerosis is a systemic disease, the prognosis of patients with clinical manifestation of chronic limb ischemia is also characterized by an increased risk of cardiovascular ischemic events or ischemic stroke [7,19]. Atherosclerosis may lead to progressive stenosis and in severe cases to the occlusion of the blood vessel or to aneurysmal dilation of the affected arteries.

Stenotic atherosclerosis of the iliac arteries and lower extremity arteries
Certain anatomic sites are more prone to be affected by atherosclerosis, e.g., the femoral artery is most frequently occluded at the adductor hiatus, where it has to bear great mechanical stress by the tendinous arch of the adductor magnus muscle [20]. The morphology of atherosclerotic lesions in the iliac artery, the femoral artery, and the popliteal artery is the same as in other arteries. The principal

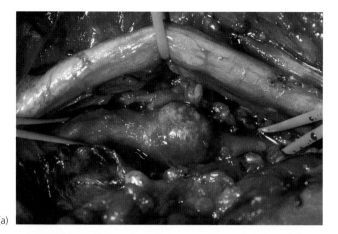

(a)

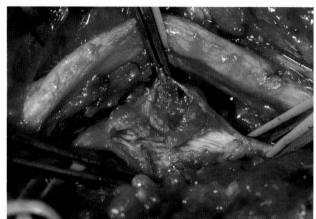

(b)

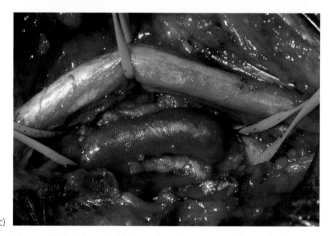

(c)

Figure 62.3 (a, b, and c) Atherosclerotic aneurysm of the popliteal artery with parietal thrombosis (a and b). Situs after aneurysm resection and surgical reconstruction. Courtesy of Professor G. Fraedrich, Department of Vascular Surgery, University of Innsbruck, Austria.

pathologic features are eccentric intimal thickening impinging on the lumen, lipid accumulation, and inflammation [21,22]. Lumen narrowing is, in part, counterbalanced by adaptive remodeling of the artery or by vessel expansion [23]. Advanced lesions of the iliac arteries and the lower extremity arteries show essentially the same complications as advanced

unstable coronary plaques, e.g., plaque rupture with intramural hemorrhage, plaque ulceration, and endothelial erosion leading to thrombosis with vessel occlusion and acute ischemia. Thrombi that are organized become incorporated into the plaque and thus lead to accelerated plaque growth. Complicating occlusive thrombosis frequently occurs at preferential sites [24] such as the aortic bifurcation (Lerich's syndrome). This leads to intermittent claudication, sexual impotence, and sometimes to pain at rest or peripheral gangrene [25].

Atherosclerotic aneurysms of the iliac arteries and the lower extremity arteries

The mean diameter of the common iliac artery, the internal iliac artery, and the femoral artery, as determined by computed tomography and arteriography show gender-specific, age-related and body size dependent differences [26–28]. The diameters of peripheral arteries increase up to 25% between the ages of 20 and 70 years. This may be due to an absolute loss of collagen and elastin of the arterial wall, which is observed with increasing age. On the other hand, the concentration of both proteins increases, indicating that there must be a considerable simultaneous loss of other components of the vessel wall, such as constituents of the extracellular matrix and/or atrophy of the smooth muscle cells [29,30]. Therefore, the diagnosis of an aneurysm should only be made by formulas that adjust for these variable parameters.

Patients with arterial aneurysms have many risk factors in common with patients with occlusive arterial disease. Isolated aneurysms of the iliac arteries are rare and represent 2–7% of all intraabdominal aneurysms [31–33] (Fig. 62.2). Most common iliac artery aneurysms are found in patients with abdominal aortic aneurysms, are bilateral, and are asymptomatic at the time of their diagnosis (Fig. 62.1). Rare complications of iliac artery aneurysms are expansive growth and rupture. Aneurysm rupture usually occurs at a diameter of 5 cm or larger whereas aneurysms with a diameter smaller than 3 cm almost never rupture [34–36].

Eighty-five percent of patients with femoral artery aneurysms and 62% of patients with popliteal aneurysms have a coexistent abdominal aortic aneurysm [37]. Most femoral artery aneurysms occur in men and are also associated with aortic and iliacal aneurysms. The natural history of extremity-artery aneurysms is characterized by thromboembolism and thrombosis.

Aneurysms of the deep femoral artery are usually found together with aneurysms of the common femoral artery. Complications of femoral artery aneurysms are related to expansion and include femoral nerve compression, venous occlusion with phlegmasia cerulea dolens, and acute ischemic syndromes due to thrombosis or thromboembolism [38–41].

Popliteal aneurysms

Popliteal aneurysms are the most frequent aneurysms of the lower extremities [42,43] (Fig. 62.3). Most of them occur in men, and approximately 50% are bilateral. Moreover, 50% of popliteal aneurysms are associated with other aneurysms, most frequently those of the aorta. Symptomatic popliteal aneurysms usually have a diameter of >2 cm and contain parietal thrombi. Forty percent of popliteal aneurysms cause clinical symptoms, such as *in situ* thrombosis or embolization to the calf or foot [44–47].

Pathogenesis and pathology of atherosclerotic aneurysms

The development of atherosclerotic aneurysms is associated with the destruction of the extracellular matrix in the media. Medial destruction in aneurysms is due to an inflammatory response within the intima, the media, and the adventitia [48]. The current view is that the inflammatory response to the injury of the vessel wall leads to an enzymatic destruction of the extracellular matrix caused by an imbalance of activated matrix metalloproteinases and their natural inhibitors [49–52]. The vessel wall can then no longer withstand the expansile forces which are imposed on the vessel wall during systole [53].

Atherosclerotic aneurysms are true aneurysms comprising all layers of the vessel wall characterized by a saccular or fusiform expansion of the artery. The morphology of atherosclerotic aneurysms is characterized by the presence of advanced atherosclerotic plaques in the intima, often complicated by parietal thrombosis. The media beneath the plaques is often atrophic and shows widespread fibrosis with a loss of elastic fibers and of smooth muscle cells, as well as an infiltration with inflammatory cells (e.g., lymphocytes and macrophages). Moreover, the adventitia often shows dense chronic inflammatory infiltration with lymph follicles and extensive scarring of the periaortic tissue. Sometimes atherosclerotic aneurysms become infected during bacteremia. This may cause suppurative inflammation which may lead to acceleration of medial destruction, and in some cases to rupture.

Degenerative diseases with dissection and rupture

Rarely, aneurysms of the iliac and femoral arteries are caused by degenerative disorders and may lead to dissection or rupture of the vessel wall. Dissections are so-called false aneurysms since the wall of the aneurysm does not comprise all layers of the vessel wall. Dissection is characterized by the penetration of blood into the arterial wall, forming a blood-filled channel. In most cases, the dissection extends from the aorta into the peripheral arteries. The histologic hallmark of degenerative disease and dissection is cystic medial degeneration (CMD) and was at first described by Erdheim in 1929 [54]. CMD comprises the accumulation of mucoid substance in pseudocysts—interrupting the network of smooth muscle cells and elastic fibers, leaving often multiple voids—focal

fibrosis with accumulation of collagen to a variable extent, and haphazardly distributed areas with loss of vascular smooth muscle cells (VSMCs). However, the current view is that the morphologic alterations of cystic medial degeneration are nonspecific, occurring during the normal aging process of the vessel wall. Nevertheless, these changes are more widespread in patients with antecedent hypertension or genetic disorders of the connective tissue. In fact, spontaneous dissections occur mainly in two age groups: first in men with antecedent uncontrolled arterial hypertension between 40 and 60 years, and second in a much younger group between 20 and 30 years with a genetically fixed disorder of the elastic fibers (e.g., Marfan's syndrome) [55–57]. By contrast, genetic abnormalities of collagen, either type I (osteogenesis imperfecta) or type III (Ehlers–Danlos type IV syndrome), lead to saccular aneurysms which may rupture. Abnormalities in the collagen reduce the ability to resist expansile force, but the tissue has a normal resistance to shear stress [58,59].

Pathology of angioplasty

For the majority of patients with intermittent claudication, interventional treatment using percutaneous transluminal angioplasty (PTA) or stent placement represent a frequently applied treatment option. Stents can be placed either as a primary or as an adjunct therapy after suboptimal results achieved with PTA [60]. Additional options are atherectomy, laser-angioplasty, cutting balloon angioplasty, thermal angioplasty, and thrombolysis. Outcomes depend on the anatomical location, the techniques used, and the clinical situation.

Balloon angioplasty

During balloon angioplasty the vessel wall is exposed to a radial force which causes endothelial denudation, plaque fracture, intimal–medial separation, along with a dissecting hematoma and stretching of the media and intima. Importantly, plaque configuration determines the response to PTA; for example, different atherosclerotic plaques respond differentially to balloon dilation. Thus, composition and configuration of the atherosclerotic lesion play a key role in the outcome of angioplasty [61].

Acute complications occurred in one study in 8% of the cases and comprised intramural hematomas, dissection, and embolism. However, surgical intervention was only necessary in 1.9% of the cases [62].

Restenosis

Restenosis with recurrent ischemia of the limb restricts the success of angioplasty, especially during the first year. Long term patency rates after PTA depend on anatomic sites and clinical factors. They are greatest for lesions in the common iliac artery and decrease distally. Patency rates also decrease with increasing length of the stenosis, multiple and diffuse lesions, impaired contrast runoff following the procedure, diabetes, renal failure, and smoking [63–78]. Restenosis occurs as part of a vascular repair process after angioplasty-induced injury with a smooth muscle cell hyperplasia of the intima [79]. In the beginning of the process, the neointima consists of loosely arranged and haphazardly oriented stellate-shaped smooth muscle cells embedded in a mucoid matrix rich in glycosaminoglycans and collagen. With time, cellularity decreases and collagen becomes more dense.

Endoluminal stents

Percutaneous implantation of balloon-expandable stents has been shown to reduce the frequency of restenosis after angioplasty [80,81]. Intravascular stents may provide a larger and more regular lumen, serving as a scaffolding to support the vessel wall after injury from balloon angioplasty. Additionally, they may limit elastic recoil as well as preventing the effects of vascular spasm, thus increasing blood flow and minimizing the risk of thrombosis [82].

Complications of stent implantation include initial failure, early thrombosis, late restenosis, and stent fracture [60,83]. Subacute stent thrombosis usually occurs 7–10 days after the stent implantation and leads to occlusion of the stented vessel.

The histologic changes induced in human arteries by stents have mainly been characterized in coronary arteries. They do not differ substantially from the alterations found in other locations. Stent implantation in combination with PTA leads to an injury of the vessel wall leading to adherence of platelets and leukocytes on the stent surface. Eventually, the struts are completely embedded in a neointima rich in vascular smooth muscle cells and collagen fibers. Finally, they are covered with endothelium. Neointimal growth in a stented vessel segment was found to be greatest at strut sites in the vicinity of medial laceration or rupture compared with struts in contact with an atherosclerotic plaque [84,85].

References

1. Gray H (1918) *Anatomy of the Human Body*. Philadelphia: Lea & Febiger.
2. Fatu C, Puisoru M, & Fatu IC (2006) Morphometry of the internal iliac artery in different ethnic groups. *Ann Anat* **188**: 541–546.
3. Ross R (1997) Cellular and molecular studies of atherogenesis. *Atherosclerosis* **13**:(1 Suppl.), S3–4.
4. Fowkes FG, Housley E, Riemersma RA, *et al.* (1992) Smoking, lipids, glucose intolerance, and blood pressure as risk factors for peripheral atherosclerosis compared with ischemic heart disease in the Edinburgh Artery Study. *Am J Epidemiol* **135**:331–340.
5. Ridker PM, Cushman M, Stampfer MJ, *et al.* (1998) Plasma concentration of C-reactive protein and risk of developing peripheral vascular disease. *Circulation* **97**:425–428.
6. Taylor LM Jr, DeFrang RD, Harris EJ Jr, *et al.* (1991) The associ-ation of elevated plasma homocyst(e)ine with progression of symptomatic peripheral arterial disease. *J Vasc Surg* **13**:128–136.
7. Criqui MH, Denenberg JO, Langer RD, *et al.* (1997) The epidemi-ology of peripheral arterial disease: importance of identifying the population at risk. *Vasc Med* **2**:221–226.
8. Kannel WB & McGee DL (1985) Update on some epidemiologic features of intermittent claudication: the Framingham Study. *J Am Geriatr* Soc **33**:13–18.
9. Smith GD, Shipley MJ, & Rose G (1990) Intermittent claudica-tion, heart disease risk factors, and mortality. The Whitehall Study. *Circulation* **82**:1925–1931.
10. Bowlin SJ, Medalie JH, Flocke SA, *et al.* (1994) Epidemiology of intermittent claudication in middle-aged men. *Am J Epidemiol* **140**:418–430.
11. Meijer WT, Hoes AW, & Rutgers D, *et al.* (1998) Peripheral arterial disease in the elderly: the Rotterdam Study. *Arterioscler Thromb Vasc Biol* **18**:185–192.
12. Kannel WB & Shurtleff D (1973) The Framingham Study: cigarettes and the development of intermittent claudication. *Geriatrics* **28**:61–68.
13. Newman AB, Siscovick DS, Manolio TA, *et al.* (1993) Ankle-arm index as a marker of atherosclerosis in the Cardiovascular Health Study. Cardiovascular Heart Study (CHS) Collaborative Research Group. *Circulation* **88**:837–845.
14. Hiatt WR, Hoag S, & Hamman RF (1995) Effect of diagnostic criteria on the prevalence of peripheral arterial disease. The San Luis Valley Diabetes Study. *Circulation* **91**:1472–1479.
15. Beks PJ, Mackaay AJ, de Neeling JN, *et al.* (1995) Peripheral arterial disease in relation to glycaemic level in an elderly Caucasian population: the Hoorn study. *Diabetologia* **38**:86–96.
16. Molgaard J, Malinow MR, Lassvik C, *et al.* (1992) Hyper-homocyst(e)inaemia: an independent risk factor for intermittent claudication. *J Intern Med* **231**:273–279.
17. Murabito JM, D'Agostino RB, Silbershatz H, *et al.* (1997) Intermittent claudication. A risk profile from The Framingham Heart Study. *Circulation* **96**:44–49.
18. Kannel WB, Skinner JJ Jr, Schwartz MJ, *et al.* (1970) Intermittent claudication: incidence in the Framingham Study. *Circulation* **41**:875–883.
19. Ness J, Aronow WS (1999) Prevalence of coexistence of coronary artery disease, ischemic stroke, and peripheral arterial disease in older persons, mean age 80 years, in an academic hospital-based geriatrics practice. *J Am Geriatr Soc* **47**:1255–1256.
20. Rodda R (1953) Arteriosclerosis of the lower limbs. *J Pathol Bacteriol* **65**:315–332.
21. Davies MJ (1996) Stability and instability: two faces of coronary atherosclerosis. *Circulation* **94**:2013–2020.
22. Libby P (1995) Molecular bases of the acute coronary syndromes. *Circulation* **91**:2844–2850.
23. Glagov S, Weisenberg E, Zarins C, *et al.* (1987) Compensatory enlargement of human atherosclerotic coronary arteries. *N Engl J Med* **316**:1371–1375.
24. Kinmonth JB, Rob CG, Simeone FA (1962) Vascular surgery. Edward Arnold London.
25. Leriche R & Morel A (1948) The Syndrome of thrombotic obliteration of the aortic bifurcation. *Ann Surg* **127**:193–206.
26. Pearce WH, Slaughter MS, LeMaire S, *et al.* (1993) Aortic diameter as a function of age, gender, and body surface area. Surgery **114**:691–697.

27. Sandgren T, Sonesson B, Ahlgren AR, *et al.* (1998) Factors predicting the diameter of the popliteal artery in healthy humans. *J Vasc Surg* **28**:284–289.

28. Sonesson B, Lanne T, Hansen F, *et al.* (1994) Infrarenal aortic diameter in the healthy person. *Eur J Vasc Surg* **8**:89–95.

29. Cattell MA, Anderson JC, & Haselton PS (1996) Age-related changes in amounts and concentrations of collagen and elastin in normotensive human thoracic aorta. *Clin Chim Acta* **245**:73–84.

30. Zeiser R, Albrecht-Bellingrath W, & Schaefer HE (2000) Age-dependent leiomuscular atrophy in vertebral arteries of individuals under low fat diet. *In Vivo* **14**:631–634.

31. Nachbur BH, Inderbitzi RG, & Bar W (1991) Isolated iliac aneurysms. *Eur J Vasc Surg* **5**:375–381.

32. McCready RA, Pailolero PC, Gilmore JC, *et al.* (1983) Isolated iliac artery aneurysms. *Surgery* **93**:688–693.

33. Sacks NPM, Huddy SPJ, Wegner T, *et al.* (1992) Management of solitary iliac aneurysms. *J Cardiovasc Surg* **33**:679–683.

34. Richardson JW & Greenfield LJ (1988) Natural history and management of iliac aneurysms. *J Vasc Surg* **8**:165–171.

35. Krupski WC, Selzman CH, Floridia R, *et al.* (1998) Contemporary management of isolated iliac aneurysms. *J Vasc Surg* **28**:1–11.

36. Kasirajan V, Hertzer NR, Beven EG, *et al.* (1998) Management of isolated common iliac artery aneurysms. *Cardiovasc Surg* **6**:171–177.

37. Graham LM, Zelenock GB, Whitehouse WM Jr, *et al.* (1980) Clinical significance of arteriosclerotic femoral artery aneurysms. *Arch Surg* **115**:502–507.

38. Cutler BS & Darling RC (1973) Surgical management of arteriosclerotic femoral aneurysms. *Surgery* **74**:764–773.

39. Roseman JM & Wyche D (1987) True aneurysm of the profunda femoris artery. Literature review, differential diagnosis, management. *J Cardiovasc Surg* **28**:701–705.

40. Levi N & Schroeder TV (1997) Blood transfusion requirement in surgery for femoral artery aneurysms. *J Cardiovasc Surg* **38**:661–663.

41. Levi N & Schroeder TV (1997) Arteriosclerotic femoral artery aneurysms: a short review. *J Cardiovasc Surg* **38**:335–338.

42. Duffy ST, Colgan MP, Sultan S, *et al.* (1998) Popliteal aneurysms: a 10-year experience. *Eur J Vasc Endovasc Surg* **16**:218–222.

43. Taurino M, Calisti A, Grossi R, *et al.* (1998) Outcome after early treatment of popliteal artery aneurysms. *Int Angiol* **17**:28–33.

44. Lowell RC, Gloviczki P, Hallett JW Jr, *et al.* Popliteal artery aneurysms: the risk of nonoperative management. *Ann Vasc Surg* **8**:14–23.

45. Schroder A, Gohlke J, Gross-Fengels W, *et al.* (1996) Popliteal aneurysms-surgical management versus conservative procedure. *Langenbecks Arch Chir Suppl Kongressbd* **113**:857–863.

46. Gifford RW Jr, Hines EA Jr, & Janes JM (1953) An analysis and follow-up study of one hundred popliteal aneurysms. *Surgery* **33**:284–293.

47. Dawson I, Sie RB, & van Bockel JH (1997) Atherosclerotic popliteal aneurysm. *Br J Surg* **84**:293–299.

48. MacSweeney ST, Powell JT, & Greenhalgh RM (1994) Pathogenesis of abdominal aortic aneurysm. *Br J Surg* **81**:935–941.

49. McMillan WD, Patterson BK, Keen RR, *et al.* (1995) In situ localization and quantification of mRNA for 92-kD type IV collagenase and its inhibitor in aneurysmal, occlusive, and normal aorta. *Arterioscler Thromb Vasc Biol* **15**:1139–1144.

50. Newman KM, Ogata Y, Malon AM, *et al.* (1994) Identification of matrix metalloproteinases 3 (stromelysin-1) and 9 (gelatinase B) in abdominal aortic aneurysm. *Arterioscler Thromb* **14**:1315–1320.

51. Thompson RW, Holmes DR, Mertens RA, *et al.* (1995) Production and localization of 92-kilodalton gelatinase in abdominal aortic aneurysms: an elastolytic metalloproteinase expressed by aneurysm-infiltrating macrophages. *J Clin Invest* **96**:318–326.

52. Brophy CM, Sumpio B, Reilly JM, & Tilson MD (1991) Decreased tissue inhibitor of metalloproteinases (TIMP) in abdominal aortic aneurysm tissue: a preliminary report. *J Surg Res* **50**:653–657.

53. Davies MJ (1998) Aortic aneurysm formation. Lessons from human studies and experimental models. *Circulation* **98**:193–195.

54. Erdheim J (1929) Medionecrosis aortae idiopathica. *Virchows Arch Pathol Anat* **273**:454–479.

55. Schlatmann TJM & Becker AE (1977) Histologic changes in the normal aging aorta: implications for dissecting aortic aneurysm. *Am J Cardiol* **39**:13–20.

56. Schlatmann TJM & Becker AE (1977) Pathogenesis of dissecting aneurysm of aorta: comparative histopathologic study of significance of medial changes. *Am J Cardiol* **39**:21–26.

57. Dietz H, Cutting G, Pyeritz R, *et al.* (1991) Marfan syndrome caused by a recurrent de novo missense mutation in the fibrillin gene. *Nature* **24**:337–339.

58. Davies MJ, Trasure T, & Richardson PD (1996) The pathogenesis of spontaneous arterial dissection. *Heart* **75**:434–435.

59. Tromp G, Wu Y, Prockop DJ, & Swarna L (1993) Sequencing of cDNA from 50 unrelated patients reveals that mutations in the triple-helical domain of type III procollagen are an infrequent cause of aortic aneurysm. *J Clin Invest* **91**:2539–2545.

60. Tetteroo E, van der Graaf Y, Bosch JL, *et al.* (1998) Randomised comparison of primary stent placement versus primary angioplasty followed by selective stent placement in patients with iliac artery occlusive disease. *Lancet* **351**:1153–1 159.

61. Waller BF (1991) Pathology of new interventional procedures. In: Silver (ed.): *Cardiovascular Pathology*, New York: Churchill Livingstone, p. 1683.

62. Gallino A, Mahler F, Probst P, & Nachbur B (1984) Percutaneous transluminal angioplasty of the arteries of the lower limbs: a five year follow-up. *Circulation* **70**:619–623.

63. Johnston KW, Rae M, Hogg-Johnston SA, *et al.* (1987) 5-year results of a prospective study of percutaneous transluminal angioplasty. *Ann Surg* **206**:403–413.

64. Lofberg AM, Karacagil S, Ljungman C, *et al.* (2001) Percutaneous transluminal angioplasty of the femoropopliteal arteries in limbs with chronic critical lower limb ischemia. *J Vasc Surg* **34**:114–121.

65. Jamsen T, Manninen H, Tulla H, *et al.* (2002) The final outcome of primary infrainguinal percutaneous transluminal angioplasty in 100 consecutive patients with chronic critical limb ischemia. *J Vasc Interv Radiol* **13**:455–463.

66. Powell RJ, Fillinger M, Walsh DB, *et al.* (2002) Predicting outcome of angioplasty and selective stenting of multisegment iliac artery occlusive disease. *J Vasc Surg* **32**:564–569.

67. Laborde JC, Palmaz JC, Rivera FJ, *et al.* (1995) Influence of anatomic distribution of atherosclerosis on the outcome of revascularization with iliac stent placement. *J Vasc Interv Radiol* **6**:513–521.

68. Capek P, McLean GK, & Berkowitz HD (1991) Femoropopliteal angioplasty: factors influencing long-term success. *Circulation* **83**(2 Suppl.):I70–80.

69. Stokes KR, Strunk HM, Campbell DR, *et al.* (1990) Five-year results of iliac and femoropopliteal angioplasty in diabetic patients. *Radiology* **174**:977–982.

70. Johnston KW (1993) Iliac arteries: reanalysis of results of balloon angioplasty. *Radiology* **186**:207–212.

71. Clark TW, Groffsky JL, & Soulen MC (2001) Predictors of long-term patency after femoropopliteal angioplasty: results from the STAR registry. *J Vasc Interv Radiol* **12**:923–933.

72. Beck AH, Muhe A, Ostheim W, *et al.* (1989) Long-term results of percutaneous transluminal angioplasty: a study of 4750 dilatations and local lyses. *Eur J Vasc Surg* **3**:245–252.

73. Palmaz JC, Laborde JC, Rivera FJ, *et al.* (1992) Stenting of the iliac arteries with the Palmaz stent: experience from a multicenter trial. *Cardiovasc Intervent Radiol* **15**:291–297.

74. Soder HK, Manninen HI, Jaakkola P, *et al.* (2000) Prospective trial of infrapopliteal artery balloon angioplasty for critical limb ischemia: angiographic and clinical results. *J Vasc Interv Radiol* **11**:102–131.

75. Sapoval MR, Chatellier G, Long AL, *et al.* (1996) Self-expandable stents for the treatment of iliac artery obstructive lesions: long-term success and prognostic factors. *AJR Am J Roentgenol* **166**:1173–1179.

76. Bakal CW, Sprayregen S, Scheinbaum K, *et al.* (1990) Percutaneous transluminal angioplasty of the infrapopliteal arteries: results in 53 patients. *AJR Am J Roentgenol* **154**:171–174.

77. Brown KT, Moore ED, Getrajdman GI, *et al.* (1993) Infrapopliteal angioplasty: long-term follow-up. *J Vasc Interv Radiol* **4**:139–144.

78. Bull PG, Mendel H, Hold M, *et al.* (1992) Distal popliteal and tibioperoneal transluminal angioplasty: long-term follow-up. *J Vasc Interv Radiol* **3**:45–53.

79. Kearney M, Pieczek A, Haley L, *et al.* (1997) Histopathology of In-Stent restenosis in patients with peripheral artery disease. *Circulation* **95**:1998–2002.

80. Fischman DL, Leon MB, Baim DS, *et al.* (1994) A randomized comparison of coronary-stent-placement and balloon angioplasty in the treatment of coronary artery disease. *N Engl J Med* **331**:496–501.

81. Serruys PW, DeJaegere P, Kiemeneij F, *et al.* (1994) A comparison of balloon-expandable-stent implantation with balloon angioplasty with coronary artery disease. *N Engl J Med* **331**:489–495.

82. Topol E (1994) Caveats about elective coronary stenting (editorial). *N Engl J Med* **331**:539.

83. Richter GM, Roeren T, Noeldge G, *et al.* (1992) Initial long-term results of a randomized 5-year study: iliac stent implantation versus PTA. *Vasa Suppl* **35**:192–193.

84. Farb A, Sangiorgi G, Carter AJ, *et al.* (1999) Pathology of acute and chronic coronary stenting in humans. *Circulation* **99**:44–52.

85. Grewe PH, Deneke T, Machraoui A, *et al.* (2000) Acute and chronic tissue response to coronary stent implantation: pathologic findings in human specimens. *J Am Coll Cardiol* **35**:157–163.

63 Interventional Treatment of Iliac and Lower Artery Disease

Dierk Scheinert & Andrej Schmidt

Parkhospital Leipzig, Medical Clinic I, Angiology, Cardiology and Heart Center Leipzig, Department of Angiology, Leipzig, Germany

Introduction

Peripheral arterial occlusive disease (PAOD) is one of the most frequent manifestations of atherosclerosis, which particularly effect patients of older age. Clinically, patients present with either intermittent claudicatio or, in a lower percentage, with critical limb ischemia due to significant reduction of arterial perfusion. In more then 90%, the lower extremity is affected. Although multilevel disease is frequent, particularly in patients with advanced disease stages, typical locations for PAOD lesions are the iliac arteries, the femoro-popliteal arteries, and the below-the-knee vessel. Although revascularization has traditionally been achieved by surgery, in recent years interventional techniques underwent a dramatic improvement, thus offering a valid treatment alternative for many patients.

Recanalization of pelvic arteries

Clinical manifestation and noninvasive workup

About one-third of the obstructive lesions in PAOD affect the aortoiliac segment. Lifestyle limiting claudicatio is the leading symptom of patients with pelvic obstructions. Whereas patients with femoral obstructions almost uniformly present with pain in the calf during exercise, the complaints of patients with aortoiliac disease may be more unspecific, with pain in the thigh or even in the back and the hips besides claudicatio of the calf. Furthermore, obstructions involving the internal iliac artery may cause claudicatio of hips and buttocks. Even though these complaints typically occur during exercise, they are frequently misdiagnosed as orthopedic or ischiadic problems.

Moreover, standard diagnostic methods, such as ankle brachial index recordings or duplex ultrasound investigations, may not be fully conclusive owing to difficulties in directly visualizing the iliac vessels and the presence of collaterals. Noninvasive imaging modalities, such as computed tomography (CT) angiography or magnetic resonance (MR) angiography are best suited to provide a reliable diagnosis.

Treatment strategies

Iliac artery obstructions have traditionally been treated by open surgery, e.g., aortofemoral or aorto-bifemoral bypass grafting. According to patency rates of 85–89% after 5 years, and 70–74% after 15 years, this treatment is highly effective. However, surgical interventions are associated with a substantial procedure-related risk for the patient, leading to aggregated mortality rates of up to 8% [1].

Percutaneous transluminal angioplasty (PTA) is a less invasive treatment alternative, and in the last years it has proven to be an effective technique for the treatment of focal iliac artery stenosis [2,3]. The reported procedural technical success rate was 85–99% (average 95%). Adjunctive stent implantation has even increased the primary success rates to 97–100% (average 99%). The patency rates of 80% to 90% after 5 years for short iliac stenoses are similar to surgical results. Furthermore, PTA is associated with a much lower complication rate, with a mortality rate of 0.2% [4–6].

The recommendations of the TransAtlantic InterSociety Consensus (TASC) attempted to define a treatment of choice, depending on the morphologic stratification of iliac lesions. Thus, interventional treatment is generally considered for focal stenoses and short occlusions (type A and B lesion). For diffuse, extensive, complex multilevel, multifocal or longer totally occluded segments of the iliac arteries (type C and D lesion) surgery is still recommended as the procedure of choice [7].

The TASC document may be a good guideline for an institution with a low volume of interventions or during the initial phase of starting the peripheral program. Completed in the middle of 1999 (TASC I), the consensus process represented the most up-to-date view at that time. However, with new endovascular devices, for experienced and well-skilled interventionalists today, the length and morphology of iliac lesions has less influence on technical success and long-term results, which

Cardiovascular Interventions in Clinical Practice. Edited by Jürgen Haase, Hans-Joachim Schäfers, Horst Sievert and Ron Waksman. © 2010 Blackwell Publishing.

Table 63.1 TASC II recommendations for the treatment of iliac obstructions (modified from reference 8).

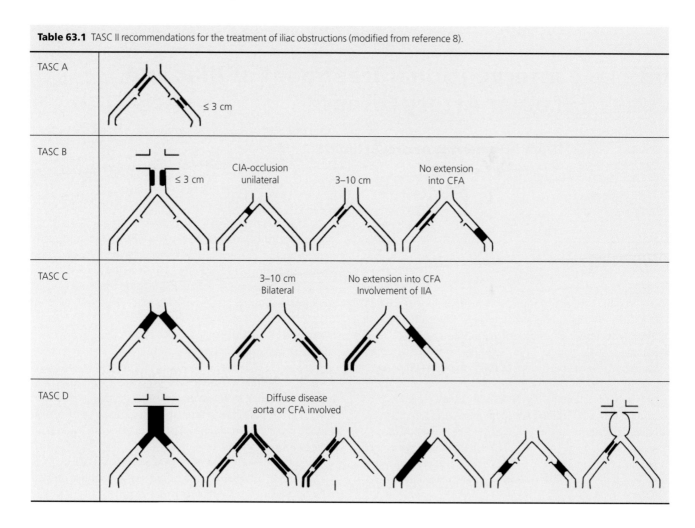

is at least partially reflected by the revised version of the TASC recommendations (TASC II), published in 2007 (Table 63.1) [8].

Interventional techniques

Angiography

Once the indication for an interventional therapy is given, intraarterial angiography will clarify the morphologic situation during the therapeutic session. Depending on the anatomical location of the lesion and the tortuosity of the iliac arteries, a single posterior–anterior projection may be insufficient. Additional lateral views may be helpful for optimal imaging of specific arterial segments (30–45° contralateral angulation for imaging of the bifurcation of the iliac artery; 30–45° ipsilateral angulation for visualization of the external iliac artery and the femoral bifurcation).

Approach to the lesion

Retrograde access

In most cases, iliac artery stenoses can be treated using the ipsilateral retrograde access. The initial passage of the stenosis

can be performed using a standard 0.018-inch or a hydrophilic 0.035-inch angled tipped guidewire. For PTA of the stenosis, the dimensions of the balloon should be chosen according to the length of the lesion and by comparison with the proximal and distal reference diameter (mostly 7–10 mm for the common iliac artery and 6–8 mm for the external iliac artery). If primary stent implantation is considered, predilation of the stenosis should be performed with an undersized balloon and low dilation pressure.

Balloon-expandable stents should be chosen for implantation in short lesions of the common iliac artery; these allow precise placement and have the potential for further expansion with larger balloons if necessary. Self-expanding stents may be considered for long, less calcified, nonostial lesions in the external iliac artery.

Antegrade iliac approach in cross-over technique

In total occlusions, an antegrade recanalization is recommended. Especially in occlusions of the common iliac artery, retrograde recanalization can lead to a dissection of the distal abdominal aorta, making stent implantation far above the aortic bifurcation necessary. Using a cross-over approach, this scenario

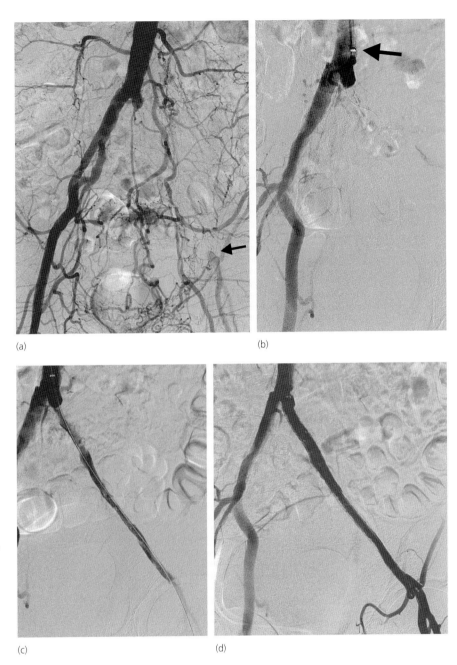

Figure 63.1 (a) Chronic total occlusion of the left common and external iliac artery (TASC D lesion). Refilling of the common femoral artery (black arrow). (b) Positioning of a 6F 90 cm sheath (Cook) via a left brachial access. Black arrow indicates the tip of the sheath at the aortic bifurcation. (c) After predilation with a 5-mm balloon. (d) Final result after stenting.

can be avoided. After retrograde puncture of the contralateral common femoral artery, a suitably shaped 5F guiding catheter (Hook, Merit Medical Systems Inc., South Jordan, USA, or Sheperd-Hook, Cordis Corporation, Miami Lakes, FL, USA) is positioned at the aortic bifurcation. The occlusion is initially passed with a stiff 0.035-inch hydrophilic guidewire, which is finally placed into the ipsilateral common femoral artery. Using this wire as a marker, the artery is punctured and a second 8F sheath is inserted. An angled shaped wire loop, introduced through the ipsilateral sheath is used for snaring and retrieving the hydrophilic wire out of the 8F sheath. After this step, the wire in cross-over position is exchanged for an ipsilateral guidewire and the dilation and stenting process is performed in a retrograde fashion.

Transbrachial approach

In some cases of chronic total occlusions of the common iliac artery, the cross-over-approach may not offer enough support for a successful recanalization. In these cases, or in bilateral iliac obstructions, the transbrachial access is an important alternative. The left brachial approach should be preferred whenever possible to avoid passage of the aortic arch with subsequent risk of cranial embolization. By advancing a 90-cm-long shuttle introducer to the aortic bifurcation, the

Table 63.2 Interventional therapy of obstructions of the aortic bifurcation with the "kissing stent" technique: technical success, complications and follow-up.

Author	n	Technical success	Complications[a]	Primary patency (%)[b]	Follow-up (months)
Scheinert et al. [10]	48	48 (100%)	0	86.8	24
Haulon et al. [11]	106	106 (100%)	0	81.1	24
				79.4	36
Mouanoutoua et al. [12]	50	50 (100%)	2 (4%)[c]	92	20

[a]Embolization, dissection, vessel rupture, death.
[b]Cumulative patency rates (Kaplan–Meier life table method).
[c]Distal embolization after recanalization of acute thrombotic occlusion.

iliac arteries are directly accessible (Fig. 63.1). In general, this approach provides the straightest access to the iliac occlusion, resulting in the highest recanalization rates.

Periprocedural treatment

During intervention, 5000 units of heparin is the standard dose. Acetylsalicylic acid (ASA) 100 mg per day for all patients and, in case of stenting, Clopidogrel 75 mg daily for 4 weeks may be given additionally.

Summary of outcome results

Iliac artery stenoses

Technical success rates of >95% and 5-year patency rates of 80–90% have been reported for balloon-angioplasty of short segment stenosis of iliac arteries. Whether iliac stenoses should undergo direct-stent implantation has been addressed in the Dutch Iliac Stent Trial [9]. Two hundred and seventy-nine patients with short iliac artery stenoses were randomly assigned to direct stent placement or primary angioplasty, with subsequent stent placement in case of a residual mean pressure gradient >10 mmHg across the treated site (stent frequency in this group, 43%). As there were no substantial differences in technical results and clinical outcomes of the two treatment strategies at short-term and long-term follow-up, provisional stenting in case of an insufficient angioplasty result can be considered as state-of-the-art treatment of focal iliac artery stenoses.

Iliac artery occlusions

Stent-supported reconstruction of the aortoiliac bifurcation
According to the TASC recommendations, complex iliac artery obstructions, particularly bilateral stenoses or total occlusions, are usually treated with aortofemoral or aortobifemoral graft surgery. Although highly effective, these surgical interventions are associated with a substantial procedure-related risk. Further development of percutaneous techniques, particularly the introduction of the "kissing stent" procedure, minimized

PTA-related complications. This technique minimizes the risk of contralateral embolism or contralateral iliac artery occlusion due to dislodgement of atherosclerotic or thrombotic material during unilateral PTA. In a series of 48 patients with obstructions of the aortoiliac segments who underwent kissing stent implantation, primary technical success was 100%. A clinical improvement of +2 to +3 Rutherford category was observed in 41 and 7 patients, respectively. The primary angiographic patency rate at 2 years was 87%. In three cases, significant restenoses were detected, which could be successfully treated by PTA. No relevant complications, particularly no embolic events or thrombotic occlusions, occurred in this series [10]. Two recently published studies, with a technical success rate of 100% (106 patients in one study and 50 patients in the other), confirmed these results (Table 63.2). In addition, the rates of restenosis and reocclusion are comparably low in both studies [11,12].

Recanalization of chronic iliac artery occlusions
Long-term patency after 3 years for PTA of complete iliac occlusions is reported to be 20% lower than with iliac stenoses [13,14]. However, using an appropriate approach, such as the cross-over or transbrachial technique, and new stent devices, long-term results might be more favorable (Table 63.3). In a study with 212 patients with unilateral chronic iliac artery occlusions, a recanalization by Excimer laser assisted angioplasty and primary stent implantation was performed [15]. A technical success could be achieved in 190 of the 212 patients (89.6%), and was associated with a marked clinical improvement of +3 or +2 grades according to the AHA guidelines in 112 (52.8%) and 67 cases (31.6%), respectively. The major complication rate in this series was 1.4%. Primary patency rates of 81.2% at two and 75.7% at four years demonstrate that this technique is a safe and effective treatment for patients with chronic iliac artery occlusions.

More recently, the transbrachial approach, which has been described above, has been implemented as a standard approach for most iliac recanalization procedures. The initial data of 45 patients, in which this approach has been used as a

Table 63.3 Stent-supported interventional therapy of iliac artery occlusions: technical success, complications and follow-up.

Author	n	Technical success	Complications[a]	Primary patency (%)[b]	Follow-up (months)
Scheinert et al. [15]	212	190 (90%)	3 (1%)	78	36
Vorwerk et al. [16]	103	82 (80%)	11 (11%)	81	36
Reyes et al. [17]	59	54 (92%)	5 (8%)	73	24

[a]Embolization, dissection, vessel rupture, death.
[b]Cumulative patency rates (Kaplan–Meier life table method).

Table 63.4 Summary of the results for transbrachial recanalization of chronic total iliac artery occlusions.

Pre- and peri-interventional data
n = 45 (primary brachial approach n = 32; secondary approach after failed femoral access n = 13)
Unilateral occlusion n = 36; unilateral occlusion + contralateral stenosis n = 5
Bilateral occlusion n = 4
Median occlusion length, 10.2 cm; number of implanted stents, 74
Primary technical success, 98% (n = 44)

Results
[a]Clinical improvement: +3 grades in 41% (n = 18) and +2 grades in 50% (n = 22)
Mean clinical follow-up of 17 months
[b]Primary patency: 97% at 9 months and 92% at 12 months
[b]Secondary patency: 100% at 12 months and 88% at 24 months

[a]Rutherford classification.
[b]Cumulative patency rates (Kaplan-Meier life table method).

primary technique (32 patients) and as a salvage technique after a failed standard recanalization attempt (13 patients), demonstrate a high technical success rate of 98%. The details of these procedures are outlined in Table 63.4.

Recanalization of the femoropopliteal tract

Introduction

More than 50% of all PAOD-lesions are localized in the femoropopliteal tract. Endovascular therapy is often challenging owing to the predominance of occlusions over stenoses (which are often extensive and typically reaching from the femoral bifurcation down to the adductors channel), the severe calcification often encountered in this arterial segment, and finally the relatively high restenosis-rate after angioplasty. Conservative treatment with walking exercise and medical therapy is often unsatisfactory and the interventional treatment-option, which is clearly less invasive than surgery, therefore highly attractive.

Indications for treatment

The recent improvements in terms of technical success and patency rate after an endovascular treatment have shifted the therapeutic approach from surgery to angioplasty as reflected in the TASC recommendations [7,8] (Table 63.5).

The decision for one of the treatment options, medical, endovascular, or surgical, should not only depend on the morphology of the obstruction, but clearly also on the clinical situation of the limb and the general patient condition. Conservative treatment would be the preferred option for patients with intermittent claudicatio with a walking capacity acceptable for the patient, even if the lesion is short and "easy-to-treat." On the other hand, endovascular treatment might be preferable over surgery also in a long occlusion (TASC D lesion) in a patient with critical limb ischemia, if surgery is risky owing to the patients condition. Finally, the TASC recommendations cannot apply for every center in the same way, because experience and availability of the treatment options are different.

Pre-interventional workup

Pre-interventional diagnostic workup should include duplex ultrasound. Owing to the superficial course of the artery, it is easily visible by sonography and several trials have demonstrated a good correlation between duplex ultrasound and digital subtraction angiography or MR [18]. CT or MR angiography play an ancillary role for planning the intervention, e.g., to rule out additional lesions in different arterial segments. Measurements of the ankle-Brachial Index (ABI) are mandatory before and after recanalization to verify the interventional success.

Digital subtraction angiography should only be performed if an endovascular treatment is intended in the same setting. In this regard, the contralateral access and cross-over-approach is of advantage because a complete angiography of the abdominal aorta down to the foot arteries on both sides can precede the treatment of the target lesion.

Techniques for femoropopliteal angioplasty

Approach to the lesion

The most frequent approaches to the femoropopliteal lesion are a retrograde contralateral puncture and a cross-over approach

Table 63.5 Shift of recommendations for treatment of fermoropopliteal lesions from TASC I (2000) to TASC II (2007).

or the ipsilateral antegrade approach. The contralateral access is of advantage if the lesion involves the proximal superficial femoral artery (SFA), if an antegrade puncture is difficult as in obese patients, or to avoid reduction of the inflow to the lesion by compression of the artery for hemostasis after the intervention. Antegrade ipsilateral access might be more easily performed in the case of significantly kinked and calcified iliac arteries and a steep aortic bifurcation. A transpopliteal approach is reserved for situations when an antegrade recanalization fails and a second retrograde attempt seems promising. A brachial approach is also possible if a femoral puncture is contraindicated, as for example after aortobifemoral or bilateral femoropopliteal bypass surgery. Anticoagulation during the intervention usually consists of the administration of 5000 IU heparin. If thrombotic material is visualized during the procedure, the additional administration of 5000 IU of heparin or glycoprotein (GP) IIb/IIIa inhibitors [19] should be considered.

Primary lesion crossing

In the case of stenosis, the passage of the lesion is fairly simple and is normally performed using a 0.018-inch or 0.035-inch guidewire. For recanalization of total occlusions, the guidewire can either be passed intraluminally through the occluded artery or via the subintimal space [20], which is also called the "percutaneous intended subintimal recanalization" (PIER) technique. The guidewire, a hydrophilic

coated 0.035-inch wire, is directed subintimally at the very beginning of the occlusion by using an angulated support catheter, such as a Judkins right, an internal mammarian artery (IMA), or a vertebral catheter. Which technique is more successful in terms of primary success or patency has never been proven. However, often, especially in highly calcified occlusions, there is no other option than to pass the guidewire within the subintimal space through the occlusion (Fig. 63.2a). Other devices to pass CTOs (chronic total occlusions) are the excimer laser (Spectranetics, Colorado Springs, CO, USA) or the Frontrunner (Cordis Corporation, Miami Lakes, FL, USA), a catheter with a jaw-like blunt tip to create a channel before further endovascular treatment.

Re-entry from the subintimal space into the true lumen distal to the occlusion can be problematic. Dedicated re-entry catheters such as the Outback (Cordis) (Fig. 63.2b) or Pioneer catheter (Medtronic, Minneapolis, MN, USA) are very successful in this regard [21,22]. These catheters harbor a bent needle, which can be directed from the subintimal space through the dissection membrane back in to the true lumen. Recanalization success, using these devices, is >95% [22] (Fig. 63.2c and d).

Angioplasty process

After wire passage, balloon angioplasty is the standard technique. Alternative balloon technologies are the cutting balloon, the cryoplasty catheter, which cools down the arterial wall to −10° Celsius by using liquid nitrous oxide for inflation of the

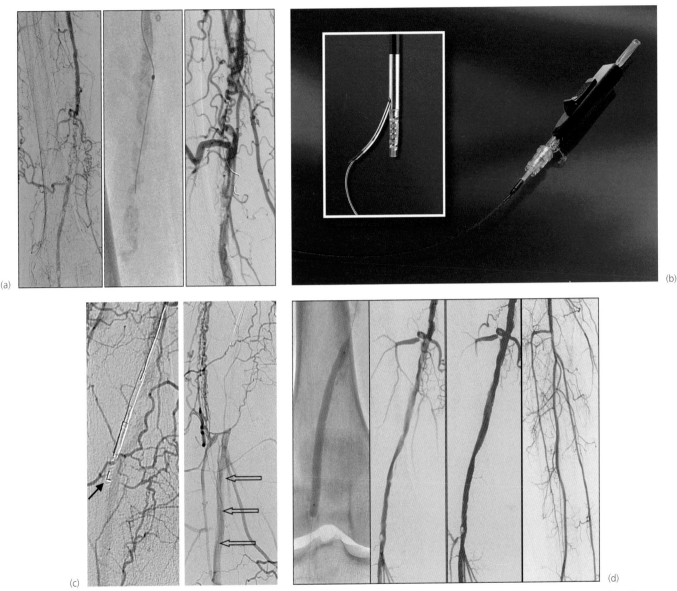

(a)

(b)

(c)

(d)

Figure 63.2 (a) Chronic total occlusion of the right distal SFA. Owing to severe calcification, guidewire passage is possible only in the subintimal space. (b) Outback catheter with bent needle to redirect the guidewire from the subintimal space back into the patent artery distal to the occlusion. (c) Outback catheter in position, black arrow indicates the L-marker of the tip to direct the needle. Open arrows: successful deployment of the guidewire into the patent distal artery. (d) Final result after ballooning and stenting.

balloon or the AngioSculpt (AngioScore, Fremont, CA, USA), a semicompliant balloon with an external nitinol shape-memory helical scoring edge [23] (Fig. 63.3), which is currently under investigation (see also chapter 35). Recently, there has been an increasing interest in another alternative to balloon angioplasty: catheter-based atherectomy. The excimer laser, which has recently undergone several changes and improvements (turbo-laser emitting higher energy, and Booster laser to ablate a larger area), the SilverHawk (ev3 Endovascular, Inc., Plymouth, MN, USA), a rotating blade to "shave" off the obstructing material and two newer rotational atherectomy-devices (Pathway [Pathway Medical Technologies Inc.,

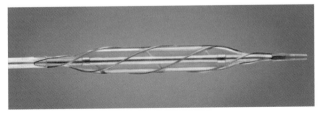

Figure 63.3 The AngioSculpt scoring balloon (AngioScore).

Kirkland, WA, USA], CSI-orbital atherectomy system [Cardiovascular Systems Inc., St. Paul, MN, USA]) are available.

Up-to-date data supporting a superiority of these alternative techniques over balloon angioplasty are lacking. Therefore, the use is restricted to lesions adjusted to the specific features of the devices, such as using a cutting balloon for lesions resistive to plain old balloon (POB) angioplasty or atherectomy for lesions for which stenting should be avoided (e.g. the popliteal artery).

Stenting of the femoropopliteal tract

Self-expanding nitinol stents are standard. A large variety of different designs is available today, with differences in radial force, flexibility, and potentially also patency rate. More flexible stents, for example with a helical design (Everfelx [ev3, Plymouth, MN, USA] or LifeStent [Bard, Murray Hill, NJ, USA]) are preferred in the popliteal region. Enhanced flexibility might be linked to lower radial force, and, after implantation of standard nitinol stents in highly calcified lesions, recoil is not infrequent. An additional implantation of a short balloon-expandable stent or nitinol stents with enhanced radial force, like the SUPERA™ stent (IDEV Technologies Inc., Webster, TX, USA) might be a solution. The latter stent with its woven construction has a fundamentally different design to the standard nitinol stents, which have a segmental design, resulting in a significantly increased radial force.

Stenting can be performed as full lesion coverage or spot stenting. In the case of intentional subintimal recanalization, stenting of the proximal "entrance" to the subintimal channel and distal re-entry into the true lumen might preserve the flexibility of the artery; however, whether the patency-rate is superior to long-segment stenting is not proven. In fact, if the artery re-occludes, entry into the occluded distal stent can be extremely difficult, and failure to re-open the artery is not infrequent.

Surveillance after superficial femoral artery angioplasty

Acute reocclusion of the superficial femoral artery (SFA) after recanalization is rare. A postinterventional anticoagulation regime including acetylsalicylic acid (ASA; 100 mg per day) after balloon angioplasty and additionally clopidogrel (75 mg per day) for 30 days after stenting is sufficient.

Late restenosis or reocclusion by intimal hyperplasia or progressive arteriosclerosis remains a relevant problem in this arterial segment. In contrast to other regions, restenosis can also emerge, even after years. Therefore, follow-up examinations are important and re-intervention should be performed, even in cases of an asymptomatic restenosis, to avoid progression to complete occlusion. Duplex-sonography is the method of choice.

Treatment of in-stent restenosis

Treatment of in-stent restenosis is technically easy to perform with balloon angioplasty; however, secondary restenosis is frequent. Solutions could be atherectomy, e.g., with the excimer laser with or without additional implantation of covered stents. These concepts are currently under investigation using the Booster laser (Spectranetics) and the Viabahn stent graft (Gore Inc., Flagstaff, AZ, USA). Another option might be the implantation of a drug-eluting stent after balloon angioplasty of the in-stent restenosis, as performed in a registry using a Paclitaxel eluting nitinol stent (Zilver-PTX, Cook Medical Inc., Bloomington, IN, USA). The results are pending.

Brachytherapy might be a solution. The need for a special radiation oncology-type room for the procedure, because of the use of gamma radiation, is a limitation and makes other techniques for treatment of restenosis more attractive.

Technical success and patency rates

The technical success rate, in terms of possibility to pass the occlusion and using available tools such as re-entry devices (Pioneer catheter, Outback catheter), is very high and up to 100% [21,22]. The ability to dilate the lesion with a maximally 30% residual stenosis might be lower, as highly calcified lesions have a tendency to recoil.

The restenosis rate after balloon angioplasty of the femoropopliteal tract is relatively high and inversely correlated to the length of the lesion (Table 63.6). At least for longer lesions, the systematic implantation of nitinol stents seems to improve the patency rate [24,25]. A superiority of one stent design over another has not yet been shown. Stents with a relatively high stiffness seem to show a higher frequency of stent fractures [26] than with more flexible stents [24]. Whether the use of other interventional tools and concepts, such as atherectomy devices (Excimer-laser, SilverHawk, ev3, Plymouth, MN, USA), alternative balloon techniques (cryotherapy, cutting balloon, scoring balloon), or the implantation of covered stents (Viabahn, GORE), are superior has not been proven. First results using a drug-eluting balloon are promising [27].

Stent fracture

The Sirocco I trial [34], a randomized comparison of drug-eluting versus bare stents in SFA lesions, revealed that fracture can occur to self-expanding nitinol stents in this arterial segment. Triggered by this observation, we investigated the occurrence and clinical impact of stent fractures in a cohort of 93 patients, with 121 legs treated with the implantation of different designs of self-expanding nitinol stents. Systematic X-ray screening was performed 10.7 months (mean) after implantation. The mean length of the stented segment was 15.7 cm. Stent fractures were detected in 37.2% of the treated legs. Fractures could be classified as: minor, a single strut fracture (48.4% of the cases); moderate, with a fracture of > 1 strut (26.6% of the cases); and severe, with complete separation of the segments (in 25.0% of the cases). The rate of stent fracture was dependent on the length of the stented vessel and was highest in lesions > 16 cm. The primary patency rate at 12 months was significantly lower for patients with stent fractures (41.1% vs. 84.3%, $P < 0.0001$) [26]. Other authors

Table 63.6 Patency rate after femoropopliteal recanalization.

Author	No. of patients	Lesion length (mm)	Treatment	Patency rate and follow-up period
Krankenberg 2007 [28]	121	45	Balloon angioplasty	61% (12 months)
Capek 1991 [29]	217	>100	Balloon	<30% (12 months)
Scheinert 2001 [30]	318	194	Excimer laser + balloon	34% (12 months)
Amighi 2008 [31]	21	20	Cutting balloon	38% (6 months)
Zeller et al. 2006 [32]	45	43	SilverHawk	84% (12 months)
Krankenberg 2007 [28]	123	45	Nitinol stent (Luminexx)	68% (12 months)
Gray 1997 [33]	55	165	Wallstent	22% (12 months)
Schillinger 2007 [25]	63	138	Nitinol stent (Dynalink/Absolute)	69% (24 months)
Duda 2006 [34]	47	83	Sirolimus-eluting nitinol stent (Smart)	77% (24 months)
Saxon 2008 [35]	97	Up to 130	Viabahn endoprosthesis	65% (12 months)
Tepe 2008 [27]	41	75	PTX-eluting balloon	83% (6 months)

confirmed these findings; however, significantly lower fracture rates using different stent designs were reported [24,25]. Published fracture rates and the impact on the patency for different stent designs are difficult to interpret, owing to differences in lesion characteristics, and need to be clarified in further trials.

Infrapopliteal angioplasty

Introduction

Angioplasty of infrapopliteal arteries was, for a long time, considered to be ineffective and hazardous. Recently, however, it has emerged as a very promising treatment option. The increasing prevalence of diabetes mellitus, frequently associated with tibioperoneal obstructive disease, improved diagnostic methods for evaluation of these small arteries and recent advances in catheter technology for infrapopliteal arteries have increased the demand and acceptance of endovascular therapy in this arterial segment. Excellent technical success rates above 90%, a low frequency of complications and a high limb salvage rate around 95% even in long segment disease justify a more widespread use of an endovascular approach in infrapopliteal obstructions.

Indications

The indication for infrapopliteal angioplasty is usually restricted to patients with critical limb ischemia (CLI), which is defined as rest pain, minor or major gangrene or ulceration, and an absolute ankle pressure ≤50 mmHg and/or toe pressure ≤30 mmHg. Angioplasty of below-the- knee lesions in patients with claudication is controversially discussed. In asymptomatic patients, also with a history of CLI, infrapopliteal PTA is not indicated.

Regarding the morphology of the lesion, the TASC recommendation, published in 2000, was very restrictive [7]; endovascular treatment was recommended only in very short lesions and bypass surgery was considered the treatment of choice for more diffuse stenosis and occlusions longer then 2 cm. CLI patients, however, are often high-risk surgical candidates, owing to their advanced age and comorbidities, thus a less invasive treatment option is more desirable. Furthermore, an unsuccessful endovascular attempt rarely hampers subsequent surgical revascularization. In fact, in several centers [36], the endovascular approach is already considered first-choice therapy, with surgery reserved for failed angioplasty, largely independent of the morphology of the lesion.

The revised version of the TASC recommendations, published in 2007 [8], also reflects the advances of endovascular therapy in this arterial segment by giving no clear recommendations for the choice of therapy with regard to the morphology and extent of the lesion.

Revascularization strategies for infrapopliteal intervention

The goal is to achieve a straight line pulsatile flow to the foot. In the case of multilevel disease, it is deemed insufficient if only the inflow to the infrapopliteal arteries is improved. At least one infrapopliteal artery should be reconstructed.

Approach to infrapopliteal lesions

In most cases, infrapopliteal obstructions can be treated by using an ipsilateral antegrade approach. Thanks to the miniaturization of the material a 4F or 5F sheath is, in many circumstances, sufficient. Antegrade access is unfamiliar to many cardiologists used to the retrograde puncture of the groin. The puncture site is somewhat higher, but still below the groin ligament. The wire tends to engage the profunda artery; therefore, a wire with a bent tip which can be directed toward the superficial femoral artery is helpful, e.g., a manually bent tip of a 0.035-inch wire (Fig. 63.4) coming with many introducer sheaths (e.g., 4F Maximum Hemostasis

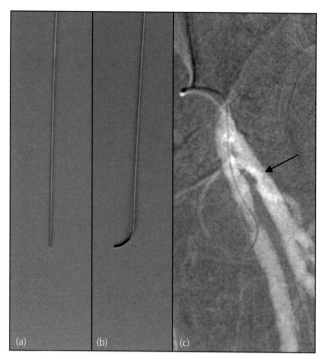

Figure 63.4 (a) Inverted tip of a 0.035-inch guidewire coming with the introducer sheath, (b) After manual bending of the tip. (c) Introduction of the wire into the SFA after antegrade puncture of the CFA.

Introducer, St. Jude Medical Inc., St. Paul, MN, USA). Optionally, the intervention can be performed using the cross-over technique. A 90-cm-long sheath, reaching down to the contralateral popliteal artery, is recommended for this approach (e.g., 6F 90 cm Check-Flo Introducer, Cook). Equipment to reach even the very distal segments of the infrapopliteal arteries in a cross-over approach is available (e.g., Amphirion Deep-balloon, shaft length 150 cm, Invatec, Roncadelle, Italy). Both approaches present advantages and disadvantages. The cross-over approach is preferred in obese patients, in whom an antegrade puncture of the common femoral artery can be impossible. It also allows to perform a complete angiographical evaluation of the lower extremity arteries before treatment, and an inflow-lesion at the level of the iliac arteries can be treated during the same session. The pushability and steerability of the angioplasty equipment, however, is reduced in cases of severely calcified and elongated iliac arteries. An optimal pushability is also desirable in severely calcified total occlusion of the infrapopliteal target lesion, and an antegrade approach in these cases is potentially more successful. In the case of inability to pass an occlusion from antegrade, a transpedal access and retrograde passage can be attempted [37]; however, this technique requires some experience.

Primary lesion crossing
Owing to the smaller caliber of below-the-knee arteries, low-profile material tracking over 0.014-inch or 0.018-inch guidewires is preferred. Shorter stenoses can easily be treated using coronary 0.014-inch guidewires and monorail percutaneous coronary intervention balloons. For more extensive lesions and total occlusions, hydrophilic coated guidewires and over-the-wire (OTW) balloons are standard. In severely calcified occlusions, coronary chronic total occlusion (CTO) guidewires such as the Miraclebros (Asahi Intec Co, Nagoya, Japan, provided by Abbott Laboratories, Abbott Park, IL, USA) can be very helpful. Support catheters (e.g., QuickCross, Spectranetics or Diver, Invatec) are helpful in CTOs; however, OTW low-profile balloons can be used instead, omitting one interventional step. As for the femoropopliteal tract, in this arterial segment either an intraluminal or subintimal guidewire passage can be performed in total occlusion, and, similar to the femoropopliteal tract, superiority of one over the other technique is not proven. For a subintimal recanalization, even 0.035-inch guidewires are utilized [38]. The risk of perforation might be higher using these wires. Re-entry devices, as for the femoropoliteal tract, to enable redirection of the guidewire back into the true lumen after passage of the occlusion do not exist for infrapopliteal arteries.

Angioplasty process
Balloon angioplasty is standard, and recently many companies have introduced balloons with a length of 120 mm, and even up to 220 mm, dedicated for infrapopliteal arteries to the market. Owing to the low profile of these balloons (e.g., Amphirion Deep, Invatec), even extensive occlusions can be passed and dilated in a high number of cases (Fig. 63.5). Other techniques for revascularization of below-the-knee lesions are the excimer-laser system or other atherectomy systems, such as the SilverHawk device (ev3).

Stenting in below-the-knee arteries
The benefit of systematic stenting of infrapopliteal obstructions has not been investigated up to now. Therefore, stenting is currently restricted to situations with unsatisfactory results after balloon angioplasty or atherectomy, like flow-limiting dissections or significant residual stenoses. Stents dedicated for infrapopliteal arteries became available only very recently and balloon-expandable coronary bare metal stents had to be used before. New stents for infrapopliteal use address the fact that infrapopliteal lesions are often long and are available in a length of up to 80 mm. Whether balloon-expandable stents (Chromis Deep, Invatec) or self-expanding stents (Xpert, Abbott; Astron Pulsar, Biotronik, Berlin, Germany; Maris Deep, Invatec) should be preferred is not clear yet.

Outcome of infrapopliteal angioplasty
To date, no randomized trials have been conducted to compare endovascular with surgical therapy exclusively of infrapopliteal lesions. Limb salvage rates achieved by endovascular treatment and published mostly as single-center registries, however, compare fairly well with surgical data (Table 63.7). Also, in a prospective multicenter trial using laser angioplasty

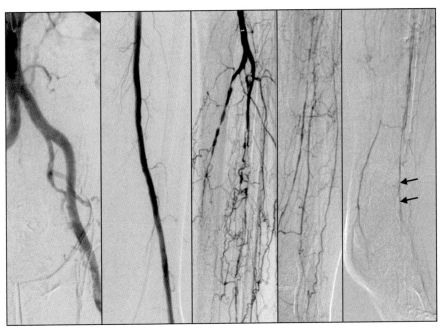

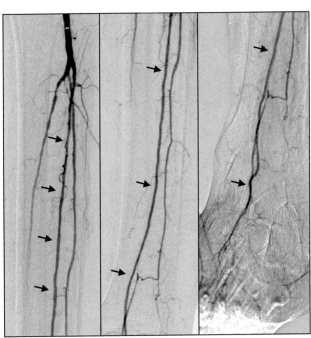

(a)

(b)

Figure 63.5 (a) Extensive infrapopliteal obstructions left leg with patent iliac and femoral arteries, typical for a diabetes patient. Black arrows indicate the distal anterior tibial artery. (b) After PTA of the anterior tibial artery (ATA) and fibular artery using a 2.5-mm/120-mm balloon (Amphirion Deep, Invatec). Black arrows indicates the ATA.

Table 63.7 Outcome of infrapopliteal angioplasty. Infrapopliteal intervention was often performed combined with inflow-lesion angioplasty.

Author	No. of patients	Treatment	Mean follow-up period (months)	Limb salvage rate (%)
Soder 2000 [40]	60	Balloon	18	80
Dorros 2001 [41]	215	Balloon	60	91
Faglia 2002 [43]	191	Balloon	14	94.8
Tartari 2007 [38]	82	Balloon	24	85
Bosiers 2006 [36]	443	Balloon, stenting, laser	12	96.6
Laird 2006 [39]	145	Laser, balloon, stenting	6	93
Feiring 2004 [44]	49	Primary stenting	12	100

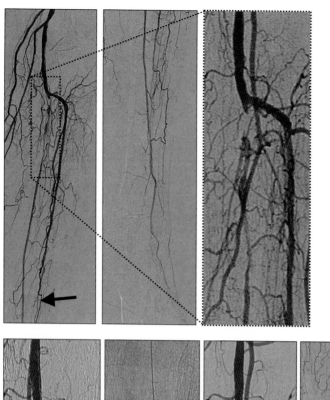

(a)

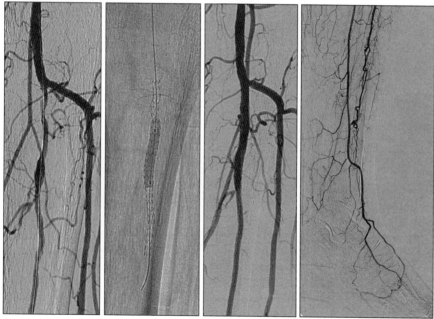

(b)

Figure 63.6 (a) Occlusion of the tibioperoneal trunk and high-grade stenosis of the proximal part of the fibular artery. Black arrow indicates the occlusion of the middle anterior tibial artery. (b) Predilation, implantation of two Cypher stents resulting in a brisk flow into the fibular artery as the only vessel supplying the foot.

and optional ballooning and/or stenting, a limb salvage rate of >90% was achieved [39]. Surgical revascularization due to early or late failure of angioplasty is reported to be rarely necessary [40,41]. The complication rate seems to favor an endovascular approach. The perioperative mortality for distal bypass procedures is typically reported to be at 2%, sometimes up to 5% and even 12% [42], whereas the mortality after an endovascular approach ranges from 0.0% to around 2% [37–41].

Lesion length treated within these registries varied greatly. Experience in extensively long infrapopliteal obstructions typical for diabetes patients is growing, and endovascular

treatment seems to be feasible and effective with a success rate of 85% [38] and limb salvage rate of 85% after 24 months in these complex lesions.

Clearly, the restenosis rate after angioplasty, especially of diffuse obstructions is higher compared with crural or pedal bypass-surgery. Revascularization is necessary to meet the increased oxygen demand, during wound healing. However, patency is considered of secondary importance after wound healing has resolved. Oxygen demand will be back to normal and recurrence of symptoms is not necessarily the consequence if restenosis after angioplasty or bypass-occlusion occurs. Therefore, follow-up is normally purely clinical, and information about the patency only of interest if CLI recurs. Still, if a higher patency rate could be achieved with new techniques, the clinical success might potentially be even higher and the need for secondary interventional treatment reduced.

Whether stenting may be beneficial in this regard is not yet clear. Balloon-expandable bare metal stents showed an angiographical binary restenosis rate of around 50% after 6 months [45,46]. First results using self-expanding stents (Xpert, Abbott) were superior [47]; however, the results are difficult to compare, owing to differences of the patient characteristics and lesion morphology. The sirolimus-eluting Cypher stent (Fig. 63.6) achieved a primary patency rate in infrapopliteal arteries of up to 100% after 6 months [45,46]. Whether the use of drug-eluting stents in CLI patients will also lead to a significantly higher limb salvage rate or lower recurrence rate of symptoms than with balloon angioplasty or bare metal stents has to be clarified in randomized trials, currently ongoing.

In summary, limb salvage after angioplasty, is in the same range as for surgical revascularization, can be performed with a potentially lower morbidity and mortality, and, finally, is relatively easy to repeat and should therefore be first choice therapy in CLI due to infrapopliteal lesions.

References

1. de Vries SO & Hunink MGM (1997) Results of aortic bifurcation grafts for aorto-iliac occlusive disease: a meta-analysis. *J Vasc Surg* **26**:558–569.

2. Tegtmeyer CJ, Hartwell GD, Selby JB, *et al.* (1991) Results and complications of angioplasty in aorto-iliac disease. *Circulation* **83**(Suppl. I):I53–I60.

3. Johnston KW (1993) Iliac arteries: reanalysis of results of balloon angioplasty. *Radiology* **186**:207–212.

4. Henry M, Amor M, Ethevenot G, *et al.* (1995) Palmaz stent placement in iliac and femoropopliteal arteries: primary and secondary patency in 310 patients with 2–4 year follow-up. *Radiology* **197**:167–174.

5. Sullivan TM, Childs MB, Bacharach JM, *et al.* (1997) Percutaneous transluminal angioplasty and primary stenting of the iliac arteries in 288 patients. *J Vasc Surg* **25**:829–838.

6. Vorwerk D, Günther RW, Schürmann K, & Wendt G (1996) Aortic and iliac stenoses: follow-up results of stent placement after insufficient balloon angioplasty in 118 cases. *Radiology* **198**:45–48.

7. Dormandy JA & Rutherford RB (2000) Management of peripheral arterial disease (PAD). TASC Working Group TransAtlantic Inter-Society Consensus (TASC). *J Vasc Surg* **31**(Suppl.):S1–S296.

8. Norgren L, Hiatt WR, Dormandy JA, *et al.* (2007) Inter-Society Consensus for the Management of Peripheral Vascular Disease (TASC II). *J Vasc Surg* **45**(Suppl. S):S5–S67.

9. Tetteroo E, van der Graaf Y, Bosch JL, *et al.* (1998) Randomised comparison of primary stent placement versus primary angioplasty followed by selective stent placement in patients with iliac artery occlusive disease. Dutch Iliac Stent Trial Study Group. *Lancet* **351**:1153–1159.

10. Scheinert D, Schröder M, Balzer JO, *et al.* (1999) Stent-supported reconstruction of the aorto-iliac bifurcation with the kissing balloon technique. *Circulation* **100**(19 Suppl.):II295–II300.

11. Haulon S, Mounier-Vehier C, Gaxotte V, *et al.* (2002) Percutaneous reconstruction of the aortoiliac bifurcation with the "kissing stents" technique: long-term follow-up in 106 patients. *J Endovasc Ther* **9**:363–368.

12. Mouanoutoua M, Maddikunta R, Allaqaband S, *et al.* (2003) Endovascular intervention of aortoiliac occlusive disease in high-risk patients using the kissing stents technique: long-term results. *Catheter Cardiovasc Interv* **60**:320–326.

13. Blum U, Gabelmann A, Redecker M, *et al.* (1993) Percutaneous recanalization of iliac artery occlusions: results of a prospective study. *Radiology* **189**:536–540.

14. Hausegger KA, Lammer J, Klein G, *et al.* (1991) Perkutane rekanalisation von beckenarterien verschlüssen: fibrinolyse, PTA, stents. Fortschr. *Roentgenstr* **155**:550–555.

15. Scheinert D, Schroeder M, Ludwig J, Braunlich S, *et al.* (2001) Stent-supported recanalization of chronic iliac artery occlusions. *Am J Med* **110**:708–715.

16. Vorwerk D, Guenther RW, Schürmann K, *et al.* (1995) Primary stent placement for chronic iliac artery occlusions: follow-up results in 103 patients. *Radiology* **194**:745–749.

17. Reyes R, Maynar M, Lopera J, *et al.* (1997) Treatment of chronic iliac artery occlusions with guide-wire recanalization and primary stent placement. *J Vasc Interv Radiol* **8**:1049–1055.

18. Schlager O, Francesconi M, Haumer M, *et al.* (2007) Duplex sonography versus angiography for assessment of femoropopliteal arterial disease in a "real-world" setting. *J Endovasc Ther* **14**:452–459.

19. Dörffler-Melly J, Mahler F, Do DD, Triller J, & Baumgartner I (2005) Adjunctive abciximab improves patency and functional outcomes in endovascular treatment of femoropopliteal occlusions: initial experiences. *Radiology* **237**:1103–1109.

20. Laxdal E, Jenssen GL, Pedersen G, & Aune S (2003) Subintimal angioplasty as a treatment of femoropopliteal artery occlusions. *Eur J Vasc Endovasc Surg* **25**:578–582.

21. Jacobs DL, Motaganahalli RL, Cox DE, Wittgen CM, & Peterson GJ (2006) True lumen re-entry devices facilitate subintimal angioplasty and stenting of total chronic occlusions: initial report. *J Vasc Surg* **43**:1291–1296.

22. Scheinert D, Braunlich S, Scheinert S, Ulrich M, Biamino G, & Schmidt A (2005) Initial clinical experience with an IVUS-guided transmembrane puncture device to facilitate recanalization of total femoral occlusions. *EuroIntervention* **1**:115–119.

23. Scheinert D, Peeters P, Bosiers M, O'Sullivan G, Sultan S, & Gershony G (2007) Results of the multicenter first-in-man study of a novel scoring balloon catheter for the treatment of infra-popliteal peripheral arterial disease. *Catheter Cardiovasc Interv* **70**:1034–1039.

24. Schillinger M, Sabeti S, Loewe C, *et al.* (2006) Balloon angioplasty versus implantation of nitinol stents in the superficial femoral artery. *N Engl J Med* **354**:1879–1888.

25. Schillinger M, Sabeti S, Dick P, *et al.* (2007) Sustained benefit at 2 years of primary femoropopliteal stenting compared with balloon angioplasty with optional stenting. *Circulation* **115**:2745–2749.

26. Scheinert D, Scheinert S, Sax J, *et al.* (2005) Prevalence and clinical impact of stent fractures after femoropopliteal stenting. *J Am Coll Cardiol* **45**:312–315.

27. Tepe G, Zeller T, Albrecht T, *et al.* (2008) Local delivery of paclitaxel to inhibit restenosis during angioplasty of the leg. *N Engl J Med* **358**:689–699.

28. Krankenberg H, Schlüter M, Steinkamp HJ, *et al.* (2007) Nitinol stent implantation versus percutaneous transluminal angioplasty in superficial femoral artery lesions up to 10 cm in length: the femoral artery stenting trial (FAST). *Circulation* **116**:285–292.

29. Capek P, McLean GK, & Berkowitz HD (1991) Femorpopliteal angioplasty. Factors influencing long-term success. *Circulation* **83**:170–180.

30. Scheinert D, Laird JR, Schroeder M, Steinkamp H, Balzer JO, & Biamino G (2001) Excimer Laser-assisted recanalization of long chronic superficial femoral artery occlusions. *J Endovasc Ther* **8**:156–166.

31. Amighi J, Schillinger M, Dick P, *et al.* (2008) De novo superficial femoropopliteal artery lesions: peripheral cutting balloon angioplasty and restenosis rates-randomized controlled trial. *Radiology* **247**:267–272.

32. Zeller T, Rastan A, Sixt S, *et al.* (2006) Long-term results after directional atherectomy of femoro-popliteal lesions. *J Am Coll Cardiol* **48**:1573–1578.

33. Gray BH, Sullivan TM, Childs MB, Young JR, & Olin JW (1997) High incidence of restenosis/reocclusion of stents in the percutaneous treatment of long-segment superficial femoral artery disease after suboptimal angioplasty. *J Vasc Surg* **25**:74–83.

34. Duda SH, Bosiers M, Lammer J, *et al.* (2006) Drug-eluting and bare nitinol stents for the treatment of atherosclerotic lesions in the superficial femoral artery: long-term results from the SIROCCO trial. *J Endovasc Ther* **13**:701–710.

35. Saxon RR, Dake MD, Volgelzang RL, Katzen BT, & Becker GJ (2008) Randomized, multicenter study comparing expanded polytetrafluoroethylene-covered endoprosthesis placement with percutaneous transluminal angioplasty in the treatment of superficial femoral artery occlusive disease. *J Vasc Interv Radiol* **19**:823–832.

36. Bosiers M, Hart JP, Deloose K, Verbist J, & Peeters P (2006) Endovascular therapy as the primary approach for limb salvage in patients with critical limb ischemia: experience with 443 infrapopliteal procedures. *Vascular* **14**:63–69.

37. Montero-Baker M, Schmidt A, Bräunlich S, *et al.* (2008) The retrograde approach for complex popliteal and tibioperoneal occlusions. *J Endovasc Ther* **15**:594–604.

38. Tartari S, Zattoni L, Rizzati R, *et al.* (2007) Subintimal angioplasty as the first-choice revascularization technique for infrainguinal arterial occlusions in patients with critical limb ischemia. *Ann Vasc Surg* **21**:819–828.

39. Laird JR, Zeller T, Gray BH, *et al.* (2006) Limb salvage following laser-assisted angioplasty for critical limb ischemia: results of the LACI multicenter trial. *J Endovasc Ther* **13**:1–11.

40. Soder HK, Manninen HI, Jaakkola P, *et al.* (2000) Prospective trial of infrapopliteal artery balloon angioplasty for critical limb ischemia: angiographic and clinical results. *J Vasc Interv Radiol* **11**:1021–1031.

41. Dorros G, Jaff MR, Dorros AM, *et al.* (2001) Tibioperoneal (outflow lesion) angioplasty can be used as primary treatment in 235 patients with critical limb ischemia: five-year follow-up. *Circulation* **104**:2057–2062.

42. Giles KA, Pomposelli FB, Hamdan AD, Blattman SB, Panossian H, & Schermerhorn ML (2008) Infrapopliteal angioplasty for critical limb ischemia: relation of TransAtlantic InterSociety Consensus class to outcome in 176 limbs. *J Vasc Surg* **48**:128–136.

43. Faglia E, Mantero M, Caminiti M, *et al.* (2002) Extensive use of peripheral angioplasty, particularly infrapopliteal, in the treatment of ischaemic diabetic foot ulcers: clinical results of a multicentric study of 221 consecutive diabetic subjects. *J Intern Med* **252**:225–232.

44. Feiring AJ, Wesolowski AA, & Lade S (2004) Primary stent-supported angioplasty for treatment of below-knee critical limb ischemia and severe claudication, early and one-year outcomes. *J Am Coll Cardiol* **44**:2307–2314.

45. Scheinert D, Ulrich M, Scheinert S, *et al.* (2006) Comparison of sirolimus-eluting vs. bare metal stents for the treatment of infrapopliteal obstructions. *EuroIntervention* **6**:169–174.

46. Siablis D, Karnabatidis D, Katsanos K, *et al.* (2007) Sirolimus-eluting versus bare stents after suboptimal infrapopliteal angioplasty for critical limb ischemia: enduring 1-year angiographic and clinical benefit. *J Endovasc Ther* **14**:241–250.

47. Bosiers M, Deloose K, Verbist J, & Peeters P (2007) Nitinol stenting for treatment of "below-the-knee" critical limb ischemia: 1-year angiographic outcome after Xpert stent implantation. *J Cardiovascular Surg (Torino)* **48**:455–461.

64 Surgical Treatment of Iliac and Lower Extremity Artery Disease

Frank E.G. Vermassen

Ghent University Hospital, Ghent, Belgium

Historical background

Although some descriptions exist of operations on the vascular system, dating from antiquity till the middle of twentieth century, these interventions were relatively simple and the results disappointing. Only ligations of bleeding vessels or aneurysms were performed with relative success, such as the well-known ligation of popliteal aneurysms by Hunter in the eighteenth century [1]. With the description of the vascular anastomosis in the beginning of the twentieth century, Alexis Carrel is generally considered as the father of vascular as well as transplant surgery [2]. Some of the problems that precluded rapid advancement of vascular procedures were, besides an insufficient insight in the pathophysiology of atherosclerosis and limb ischemia, the absence of an effective method to prevent clotting, the unavailability of a useful substitute, and the high risk for infection. Only in the 1930s did solutions for some of these problems become available, with the introduction of heparin into clinical practice and the first translumbar aortography performed by Dos Santos in 1929 [3].

The modern era of vascular surgery started after the second world war with the first femoral endarterectomy by Dos Santos in 1947 and the first femoro-popliteal bypass with saphenous vein by Kunlin in 1949 [4]. In the aortoiliac system endarterectomy was introduced by Wylie, and Dubost performed the first resection and allograft replacement of an abdominal aortic aneurysm in 1951 [5]. The first similar operation for obstructive disease was performed 1 year later by Oudot [6]. However, the further development of reconstructions in the aortoiliac system suffered from the unavailability of suitable prosthetic material, as homografts proved to be less reliable in the long run. After the first description of a successful implant of a prosthesis made of Vinyon N by Voorhees in 1949 [7], Dacron (a polyester fabric) soon proved to be a very useful and biocompatible material, enabling a rapid and huge expansion of the number of procedures.

Cardiovascular Interventions in Clinical Practice. Edited by Jürgen Haase, Hans-Joachim Schäfers, Horst Sievert and Ron Waksman. © 2010 Blackwell Publishing.

In the following decades, diagnostic methods (invasive as well as noninvasive) were improved, the techniques were refined, enabling interventions on smaller vessels, and indications extended to reconstructions on the carotid arteries, the visceral branches of the aorta and the infragenual blood vessels. Efforts were made to diminish the thrombogenicity and improve the long-term results of prosthetic grafts, especially in smaller vessel reconstructions. All these evolutions resulted in a gradual improvement of the results and expansion of the indications.

From the 1980s and onward, endovascular techniques started to develop, opening blood vessels intraluminally with wires, balloons, and stents. This technique has the major advantage of being less invasive and has gradually taken over, parallel to the development of better materials; many indications that are classically treated with open surgical techniques. One should not consider both of these approaches as competitive to each other but rather as complementary. Easier and shorter lesions are now treated endovascularly but the more difficult and more extensive indications remain for open surgery. This inevitably will have its influence on the type of surgical reconstructions, the case mix, and the caseload of the vascular surgeon in the future.

Pathophysiology

Most lesions that cause limb ischemia are, at least in the Western world, due to atherosclerosis. They can progress continuously or stepwise to varying degrees of stenosis, and eventually thrombosis of the diseased blood vessel. The symptoms caused by these stenoses will depend on their severity, extent, and number, as well as on the presence and quality of the collaterals. The hemodynamic significance of a lesion is function not only of the percentage stenosis, but also of the flow velocity across the lesion [8]. At rest, a lesion in the femoral artery will only become hemodynamically significant when it is about 90% occlusive. When exercising, the flow velocity in the artery will increase and the stenosis can become hemodynamically significant and impair blood flow at approximately 50%. The obstructed blood flow in the

Table 64.1 Classification of peripheral arterial disease: Fontaine's stages and Rutherford's categories.

Fontaine		Rutherford	
I	Asymptomatic	0	Asymptomatic
IIa	Mild claudication	1	Mild claudication
IIb	Moderate to severe claudication	2	Moderate claudication
		3	Severe claudication
III	Ischemic rest pain	4	Ischemic rest pain
IV	Ulceration or gangrene	5	Minor tissue loss
		6	Major tissue loss

main vessel can partially or totally be overtaken by the development of collaterals. Lesions at multiple levels will have a cumulative effect and result in more severe symptoms.

Some blood vessels are more prone to the development of atherosclerosis and stenotic lesions show a predilection for certain locations. Examples are the divisions of blood vessels, such as the aortic or femoral bifurcation. The predilection of plaque formation at these sites can be explained by the disturbance of laminar flow and its hemodynamic consequences [9]. The superficial femoral artery is the artery most often affected by atherosclerotic lesions. This probably has to do with the structure of this artery and its relatively low flow. Especially at the level of the adductor hiatus, lesions are frequent [10]. Although not absolute, the pattern of lesions is also influenced by the risk factors that contribute to the development of atherosclerosis: smoking predominantly affects the more proximal arteries, whereas, in older and diabetic patients, the infragenual arteries are more often affected [11].

Indications

Symptoms related to peripheral arterial disease (PAD) and chronic limb ischemia are categorized according to the Fontaine or Rutherford classification (Table 64.1) [12]. In asymptomatic patients there is generally no indication for invasive treatment. An exception can be made for the treatment of an inflow or anastomotic lesion to preserve the flow and patency of a previously inserted bypass.

The majority of patients with symptoms of PAD have limited exercise capacity and walking ability. They have sufficient blood flow at rest, but with exercise the arterial lesions limit the increase in blood flow and cause a mismatch between the oxygen supply and the metabolic demand of the exercising muscle. In these patients with intermittent claudication (Rutherford categories 1–3) risk factor modification, antiplatelet drugs and regular walking exercise are the cornerstones of primary treatment. These are aimed at reducing the overall cardiovascular risk, which is significantly elevated in these

patients, as well as at improving their walking distance. The decision to consider a patient for invasive treatment is made by balancing the disability caused by the impaired walking capacity in a particular patient against the procedural risks and likelihood of long-term success of the intervention [13]. Nowadays, most patients with claudication, due to the less severe degree of their arterial lesions, can be treated with endovascular procedures.

Patients with chronic ischemic rest pain, ulcers, or gangrene attributable to objectively proven arterial occlusive disease (Rutherford categories 4–6) are considered to have "critical limb ischemia" [14]. In these patients, invasive therapy to improve blood supply to the leg or foot is mandatory; with conservative therapy 75–95% of these patients will die or loose their leg within 1 year [15].

The choice between endovascular and open surgical treatment is made depending on the location, degree of obstruction, and extension of the lesions. In the Transatlantic Intersociety Consensus (TASC) documents, the authors tried to organize the lesions into four categories guiding the choice between these two treatment options. The difference in categorization between the two versions of this document published in 2000 and 2007 [13,14] illustrates the increasing capacities and improving results with endovascular techniques related to the development of new materials.

Acute limb ischemia is to be differentiated from chronic limb ischemia. It is defined as a sudden decrease or worsening in limb perfusion, causing a potential threat to extremity viability [13]. Causes for acute limb ischemia are embolism, thrombosis superimposed on a pre-existing atherosclerotic lesion or of a previously implanted bypass, and less frequent pathologies such as dissection or trauma. In the assessment of a patient with acute limb ischemia, the viability of the limb should be evaluated to guide the treatment. A difference has to be made between patients with a viable limb, a limb with threatened viability, and a limb with irreversible ischemic damage. The viability is considered as threatened when sensory or motor deficits are present. Within this group, a difference is made between marginally threatened (limited sensory deficit, no persistent ischemic pain, no motor deficit) and immediately threatened limbs (persistent ischemic pain, motor deficit) [12,16].

In an immediately threatened limb, prompt revascularization by surgical intervention is indicated. This will consist of clot removal through a surgical thrombectomy or creation of a bypass. A completion angiography after removal of the thrombus is mandatory to identify any residual occlusion or critical underlying lesion requiring further treatment.

In a marginally threatened limb, and when no contraindications are present, catheter-directed thrombolysis is preferred [13]. After prolonged or severe acute ischemia, a reperfusion injury with swelling of the leg is the rule. In order to prevent the development of a compartment syndrome and myonecrosis, a fasciotomy should be considered. After restoration of blood flow, efforts should be made to identify and treat the underlying cause such as the source of emboli or a critical stenosis.

Instead of stenosis and obstruction the atherosclerotic inflammatory process can also result in dilation of blood vessels. Once an artery is dilated to more than twice its normal diameter, this is called an aneurysm. Aneurysms can occur at many places in the human body, but the most frequent are: infrarenal aorta (with or without extension into the iliac arteries), thoracic aorta, popliteal arteries, and femoral arteries. The risks related to the presence of an aneurysm are rupture with bleeding, embolization, thrombosis, and compression of adjacent structures. Abdominal aortic aneurysms (AAA) mostly present with rupture as the first symptom when not treated timely, whereas in popliteal aneurysms embolization and thrombosis with acute limb ischemia are the major complication.

Because of the high mortality related to ruptured AAA it is important to treat these aneurysms before this catastrophe occurs. In deciding when this elective repair should be performed, a balance has to be made between the risk of rupture and the risk of the operation. Some large randomized studies comparing a "watchful waiting policy" to immediate intervention concluded that the threshold for elective treatment of AAA is around 55 mm in men and 50 mm in women [17]. Nowadays, 60–70% of AAA can also be treated endovascularly. In two randomized studies comparing endovascular treatment with open treatment, endovascular treatment showed an advantage in peri-operative mortality and morbidity. However, this advantage had disappeared after 2 years of follow-up and more secondary interventions were necessary after implantation of an endoprosthesis [18,19].

Popliteal aneurysms are less prone to rupture but easily cause embolization resulting in occlusion of the tibial vessels or thrombosis of the aneurysm itself. Once a diameter of 2 cm is reached and/or embolization has occurred, exclusion of the aneurysm combined with a bypass procedure is indicated [20]. Endovascular treatment can be an alternative when no good-quality saphenous vein is available to perform the bypass [21].

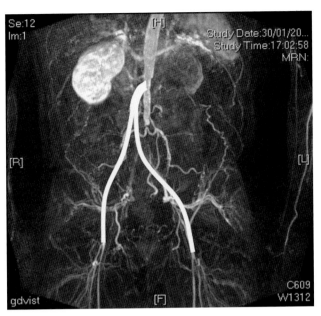

Figure 64.1 Extensive aortoiliac lesions. Treatment with aortobifemoral bypass.

Surgical treatment

Introduction

The primary aim of revascularization in patients with peripheral artery disease (PAD) is to restore blood flow to a sufficient level to relieve the symptoms (claudication or critical limb ischemia). The treatment will consist in removing the blockage or providing a new conduit for the blood flow through a bypass procedure. In patients with single-level disease, the choice of the procedure is often obvious. In patients with multilevel disease, elimination of the most proximal obstruction might be sufficient to achieve this goal and should be the first step in any procedure. However, in patients with critical limb ischemia, and certainly in those with tissue loss, complete revascularization with restoration of direct pulsatile blood flow to the affected area is often necessary.

Aortoiliac reconstructions

Procedures

Aorto(bi)femoral bypass
An aorto(bi)femoral bypass (ABF) (Fig. 64.1) can be considered as the standard of therapy in patients with extensive involvement of the aorta and/or both iliac arteries [14]. It is generally performed through a midline laparotomy with dissection of the infrarenal aorta after mobilization of the intestines and opening of the retroperitoneum. Alternative approaches, such as a transverse or retroperitoneal incision, can be used also and might be preferable in patients with impaired pulmonary function. During the last decade there has been

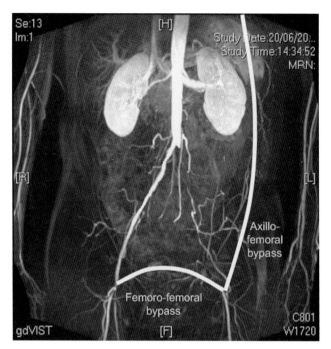

Figure 64.2 Unilateral iliac occlusive disease. Treatment with extraanatomic reconstruction.

growing interest in a minimally invasive and laparoscopic approach [22]. The technical difficulties and learning curve with this technique still prevent its widespread use.

The proximal anastomosis of an ABF is constructed at the level of the infrarenal aorta proximal to the obstruction (Fig. 64.1). When the occlusion extends to the level of the renal arteries the obstruction can partially be removed of the aorta or an alternative extraanatomic technique can be chosen. The proximal anastomosis can be made in an end-to-side or end-to-end fashion. Patency rates are not different between both of these techniques. Factors that can guide the choice are: the presence of aneurysmal dilation, preservation of inferior mesenteric or (internal) iliac arteries, and exclusion of embolic foci. Distal anastomoses are performed on the common femoral arteries through an end-to-side anastomosis. When the common femoral arteries are diseased, this procedure can easily be combined with a femoral endarterectomy. As a conduit, a bifurcated coated Dacron graft is generally used [23].

In open aneurysm treatment, when the aneurysm is confined to the infrarenal aorta, implantation of a straight tube graft between the infrarenal neck of the aneurysm and the aortic bifurcation is the preferred option. After clamping and incision of the aneurysm, both anastomoses are performed in an end-to-end fashion and the aneurysmal sack is closed again over the prosthesis. When the aneurysm extends into the iliac arteries or is combined with stenotic lesions in these vessels, an aortobiiliac or aortobifemoral graft will be performed.

The excellent results with aortobifemoral grafting and the growing use of endovascular techniques decrease the place for aortoiliac endarterectomy for which only a few indications remain [24].

When only one iliac axis is affected and the patient cannot be treated endovascularly, a unilateral aortofemoral or iliofemoral bypass (using the proximal part of the common iliac artery as inflow) can be performed. A retroperitoneal approach can diminish the peri-operative complications related to laparotomy in this indication. For this reason, a unilateral revascularization in combination with a femorofemoral cross-over bypass is sometimes preferred in patients with bilateral disease.

Extraanatomic bypasses

Thoracofemoral bypass
When the abdominal aorta cannot be used for inflow in a patient in otherwise good general condition, the lower part of the descending aorta can be an alternative. This is accessed through a small lower thoracotomy and the graft is retroperitoneally tunneled to both groins. Indications for this intervention remain scarce.

Axillofemoral bypass
In patients with contraindication for an abdominal approach (infections, multiple previous abdominal interventions, etc) or elevated surgical risk due to comorbidities, an axillofemoral bypass can be preferred (Fig. 64.2). In these cases, the axillary artery is used as the inflow source. An externally supported prosthesis is used that is tunneled subcutaneously from the infraclavicular crest to the groin. Preoperative assessment of the subclavian and axillary artery is mandatory to exclude the presence of an inflow stenosis. In the case of bilateral involvement, a bilateral axillofemoral or an axillobifemoral bypass can be performed.

Femorofemoral bypass
When one iliac axis is widely patent and an abdominal approach is to be avoided a femorofemoral cross-over bypass might be a good alternative (Fig. 64.2). When the donor artery shows focal stenosis, this procedure can be combined with percutaneous transluminal angioplasty with or without stenting of this iliac axis. However, in this situation alternatives should also be considered. In recent years femorofemoral bypasses have been increasingly performed in conjunction with aortouniiliac endoprostheses in the treatment of abdominal aortic aneurysms.

Complications
Aortobifemoral reconstructions yield excellent results in the long term also but have a non-negligible morbidity, at least in compromised patients. General complications, such as myocardial infarction and renal as well as pulmonary insufficiency,

are related to the cardiovascular status and occur with a frequency of up to 5%. Perioperative mortality is around 1–3% in most series [25].

Acute limb ischemia occurring shortly after operation is generally attributable to acute thrombosis of one of the limbs, owing to technical problems or deficiencies. It can also occur as a result of intraoperative thromboembolic events. Early reintervention is necessary to correct the cause and restore blood flow. Late limb occlusion is usually related to impaired outflow due to progression of atherosclerotic disease.

Local complications, such as wound infection or lymphatic fistula, mostly occur at the femoral incisions and should be treated vigorously to prevent graft infection. Graft infection is a dreadful complication that can occur early after the intervention or late after an episode of bacteremia. Treatment of aortic graft infection is challenging. In a few cases the infection can be treated with local debridement and irrigation with antibiotics, but, in general, graft excision will be necessary. After excision, extensive retroperitoneal debridement must be done. Classicaly, blood flow was restored with extraanatomic bypasses (bilateral axillofemoral or axillopopliteal bypass). Nowadays, *in situ* replacement techniques are used increasingly. A number of reports describe direct *in situ* replacement with a rifampicin-soaked or silver impregnated graft, but the use of this technique is usually limited to indolent infections with less virulent germs. Homografts have the advantage of being more resistant toward infection and allow a relatively easy *in situ* reconstruction. Questions remain with regard to their long-term durability [26]. Autogenous reconstruction with femoral veins is a good alternative technique, with good resistance to infection, but is a lengthy and tedious operation [27].

An aortoenteric fistula is a fistula between the graft and the intestines, mostly occurring between the proximal anastomosis and the duodenum. Causes are infection or erosion of intestines that lie in direct contact with the graft. The therapy is similar to that of an infected graft, together with closure of the intestinal fistula. Mortality is high.

Pseudo-aneurysm (anastomotic false aneurysm) formation is a late complication that occurs in up to 5% of anastomoses at the femoral level. It is less frequent at the proximal anastomosis. Frequency is decreasing as a result of better materials and surgical techniques. Treatment consists of excision and reconstruction.

Extraanatomical bypasses are less invasive operations, and therefore usually have less general complications. The major complication after femorofemoral or axillofemoral bypass are wound problems and graft infection due to the more superficial location of these grafts. When an anastomosis is involved, prompt reconstruction with removal of the bypass is indicated owing to the risk of anastomotic dehiscence and bleeding.

Results

The results of aortobifemoral grafting are among the best one can possibly achieve with vascular reconstructions. Patency rates are as high as 91% after 5 years in patients with claudication and 87% in critical limb ischemia [25]. Most patients are rendered asymptomatic and 80% remain so after 5 years. Unilateral aorto- or iliofemoral grafts have similar patency rates after 3 years [23]. Axillofemoral grafts have a patency of around 60–70% after 5 years, depending on the indication and outflow. Similar results are described with femorofemoral bypasses if the inflow artery is of sufficient quality [14].

Infrainguinal reconstructions

Procedures

Inguinal reconstructions

The location of the common femoral artery in the flexion area of the groin, and the presence of its bifurcation in deep and superficial femoral artery makes this artery less suitable for endovascular treatment. On the other hand, its superficial location makes it ideally suited for an open approach. As most of the lesions are located at or involve the origin of its branches, the procedure most commonly performed in this artery is an endarterectomy with patch angioplasty. When the origin of the deep femoral artery is de-obstructed or enlarged this is also called a profundoplasty.

In this procedure, the common femoral artery and its branches are dissected from the level of the inguinal ligament till the first centimeter of both superficial and deep femoral artery. A longitudinal arteriotomy is performed and the obstructive plaque is removed in a plane within the media of the blood vessel. A proximal extension in the external iliac artery can often be removed blindly by gentle traction or the use of special devices. Distally, care is taken to obtain a good end point without flap formation. If necessary, the distal intimal flap can be tacked to the wall. When no good end point can be obtained, the incision should be furthered within the deep and/or superficial femoral artery. Taken into account the importance of the deep femoral artery as collateral blood flow provider all efforts should be made to obtain a good inflow in this artery and its branches. The arteriotomy is closed with a venous or prosthetic patch.

In some cases the atherosclerotic plaque cannot easily be removed or the endarterectomy results in a severed blood vessel. In these cases, a short interposition graft between the external iliac artery and the bifurcation of the femoral artery is preferred.

Above-knee reconstructions

Thanks to the collateral blood supply, originating from the branches of the deep femoral artery, isolated lesions of the superficial femoral artery usually only cause symptoms of claudication and not critical limb ischemia. This collateral circulation is also the reason why exercise therapy is often successful in these patients. When invasive treatment is indicated, a growing number of cases can now be treated endovascularly with improving results. For this reason, the number of surgical procedures for isolated lesions of the superficial femoral artery (SFA) is decreasing. The classical surgical intervention in this area is the supragenual femoropopliteal bypass (Fig. 64.3) between the common femoral artery and the supragenual popliteal artery. The latter is accessed through a medial incision just above the knee. The popliteal artery is easily found distally from the adductor's canal where it lies under the fascia, beneath the femur and above the gracilis muscle. Both the proximal and distal anastomoses are mostly performed in an end-to-side fashion. For this conduit, both saphenous vein and prosthetic materials can be used. Best patency rates are obtained with saphenous vein grafts. Prosthetic materials have the advantage of leaving the saphenous vein for later, more distal, or coronary interventions and make the operation easier and faster [28]. Both Dacron and polytetrafluoroethylene (PTFE) grafts can be used for this indication [29]. Heparin-coated PTFE grafts show promising preliminary results with regard to improvement of patency.

A direct relation can be observed between the long-term patency of these grafts and the number of infragenual outflow arteries. Nevertheless, also in the presence of an isolated popliteal artery with sufficient collateral outflow a bypass to this artery can be performed and is indicated when no better, more distal, outflow vessel is present or this vessel cannot be reached due to insufficient available vein [30].

As an alternative to bypass grafting, some propose an endarterectomy of the SFA performed as an open or semi-closed procedure. Results with this procedure are less consistent then with a bypass procedure [31].

Below-knee reconstructions

Owing to the difficult collateralization around the bony knee, isolated lesions of the popliteal artery often cause severe symptoms. However, these isolated lesions are not common, and mostly popliteal lesions are combined with or are extensions of lesions of the superficial femoral artery. In these cases an infragenual femoropopliteal bypass (Fig. 64.3) is indicated. The distal anastomosis is performed on the infragenual popliteal artery that is accessed through a medial incision below the knee, just dorsal of the inferior border of the tibia. After division of the fascia, the artery can be found dorsal from the tibia just behind the popliteal vein. The proximal anastomosis is mostly performed on the common femoral artery, but also the distal superficial femoral artery and the deep femoral artery can be used as inflow sources provided that they are free from inflow lesions. In infragenicular reconstructions, as a conduit, the saphenous vein should always be preferred whenever it is available and suited for use [32] (diameter >3–4 mm, no extreme varicosities or fibrotic areas). The saphenous vein can be used according to the *reversed* or the *in situ* technique.

In the *reversed* technique, the saphenous vein is harvested and inserted in an upside-down fashion with the distal part of the vein at the proximal anastomosis and vice versa. In the *in situ* technique, the vein is left in place and the valves are destroyed using a valvulotome. The side branches are looked up by angiography or duplex and ligated. The advantages of the reversed technique are that the valves need not be destroyed and that the intervention is technically somewhat simpler. Advantages of the *in situ* technique are the better congruence of the vein with the donor and acceptor artery (larger part of the vein at the proximal anastomosis and vice versa) and the fact that less incisions need to be made. Results with both techniques with regard to patency or late complications are similar [33]. After every below-the-knee bypass, a completion angiogram to exclude technical imperfections is mandatory.

In 20–25% of patients in need of an infragenual reconstruction, no or insufficient saphenous vein is available. In such cases another conduit is required. When the other leg

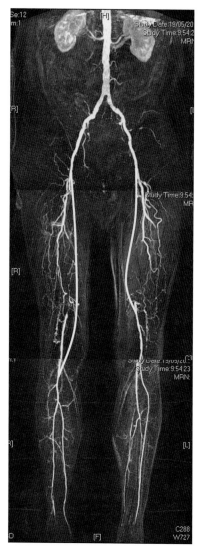

Figure 64.3 Extensive lesions of superficial femoral artery. Treatment with supra- or infragenual femoropopliteal bypass.

is not in danger of developing critical limb ischemia, the contralateral saphenous vein can be used. The lesser saphenous vein or arm veins might also provide a solution in some of these patients. However, these are often of insufficient quality and length when a long bypass is needed and difficult to harvest. Prosthetic materials yield less good results, with regard to patency, than venous grafts and should only be used when no autologous veins are available [32].

Composite grafts consisting of a proximal prosthetic part and a distal venous part are sometimes preferred when only a limited amount of venous material is available [14,34]. However, although in some studies a trend toward better results compared with totally prosthetic grafts can be observed, no randomized data are available comparing all prosthetic to composite grafts.

When the infragenual popliteal artery or the proximal segments of the tibial vessels are also stenosed or occluded, a tibial bypass can be preformed. Taking into account the less durable results with these bypasses in the long run, these reconstructions are, with a few exceptions, only indicated in patients with critical limb ischemia [23].

Although in most reconstructions the common femoral artery will be used, every proximal artery with unobstructed inflow can be used as an inflow source. Short bypasses originating from the distal SFA have the advantage of less venous material being required for a total venous bypass graft [35]. For an outflow artery, the best of the three tibial arteries (posterior tibial, anterior tibial, and peroneal) should be chosen. Direct outflow to the foot is an important criterium to guide the choice. Different studies have shown the importance of an open pedal arch in predicting the success of a tibial bypass procedure. Nevertheless, also the fibular artery can serve as an adequate outflow artery [36].

As in every below-the-knee procedure, the saphenous vein is the preferred conduit also in tibial reconstructions. Prosthetic materials are only indicated when no sufficient autologous vein is available. Whether heparin coating, to diminish the thrombogenicity of the graft, has a positive influence on results remains to be determined.

Different adjuvant procedures have been tried out to improve the patency of tibial reconstructions:
• The use of a venous patch or cuff at the distal anastomosis has been proposed by several authors [37,38]. The main purpose of these cuffs is to provide a venous interface between the graft and the artery, decreasing the compliance mismatch between both, and to create a hemodynamically more favorable situation at the distal anastomosis between the larger prosthetic graft and the smaller artery. Conflicting results have been obtained with this technique in randomized studies at different levels but at least at the crural level there seems to be an advantage with the use of a vein cuff in the long term [39]. Some companies have tried to mimic the hemodynamic alterations, creating less vortex, caused by the cuff and altered the design of the graft producing a pre-cuffed prosthetic graft. Results with these grafts compared with regular grafts are equivocal [40].
• Creation of an arteriovenous fistula at the distal anastomosis to decrease vascular resistance and increase flow in the graft without creating a hemodynamically significant steal phenomenon is another adjuvant technique. A randomized study showed no difference in results with or without the use of this technique [41], and, although theoretically attractive, this technique has largely been abandoned.

Cryopreserved homologous veins have also been tried out as an alternative to prosthetic grafts for this indication. They are easier to handle and are infection resistant compared with prosthetic grafts. However, some immunosuppressive, to avoid rejection and early occlusion, needs to be administered to obtain equivalent results to those obtained with synthetic grafts [42].

Especially in diabetic patients, the tibial arteries are often diffusely diseased, whereas the pedal arteries are relatively spared. In these patients a bypass to the pedal arteries (dorsal pedal or posterior tibial at ankle level or even plantar arteries) can, in the presence of nonhealing ulcers or minor gangrene be indicated. Often, thanks to the specific pattern of disease in diabetics, the infrapopliteal artery can be used as inflow source (Fig. 64.4). Venous material should be used at any effort. The results of these bypasses are similar to the results with tibial reconstructions, and limb salvage can be obtained in a considerable number of patients [43].

Complications

Complications of reconstructions in the groin are mostly related to local problems, such as wound infection or lymphatic fistula. The most frequent complications after infrainguinal reconstructions are the general complications related to the cardiovascular comorbidity and high age present in a considerable number of these patients. Certainly in below-the-knee reconstructions many patients are diabetics and/or of advanced age and their blood vessels in other territories are affected as well [44]. Local complications are mostly related to wound problems, especially in diabetic and in obese patients, in whom wound healing can be significantly impaired. Meticulous dissection without creation of flaps and tension-free closure are helpful in preventing this complication.

Saphenous nerve neuralgia is a frequent but mostly temporary complication. Graft infection is limited to prosthetic grafts that are less commonly used in this indication.

Leg swelling is common after a successful distal revascularization. Reasons for this are the increased lymph production during postoperative reactive hyperemia and disruption of lymph vessels along the path of vein harvest or in the groin.

Early graft occlusion is mostly attributable to technical failure or insufficient outflow. A completion angiogram or a duplex or flow measurement is indicated after every distal revascularization to reduce the incidence of this complication.

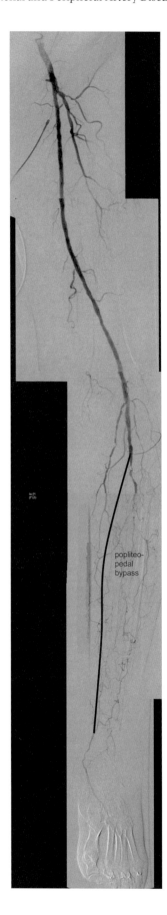

In saphenous vein grafts, focal stenosis can develop, especially during the first 2 years after implantation. As these can lead to occlusion of the bypass surveillance of the graft by means of regular duplex, examination is indicated to identify and treat flow-limiting stenoses before complete occlusion of the conduit [13].

Results

A profundoplasty as an isolated procedure is often sufficient to relieve the symptoms of claudication or rest pain, but, in the presence of ischemic lesions and more distal arterial obstructions, a more extensive revascularization is often necessary [45].

The patency rates for supra- and infragenual femoropopliteal bypass depend on the indication, localization of the distal anastomosis, and quality of the outflow and graft material that can be used. In patients with claudication the 5-year patency rates in above-knee reconstructions are as high as 70–80% when saphenous vein can be used, and 10% lower with the use of PTFE-grafts. In below-knee reconstructions 5-year patency rates are around 60% with venous grafts and 40% with prosthetic grafts. When the indication for intervention is critical limb ischemia, these results fall to 66% after 5 years with vein grafts, and 47% and 33% for above-knee and below knee prosthetic grafts, respectively [46,47].

The 5-year results with tibial venous grafts are around 50–60%, with limb salvage rates of up to 80%. With prosthetic grafts, patency after 5 years is <35% [48]. Pedal bypass grafts have similar results as tibial bypasses and are indicated in critical limb ischemia also when limited gangrene is present. Diabetes does not have a negative impact on results [43].

These results with open surgery remain better than results obtained with percutaneous intervention, certainly with regard to patency. Nevertheless, the minimal invasive character and the possibility to repeat the procedure easily as well as the comorbidity and limited survival in this patient group increased the tendency to prefer endovascular treatment also in this area. However, we should not forget that there is still a surgical alternative with good results (patency rates that are predictably 20% or more above those with percutaneous transluminal angioplasty).

Conclusion

In extensive aortoiliac lesions, and when the patient is in good condition, an aortobifemoral bypass is the preferred intervention. Results with this technique are excellent in the long term also. In patients with hostile abdomen or important comorbidity, extraanatomic reconstructions can be an alternative.

Figure 64.4 (*left*) Lesions of infragenicular vessels in a diabetic patient. Treatment with pedal artery bypass.

Extensive lesions of the femoral and popliteal arteries can be treated successfully with a supra- or infragenual femoropopliteal bypass. When the distal popliteal artery or tibial arteries are also involved, a femorotibial bypass can be performed. Particularly in diabetic patients with nonhealing ulcers, a bypass to the pedal arteries can be very useful to save the limb. The autogenous saphenous vein is the preferred conduit for all reconstructions with distal anastomosis on the infragenicular vessels. All these reconstructions have acceptable patency rates and even higher limb salvage rates, superior to those that can be obtained with endovascular treatment, all be it at the cost of a higher morbidity.

Although during the last decades a clear tendency toward endovascular treatment could be observed in patients with iliac and lower extremity arterial disease, there is still a place for open surgery in this patient group. Some lesions cannot be treated endovascularly, and in others the results with open surgical techniques remain superior. Nevertheless, open surgical and endovascular techniques used in the treatment of PAD should not be considered as competitive but rather as complementary to each other. In many instances, a combination of both will be the best solution.

References

1. Galland RB (2007) Popliteal aneurysms: from John Hunter to the 21st century. *Ann R Coll Surg Engl* **89**:466–471.
2. Carell A (1908) Results of the transplantation of blood vessels, organs and limbs. *JAMA* **51**:1662.
3. Dos Santos R, Lamas A, & Pereira CJ (1929) L'artériographie des membres de l'aorte et ses branches abdominals. *Bull Soc Nat Chir* **55**:587.
4. Kunlin J (1949) Le traitement de l'artérite oblitérante par la greffe veneuze. *Arch Mal Cooeur* **42**:371.
5. Dubost C (1951) A propos du traitement des aneurysmes de l'aorte; ablation de l'aneurysme: rétablissement de la continuité par greffe d'aorte conservé. *Mem Acad Chir* **77**:381.
6. Oudot J (1951) La greffe vasculaire dans les thromboses du carrefour aortique. *Presse Med* **59**:234.
7. Voorhees AB, Jaretzki A, & Blakemore AW (1952) The use of tubes constructed from Vinyon N cloth in bridging arterial defects. *Ann Surg* **135**:332.
8. Young DF, Cholvin NR, Kirkeeide RL, *et al.* (1977) Hemodynamics of arterial stenosis at elevated flow rates. *Circ Res* **41**:99–107.
9. Zarins CK, Giddens DP, Bharadvaj BK, *et al.* (1983) Carotid bifurcation atherosclerosis: quantitative correlation of plaque localization with flow velocity profiles and wall shear stress. *Circ Res* **53**:502.
10. Blair JM, Glagov S, & Zarins CK (1990) Mechanism of superficial femoral artery adductor canal stenosis. *Surg Forum* **41**:359.
11. Diehm N, Shang A, Silvestro A, *et al.* (2006) Association of cardiovascular risk factors with pattern of lower limb atherosclerosis in 2659 patients undergoing angioplasty. *Eur J Vasc Endovasc Surg* **31**:59–63.
12. Rutherford RB, Baker JD, Ernst C, *et al.* (1997) Recommended standards for reports dealing with lower extremity ischemia: revised version. *J Vasc Surg* **26**:517–538.
13. Anon (2000) Management of peripheral arterial disease (PAD). TransAtlantic Inter-Society Consensus (TASC). *J Vasc Surg* **31**: S1–S288.
14. Norgren L, Hiatt WR, Dormandy JA, *et al.* (2007) Inter-Society consensus for the management of peripheral arterial disease (TASC II). *J Vasc Surg* **45**:S5–S67.
15. Wolfe JHN & Wyatt MG (1997) Critical and subcritical ischemia. *Eur J Vasc Endovasc Surg* **13**:578–582.
16. Working party on thrombolysis in the management of limb ischemia (1998) Thrombolysis in the management of lower limb peripheral arterial occlusion—a consensus document. *Am J Cardiol* **81**:207–218.
17. Powell JT, Brown LC, Forbes JF, *et al.* (2007) Final 12 year follow-up of surgery versus surveillance in the UK small aneurysm trial. *Br J Surg* **94**:702–708.
18. EVAR trial participants (2005) Endovascular aneurysm repair versus open repair in patients with abdominal aortic aneurysm (EVAR trial 1): randomized controlled trial. *Lancet* **365**:2179–2186.
19. Blankensteijn JD, Sjors ECA, de Jong MD, *et al.* (2005) Two-year outcomes after conventional or endovascular repair of abdominal aortic aneurysms. *N Engl J Med* **352**:2398–2405.
20. Davies RS, Wall M, Rai S, *et al.* (2007) Long-term results of surgical repair of popliteal aneurysm. *Eur J Vasc Endovasc Surg* **34**:714–718.
21. Tielliu IF, Verhoeven EL, Zeebregts CJ, *et al.* (2007) Endovascular treatment of popliteal artery aneurysms: is the technique a valid alternative to open surgery. *J Cardiovasc Surg* **48**:275–279.
22. Coggia M, Javerliat I, Di Centa I, *et al.* (2004) Total laparoscopic bypass for aorto-iliac occlusive lesions: 93 case experience. *J Vasc Surg* **40**:899–955.
23. ACC/AHA (2005) Practice guidelines for the management of patients with peripheral arterial disease. *Circulation* **113**:463–654.
24. Naylor AR, Ah-See AK, & Engeset J (1990) Aorto-iliac endarterectomy: an 11 year review. *Br J Surg* **77**:190–193.
25. De Vries S & Hunink M (1997) Results of aortic bifurcation grafts for aorto-iliac occlusive disease: a meta-analysis. *J Vasc Surg* **26**: 558–569.
26. Kieffer E, Bahnini A, Koskas F, *et al.* (1993) In situ allograft replacement of infected infrarenal aortic prosthetic grafts: results in forty-three patients. *J Vasc Surg* **17**:349–356.
27. Clagett GP, Valentine RJ, & Hagino RT (1997) Autogenous aortoiliac/femoral reconstruction from superficial femoral-popliteal veins: feasibility and durability. *J Vasc Surg* **25**:255–270.
28. Quinones-Baldrich WJ, Busuttil RW, *et al.* (1988) Is the preferential use of poly-tetra-fluoroethylene grafts for femoropopliteal bypass justified? *J Vasc Surg* **8**:219–228.
29. Abbott WM, Green RM, Matsumoto T, *et al.* (1997) Prosthetic above-knee femoropopliteal bypass grafting: results of a multicenter randomized prospective trial: Above-Knee Femoropopliteal Study Group. *J Vasc Surg* **25**:19–28.
30. Kram HB, Gupta SK, Veith FJ, *et al.* (1991) Late results of two hundred seventeen femoro-popliteal bypasses to isolated popliteal artery segments. *J Vasc Surg* **14**:386–390.
31. Derksen WJ, Gisbertz SS, Pasterkamp J, *et al.* (2008) Remote superficial femoral artery endarterectomy. *J Cardiovasc Surg* **49**:193–198.
32. Veith FJ, Gupta SK, Asher E, *et al.* (1986) Six-year prospective multicenter randomized comparison of autologous saphenous

vein and expanded polytetrafluoroethylene grafts in infragenual arterial reconstructions. *J Vasc Surg* **3**:104–114.

33. Moody AP, Edwards PR, & Harris PL (1992) In situ versus reversed femoropopliteal vein grafts: long-term follow-up of a prospective, randomized trial. *Br J Surg* **79**:750–752.

34. Londrey GL, Ramsey DE, Hodgson KJ, *et al.* (1991) Infrapopliteal bypass for severe ischemia: comparison of autogenous vein, composite and prosthetic grafts. *J Vasc Surg* **13**:631–636.

35. Shah DM, Darling RC, Chang BB, *et al.* (1995) Durability of short bypasses to infragenicular arteries. *Eur J Vasc Endovasc Surg* **10**:440–444.

36. Darling RC, Chang BB, Shah DM, *et al.* (1995) Choice of peroneal or dorsalis pedis artery bypass for limb salvage. *Semin Vasc Surg* **8**:225–235.

37. Miller JH, Foreman RK, Ferguson L, *et al.* (1984) Interposition vein cuff for anastomosis of prosthesis to small artery. *Aust NZ J Surg* **54**:283–285.

38. Tyrell MR & Wolfe JHN (1991) New prosthetic venous collar anastomotic technique: combining the best of other procedures. *Br J Surg* **78**:1016–1017.

39. Stonebridge PA, Prescott RJ, & Ruckley CV (1997) Randomized trial comparing infrainguinal polytetrafluoroethylene bypass grafting with and without vein interposition cuff at the distal anastomosis. *J Vasc Surg* **26**:543–550.

40. Paneton JM, Hollier LH, & Hofer JM (2004) Multicenter randomized prospective trial comparing a pre-cuffed polytetrafluoroethylene graft to a vein cuffed polytetrafluoroethylene graft for infragenicular arterial bypass. *Ann Vasc Surg* **18**:199–206.

41. Hamsho A, Nott D, & Harris PL (1999) Prospective randomised trial of distal of distal arteriovenous fistula as an adjunct to femoro-infrapopliteal PTFE bypass. *Eur J Vasc Endovasc Surg* **17**:197–201.

42. Albers M, Romiti M, Pereira CA, *et al.* (2004) Meta-analysis of allograft bypass grafting in infrapopliteal arteries. *Eur J Vasc Endovasc Surg* **28**:462–472.

43. Pomposelli FB, Marcaccio EJ, Gibbons GW, *et al.* (1995) Dorsalis pedis arterial bypass: durable limb salvage for foot ischemia in patients with diabetes mellitus. *J Vasc Surg* **21**:375–384.

44. Conte M, Belkin M, Upchurch G, *et al.* (2001) Impact of increasing comorbidity on infragenual reconstruction. A 20 year perspective. *Ann Surg* **233**:445–452.

45. Diehm N, Savolainen H, Mahler F, *et al.* (2004) Does deep femoral artery revascularization as an isolated procedure play a role in chronic critical limb ischemia. *J Endovasc Ther* **11**:119–124.

46. Hunink MG, Wong JB, Donaldson MC, *et al.* (1989) Patency results of percutaneous and surgical revascularization for femoropopliteal arterial disease. *Med Dec Makining* **14**:71–81.

47. Pereira CE, Albers M, Romiti M, *et al.* (2006) Meta-analysis of femoropopliteal bypass graft for lower extremity arterial insufficiency. *J Vasc Surg* **44**:510–517.

48. Albers M, Batistella V, Romiti M, *et al.* (2003) Meta-analysis of polytetrafluoroethylene bypass grafts to infrapopliteal arteries. *J Vasc Surg* **37**:1263–1269.

Index

Index

Index